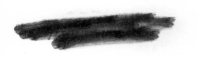

EQUINE MEDICINE AND SURGERY

THIRD EDITION

VOLUME TWO

Edited by

R.A. MANSMANN, VMD, PhD
Santa Barbara Equine Practice
Goleta, California

E.S. McALLISTER, VMD, MS
Diplomate, American College of
Veterinary Internal Medicine
Centre Equine Practice
Centre Hall, Pennsylvania

P.W. PRATT, VMD
Book Editor
American Veterinary Publications
Santa Barbara, California

AMERICAN VETERINARY PUBLICATIONS

DRAWER KK, SANTA BARBARA, CALIFORNIA

1982

Library of Congress Catalog Card No. 81-70196

ISBN   0-939674-04-1

PRINTED IN THE UNITED STATES OF AMERICA

PREFACE

In the 10 years since publication of the preceding edition of this book, the practice of equine medicine and surgery has expanded in many regards. New drugs have been approved for use in horses, research curiosities have evolved into commonly used modes of treatment, and the numbers of horses, as well as the people who care for them, have increased. Sophisticated research programs have contributed reams of new information to the rapidly expanding pool of information available to students, practitioners and researchers.

It is often said that medical texts are "out of date" by the time they appear in print. We hope this third edition of *Equine Medicine and Surgery* is an exception in that regard. Each chapter is strongly oriented toward the *management* of various diseases so that even though the specific technics and drugs used may change, the general therapeutic principles advocated should be applicable for years to come.

The book's practical orientation is attributable to its authors, most of whom are engaged in institutional or private equine practice. We are indebted to them for their outstanding contributions and their patience during production of the book.

The Editors

AUTHORS

R. ALLEN, JR.
General Manager, Silver Creek Ranch, Montecito, CA

H.E. AMSTUTZ, DVM
Professor, School of Veterinary Medicine, Purdue University, West Lafayette, IN

A.L. ARONSON, DVM, MS, PhD
Professor, School of Veterinary Medicine, North Carolina State University, Raleigh, NC

A.C. ASBURY, DVM
Associate Professor, College of Veterinary Medicine, University of Florida, Gainesville, FL

E.M. BAILEY, JR., DVM, PhD
Associate Professor, College of Veterinary Medicine, Texas A & M University, College Station, TX

G.J. BAKER, BVSc, MRCVS, PhD
Senior Lecturer, Veterinary School, University of Glasgow, Glasgow, Scotland

J.L. BAUM, DVM
Assistant Professor, College of Veterinary Medicine, University of Illinois, Urbana, IL

T.R. BELLO, DVM
Practitioner, Southern Pines, NC

L.R. BRAMLAGE, DVM, MS
Assistant Professor, College of Veterinary Medicine, Ohio State University, Columbus, OH

C.F. BROWNIE, DVM, PhD
Assistant Professor, College of Veterinary Medicine, University of Florida, Gainesville, FL

W.B. BUCK, DVM, MS
Professor, College of Veterinary Medicine, University of Illinois, Urbana, IL

J.F. BULLARD, DVM, MS (retired)
Professor, School of Veterinary Medicine, Purdue University, West Lafayette, IN

C.H. BURGER, DVM, MS
Practitioner, Bakersfield, CA

J.H. CANNON, DVM
Practitioner, Sierra Madre, CA

G.P. CARLSON, DVM, PhD
Associate Professor, School of Veterinary Medicine, University of California, Davis, CA

M. COHEN, VMD
Visiting Lecturer, School of Veterinary Medicine, University of California, Davis, CA

P.T. COLAHAN, DVM
Assistant Professor, College of Veterinary Medicine, University of Florida, Gainesville, FL

H.S. CONBOY, DVM
Practitioner, Lexington, KY

L.E. DAVIS, DVM, PhD
Professor, College of Veterinary Medicine, University of Illinois, Urbana, IL

D.A. DEEM, DVM
Lecturer, School of Veterinary Medicine, University of Pennsylvania, Philadelphia, PA

A. deLAHUNTA, DVM, PhD
Professor, New York State College of Veterinary Medicine, Cornell University, Ithaca, N.Y.

M.D. DEVOUS, SR., PhD
Nuclear Medicine Center, Southwestern Medical School, University of Texas, Dallas, TX

D.C. DODD, BVSc
Pathologist, G.D. Searle & Co., Chicago, IL

K.J. EASLEY, JR., DVM
Assistant Professor, Virginia-Maryland Regional College of Veterinary Medicine, Blacksburg, VA

W.C. EDWARDS, DVM
Toxicologist, Oklahoma Animal Disease Diagnostic Laboratory, Stillwater, OK

G.C. FARNBACH, VMD, PhD
Assistant Professor, School of Veterinary Medicine, University of Pennsylvania, Philadelphia, PA

D.L. FELLER, DVM
Veterinary Consultant, Ralston Purina Co., St. Louis, MO

G.L. FERRARO, DVM
Practitioner, Del Mar, CA

D.V. FLYNN, VMD
Practitioner, Charlottesville, VA

M.E. FOWLER, DVM
Professor, School of Veterinary Medicine, University of California, Davis, CA

D.E. FREEMAN, MVB, MRCVS
Assistant Professor, School of Veterinary Medicine, University of Pennsylvania, Philadelphia, PA

G.F. FREGIN, VMD
Assistant Professor, School of Veterinary Medicine, University of Pennsylvania, Philadelphia, PA

A.M. GALLINA, DVM, PhD
Professor, College of Veterinary Medicine, Washington State University, Pullman, WA

K.N. GELATT, VMD
Professor, College of Veterinary Medicine, University of Florida, Gainesville, FL

W.J. GIBBONS, DVM, MS (deceased)
Professor, School of Veterinary Medicine, Auburn University, Auburn, AL

D.O. GOBLE, DVM
Associate Professor, College of Veterinary Medicine, University of Tennessee, Knoxville, TN

B.D. GRANT, DVM, MS
Associate Professor, College of Veterinary Medicine, Washington State University, Pullman, WA

R.P. HACKETT, DVM, MS
Assistant Professor, New York State College of Veterinary Medicine, Cornell University, Ithaca, NY

E.P. HAMMEL, VMD
Associate Professor, School of Veterinary Medicine, University of Pennsylvania, Philadelphia, PA

D.V. HANSELKA, DVM, MS
Professor, College of Veterinary Medicine, Texas A & M University, College Station, TX

P.F. HAYNES, DVM, MS
Associate Professor, School of Veterinary Medicine, Louisiana State University, Baton Rouge, LA

R.B. HEATH, DVM, MSc
Professor, College of Veterinary Medicine, Colorado State University, Fort Collins, CO

C.D. HEINZE, DVM
Practitioner, West Lafayette, IN

R.C. HERSCHLER, DVM, PhD
Syntex Corporation, Palo Alto, CA

H.F. HINTZ, PhD
Professor of Animal Nutrition, New York State College of Veterinary Medicine, Cornell University, Ithaca, NY

D.C. HIRSH, DVM, PhD
Associate Professor, School of Veterinary Medicine, University of California, Davis, CA

J.A. HUBBELL, DVM
Assistant Professor, College of Veterinary Medicine, University of Florida, Gainesville, FL

J.H. JOHNSON, DVM
Practitioner, Lexington, KY

L.E. JOHNSON, DVM, MSc (retired)
Professor, College of Veterinary Medicine, Ohio State University, Columbus, OH

E.W. JONES, MRCVS, PhD
Vice Dean, College of Veterinary Medicine, Mississippi State University, Mississippi State, MS

J.R. JOYCE, DVM
Professor, College of Veterinary Medicine, Texas A & M University, College Station, TX

F.A. KALLFELZ, DVM, PhD
  Professor, New York State College of Veterinary Medicine, Cornell University, Ithaca, NY

M.D. KINGSBURY, DVM
  Practitioner, Ashland, VA

L. KLEIN, VMD
  Assistant Professor, School of Veterinary Medicine, University of Pennsylvania, Philadelphia, PA

H.D. KNIGHT, DVM, PhD (deceased)
  Professor, School of Veterinary Medicine, University of California, Davis, CA

R.C. KNOWLES, DVM
  Chief Staff Veterinarian, Equine Diseases National Program Planning Staffs, US Department of Agriculture, Hyattsville, MD

D.B. KOCH, DVM
  Practitioner, Bedford Hills, NY

L.M. KOGER, DVM
  Professor Emeritus, College of Veterinary Medicine, Washington State University, Pullman, WA

C.W. KOHN, VMD
  Assistant Professor, College of Veterinary Medicine, Ohio State University, Columbus, OH

R.E. LARSEN, DVM, PhD
  Assistant Professor, College of Veterinary Medicine, University of Florida, Gainesville, FL

M. LEITCH, VMD
  Practitioner, Cochranville, PA

I.K.M. LIU, DVM, PhD
  Assistant Professor, School of Veterinary Medicine, University of California, Davis, CA

W.E. LLOYD, DVM, PhD
  Toxicologist, Veterinary Diagnostic Laboratory, Iowa State University, Ames, IA

R.J. MACKAY, BVSc
  Graduate Student, College of Veterinary Medicine, University of Florida, Gainesville, FL

M.P. MACKAY-SMITH, DVM, MS
  Practitioner, Cochranville, PA

R.A. MANSMANN, VMD, PhD
  Practitioner, Goleta, CA

R.J. MARTENS, DVM
  Associate Professor, College of Veterinary Medicine, Texas A & M University, College Station, TX

I.G. MAYHEW, BVSc, PhD
  Associate Professor, College of Veterinary Medicine, University of Florida, Gainesville, FL

E.S. McALLISTER, VMD, MS
  Practitioner, Centre Hall, PA

J.J. McCLURE, DVM, MS
  Assistant Professor, School of Veterinary Medicine, Louisiana State University, Baton Rouge, LA

T.C. McGUIRE, DVM, PhD
  Professor, College of Veterinary Medicine, Washington State University, Pullman, WA

C.W. McILWRAITH, BVSc, MS, PhD, MRCVS
  Assistant Professor, College of Veterinary Medicine, Colorado State University, Fort Collins, CO

W.C. McMULLAN, DVM, PhD
  Professor, College of Veterinary Medicine, Texas A & M University, College Station, TX

A.M. MERRITT, DVM, MS
  Professor, College of Veterinary Medicine, University of Florida, Gainesville, FL

D.W. MILNE, DVM, MS
  Practitioner, Pittstown, NJ

W.M. MOULTON, VMD
  Chief, International Operations, Animal Health Programs, US Department of Agriculture, Hyattsville, MD

W.W. MUIR, DVM, PhD
  Associate Professor, College of Veterinary Medicine, Ohio State University, Columbus, OH

R.D. NORRIE, DVM
  Practitioner, Windsor, CA

G.L. NORWOOD, DVM
  Practitioner, Metairie, LA

J.E. PALMER, VMD
  Lecturer, School of Veterinary Medicine, University of Pennsylvania, Philadelphia, PA

R.J. PANCIERA, DVM, MS, PhD
Professor, College of Veterinary Medicine, Oklahoma State University, Stillwater, OK

C.W. RAKER, VMD
Professor, School of Veterinary Medicine, University of Pennsylvania, Philadelphia, PA

M.H. RATZLAFF, DVM, PhD
Associate Professor, College of Veterinary Medicine, Washington State University, Pullman, WA

J.T. ROBERTSON, DVM
Assistant Professor, College of Veterinary Medicine, Ohio State University, Columbus, OH

N.E. ROBINSON, BVSc, PhD
Professor, College of Veterinary Medicine, Michigan State University, East Lansing, MI

J.R. ROONEY, DVM
Pathologist, ICI Americas, Wilmington, DE

R.D. SANDE, DVM, MS, PhD
Professor, College of Veterinary Medicine, Washington State University, Pullman, WA

O.W. SCHALM, DVM, PhD
Professor Emeritus, School of Veterinary Medicine, University of California, Davis, CA

R.K. SCHNEIDER, DVM, MS
Assistant Professor, College of Veterinary Medicine, University of Florida, Gainesville, FL

S.J. SELWAY, DVM
Practitioner, Pembroke Pines, FL

J.L. SHUPE, DVM, MS
Professor, Utah State University, Logan, UT

R.T. SKARDA, DMV
Assistant Professor, College of Veterinary Medicine, Ohio State University, Columbus, OH

E.P. STEFFEY, VMD, PhD
Associate Professor, School of Veterinary Medicine, University of California, Davis, CA

B.C. TENNANT, DVM
Professor, New York State College of Veterinary Medicine, Cornell University, Ithaca, NY

J.C. THURMON, DVM, MS
Professor, College of Veterinary Medicine, University of Illinois, Urbana, IL

T. TOBIN, DVM, PhD
Professor, College of Agriculture, University of Kentucky, Lexington, KY

A.S. TURNER, BVSc, MS
Associate Professor, College of Veterinary Medicine, Colorado State University, Fort Collins, CO

G.A. VAN GELDER, DVM, PhD
Toxicologist, Shell Development Corporation, Houston, TX

J.T. VAUGHAN, DVM
Dean, School of Veterinary Medicine, Auburn University, Auburn, AL

P.C. WAGNER, DVM, MS
Assistant Professor, College of Veterinary Medicine, Washington State University, Pullman, WA

E. WALDRON-MEASE, VMD
Sports Medicine Consultant, Berwyn, PA

R.H. WHITLOCK, DVM, PhD
Associate Professor, School of Veterinary Medicine, University of Pennsylvania, Philadelphia, PA

R.P. WORTHMAN, DVM, MS
Professor, College of Veterinary Medicine, Washington State University, Pullman, WA

CONTENTS

ix

20. THE SKELETAL SYSTEM

15

The Respiratory System

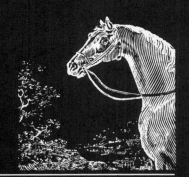

RESPIRATORY PHYSIOLOGY
by N.E. Robinson

The major function of the respiratory system is gas exchange. The respiratory tract also filters inhaled air and the blood, and performs a variety of metabolic functions. Adequate gas exchange requires ventilation of the lung, distribution of gas among lung lobules, perfusion of lobules, and diffusion of gases between air and blood. Since diffusion only occurs when air and blood are in close proximity, matching of ventilation and blood flow is an essential component of gas exchange.

Mechanics of Ventilation

Ventilation is the movement of gases through conducting airways into and out of the acini, where gas exchange occurs. Conducting airways, which include the nasopharynx and tracheobronchial tree to the level of the respiratory bronchioles, do not participate in gas exchange and are anatomic deadspace. Gas exchange occurs in the acinus, which consists of respiratory bronchioles, alveolar ducts and alveoli.

In most species at rest, inhalation is active and exhalation is passive. The resting horse exhibits a rather unique biphasic inhalation and exhalation, which may indicate active and passive components of inhalation and exhalation.[1,2] Inspiratory muscles enlarge the thorax during inhalation, thereby decreasing pleural pressure from its resting value of -5 cm H_2O to an end-inspiratory value of about -10 cm H_2O. This change in pleural pressure stretches the lung and generates flow through the conducting airways. During exhalation, the elastic recoil of lungs and thorax forces air out of the respiratory system. A second peak expiratory flow occurs late in exhalation and may be due to forced exhalation brought about by contraction of abdominal muscles. In the resting horse, an accentuated abdominal effort during exhalation indicates severe airway obstruction, as in heaves.

Pulmonary Elasticity: The elasticity of the lungs is due to elastion and collagen fibers in the lung parenchyma and surface tension forces in the air-liquid interface lining the alveoli. Surface tension, which tends to collapse the lung, is reduced by pulmonary surfactant. Surfactant contains dipalmitoyl lecithin and stabilizes the lung, slows the development of atelectasis and reduces the work of breathing. Sighing reactivates surfactant. Anesthesia and painful lesions of the thorax and abdomen can eliminate sighing and enhance the development of atelectasis. Anesthetized horses should be given deep breaths (airway pressure of 25-35 cm H_2O) by positive-pressure ventilation every 5 minutes to prevent atelectasis and maintain gas exchange.

Intracellular lamellated osmiophilic bodies representing intracellular surfactant are first observed in type-II alveolar epithelial cells at 150 days of gestation, but surfactant is not fully developed until 300 days or even later.[3] The conditions causing inadequate surfactant in some foals at term are not well understood. Inadequate surfactant is one cause of newborn respiratory distress.[4] Lack of surfactant results in atelectasis and increased work of breathing. A foal surviving prolonged delivery may have adequate surfactant to breathe normally; however, failure of surfactant production may lead to the development of respiratory distress.

Pulmonary elasticity is evaluated by measurement of lung compliance. Decreased compliance ("stiff lungs") can result from surfactant deficiency, edema, consolidation (*eg*, in pneumonia), or increased connective tissue in lung parenchyma. Decreased lung compliance makes lung inflation more difficult and increases the work of breathing, which appears clinically as inspiratory dyspnea. Other diseases that restrict inflation include pleural effusion, intrathoracic masses and abdominal distension.

Airway Resistance: In addition to stretching the lungs, respiratory muscles cause airflow through the nasopharynx and tracheobronchial tree. The resistance to airflow created by these conducting airways is determined primarily by their cross-sectional area, which varies with a variety of physiologic stimuli and disease processes.

Upper Airway Resistance: The horse is an obligate nose-breather yet must generate high airflow rates during exercise. Other species mouth-breathe during exercise to reduce upper airway resistance. If the energy used in breathing is not to be excessive, the exercising horse must decrease the resistance of the nasopharynx. Upper airway (nasopharynx) resistance reportedly ranges from 20-80% of total airway resistance.[5,6] The higher figure is more in agreement with values reported in other species, although it is tempting to speculate that a low nasal resistance might be an adaptation for nose-breathing.

Within the nasopharynx, most resistance is provided by the external nares. The turbinate region, pharynx and larynx provide only a small resistance. Decreased upper airway resistance during exercise probably results from dilation of the external nares, vasoconstriction in erectile tissue of the nasal mucosa, straightening the pharynx, and dilation of the larynx.

Within the upper airway, the external nares and pharynx are collapsible, while the turbinate portion is prevented from collapsing by a bony skeleton. The larynx is collapsible but is supported by cartilage plates and the trachea is supported by fairly rigid cartilage rings. During inhalation, poorly supported parts of the extrathoracic airway tend to collapse because pressure within the airway is subatmospheric. During exhalation, positive pressure within the upper airway causes passive dilation. Collapse of the external nares and larynx during inhalation is prevented by the dilator muscles of the alae nasi and abductor muscles of the larynx.

Inspiratory collapse of the upper airway is most likely to occur at points where airflow velocity is greatest since, at such points, energy is converted into kinetic energy, resulting in decreased intraluminal pressure. Airflow velocity is probably greatest at the external nares and larynx, which are the narrowest points of the upper airway.[5] Abduction of the alae nasi and dilation of the larynx during exercise not only decrease total resistance but, by increasing cross-sectional area, also prevent excessive increases in airflow velocity resulting from increased ventilation. If the horse is unable to dilate the larynx during inhalation, as in laryngeal hemiplegia, airflow velocity through the larynx is greater than normal. This increased velocity decreases pressure in the lumen of the larynx, which further collapses the airway and increases resistance and airflow velocity during inspiration.

In upper airway collapse, flow limitation develops during inhalation. Xylazine relaxes the facial muscles and prevents abduction of the alae nasi. Before the administration of xylazine, inspiratory flow increases progressively with increased exercise; however, after xylazine administration, inspiratory flow plateaus because the nares collapse as the horse makes increased inspiratory efforts. A horse with pharyngeal edema and right-sided laryngeal hemiplegia has a normal pressure flow curve at rest. As flow rates increase after injection of doxapram HCl, inspiratory flow is limited.

Although extensive recordings of laryngeal pressure-flow relationships have not been made in exercising horses with laryngeal hemiplegia, increased air flow velocity may cause collapse of the paralyzed side of the larynx to result in flow limitation and the characteristic roaring or whistling noise.

Tracheobronchial Tree Resistance: The tracheobronchial tree divides repeatedly between the trachea and alveoli (10-24 times in humans). The total cross-sectional area of the airways does not change in the first 4-7 divisions but increases dramatically at the level of the bronchioles. In humans the total cross-sectional area of the twentieth generation is a thousand times the total cross-sectional area of the trachea.[7] If similar figures apply to horses, approximately 80% of the resistance of the tracheobronchial tree is in airways greater than 2-3 mm in diameter. Because of the large total cross-sectional area of the bronchioles, bronchiolar obstruction must be extensive to produce dyspnea. In contrast, modest decreases in the diameter of larger airways produces severe dyspnea.

Airways larger than 1-2 mm in diameter are known as bronchi and have cartilaginous plates to provide some support. Airways less than 1 mm in diameter (bronchioles) have no rigid support but are kept patent by the tethering action of surrounding lung parenchyma. Smooth muscle is found in the walls of airways from the trachea to the alveoli. The innervation of this smooth muscle has not been investigated in horses, but in dogs vagal parasympathetic fibers innervate the large and small airways.

Airway resistance changes in response to a variety of causes. Because intrapulmonary airways are tethered by surrounding lung parenchyma, they dilate and narrow as lung volume increases and decreases, respectively. The narrowing of small airways explains why rhonchi are loudest at the end of expiration. Because emphysema destroys lung parenchyma, the tethering of airways by adjacent tissue is reduced and airways narrow. However "emphysema" in horses is usually bronchiolitis rather than the extensive tissue destruction observed in humans.[8]

Increases in smooth-muscle tone increase airway resistance. Bronchoconstriction can result from a vagal reflex induced by stimulation of irritant receptors by physical agents, eg, dust or chemical mediators such as histamine. Chemical mediators may also stimulate smooth muscle directly.[9]

In horses the bronchoconstrictor role of chemical mediators released from mast cells is not known. In other species mast-cell mediator release is controlled by a variety of stimuli including immune responses and stimulation of adrenergic or cholinergic receptors. Agents capable of stimulating adenylate cyclase, such as beta-adrenergic agonists and certain prostaglandins, increase tissue concentrations of cyclic AMP, which inhibits mediator release and results in bronchodilation. Phosphodiesterase metabolizes cyclic AMP, and substances that inhibit phosphodiesterase, eg, aminophylline, cause accumulation of cyclic AMP and inhibit mediator release. In contrast, other prostaglandins, such as PGF_2alpha, decrease cyclic AMP levels and enhance mediator release. Cholinergic stimulation of most cells results in accumulation of cyclic GMP, which enhances mediator release and causes bronchoconstriction.[9]

In addition to histamine, chemical mediators, such as slow-reacting substance of anaphylaxis (SRSA), kinins, prostaglandins and eosinophilic chemotactic factor, are released from target cells in antigen-antibody reactions. Histamine, SRSA, and PGF_2alpha are bronchoconstrictors. The effect of other mediators on bronchial smooth muscle is not known. Drugs such as cromolyn sodium, diethylcarbamazine and meclofenamic acid block the synthesis and release of mediators and can therefore be used to prevent bronchoconstriction.

As stated earlier, some mediator-induced bronchoconstriction is vagally mediated and can be blocked by atropine. However, mediators also act directly on airway smooth muscle.

Clinical signs of increased airway resistance (airway obstruction) vary from reduced exercise tolerance to expiratory dyspnea in resting horses. In addition to bronchoconstriction resulting from mediator release and vagal stimulation of smooth muscle, airway obstruction can result from masses impinging on the airway (as in hilar lymphadenopathy), airway foreign bodies and accumulation of secretions. Intrathoracic airway obstruction results in prolonged or forced exhalation and increased resting volume of the thorax (functional residual capacity). Increased functional residual capacity results when passive exhalation cannot occur in a normal timespan and subsequent exhalations begin at a higher lung volume. The increased lung volume passively dilates the airways so that exhalation can occur more rapidly. Should the increased functional residual capacity fail to allow passive exhalation, expiratory muscles are used.

Tracheostomy tubes are frequently used to bypass upper airway obstructions. Damage to the mucociliary escalator by tracheostomy allows accumulation of secretions and leads to severe airway obstruction unless the tracheostomy wound is cleaned regularly. Tracheostomy tubes must be large enough so that they do not themselves cause obstruction.

Intrathoracic airway diameter is greatly decreased during forced exhalation because the high intrapleural pressure results in airway compression. This intrathoracic airway compression determines a maximal limit to expiratory flow rates. Airway compression during forced exhalation normally occurs in the larger airways and peak flow rates exceed the maximal flow rate attained during exercise. In the presence of extensive small airway (bronchiolar) obstruction, as in heaves, intrathoracic airway compression may occur extensively throughout the tracheobronchial tree, and the maximal limits of expiratory flow may severely limit the exercise abilities of the horse.[10] In heaves, forced exhalation may further obstruct already severely obstructed airways. Collapse of the extrathoracic airways occurs during forced inspiratory efforts and extrathoracic airways obstructions cause primarily inspiratory dyspnea.

Airway Closure: Because small airways (bronchioles) are tethered by surrounding lung parenchyma, their diameters decrease as lung volume decreases and at low lung volumes they may close. Airway closure limits ventilation to alveoli distal to the point of closure and therefore leads to hypoxemia. Although airway closure has not been demonstrated conclusively in horses, it probably occurs when the volume of any part of the lung decreases below functional residual capacity. This probably occurs in the dependent portions of the anesthetized horse lung and may also occur with pleural effusions.[11] Airway closure can be prevented by maintaining a normal functional residual capacity. This requires regular sighing to reactivate surfactant, removal of pleural effusions and positioning to avoid compression of the lung by abdominal contents.

Gas Distribution

In an ideal lung, air and blood are evenly distributed to the many gas exchange units. Due to gravity, healthy lungs have some uneven distribution of ventilation and blood flow, resulting in less than ideal gas exchange. The magnitude of the gravitational effect on the distribution of ventilation and blood flow in horse lungs is not known. In sternally recumbent horses, distribution of ventilation is much more uniform than in laterally recumbent or supine horses, probably because the sloping diaphragm of the horse prevents undue compression of the lungs by abdominal contents in the upright animal.[11]

In lung disease, regional variation in airway resistance and lung compliance increases uneven distribution of ventilation. Air is preferentially delivered to regions of high compliance served by airways with low resistance.

Airway obstruction by foreign bodies and exudate, and bronchoconstriction result in regional variations in increased airway resistance. Uneven distribution of ventilation due to local increases in airway resistance is accentuated by increased respiratory frequency. Whereas regions served by partially obstructed airways have time to fill with air when the horse breathes slowly, there is insufficient time for filling when the horse ventilates rapidly. As a result, horses with bronchiolitis may show few signs of lung disease at rest but have poor exercise tolerance because of increasingly uneven distribution of ventilation.

Localized inflammatory processes, edema and fibrosis all result in local variations in lung compliance, which restrict the delivery of air to certain parts of the lung. Pleural effu-sions and local restrictions in thoracic cage mobility may also cause uneven distribution of ventilation.

In species with unlobulated lungs, such as dogs, collateral ventilation may reduce some inequalities in ventilation distribution. Horses have poor collateral ventilation that may add little to gas exchange maintenance.[12]

Pulmonary Circulation

The pulmonary circulation delivers blood to the lungs for gas exchange, acts as a filter for venous blood, supplies nutrients to the lung parenchyma, acts as a reservoir for the left ventricle, provides a large surface area for the absorption of liquids from the alveoli, and modifies many vasoactive agents. The lung is also supplied by the bronchial circulation, a branch of the systemic circulation. In the horse, the bronchial circulation also supplies the bronchi and visceral pleura, and subsequently drains into the pulmonary veins.[13]

Mean pulmonary arterial pressure averages 25 mm Hg and left atrial pressure is 8 mm Hg, to give a driving pressure for pulmonary blood flow of only 17 mm Hg, compared to the pressure differential of 100 mm Hg in the systemic circulation. Since blood flow in the pulmonic and systemic circulations is equal, it is apparent that the pulmonary circulation has a very low resistance. In all species studied, pulmonary vascular resistance decreases even further during exercise because of distension of perfused vessels and recruitment of previously unperfused vessels. In this way blood flow may increase greatly without doubling the pressure differential across pulmonary circulation.

Pulmonary vascular resistance can change in response to a variety of passive and active factors, but one of the most potent pulmonary vasoconstrictors is alveolar hypoxia.[15] Hypoxic vasoconstriction directs blood away from poorly ventilated lung and may help maintain gas exchange in the presence of airway obstruction. However, this system is not very efficient and fails to compensate in the presence of diffuse lung disease. In fact, diffuse lung disease may cause generalized vasoconstriction, which can lead to right heart failure (cor pulmonale).

Blood flow through the pulmonary capillaries depends on the relative magnitudes of alveolar pulmonary arterial and pulmonary venous pressures. As a result of gravity, intravascular pressures probably increase from the uppermost to the dependent portions of the lung, so that blood flow is least in the uppermost lung and greatest in dependent portions of the lung.

Increased pulmonary venous pressure (as in left heart failure) and increased pulmonary arterial pressure (as in exercise or patent ductus arteriosus) raise capillary pressure, which increases vascular volume throughout the lung. Vascular engorgement may be observed radiographically as arterial and/or venous enlargement. In contrast, decreased pulmonary venous pressure (as in shock) or decreased pulmonary arterial pressure (as in anesthesia) and increased alveolar pressure (as in positive-pressure ventilation) produce a hypoperfused lung. Because both decreased vascular pressures and positive-pressure ventilation tend to hypoperfuse the lung, it is important in surgical patients to maintain vascular volume and to keep the inspiratory phase of ventilation as short as possible.

Gas Exchange

A clinician evaluates gas exchange by examination of the mucous membranes for cyanosis or by determination of arterial O_2 and CO_2 tensions (PaO_2, $PaCO_2$). These evaluations show the result of gas exchange processes, including alveolar ventilation, diffusion between the alveoli and capillaries, and coordinated ventilation and blood flow.

Alveolar Ventilation: The volume of air breathed per minute is known as minute ventilation and is the product of tidal volume and respiratory rate. In a conscious animal, approximately 75% of minute ventilation enters the exchange area of the lung and is involved in gas exchange. This portion is known as alveolar ventilation, while the remainder, deadspace ventilation, enters the conducting airways and does not participate in gas exchange. Alveolar ventilation is normally matched to the body's rate of CO_2 production so that, as tissue metabolism increases, there is a similar increase in alveolar ventilation, causing $PaCO_2$ to remain at the normal 40 mm Hg.

The $PaCO_2$ decreases when alveolar ventilation is large in relation to tissue CO_2 production. This hyperventilation occurs in cardiopulmonary disease in an attempt to compensate for low $PaCO_2$, in metabolic acidosis to help to return body pH to normal, and especially in excited animals.

The $PaCO_2$ rises when alveolar ventilation fails to keep pace with the body's CO_2 production. This situation is known as alveolar hypoventilation or respiratory failure and is observed in some horses with severe heaves.[14] It also occurs when ventilation is severely compromised by upper airway obstruction, abdominal distension or trauma to the thoracic cage. To prevent severe acidosis, alveolar ventilation should be restored by removing the cause of the hypoventilation whenever possible. While O_2 administration elevates PaO_2 depressed by hypoventilation, it does not assist in the elimination of CO_2 and correction of acidosis.

The surgeon should be aware that anesthetized horses are frequently acidotic due to hypoventilation. A means of positive-pressure ventilation should therefore be available for use in deeply anesthetized horses or where acid-base homeostasis is endangered by other disease processes such as intestinal obstruction. It is also important to ensure that anesthetic equipment never contributes to deadspace, which is accomplished by the use of endotracheal tubes of proper length with non-rebreathing systems.

Diffusion: When barometric pressure is 760 mm Hg, the 21% O_2 content of air results in O_2 tension (pO_2) of 160 mm Hg. In the upper respiratory tract, water vapor is added to the air and in the alveoli O_2 diffuses into the capillary bed and CO_2 diffuses into the alveoli so that alveolar O_2 tension averages 100 mm Hg. The pO_2 and pCO_2 of venous blood returning to the lungs averages 40 and 46 mm Hg, respectively, so that the pressure gradient for O_2 between the alveolus and capillary blood is 60 mm Hg and the pressure gradient for CO_2 between blood and the alveolus averages 6 mm Hg. Because CO_2 is so much more diffusible than O_2, approximately equal volumes of these 2 gases diffuse across the alveolar capillary membrane per minute despite differences in the pressure gradient.

The rate of gas diffusion across the alveolar capillary membrane is determined by the available capillary surface area and the pressure gradient, and is also inversely proportional to the membrane thickness. The rate of gas diffusion can be reduced by diseases that increase the thickness of the alveolar capillary membrane (*eg*, edema), by reduction of the alveolar surface area available for diffusion (as in atelectasis), or by reduction in capillary surface area resulting from hypoperfusion of the lung (as in shock). Because CO_2 is so much more diffusible than O_2, diffusion barriers cause hypoxemia but not hypercarbia (increased $PaCO_2$).

Matching of Ventilation and Blood Flow: The most common cause of low PaO_2 in horses is probably mismatched ventilation and blood flow. If the healthy horse is like other species, most alveolar ventilation and pulmonary blood flow is delivered to gas-exchange units with a ventilation: blood flow ratio close to 1.0. Some alveoli in the upper part of the lung may receive more ventilation than blood flow and some in the lower parts of the lung may receive relatively more blood flow than ventilation. This normal distribution of ventilation to blood flow ratios results in normal arterial blood gas values (PaO_2 = 85-100 mm Hg, $PaCO_2$ = 40 mm Hg).[6,14] In animals with lung disease, the normal distribution of ventilation and blood flow is severely disturbed so that some groups of alveoli receive very little ventilation but continue to receive blood flow, while others receive ventilation but no blood flow.

Bronchitis, bronchiolitis, bronchoconstriction, airway closure of local restriction of lung movement results in reduced ventilation to portions of the lung. If these portions of lung continue to receive normal blood flow, they can be said to have a low ventilation: blood flow ratio and the blood leaving such areas has a low-O_2, high-CO_2 content. The extreme case of a low ventilation: blood flow ratio is a right-to-left vascular shunt, in which blood passes from the right to the left ventricle without contacting ventilated alveoli. Such shunts occur in congenital cardiac defects, such as tetralogy of Fallot, and through areas of atelectasis and consolidation within the lung.

If areas of lung have reduced blood flow because of emboli or decreased pulmonary arterial pressures (as in shock) but continue to receive ventilation, these units are said to have a high ventilation: blood flow ratio. Blood leaving such units has a high pO_2 and a low pCo_2. However, because of the sigmoid shape of the oxyhemoglobin-dissociation curve, the high pO_2 produced by these units does not significantly increase the O_2 content of blood. In contrast, the low pO_2 produced by poorly ventilated lung units lowers O_2 content. Combining blood from high- and low-ventilation: blood flow ratio regions of the lung results in a low arterial O_2 content and low PaO_2. Because of the almost linear CO_2 dissociation curve, high ventilation: blood flow ratios compensate for low ventilation: blood flow ratios in CO_2 elimination so that $PaCO_2$ is often normal or below normal.

Hypoxemia from ventilation-perfusion inequalities can be corrected by the administration of O_2, which increases the rate of O_2 delivery to poorly ventilated alveoli. However, O_2 administration does not significantly increase PaO_2 in horses with large right-to-left shunts because poorly oxygenated blood bypasses the lungs completely. Right-to-left shunt should therefore be suspected in any horse that remains cyanotic after administration of O_2.

Gas Transport

Arterial O_2 tension averages 85-100 mm Hg and alveolar O_2 tension averages 100-110 mm Hg in horses.[6,14] The difference between arterial and alveolar O_2 tensions results from admixture of venous blood from the bronchial and coronary circulations into the oxygenated blood leaving the lungs, and also from ventilation-perfusion inequalities. Foals have a lower O_2 tension than do older horses, probably because of increased ventilation-perfusion inequalities resulting from the immature state of the lung.[4]

Hemoglobin (Hb) is necessary for the transport of O_2 because O_2 has a low solubility in plasma. Each gram of Hb can carry 1.34 ml O_2, so that blood with an average of 15 g Hb/dl has an O_2 capacity of 21 ml/dl blood or 21 volumes %. Because O_2 capacity is dependent on the amount of Hb in the blood, O_2 capacity decreases in anemia and increases with the polycythemia of exercise.

The combination of O_2 and Hb depends mainly on pO_2 but is also affected by pH, pCO_2, temperature and the levels of 2,3-diphosphoglycerate (2,3-DPG) within the RBC. Hemoglobin is almost fully saturated with O_2 when blood pO_2 exceeds 85 mm Hg; raising pO_2 further by O_2 therapy or hyperventilation adds little O_2 to Hb and only a small amount into solution in the plasma. This plateau in the oxyhemoglobin-dissociation curve allows saturation of Hb when PaO_2 is slightly reduced by altitude or cardiopulmonary disease.

The slope of the oxyhemoglobin-dissociation curve is steep in the range of tissue pO_2 allowing rapid unloading of O_2. Unloading of O_2 is enhanced by increased pCO_2 and decreased pH of tissues. Approximately one-third of O_2 is removed from Hb by the tissues in a resting animal, which allows an O_2 reserve for increased activity. The unloading of O_2 is also enhanced by increased RBC levels of 2,3-DPG, which occur with chronic hypoxemia and increased metabolic rates from thyroid activity. The reduction in 2,3-DPG levels in stored blood prevents the release of O_2 to the tissues when this blood is transfused into an animal. Twenty-four hours may be required to restore normal, 2,3-DPG levels in transfused blood.

Observation of the oxyhemoglobin-dissociation curve reveals several clinically important facts. The administration of pure O_2 does not provide an O_2 store because Hb is already saturated at a pO_2 of 100 mm Hg. The additional O_2 adds only a small amount in solution in plasma. This small O_2 reserve is rapidly depleted when O_2 administration is discontinued.

Anemic animals with healthy lungs have a normal PaO_2 and all available Hb is saturated. These animals need Hb, not treatment with O_2. Animals with lung disease have a low PaO_2 and usually have normal Hb levels. Low PaO_2 results in unsaturation of Hb and O_2 therapy is needed to elevate PaO_2 to 100 mm Hg. In many cases, pure O_2 is not necessary and 40-60% O_2 will suffice. High levels of O_2 given over several hours result in O_2 toxicity and lung damage.

Since PaO_2 must decrease below 60 mm Hg to significantly reduce O_2 content or the percent saturation of Hb, PaO_2 is a better measure of gas exchange than is O_2 content or Hb saturation. Mixed venous pO_2 is useless as an indicator of gas exchange since it is affected by tissue metabolism, blood flow and PaO_2. Cyanosis results from the presence of unsaturated Hb and is a sign of severely impaired gas exchange. It is important to remember that cyanosis also results from local decreases in the blood flow: metabolism ratio and from severe lung disease.

In contrast to O_2, CO_2 is very soluble and large amounts are transported in solution in plasma or within the RBC. Carbon dioxide is also transported as bicarbonate ion and as carbamino compounds formed by the combination of proteins and CO_2. The transport of CO_2 is accompanied by production of hydrogen ions, which are buffered by Hb, plasma proteins and phosphates. Since there are large reserves of buffer in the body, blood does not become saturated with CO_2 in the same way it becomes saturated with O_2.

Contol of Ventilation

Groups of inspiratory and expiratory neurons in the medulla provide neural input to the respiratory muscles. These neurons generate a rhythmic but somewhat erratic pattern of ventilation; however, input from higher brain centers, chemoreceptors and mechanoreceptors is necessary to maintain normal alveolar ventilation at a minimal energy cost to the horse.

If the horse is like other mammals, ventilation is modified by the apneustic and pneumotaxic centers in the pons, by the thermoregulatory center in the hypothalamus, and by the cerebral cortex. The medullary respiratory neurons and pontine centers share responsibility for providing rhythmic ventilation. The thermoregulatory center induces changes in respiration necessary for heat loss, and the cerebral cortex temporarily overrides other controls during vocalization, defecation and parturition.

Chemoreceptors are located in the medulla, and carotid and aortic bodies. Ventilation is normally regulated by the medullary chemoreceptor, located behind the blood-brain barrier and probably bathed by tissue fluid with a composition close to that of CSF. When $PaCO_2$ increases, CO_2 diffuses across the blood-brain barrier and lowers CSF pH, which in turn stimulates the chemoreceptoer to increase ventilation. Conversely, when $PaCO_2$ is low, CSF pH increases and ventilation decreases. Because the blood-brain barrier is only slightly permeable to hydrogen and bicarbonate ions, peripheral chemoreceptors are primarily responsible for the ventilatory response to metabolic acidosis and alkalosis.

Peripheral chemoreceptors (carotid and aortic bodies) are the only mechanism for detection of hypoxemia, but can also detect increases in $PaCO_2$ and decreases in pH.[16,17] Ponies hypoventilate when their carotid bodies are denervated, suggesting that peripheral chemoreceptors are essential for normal ventilation.[16] However, PaO_2 must decrease to less than 60 mm Hg before hypoxia significantly increases ventilation.[18] The carotid and aortic bodies probably play only a small role in ventilatory control in awake animals, but may become important during anesthesia since their functions are not depressed by anesthetics. This is in contrast to the medullary (central) chemoreceptor, which is depressed by anesthetic agents.

Mechanoreceptors are found within the respiratory tract and in joints, and can affect ventilation. Lung inflation stimulates stretch receptors within the airways and diminishes the inspiratory effort. These receptors may be responsible for adjusting tidal volume and frequency to minimize the work of breathing.

As stated earlier, there are irritant receptors within the airways that can be stimulated by physical agents, such as dust, and by some chemical mediators such as histamine. Stimulation of irritant receptors causes coughing and reflex bronchoconstriction. A third type of chemoreceptor in the lung is the J receptor, which apparently detects increased levels of interstitial fluid and may be responsible for the pattern of respiration observed in pulmonary edema. Mechanoreceptors in the joints are thought to be partially responsible for the increase in ventilation during exercise.

References

1. Amoroso, EC et al. Proc Roy Soc London **159** (1962) 325.
2. Derksen, FJ and Robinson, NE. Am J Vet Res **41**(1980) 1756.
3. Pattle, RE et al. J Repro Fert **23** (1975) 651.
4. Rossdale, PD. Vet Clin No Am **1** (1979) 203.
5. Robinson, NE et al. Proc 21st Ann Mtg Am Assoc Eq Pract, 1975. p 11.
6. Willoughby, RA and McDonnell, WN. Vet Clin No Am **1** (1979) 219.
7. Weibel, ER: Morphometry of the Human Lung. Springer-Verlage, Berlin, 1963.
8. Breeze, RG. Vet Clin No Am **1** (1979) 219.
9. Drazen, JM and Austen, KF. J Clin Invest **53** (1974) 1679.
10. Leith, DE and Gillespie,JR. Fed Proc **30** (1971) 556.
11. Sorenson, PR and Robinson, NE. J Appl Physiol. In press, 1981.
12. Robinson, NE and Sorenson, PR. J Appl Physiol **44** (1978) 63.
13. McLaughlin, RF et al. Am J Anat **108** (1961) 149.
14. Gillespie, JR et al. Am J Physiol **207** (1964) 1067.
15. Bisgard, GE et al. Am J Vet Res **36** (1975) 49.
16. Bisgard, GE et al. J Appl Physiol **40** (1976) 184.
17. Forster, HV et al. J Appl Physiol **41** (1976) 878.
18. Muir, WW et al. Am J Vet Res **36** (1975) 155.

RESPIRATORY SYSTEM DEFENSE MECHANISMS
by R.A. Mansmann

Many defense mechanisms are required in the respiratory system since the lungs are exposed to the external environment. Inhaled particles have the potential to cause respiratory disease. Particles larger than 10μ in diameter generally lodge in the upper airway. Those from 0.2-5μ can penetrate as far as the alveolae, and those less than 0.2μ pass in and out of the airway without impaction.

Mechanical factors, surface fluids and cellular components comprise the defense mechanisms of the respiratory system. Mechanical factors are generally related to airway anatomy (Fig 1). The nasal turbinates produce turbulence in the inspired air, which stabilizes the temperature and humidifies the air to prepare large particles for impaction in the nasopharynx. Particle impaction in the pharynx occurs primarily in the dorsal pharyngeal wall due to the sharp change in direction of the airflow as it enters the larynx. As air moves into the lung, impaction of particles occurs at each of approximately 22 bronchial branches.

Particle impaction may play a significant role in the pleuropneumonia complex in race horses. Many cases of pleuropneumonia involve primarily the right apical lobe area. The bronchus to the right apical lobe of the lung leaves the trachea at a 90° angle just cranial to the bifurcation of the mainstem bronchi (Fig 1). The cranial location and acute angle of bifurcation of the right apical lobe permit easier entrance of inhaled particles than in more caudal parts of the lung and may make particle removal more difficult.

Cilia on respiratory epithelial cells are another important aspect of the mechanical defense system. Cilia are present on epithelial cells from the nares caudal to the bronchioles. Each ciliated cell has approximately 200 cilia that beat in waves to force exudates and debris craniad. The rate of transit of particles on the mucociliary blanket in equine species is about 1 cm/minute.[1] Particles on any part of the mucociliary blanket are normally removed within 24 hours of impaction. Noxious gases, such as nitrous oxide and sulfur dioxide, are ciliotoxic.[2] Chronic pulmonary disease also alters the motion of cilia on respiratory epithelial cells.[3]

Gravity affects particle impaction in the lung periphery, where airflow velocity falls to nearly zero. The cranioventral location of bacterial pneumonia in foals is related to the effect of gravity on bacteria, since the dependent lung lobes are parallel to the ground.

The second important defense mechanism of the respiratory system is the surface fluids of the airway. The main portion of the surface fluid is the mucociliary blanket, which is a double layer of water and mucus produced by the submucosal glands and goblet cells. Virus particles can attack respiratory epithelial cells if the mucociliary blanket is not intact. Dehydration may cause the blanket to become viscous, causing separations.[4]

Nonspecific soluble factors normally aid the mucociliary blanket defense mechanism. Lactoferrin, lysozymes from WBC, interferon, antibodies from submucosal lymphocytes, and IgA are all important parts of surface fluids. The last has been called the "antiseptic paint" of the respiratory and GI tract surfaces. The exact function of IgA in relation to prevention of disease and the ultimate stimulation by vaccines in the prevention of disease are obscure. At the mucosal surface, IgA acts by limiting the absorption of antigen, which prevents bacterial colonization on the mucous membranes. Small amounts of IgG may also be important in preventing disease in respiratory secretions of normal horses. During disease in which the mucous membranes have been altered, increased levels of serum IgG neutralize infectious antigens in the airways.

Surfactant is another important ingredient of surface fluid and is produced by type-II alveolar cells. Surfactant regulates surface tension to prevent the lung from completely collapsing at the end of expiration. In premature foals, lack of surfactant may be an important factor in the development of acute respiratory distress and subsequent infectious pneumonia. Surfactant development is markedly increased late in fetal life by the effects of endogenous corticosteroids.

The final defense mechanism of the lung is the variety of cells lining the respiratory tract. Ciliated columnar epithelial cells line the airway to the level of the bronchioles. Goblet cells produce mucus for the mucociliary blanket and increase in number during chronic irritation such as chronic bronchitis. Three types of cells line the alveolus. Type-I alveolar cells are thin and transport O_2 into the bloodstream. Type-II alveolar cells are larger and are thought to produce surfactant. Alveolar macrophages remove particulate matter from the alveolus, which may take up to 100 days.

Other immunologically important airway cells, primarily in the submucosa, are lymphocytes that produce IgA, IgG and IgE. The only known function of IgE is sensitization of mast cells for subsequent release of chemical mediators of inflammation, such as histamine and the slow-reacting substance of anaphylaxis. Some forms of chronic lung disease may increase the number of IgE-containing cells. Mast cells primarily provide chemical mediators of smooth muscle contraction and inflammation. Eosinophils in the submucosa act primarily as phagocytes.

Many environmental factors promote disease. The area in which horses are stabled is important. In a study of transtracheal aspirations from horses in a hospital environment vs those from horses in an old, wooden barn, the character of the flora isolated depended on the environment. Twice the number of bacterial species were isolated from horses in the hospital environment, and over 7 times the number

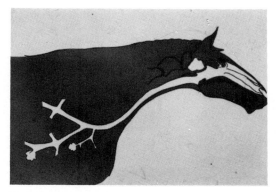

Fig 1. Particle impaction points in the equine respiratory system.

of fungi were isolated from horses in wooden barns.[5] Hay, presumably containing many fungal spores, was stored above the horses in the wooden barn. In an English study of 200 samples of hay, 90 species of fungi and 15 species of actinomycetes were isolated.[6] When moldy hay was shaken in the experimental stall, spore content of the air increased 300-fold. Twenty minutes later spore content of the air was still 30 times the resting level. These studies indicate that horses housed in average stall surroundings and fed hay are constantly bombarded by infectious organisms, irritants and potential allergens.

Other environmental inhalants, such as smog, Pb and sulfur dioxide, can modify respiratory tract defense mechanisms. Starvation, chilling, acidosis and corticosteroids also diminish respiratory tract resistance to infection.[4]

References

1. Albert, RE *et al*. Arch Envrn Hlth **17** (1968) 50.
2. Green, GM. Am Rev Resp Dis **102** (1970) 691.
3. Sturgess, JM *et al*. N Engl J Med **300** (1979) 53.
4. Hjerpe, CA. Proc Ann Mtg Am Coll Vet Int Med, 1978. p 1.
5. Mansmann, RA and Strouss, AA. JAVMA **169** (1976) 631.
6. Lacey, J. Proc 4th Int Symp Aspergillosis and Farmer's Lung, 1971. p 16.

EXAMINATION OF THE RESPIRATORY SYSTEM
by R.A. Mansmann and E.S. McAllister

History

The history is one of the most important aspects in the examination of any body system. It must be as complete as possible and carefully evaluated in regard to its credibility. Each clinician should develop a protocol when obtaining the history and should remember that history-taking is a continual process as the workup of the case progresses. The age, sex, breed, type of exercise and environment of the horse should be noted.

A history can be broken into 2 major areas: the animal's past and present. The horse's origin, its various environments, and preventive medication given during its life may be important. Recent changes in environment and routine should be noted.

Current history begins with a discussion of the presenting clinical signs. The clinician must determine the primary complaint and its duration. Is it progressing, regressing or static? Complaints related to the respiratory system include coughing, nasal discharge, altered breathing patterns, abnormal respiratory sounds and asymmetric swellings of the head, neck or chest. Each of these signs should be defined in as much detail as possible. Are the clinical signs continuous, related to exercise or eating, or altered by environmental changes? Is the cough dry, hacking and nonproductive, or moist and productive? Is the nasal discharge bilateral or unilateral, does it change with repositioning of the head, and is it constant or intermittent? Is the discharge serous, mucoid, purulent, sanguineous or a combination of these? Is there food in or a smell related to the nasal discharge? Are the altered breathing patterns inspiratory, expiratory or both? Are abnormal respiratory sounds inspiratory or expiratory, high- or low-pitched, barking or otherwise described by the owner? Have any swellings changed position or size? Nonspecific signs closely related to the respiratory system include fever, anorexia, depression, lethargy and weight loss.

Some histories may be very confusing. For example, severe pain anywhere in the horse may mimic colic signs, and chest pain may mimic lameness. Reluctance to gallop may be related to respiratory, cardiovascular or orthopedic problems.

A final consideration related to history is the type of medication the horse has received and its response to that medication. Additional information may be obtained as the clinician proceeds through the physical examination.

Physical Examination

The general examination of the respiratory system should always include observation, palpation, percussion and auscultation. The history may be confirmed and clarified during the examination as needed. All diagnostic findings should be compatible with the findings of the physical examination and history.

Observation: The examination is initiated by observing the horse in its stall. In this way, the clinician can judge the horse's environment, general condition, attitude, appetite and bodily functions. The temperature should be taken prior to removing the animal from the stall. The pattern, rate and depth of respiration are noted while the temperature is taken. Are the nostrils flaring and moving excessively? Does the horse have respiratory noise at rest? Is the abdominal wall used as an aid to inspiration, expiration or both? The clinician should also look for any discharges from the nostrils or other areas about the head and neck, and note any discharges on the stall walls.

Mucous membrane color and capillary refill time should be observed. Cyanosis is a very grave sign and the degree of cyanosis is generally related to the gravity of the condition. The animal should be moved around the stall and taken outside to observe its response to movement. Horses with pleural disease are often very reluctant to move. In some instances, the primary complaint may be that of lameness rather than respiratory disease.

Palpation and Percussion: Palpation and percussion of the respiratory system are valuable diagnostic aids. The entire respiratory system should be examined from the nostrils to the chest. Palpation of the nostrils reveals the size of the external nares and the presence of defects or redundant tissue. The quantity, quality and odor of any nasal discharge should be noted.

Next, the clinician should palpate and percuss the area over the paranasal sinuses. Percussion of normal paranasal sinuses produces a resonant sound. Percussion produces a dull, low-pitched sound if one or more sinuses is filled with fluid or solid material. Both sides of the face should be palpated and percussed for comparison and the animal observed for signs of pain. Most paranasal sinus abnormalities are unilateral.

After percussing the paranasal sinuses, the face and head should be observed for symmetry. The submandibular area should be examined for any abnormal swelling or sensitivity. Horses suffering from infectious diseases may have some degree of lymphadenopathy. Individuals affected with *Streptococcus equi* often have a dramatic lymphadenopathy, whereas animals suffering from viral diseases usually have a moderate to minimal lymphadenopathy. Some animals may resent palpation of the submandibular area.

The larynx should be palpated externally. Atrophy of the cricoarytenoideus dorsalis muscle is evident in advanced cases of laryngeal hemiplegia. The larynx may be manually collapsed in some cases of advanced laryngeal hemiplegia. Asymmetry scars or other irregularities should be noted. A cough can usually be induced in all animals by applying firm pressure to the cricotracheal space. In normal animals usually 1 or 2 nonproductive coughs can be elicited. A paroxysm of coughs can often be elicited in animals suffering from inflammation of the respiratory tract. The quality of the cough may vary, depending on the nature of the disease.

The caudal border of the mandible and the parotid salivary gland should be palpated to the base of the ear. Animals suffering from acute guttural pouch disease may resent palpation in this area. The degree of nasal discharge may be increased by applying pressure in this area. If swelling is present, percussion can be helpful in determining if there is fluid or air in the pouches. The entire neck should be palpated for evidence of asymmetry. The trachea should be carefully examined for abnormalities. Scars or irregularities on the tracheal wall should be noted.

Palpation of the chest can be helpful in some situations. The animal with advanced lower respiratory or pleural disease may resent pressure along the thoracic wall. Percussion of the chest is best accomplished through the use of a plexor and pleximeter (Fig 2). The technic requires some practice, but the time spent mastering it is worthwhile. It is useful to detect fluid levels and consolidated areas of pulmonary parenchyma (Fig 3).

Auscultation: Auscultation is a valuable diagnostic aid in the examination of the respiratory system and should be carefully performed in a thorough routine developed by each clinician. The type of stethoscope used is not critical as long as the instrument is clean and properly functioning. Most errors in auscultation of the equine thorax are related to inability of the operator to properly interpret what is heard. Auscultation of the respiratory system should include the larynx, trachea and both sides of the thorax, and should be performed in a quiet stall or examining room.

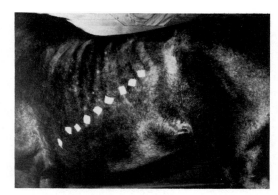

Fig 2. Normal margins of the thorax as defined by percussion.

It is probably beneficial to force the horse to breathe hard. One of the difficulties in auscultating a resting adult horse without overt disease is that there may not be enough air moving through the respiratory system to produce sound through the thick chest wall. The veterinarian should encourage the horse to breathe deeply by holding off both nostrils for 30-45 seconds. This is usually followed by at least 4 deep breaths. Another method is to place a bag over the horse's mouth and nostrils so that it breathes deeply into the bag. A final method is to exercise the horse for a few minutes and listen to the chest immediately after exercise. Complete auscultation should include both sides of the thorax before and after deep breaths have been induced.

Respiratory sounds can be classified in a number of ways.[1] Tracheal sounds are the normal, semiharsh inspiratory sounds heard over the trachea and generated by the movement of air through the trachea. Vesicular sounds are soft, blowing sounds heard primarily on inspi-

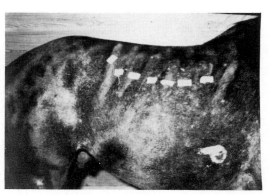

Fig 3. Margins of the thorax, as defined by percussion, when the pleural space is occupied by fluid.

ration and produced by air moving through the lower pulmonary tree. Bronchovesicular sounds are characterized by a soft, blowing sound heard on both inspiration and expiration; they are generally more intense on expiration.

Rales are produced by the movement of air through a fluid medium to produce a bubbling sound characterized as coarse, medium or fine. Coarse rales may be heard over the trachea of horses with large amounts of exudate within the trachea. Fine rales are very soft, crepitous sounds heard over the thorax of horses with pulmonary edema. Rhonchi (dry rales) are produced by air moving through narrowed conducting airways and may be characterized as either sonorous or sibilant, depending on their pitch and character. Sonorous rhonchi are very low-pitched and coarse, while sibilant rhonchi are often high-pitched and somewhat musical in nature.

A sound rarely heard in horses is a pleural friction rub, which is usually generated by inflamed pleural surfaces rubbing against each other as the animal breathes. They may be described as a scratching, squeaking sound, but their interpretation may be somewhat complicated. Most clinicians feel that any signs of rales or rhonchi are definitive evidence of respiratory disease.

Tracheal and vesicular sounds are generally thought to be normal in most individuals. Bronchovesicular sounds may be normal or abnormal, depending on their intensity and character, and the size of the animal. As stated earlier, many normal adult horses in good flesh have no audible sounds when resting. Vesicular sounds can usually be heard in these horses at increased respiratory rates. Bronchovesicular sounds may be heard if the animal is forced to exercise severely. Normal thin horses and foals produce bronchovesicular sounds because the size and thickness of their body wall allow easy transmission of sound. Bronchovesicular sounds in resting adult horses may indicate disease.

A lack of audible respiratory sounds is as significant as rales, rhonchi, etc. If a concerted effort has been made to have the animal breathe heavily and no air movement is detected, some abnormality exists. Most pleural disease is characterized by an absence of sounds rather than by pleural friction rubs because an effusion insulates the pulmonary parenchyma from the body wall. Severe, rapidly progressing pulmonary air movement heard on one side of the thorax and not on the other warrants concern.

Diagnostic Aids

The initial examination must be conducted systematically. Exercise to enhance air movement should be performed after observation, palpation, percussion and initial auscultation. The animal can then be moved from the stall or examining room and jogged or ridden for further observations. If no diagnosis has been reached at this point in the examination, the

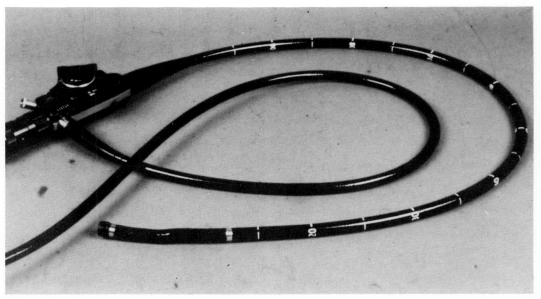

Fig 4. Flexible fiberoptic endoscope.

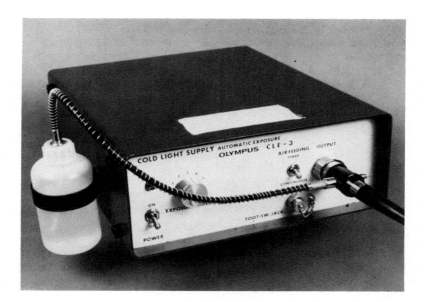

Fig 5. Light source for a fiberoptic endoscope.

clinician should decide which diagnostic aids are required.

Endoscopy: As endoscopic equipment has improved, clinicians have been better able to use it to evaluate more cases of respiratory disease. Endoscopy is generally a simple procedure with few adverse effects.

Animals with persistent signs of upper respiratory disease, such as chronic nasal discharge, abnormal respiratory sounds or regurgitation of food, are candidates for rhinolaryngoscopic examination. As the capability of the instruments improves, patients with lower respiratory tract disease may be subjected to thorough endoscopic examination. Animals with recurrent epistaxis should be examined with an endoscope before and after exercise. Uses of the endoscope will become apparent as specific disease entities are discussed in the remainder of this chapter.

Two basic types of endoscopes are available to equine practitioners for visualization of the respiratory tract (Figs 4-6). Rigid endoscopes have been used in veterinary medicine for many years for initial observations of the upper respiratory tract. These instruments have been successful but have several limitations. In the past 12 years, flexible fiberoptic systems have been very helpful in the diagnosis of upper and lower respiratory tract disease in horses.[2] Endoscopes are sophisticated instruments that require careful handling, which is one of the drawbacks of their use in equine practice. However, the advent of effective tranquilizers and sedatives has made endoscopy much easier.

The clinician should develop a systematic routine for use of the endoscope so that he or she neither overlooks nor produces any lesions.[3] The patient should be appropriately restrained and provisions made to protect the instrument. The nasal septum and nasal turbinates should be initially examined and, if a flexible system is used, the ventral and middle meati examined. Both nasal passages should be observed. The nasomaxillary opening of the caudal maxillary sinus may or may not be directly visualized. However, any abnormal secretions exiting this opening may be seen as they drain into the middle meatus. The ethmoid turbinates should be inspected on both sides if there is any question as to source of a lesion. Some horses resent the examination of this area even if a flexible system and adequate restraint are used. Examination of this area is

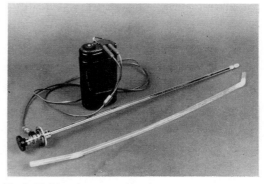

Fig 6. Rigid endoscope with a battery power pack.

often easier if performed at the end of the endoscopic examination.

The endoscope should be advanced into the nasopharynx and the pharyngeal walls examined for color, contour and evidence of secretions. The nasopharyngeal openings of the eustachian tubes should be examined and evidence of secretions noted. The dorsal recess of the nasopharynx should be inspected and abnormalities noted.

The endoscope can also be used to visualize the larynx and surrounding areas while in the nasopharynx. The arytenoid cartilage and vocal folds should be examined for symmetry and movement. The triangular shape and scalloped borders of the epiglottis should be observed. Failure to visualize the epiglottis may be due to displacement of the soft palate in some instances. The soft palate should be observed for color, contour and evidence of secretions. In normal individuals the caudal edge should lie ventral to the epiglottis. Some animals undergoing endoscopy displace the palate dorsad; however, this does not signify a functional abnormality of the soft palate. If the animal is encouraged to swallow, the soft palate usually returns to its normal position.

Flexible endoscopes can usually be passed through the larynx into the upper portion of the trachea in conscious horses. There may be some coughing and gagging but most horses tolerate the procedure. The inner aspects of the trachea can then be evaluated for color, symmetry and presence of secretions. The length of the trachea examined depends upon the length of the endoscope used and the size of the horse. In some cases, an appropriately sized endoscope can reach the tracheal bifurcation and even pass into primary and secondary bronchi.

An endoscope may also be passed into the guttural pouch of most adult horses. This technic is easy to describe, but may be very difficult to perform, and requires training and experience to master. In this procedure the rigid endoscope has an advantage over the flexible system because the rigidity allows easier passage through the nasopharyngeal orifice into the guttural pouch. However, the flexible system generally allows better visualization and exploration of the pouch. The use of a bent-tipped catheter or extension of the endoscope as a guide facilitates entry into the guttural pouch. Horses displaying signs of respiratory disease only on exercise should be examined with the endoscope before and immediately after strenuous exercise.

Radiography: Radiographic equipment and technic for evaluating the head and guttural pouch have been thoroughly described.[4,5] In certain cases, radiography can be used to definitively diagnose a respiratory problem. Radiography of the head and paranasal sinuses often reveals disease in those areas more readily than do other diagnostic tools. For example, infected teeth and sinus tumors are best defined with radiographs. Abnormalities of the nasal turbinates and nasal septum can be confirmed and often the severity and extent of the lesion determined with radiography. Guttural pouch abnormalities, such as the presence of fluid, air, foreign bodies or combinations of all 3, can be detected. Tracheal defects can also be identified.

Regardless of what type of radiographic equipment a clinician uses, several basic procedures should be followed. Two views at 90° to each other should be obtained whenever possible. However, this may be difficult when trying to obtain radiographs of the head and neck in standing horses. It is possible in most instances to obtain 2 views of the nasal passages and paranasal sinuses. Two views of the guttural pouch and cervical area may be difficult even with the best of equipment. If one is unable to obtain 2 views at 90° to each other, that fact should be considered when the films are interpreted.

As larger radiographic machines become available, the quality and usefulness of equine thoracic radiographs should improve. It is very difficult, except in very small horses, to obtain 2 views at 90° regardless of the animal's position. Although not as useful as in smaller animals, thoracic radiography in horses may be valuable in prognosis. For example, one should be able to recognize fluid in the chest in most cases through the use of other diagnostic aids. One should be able to diagnose pneumonia in most situations without the use of radiographic equipment. However, in cases of large masses in the thorax or pneumonia with overt abscesses that are apparent radiographically, the prognosis may be affected greatly. Thoracic radiography should be performed by those experienced in radiographic technic and interpretation of films of the thorax. Repeated use of thoracic radiography eventually produces consistent results.

Exercise and Observation: As mentioned earlier, exercise is a valuable tool for evaluation of the respiratory system through auscultation. It may be valuable for the clinician to listen for respiratory noises as the horse is strenuously exercised. In some cases, this may require the veterinarian to be at the rail of a race track as the horse is worked. The sounds should be classified as inspiratory, expiratory or both. It is best if the clinician can be stationed at the end point of the horse's exercise to hear the animal as exercise peaks and ceases. Riding or driving the animal may be unrewarding because of interfering sounds of the horse's feet and/or equipment. Listening to the horse at exercise may be the only time when abnormalities are detected.

It may be beneficial to repeat various portions of the examination immediately after exercise. These include auscultation, percussion, palpation and endoscopy. Observing the horse at exercise also allows the clinician to evaluate other body systems, especially the musculoskeletal and nervous systems, to determine if they have any relationship to the presenting complaint.

Nasopharyngeal Sampling: Collecting material from the external nares is of little benefit in most situations. The horse's environment is so contaminated that reliability of cultures is very limited and, even if cytologic examination is used, the chance of contamination from the environment is very great. Samples obtained by nasal swab should be collected from the nasopharynx using a guarded swab, which should be flexible to avoid damage to the nasal turbinates and other structures in the nasopharyngeal area (Fig 7).

A swab passed blindly through the ventral meatus of the nasal passage to the nasopharynx usually engages the dorsal pharyngeal recess, which feels firm and hard. Samples collected from this area must be interpreted very carefully because studies have shown that a wide variety of bacterial, fungal and viral agents normally inhabit the upper respiratory tract of healthy horses.[6,7] The environment of the animal largely determines the normal flora of the upper respiratory tract. The isolation of an apparent pathogen, such as *Streptococcus*, does not always mean the agent is producing disease. Cytologic examination of nasal swab samples is of more value than bacterial cultures. The detection of intranuclear inclusion bodies in adenovirus or equine rhinopneumonitis infections may be an aid in diagnosis.

Guttural Pouch Sampling: Sampling of the guttural pouch can produce very unreliable results, since the guttural pouch is simply an extension of the upper respiratory tract and contains contaminants common to the rest of

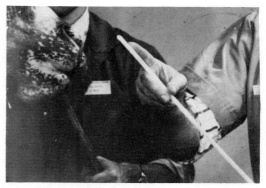

Fig 7. Culture rod used for nasopharyngeal sampling.

the tract. It is often extremely difficult to obtain uncontaminated samples from the guttural pouch for culture and cytologic examination. Various technics can be used to sample the guttural pouch. A guarded swab may be passed into the pouch during visualization with a rhinolaryngoscope. Alternatively, a catheter may be passed into the pouch and washings obtained with the use of a sterile physiologic solution free of preservatives. The catheter may be sutured in place for therapeutic lavage.

In cases of distention of the guttural pouch with air and/or fluid, the pouch may be sampled by percutaneous aspiration. The swelling is delineated by palpation and percussion. After a small area is clipped and aseptically prepared, a sterile needle attached to a syringe is inserted into the pouch for aspiration. This method avoids the possibility of contamination from the upper respiratory tract and is often much easier to perform than swab sampling. The clinician must exercise caution since the parotid salivary gland, external maxillary vein and common carotid artery are near the guttural pouch.

When evaluating culture results of the nasopharynx or guttural pouch, the clinician should look closely at the types, quantity and rate of bacterial growth and be aware that anerobic bacteria can be present in the upper respiratory tract.

Paranasal Sinus Sampling: Sampling of the paranasal sinuses is probably more reliable than that of the nasopharynx and guttural pouch, and has been described by others.[8] It can be performed unilaterally or bilaterally as indicated. The caudal maxillary sinus is most often sampled since it communicates with 3 of the other 4 paranasal sinuses. Sepsis of either the rostral or caudal maxillary sinus erodes

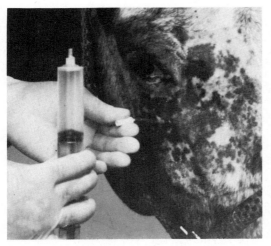

Fig 8. Catheter positioned in the caudal maxillary sinus in preparation for sinus lavage and aspiration.

the dividing septum to form a communication among all of the paranasal sinuses. The sinuses may be sampled with a minimum of instruments in standing patients. Trephination and catheterization of the maxillary sinus can be used to diagnose sinusitis, obtain material for culture and treat the sinus.

One should review the borders of the maxillary sinus before starting the procedure. The dorsal border runs from the medial canthus of the eye to the infraorbital foramen. The rostral border arises at the infraorbital foramen and proceeds to the rostral edge of the facial crest. The ventral border is the facial crest to below the middle of the eye, and the caudal border from the middle of the eye to the facial crest.

The sinus should be entered approximately 2 cm dorsal to the facial crest and 2 cm rostral to the middle of the eye. One must be careful not to interfere with the nasolacrimal duct,

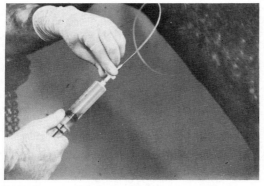

Fig 9. The site is prepared and the catheter is in position for transtracheal aspiration.

which runs from the medial canthus of the eye to the nostril. A small area should be aseptically prepared and local anesthesia applied intradermally and down to the periosteum. A small stab incision is made and a ¼-inch Steinmann pin used to trephine the sinus wall. Tubing is then inserted into the sinus and attached to a syringe for flushing (Fig 8). If the nasomaxillary opening is patent, discharge from the nostril should be evident after 35-50 ml solution are flushed into the sinus. Purulent material is flushed through the nasomaxillary opening if sinusitis is present. The material may also be aspirated for culture and cytologic examination. There is no drainage from the nostril if the nasomaxillary opening is occluded either by inspissated material or soft tissue occlusion and the material regurgitates around the catheter. Food material may be observed in the exudate if severe tooth disease is present.

It must be emphasized that the material obtained from sinus aspiration should be examined carefully by cytologic methods to determine the presence of fungal disease or neoplasia within the sinus. The recovery of one organism in pure culture is probably of much greater significance than if a variety of organisms are cultured from the sinus.

Although sinus aspiration is used in diagnosis, it may also be used in therapy. The tubing can be sutured to the skin, a bandage placed over the area and the catheter used to infuse the sinus with antiseptic or antibiotic solutions.

Transtracheal Aspiration: Transtracheal aspiration has allowed great advances in the diagnosis of lower equine respiratory disease. The technic is easy to perform, has few complications and can be performed on any size of horse with the appropriate restraint. A foal may be more easily examined by placing it with the dam in the stall, with a bale of hay or straw before it. Light sedation may be beneficial; however, one should avoid heavy sedation because the animal may become ataxic and lower its head, making the procedure difficult.

A 6-cm² area, halfway between the head and the thoracic inlet, on the ventral midline of the cervical region should be clipped and scrubbed. A local anesthetic is infiltrated in the skin and underlying muscle down to the trachea. Using aseptic technic, a syringe is filled with 20-40 ml sterile solution free of preservatives. An over-the-needle IV catheter is inserted through the skin into the trachea and the needle is removed to prevent cutting the catheter. Tubing, such as #5 polypropylene tubing, is passed through the catheter into the trachea and primary bronchi (Fig 9). The syringe is then attached and the sterile solution flushed into the lower respiratory tract. Injection of the fluid induces coughing, which forces material up to an area where it can be aspirated, and dilutes or dissolves secretions so they can be aspirated. The clinician should attempt to aspirate material from the lower respiratory tract as the catheter is withdrawn. The IV catheter protects the subcutaneous tissues from contamination or emphysema as the tubing is withdrawn.

The aspirate should be submitted for cytologic examination and, if infection is suspected, culture. Cytologic examination often aids diagnosis of chronic respiratory conditions. A gram stain of the aspirate from acutely infected horses aids in the rational selection of antibiotics for initial therapy.

Thoracentesis: Thoracentesis is easily performed and requires minimal equipment. The procedure is usually performed on the standing patient from the right side unless aspiration on the left side is indicated. The thorax should be entered at the sixth or seventh intercostal space at the level of the point of the elbow. The lateral thoracic vein, which courses along the chest wall in this area, should be avoided.

A 6-cm² area is surgically prepared and a local anesthetic is infiltrated into the skin and subcutaneous tissue. Using aseptic technic, a stab incision is made in the skin and a 2- to 3-inch, open-sided teat cannula is forced through the thoracic wall at a level different from that of the skin incision (Fig 10). A distinct popping is usually felt as the cannula penetrates the parietal pleura. Entry into the thorax is sig-

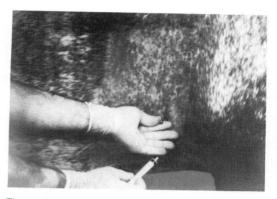

Fig 10. Cannula positioned for thoracentesis.

naled by air rushing in through the cannula on inspiration. If the point of entry is ventral to the lateral thoracic vein, a small amount of fluid may exit the cannula. Fluid obtained from entry dorsal to the lateral thoracic vein can be assumed to the abnormal.

If air is aspirated into the chest upon entry of the cannula, the thoracic cavity is either normal or does not contain a large quantity of effusion. If air is not aspirated and no effusion exits the cannula, the thoracentesis should be repeated because the cannula may be blocked by tissue or fibrin. A small syringe should be used to collect fluid or to stop the influx of air. Repeated attempts should be made if signs of thoracic entry are not evident. In rare instances, one may neither recover fluid nor note inrushing of air. If the thoracic wall is properly penetrated, there is usually little worry of air leaking into the thorax. On retraction of the cannula, the overlying skin seals the wound in the chest wall (Fig 11). A simple suture may be placed in the stab incision if desired.

Fig 11. A. An open-sided teat cannula is inserted through a stab incision in the skin. B. The cannula is pulled dorsad and forced through the thoracic wall and parietal pleura. C. The overlying skin seals the wound in the thoracic wall after retraction of the cannula.

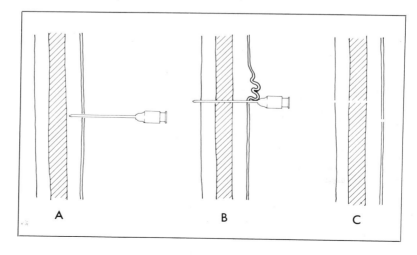

A   B   C

The fluid obtained from the thoracic cavity of a normal horse is usually slightly yellow-tinged yet transparent, and has the characteristics of a transudate. Abnormal fluid should be submitted for culture and cytologic evaluation (Table 1, p. 774).

The most commonly encountered complication is hemorrhage due to laceration of the lateral thoracic vein or an intercostal vessel entering the chest. This hemorrhage is usually self-limiting but can be controlled by simple pressure. If thoracentesis of the left side of the thorax is necessary, the region of cardiac dullness should be avoided, since it is possible to lacerate the myocardium. The eighth or ninth intercostal space at a level 2-3 inches above the elbow should be used if thoracentesis of the left side of the thorax is indicated.

Laboratory Procedures

Laboratory determinations can be extremely helpful to equine clinicians when dealing with disease of the respiratory system.

Hematologic Examination: Hematologic examination is beneficial in the diagnosis of infectious and noninfectious disease of the respiratory tract. Samples should be collected prior to patient stimulation or exercise. Chapter 11 has details on hematologic examination.

Blood-Gas Analysis: The use of blood-gas determinations as a diagnostic aid is justified in certain cases of respiratory disease. In most cases, blood-gas determinations are primarily used as a prognostic aid rather than as a definitive diagnostic tool

Microbiologic Examination: Microbiologic examination is a valuable aid in the diagnosis of equine respiratory disease. The proper handling of specimens for culture is imperative. The fact that a large population of anaerobic organisms is present in the normal equine respiratory tract should be considered when interpreting culture results. Microbiology laboratories may also be helpful in the diagnosis of certain mycotic diseases of the equine respiratory tract.

Virologic Examination: Virologic examination may be beneficial in the definitive diagnosis of certain abnormalities of the respiratory system. A detailed history and description of the case helps the laboratory isolate various viral agents. Three methods are generally available to diagnose viral disease.[9] The first is the isolation and identification of the viral agent. In most cases this is the least rewarding method, since the period of viremia varies and may actually be over before the animal is rec-ognized as ill. Virus isolation requires precise collection and handling of specimens to identify the virus. Laboratory requirements for virus isolation and identification are often exacting. The percentage of isolations per number of samples collected is often quite low.

Immunofluorescence is the second diagnostic method used in the diagnosis of viral disease. Immunofluorescence has limitations but can provide rapid results. The technic can be used on biopsies, smears or necropsy samples. The reliability of results is usually related to the abilities of laboratory personnel.

Serologic examination probably has the most application in the diagnosis of viral disease. Serum is easily collected, frozen and shipped to the laboratory. Also, samples need not be taken during viremia. It is absolutely imperative that 2 samples be collected from each horse 10-14 days apart so that any change in titer can be identified. One serum sample, whether at the beginning or the end of the disease process, is usually of little value. Horses with past viral diseases or those vaccinated have titers to a variety of viral agents. Unless a rising titer can be documented in the period after signs of infectious disease, little can be said other than that the horse has been exposed to the specific viral agent some time in the past.

Percutaneous Biopsy

A biopsy may be performed in cases of obscure lower respiratory tract disease such as chronic fibrotic pneumonia. Radiography and auscultation-percussion may help localize the best area for biopsy. Although large biopsy instruments, such as a liver biopsy cannula or alligator uterine biopsy forceps, have been used to obtain lung specimens, the risk of fatal hemothorax from pulmonary vessel laceration is greater than when small instruments are used.[10,11] The safest instrument for percutaneous lung biopsy is a disposable 8-inch biopsy needle (Tru-Cut: Travenol Labs).

Necropsy

Postmortem examinations should always be performed on horses with fatal respiratory disease when other horses have been exposed to affected animals. Necropsy specimens can be obtained and cultures performed to determine the etiology in cases where acute death precluded ante mortem diagnosis. A technic for postmortem examination of the upper respiratory tract, originally performed in sheep, can be adapted to horses.[12] Chapter 1 contains a discussion of necropsy technic.

References

1. Beech, J. Vet Clin No Am **1** (1979) 43.
2. Cook, WR. Vet Rec **94** (1974) 533.
3. Cook, WR. Eq Vet J **2** (1970) 137.
4. Cook, WR. J Am Vet Rad Soc **11** (1970) 35.
5. Cook, WR. J Am Vet Rad Soc **14** (1973) 51.
6. Floia, W *et al*. Dtsch Tier Wschr **80** (1973) 49.
7. Mansmann, RA and Strauss, AA. JAVMA **169** (1976) 631.
8. Mansmann, RA and Wheat, JD. Proc 18th Ann Mtg Am Assoc Eq Pract, 1972. p 375.
9. Coggins, L and Keman, MJ. JAVMA **166** (1975) 80.
10. Mansmann, RA. Doctoral thesis, Univ Calif, 1972.
11. Hughes, JP. Am J Vet Res **23** (1962) 1111.
12. Winter, H: Postmortem Examination of Ruminants. Univ Queensland Press, Australia, 1966.

Pulmonary Function Tests
by N.E. Robinson

Pulmonary function tests measure the extent of lung damage and the lung's response to treatment. Ideally, function tests provide information on gas exchange, the mechanical properties of the lungs and pulmonary blood flow. However, most tests require sophisticated equipment available only in research laboratories and are difficult to adapt for use in conscious horses. The technics of function testing have been reviewed;[1] this section provides only a brief overview of what is available.

Gas Exchange

Evaluation of gas exchange in horses at rest, during exercise and after exercise is the most valuable lung function test. The clinician evaluates gas exchange by observing the rate and depth of breathing and the rate of return to normal respiration after exercise. More objective information is obtained by measurement of arterial O_2 and CO_2 tensions (PaO_2, $PaCO_2$). Venous samples are useless for measurement of gas exchange.

Arterial samples are obtained by direct puncture of the carotid, facial, submandibular or digital artery.[1] The sample is withdrawn anaerobically into 3-ml syringes moistened with heparin (1000 IU/ml). Syringes sealed with a special cap or by folding the needle at the hub are stored in ice until the sample is analyzed. If blood is to be stored more than 20 minutes, it is advisable to collect samples in glass syringes, in which blood can be stored for up to 3 hours. Following sample collection the artery is manually compressed to prevent hematoma formation.

The PaO_2, $PaCO_2$ and pH are measured with blood-gas analyzer available in many clinical laboratories. The calibration of the machine must be questioned if the PaO_2 plus $PaCO_2$ totals more than 140 mm Hg when a horse breathes air. The PaO_2 plus $PaCO_2$ frequently total less than 150 mm Hg, particularly in animals with lung disease.

The normal $PaCO_2$ is 40-45 mm Hg.[1,2] Increased $PaCO_2$ indicates alveolar hypoventilation due to CNS depression, damage to the thoracic cage, or increased work of breathing from respiratory disease. Decreased $PaCO_2$ results from increased alveolar ventilation. This may be a response to hypoxemia or metabolic acidosis. Because CO_2 is more diffusible than O_2 and because of the shape of the oxyhemoglobin-dissociation curve, CO_2 can be eliminated when O_2 exchange is impaired. Only in severe respiratory distress is CO_2 retained.

In hypoventilation, a decreased PaO_2 approximates the elevation in $PaCO_2$. In such cases, increasing the alveolar ventilation eliminates CO_2 and restores O_2 exchange to normal. Hypoventilation is rarely the sole cause of hypoxemia; usually the PaO_2 is depressed more than can be explained by any elevation in $PaCO_2$. The hypoxemia of respiratory disease usually results from a combination of ventilation/perfusion inequalities and diffusion problems, and less commonly from hypoventilation.

When horses are breathing supplemental O_2, evaluation of gas exchange from PaO_2 and $PaCO_2$ measurements is difficult unless the exact composition of the inhaled or alveolar gas is known. This is usually only possible in clinical practice if a horse if breathing pure O_2 via an endotracheal tube and closed anesthetic system. Otherwise, measurement of alveolar gas composition requires collection and analysis of a 3-minute sample of expired gas. Once alveolar O_2 tension is calculated, the alveolar-arterial O_2 difference can be determined.[3] This excellent indicator of lung function measures the efficiency of O_2 exchange in the lung.

Mechanics of Ventilation

Respiratory muscles stretch the lung and generate flow through airways during breathing. Disease alters lung elasticity (compliance) or increases airway resistance. Lung compliance can be calculated in conscious horses (dynamic compliance) by simultaneously measuring tidal volume and the change in pleural pressure between the beginning and end of either inhalation of exhalation.[1,4] Dynamic compliance is more commonly decreased by small airway obstruction than by stiffening of lung parenchyma. Evaluation of lung elasticity requires measurement of static or quasi-static lung compliance and necessitates anesthesia.[5] Pulmonary resistance (primarily airway resistance) can be measured during breathing using equipment required for measurement of dynamic compliance.[1]

Lung Volume

Most clinicians want to measure lung volumes when first thinking of pulmonary function tests. Lung volumes are affected by the size and conformation of the horse, exercise and training, and probably also by the state of excitement of the horse. Lung volumes are also altered by disease processes. In conscious horses it is possible to measure tidal volume and minute ventilation using pneumotachography and functional residual capacity by gas-dilution technics.[1,4] Measurements of total lung capacity, vital capacity or residual volume require anesthesia, which in itself alters lung volumes.[5,6]

Distribution of Ventilation

The N_2-washout test has been used for evaluation of distribution of ventilation in horses.[1,7] In this test, the rate of elimination of N_2 from the lung is monitored while the horse breathes O_2 via a face mask-valve assembly. Washout of N_2 is prolonged by lung disease that obstructs small airways.

The problem with a single measurement of dynamic compliance, pulmonary resistance, lung volumes or N_2 washout in conscious horses is that the range of normal is very great. Only when a horse has clinically obvious dyspnea do the values exceed normal. However, these tests may be useful when multiple measurements are made to assess the response to treatment.

Pulmonary Vasculature

The pulmonary vasculature is evaluated by measurement of pulmonary arterial and left atrial pressures, and cardiac output.[8,9] Elevated arterial pressure in the presence of normal cardiac output results from increased vascular resistance, which can be due to destruction of vasculature, but more commonly results from alveolar hypoxia. The distribution of pulmonary blood flow, an important determinant of gas exchange, must be evaluated by isotopic scanning of the lung.

In summary, pulmonary function tests in horses are difficult to perform and generally require sophisticated equipment. However, pulmonary medicine would be improved vastly by more routine measurement of blood-gas tensions. These measurements are not out of the realm of modern equine practice.

References

1. Willoughby, RA and McDonnell, WN. Vet Clin No Am (Lg Anim) 1 (1979) 171.
2. Gillespie, JR et al. Am J Physiol 207 (1964) 1067.
3. West, JB: Respiratory Physiology. 2nd ed. Williams & Wilkins, Baltimore, 1971.
4. Gillespie, JR et al. J Appl Physiol 21 (1966) 416.
5. Sorenson, PR and Robinson, NE. J Appl Physiol. In press, 1981.
6. McDonell, WN and Hall, LW. Br J Anaesth 46 (1974) 802.
7. Muylle, E et al. Zbl Vet Med A 19 (1972) 310.
8. Muir, WW et al. Am J Vet Res 37 (1976) 697.
9. Milne, DW et al. Am J Vet Res 36 (1975) 1431.

RESPIRATORY TRACT SURGERY
by C.W. Raker

Tracheotomy

Emergency tracheotomy is often required in life-threatening respiratory obstruction and is an operation that "opens the doors of breath."[1] Concurrent elective tracheotomy is used prophylactically by some surgeons to provide a patent airway after surgical procedures to relieve partial upper airway obstruction. Tracheotomy is also used less frequently to bypass mechanical obstructions of the upper airway in diseases such as nasal septal deformities, fractures of the paranasal sinuses and turbinate bones, tumors of the nasal passages, pharynx or larynx, bilateral laryngeal hemiplegia, unilateral and bilateral arytenoid cartilage deformities, acute laryngeal edema, and after smoke inhalation and snakebites.

Tracheotomy is not a totally innocuous procedure and, therefore, should not be used on a routine basis in conjunction with elective upper airway surgery unless the airway has been occluded, as in tamponage of the nasal passages following removal of the nasal septum or an ethmoid hematoma, extensive repair of fractured facial bones, and in some cases of radical laryngeal surgery. Some disadvantages and complications of tracheotomy are loss of function of the nasal filter and warming of inspired air, loss of efficient coughing to clear the trachea and lungs of exudates, and the inherent risk of necrotizing tracheitis, with cicatrization and stenosis.

Tracheotomy may be either temporary or permanent. Permanent tracheotomy (tracheostomy) is seldom used in the US and is generally reserved to prolong the useful life of horses with an uncorrectable upper airway obstruction. Broodmares, stallions and retired or pet horses may benefit from this procedure. Horses are not permitted to compete in events in the US with a tracheotomy but may do so in some other countries.[2]

Tracheotomy is frequently performed as an elective or emergency procedure. In an emergency, a tracheotomy tube may be fashioned from any tubing, even a short section of stomach tube or the neck of a soda pop bottle. The tubes usually used are metal or plastic. Cuffed tubes have not been used in horses but should be adaptable. The temporary tracheotomy tube is a right-angled, ovoid tube with an external flange. The flange contains openings to permit the tube to be tied to the neck or sutured to the skin. Being ovoid, it can be placed between 2 opposing tracheal rings after incision of the tracheal annular ligament. Tubes used in tracheostomy are usually self-retaining and consist of male and female interlocking cannulae. These are available in ovoid shape as the right-angle temporary tube described above; however, most permanent tubes are cylindric, and therefore much larger, and require partial or complete removal of a segment of one or more tracheal rings. Complete excision of a segment of one or more tracheal rings should be avoided since the risk of tracheal stenosis is greatly increased. As one author stated, "One of the cardinal sins of surgery is excision of a segment of the tracheal cartilages because this lack of structural support results in obligatory narrowing of the trachea."[3]

Tracheotomy may be performed with the sedated horse standing, employing local anesthesia, or under general anesthesia with the horse in dorsal or lateral recumbency. Except for some emergencies, it is best to operate under general anesthesia with the patient intubated to provide good anesthetic control and an open airway. Hemorrhage is also more easily controlled and good surgical technic can be applied. While operating upon some upper airway obstructions, it may be desirable to relocate the endotracheal tube from the operative site. Under these circumstances, a tracheotomy is performed and the endotracheal tube is withdrawn from the mouth and replaced with a suitably sized tube inserted into the trachea, through which anesthetic gas administration is continued. If postsurgical upper airway obstruction is anticipated, a tracheotomy is performed during or at completion of the procedure and before recovery from anesthesia. Airway obstruction during or soon after recovery from anesthesia is relieved by inserting a standard tracheotomy tube or a suitably sized endotracheal tube into the laryngotomy, provided the wound has not been closed. Within a short time, most of these obstructions are overcome, especially when swallowing reflexes return. If signs of obstruction persist, an elective standing tracheotomy can be performed if the patient is comfortable and not thrashing about.

The tracheotomy technic is the same whether done on the standing or recumbent horse. The rostroventral half of the neck is prepared for aseptic surgery, except in a life-threatening emergency, when skin preparation and anesthesia are dispensed with. In a suffocating horse, a skin incision must be made as quickly as possible to insert a tube of any type or to dilate the incised tracheal annular ligament with a finger to establish an airway.

If the procedure is performed standing, local anesthesia is induced by SC and deep infiltration to the level of the trachea. The preferred site is the junction of the rostral and middle thirds of the neck over the ventral midline. This location allows reinsertion of the tube farther caudad if stenosis develops in situations that require long-term tracheostomy. Local anesthesia is placed on a line 10 cm long and a 7- to 8-cm skin incision is made. The sternothyrohyoideus muscle is bluntly separated on the midline to expose the tracheal rings.

After selection of a convenient site to enter the tracheal lumen, a cartilage knife or one-piece scalpel is placed transversely between 2 opposing cartilaginous rings and the tracheal annular ligament is incised. A one-piece scalpel is required to avoid detachment of the cutting blade of a conventional scalpel. The incision of the annular ligament should extend approximately 180°, or from 9 o'clock to 3 o'clock, to provide sufficient space for introduction of the tracheotomy tube. Placement of the tube is assisted by dilating the incision with the index finger and directing the tube into the tracheal lumen. If a temporary right-angle tube is used, it is tied securely to the neck or secured to the skin with sutures. Two ties, one directed craniad and the second caudad are helpful. A secondary tie to the mane increases fixation.

If a larger cylindric tube, usually the interlocking, self-retaining type, is used it may be necessary to increase the size of the surgical opening by grasping the free border of one tracheal ring with a towel clamp or Allis tissue forceps and placing it close to the free border. With scissors or a one-piece scalpel, a cresent-shaped section of cartilage is excised. The section excised should not extend more than halfway through the tracheal ring. The same procedure is repeated on the border of the opposing tracheal ring to create a window and the interlocking tube is then inserted.

The tracheotomy tube should be checked at frequent intervals during the first 24 hours to determine if it has been dislodged by movement and to ensure patency and should be replaced with a sterile tube one or more times daily. A second sterile tube should be inserted as soon as the soiled one has been removed for cleaning. Infection of the tracheotomy wound is controlled by repeated applications of antibiotic ointment. Any excessive granulation tissue is controlled by application of 1% hydrocortisone ointment or other suitable ointment.

The best method to evaluate upper airway patency following a tracheotomy is to plug the opening to the tube with the finger for several minutes or to seal it with adhesive tape. The sealed tube is left in place for whatever time necessary to evaluate adequate airflow.

It is best to let a tracheotomy wound heal by granulation. Tracheotomy wounds have been sutured but are generally contaminated or in the initial stages of granulation by the time the tube is removed. Furthermore, if they are closed, great detail must be directed to obtaining an airtight closure to avoid subcutaneous emphysema, which at times may extend to cover the entire body. This may be frightening but is rarely a serious complication.

The major complication following tracheotomy is necrotizing or granulomatous tracheitis, terminating in stenosis of the trachea. By maintaining the structural integrity of the tracheal rings and providing good wound care on a regular basis, risk of this complication can be minimized but not eliminated. Other less frequent complications are hemorrhage, with blood gravitating to the lungs, and a less effective cough reflex that, if food is aspirated into the trachea, may lead to foreign-body pneumonia. Pneumothorax is rare but pneumomediastinum has been reported as a complication of transtracheal aspiration.[4]

Surgical Approaches to the Larynx and Nasopharynx

Surgical approach to the nasopharynx through the nasal passage has been used to obtain pharyngeal biopsies, for chemical or cryosurgical cautery, for cyst or polyp removal and similar procedures. Visualization of the surgical area is achieved with an endoscope, preferably a flexible fiberoptic system.

Oral approach to the nasopharynx is difficult and often unrewarding because it leads to the oropharynx and the soft palate limits access to much of the nasopharynx. Cysts originating from the ventral aspect of the epiglottis can be palpated and subsequently removed successfully with a snare. Entrapment of the epiglottis has likewise been corrected using this approach. However, the surgery is essentially done blind or by feel since the operator's hand obscures vision of the surgical site. Furthermore, introduction of the hand and forearm through the mouth is at times difficult and laceration to the operator's hand and arm by the teeth is common.

Laryngotomy may be used for surgery on lesions of the dorsal wall of the pharynx and larynx, epiglottis and soft palate, for laryngeal sacculectomy and arytenoidectomy, and for removal of cysts, polyps and adhesions.

The procedure can be performed on an unanesthetized, standing horse. However, due to poor visibility of the surgical field, this approach is generally limited to laryngeal sacculectomy or exploration. As most laryngotomies are done under general anesthesia with the horse in dorsal recumbency, this approach will be described.

Preoperative preparation consists of withholding feed and muzzling the horse at least 12 hours prior to surgery. Two grams of phenylbutazone are administered IV 2-4 hours before surgery. No significant detrimental effect on blood clotting has been noted with this program, and postoperative inflammation and edema are effectively controlled and tracheotomy seldom required. Prophylactic antibiotic treatment is not used unless complications are expected. If employed, antibiotic therapy should be initiated in sufficient time to allow a therapeutic serum level of the drug by the time of surgery. Antibiotics should be administered for at least 4 days after surgery unless a change in medication is indicated based on the condition and response of the patient. Penicillin alone or combined with dihydrostreptomycin is usually adequate for initial prophylactic therapy.

Clipping the surgical site before preanesthetic preparation of the patient saves anesthesia time and permits scrubbing and preparation of the surgical site to begin as soon as the horse is positioned in dorsal recumbency.

Any acceptable general anesthetic program may be used but the advantages of halothane anesthesia with endotracheal intubation make this the method of choice. The endotracheal tube must be withdrawn to expose some of the lesions, but it can be replaced as indicated and additional anesthetic administered, or it can be supplemented by appropriate IV doses of a short-acting barbiturate or a combination of a barbiturate and a muscle relaxant as required. Prolonged administration or numerous repetitive doses of these agents should be avoided.

Several guides are used to establish the location of the ventral laryngeal skin incision in a horse in dorsal recumbency, with the head extended. An imaginary transverse line is drawn at the point where the ramus of the mandible disappears at the level of the parotid gland and the insertion of the sternocephalicus muscle. From this line the ventral surface of the throat is continuously palpated caudad toward the trachea. The first firm palpable transverse ring is the cricoid cartilage, followed by the first tracheal ring. Palpation of the cricoid and the first tracheal ring may also be accomplished by flexing the neck temporarily. The body of the thyroid cartilage is seldom palpable, especially with the head extended.

An 8- to 10-cm incision is made through the skin on the ventral midline, terminating at the cricotracheal space (Fig 12). The subcutaneous connective tissue is carefully incised by sharp dissection to expose the paired sternothyrohyoideus muscles. The septum between these muscles is identified and bluntly separated with dissecting scissors, being careful to stay within the septum. If the muscles are invaded, all loose tags should be excised to reduce postoperative edema and infection. A second layer of connective tissue fascia on the opposite (dorsal) side of these muscles, when incised, exposes the ventral surface of the larynx.

The length of the incision is increased as required for unhampered exposure. The muscles are retracted with a self-retaining blade retractor, such as the Adson (Sklar Manufacturing, Long Island City, NY), providing good exposure of the ventral surface of the larynx (Fig 13). The cricothyroid membrane occupies the space bounded by the transversely positioned ventral ring of the cricoid cartilage cau-

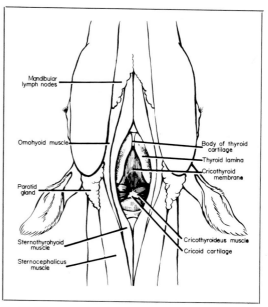

Fig 12. The ventral laryngeal region, with pertinent anatomic structures for laryngotomy.

dad and the thin ventral margins of the lamina of the thyroid cartilage on each side; it courses obliquely rostrad to join on the midline to form the body of the thyroid cartilage. The interlying space forms a triangle with the body of the thyroid cartilage as the apex, the lamina of the thyroid cartilage as the sides, and the cricoid cartilage as the base. The cricothyroid mem-

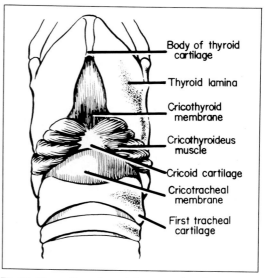

Fig 13. Deep dissection of the ventral surface of the larynx.

brane is incised by a stab incision with the scalpel. A scalpel with a detachable blade is acceptable; however, it should never be used when performing a standing laryngotomy or tracheotomy as the blade may detach.

Gentle incision leads to separation of the underlying mucosa from the cricothyroid membrane and creates deadspace that is detrimental to healing. With a stab incision, the membrane and mucosa are incised together. The scalpel should not be removed at once but rather left in place and incision of the membrane and mucosa extended to the body of the thyroid cartilage and cricoid cartilage. The incision should be as close to the ventral midline of the cricoid cartilage as possible. The ventral midline is determined by locating the right and left cricothyroideus muscles along the rostral margin of the cricoid. The small space between these 2 muscles is the ventral midline. If a previous laryngotomy has been performed, these muscles may not be easily found; however, the scar from the earlier incision should be apparent. Note is made of this landmark since the endotracheal tube or position of the head may cause rotation of the larynx and trachea from their usual anatomic position. Paramedian incision into the larynx is to be avoided since the vocal fold may be severed and healing complicated.

A small vessel transverses the cricothyroid membrane near its middle. Hemorrhage can be controlled by clamping, twisting and snapping the vessel from its tissue bed. Transection of the cricoid cartilage should be avoided since it may lead to complications. In young horses the resistance encountered to sectioning the cricoid cartilage is not significantly greater than when sectioning the cricothyroid ligament.

The retractor is then removed and placed within the larynx. Great care should be taken to ensure inclusion of the incised mucosal edges of the cricothyroid membrane within the blades of the retractor. Failure to do so may cause separation of the mucosa from the floor of the larynx and unnecessary trauma.

If additional access to the surgical site is required, as in a pony or a small or young horse, the body of the thyroid cartilage is incised with a small bone cutter or a scalpel. Severing the body of the thyroid cartilage in a mature horse with a scalpel is more difficult since the cartilage becomes more firm with age. The body of the thyroid cartilage is approximately 1 cm thick and continuous with the base of the epiglottis. Therefore, the body of the thyroid cartilage should be incised with care. Bleeding

from the severed cartilage rarely persists and is best controlled by packing with sterile gauze. Cautery of these vessels may lead to complications; one horse subjected to cautery of these bleeders later developed ossification of the cartilages of the left side of the larynx. Whether this was related to the cautery is unknown. As the surgeon gains experience with upper airway surgery, the need to incise the body of the thyroid cartilage decreases.

A laryngotomy may also be performed on unanesthetized standing horses. This procedure is extensively used by some surgeons for laryngeal sacculectomy and less frequently for digital exploration of the larynx. Successful laryngeal sacculectomies have been done for many years by surgeons experienced with the technic. Sedation is seldom required but may be used in nervous or fractious horses. Oversedation is to be avoided.

The procedure should be performed in a quiet area, preferably with the horse confined in stocks. After clipping the hair from the ventral aspect of the skin over the larynx and preparation of the surgical site, anesthesia is induced by SC infiltration of a local anesthetic along the proposed incision line. Additional injections are deposited at intervals about 2 cm apart between the sternothyrohyoid muscles to the level of the cricothyroid ligament. The skin is incised 8-10 cm on the ventral midline of the larynx. The sternothyrohyoid muscles are bluntly separated with scissors and the fingers to expose the cricothyroid space and membrane. The membrane is incised by stabbing a cartilage knife (one-piece scalpel) into the laryngeal airway, preferably during inspiration. The stab incision is required to incise both the membrane and the underlying mucosa simultaneously and should be on the midline.

The incision is continued rostrad to the body of the thyroid cartilage and caudad to the cricoid cartilage. Caution is required not to transect the cricoid cartilage. Introduction of a finger elicits a cough and swallowing. Anesthesia of the laryngeal mucosa is induced with a topical anesthetic applied by spray or moistened swabs. Anesthetic ointments are inconvenient and generally ineffective.

After completion of the surgery, the laryngotomy wound is handled in one of several ways. It is customary to leave the incision open to heal by second intention or granulation. This method is acceptable since healing is complete in about 3 weeks, leaving no significant scar. Alternately, the laryngotomy is carefully closed, using standard acceptable suture materials and patterns.

Postoperative management consists of close observation during the first 12-24 hours for signs of protracted hemorrhage or airway obstruction. Tracheotomy should be performed if indicated. Some surgeons routinely perform a tracheotomy when operating on the upper respiratory tract. The administration of 2 g phenylbutazone IV 2-4 hours before surgery significantly reduces the incidence of serious airway obstruction and the need for tracheotomy. An emergency tracheotomy set should accompany the patient from the operating room to recovery and to the horse's stall. In the event of the need for emergency tracheotomy, the tracheotomy tube or an endotracheal tube is inserted and retained through the laryngotomy incision. This is suitable for short terms; for prolonged intubation, the tube should be placed within the trachea (see Tracheotomy).

The horse should not be allowed free access to food or water during the first 12 hours or at least until good swallowing reflexes have returned. This is accomplished by use of a muzzle or cross-ties in a stall. Water from a bucket is allowed, but the bucket should be held by an attendant at knee level or set on the ground. This causes the horse to lower the head sufficiently so that if difficulty in swallowing is experienced, as is often the case initially, the water runs from the laryngotomy incision to lessen the chance of aspiration. Free access to food and water is allowed the day after surgery. The horse should be closely observed initially to determine the ability to swallow. Some coughing or choking may be apparent but generally subsides within a few hours to a day. Severe coughing with the potential to aspirate food or water is an indication to continue appropriate doses of nonsteroidal anti-inflammatory drugs and perhaps for tracheotomy. A bland diet of moistened feed pellets or wet oats with bran and good-quality hay should be fed.

If the laryngotomy has not been sutured, the incision should be gently cleaned 1-2 times a day, depending upon the amount of exudate. Gentle handling of the tissues is stressed to allow healing to progress without severe gaping of the skin edges or the production of excess granulation tissue. Application of any acceptable surgical scrub is adequate, followed by a saline rinse. Mild, nonirritating antibacterial drugs may be applied but are not essential to healing. Should excess granulation tissue develop or if the skin edges show marked retrac-

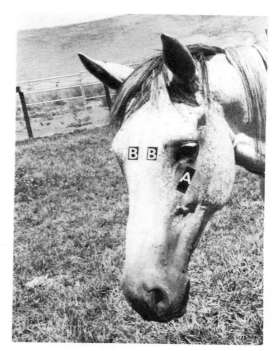

Fig 14. Landmarks for maxillary sinus (A) and frontal sinus (B) surgery.

tion, daily application of an antibacterial ointment with 1% hydrocortisone effectively controls these signs.

Paranasal Sinus Flap*

Paranasal sinus flap surgery is indicated in cases of diffuse sinus disease, disease of the roots of several upper teeth, and when exposure of the caudal nasal passage or ethmoid turbinate area is required.[5]

Maxillary Sinus: The horse is anesthetized and placed in lateral recumbency with the affected side up. After the surgical site is clipped and aseptically prepared, a skin incision is made over the rostral, ventral and caudal borders of the maxillary sinus (Fig 14). The skin and subcutaneous tissue are reflected dorsad, and the levator nasolabialis muscle is partially reflected from its origin, so it too can be reflected dorsad.

The periosteum is incised on the same 3 sides as the skin incision and is retracted 5 mm in from the edges of the incision. The bone is then cut along the same margins using a burr attached to a surgical air drill. The bone incision is made slightly oblique, rather than perpendicular to the bone surface, to create a dovetail pattern for flap security upon closure.

*by E.S. McAllister

After the bone is incised on the 3 margins, the bone is carefully elevated to fracture the flap along the dorsal margin, using the intact periosteum as a hinge. During this step of the procedure, care must be taken to avoid damaging the osseous nasolacrimal duct, which lies dorsal to the maxillary sinus.

After the appropriate exploration and treatments are performed in the maxillary sinus, the bone flap is repositioned and the periosteum sutured with simple-interrupted absorbable sutures. If the bone has been properly cut and the periosteum properly sutured, no other flap fixation is required. Wire sutures can be placed at the corners if the bone flap is unstable. The subcutaneous tissue and skin are closed with absorbable and nonabsorbable sutures, respectively.

A catheter can be placed through the flap into the sinus if postoperative irrigation is necessary. A nonadhesive dressing is placed over the site and several gauze sponges are placed over the dressing. The dressing is held in place by an elastic bandage (eg, Elastikon), that encircles the head.

Frontal Sinus: The above technic can be used if exposure of the frontal sinus or caudal turbinate area is indicated (Fig 14). The size and location of the flap depend on the lesion involved. The flap should be created as atraumatically as possible since excessive tissue damage causes hemorrhage and makes exploration of the area very difficult. Some hemorrhage occurs even under the best circumstances. Postoperative closure and dressing is similar to that used in maxillary sinus surgery.

References

1. Beatrous, WP. Laryng **78** (1968) 3.
2. Baker, in Catcott: Equine Medicine and Surgery. 2nd ed. American Veterinary Publications, Santa Barbara, 1972.
3. Webb, WR et al. Ann Surg **179** (1974) 819.
4. Farrow, CS. Am J Vet Res **17** (1976) 192.
5. Wheat, JD. Proc 19th Ann Mtg Am Assoc Eq Pract, 1973. p 171.

THERAPEUTIC PRINCIPLES
by R.A. Mansmann and E.S. McAllister

Signs of Respiratory Infection

The respiratory system is directly exposed to the environment and potentially pathogenic organisms. When respiratory tract infection occurs, definitive diagnosis often cannot be made only from clinical signs and is often only made long after the disease outbreak has occurred. In most clinical situations, therapy is initiated without knowledge of the etiologic agent. This is not to lessen the importance of a definitive diagnosis, which is often valuable in designing a vaccination program and preventing disease on the farm.

General signs of respiratory tract infection are multiple and varied, and in some cases not specific for respiratory tract abnormalities. In many instances, the initial sign of infectious disease is a change in attitude and loss of appetite. Many affected horses become depressed or at least are quiet, docile and less active. As the horse's condition worsens, there may also be partial or complete anorexia. Many infectious agents also produce a febrile response. The degree and duration of the fever can vary, depending upon the individual and the agent responsible for the disease. In certain situations, the degree of depression and appetite loss may or may not be noticed by a casual observer. The observer may note a nasal discharge and cough as the disease progresses. In many viral diseases the nasal discharge is serous unless complicated by secondary bacterial infection. The cough is often dry, harsh and nonproductive. The cough may become moist and productive if secondary bacterial invasion occurs. Secondary bacterial invasion is a result of disruption of the mucociliary blanket by viral agents.

Other signs of respiratory infection include labored breathing and an elevated respiratory rate. Close observation reveals "pumping" of the thoracic and abdominal muscles, which indicates diffuse involvement of the respiratory tract. Swelling of the head and neck may occur. Some viruses cause swelling of the eyelids, conjunctivitis and excessive lacrimation. Some bacterial diseases, such as *Streptococcus equi* infection, may produce marked swelling in the submandibular and retropharyngeal area. In cases of viral respiratory disease, lymphadenopathy may be minimal; however, the lymph nodes may be quite tender. Many viruses affecting the respiratory tract also affect other body systems. Concurrent signs may include enteritis, edema of the ventral abdomen and distal extremities, and reluctance to move. These signs should alert the clinician of some infectious agent.

As mentioned earlier, determining if a virus is involved is often difficult because the patient has usually recovered by the time the virus is identified. Prior knowledge of the incidence of certain organisms in a particular area may be beneficial in handling the disease. However, in many cases there is no indication of the exact etiologic agent.

The clinician must first determine if a virus, bacterium or a combination of both is involved. Next it should be determined if there is primarily upper respiratory tract involvement, lower respiratory tract involvement, or both. Therapy is based on these basic observations. The horse may be treated very conservatively if it shows few signs of bacterial infection and there is no significant lower respiratory tract involvement. Therapy must necessarily be very vigorous if significant bacterial infection is suspected and there is massive lower respiratory tract involvement.

General Therapeutic Principles

Preventive Management

Stress should be prevented or reduced in all animals suffering from infectious respiratory disease. This is especially important in foals with pneumonia and athletic horses with viral respiratory disease. The horses should not be shipped, forcibly exercised or used to compete when suffering from infectious disease.

Vaccines against locally prevalent respiratory diseases should be used at least twice annually and possibly more often if warranted.[1] Proper parasite control should be instituted and maintained to help reduce background irritation of the lungs. This is especially important in young horses.

Environmental Control

All horses should be stabled in well-ventilated barns. Good-quality grain, hay and bedding should be used to keep mold and dust to a minimum. Stable maintenance to remove dust and cobwebs, and watering small paddocks in dry environments are also important.

Horses with chronic respiratory disease may benefit from the elimination of hay as a feed. Even high-quality hay contains some dust and mold particles, which can be inhaled when the horse eats. This situation can be controlled by thoroughly dampening the hay with water, replacing baled hay with cubed or pelletized roughage, or using beet pulp as a source of bulk in their diet.

Horses with chronic respiratory disease should not be stabled in stalls under hay mows or next to dusty arenas. These horses may ben-efit from painting the stalls with varnish containing a fungicide, and spraying the floors with a fungicide, such as trisodium phosphate. Coarse wood shavings or chips, sprayed with 1 gal of mineral oil per 10 x 10-ft stall, make an ideal bedding for these animals.

Drug Therapy

Antibiotics: Penicillin is effective against all species of *Streptococcus* associated primarily or secondarily with equine respiratory disease. Penicillin is the authors' drug of choice in routine, uncomplicated respiratory tract infections. Sulfanilamides and tetracyclines may also be useful in nonspecific infections. Kanamycin and gentamicin are the drugs most suitable for gram-negative infections. These drugs are expensive, pose greater risks of adverse effects, and should only be used when indicated by culture and sensitivity tests.[2]

Antipyretics: Phenylbutazone, dipyrone, flunixin meglumine and aspirin can be helpful in making an animal more comfortable by reducing fever. However, fever is an important clinical sign that can aid the clinician in assessing the course of disease. Antipyretics should be given every other day so the degree of fever can be evaluated.

Corticosteroids: Corticosteroids are contraindicated in bacterial and viral pneumonia in foals, pleuropneumonia and routine upper respiratory viral and bacterial infections. Corticosteroids may make the animal appear better; however, the immune response can be depressed, causing prolongation of disease or secondary invasion by other organisms.

High corticosteroid dosages, such as prednisolone at 1-2 mg/lb daily for 3-5 days, may be life-saving in aspiration pneumonia and help reduce severe pulmonary inflammation.

Corticosteroids may be indicated in secondary pharyngeal paralysis due to *Streptococcus equi* infection to reduce neuritis in the guttural pouch. Penicillin should also be given.

Purpura hemorrhagica secondary to strangles infection may respond to high levels of corticosteroids and penicillin.

Alternate-day therapy, using prednisolone at 0.25-0.5 mg/lb every other day, is beneficial in treating chronic bronchiolitis and possibly chronic bronchitis in horses.[3] Antibiotics may or may not be given, depending on clinical signs and culture results.

Cough Suppressants, Decongestants, Bronchodilators: A moderate cough response helps expel mucus and thickened exudates. Coughing should not be suppressed in lower respiratory disease. Prolonged coughing from upper respiratory disease, such as tracheitis, is best treated by reducing upper airway irritation with iodides and antihistamines combined with bronchodilators.

Bronchodilation may be helpful in the treatment of chronic obstructive lung disease. Atropine at 2-4 mg/450 kg or isoproterenol at 0.1-0.2 mg/450 kg are useful in that regard. Horses with acute pneumonia may benefit from aminophylline given PO, IM or by rectal suppository. The diuretic effect of aminophylline may be valuable in the treatment of acute pulmonary edema. Prolonged therapy with bronchodilators has not been very beneficial in horses.

Nebulization

Nebulization is beneficial only if the animal is not stressed during treatment. Masks may stress some foals and young horses. In such cases, an ultrasonic nebulizer may be placed in a plastic-draped stall to humidify the animal's environment. Nebulizing equipment must be kept clean to prevent iatrogenic contamination of the horse's lungs.

References

1. Am Assoc Eq Pract Newsletter **2** (1980) 49.
2. Knight, HD and Hietala, S. Proc Ann Mtg Am Coll Vet Int Med, 1978. p. 120.
3. Beech, J. Vet Clin No Am **1** (1979) 73.

VIRAL RESPIRATORY INFECTIONS
by E.S. McAllister

At this writing 9 viruses have been associated with disease of the equine respiratory tract.[1] Several are also capable of producing disease of other body systems. The following is a review of all viruses associated with respiratory tract disease in horses.

Influenza

Although the terms "influenza" or "flu" have been used indiscriminately for many years in the literature, equine influenza produced by a myxovirus was first documented in 1956.[2]

Cause: Influenza in horses is caused by 2 subtypes of myxovirus: A-equi-1 and A-equi-2.[3] These myxoviruses are RNA viruses containing 2 types of antigens. The type-specific antigen is associated with the protein coat of the RNA genome. No protection is obtained from type-specific antigen-antibody reaction. The strain-specific antigen is associated with hem-

agglutinin spikes that protrude from the protein envelope of the virus, which allow the virus particle to attach to susceptible cells. Antibodies from strain-specific antigen reactions confer immunity and allow laboratory identification of the strains of influenza.[2] No cross-species infections have been documented among horses and other animals, including humans.

The influenza virus attacks the ciliated columnar epithelial cells lining the respiratory tract. Disruption of the respiratory track lining and alteration of the mucociliary blanket allows secondary bacterial invasion. Uncomplicated cases of influenza require 3 weeks for regeneration of normal respiratory tract epithelium. Influenza virus infects the entire lining of the respiratory tract and it is not limited to the upper portion of the tract.

Clinical Signs: Clinical signs of equine influenza vary greatly. Populations with no prior exposure are most susceptible and young horses are chiefly affected. However, all ages are susceptible. The disease may spread explosively throughout a susceptible herd.

Infection usually produces fever, which may be biphasic and as high as 41.1 C (106 F). Most affected animals have some degree of lethargy and anorexia. A cough, which is dry and nonproductive unless complicated by bacterial infection, may last several weeks after all other signs are gone. Nasal discharge is serous unless the disease is complicated by secondary bacterial infection.

Palpation of the submandibular and retropharyngeal area may elicit pain and coughing, but only minimal lymph node enlargement may be noted. Auscultation of the trachea and thorax may reveal rales or rhonchi. Coarse rales may be quite evident if bacterial invasion has occurred. Some animals may have a "pumping" respiration, which usually indicates lower respiratory tract involvement. Severely affected animals may have altered heart, liver, gut and musculoskeletal function.

Hematologic examination in uncomplicated early cases reveals leukopenia. As the disease progresses and secondary bacterial invasion occurs, the hemogram is often characterized by neutrophilic leukocytosis.

Treatment: Exercise should be minimized for 3 weeks and phenylbutazone may be given every other day while the body temperature is monitored. The use of antibiotics is warranted in cases of secondary bacterial infection.

Control: Prevention of influenza is best achieved through proper vaccination. All vaccines produced in the US are killed-virus vaccines that contain both strains of influenza virus. A primary immunization series of 2 IM injections, followed by a single annual booster, is recommended by vaccine manufacturers. The effectiveness of either natural or acquired immunity appears good; however, the effective duration of immunity is not precisely known.[1] Many researchers advocate influenza vaccination more often than annually. Data studies indicate that hemagglutination-inhibition titers fall to low levels 3-4 months after vaccination.[1] Clinical observations of horses in high-risk populations support a vaccination schedule of every 3-6 months.

Vaccination programs for influenza probably should be individualized for specific populations, depending on the risk. All foals should receive a primary immunization series beginning at 3 months of age. All horses in a particular population should be vaccinated, if possible, to maintain a high level of immunity.

Herpesvirus-1 Infection

Equine herpesvirus-1 (EHV-1) infection has several synonyms, the most common of which are rhinopneumonitis and viral abortion. The virus causes respiratory disease, abortion or neurologic disease, all of which may be present in an outbreak.

Cause: The EHV-1 particle is a DNA virus that cannot survive long outside the host. Close contact among individuals or with fresh secretions is usually necessary for transmission of the organism.

Clinical Signs: The respiratory form of EHV-1 infection is usually mild, transient and limited to weanlings and yearlings. It is one of the most common upper respiratory diseases in young horses. The incubation period is 2-10 days. Spread of the disease is often rapid, with high morbidity and low mortality.

The initial signs include serous nasal discharge and fever as high as 41.1 C (106 F). Depression, anorexia, cough and slight mandibular lymph node enlargement may also be observed. In uncomplicated cases recovery is usually spontaneous in 5-7 days. In many instances the respiratory form of the disease is mild and unnoticed unless other forms of the disease manifest themselves.

Hematologic examination of affected horses may reveal an initial leukopenia due to a decrease in neutrophils and lymphocyte numbers.[4] As the disease progresses, lymphocyte numbers and then neutrophil numbers return

to normal. Reinfection can occur but subsequent infections are often subclinical.

Diagnosis: The virus can be isolated from nasal swabs collected in the acute febrile period. Serologic examination may reveal complement-fixation or serum-neutralizing antibodies. Fluorescent microscopy of infected material collected from the upper respiratory tract may reveal EHV-1 particles.

Treatment: Treatment is usually unnecessary unless the disease is complicated by secondary bacterial infection.

Control: Modified-live and killed vaccines are available in the US. To prevent respiratory disease, foals should be vaccinated initially at 3 months of age, and then every 3 months until 2 years of age.[1] Depending upon the use of the animal and the risk of infection, older horses may be vaccinated less frequently thereafter.

Herpesvirus-2 Infection

Synonyms for equine herpesvirus-2 (EHV-2) infection include cytomegalovirus infection and slow-growing herpesvirus infection. The significance of EHV-2 in the pathogenesis of respiratory tract infection is unknown. Several strains have been isolated from the respiratory tract of horses with clinical disease.[5-7] Surveys have shown that almost all horses have evidence of current or past EHV-2 infection.[8] The apparent ubiquitous nature of the virus makes it difficult to determine its significance. One investigator recovered virus particles from the nasal cavity of 3 horses for 418 days after experimental infection.[9]

Clinical signs are very mild. The development and persistence of lymphoid follicular hyperplasia in young foals infected with EHV-2 may be significant. The fact that the virus persists for long periods may explain the persistent but mild signs of upper respiratory disease.[10]

The lack of animals unexposed to EHV-2 makes it difficult to do controlled or field trials with this agent. Little documentation of the significance of EHV-2 is available, but practitioners should be aware of the virus.[11]

Adenovirus Infection

The first adenovirus isolation from a horse was made in 1969.[12] Initially adenoviruses were thought to cause a fatal disease in Arabian foals;[13] however, further work indicated this virus as an opportunist in immunologically incompetent animals.[14]

The syndrome produced by adenovirus infection in experimental studies is nonspecific and mild in immunocompetent horses. Equine adenovirus is probably one of the viral agents that contributes to nonspecific upper respiratory signs in young animals.

Viral Arteritis

Equine arteritis virus sporadically affects a number of body systems. Although most horses have been exposed to the virus, few outbreaks of the disease have been reported.

Cause: The name of the virus was derived from the lesion produced in the media of small arteries. The incubation period of viral arteritis is 2-10 days.

Clinical Signs: Clinical signs vary and include fever, depression, muscular weakness, congestion of the nasal mucosa, serous nasal discharge, lacrimation and cough. Many horses have painful edema of the eyelids, ventral abdomen and extremities. Severely affected horses may develop colic, diarrhea, dehydration and weight loss. Abortions may be caused by this virus and usually occur within 7-14 days of infection. Hematologic examination at the onset of disease may reveal leukopenia.

Diagnosis: Diagnosis may be difficult if based only upon clinical signs. Virus isolation and serologic examination, using serum neutralization, can be used for definitive diagnosis. Microscopic lesions in the arteries are rather specific for this virus and include necrosis of smooth muscle cells and replacement with eosinophilic hyaline material. Subsequently there is edema and accumulation of lymphocytes in the arterial adventitia and media.[16]

Treatment: Treatment is supportive and directed toward alleviation of clinical signs.

Control: A modified-live virus vaccine was developed against viral arteritis but is not commercially available.

Rhinovirus Infection

The clinical signs associated with rhinovirus infection are those of mild upper respiratory tract disease: mild fever, serous nasal discharge and cough, which may be persistent. Morbidity can be high but recovery is usually uncomplicated.

The relationship between antibody levels and disease protection has not been established but it is thought that recovered horses have lifelong immunity. Serologic surveys showed a high percentage of horses over 6 years of age have antibodies against rhinovirus.[17]

Subclinical infections may help disseminate the virus. No vaccine is available to prevent equine rhinovirus infection.

Parainfluenza-3 Infection

This viral agent has been associated with equine upper respiratory disease. Its importance in the production of epizootics of respiratory disease in horses is not known. The upper respiratory signs produced by this agent in one disease outbreak were nonspecific.[18]

BACTERIAL RESPIRATORY INFECTIONS
by E.S. McAllister

Streptococcus Equi Infection

Streptococcus equi can produce infection without other initiating agents. "Strangles" is a term used by most lay people to describe the clinical syndrome produced by *S equi* infection. This disease has been recognized as a problem of horses since 1600.[19]

Cause: Streptococcus equi is a beta-hemolytic gram-positive organism. More than one strain may exist, which may account for some of the variable clinical signs and responses to vaccination observed by some investigators.[21]

Clinical Signs: Clinical signs produced by *S equi* infection can vary. The classic description includes signs primarily referable to abnormalities of the upper respiratory tract. However, in certain instances, a variety of systemic signs may be observed. Clinical signs most often observed include fever (102-106 F), varying degrees of depression and anorexia, and a nasal discharge, which may be serous or mucoid initially but quite purulent as the disease advances. Affected animals cough and are usually dyspneic to some degree. Many affected animals may resist palpation of the submandibular and retropharyngeal area (Fig 15). In most individuals the organism spreads to cause abscesses in the retropharyngeal or mandibular lymph nodes 10-14 days after the initial onset of signs.

The disease is most commonly transmitted through infective secretions. Once the disease establishes itself on a farm or ranch, it often becomes a persistent, recurrent problem even though there may be long periods when no resident horses have clinical signs of the disease. Once the organism establishes itself in a susceptible population, morbidity is generally quite high and often approaches 100%. However, mortality in most uncomplicated cases is low. Listlessness and rapid spread are also common. Most uncomplicated cases are confined to the upper respiratory tract; however, involvement of the lower respiratory tract can cause pneumonia. In some horses the organism localizes in the guttural pouch or paranasal sinuses and is a constant source of purulent discharge. Persistent drainage from the submandibular or pharyngeal areas occurs in some cases. Cranial nerve dysfunction may occur in cases of retropharyngeal abscesses affecting the recurrent laryngeal nerve. In horses with the most severe form of systemic *S equi* infection, any part of the body or viscera may be affected, including the heart.[22]

Diagnosis: A diagnosis of *S equi* infection can only be confirmed by isolation of the bacterium from lesions. Although most clinicians may suspect strangles because of clinical signs, other organisms can produce similar lesions. Obviously if the organism has been isolated previously on the premises, the index of suspicion should be raised.

Treatment: Streptococcus equi is quite susceptible to penicillin and there are no documented reports of resistance to that drug. Because the use of penicillin in the treatment of strangles has been controversial, only guidelines to therapy will be discussed.

Chemotherapy is unwarranted if the horse is alert, has a reasonably good appetite and has no dyspnea or dysphagia. Good nursing care and minimization of stress are important in all cases. A palatable diet and dry, comfortable surroundings should be provided. If warranted and practical, application of hotpacks or poultices helps promote maturation of abscesses. Mature abscesses should be lanced ventrally for good drainage.

Severely affected horses may require intensive supportive therapy, including IV fluids, feeding by nasogastric tube and tracheotomy. The use of penicillin is indicated if the temperature remains elevated for a long period, the horse is severely depressed and lethargic, and the pharyngeal and retropharyngeal areas are severely affected. Although some clinicians argue against the use of penicillin before abscesses have matured, administration of penicillin at the proper dosage for an adequate period is unquestionably beneficial. The recommended dosage in such cases is 10,000-20,000 IU/lb daily for a period to include 5-7 days after the last abscess has drained. Administration of penicillin in small doses or intermittently should be avoided.

The decision to administer penicillin should be closely evaluated if young animals or many animals on a farm are affected. In some cases the stress of rounding up and restraining af-

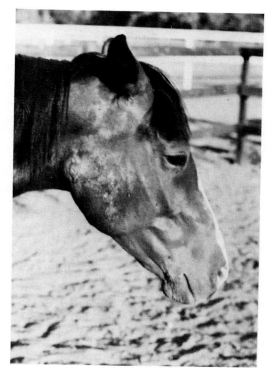

Fig 15. *Streptococcus equi* abscess in the submandibular area.

fected animals to administer penicillin outweighs the benefits of therapy. Other antibiotics should only be used if indicated by culture and sensitivity tests.

Control: If recognized early, an outbreak can be contained by isolation of affected horses and strict hygiene by handlers. Although vaccines have been developed, their efficacy has been questioned.[19,23,24] Difficulties in vaccine development stem from the relatively low immunogenicity of the bacterium and a lack of serologic tests to measure the immune response to *S equi* infection.[25,26] In view of the paucity of information on vaccine efficacy, it is difficult to recommend the use of strangles vaccine at this time. Although infrequent, systemic reactions to vaccination may also occur.

If a persistent severe problem with *S equi* exists on a farm, the use of the vaccine may be beneficial. The owner and clinician must be aware of the potential failures and adverse reactions if use of the vaccine is elected. Local reactions and abscesses at the injection site can occur from use of vaccines presently available. In most younger animals, especially those intended for racing, this is probably of little consequence. However, an injection reaction in a young horse being groomed for show purposes can be unsightly and cause the animal to be removed for competition for several weeks.

The use of autogenous vaccines has been advocated in cases of protracted, persistent outbreaks of strangles on a farm. In such instances autogenous vaccines may be more beneficial than commercial vaccines; however, care must be taken to prevent contamination in preparation of the vaccine. Although autogenous vaccines may be valuable in some situations, use of the vaccine in clinically affected individuals may result in a higher incidence of adverse reactions.[27]

Streptococcus Zooepidemicus Infection

Streptococcus zooepidemicus is the most common secondary bacterial invader of the equine respiratory system. Epidemiologic surveys of normal equine respiratory tracts indicate this organism is present in a high percentage of healthy horses. The organism probably cannot invade normal tissue and must rely on another agent to damage the respiratory epithelium before it can become established.[27] It is the most common secondary bacterial invader of either the upper or lower respiratory tract.

The organism, like *S equi*, is a beta-hemolytic streptococcus. It can be differentiated from *S equi* based on its production of acid and reduction of certain sugars.[29] However, unlike *S equi*, it does not tend to produce the severe abscesses of lymphoid tissue. It can produce purulent exudate but does not cause large submandibular or retropharyngeal abscesses.

Streptococcus zooepidemicus is sensitive to penicillin therapy. However, large abscesses may be refractory to antibiotic therapy. In uncomplicated secondary bacterial infections of

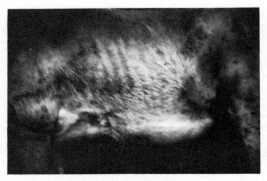

Fig 16. *Corynebacterium pseudotuberculosis* abscess along the ventral abdominal wall.

the respiratory tract, it is reasonable to assume that *S zooepidemicus* is involved unless otherwise indicated by culture.

Host response to infection by this organism is poorly understood. Most horses are susceptible to reinfection by this agent, perhaps due to lack of formation of immunity to the organism or due to the wide variety of antigenic strains. No commercial vaccine is available for prevention of *S zooepidemicus* infection.

Corynebacterium Equi Infection

Another common opportunist of the equine respiratory tract is *Corynebacterium equi*. It is not considered a primary pathogen, but rather requires some prior debilitating condition of the respiratory tract to cause disease. The organism apparently is not transmitted directly from animal to animal.[30] An Australian report indicated *C equi* was very common in the equine environment and was recovered from the feces of 72% of horses sampled.[31]

The organism most commonly affects the lower respiratory tract, but can cause disease in other areas. It is most commonly seen in young foals but may occur in adults as well. The organism has a propensity for producing abscesses that become quite large and involve extensive areas of pulmonary parenchyma. Infection by *C equi* is often insidious in onset and may be quite advanced before clinical signs are apparent.[30] Some horses may be near death from abscesses associated with *C equi* infection before the cause is apparent.

Chemotherapy should be guided by culture and sensitivity tests. Although this gram-positive organism may be susceptible to many antibiotics *in vitro*, it seems to develop resistance rapidly or show no response when treated in a clinical situation. This may be due to the inability of the antibiotic to reach effective concentrations in the plasma or the organism's ability to easily become resistant to a drug. Although many drugs have been used, gentamicin provides the best clinical response. Early diagnosis of the infection is imperative and good nursing care is extremely important.

Corynebacterium Pseudotuberculosis Infection

This organism can produce a wide variety of clinical signs in horses and is included here because of its ability to cause submandibular or cervical abscesses. Horses in California and surrounding states are most often affected.

Horses with submandibular abscesses from *C pseudotuberculosis* rarely have any signs of illness other than the firm, painful swelling, in contrast to the systemic signs observed in *S equi* infection. Abscesses from *C pseudotuberculosis* mature in 10-14 days. They may form in any location but are most commonly found in the pectoral region, along the ventral abdominal wall and on the extremities (Fig 16).[32]

Diagnosis of *C pseudotuberculosis* infection is by culture and isolation of the organism. Therapy is generally limited to local treatment of abscesses with hot packs, poultices and ventral drainage. Abscesses generally heal rapidly once drained. Systemic antibiotic therapy is of little value in cases of unopened abscesses. Penicillin is the drug of choice, unless sensitivity tests indicate otherwise, and should be administered for at least 7 days.

Other Bacterial Infections

A variety of other bacteria can secondarily invade the equine respiratory tract, including *Actinobacillus equuli, Bordetella bronchiseptica, Pasteurella, Klebsiella, Pseudomonas* and *Salmonella*. It is difficult to identify definitive clinical signs associated with infection by any of these bacteria. Culture and sensitivity tests should be performed in cases of persistent, unresponsive respiratory tract infection.

Mycotic and Protozoal Infections

Aspergillus is a fungus commonly isolated from the guttural pouch.[33] Although originally thought to be pathogenic, *Aspergillus* is now considered an opportunist. The organism was present in 10% of guttural pouch samples from normal horses.[34] *Aspergillus* has also been isolated from pulmonary parenchyma of horses with chronic lung disease or those subjected to intensive antibiotic therapy. The diagnosis of aspergillosis is based upon histologic examination and mycotic culture.

Rhinosporidium seeberi is classified as a fungus but has never been cultured. Infection by this organism is rare and characterized by soft-tissue masses on the nasal septal mucosa and nasal turbinates. Diagnosis is by histopathologic examination of excised tissue. Treatment involves complete excision of lesions, which may be combined with chemotherapy.[35]

Pneumocystis carinii is a protozoan that is probably an opportunist rather than a pathogen. The agent has affected immunosuppressed animals or those receiving protracted courses of antibiotic and/or corticosteroid therapy. Infection by *Pneumocystis carinii* should be suspected in foals with unresponsive pneumonia.[36] Diagnosis is by histologic examination of lung tissue, usually obtained at necropsy, stained with methenamine silver. No successful treatment has been reported in horses.

References

1. Proc Workshop Eq Viral Resp Dis, 1980. p 49.
2. Bryans and Gerber, in Catcott: Equine Medicine and Surgery. 2nd ed. American Veterinary Publications, Santa Barbara, 1972.
3. Waddell, GH et al. JAVMA **143** (1963) 587.
4. Doll, in Catcott: Equine Medicine and Surgery. 2nd ed. American Veterinary Publications, Santa Barbara, 1972.
5. Turner, AJ and Studdert, MJ. Aust Vet J **46** (1970) 581.
6. Roberts, AW et al. Am J Vet Res **35** (1974) 1169.
7. Rose, MA et al. Vet Rec **95** (1974) 484.
8. McGuire, TC et al. Am J Vet Res **35** (1974) 181.
9. Turner, AJ et al. Aust Vet J **46** (1970) 90.
10. Blakeslee, JR et al. Can J Microbiol **21** (1975) 1940.
11. Studdert, MJ. Cornell Vet **64** (1974) 94.
12. Todd, JD. JAVMA **155** (1969) 387.
13. McClosney, AE et al. Path Vet **7** (1970) 547.
14. McGuire, TC et al. JAVMA **164** (1974) 70.
15. McCallum, WH and Swerczek, TW. J Eq Med Surg **2** (1978) 293.
16. Doll, in Catcott: Equine Medicine and Surgery. 2nd ed. American Veterinary Publications, Santa Barbara, 1972.
17. Coggins, L and Kemen, MJ. JAVMA **166** (1975) 80.
18. Ditchfield, WJF. JAVMA **155** (1969) 384.
19. Todd, AG. J Comp Path Therapeut **28** (1910) 212.
20. Woolcock, JB. Res Vet Sci **19** (1975) 115.
22. Bergsten, G and Persson, S. Proc. 1st Int Conf Eq Infect Dis, 1966. p 76.
23. Bayeley, PL. Aust Vet J **10** (1942) 141.
24. Bryans and Moore, in Wannamaker and Matsen: Streptococci and Streptococcal Diseases. Academic Press, New York, 1972.
25. Woolcock, JB. Infect Immun **10** (1974) 116.
26. Woolcock, JB. Aust Vet J **51** (1975) 554.
27. Bryans, in Catcott: Equine Medicine and Surgery. 2nd ed. American Veterinary Publications, Santa Barbara, 1972.
28. Woolcock, JB. Res Vet Sci **18** (1975) 113.
29. Moore, BO and Bryans, JT. Proc 2nd Int Conf Eq Infect Dis, 1969. p 231.
30. Knight, in Catcott: Equine Medicine and Surgery. 2nd ed. American Veterinary Publications, Santa Barbara, 1972.
31. Woolcock, JB et al. Res Vet Sci **28** (1980) 87.
32. Miers, KC and Ley, WB. JAVMA **177** (1980) 250.
33. Cook, WR et al. Vet Rec **83** (1968) 422.
34. Floer, W et al. Dtsch Tier Wschr **80** (1973) 49.
35. Bridges, in Catcott: Equine Medicine and Surgery. 2nd ed. American Veterinary Publications, Santa Barbara, 1972.
36. Shively, JN et al. JAVMA **162** (1973) 648.

OBSTRUCTIVE UPPER RESPIRATORY DISEASE
by E.S. McAllister

The External Nares and Nasal Passages

This portion of the respiratory tract is least often affected by disease, but some conditions can cause dramatic signs. Abnormalities are often detected by observation or palpation. Unequal airflow, facial swelling or inspiratory noise can occur with lesions in the nasal passages. Endoscopy and radiography are the most useful diagnostic aids to evaluate disease in this area.

Atheroma

Atheromas are sebaceous cysts that form in the nasal diverticulum. These fluctuant, nonpainful swellings occur unilaterally or bilaterally, primarily in young horses. Their clinical significance is generally only related to cosmetic appearance but they are occasionally large enough to obstruct airflow.

Atheromas are easily treated by incision and drainage. For cosmetic reasons the incision is usually made ventrad through the false nostril, with the sedated horse standing. The nasal cartilage should be handled carefully to avoid chondroma formation. The cyst is drained and packed with iodine-soaked gauze. The pack is removed in 24-48 hours and the cystic cavity is flushed daily with povidone iodine.

Atheromas also can be completely excised, with the horse under general anesthesia and in lateral recumbency. The area is aseptically prepared and an incision made only through the skin overlying the cyst. The cyst is then carefully dissected from surrounding tissue. After the cyst is removed, the skin edges can be trimmed to remove redundant tissue and the incision is closed with absorbable sutures.

Alar Fold Stenosis

Stenotic alar folds have caused respiratory noise in young horses. However, stenotic alar folds rarely impair exercise tolerance. Alar fold stenosis can be diagnosed by temporarily retracting the folds with sutures over the nasal bones.[1] The horse is then exercised to determine if retraction of the folds reduces respiratory noise.

The alar folds can be resected if the respiratory noise is objectionable or if exercise tolerance is impaired. With the horse under general anesthesia and in dorsal recumbency, the fold is uncurled and resected along its longitudinal limits, from the alar cartilage to the cartilaginous portion of the ventral turbinates. The mucosal edge is joined to the corresponding skin edge with a continuous pattern of absorbable sutures. Work can be resumed in 2 weeks.

Lacerations of the Nares

Lacerations of the external nares often result in unsupported flaps that can occlude the airway upon inspiration. Attempts should be made to surgically correct instability of such flaps if they cause respiratory distress or objectionable noise. However, such attempts are often futile because of the difficulty in preventing motion in the area. Attempts at reconstruction may result in narrowing of the airway through scarification.

The most practical therapy for correction of unstable tissue flaps associated with lacerations is careful trimming to open the airway. Although the cosmetic aspects of this treatment may be undesirable, it is often superior to attempts at reconstruction.

Distortion of the Premaxilla

Congenital shortening and twisting of the premaxilla and nasal bones have been observed (Figs 17, 18).[2] No improvement has been noted in affected horses kept for 3 years. Although surgical correction of the condition has been reported, such radical cosmetic surgery seems unwarranted. In cases where an affected animal is to be salvaged, good nursing care should be provided in the first weeks of life until the risks of plastic surgery are lessened.

Narrowed Nasal Passages

Narrowing of the nasal passages may first be suspected when difficulty is encountered in passage of a nasogastric tube. The condition is generally diagnosed during initial training because of exercise intolerance and a stenotic inspiratory sound.

Affected horses have a narrow face and a very narrow intermandibular space. Passage of a stomach tube or an endoscope in affected horses is difficult and sometimes not possible.

Although horses have been treated for this condition by removal of the nasal septum (see Nasal Septal Disease), they are poor candidates for sustained exercise regardless of the treatment given.

Nasal Septal Disease

The nasal septum longitudinally divides the nasal cavity. The nasal septum should be palpated for thickness and symmetry when the respiratory tract is examined. Several conditions

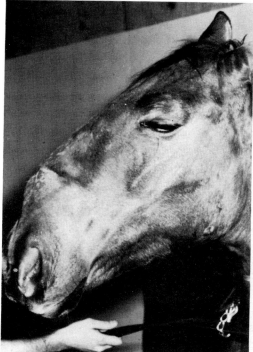

Fig 17. Congenital distortion of the maxilla in a 3-year-old horse.

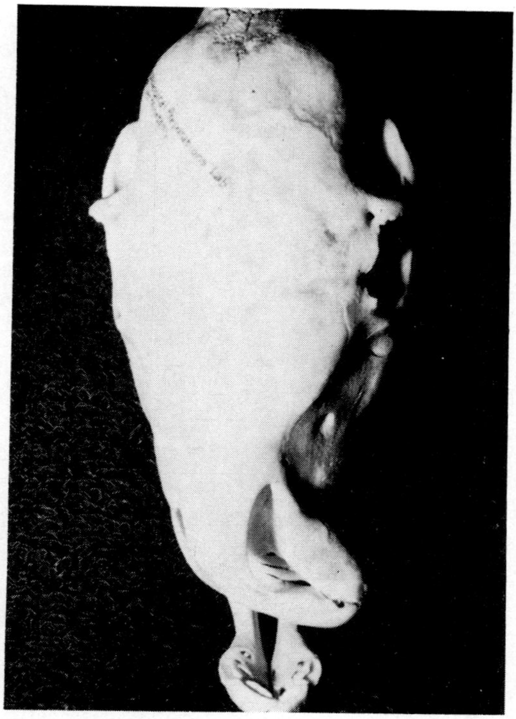

Fig 18. Skull of a foal with congenital deviation of the maxilla.

affect the nasal septum, including thickening, cystic dilations, hematomas, abscesses, mycotic granulomas, neoplasia, traumatic chondritis, fractures and deviations (Fig 19). All of these conditions can produce similar signs such as uneven airflow, inspiratory sound, facial distortion and nasal discharge. Endoscopy and radiography, with exact DV positioning, can be very helpful in evaluating the nasal septum.

All of the above conditions require removal of the nasal septum to improve airway patency. One must be sure there are no complicating factors before deciding to remove the septum. The chances of a successful surgery are poor if infection or neoplasia is diffusely spread through the nasal passage or paranasal sinuses. Removal of the nasal septum requires thorough preoperative preparation. A hemogram should be obtained and clotting functions evaluated. Blood transfusions are usually not necessary but an appropriate donor should be available and all the necessary equipment for blood transfusion assembled.

With the horse under general anesthesia and in lateral recumbency, a tracheotomy (see Tracheotomy) is performed to maintain anesthesia and provide a patent airway in the postopera-

tive period. After the tracheotomy has been completed, the horse is kept under anesthesia with the endotracheal tube passed through the tracheotomy.

The nasal bones are palpated where they diverge rostrad and a 10-cm curved skin incision is made over the nasal septum (Fig 20). The skin and subcutaneous tissue are reflected and a 1-inch trephine is used to make a hole directly on the midline where the nasal bones di-

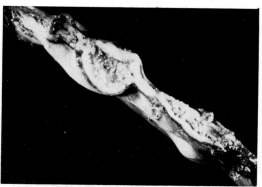

Fig 19. *Streptococcus equi* abscesses in the nasal septum.

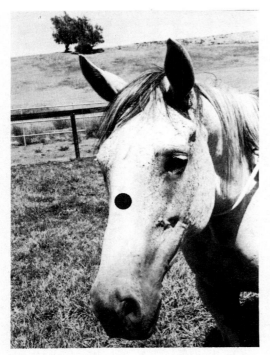

Fig 20. Site of skin incision to expose the nasal septum.

verge. Rochester-Pean forceps are then placed through the trephine opening and around the septum. An incision is made in the rostral aspect of the septum, 2 cm caudal to its rostral edge from the dorsal to the ventral limit of the septum. It is important that a portion of the rostral limit of the septum remain intact to maintain stability of the external nares.

A guarded chisel is then used to incise the septum along its dorsal and ventral limits, from the rostral incision to the forceps applied to the caudal aspect of the septum.[2] The surgeon must be prepared to work rapidly and efficiently at this point since considerable hemorrhage is usually encountered. The septum is then incised along the rostral aspect of the applied forceps to free it. A towel clamp or other heavy forceps is then used to grasp the rostral edge of the cut septum, which is pulled out through the nostril. The nasal passage is then tightly packed with gauze soaked in nitrofurazone solution to control hemorrhage. The skin flap is sutured with interrupted sutures of nonabsorbable material.

The horse must be monitored closely in the postoperative period for evidence of hemorrhage or respiratory difficulty. The gauze pack is removed from the nasal passage 24-36 hours after surgery and the tracheotomy tube 48-72 hours postoperatively. The nasal passage usually develops a profuse, foul-smelling discharge and should be irrigated daily with antiseptic solution until the odor is gone and the discharge minimal. Performance horses can return to work in 6 weeks if there are no complications.

Nasal Polyps

Nasal polyps are soft masses, usually pedunculated, that arise from the nasal mucosa. The cause of the polyps is unknown but chronic inflammatory response has been suggested.

Polyps not visible externally can be identified by endoscopy. A typical polyp is a smooth, nonulcerated mass filling a variable amount of the nasal passage. When examining a horse with a nasal polyp, one should attempt to identify the base of the polyp so the proper surgical approach can be planned for removal.

The clinical signs associated with nasal polyps vary depending on the size. Large polyps can be seen at the external nares. Affected horses have unequal airflow, inspiratory noise at exercise and/or rest, and possibly exercise intolerance.

Polyps in the rostral nasal passage can be reached through the external nares; however, most polyps seem to have their origin in the caudal portion of the nasal cavity. In these cases a trephine opening or bone flap is made over the affected nasal passage and the passage carefully entered. The base of the polyp is cut with scissors and the polyp removed through the nares. The base of the polyp is thoroughly debrided and treated with chemical cauterization or cryotherapy. The affected nasal cavity must usually be packed to control hemorrhage. If the cavity is packed, one should carefully watch for signs of respiratory distress and be prepared to perform a tracheotomy.

Nasal polyps have been removed using a snare introduced through the nares and the surgeon's hand through the mouth.[3] The soft palate is incised and the hand moved into the ethmoid region to guide the snare in removal of the polyp.

Neoplasia

The most commonly observed nasal tumor is squamous-cell carcinoma of the turbinates. Fibrosarcoma and lymphosarcoma also affect the area. Localized tumors can be resected; however, most tumors are too far advanced by the time they are detected. Chemotherapy and radiation therapy may be attempted where economics allow, but such treatment is usually only palliative.

Progressive Ethmoidal Hematoma

This condition can affect the turbinates, sinuses or both. The lesion resembles a neoplasm but has not been precisely classified. The masses are encapsulated in fibrous tissue and are composed of blood, fibrous tissue, macrophages, multinucleate giant cells and hemosiderin.[4] Progressive hematomas can become quite large; some are visible at the external nares, fill the entire nasal passage, nasopharynx and paranasal sinuses, and cause facial distortion.

A variety of clinical signs may occur but the most consistently observed is a hemorrhagic or serosanguineous unilateral nasal discharge.[5] Affected horses may have respiratory noises at rest, unequal airflow, and fetid breath.

When examined endoscopically, the hematoma appears as a mass with a granular surface in varying shades of green, yellow and red (Fig C1). The masses bleed easily if traumatized. Radiography is valuable in determining the extent and location of the lesion, especially with regard to the paranasal sinuses.

Treatment of progressive hematomas is usually initiated with surgery.[5] After the extent and location of the lesion are determined, a large bone flap is made in the appropriate area. For lesions in the ethmoid turbinate area the flap is made over the rostral aspect of the frontal sinus. The turbinate portion of the frontal sinus is then opened to reveal the ethmoid turbinates. The hematoma is usually friable and should be handled carefully. It should be bluntly dissected free in a wide area from its attachments. Hemorrhage is controlled by pressure and packing. Cryotherapy at the site of excision may help prevent recurrence.

The area is packed with nitrofurazone-soaked gauze after surgery and the tail of the pack brought to the external nares. The pack is removed 48-72 hours after surgery. The horse is closely observed for postoperative hemorrhage and respiratory distress. Performance horses can return to work in 6 weeks if no complications occur. The animal should be examined at least every 6 months following surgery for evidence of recurrence.

Success rates for treatment by surgery-cryotherapy have been variable. The most complete report of ethmoid hematomas indicated recurrence in 5 of 13 horses.[5] The prognosis depends on the extent of the lesion when diagnosed, ability to entirely remove the hematoma, and ability to control hemorrhage during surgery.

The Paranasal Sinuses

Horses have 4 pairs of paranasal sinuses: maxillary, frontal, sphenopalatine and ethmoidal. The maxillary sinus is divided into a rostral and a caudal compartment by a thin septum. All sinuses on each side communicate and drain to the nasal passage through the nasomaxillary opening. This opening is present between the caudal maxillary sinus and the middle meatus of the nasal turbinates. The maxillary and frontal sinuses are most often involved with disease processes.

Follicular Cysts

The most common congenital defects of the paranasal sinuses are follicular cysts, which occur most often in the maxillary sinus. They are an abnormal development from the tooth follicle, a form of odontoma, and are typically filled with honey-like fluid. Early recognition of a follicular cyst is important because cyst growth causes permanent stenosis of the airway by distortion of the nasal septum.[6] Secondary infection of a follicular cyst has been observed in an older horse.[7]

Follicular cysts should be considered in the differential diagnosis of any facial swelling in foals 2-3 months of age (Fig 21). The diagnosis can usually be confirmed by radiography.

Successful treatment requires removing the entire cyst and its lining from the maxillary sinus by creating a bone flap. Additional benefit may be obtained in some patients by creating or enlarging an opening from the affected sinus into the nasal passage using a seton bandage. This is done by pushing nitrofurazone-soaked gauze through the medial aspect of the affected sinus into the nasal passage. Sponge forceps or a similar instrument is then passed up the nasal passage to grasp the gauze end and pull it to the exterior. The other end of the gauze is brought to the exterior as the surgical site is closed and the free ends are tied together over the face. This seton bandage establishes a permanent fistula between the sinus and the nasal passage. The bandage should remain in place for 10-14 days after surgery and is changed daily or every other day. Most animals strongly resent changing of the bandage and become difficult to handle. Adequate assistance should be available when per-

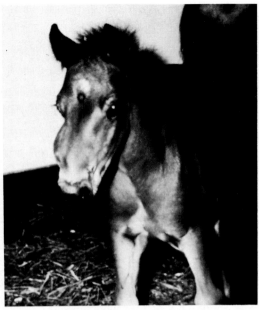

Fig 21. Two-month-old foal with typical swelling associated with a follicular cyst of the maxillary sinus.

forming this procedure and sedation used as needed.

Facial Trauma

Trauma to the facial region can cause sinus damage. Fractures can often be identified by physical examination. Radiographs are valuable in determining the extent of the fractures and at times may be essential for the definitive diagnosis.

Closed fractures with minimal displacement can be treated conservatively. Surgery is usually necessary to restore facial contours in cases of severe fragment displacement or comminution.[8] Sinuses opened by compound fractures should be kept as clean as possible. The

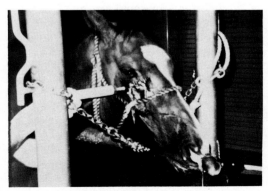

Fig 22. Sinus lavage in a horse with septic sinusitis.

wound should be carefully cleaned and debrided. All bone fragments should be examined carefully and either securely stabilized or removed if not vital. The sinus should be flushed, directly or via catheter, with antibiotic or antiseptic solutions. Systemic antibiotics can be used when indicated. The wound should be covered with nonadhesive dressings held in place by elastic tape. Wounds in this area heal rapidly if sepsis is controlled and nonviable bone fragments are removed.

Septic Sinusitis

Septic sinusitis is the most common form of sinus disease in horses. It occurs most often in the maxillary sinus secondary to dental disease in middle-aged horses. Septic sinusitis also may occur as a sequel to viral or bacterial upper respiratory infections and sinus trauma.

Clinical Signs: Signs of septic sinusitis include purulent nasal discharge, fetid breath, dullness and pain on percussion of the affected sinus, facial swelling, and fistula formation. A careful oral examination should be performed if these signs are present.

Diagnosis: The diagnosis of septic sinusitis can be confirmed by sinus aspiration, as described earlier. Dental disease should be considered as a primary cause if food-stained exudate is obtained. Radiography can also confirm the presence of septic sinusitis. Fluid lines, increased density within the sinus and destruction of the alveolar wall around affected teeth are radiographic signs suggestive of sinusitis and dental disease.

Treatment: Septic sinusitis may be treated medically or surgically. Sinusitis secondary to infectious disease or trauma can usually be managed by insertion of an indwelling catheter and irrigation with an antiseptic or antibiotic solution (Fig 22). The sinus should be flushed 2-3 times daily for 5-7 days. Surgery is required for treatment of septic sinusitis secondary to dental disease or long-standing bacterial disease (see Chapter 13). Surgical exposure is best made with a bone flap in cases of long-standing disease or multiple tooth involvement. This allows good visualization of the sinus and gives the surgeon an opportunity to evaluate the extent of the disease process. After the surgery is completed, an indwelling catheter can be placed for postoperative irrigation.

Tooth or bone fragments can act as sequestra within the sinus to cause persistent postoperative drainage. These may be identified on postoperative radiographs. Small fragments may gradually break down and be flushed from the sinus. Surgical removal of large fragments is usually required for satisfactory healing. Radiographs obtained just after surgery ensure that all fragments have been removed.

Other complications of septic sinusitis include the development of fistulous tracts around the lavage catheter or cellulitis in the subcutaneous tissue over the surgical site. These can usually be managed by vigorous irrigation, hot packs, removal of all foreign material and careful attention to bandaging of the surgical area.

Neoplasia

Tumors of the paranasal sinuses may be primary or associated with tumors in other portions of the upper airway. Masses involving the sinuses often have a poor prognosis because of the strong possibility of recurrence. The most common and potentially locally invasive tumor is squamous-cell carcinoma. Other invasive tumors include fibrosarcoma, adenocarcinoma, osteosarcoma and lymphosarcoma.[6]

Neoplasia should be considered in cases of a fetid odor about the head in the absence of dental disease. Radiographic, cytologic and histopathologic examination aid the diagnosis.

Poorly defined masses, such as ethmoidal hematomas and granulomas, have been treated by surgical excision and cryotherapy.[5,6] Solid, noninvasive neoplasms, such as osteomas, cementomas, adamantinomas and odontomas, have been surgically removed without recurrence (Fig 23). Early removal is usually easier, and lessens the chance of recurrence and permanent nasal cavity distortion. The prognosis is usually poor in cases of invasive tumors.

The Guttural Pouch

The guttural pouch is a structure unique to equidae. The paired pouches are ventral diverticula of the eustachian tubes situated ventral to the base of the cranium and atlas, and opposing each other mediad. The pouches lie dorsal to the nasopharynx and are bounded laterad by the vertical ramus of the mandible and the parotid salivary gland.

Each pouch is divided into a medial and lateral compartment by the great cornu of the hyoid bone and has a capacity of approximately 300 ml. The pouches are lined with ciliated epithelium and are supplied with glands chiefly of the mucous type. Coursing through the wall of each guttural pouch are cranial nerves VII and IX through XII, the cranial sympathetic trunk, and the internal and external carotid

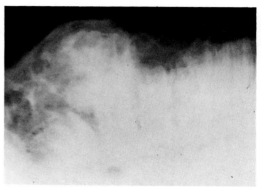

Fig 23. Radiographic appearance of an odontoma in a 4-year-old Thoroughbred mare.

arteries. Each pouch communicates with the nasopharynx through the nasopharyngeal orifice of the eustachian tube.[10] The function of the guttural pouch, although not completely understood, is probably to assist in equalizing pressure across the tympanic membrane.[11]

Diagnosis of guttural pouch disease depends on the history, physical examination, endoscopy and radiography. The ease of diagnosis depends on the disease involved and clinical signs. There is often a history of previous exposure to an infectious respiratory disease, such as *Streptococcus equi* infection.

The 2 classic and most consistently observed signs of guttural pouch disease are nasal discharge, especially unilateral, and swelling in the region of the parotid salivary gland. The nasal discharge is often purulent, but serous, hemorrhagic or food-stained discharges may also be observed. The rate of discharge may increase when the head is lowered or pressure is applied to the parotid salivary gland region. Swelling in the parotid region varies in size and may be firm, fluctuant or tympanic on palpation (Fig 24). Other clinical signs include in-

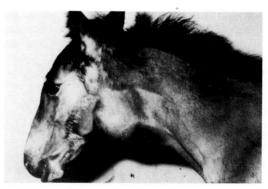

Fig 24. Weanling with tympany of the guttural pouch.

creased respiratory noise, soft palate paresis, laryngeal hemiplegia and dysphagia.

Clinical signs of the diptheritic form of guttural pouch infection include pain over the parotid area, abnormal head posture, head shyness, sweating, shivering, Horner's syndrome, conjunctivitis, lacrimation, corneal opacity, colic and facial paralysis.[12]

Endoscopy allows the examiner to confirm the presence of guttural pouch disease. If a rigid endoscope is used, a curved end aids introduction into the pouch. If an endoscope with a curved end is not available, any bent-tipped catheter, such as a mare urinary catheter or a Chambers catheter, can be used to open the cartilage flap at the nasopharyngeal orifice. The endoscope is then passed along the ventral aspect of the guiding instrument and inserted into the pouch, and the guiding instrument withdrawn (Fig C2). If a fiberoptic endoscope is used, more difficulty may be encountered because of the instrument's diameter and flexibility.[13] The fiberoptic endoscope tip is inserted into the guttural pouch with the use of a bent-tipped guide as previously described. The fiberoptic system allows visualization of the nasal passages as the scope is inserted and aids entry to the pouch.

Endoscopy of the upper airway may reveal several abnormalities. Guttural pouch disease should be considered as a potential cause of laryngeal hemiplegia, especially right-sided. Evidence of soft-palate or pharyngeal paresis, nasopharyngeal compression and purulent or hemorrhagic drainage from the nasopharyngeal orifice are indications of guttural pouch disease (Fig C3). Endoscopic evidence of exudate, concretions, diphtheritic membranes or masses within the pouch confirms a diagnosis of guttural pouch disease.

Radiography is useful in animals that cannot be endoscopically examined or in which a different perspective of the guttural pouch is desired. Fluid, concretions and abnormal amounts of air may be evident on radiographs.

Empyema

Guttural pouch empyema occurs most commonly after upper respiratory infection, especially that caused by *Streptococcus equi*. It can occur at any age but is most commonly observed in young horses. Clinical signs vary with the degree of pus accumulation. Chronic cases of empyema can lead to chondroid formation, which are thought to form from inspissated purulent exudate. Most cases of empyema

are caused by infection by beta-hemolytic *Streptococcus* but cultures should always be performed on material obtained from individuals with this condition. A small amount of serous or seromucoid discharge from the nasopharyngeal orifice of the guttural pouch is not a reliable sign of guttural pouch disease and may only be an extension of a nonspecific respiratory tract irritation.[14]

Tympany

Guttural pouch tympany is uncommon and seen most frequently in young animals. Most cases are unilateral but bilateral cases have been observed.[11] Guttural pouch tympany is thought to be caused by an abnormality of the mucosal flap of the nasopharyngeal orifice, which acts as a one-way valve that traps air in the pouch as the nasopharyngeal orifice opens and closes. The pouch may become severely distended to produce a tympanic swelling, dysphagia and respiratory distress. Confirmation of this condition can be made with radiographs, or the alleviation of signs by decompression through the nasopharyngeal orifice or percutaneous aspiration.

Horses with empyema may develop tympany because of inflammation of the mucosal flap, which may temporarily act as a one-way valve to trap air in the guttural pouch. Alternatively, tympany causes guttural pouch distension and prevents normal secretions from escaping. Accumulation of these secretions creates an ideal environment for proliferation of opportunistic organisms normally found in the pouch, resulting in empyema.[15] If empyema and tympany occur simultaneously, the horse's age and history should be closely evaluated to determine the primary disease entity.

Diphtheria

Guttural pouch diphtheria produces a great variety of clinical signs, depending on which vessels or nerves are affected. Diphtheria was initially thought to be due to mycotic infection;[16] however, recent evidence suggests that thrombosis and dilation of the internal carotid artery occur initially and subsequently allow development of a mycotic plaque.

Endoscopic inspection reveals a dark brown, black or yellow pseudomembrane, with irregular contours in the caudodorsal portion of the medial compartment of the pouch. The extent of the lesion may vary (Fig C4). Although guttural pouch diphtheria usually produces no distension, exudate may accumulate within the pouch.

Neoplasia

Guttural pouch neoplasia is extremely rare. Round-cell sarcoma, sarcoma, carcinoma and fibroma have been reported.[17,18]

Treatment of Guttural Pouch Disease

Treatment of guttural pouch disease may be medical or surgical. Medical therapy includes local and systemic treatment. Drainage and local irrigation of the guttural pouch can be rewarding in cases of empyema. In a cooperative patient the pouch may be repeatedly flushed and drained through the nasopharynx with a mare urinary catheter or Chambers catheter. The author prefers to use a #10 male-dog urinary catheter placed in the pouch and secured to the false nostril with nonabsorbable sutures (Fig 25). Once the catheter is secured, the pouch may be treated as often as necessary. The pouch can be irrigated with antibiotic or antiseptic solutions (Fig C5). One must be careful that the solutions used are not irritating since cranial nerve neuritis can result from the use of irritating solutions. When irrigating the pouch, the head should be lowered, manually or through the use of sedatives, to prevent aspiration of fluid.

Initial therapy of empyema involves flushes with 250-500 ml of solution 2-3 times daily for 5 days. A 25% povidone iodine solution may be used until culture and sensitivity results are obtained. If the guttural pouch size returns to normal and the exiting solution is free of exudate, treatment should be stopped and the pouch re-examined in 3-5 days for recurrence.

Unresponsive cases of empyema are those in which the pouch is greatly distended and fails to contract to normal size after treatment. Secretions reaccumulate and empyema returns. Surgery is indicated in such cases and in those with chondroid formation. Systemic antibiotics may be beneficial in treating empyema but adequate drainage and local therapy are of primary therapeutic importance.

Medical treatment of guttural pouch diphtheria may be attempted, but the typical location of the lesion makes application of medication difficult in standing horses. If vascular disease is the underlying cause for the diphtheritic lesion, little benefit is gained from topical therapy. Treatment of guttural pouch tympany by catheterization or percutaneous aspiration is helpful initially to decrease respiratory distress but is only palliative since the pouch usually refills after decompression.

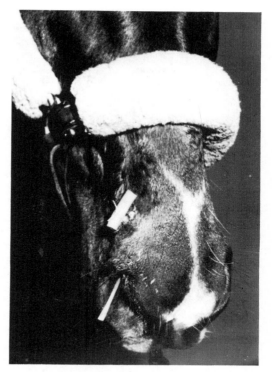

Fig 25. Catheter inserted into the guttural pouch is secured with a stay suture in the false nostril.

Surgery, which is necessary in cases of tympany and chondroid formation, is sometimes indicated in persistent empyema and seems to be the most reasonable approach to treatment of diphtheria. Three surgical approaches to the guttural pouch have been described.[20-22] The Dieterich approach is difficult to justify in any case because of the dorsal approach, minimal exposure and close contact with important anatomic structures.

The Whitehouse approach is superior because it offers the greatest exposure of all areas of the pouch, allows optimal ventral drainage and enables entry of both pouches through one incision if necessary. The Whitehouse approach is performed with the horse under general anesthesia and in dorsal recumbency. A 10- to 15-cm incision is made on the ventral midline, centered over the caudal border of the larynx. The sternothyrohyoideus muscles are separated on the midline, and the larynx and proximal trachea are retracted to one side. A guttural pouch distended with air or pus is easily identified after some blunt dissection in a dorsal direction; however, an undistended pouch may be difficult to identify and may require endoscopy for identification. The pouch is carefully opened with scissors while avoiding associated nerves and vessels. The pouch is explored after it is emptied. The lining of the pouch should be handled gently to avoid postoperative cranial nerve neuritis.

The third approach to the guttural pouch is through Viborg's triangle, which is the area bounded by the vertical ramus of the mandible, external maxillary vein, and the tendon of insertion of the sternocephalicus muscle. The triangle is usually obvious in cases of guttural pouch distension. The distended guttural pouch can be entered with the sedated horse standing. A horizontal skin incision is made within the limits of the triangle and the pouch is located by careful blunt dissection. The horse should be anesthetized and placed in lateral recumbency if the pouch is not distended. As in the Whitehouse approach, an endoscope may aid location of the pouch. The approach through Viborg's triangle offers limited exposure of an undistended pouch because of the anatomic boundaries of that area.

Regardless of the surgical approach used, a distended pouch should be packed with sterile gauze soaked in nitrofurazone solution. Incisions into the pouch should be allowed to heal by second intention if no evidence of sepsis exists; second-intention healing is rapid, with little or no cosmetic abnormalities.

Guttural pouch tympany can be treated by trimming the mucosal flap on the inner aspect of the nasopharyngeal orifice to remove redundant tissue or by fenestration of the medial septum between the 2 pouches. Fenestration can only be performed in cases of unilateral disease. Medial septum fenestration, using an electrocautery device introduced through the nasopharyngeal orifice in the standing horse, has been described.[13]

In cases of bilateral tympany the mucosal flap of the nasopharyngeal opening can be trimmed and the medial septum fenestrated, or the mucosal flap from both nasopharyngeal openings can be trimmed.

Persistent empyema or chondroid formation is treated by drainage and removal of septic material. The pouch is usually irrigated postoperatively through a drain in one of the ventral incisions. The alternative is to place a catheter in the pouch via the pharynx.

Surgery is the best treatment for guttural pouch diphtheria. The main thrusts of surgery are ligation of the internal carotid artery to prevent necrosis and subsequent rupture of that vessel, and removal of the diphtheritic membrane. One approach is to ligate the internal carotid artery proximal and distal to the diphtheritic lesion. However, it is not possible to place a distal ligature if the diphtheritic lesion is on the dorsal aspect of the pouch. If the vessel ruptures in such cases, fatal hemorrhage can occur via collateral circulation from the circle of Willis. A technic has been reported involving insertion of a balloon-tipped catheter into the internal carotid artery to induce thrombus formation in the diseased portion.[22,23] Although postoperative complications developed in the 2 cases reported, the technic appears promising.

Present knowledge suggests that removal of the diphtheritic membrane may not be necessary. However, if the membrane is removed, manipulations should be cautious because of the closely associated cranial nerves and internal carotid artery.

The potential for complications in guttural pouch disease is significant because of the close association of major vessels and cranial nerves. The most serious sequelae include permanent cranial nerve damage and fatal epistaxis. Pharyngeal and soft-palate paresis can also result in aspiration pneumonia. Other less ominous complications of guttural pouch disease are laryngeal hemiplegia, facial nerve paralysis, permanent distension of the guttural pouch, and fibrosis of the pouch.

The prognosis for guttural pouch empyema or tympany is generally favorable if the condition is recognized promptly. Guttural pouch diphtheria has a guarded prognosis. A review of 32 cases indicated a recovery rate of 47%.[12] Severe epistaxis associated with guttural pouch diphtheria warrants a poor prognosis.

References

1. Boles, CL. Vet Clin No Am (Lg Anim) 1 (1979) 89.
2. Boles, CL. Vet Clin No Am (Lg Anim) 1 (1979) 127.
3. Stickle, RL and Jones RD. VM/SAC 71 (1976) 1453.
4. Platt, H. J Path 115 (1975) 51.
5. Cook, WR and Littlewort, MCG. Eq Vet J 6 (1974) 101.
6. Leyland, A and Baker, JR. Br Vet J 131 (1975) 339.
7. Cannon, JH et al. JAVMA 169 (1976) 610.
8. Levine, SB. J Eq Med Surg 3 (1979) 186.
9. Peterson, FB et al. J Eq Med Surg 2 (1978) 279.
10. Sisson and Grossman: Anatomy of the Domestic Animals. 4th ed. WB Saunders, 1953.

11. Johnson, JH and Raker, CW. Proc 16th Ann Mtg Am Assoc Eq Pract, 1970. p 267.

12. Cook, WR. Vet Rec 83 (1968) 336.

13. Cook, WR. Vet Rec 94 (1974) 533.

14. McAllister, ES. Proc 23rd Ann Mtg Am Assoc Eq Pract, 1977. p 251.

15. Floer, W and Deegan, E. Berl Mnch Tier Wschr 86 (1973) 381.

16. Cook, WR et al. Vet Rec 83 (1968) 422.

17. Cook, WR. Vet Ann 16 (1971) 12.

18. Merriam, JG . JAVMA 161 (1972) 487.

19. Moller and Dollar: Regional Veterinary Surgery. WR Jenkins, New York, 1906.

20. O'Conner: Dollar's Veterinary Surgery. 4th ed. Williams & Wilkins, Baltimore, 1950.

21. Holmes, RA. Mod Vet Pract 43 (1962) 45.

22. Freeman, DE and Donawick, WJ. JAVMA 176 (1980) 232.

23. Freeman, DE and Donawick, WJ. JAVMA 176 (1980) 236.

The Nasopharynx*

The nasopharynx is separated from the oropharynx by the soft palate; the free border of the soft palate lies under the epiglottis except during swallowing. This arrangement establishes an unobstructed airway from the nasal passages to the larynx. Considerable turbulence develops as air passes through the pharynx; lesions obstructing the airway increase the turbulence, and restrict airflow.

The soft palate is a musculomembranous shelf arising from the lateral walls of the pharynx.[1] The mucosa of the oral surface is continuous with the hard palate and is attached to the base of the tongue by paired thick folds known as the rostral pillar of the soft palate. The mucosa of the pharynx is continuous with that of the nasal cavity. The free border is concave and continues as mucosal folds attached to the lateral walls of the pharynx to unite over the apex of the corniculate processes of the arytenoid cartilages and the opening to the esophagus, thereby forming the palatopharyngeal arch or caudal pillar of the soft palate. This anatomic arrangement results in a somewhat circular opening through which, except during swallowing, the epiglottis and the corniculate processes of the arytenoid cartilages protrude to form the laryngeal orifice. During deglutition the airtight seal around the laryngeal orifice is broken as the soft palate is elevated, permitting food to leave the oropharynx and pass over the occluded laryngeal orifice into the esophagus.

The internal and external maxillary arteries provide blood to the soft palate and lymph drains

*by C.W. Raker

to the pharyngeal lymph glands. The soft palate is innervated by cranial nerves V, IX and X.

Normally there is no significant restriction of air passage through the nasopharynx.[2] However, abnormalities of the soft palate or pharyngeal walls may lead to malfunction and obstructive airway disease.

The nasopharynx is an important segment of the upper airway and a frequent site of obstructive lesions. The most pertinent clinical signs associated with disease in this segment of the upper airway are respiratory noise, intolerance for work, choking-up, dysphagia, coughing and nasal discharge.

Common obstructive lesions of the nasopharynx include defects or disease of the soft palate, pharyngeal cysts, inflammation, neoplasia, mucosal trauma, and pharyngeal collapse.

Acute Pharyngitis

Pharyngitis is a common cause of obstructive upper airway disease. Acute pharyngitis is associated with bacterial or viral infections such as strangles, rhinopneumonitis, influenza and similar infections. In addition to the usual systemic signs associated with these diseases, those closely related to the pharynx are dysphagia, dyspnea and coughing. Dyspnea and hypoxia become more obvious with exercise. Swelling of the regional lymph nodes may be apparent externally. Endoscopy reveals the acutely inflamed mucosa and varying quantities of mucous or mucopurulent exudate. The size of the airway decreases commensurate with the extent of the inflammatory reaction and involvement of the guttural pouches and retropharyngeal lymph glands. Pain associated with acute pharyngeal and oropharyngeal inflammation causes dysphagia.

Acute inflammation of the nasopharynx may also follow the administration of irritant drugs, such as chloral hydrate, turpentine and carbon disulfide, by mouth or nasogastric tube if reflux around the tube occurs. Acute pharyngitis may also result from trauma caused by improper passage of a nasogastric tube or the introduction of foreign objects such as rigid endoscope or nasopharyngeal swabs. Localized areas of submucosal hemorrhage are commonly seen endoscopically and are probably the result of blunt trauma induced by endoscopy. These tissues are very susceptible to trauma and it is surprising that similar lesions are not seen more often after strenuous work. Because they are localized, they do not present a serious problem and heal rapidly without treatment.

Pharyngeal wall abscesses are rare. Trauma may lead to secondary infection and abscess formation. Abscesses involving the mucosae of the aryepiglottic folds and underlying the epiglottis may be seen at endoscopy. Local treatment with antibiotics alone or combined with low levels of corticosteroids can be effectively applied by nasopharyngeal spray several times a day. Recovery is usually satisfactory but rarely may be complicated by adhesions, which limit the function of the epiglottis or obstruct the airway.

On rare occasions retropharyngeal or pharyngeal lymph node abscesses may rupture and drain into the nasopharynx. Treatment involves systemic administration of antimicrobials and local application of medication through a nasopharyngeal tube, if indicated. Disease of the guttural pouches may likewise extend into the nasopharynx.

A nasopharyngeal tube for application of medication to the nasopharyngeal mucosa can be fashioned from a plastic tube of adequate size to deliver 10-15 ml fluid rapidly. A piece of flexible tubing of suitable length to reach the nasopharynx is obtained. One end is sealed by heating with a flame and then immediately crushed. Rough edges should be removed. With an 18- or 20-ga needle, 8-12 holes are made close to the sealed end. These openings are staggered around the circumference of the tube in a pattern to deliver a stream of medication in all directions and must be large enough to allow rapid delivery of the contents of the attached syringe. Rigid plastic tubing can be used but is subject to breaking should the horse move. A semi-rigid tube is preferred.

Chronic Pharyngitis

Chronic pharyngitis (pharyngeal lymphoid hyperplasia, lymphoid follicular pharyngitis) is a common cause of upper respiratory obstruction, especially in 2- and 3-year-old race horses.[3-7] Obstruction of the nasopharyngeal airway results from the proliferation of lymphoid tissue. The presence of a lymphoid follicles is normal in the nasopharynx of young horses. Decreased exercise tolerance may become apparent with proliferation and hyperplasia of this lymphoid tissue.

Cause: The etiology and pathogenesis of chronic pharyngitis is poorly understood. As previously stated, lymphoid follicles arising from the nasopharyngeal mucosa, especially from the dorsum, are found in nearly all young horses, especially those 2-3 years of age. The highest incidence of infectious upper respiratory disease reportedly occurs in 2- and 3-year-olds.[18] The follicles normally undergo natural regression at 4-5 years of age or soon thereafter unless chronically stimulated by unknown factors. Clinically significant chronic pharyngitis with airway obstruction may result from exposure to one or more respiratory viruses, such as herpesviruses, myxoviruses and possibly others.[3] Environmental factors, particularly air pollutants, may also play a significant role in this disease. It is interesting to postulate on the last as many trainers, owners and some veterinarians report a high incidence of chronic pharyngitis in horses stabled at race tracks close to industrial centers.

Clinical Signs: The clinical signs of chronic pharyngitis are decreased exercise tolerance, inspiratory and expiratory "blowing" noises of varying intensity, and occasionally coughing, especially at the beginning of or soon after a strenuous workout. A serous nasal discharge may be seen in some cases. Limited studies conducted at the University of Pennsylvania have not shown a direct relationship between chronic pharyngitis and hemorrhage from the respiratory tract; however, there may be a connection in some cases.

Diagnosis: Diagnosis of chronic pharyngitis can only be established by endoscopic examination of the nasopharynx. A system to grade chronic pharyngitis at endoscopy based upon the number, size, appearance and area of distribution of lymphoid follicles has been developed.[5] Grade I involves a relatively small number of white follicles scattered over the dorsal wall of the pharynx (Fig C10). Most of the follicles are small and inactive, which is normal in horses of all ages, particularly young horses. Grade II consists of many small, white follicles with numerous larger edematous, pink follicles on the dorsal wall of the pharynx and near the level of the pharyngeal orifices of the guttural pouches (Fig C11).

Grade III is characterized by the presence of many large, pink follicles interspersed among a few shrunken white follicles on the dorsal and lateral pharyngeal walls (Fig C12). The follicles may extend into the pharyngeal diverticulum, eustachian tubes and onto the dorsal surface of the soft palate. In addition to the findings noted in Grade III, Grade IV has even more large, pink follicles closely packed together all over the pharyngeal mucosa, including the pharyngeal diverticulum, dorsal surface of the soft palate and occasionally the eustachian tube, guttural pouches and epiglottis (Fig C13). Variably sized masses of lymphoid tissue resembling polyps are common, especially on the dorsal wall of the pharynx and in the region of the pharyngeal diverticulum.

Grade I is seldom accompanied by clinical signs of upper airway obstruction unless associated with a narrow pharyngeal airway, pharyngeal collapse, elevation of the soft palate or similar defects. Thus, Grade I is usually considered normal. Grade II may cause clinical signs of airway obstruction in a few horses, but is not generally significant unless accompanied by another abnormality. Grades III and IV are more likely to cause clinical signs compatible with airway obstruction and decreased performance. However, to conclude that Grade III or IV chronic pharyngitis is the cause of respiratory distress can lead to misdiagnosis unless all other potential diagnoses have been ruled out. Horses have been known to perform satisfactorily in spite of advanced (Grade III-IV) chronic pharyngitis. Horses have also been subjected to treatment for pharyngitis when the cause of the clinical signs was unquestionably the result of some other lesion.

Hyperplastic lymphoid follicles in the nasopharynx act as space-occupying lesions, decreasing the size of the airway and increasing air turbulence. The increased negative pressure that accompanies the obstruction may elevate the soft palate and collapse the lateral and dorsal walls of the nasopharynx. Additional airway obstruction may occur from contraction of throat muscles if the horse is tense from flexion of the neck at the poll as when the rider or driver takes a firm hold to restrain the animal. These events may be accompanied by caudal movement of the tongue, thereby elevating the soft palate to add to the nasopharyngeal airway obstruction.

Biopsies of acute lymphoid follicles reveal aggregates of lymphocytes, with infiltration by fibrous tissue. Biopsies of subacute or chronic white follicles are similar but contain more fibrous tissue and fewer lymphoid cells.

Cultures of the nasopharynx have not been particularly helpful in diagnosis and treatment. A variety of bacteria has been isolated and it has been difficult to relate these organisms to the disease. Treatment based upon culture findings has not been rewarding.

Treatment: A variety of treatments for chronic pharyngitis has been tried. Rest for 30-60 days may result in partial regression in the number, size and state of activity of the lymphoid follicles. However, when the animal returns to work, the lymphoid follicles often increase in size, number and area of involvement. This is especially true in young race horses. A few cases, however, have shown more prolonged regression.

Systemic or topical administration of a variety of antimicrobial drugs has been used alone or in combination with anti-inflammatory drugs, such as corticosteroids. The response to antimicrobials has been variable and generally unrewarding except for a few horses, in which initial regression was followed by recurrence when work was resumed. The response to antibiotic therapy has been difficult to assess but may be of limited value. In many cases there appears to be significant response to the administration of corticosteroids. This elevation, however, is subjective and the effect seems to last only as long as the drug is given. Topical application of medication through a nasopharyngeal spray seems to be as effective, if not more so, than using the same drugs systemically; however, the improvement often depends upon continuation of the treatment.

Iodides have been used empirically to treat chronic pharyngitis. Clinical evidence suggests they may be beneficial, but definitive data are not available. They should be administered in the feed or parenterally until signs of iodine toxicity are apparent. Many horses receiving iodide therapy are also rested while being treated. The nasopharynx may be directly treated 1-3 times daily with 10-15 ml of a mixture of 375 ml nitrofurazone solution and 125 ml DMSO (90%), to which has been added 1 g prednisolone acetate. Some horses with chronic pharyngitis respond to one massive oral dose of griseofulvin.[8,9] The general efficacy of this treatment is not known.

Hyperimmunization by repeated administration of influenza vaccine at relatively short intervals has also been tried. The results of these field trials are not available but may bear close observation. Recurrent lymphoid pharyngitis affecting the tonsils, lateral pharyngeal lymphoid bands and lymphoid follicles on the caudal pharyngeal wall is an immunologic entity in humans.[10] These patients lacked resistance to normal pharyngeal and nasopharyngeal flora. Treatment with a mixed respiratory bacterial vaccine reportedly improved resistance.

Changes in environment may also be helpful. Some horses improve cinically when moved from one race track to another or from one section of the country to another. Data to support these claims, particularly endoscopic evaluation, are limited. Other management changes, including good ventilation, air and feed, and avoidance of dust, are important.

Chronic pharyngitis has been effectively treated by cautery using a 50% solution of trichloroacetic acid swabbed onto the lymphoid follicles under observation through a fiberoptic endoscope passed through the contralateral nasal passage.[3] Satisfactory results were obtained when the treatment was repeated daily for 3-5 days or until the follicles sloughed.

Cryosurgery has also caused sloughing of the lymphoid follicles.[11] This treatment was applied through the nasal passage with a specially developed applicator while observing the nasopharynx through an endoscope. Cryosurgery has also been successful when applied to an anesthetized horse through a laryngotomy to expose the dorsal wall of the pharynx.

Electrocautery is another effective method of treating chronic pharyngitis.[5] A laryngotomy is performed after the horse is anesthetized and placed in dorsal recumbency. The endotracheal tube is removed when a surgical plane of anesthesia is achieved. The soft palate is then elevated with sponge forceps and all of the follicles within reach are cauterized. Cautery should be applied with a ball-tipped applicator until the follicles turn a light copper color. Excessive cauterization may cause adhesions and scarring. The arytenoid cartilages should be retracted to avoid damaging them.

A deep surgical plane of anesthesia must be maintained throughout the procedure to abolish the swallowing reflex and thereby maintain good visualization of the field. Topical anesthetic agents applied directly to the mucosa are of some value but may not totally eliminate the reflex. Cauterization is continued rostrad to the pharyngeal diverticulum and laterad to the level of the openings to the guttural pouches even though visualization of these areas is minimal.

Adjustment of the cautery unit is important for good cauterization. The settings can be determined by experience or by trials on the pharynx of a fresh cadaver. Allowing a coating of cauterized tissue to accumulate on the applicator is useful as it allows cauterization to proceed more rapidly by stroking the applicator over the affected tissue.

Electrocautery results in a regression of all accessible lymphoid follicles adequately cauterized and increased airway size. As some follicles may be inaccessible to cautery, total regression may not occur. However, since the largest number of the follicles involve the dorsal wall of the pharynx, a Grade-III or -IV chronic pharyngitis may revert to Grade I or II, and exercise tolerance is not noticeably impaired.

Postoperative management of the surgical site is as described for laryngotomy. Antibiotics are not given unless the presurgical workup or postsurgical complications indicate such. Endoscopic evaluation is performed 1-2 days after surgery and additionally as indicated. A necrotic exudate should cover the cauterized area within 1-2 days and become less apparent as healing progresses through 14 days. The horse is rested in a stall and walked daily for 30 days. Endoscopic evaluation is made at 30-45 days. Training can be resumed if the nasopharyngeal mucosae appear fairly normal.

Pharyngeal Cysts

Cysts in the pharynx are an infrequent cause of upper airway obstruction.[12] They have been diagnosed predominantly in the Standardbred and Thoroughbred but also occur in other breeds. Pharyngeal cysts frequently arise ventral to the epiglottis and are probably remnants of the embryonic thyroglossal duct.[4,12,13] Cysts arising from the dorsal pharyngeal wall are less common and may be remnants of the embryonic craniopharyngeal duct.[4,12,13] Cysts that arise from other areas of the nasopharynx are rare.

Cause: Pharyngeal cysts are most frequently diagnosed in stressed 2- and 3-year-old race horses. However, as pharyngeal cysts are probably congenital, they may have been present much earlier in life without producing apparent signs of obstruction until the animal was subjected to strenuous exercise. One case was effectively treated by the author in a 1-day-old Standardbred foal.

Clinical Signs: The clinical signs are those usually seen in upper airway obstruction and include intolerance for work, dyspnea, and an abnormal respiratory noise on both inspiration and expiration at work. Some affected horses may "choke up" and cough repeatedly as though severely obstructed. Less frequently observed clinical signs are difficulty in swallowing and nasal discharge. Two horses were referred to the University of Pennsylvania clinic with a history of gradual enlargement of a subepiglottal cyst and concurrent increase in the intensity of clinical signs; after the cyst apparently ruptured spontaneously, clinical signs disappeared. This course of events continued repeatedly until the cyst was surgically excised.

Diagnosis: Diagnosis is made by endoscopic examination. Pharyngeal cysts usually arise from the subepiglottal tissues and appear as a variably sized white or grey-white mass (Fig C6). Under bright illumination the surface may glisten and a fine vascular network is at times apparent. The cyst elevates the epiglottis to one side and infrequently the cyst and epiglottis are partially or totally occluded by dorsal displacement of the soft palate. Repeated stimulation of swallowing may return the soft palate to its normal position.

Treatment: The most effective treatment of pharyngeal cysts is surgical excision through the mouth or a laryngotomy. The laryngotomy approach is preferred. Removal of a cyst with a snare introduced through the mouth is not only more difficult for the reasons previously cited (Surgical Approaches), but the subsequent development of adhesions may interfere with swallowing.

A laryngotomy is performed with the horse under general anesthesia and in dorsal recumbency. To expose a subepiglottal cyst, the epiglottis must be rotated caudad 180° from the nasopharynx into the laryngeal airway, thereby presenting the cyst on the oral surface of the epiglottis into the laryngotomy field. Rotation of the epiglottis is accomplished by grasping the aryepiglottic fold on the lateral wall of the pharynx between the base of the epiglottis and the corniculate process of the arytenoid with a sponge forceps. Traction initiates caudal rotation and, by interchanging the position of 2 sponge forceps repeatedly, complete rotation into the larynx is effected. A sponge forceps applied to the apex of the epiglottis retains it in position. Gentle traction on the cyst also everts the epiglottis; however, extreme care should be exercised to avoid rupture of the capsule, which makes excision extremely difficult. The application of a sponge forceps or similar nonpenetrating instrument to the epiglottis is preferred to one that holds by puncturing the cartilage, *eg*, a towel clamp. The latter has been used in a few cases and has caused some serious, irreversible deformities of the epiglottis. Clamping the epiglottis for a short time traumatizes the epiglottic cartilage and its mucosal covering, but no serious complications

have been observed. Rotation of the epiglottis into the laryngeal airway has not caused obvious problems; however, the epiglottis should probably not be retained in this position longer than necessary to complete the surgery.

The cyst mucosa is carefully stabilized with Allis tissue forceps or hemostats, incised, and dissected from surrounding tissue by blunt dissection with scissors. Careful dissection is necessary to avoid cyst rupture. Should rupture occur, the hole may be occluded with mosquito forceps. Excess mucosa may be trimmed, but this is not essential. The wound may be left open to heal by granulation or can be closed with 00 or 000 chromic catgut or polyglycolic acid sutures, buried to lessen the chance of wound granulomas.[12]

If the cyst is inadvertently ruptured, total excision may not be possible. Failure to excise all secretory tissue may lead to recurrence. In these cases the depths of the cyst cavity can be swabbed with a cautery preparation, such as strong iodine solution. Care should be taken to confine application of the chemical to the cyst to avoid trauma to the surrounding mucosa.

Cysts that arise from the dorsal wall of the pharynx are more accessible and are excised in the same way as for a subepiglottal cyst. If the cyst arises from an area where surgical dissection cannot be readily carried out, it can be grasped and stabilized with Allis tissue forceps and, under moderate traction, removed with scissors. However, a larger defect is created due to the removal of more mucosa. Access to the wound for closure is limited, so it generally is not sutured.

The prognosis is favorable and complications are seldom encountered. Some horses develop adhesions, resulting in displacement of the epiglottis to one side; however, noticeable interference with swallowing or ventilation has not been observed. The effectiveness of the surgery is evaluated by endoscopic examination 1-2 days after surgery and thereafter as indicated. After a rest of 4-6 weeks, work can be resumed if healing is complete.

Soft Palate Defects

Functional obstruction of the nasopharyngeal airway by the soft palate is an important cause of decreased exercise tolerance and is commonly referred to as "choking up" or "swallowing the tongue." While the condition has been diagnosed in all breeds, it is a clinically significant cause of pharyngeal airway obstruction in race horses. The etiology and pathogenesis of soft palate defects are poorly understood. The clinical defects most often discussed in relation to abnormal function or position of the soft palate are dorsal (rostral) displacement, elongation with elevation, and paresis or paralysis. In functional abnormality of the soft palate resulting in obstruction of the nasopharyngeal airway, no organic lesions are demonstrable.[16,19] The term "functional pharyngeal obstruction" has been suggested to distinguish the syndrome from cases with obvious signs of paralysis or lesions of the soft palate.

While the etiology and pathogenesis of the syndrome are unclear, several factors may predispose to nasopharyngeal airway obstruction. In reports of several horses with respiratory noise and "choking up" while racing, dorsal displacement of the soft palate over the pharyngeal surface of the epiglottis was thought to be the cause of clinical signs.[14,15]Some horses had clinical evidence of concurrent laryngeal hemiplegia. From these observations it was concluded that the same factors that caused paralysis of the recurrent laryngeal nerve were responsible for paralysis of the pharyngeal branch of the vagus nerve, leading to paralysis and dorsal displacement of the soft palate. However, this hypothesis has not been substantiated. Similarly, there is no evidence to support a relationship between laryngeal hemiplegia and functional soft palate pharyngeal obstruction or the high incidence of soft palate displacement in horses without laryngeal paralysis. Mechanical and physical factors associated with soft palate displacement include fatigue, neck flexion, tenseness or excitability, mouth-breathing, retraction of the tongue, fighting the bit, increased negative-inspiratory pressure from respiratory infections, chronic pharyngitis, laryngeal hemiplegia, and defects of the epiglottis.

The horse is an obligatory nose-breather because the soft palate seals the nasopharynx from the oropharynx except during deglutition. Negative pressure develops in the upper respiratory tract during inspiration and factors that increase this negative pressure further restrict the flow of air. During endoscopic examination the effects of functional pharyngeal airway obstruction can be evaluated by occluding the horse's nostrils with the hand. As efforts to inspire continue, the dorsal wall of the pharynx moves ventrad, the soft palate moves dorsad, the walls of the pharynx begin to move mediad, and the larynx is pulled caudad. Flexion of the neck at the poll accentuates

these movements. The state of fitness for the work performed is important since fatigue is accompanied by increased respiratory effort and increased negative-inspiratory pressure.

If the mouth is opened, the airtight seal of the soft palate may be broken as the soft palate is displaced. When access to air is restored with the seal broken, the soft palate flutters on inspiration and expiration, and makes a gurgling or rattling noise often heard during expiration. Fighting a bit may cause a horse to mouth-breathe. A nervous horse may retract the tongue and elevate the soft palate to break the airtight seal. Retraction of the larynx assists in breaking the seal. Other diseases that partially obstruct the airway to increase the negative-inspiratory pressure include pharyngeal lymphoid hyperplasia, epiglottic entrapment, empyema of the guttural pouch, and epiglottic, thyroid and arytenoid cartilage defects.

Dorsal displacement of the soft palate occurs frequently in association with epiglottic hypoplasia, with or without concurrent entrapment, and is more frequent after successful surgical correction of epiglottic entrapment. A hypoplastic epiglottis may enable the soft palate to separate from the laryngeal orifice easily, whereas an entrapped hypoplastic epiglottis presents a larger contact area to retain the soft palate in position.

Soft palate elongation is thought to cause functional pharyngeal obstruction. Endoscopic examination of a resting horse may reveal the soft palate bulging dorsad into the nasopharyngeal airway (Fig C14, C15). Nasal occlusion significantly increases the elevation of the soft palate and may totally occlude the airway. During this maneuver the intrapharyngeal orifice of the soft palate may become dislodged from the laryngeal orifice. This is especially true should the horse begin to mouth-breathe or retract the larynx.

Dorsal bulging of the soft palate may be associated with tenseness, as when a twitch is applied to facilitate endoscopic examination. The muscle contraction associated with twitch application often encourages retraction of the tongue to elevate the soft palate, retraction of the larynx, excessive neck flexion and mouth-breathing. If possible, the twitch should be removed and endoscopic evaluation repeated. The administration of tranquilizers or other chemical restraint should be avoided if possible because these drugs often alter the results of endoscopic examination.

There is no evidence to support the hypothesis that a long soft palate is a cause of airway obstruction. The endoscopic diagnosis of an elongated soft palate is subjective. The soft palate may be of normal length but, due to other factors, elevated into the nasopharynx. There may be other as yet unrecognized defects of the nasopharynx or larynx, such as laryngeal cartilage defects, or anatomic differences in these segments of the airway that lead one to suspect soft palate elongation.

Displacement of the soft palate is a major cause of partial or complete upper airway obstruction and renders the horse unsuitable for work.[13,16,17,19] Some horses have a history fully compatible with the typical clinical signs of soft palate displacement but the diagnosis cannot be confirmed by endoscopic examination. Perhaps the clinical factors necessary to initiate the displacement cannot be induced during examination.

Soft palate paralysis is associated with disease of the vagus nerve. Botulism, moldy-corn poisoning, forage poisoning and guttural pouch disease are among those conditions most likely to be accompanied by pharyngeal paresis or paralysis. Dysphagia is a common clinical sign, and both food and water may exit the nostrils. Other clinical signs include choking, coughing and occasionally aspiration pneumonia.

Soft palate displacement can be observed during endoscopy and may be intermittent or permanent. Food, saliva and inflammatory secretions may be seen in the nasopharynx, nasal passages and occasionally within the larynx and trachea. A diagnosis of paresis or paralysis of the soft palate in the presence of these findings is reasonable. However, most horses with intermittent soft palate displacement do not have food or secretions in the nasopharynx, nasal passages, larynx or trachea. There is seldom a history of water exiting the nares. Paresis of the soft palate in these horses is therefore in doubt and the displacement must be the result of other causes. Infrequently the history contains information of coughing and choking while eating and drinking, with feed and water exiting the nostrils; however, these signs are usually intermittent and apparently only when the soft palate is dorsally displaced. Most horses with a soft palate defect or displacement do not show these signs.

Clinical signs of a dorsal displacement of the soft palate over the epiglottis closely mimic those observed in brachycephalic dogs. The owner frequently reports the horse makes a rattling or gurgling noise at work and may choke-up and rapidly slow its pace or stop. Rattling, gurgling, coughing and choking may also be heard when the horse is eating or drinking. The history may further indicate that clinical signs of airway obstruction disappear when the horse swallows. A similar noise is frequently heard during recovery from general anesthesia when the endotracheal tube has been removed before the swallowing reflex is restored.

A history of a horse that races normally, but on occasion chokes up, makes a rattling noise, staggers, becomes cyanotic and stops or falls down on the race track strongly suggests dorsal displacement of the soft palate. A detailed history should be obtained concerning when and under what circumstances clinical signs became apparent, the type of bit used, whether the tongue was tied, or the horse was excited, tried to mouth-breathe, "swallowed the tongue" or was tired.

The diagnostic endoscopic feature of dorsal displacement is observation of the soft palate lying over the pharyngeal surface of the epiglottis. Repeated stimulation of swallowing during endoscopic examination is used to evaluate the function of the soft palate. In carrying out this procedure, the endoscope should not be placed directly on the epiglottis since it may interfere with the return of the soft palate to the laryngeal orifice and lead to misdiagnosis. Under these conditions, especially if the endoscope has been retracted a short distance, the horse seems to be aware of the malposition of the soft palate and almost immediately swallows and the soft palate returns to its normal position ventral to the epiglottis. This finding must be carefully assessed so as not to confuse it with a "true" displacement.

A complete evaluation of the upper respiratory tract by inspection, palpation and percussion is essential. Signs of cranial nerve damage, swelling, muscle atrophy, exudates and other abnormalities should be noted. Endoscopic examination is essential to establish a diagnosis. The possibility of other diseases of the upper respiratory tract must be eliminated. In particular, disease of the guttural pouch with cranial nerve damage, defects of the epiglottis or other laryngeal cartilages, "elongated" soft palate and infections should be ruled out. The possibility of an association between laryngeal hemiplegia and dorsal displacement of the soft palate has been reported.[15,16]

Induction of swallowing during endoscopic examination is accomplished by forcing a spray of water through the endoscope onto the epiglottis. If swallowing does not occur, air under pressure is applied to blow the remaining water forcefully onto the epiglottis. Persistence with this technic causes the horse to swallow. This should be repeated a number of times to assess function. Generally, if the horse swallows 8-10 times and no abnormality is noted, there is little advantage in continuing. However, if the soft palate is displaced several times, a soft palate defect should be suspected, especially if the horse makes no immediate attempt to replace the soft palate by additional swallowing or if such attempts are ineffective. Occasional displacement with almost immediate replacement is of questionable diagnostic value, whereas repeated or continued displacement is probably significant.

During endoscopic examination, air should be withheld by nostril occlusion. Normal horses cannot breathe through the mouth with the nostrils occluded. While this test is not totally reliable, it is very useful. The nostrils should be occluded, with the fiberoptic endoscope in place and observations continued. As inspiratory efforts increase, the laryngeal orifice may be briefly occluded, the walls of the pharynx are drawn into the airway, the laryngeal orifice opened, the larynx is retracted and the soft palate may be displaced.

If dorsal displacement of the soft palate repeatedly occurs with minimal withholding of air and discomfort to the horse, the same events may take place while the horse is racing or performing strenuous work. Induction of displacement of the soft palate may be aided by removal of the twitch. Also, a twitch may cause some horses to begin to mouth-breathe due to retraction of the tongue and larynx, not unlike that which may occur during a race.

Repeated examinations are often helpful at rest and as soon as possible after strenuous work. Abnormal respiratory noise during work is noted and characterized as to type and when it occurs. Inspiratory noise may be confused with laryngeal hemiplegia or similar problems. The typical noise produced by dorsal displacement of the soft palate is an expiratory flutter or rattle. Inspiratory noise may also be heard, especially in those cases with a dorsal bulging or "elongated" soft palate without dorsal displacement.

Displacement may or may not occur with an "elongated" soft palate. However, the dorsal bulging of the soft palate into the nasopharyngeal airway, which may be observed before or while air is being withheld, is probably a significant cause of functional airway obstruction. Clinical signs associated with an "elongated" soft palate can be accentuated by flexing the neck and lessened by elevating the head.

Approximately 50-60% of the cases diagnosed as soft palate "elongation" with dorsal bulging or displacement respond favorably to surgical trimming of a small portion from the free margin of the soft palate underlying the epiglottis. Trimming the soft palate is less effective in managing paresis and paralysis. Other successful corrective procedures include injection of a sclerosing agent into the free border of the soft palate to shorten and tighten the free border, and cauterization of the free border with multiple penetrations of a fine cautery needle to induce a similar reaction.[30]

Excision of a small segment from the free border of the soft palate has been effective in most cases and is the author's treatment of choice. A new technic being evaluated is myectomy of the sternothyrohyoideus and omohyoideus muscles close to their insertion onto the larynx and hyoid bone. The function of the larynx and pharynx in 10 horses with clinical signs of pharyngeal airway obstruction compatible with dorsal displacement of the soft palate has been described.[19] Contraction of the sternothyrohyoideus and omohyoideus muscles causes caudal retraction of the larynx. If the soft palate seal around the laryngeal orifice is broken, the soft palate can be displaced and mouth-breathing occurs. These same events may occur in a horse at hard work due to the increased inspiratory effort, negative pressure and other contributory factors previously noted. This suggested that myectomy of the omohyoideus and sternothyrohyoideus muscles close to their insertion might prevent laryngeal retraction and resultant dorsal displacement of the soft palate.[19] Myectomy of these muscles has been successfully used to treat horses with dorsal displacement of the soft palate.[20] Some horses failed to respond to trimming the soft palate but responded favorably to myectomy.

Trimming a small section from the free border of the soft palate is performed with the horse under general anesthesia and in dorsal recumbency. A deep plane of anesthesia is induced and the endotracheal tube is withdrawn into the mouth. The soft palate is approached through a laryngotomy. The free border of the soft palate is then apparent in the nasopharyngeal airway. If additional exposure to the soft palate is necessary, the body of the thyroid cartilage is severed (see Surgical Approaches). The soft palate should be carefully examined for signs of ulcers or other obvious defects and the degree of flaccidity evaluated. In some horses the soft palate is taut but is very flaccid in others. The significance of this difference is not understood.

The length of the soft palate should also be determined. There is a distinct difference in the length and outline of the free border of the soft palate from horse to horse, and the size of the segment excised depends upon this appearance. As an aid to determine the size of the section to be removed, a classification of length and appearance of the border of the soft palate was developed (Fig 26). Graduations among these 3 configurations occur.

Excision is assisted by placing sponge forceps in the center of the margin of the free border to tighten and stabilize the soft palate during trimming. The sponge forceps also serve as a guide to the size of the section to be removed. No firm criteria are available as to how much of the soft palate should be trimmed, but the rule of thumb is not to remove more than 2.5 cm of the tensed palate centrally, tapering the incision on both sides toward the caudal pillar. The jaws of the sponge forceps serve this purpose well (Fig 27). The soft palate is trimmed with double-curved Satinsky thoracic scissors or long-handled Mayo dissecting scissors. Hemorrhage is usually minimal and requires no special attention. Large bleeders are cauterized or clamped.

The soft palate may also be trimmed with an electrosurgical scalpel. This method effectively controls hemorrhage but requires a deep plane of anesthesia to abolish the swallowing reflex. Care should be taken to avoid cutting the arytenoid cartilages should the horse swallow.

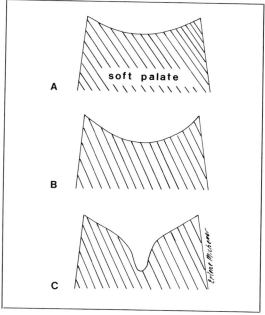

Fig 26. Classification of soft palate defects. In type A, the free border of the soft palate is concave but not excessively so. In type B, the free border is markedly concave. The free border of a type-C soft palate has a deep rostral concavity.

Granulomas of the arytenoid cartilage have occurred after use of an electrosurgical unit.

Moderate traction is applied to the sponge forceps to tighten and manipulate the soft palate. The incision is initiated on the caudal pillar of the soft palate on one side rostral to the arytenoid and is continued rostrad to the leading edge of the sponge forceps jaws. A second corresponding incision is made in the opposite caudal pillar. If the 2 incisions have not joined to free the trimmed segment of the soft palate, a third incision is made immediately rostral to

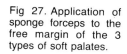

Fig 27. Application of sponge forceps to the free margin of the 3 types of soft palates.

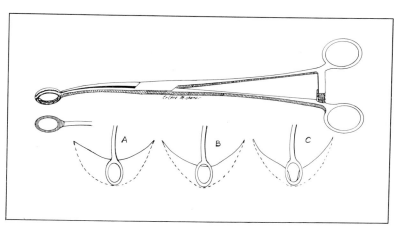

the forceps to free the segment. The surgical field is sponged free of blood and observed until hemorrhage is adequately controlled. Bleeding can be controlled by electrocautery.

The laryngotomy wound is managed as previously described. The nasopharynx is examined through the endoscope 1-2 days after surgery. If the soft palate lies in its normal position ventral to the epiglottis, the area of excision may not be visible. The points where the incisions were initiated in the caudal pillar of the soft palate are often very edematous and red; however, this inflammatory response usually subsides within 2-4 days. The most serious and disturbing complication in about 40% of operated cases is a persistent or frequent dorsal displacement of the soft palate despite the trimming. Fortunately, most postoperative dorsal displacement is intermittent. A small number (1-4%) of the cases operated have a persistent dorsal displacement accompanied by coughing, especially when drinking and eating, food in the nares and larynx, and the serious potential for developing aspiration pneumonia.

A guarded prognosis is issued in all cases until the horse resumes training at 30-45 days. Pretraining endoscopic examination is advised to evaluate the position of the soft palate and stage of healing. Training should not commence until healing is complete. The success of the surgery can be more completely evaluated by the ability of the horse to perform without demonstrating clinical signs. The owner should always be advised of the potential for serious complications.

Because trimming the soft palate may lead to more serious problems, it should not be undertaken lightly and only when diagnosis is reasonably or totally certain. Removal of an additional section from the soft palate should be done only after obtaining approval of the owner. Very few horses improve after removal of additional soft palate, and extreme caution is advised.

Pharyngeal Paralysis

Pharyngeal paralysis is characterized by dysphagia.

Cause: Acute pharyngitis, often associated with *Streptococcus equi* infection, can cause pharyngeal paralysis due to the inflammation and pain associated with the intense inflammatory reaction. These signs subside as the acute pharyngitis regresses and produce no lasting effects. Smoke inhalation, acute viral respiratory infections and chemical burns may produce similar clinical signs.

Cranial nerve disease, as in botulism and forage poisoning, is probably the most frequent cause of pharyngeal paralysis. Another common cause is mycosis of the guttural pouch.[21]

Pharyngeal paralysis occurred after irrigation of the guttural pouch with a solution of iodine and hydrogen peroxide in several horses. Irrigation with strong irritants should be undertaken with extreme caution or avoided.

The prognosis is poor, especially in those horses with damage to nerves within the wall of the guttural pouch. Botulism and forage poisoning likewise present a poor prognosis, although a few horses recover.

Clinical Signs: Clinical signs include choking, coughing and discharge of water and food from the nostrils. Endoscopic examination reveals dorsal soft palate displacement and feed within the nasal passages, nasopharynx, larynx and trachea. The potential for aspiration pneumonia is great.

Treatment: Treatment of pharyngeal paralysis involves continuous monitoring of the patient and maintaining an adequate level of nutrition and hydration by frequent feeding both IV and through a nasogastric tube. Local treatment, as described for disease of the guttural pouch, should be performed. In general, therapy is supportive to allow time for reversal of nerve damage. Even so, many horses do not survive. Surgical trimming of the soft palate has been employed with limited success.

Nasopharyngeal Tumors

Tumors of the equine nasopharynx are rare. A review of records at the University of Pennsylvania (approximately 10,000 accessions) revealed no cases of equine nasopharyngeal neoplasia. Tumors originating in adjacent tissues may invade the nasopharynx. One horse with hemangiosarcoma of the guttural pouch had a history of a rapidly developing mass in the supraorbital region and unilateral epistaxis. Endoscopic examination showed blood draining from the pharyngeal orifice of the affected guttural pouch. The guttural pouch was distended and protruded into the dorsal wall of the nasopharynx.

A carcinoma of the tonsil was recently diagnosed at necropsy in our hospital. This tumor was very large, occupied an extensive area on the floor of the oropharynx, and began to invade the nasopharynx. The soft palate was dorsally displaced and advanced obstruction of the airway had occurred.

Granulomas arising from the walls of the nasopharynx after electrocautery for pharyngeal lymphoid hyperplasia have been reported.[5] All 3 granulomas regressed without treatment.

Grade-IV pharyngeal lymphoid hyperplasia is often accompanied by masses of proliferating lymphoid tissue that project from the walls of the nasopharynx, particularly from the dorsal wall. The pharyngeal diverticulum is also a common site for these masses. Biopsy reveals primarily aggregates of lymphoid tissue.

Pharyngeal Collapse

Collapse of the pharynx is usually secondary to space-occupying obstructive lesions. Tumors, empyema and tympanites of the guttural pouches, acute infection, dorsal bulging or displacement of the soft palate, and "swallowing of the tongue" may contribute to pharyngeal collapse.

Primary lesions leading to collapse of the pharynx have not been defined. During endoscopic examination of the nasopharynx, some horses have a smaller than normal nasopharyngeal airway with no detectible lesions to explain the apparent decreased size. The dorsal pharyngeal wall may appear flat rather than slightly concave. The possibility of retropharyngeal lesions must be considered. The lateral nasopharyngeal walls may appear flat and compressed, thereby narrowing the airway. Whether these subjective findings represent a congenital defect or result from some unidentified primary lesion is unknown.

No treatment is effective in alleviating pharyngeal collapse, aside from that indicated to remove the primary cause.

The Larynx*

The larynx is that section of the upper respiratory tract that connects the nasopharynx with the trachea. Its primary functions are to deliver and regulate the volume of air during respiration, to prevent aspiration of foreign materials and to assist in phonation.

The larynx is made up of several cartilages that render it semirigid (Fig 28). The cricoid cartilage is shaped like a signet ring, with a broad and relatively flat dorsal lamina and an irregular dorsal median longitudinal ridge. It continues laterad as curved arches that join ventrad, where they are narrowest. The slight concavities of the lamina on either side of the dorsal median ridge contain the dorsal cricoarytenoideus muscles. The cricoid cartilage articulates rostrad with the arytenoid cartilages and caudad with the caudal cornu of the thyroid cartilage.

The thyroid cartilage is made up of 2 lateral laminae that join rostroventrad to form the body. The body of the thyroid cartilage is dorsal to the base of the epiglottis, to which it is attached by a ligament. The laminae are large, form a major part of the lateral laryngeal walls, and bear a cornu at each end that articulates with the cricoid cartilage. The rostral border articulates with the hyoid bone by the thyrohyoid membrane.

The epiglottis lies dorsal to the thyroid cartilage, with which it articulates at its base. It is shaped somewhat like a triangle, with its rostral apex curved ventrad. The dorsal surface is convex, the ventral surface is concave, and

*by C. W. Raker

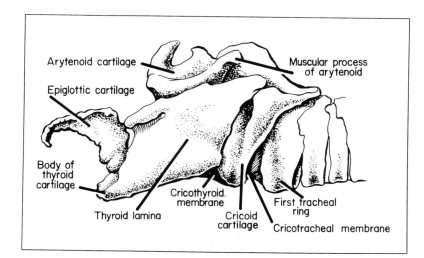

Fig 28. Lateral aspect of the larynx, showing the relationship of the laryngeal cartilages.

Arytenoid cartilage

Muscular process of arytenoid

Epiglottic cartilage

Body of thyroid cartilage

Thyroid lamina

Cricothyroid membrane

Cricoid cartilage

First tracheal ring

Cricotracheal membrane

the margins are slightly scalloped. The cuneiform processes extend dorsad and caudad from each side. Two prominent branching blood vessels on the dorsal surface pass from its base toward the apex.

The paired arytenoid cartilages lie on either side, rostral to the cricoid cartilage and medial to the laminae of the thyroid cartilage, and present 3 prominent projections. The rostral corniculate process curves dorsad and caudad. This is the portion clearly seen during endoscopic examination. The vocal process to which the vocal ligament attaches is formed by convergence of the rostral and caudal borders. The muscular process projects dorsad from the lateral surface, articulates with the cricoid cartilage, and serves as the point of attachment for the dorsal cricoarytenoideus muscle.

The laryngeal cartilages are hyaline except for the epiglottis and the corniculate and vocal processes of the arytenoids, which are elastic. The recurrent laryngeal nerve passes between the cricopharyngeus and cricoarytenoideus dorsalis muscles, and enters the larynx on the medial side of the thyroid cartilage lamina. It innervates all of the intrinsic laryngeal muscles except the cricothyroideus.[22] The cricoarytenoideus dorsalis is the only dilator of the glottis.[22] Sensory innervation of the laryngeal mucosa is through the cranial laryngeal nerve.

The cricopharyngeus muscle arises from the lateral rostral surface of the ventral arch of the cricoid cartilage and passes rostrodorsad over the side of the larynx to insert dorsad on the median pharyngeal raphe. The thyropharyngeus lies rostral to the cricopharyngeus and arises from the lateral surface of the thyroid lamina, which it covers as it passes dorsomediad to insert on the pharyngeal raphe. These 2 muscles play a significant role as pharyngeal constrictors.

Laryngeal Hemiplegia

Laryngeal hemiplegia is a common cause of upper airway obstruction and is clinically significant in performance horses. It is commonly known as "roaring," which is derived from the noise heard when affected horses exercise. The condition has been diagnosed in all breeds but is especially common in large, long-necked horses. The incidence of laryngeal hemiplegia increases with maturity.[23]

The left recurrent laryngeal nerve is involved in approximately 90% of affected horses. Less frequently the right recurrent laryngeal nerve alone is involved; many of these cases have an iatrogenic origin, *ie*, nerve damage is from thrombophlebitis and trauma to surrounding tissues following injection of a drug into or outside of the jugular vein. Bilateral laryngeal paralysis is rare.

Cause: The cause of left recurrent laryngeal nerve damage has not been definitively identified. Many causes have been suggested, including lead poisoning, plant poisoning, jugular thrombophlebitis, aortic arch pulsations, damage from cervical movement, thiamin deficiency and genetics.[16,23-27]

Clinical Signs: The major clinical sign of laryngeal hemiplegia is inspiratory dyspnea, which results from the decreased size of the airway. Inadequate ventilation leads to hypoxia and early tiring. The inspiratory noise is produced by the airway obstruction and vibration of the flaccid vocal fold. The intensity of the noise and dyspnea are increased in bilateral paralysis.

Diagnosis: The history is important in establishing a diagnosis and suitable questions should be asked to elicit information as to when clinical signs appear and the character of the abnormal respiratory noise. Multiple obstructive airway lesions, such as laryngeal hemiplegia and soft palate displacement, may coexist.[28] A complete physical examination of the upper respiratory tract is essential and should include inspection, palpation and percussion of the head for signs of disease of the paranasal sinuses, nares and rostral segment of the nasal passages, turbinates, alar folds, nasal diverticulum and nasal septum.

The width of the space between the cricoid cartilage and the first tracheal ring should be about 1-2 cm. If this space is considerably wider, the mucosa may be drawn into the airway during periods of increased respiratory-negative pressure, especially with the neck flexed. The trachea should be examined for evidence of stenosis or collapse, and the horse worked to characterize the noise and the onset of dyspnea.

Endoscopic examination of the upper airway provides definitive evaluation of laryngeal function and is the most effective method to detect obstructive lesions and to define the cause. Endoscopic findings in laryngeal hemiplegia vary, depending upon the degree of nerve involvement and the extent to which the laryngeal airway has collapsed. The appearance of the laryngeal orifice should be carefully studied for asymmetry and medial displacement of the arytenoid cartilage on the affected side.

The opening to the laryngeal ventricle on the affected side is dilated due to relaxation and displacement of the vocal fold and at times contains exudate or foreign debris. As these observations depend to a degree on the examiner's evaluation of laryngeal dynamics, abnormal function is more apparent if air is withheld by nasal occlusion. During this time laryngeal function should be observed for the capability of the arytenoid cartilages to abduct and adduct and, when access to air is allowed, how fast and to what extent they are abducted. Impaired function causes the arytenoid cartilage on the affected side to "tremble" or "shiver" as it is slowly or incompletely retracted. With complete paralysis the affected arytenoid cartilage does not move from its medial position and may be further adducted with deep inspiratory effort when air is withheld or after strenuous work.

Induction of swallowing during observation of the larynx through a fiberoptic endoscope is also useful to evaluate abduction of the arytenoid cartilages. During swallowing there is momentary occlusion of the endoscope as the soft palate elevates and the pharynx contracts. This is followed by abduction of the arytenoids as the soft palate returns to its position beneath the epiglottis. Any malfunction of the larynx is often observed at this time. The swallowing maneuver is likewise of value in evaluating function of the soft palate.

The "grunt test" may be used as an aid in diagnosis of laryngeal hemiplegia; however, it is difficult to evaluate the results of this test. A positive "grunt test" may suggest abnormal laryngeal function. The induced expiratory grunt or prolonged groan results from failure to completely adduct the arytenoid cartilages.

Treatment: Many surgical procedures have been developed to correct laryngeal hemiplegia, including anastomosis of the recurrent laryngeal and vagus nerves, resection of the arytenoid cartilage, resection of the vocal cord, combinations of arytenoidectomy and cordectomy, and laryngeal ventriculectomy.[23,29-33] Laryngeal ventriculectomy is the most effective and involves the removal of the laryngeal saccule mucosa on the affected side.[31,32] The space within the saccule is eventually replaced by granulation tissue, which retracts as it matures and stabilizes the vocal fold and to a lesser extent the arytenoid cartilage, to increase airway size.

Laryngeal sacculectomy is successful in 60-70% of the cases operated. These figures are the subject of considerable discussion and disagreement and are based entirely on the author's follow-up observations of operated cases. The criterion used to determine the success of laryngeal sacculectomy is the ability of the horse to perform to the owner's satisfaction. In studies of sacculectomy success rates, only 10% were deemed successful when criteria for success were the degree of vocal fold and arytenoid cartilage abduction and the postoperative size of the airway.[23,33]

Some horses have had good clinical response to laryngeal ventriculectomy for 1-3 years, after which signs of noise and airway obstruction recurred. Endoscopic examination of these horses usually reveals marked displacement of the affected arytenoid cartilage and vocal fold into the laryngeal airway, with no evidence of function. The reasons for recurrence may be the result of repeated or continued tension placed upon the adhesions within the saccule from increased negative pressure during strenuous work.

An improved surgical procedure to correct laryngeal hemiplegia involves the insertion of an elastic prosthesis to replace the atrophied, nonfunctional cricoarytenoideus dorsalis muscle.[23,33] An elastic suture is inserted through the muscular process of the arytenoid cartilage and anchored around the caudodorsal margin of the cricoid cartilage. The ends of the prosthesis are tied under tension to abduct and retain the arytenoid cartilage in permanent retraction. Placement of the prosthesis is followed by a unilateral laryngeal sacculectomy on the paralyzed side.

Laryngeal prosthesis placement significantly improved the prognosis to effectively relieve the airway obstruction caused by laryngeal hemiplegia. The rate of success with this procedure, when properly performed, is 80-90%. Several complications are associated with the technic, the most serious of which is a chronic cough. Coughing while eating or drinking occurs rather frequently and, in some horses, food and water are blown from the nostrils. Coughing may also be accompanied by choking and gagging, and may occasionally progress to a chronic and sometimes fatal aspiration pneumonia. This complication seems to be associated with "over-correction" or extreme retraction of the arytenoid cartilage by the prosthesis. Permanent retraction of the arytenoid cartilage to a fully abducted position beyond that of retraction by a functional cricoarytenoideus muscle may lead to patency of the laryngeal orifice on the retracted side during swallowing. Caudodorsal elevation of the epiglottis ineffectively covers the remaining patent airway, which allows food and water to enter the larynx or be retained in the lateral food channels. Intralaryngeal granuloma formation secondary to penetration of the airway by the prosthesis is a less frequent cause of chronic coughing.

A second complication associated with elastic prosthesis placement is delayed wound healing, as evidenced by an extensive inflammatory reaction and occasional drainage from the suture line from rejection of the material used as a prosthesis. Cultures of such wound exudates revealed infection in some cases. The incidence of this complication is less than 5%.

Laryngeal ventriculectomy may be performed by experienced surgeons with the horse standing and sedated as necessary. Over-sedation should be avoided since the horse's response to stimuli may be unpredictable. Most laryngeal ventriculectomies are performed with the horse under general anesthesia.

A standing laryngeal ventriculectomy is done through a ventral laryngotomy as previously described. The index finger is introduced through the incision in the cricothyroid membrane to the first joint. At this level the vocal fold can be palpated on the wall of the airway as it passes dorsal to the vocal process of the arytenoid cartilage. Introduction of the finger and contact with the mucosa within the airway before the application of a topical anesthetic stimulates coughing and/or swallowing. The finger is then directed to the rostral border of the vocal fold where it enters the opening into the laryngeal saccule. As the finger is directed caudodorsad, it enters the depths of the saccule. Failure of the ventricle to contract over the finger is a useful aid to confirm the clinical diagnosis.

After application of a topical anesthetic to the mucosa of the accessible laryngeal airway, the saccule mucosa is removed with a laryngeal burr inserted into the saccule and twisted to firmly grasp the mucosa. With the burr held firmly in this position, gentle traction is applied to evert the mucosa out of the ventricle. A curved hemostat or other suitable curved forceps is then applied to the everted saccule between the burr and the opening to the ventricle and the lining of the saccule is excised with long, curved dissecting scissors. In lieu of applying forceps to stabilize the everted tissue, the saccule can be excised while traction is maintained with the laryngeal burr. The mucosa can be everted with Allis tissue forceps or rolled-up gauze in the jaws of an Allis tissue forceps. After the saccule mucosa is excised, it should be stretched over a finger to determine if the entire lining has been removed. Total excision is essential to obtain good results. Remaining tags of tissue within or at the margin of the saccule should be excised.

A modification of the standing laryngeal sacculectomy technic is the "finger technic," in which the lining of the saccule is incised, stripped from its submucosal attachments and everted for excision with the index finger. Right-handed surgeons prefer to perform this procedure with the index finger of the left hand since it allows excision of the everted lining with scissors held by the right hand. The mucosa is incised by placing the end of the finger on the border of the opening of the laryngeal ventricle along its dorsal margin immediately rostral to the insertion of the vocal fold onto the vocal process of the arytenoid cartilage. The finger is placed in a position where the nail (gloves cannot be used) is stabilized against the border of the opening so that firm pressure is applied to the mucosa. The mucosa is incised with a backward and forward motion of the finger and the opening enlarged by gently pushing the finger dorsad into the incision. The mucosa is then separated from the submucosa with the finger by gentle blunt dissection up the medial wall of the saccule to its base, where it is flexed and traction applied to allow the finger to pass down the lateral wall of the saccule. Extreme care is required to avoid unnecessary trauma to underlying tissues. The ventricle is approximately as deep as the distance from the tip of the finger to the first joint.

Retraction of the mucosa with the finger is continued rostroventrad toward the pharynx to complete eversion of the lining. Eversion cannot be effectively accomplished in any other direction since the vocal fold deters caudal eversion. The flexed finger is slowly rotated 180° within the laryngeal orifice while retaining the everted lining and is manipulated to present the finger and lining of the saccule into the laryngotomy incision, where it can be stabilized by pressing the thumb against the index finger. Excision of mucosa is completed with scissors. An alternative step is to clamp the everted lining with a curved hemostat so the finger can be removed and excision completed. The margins of the opening to the ventricle should always be thoroughly palpated for the presence of mucosal tags, which should be removed. If not removed, airway obstruction may occur as tissue tags become edematous and protrude into the airway. The postoperative management of the wound has previously been described (see Surgical Approaches).

Laryngeal ventriculectomy is frequently done under general anesthesia. With the horse in dorsal recumbency, a laryngotomy is performed as previously described. The lining of the laryngeal saccule is removed, as described under the standing approach, with a laryngeal burr, Allis tissue forceps, ball of gauze or the finger. The mucosa is incised with a scalpel by cutting along the border of the opening to the saccule. The major advantages of this approach to ventriculectomy are good patient control, good visualization of the surgical field and less chance of unnecessary tissue trauma. Suturing the opening to the laryngeal saccule after removal of its lining has also been suggested.[29,30,44]

Laryngeal prosthesis, in combination with laryngeal ventriculectomy, stabilizes the non-functional arytenoid cartilage into an abducted position and retracts the vocal fold to the side of the laryngeal airway.[23,33] Insertion of a laryngeal prosthesis is not essential to effectively treat all cases of laryngeal hemiplegia. Thus, cases for laryngeal prosthesis placement should be carefully selected and the procedure reserved for those that require this technic for successful correction of the defect. This also circumvents the inherent complications of the procedure, which can be serious.

Laryngeal ventriculectomy alone is successful in a large number of cases where the affected arytenoid cartilage lies in a median position, ie, neither adducted nor abducted (Fig C16). Stabilization of the arytenoid in this position and retraction of the vocal fold by adhesions in the saccule are often adequate for good performance, at least for the first several years. In contrast, if the affected arytenoid cartilage has been displaced medial to cause significant laryngeal airway obstruction, laryngeal ventriculectomy, while it may stabilize the arytenoid, does not result in enough abduction to provide an adequate airway (Fig C17). Therefore, use of both procedures is recommended. Insertion of a laryngeal prosthesis should always be accompanied by laryngeal ventriculectomy except in those cases with a history of a previous successful ventriculectomy. A previous unsuccessful laryngeal ventriculectomy, however, should be reoperated if there is endoscopic evidence of a correctable lesion. In contrast, other investigators believe a laryngeal prosthesis, without ventriculectomy, is equally effective.[34]

For prosthesis placement, the horse is placed on its right side, under general anesthesia with the head extended. The surgical site over the left side of the larynx is prepared and a 12-cm skin incision is made ventral and parallel to the external maxillary and jugular veins from the rostral border of the larynx to near the second tracheal ring. Hemorrhage is controlled by clamping and ligation. Deep blunt and sharp dissection with scissors are continued close to the external maxillary vein to separate the omohyoid muscle from the vein. Care should be exercised to locate and spare the ventral branch of the second cervical nerve, which enters the omohyoid muscle and the blood vessels to the thyroid gland. Liberal dissection around these structures frees them so they can be moved within the operative field as necessary. Blood vessels to the thyroid gland have been compromised in a few horses without any observable clinical sequelae. Blunt dissection is continued with the fingers to completely expose the entire left side of the larynx and proximal trachea. Further blunt dissection over the left dorsal surface of the larynx reveals the muscular process of the arytenoid cartilage and the lamina of the cricoid cartilage. Blunt dissection is continued until the esophagus and carotid artery are identified and the dorsal longitudinal median ridge of the cricoid is palpated.

The prosthesis is made from a 40-inch strand of #2 mersilene (Johnson & Johnson) connected to a #2, #3 or #4 full-curve, trocar-point needle. The laryngeal cartilages of a 2-year-old horse are more easily penetrated than are those of a more mature horse, in which a large, strong needle may be required. The mersilene is doubled and the free ends securely tied to provide a double-strand prosthesis. Alternatively, a single strand of #5 Ethibond (Johnson & Johnson) may be used. The notch on the caudodorsal border of the cricoid cartilage lamina is palpated and the needle and prosthesis inserted 1 cm lateral to the notch. Extreme care is required in placing the prosthesis around the caudal edge of the cricoid cartilage to avoid invading the laryngeal airway, which may lead to a granulomatous foreign-body reaction and chronic coughing. Penetration of the airway can be avoided if the center of the needle is laid on the cricoid cartilage rostral to its caudal border. The needle is then slowly rotated caudad, following the curve of the needle, until the point slips off the border of the cricoid, when it is rotated rostrad, still following the curve of the needle. It emerges from the dorsal surface of the cricoid cartilage 1.5-2 cm rostral to its point of insertion. Ample cricoid cartilage should be incorporated in the suture to assure a stable anchor.

The cricopharyngeus and thyropharyngeus muscles are identified on the left laryngeal wall. The muscular process of the arytenoid cartilage lies on the dorsolateral wall of the larynx beneath the cricopharyngeus muscle and is palpable as a pinnacle of cartilage. The septum between these 2 muscles is incised with scissors and the muscles separated by blunt dissection. The cricopharyngeus muscle is freed from its attachments to the laryngeal wall, and a needle holder is passed under the muscle to emerge close to the point of emergence of the prosthesis. The prosthesis is pulled rostrad beneath the muscle. Placing the point of the needle in the jaws of the needle holder greatly eases its passage.

To avoid crossing the prosthesis, the trailing end is not handled at this time. The prosthesis is inserted through the muscular process of the arytenoid cartilage using standard suture placement technic. The larynx is rotated to the left by traction with a finger placed over the proximal border of the lamina of the thyroid cartilage. A small, blunt blade retractor has also been used effectively to rotate the muscular process of the arytenoid to a point where it can be easily observed and palpated. The needle holder and needle are placed under the cricopharyngeus muscle with a backhand motion to elevate and retract it. If the cricopharyngeus muscle has been well dissected from its underlying attachments, the needle is easily passed through the muscular process from medial to lateral. It should be directed as parallel to the caudal border of the cricoid as possible and not directed acutely rostrad.

The needle is placed deep into the muscular process to provide the second firm anchor point for the prosthesis. The prosthesis is then pulled through the muscular process until it is under tension when the trailing end of the suture is grasped and pulled rostrad under the cricopharyngeus muscle to form a mattress suture. Care should be taken to avoid crossing the suture. The free ends of the prosthesis are grasped and traction is applied to each end. This tightens the prosthesis. The degree of tension is repeatedly checked by feeling the dorsal strand

and traction is maintained until the suture lies flat against the cricoid cartilage and the finger cannot be forced beneath it. The tension applied on a 2-year-old is slightly less than that applied to horses 3 years of age and older because the laryngeal cartilages in a 2-year-old horse are less rigid. It is doubtful that sufficient tension can be applied to a mersilene prosthesis in a horse 4 years of age or older to over-correct the defect.

A surgeon's knot is placed in the prosthesis, which is pulled down so that it lies flat on the wall of the larynx under tension. It is temporarily clamped with a mosquito forceps and the tension and placement of the prosthesis are re-evaluated and corrections made if indicated. A second knot is pulled onto the first as the forceps are removed. Two or 3 additional knots are placed and the ends are cut approximately 0.5 cm from the knot. The incision between the cricopharyngeus and thyropharyngeus muscles is closed with several simple-interrupted sutures of 00 chromic catgut or polyglycolic acid.

A Penrose drain may be placed for drainage of the deadspace on the left side of the larynx and, while a drain may not be necessary, it helps control postoperative swelling and edema. I prefer to insert the drain through stab incisions rostral and caudal to the skin incision, although other methods may be used. The exposed drain end(s) should be securely anchored to the skin.

The omohyoideus muscle is sutured to the loose connective tissue along the margin of the external maxillary vein with simple-interrupted sutures of 00 chromic catgut or polyglycolic acid. As there is little tension on the suture lines in the standing horse, a layer of subcuticular sutures is not essential to first-intention healing. The skin incision is closed with simple-interrupted or horizontal mattress sutures of nonabsorbable material.

Endoscopic examination during or immediately following insertion of the prosthesis has not been useful to evaluate the degree of correction. General anesthesia and the lateral position of the horse on the operating table probably preclude accurate assessment of the position of the arytenoid.

The horse is then placed in dorsal recumbency and, through a laryngotomy, the lining of the left laryngeal saccule is excised. The endotracheal tube may be withdrawn to perform the sacculectomy but is usually not necessary. The degree of traction on the left arytenoid cartilage can be determined if the endotracheal tube is withdrawn, but the degree of retraction cannot be critically determined.

The laryngotomy incision is managed as previously described (see Surgical Approaches). The drain is carefully manipulated daily to maintain good drainage and removed on the third to fifth postoperative day, depending upon the quantity of exudate. Skin sutures are removed in 7-10 days. Nonsteroidal anti-inflammatory drugs may be administered daily but are seldom required. One or more skin sutures may be removed to provide drainage if complications in healing develop.

Endoscopic examination is conducted 1-2 days after surgery when the degree of retraction of the arytenoid cartilage can be accurately determined. Retraction of the arytenoid cartilage into a position of moderate to full abduction indicates good correction. If the arytenoid cartilage is neither abducted nor adducted, the correction is less satisfactory. In cases where the arytenoid cartilage has been retracted to a position of extreme abduction, especially if a distinct break or notch is apparent in the dorsal third of the corniculate process, complications of coughing, choking, regurgitation and aspiration are likely. The corniculate process of the arytenoid cartilage should be arched, with no sign of a distinct notch, and should not be retracted to the extent that it cannot be seen through the endoscope.

Those cases with no apparent retraction of the arytenoid cartilage represent a surgical failure, and improved performance is unlikely. Failure of the laryngeal prosthesis to effectively retract the arytenoid cartilage may be due to improper insertion, insufficient traction, deformity of the arytenoid cartilage or disruption of the points of fixation. Signs associated with over-correction may become less noticeable or disappear in a few days or weeks but may persist. Such affected horses are incapable of satisfactory performance and may develop aspiration pneumonia. Owners of horses subjected to this procedure should be forewarned of possible complications to minimize chances of litigation.

A granuloma on the dorsal laryngeal airway resulting from prosthesis placement that penetrated the airway may cause clinical signs similar to those of over-correction. This complication is uncommon but must be considered as a possible cause of inadequate performance.

Enforced stall rest for 2 weeks postoperatively is required. Daily walking in hand is permitted throughout the second 2 weeks. During the second month the horse can be turned loose in a small paddock or walked in hand to control exercise. Training may be resumed in 2 months.

An alternative material for prosthetic use is 3300 Denier Lycra (du Pont).[23,33] No rejections were observed in over 200 horses over a period of 4 years of observation. However, the author has encountered wound infection and clinical signs compatible with impending rejection with use of a Lycra prosthesis. In comparison, wound healing with a mersilene prosthesis is rarely prolonged, infection is rare and there is a significant reduction in the extent and presistence of inflammation and edema.

Laryngeal prostheses have failed several weeks, months or years after placement. The incidence of failures in horses operated upon at the University of Pennsylvania is about 3%. However, the number of failures referred to us for a second operation has been somewhat higher. The reasons for failure have not been fully determined. Upon reoperation, the prosthesis was found, in some cases, to have pulled out of the muscular process of the arytenoid cartilage. Less frequently the prosthesis had pulled through the caudal border of the cricoid cartilage lamina. These failures probably were the result of inadequate inclusion of cartilage or placement of the prosthesis at the anchor points. Some failures involved Lycra prostheses and others mersilene. Therefore, care must be exercised in placing the prosthesis to increase the rate of success.

Insertion of a second laryngeal prosthesis is difficult. The surgical field is vascular and the planes of dissection are obscured by extensive adhesions. In spite of these problems, insertion of a second prosthesis is often successful. If the failed prosthesis can be located quickly with little trauma, it is removed; otherwise, it is left and an additional one inserted. The surgery should not be unduly prolonged or tissue damaged by attempts to remove a failed prosthesis.

There is no justification for an arytenoidectomy to supplant laryngeal ventriculectomy in laryngeal hemiplegia. If the arytenoid cartilage is defective, it can be excised as described later. Total arytenoidectomy may lead to chronic coughing and aspiration pneumonia. The objective of surgical correction of uncomplicated laryngeal hemiplegia may be met with laryngeal ventriculectomy alone or, when indicated, combined with laryngeal prosthesis.

There is also no advantage to suturing the edges of the opening to the laryngeal saccule if the lining has been totally removed. The same is true for excision of the vocal folds, except in horses with a defect of the folds or a very narrow laryngeal airway associated with undetermined anatomic defects, chondroma or chondritis of the laryngeal cartilages.

Laryngeal Trauma

Trauma to the larynx is infrequent but may result from endotracheal or nasogastric tube passage into the larynx. Areas of acute inflammation are frequently seen at endoscopic examination within hours after this type of trauma. Small areas of submucosal hemorrhage may be evident. Such lesions usually disappear within 1-2 days after the insult and leave no apparent signs of permanent damage. Extensive trauma may lead to infection, chondritis or chondroma formation.

Laryngeal Tumors

Granulomas, chondromas and polyps are the most common growths involving the larynx. Chondromas have been discussed previously. Granulomas develop from trauma to the laryngeal mucosa or from localized chronic infection. Polyps may develop at any location within the laryngeal airway but most frequently arise from the laryngeal airway surface of arytenoid cartilages or vocal folds.

Surgical excision of the tumors is the treatment of choice. Polyps of the vocal folds occasionally recur after surgery.

The Epiglottis*

Epiglottic Entrapment

Epiglottic hypoplasia is a common deformity often accompanied by epiglottic entrapment.[7,36-39] Entrapment of an apparently normal epiglottis by the aryepiglottic folds and continuous mucosa occurs infrequently. Deformities of the epiglottis have been observed principally in Standardbred and Thoroughbred race horses. Other affected breeds include the Appaloosa, Arab and Grade. Since the clinical signs are primarily stress-related, the incidence may be higher than is presently recognized in horses used for work less strenuous than racing.

Cause: Acquired defects of the epiglottis have not been documented. Acquired epiglottic defects are thought to occur since some horses perform well for many years without apparent signs of airway distress. However, a deformity may have been present during that time but, for unknown reasons, did not produce signs of

*by C.W. Raker

obstruction. It is also possible that previous owners failed to observe clinical signs of obstruction or decreased performance. Among potential causes of acquired epiglottic deformity is trauma induced by passage of a nasogastric or endotracheal tube. Primary or secondary infections as from foreign bodies are also causes.

The normal epiglottis as seen through the endoscope is a distinct, rigid, triangular cartilaginous structure projecting rostrad from the laryngeal orifice into the nasopharynx. The base is continuous with the laryngeal airway and the apex is directed rostrad and often curves ventrad to the left or right. The borders are distinct and scalloped. The aryepiglottic folds of mucosa are loosely attached to the oral surface of the epiglottis and extend to its free border. They pass caudad, where they blend into the mucosa of the corniculate process of the arytenoid cartilages. From the base of the epiglottis to the base of the corniculate process of the arytenoid, the aryepiglottic folds form the laryngeal orifice and appear as distinct raised bilateral folds of tissue.

Displacement of the aryepiglottic folds dorsal to the borders of the epiglottis constitutes entrapment (Fig C18). The extent to which the folds have been displaced determines partial or total entrapment. A total epiglottic entrapment may be permanent, whereas partial entrapment is often intermittent. Ulcers on the entrapping mucosal folds are often seen near the apex of the epiglottis and less frequently along the free border. Ulcers at the apex of the epiglottis may, with erosion, allow the apex to protrude through the opening while a collar of mucosa partially covers the epiglottis. Intermittent epiglottic entrapment is more likely immediately after the horse swallows.

Preliminary studies of a small number of the cases seen at the University of Pennsylvania suggest epiglottic hypoplasia may be inherited. Epiglottic hypoplasia without epiglottic entrapment has been diagnosed in many horses during endoscopic examination. The epiglottis appeared smaller than normal. The main endoscopic feature was an apparent lack of normal substance to the epiglottic cartilage (Fig C19). It seemed flaccid and soft, with a suggestion that the borders curled dorsad and the pharyngeal surface was slightly concave. The scalloped edges were not as prominent as usual or were absent. The aryepiglottic folds bulged beyond the borders of the cartilage, as opposed to being occluded by the epiglottis. The epiglottis and aryepiglottic folds quivered on the soft palate much like a bowl of gelatin. Forceful, deep inspiration after withholding air caused the epiglottis to become further embedded within the pharyngeal surface of the soft palate; occasionally the soft palate was displaced. While entrapment was not seen in these horses, the potential for intermittent entrapment and dorsal displacement of the soft palate existed.

Epiglottic entrapment is frequently accompanied by dorsal displacement of the soft palate. Since the displaced soft palate usually completely covers the epiglottis, the entrapment may be hidden. Several horses have been examined endoscopically in which the borders of both the displaced soft palate and entrapping aryepiglottic folds were seen. Since dorsal displacement of the soft palate is frequently associated with entrapment of a hypoplastic epiglottis, attention is directed to the soft palate during surgical correction of entrapment.

A second specific deformity of the epiglottis has been seen in 3 young Standardbreds 1-3 years old. The epiglottis in these horses was not noticeably hypoplastic, but the longitudinal axis was flat to slightly concave, and the apex curved and elevated dorsad. The outline of the epiglottis resembled a spoon and the serrated margins and blood vessels were absent.

Another deformity associated with epiglottic entrapment was pronounced enlargement of the epiglottic apex. This firm, cartilaginous, papilla-like protuberance projected dorsad into the airway in numerous horses but is not always accompanied by entrapment.

Clinical Signs: The major clinical signs of epiglottic entrapment are a decreased tolerance for work and an abnormal respiratory noise. The noise is characterized as a loud inspiratory and expiratory blowing noise usually heard only during hard work. The expiratory component of the noise is usually loud and of a low pitch; in some cases it is described as a gurgle, rattle or flutter. Epiglottic entrapment partially obstructs or reduces airway size during inspiration; however, air may become trapped in these mucosal folds during expiration and expand them like a balloon to produce a more pronounced obstruction.

As mentioned previously, many horses with an entrapped epiglottis also displace the soft palate dorsal to the epiglottis and further restrict air passage. In view of these observations, one may speculate if secondary soft palate displacement is not the more significant factor that leads to critical airway obstruction. This hypothesis gains support when one considers that some horses with epiglottic entrapment have no signs of significant airway obstruction until 5 years of age or older and perform satisfactorily up to that time. Epiglottic entrapment may have been present for a much longer time but did not produce noticeable signs until accompanied by displacement of the soft palate. Coughing and choking are frequently observed soon after exercise is stopped or less frequently while eating or drinking, when food and water may be regurgitated from the nostrils.

Diagnosis: Endoscopic examination is essential to diagnosis. The epiglottis, if totally entrapped, retains its basic triangular shape; however, the blood vessels and the serrated borders are obscured. The epiglottis appears thicker and its apex more round due to the entrapping mucosal folds. Total epiglottic entrapment is often confused with dorsal displacement of the soft palate, whereas a partial entrapment is more easily diagnosed since a good portion of the dorsal surface of the epiglottis with the attendant blood vessels and the rim of the entrapping mucosal folds are evident. With dorsal displacement of the soft palate, the epiglottis cannot be seen and only rarely is its presence suggested by a slight central triangular shaped elevation of the soft palate. Induction of swallowing may assist diagnosis as the soft palate is replaced and the entrapped epiglottis is seen. Ulcers in the entrapping folds occur frequently and pressure necrosis of the folds at the epiglottic apex may permit the apex to protrude through the opening.

Treatment: Effective treatment of epiglottic entrapment consists of trimming the aryepiglottic folds through an oral approach.[36,37,40] When a surgical plane of anesthesia is reached, the endotracheal tube is withdrawn and a mouth speculum inserted. The deformity is manually palpated and the entrapping folds excised with scissors close to the epiglottis. A 24-inch rotating biopsy forceps has also been used to remove small portions of the entrapping folds to prevent further entrapment.[36] A simple relief incision of the entrapping folds at the apex of the epiglottis has been used, often unsuccessfully. Entrapment has recurred due to healing of the incision or the associated inflammation and edema.

Epiglottic entrapment has also been approached through a ventral pharyngotomy but this involves more extensive surgery and has no advantages over the laryngotomy approach.[37]

Correction of epiglottic entrapment through a laryngotomy has been effective and provides good visualization of the defect. The surgery is performed under general anesthesia with the patient in dorsal recumbency. With the endotracheal tube in place the entrapped epiglottis is inspected by elevation with a closed sponge forceps applied to its pharyngeal surface. Infrequently the entrapment may have been corrected when the endotracheal tube was introduced. To facilitate inspection, the endotracheal tube is withdrawn and both the soft palate and entrapping folds are observed. A sponge forceps or Allis tissue forceps is passed rostrad and securely attached to the entrapping folds near the apex of the epiglottis. We prefer not to grasp the epiglottis with a towel clamp, as previously noted.[38]

Traction on the sponge forceps rotates and everts the epiglottic apex into the laryngotomy site. The body of the thyroid cartilage is not incised unless essential to obtain increased exposure to the epiglottis. The tensed mucosal folds are trimmed with scissors. Satinsky thoracic scissors have been very helpful because of their "S" curvature. Extensive trimming of the entrapping folds should be avoided.

The tensed mucosal folds are cut with scissors 1 cm from the borders of the epiglottis. With the entrapping folds extended and held with sponge forceps, the first cut is started along the sponge forceps at the apex and continued to the base of the corniculate process of the arytenoid cartilage. A second similar cut removes the fold on the opposite side. A third cut caudal to the sponge forceps completes the trimming of the folds and the epiglottis returns to its normal position in the nasopharynx. Hemorrhage is minimal. The laryngotomy is left open to heal by granulation.

Endoscopic examination on the day after surgery reveals that the epiglottis is inflamed and edematous. Additional endoscopic examinations are conducted as indicated and at the end of a 4- to 6-week rest.

Because of the increasing frequency of soft palate displacement, trimming of the soft palate at the same time the epiglottic entrapment is corrected is recommended. Statistics to substantiate or refute the value of this procedure are not available. However, clinical impressions are that fewer horses have recurrent signs of soft palate displacement and the rate of successful performance has improved.

by *C.W. Raker

The Thyroid Cartilage*

Reports of thyroid cartilage deformity are few. Rostral displacement of the palatopharyngeal arch, partially covering the corniculate processes of the arytenoid cartilages, has been reported in 3 horses.[7] Clinical signs included air in the esophagus, dysphagia, nasal discharge of food, chronic cough and an abnormal inspiratory noise at work. The inspiratory noise may have been the result of a bilateral laryngeal paralysis.

A single case of rostral displacement of the palatopharyngeal arch has been reported.[41] Clinical signs included decreased tolerance for work, a pronounced inspiratory noise and a less pronounced expiratory noise. Endoscopic examination revealed rostral displacement of the palatopharyngeal arch, which obscured the apices of the corniculate processes of the arytenoid cartilages. There were no signs of laryngeal paralysis. Radiographs revealed increased density of the thyroid cartilage compatible with calcification. At necropsy, deformity of the thyroid cartilage and absence of both cricopharyngeus muscles were confirmed, with only vestiges of the thyropharyngeus muscles.

Surgical correction has been attempted in several of these cases, but the result was generally unsatisfactory.

Chondritis and chondromas of the thyroid cartilage have been encountered. Endoscopic examination revealed marked stenosis of the laryngeal airway due to a thickened thyroid and/or arytenoid cartilage. Clinical signs were of airway obstruction.

The Arytenoid Cartilages

Arytenoid Cartilage Deformity

In the author's experience, the incidence of arytenoid cartilage deformity is second only to epiglottic deformity. The incidence of arytenoid cartilage deformity has increased during the past 5 years, probably due to increased use of fiberoptic endoscopy. Since clinical signs are related to work, these deformities are diagnosed most frequently in 2- and 3-year-old race horses. The diagnosis may be easily confused with unilateral or bilateral laryngeal paralysis. The right arytenoid may be affected more commonly than the left. A few horses have bilateral arytenoid cartilage deformities.

Chondritis and chondromas are common diseases of the arytenoids. Less frequently, primary granulomas and polyps, which arise from the surface of the arytenoids, protrude into the laryngeal airway. Secondary growths are often found in conjunction with chondritis or chondroma (Fig C20). A deformed arytenoid cartilage is firm, thick, and may undergo ossification. Progressive deformation of the arytenoid cartilages establishes contact at the apices of the corniculate processes to cause pressure necrosis, ulceration and granulation of the mucosa. A variably sized granuloma or polyp may develop. Polyps arising from the airway surface of the arytenoid cartilages or vocal cords may also be primary, ie, not associated with endoscopic signs of arytenoid deformity. A deformed arytenoid cartilage loses its elasticity and cannot be abducted. This change, combined with the enlarged cartilage, causes more or less constant contact with the opposing arytenoid. The endoscopic appearance may be confused with unilateral or bilateral laryngeal paralysis and differentiation is at times difficult.

The endoscopic appearance of the corniculate process of the deformed arytenoid cartilage is frequently altered. The apex and at times the base are somewhat "squared off." The overall shape of the corniculate process is rectangular and, while this altered appearance has not been seen in all cases, when present has assisted in diagnosis. In addition to the marked stenosis of the laryngeal orifice, other alterations observed during endoscopic examination include stenosis of the laryngeal airway and partial or total obscurity of the opening to the laryngeal saccule and the vocal fold.

Cause: The cause of arytenoid cartilage deformities has not been defined. Histopathologic diagnoses of chondritis and chondroma have been made from biopsies collected during partial submucous arytenoidectomy. A chondroma in a 4-year-old Thoroughbred filly has been reported.[7] While previous laryngeal surgery may result in chondritis, not all horses with chondritis have had laryngeal surgery. Other possible causes of arytenoid cartilage deformity include trauma and infection from foreign objects, or extension of infection from paralaryngeal tissues. Most biopsy samples from young horses with arytenoid deformity are diagnosed as chondritis, whereas those from older horses are usually reported as chondromas.

Clinical Signs: Arytenoid cartilage defects produce an intolerance for work and a stertorous noise on both inspiration and expiration. Coughing is also an occasional clinical sign. As the condition has been diagnosed most frequently in 2- and 3-year-old race horses, clinical signs seem related to the stress of exercise.

The incidence of chondritis and chondromas of the arytenoid cartilages may be more frequent than previously recognized. Many cases in the past were incorrectly diagnosed as unilateral or bilateral laryngeal paralysis, especially those without concurrent ulcers, granulomas or polyps at the apices of the arytenoids. Furthermore, the possibility that some of these deformities have a congenital or inherited origin cannot be discounted. The high incidence in young horses supports this hypothesis.

Treatment: Arytenoid cartilage deformities have been successfully treated by submucosal arytenoidectomy.[42,43] The mucosa of the laryngeal saccule, vocal fold and entire arytenoid, excluding the muscular process, was removed. The surgery is performed under general anesthesia employing a laryngotomy. The endotracheal tube is removed to expose the laryngeal airway. Anesthesia is maintained by placing the endotracheal tube through a tracheotomy or by intermittent reinsertion of the endotracheal tube to re-establish a surgical plane of anesthesia. Alternatively, anesthesia can be maintained by IV agents. If necessary, the thyroid cartilage can be incised to increase surgical exposure. Sharp incision of the mucosa on the airway surface of the arytenoid is started approximately 1 cm caudal to the rostral border of the apex of the corniculate process. The incision is directed obliquely toward the vocal process and is not routinely extended around the opening to the laryngeal saccule unless the vocal process is to be removed. Near the center of this primary incision, a second sharp incision is directed caudodorsal to the vocal process over the arytenoid and, if required for good exposure, a third incision is directed rostrad at the same level.

To facilitate elevation of the mucosa, 1:10,000 epinephrine is injected into the submucosa. The mucosa is carefully elevated by blunt dissection to expose the cartilage. The cartilage is removed in segments by sharp incision and the incised segments are removed with rongeur forceps. Some of the corniculate process is left intact, if not obviously abnormal, to add stability to the corniculate process and assist in more effective closure of the laryngeal orifice during swallowing. Likewise, the vocal process and fold are not removed unless deformed.

The mucosal lining of the laryngeal saccule is always removed and the muscular process of the arytenoid is left intact to facilitate abduction of the arytenoid cartilages. The edges of the incised mucosa are trimmed as required for good closure and sutured with 00 polyglycolic acid or catgut in a series of inverted simple-interrupted or inverted simple-continuous sutures. Closure with an inverted suture pattern is preferred to avoid the risk of suture granulomas and increased scarring. While some surgeons do not advocate suturing the mucosa, it assists in hemorrhage control and lessens the chance for granulation tissue formation.

Because the surgery induces an intense local inflammatory reaction, close postoperative monitoring of the patient for the first 24-48 hours is mandatory. An emergency tracheotomy pack should be near the horse continuously until it is determined that the risk of respiratory emergency has passed. Since the laryngotomy incision remains unsutured, the tracheotomy tube can be inserted through this site in an emergency to provide a patent airway while a standard tracheotomy is performed. Nonsteroidal anti-inflammatory drugs are always given preoperatively and additional doses given daily as required.

Postoperative endoscopic examination reveals a reasonably normal corniculate process. Partial or full ability to abduct the arytenoid cartilages is often retained if the muscular process is left intact. A few cases have been complicated by coughing and choking while eating or drinking, but life-threatening complications have not been encountered. Three horses with partial bilateral arytenoidectomy have subsequently raced to expectation, while 6 horses with partial unilateral arytenoidectomy have subsequently raced successfully.

The Trachea*

Widened Cricotracheal Space

As a part of the physical examination of the respiratory tract, the cricotracheal space should be palpated and its width noted. The width of the cricotracheal space in presumably normal horses is 1-1.5 cm. In some horses the cricotracheal space approaches 2-3 cm. The clinical significance of this variation in width is difficult to assess. However, a "wider than normal" cricotracheal space is not a frequent cause of upper airway obstruction in horses.

One investigator anchored 2 wire sutures in the cricoid cartilage through the cricotracheal membrane rostral to the first tracheal ring on the ventral surface of the trachea to narrow the space.[44] The placement of sutures through a lar-

*by C.W. Raker

yngeal cartilage may lead to chondritis or chondroma formation and airway stenosis. If an incised cricoid cartilage is left unsutured, it may not heal or, if healing occurs, it may result in partial airway stenosis. Failure of the cricoid to heal may cause dorsal bulging of the membrane during forced inspiration. For these reasons, the cricoid cartilage should not be incised.

Surgery to correct a dorsal bulging of the membrane in a "wide" cricotracheal space is performed under general anesthesia. The area over the ventral larynx and proximal trachea is exposed and the neck is slightly flexed to relieve tension. The membrane is grasped with Allis tissue forceps and everted. A series of horizontal mattress sutures is placed in a staple pattern to form a pleat close to the base of the everted membrane with absorbable sutures. If necessary, several towel clamps are placed rostral to the intact cricoid cartilage and caudal to the first tracheal ring to relieve tension. If a laryngotomy has not been performed, the incision is closed in the usual manner with absorbable suture material.

Tracheal Stenosis

Tracheal stenosis occurs infrequently but is not rare. The trachea should always be palpated during physical examination to detect flattening, scars or similar deformities. The rigidity of the tracheal rings should be determined. Auscultation of the trachea may reveal signs compatible with restricted airflow.

Cause: There are many causes of tracheal stenosis. Prolonged intubation with a cuffed endotracheal tube frequently causes tracheal stenosis in humans.[45] Tracheal collapse from weakened or deformed rings has been observed in dogs, cattle and horses.[46-51] Blunt or penetrating trauma from ropes, mangers, fences and horned cattle are also frequent causes of tracheal stenosis.[52] Trauma may be accompanied by fracture of one or more tracheal rings. Stenosis frequently follows emergency tracheotomy, especially when one or more of the tracheal rings is severed or a segment excised.

Insertion of a tracheotomy tube in a foal with strangles is frequently necessary to maintain an adequate airway. Generally a pediatric-sized tube is not available and an adult-sized tracheotomy tube is inserted. The relatively large size of this tube often requires incision of one or more tracheal rings or removal of a segment to provide sufficient space for insertion. As healing progresses after tube removal, scar tissue and wound contracture may produce stenosis (Fig C21). For this reason, transection of tracheal rings or removal of a segment should be avoided, especially in foals, and efforts should be made to insert the tube between 2 rings. Use of a pediatric endotrachael tube is strongly recommended.

Tracheitis and infection of the tracheal mucosa may incite a chronic inflammatory reaction to result in the deposition of scar tissue. Peritracheal abscesses have also been reported as a cause of tracheal stenosis.[53] These abscesses may follow an attack of strangles and frequently involve the mediastinal lymph nodes; less frequently involved locations are along the cervical trachea, especially in the segments near the larynx.

Tumors and a granulomatous response to intratracheal parasites are infrequent causes of tracheal stenosis.

Clinical Signs: Clinical signs include decreased tolerance for work and a sometimes stertorous noise on inspiration and expiration. The intensity of clinical signs varies with the degree of stenosis. With advanced stenosis, noise is heard at rest and exercise may lead to collapse. Diagnosis is facilitated by endoscopic examination and radiography.

Treatment: Deformities seldom involve more than 2-5 tracheal rings and have been repaired successfully. A coated coil spring prosthesis placed around the trachea of a young horse provided an adequate airway for 3 months.[54] The spring was first covered with polyethylene, followed by a coating of silicone. The spring was spiralled around the deformed segment of the trachea and stabilized with sutures under tension to dilate the lumen. The sutures did not penetrate the tracheal mucosa.

A second procedure has been successfully used on several horses. After exposing the deformed segment of the trachea, multiple incisions are made 1 cm apart through the ventral surface of the affected tracheal rings extending 180° around the circumference, without penetration of the lumen. Sutures of 00 monofilament nylon are placed through the skin to encircle the cut segments of the tracheal rings without invading the mucosa. The wound is continuously closed as these sutures are put into place. At completion of the closure, the ends of each suture are tied under tension over a button.

Treatment of small tracheal deformities by resection and end-to-end anastomosis has been reported.[55] Up to 5 tracheal rings have been resected without developing postoperative airflow obstruction from formation of intraluminal scar tissue.

Tracheal Collapse

Tracheal collapse is caused by a lack of rigidity of the cartilaginous rings and dorsoventral flattening of the trachea. The dorsal fibroelastic membrane is thin and stretched, resulting in a lunate lumen. The etiology of the deformity has not been well defined.

The major clinical sign is a principally inspiratory noise similar to that produced by advanced laryngeal hemiplegia. Coughing and nasal exudation occur in some cases, which can cause the condition to be confused with pulmonary disease.

Palpation and endoscopic examination of the cervical trachea reveal dorsoventral flattening and decreased rigidity. Tracheal auscultation may reveal harsh respiratory sounds, especially when the trachea is compressed. Lateral radiographs reveal the altered outline and extent of involvement.

Numerous surgical procedures have been used to correct tracheal collapse. Tracheal prosthesis placement in a calf has been reported.[49] The prosthesis was a coil spring slightly longer and greater in diameter than the deformed tracheal segment. The spring was covered with polyethylene tubing and the ends sealed. After the collapsed segment of the trachea was isolated, the open-ended coil prosthesis was spiralled onto the exterior of the trachea. The trachea was then expanded by a series of simple interrupted mersilene sutures placed from the wall of the trachea to the prosthesis. The calf recovered and the prosthesis was removed 4 months later.

Another tracheal prosthesis was fashioned from a 35-ml polypropylene syringe case cut in half longitudinally.[52] The prosthesis was long enough to include a normal tracheal ring at each end of the collapsed segment. Holes were drilled along each border and the autoclaved prosthesis was sutured to the collapsed tracheal segment with wire. The sutures encircled each tracheal ring but did not penetrate the tracheal mucosa.

There is only one report of a prosthesis used for tracheal collapse in the horse.[50] The investigators inserted a reinforced polyvinylchloride corrugated hose to replace the resected segment of collapsed trachea. The horse progressed well for 3 months but was eventually euthanized due to complications.

Tracheitis

Tracheitis is frequently associated with viral or infectious respiratory tract disease. It subsides as the infection clears and usually has no sequelae. Local tracheitis of short duration is often seen following endotracheal intubation for the administration of gas anesthesia. No serious damage has been reported as a result of cuffed endotracheal tube use in horses.

Smoke inhalation may produce extensive tracheitis. Tracheotomy is the most frequent cause of a local or diffuse tracheitis. The inflammatory response is usually of short duration, leaving no permanent sequelae to obstruct the airway. Large mucosal and submucosal thickenings, probably the result of infection of the tracheotomy wound or an immune response to the tracheotomy tube, may significantly restrict the flow of air.

References

1. Getty: Sisson and Grossman's Anatomy of the Domestic Animals. 5th ed. WB Saunders, Philadelphia, 1975.
2. Robinson, NE and Sorensen, PR. JAVMA 172 (1978) 299.
3. McAllister, ES and Blakeslee, JR. JAVMA 170 (1977) 739.
4. Raker, CW. Mod Vet Pract 57 (1976) 396.
5. Raker, CW and Boles, CL. J Eq Med Surg 2 (1978) 202.
6. Von Boening, KJ. Prak Tier 4 (1978) 300.
7. Cook, WR. Vet Rec 94 (1974) 533.
8. Churchill, EA, Chesapeake City, MD: Personal communication, 1975.
9. Tiegland, MB, Hialeah, FL: Personal communication, 1975.
10. Goldman, JL. Ann Oto Rhin Laryn 87 (1978) 663.
11. Harthill, A. Horseman's J 30 (1979) 64.
12. Koch, DB and Tate, LP. JAVMA 173 (1978) 860.
13. Harvey, CE et al. Arch Am Coll Vet Surg 2 (1973) 15.
14. Quinlan, J and Morton, DD. J So Afr Vet Assoc 28 (1957) 63.
15. Quinlan, J. J So Afr Vet Assoc 28 (1957) 291.
16. Cook, WR. Proc Ann Mtg Br Vet Assoc, 1964. p 18.
17. Raker, CW. Mod Vet Pract 57 (1976) 471.
18. Sherman, J et al. Can J Comp Med 43 (1979) 1.
19. Heffron, CJ and Baker, GJ. Eq Vet J 11 (1979) 142.
20. Heffron, CJ, Univ Glasgow: Personal communication, 1977.
21. Cook, WR. Vet Rec 83 (1968) 336.
22. Sack and Habel: Rooney's Guide to Dissection of the Horse. Veterinary Textbooks, Ithaca, NY, 1977.
23. Marks, D et al. Eq Vet J 2 (1970) 159.
24. Marks, D et al. JAVMA 157 (1970) 429.
25. Cole, CR. Am J Vet Res 7 (1946) 69.
26. Rooney, JR and Delaney, FM. Eq Vet J 2 (1970) 35.
27. Cymbaluk, NF et al. Vet Rec 101 (1977) 97.
28. Quinlan, J. J So Afr Vet Assoc 28 (1957) 291.
29. Baker, in Catcott: Equine Medicine and Surgery. 2nd ed. American Veterinary Publications, Santa Barbara, 1972.
30. Schneider, in Oehme and Prier: Textbook of Large Animal Surgery. Williams & Wilkins, Baltimore, 1974.
31. Williams, WL. Am Vet Rev 32 (1907) 333.
32. Hobday, FTG. No Am Vet 17 (1936) 17.
33. Marks, D. JAVMA 157 (1970) 157.
34. Speirs, VC. Aust Vet J 48 (1972) 251.
35. Johnson, JH. VM/SAC 35 (1970) 347.
36. Boles, CL et al. JAVMA 172 (1978) 338.
37. Speirs, VC. J Eq Med Surg 1 (1977) 267.
38. Fretz, PB. Can Vet J 18 (1977) 352.
39. Ordridge, RM. Vet Rec 100 (1977) 365.
40. Wheat, JD. Proc 5th Ann Cong Br Eq Assoc, 1966. p 63.
41. Goulden, BE et al. Eq Vet J 8 (1976) 95.
42. Wheat, JD. Paper presented at 5th Ann Surg Forum, 1978.
43. White, NA and Blackwell, RB. Vet Surg 9 (1980) 5.
44. Pouret, E. Proc 12th Ann Mtg Am Assoc Eq Pract, 1966. p 207.
45. Miller, DR and Sethi, G. Ann Surg 171 (1970) 283.
46. Leonard, HC. JAVMA 158 (1971) 598.
47. Bojrab, MJ and Nafe, LL. JAAHA 12 (1976) 622.
48. Hobson, HP. JAAHA 12 (1976) 822.
49. Horney, FD. JAVMA 167 (1975) 463.
50. Carrig, CB et al. J Am Vet Rad Soc 15 (1973) 32.
51. Hanselka, DV. VM/SAC 68 (1973) 859.
52. Boyd, CL and Hanselka, DV. JAAHA 12 (1976) 829.
53. Randall, RW and Myers, VS. VM/SAC 68 (1973) 264.
54. Evans, LH, Univ Penn: Personal communication, 1979.
55. Tate, LP. Paper presented at 14th Ann Mtg Am Coll Vet Surg, 1979.

LOWER RESPIRATORY TRACT DISEASES
by R.A. Mansmann

Foal Pneumonia

Foal pneumonia is an economically important disease with multiple precipitating causes and no pathognomonic signs.[1] Foals may be initially affected at 4-12 weeks of age when passive maternal antibody levels are waning and endogenous immunoglobulins only beginning to be produced.

Cause: Numerous organisms may act alone or in combination with others to cause pneumonia in foals. Although viruses, such as EHV-1 and influenza virus, cause upper respi-

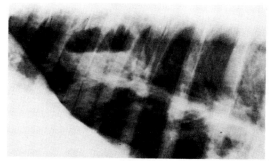

Fig 29. Thoracic radiograph of a weanling with a chronic *Streptococcus equi* infection. A cavitating abscess is evident on the upper left.

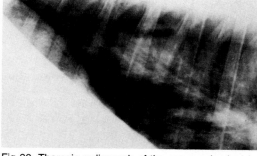

Fig 30. Thoracic radiograph of the same animal as in Figure 29 after 30 days of penicillin therapy. The size of the abscess is considerably reduced.

ratory infection and pneumonitis, their most important role is weakening pulmonary defense mechanisms, allowing secondary bacterial infection.

Helminth migration causes mild pneumonitis and allows secondary bacterial infection.

Numerous types of bacteria have been implicated in foal pneumonia. Because 2 or more organisms may simultaneously infect a foal, the course of disease and results of therapy should be monitored with more than one culture. The most commonly involved bacteria are beta-hemolytic streptococci, principally *Streptococcus zooepidemicus* and occasionally *Streptococcus equi*.[2] *Streptococcus equi* infection (strangles) causes the only distinctive signs related to foal respiratory problems, that of retropharyngeal and mandibular lymph node enlargement. Pneumonia may be part of a strangles problem on some farms and may be difficult to treat. *Streptococcus* can also form pulmonary abscesses that require lengthy treatment (Figs 29, 30).

The most severe type of bacterial pneumonia is caused by *Corynebacterium equi*. The organism is a soil contaminant that can inhabit farms for long periods and may reappear on the farm on an annual basis. In an Australian study, *C equi* was isolated from the feces of horses of all ages on all farms tested, but only 1 of 12 farms had a problem with *C equi* pneumonia in foals.[3] *Corynebacterium equi* can produce small or large pulmonary abscesses before clinical signs are evident to the farm manager and the veterinarian (Fig 31). The organism also has a propensity to change its sensitivity to antibiotics and normally requires extremely long periods of antibiotic therapy.

Actinobacillus equuli has been related to neonatal joint infections and may cause pneumonia in foals less than 7 days of age. The

organism has also been isolated in foals with chronic pneumonia.

Klebsiella pneumoniae has also been implicated in cases of chronic pneumonia. *Salmonella*, principally *S typhimurium* infection, is usually manifested as systemic disease that may include pneumonia. *Bordetella bronchiseptica* has also been isolated from pneumonic lungs. Cultures are important because each of these organisms has its own specific antibiotic sensitivity.

Clinical Signs: Labored breathing may be the earliest sign of pneumonia. Other signs include lethargy, reluctance to nurse, fever, mucopurulent nasal discharge and cough. Irritants, such as dust or ascarid larvae, may cause a slightly elevated respiratory rate, increased bronchovesicular sounds or sibilant rhonchi. The degree of dyspnea usually parallels the severity of rales. Moist rales indicate pneumonia.

Diagnosis: The clinician should obtain a thorough history, including information on

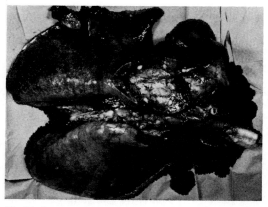

Fig 31. Large pulmonary abscess from *Corynebacterium equi* infection in a 3-month-old colt.

other cases of foal pneumonia on the farm. Physical examination should include careful thoracic auscultation, percussion and observation of respiratory patterns.

A blood sample for a CBC should be obtained before the foal is stressed. Mild leukocytosis (10,000-20,000 WBC/mm³) may indicate bacterial pneumonia or involvement of irritants. Severe neutrophilic leukocytosis (20,000-50,000 WBC/mm³) indicates mild to severe bacterial pneumonia. Mild lymphopenia indicates viral infection and marked lymphopenia (< 500 lymphocytes/mm³) may indicate immunodeficiency. Eosinophilia is relatively uncommon and may indicate parasitic infection. Repeated CBCs may be indicated to monitor the foal's progress.

A culture should be obtained before treatment is instituted. Transtracheal aspiration is relatively easy in foals and should be performed in individual cases or in the first case of a potential herd outbreak. Knowledge of the organism involved is of obvious prognostic value. Nasal swabs may be used to obtain subsequent cultures to monitor changes in antibiotic sensitivity or to confirm subsequent cases in a herd outbreak. Another transtracheal aspiration is indicated if the nasal swab results are questionable or if there is a change in the type of organism isolated. Antibiotic sensitivity and minimal inhibitory antibiotic concentrations can be determined from transtracheal aspiration cultures. Gram-staining can determine which group of antibiotics to use until culture and sensitivity results are returned. Cytologic examination of the aspirate is also useful in some cases.

Other diagnostic technics include immunoglobulin quantitation, fecal examination and paired serum samples for virus titer evaluation. Thoracic radiographs aid in the diagnosis, prognosis and monitoring of therapy of patients with pulmonary abscesses.

Treatment: Antibiotic therapy is unwarranted if only upper respiratory disease is involved. Upper respiratory disease usually resolves without treatment in normal, well-managed, unstressed foals. The stress of handling during therapy for upper respiratory disease may undermine the benefits of treatment.

Appropriate antibiotics, as determined by culture and sensitivity tests, are the most important therapeutic agents. A study of referred equine cases showed that 50% of foals were infected with penicillin-resistant organisms.[4]

However, *Streptococcus zooepidemicus*, the most common cause of foal pneumonia, responds to penicillin therapy. Although *S zooepidemicus* has never been reported as penicillin-resistant, penicillin dosage may have to be increased to achieve good results. Occasionally *Streptococcus* is initially cultured and the foal is treated with penicillin but relapses occur. Repeat cultures often reveal *Corynebacterium equi* or some other penicillin-resistant organism. Penicillin can be used until culture and sensitivity results are returned, at which time the appropriate antibiotic may be administered. Affected foals should receive penicillin until 5-7 days after abnormal chest sounds have disappeared. Although corticosteroids have been used in foal pneumonia to improve an animal's spirits, they suppress the inflammatory and immune responses. For this reason, foals should be carefully evaluated before and after corticosteroids are administered.

Nebulization may be of value, but the stress of administering that therapy to the foal must be considered. An ultrasonic nebulizer placed in an enclosed stall with the mare and foal considerably reduces the stress of nebulization therapy. Bronchodilators, mucolytic agents and antibiotics may be used in the nebulizer.

Intratracheal injection of suitable agents has been used with varying success. Bronchodilators, such as aminophylline, may be helpful, especially in the initial treatment of foal pneumonia. Antipyretics, such as phenylbutazone and aspirin, may be useful in the first 4-5 days of treatment to encourage the foal to resume nursing without altering the immune response. Antipyretic therapy should be withheld after 2 days and the foal's response assessed. Isoniazid, given IM at 11 mg/kg, may also be useful, especially in foals with large pulmonary abscesses.

Pneumocystis carinii has been isolated from foals and humans subjected to excessive use of antibiotics and corticosteroids.[5,6] Treatment in such individuals has consisted of reducing immunosuppression and administering trimethoprim (20 mg/kg QID) and sulfamethoxazole (100 mg/kg QID).

Therapy for foal pneumonia may be unsuccessful for a variety of reasons. Failure to determine the causative agent and its chemotherapeutic sensitivity, coupled with trial-and-error antibiotic therapy, may lead to chronic or fatal pneumonia. Inappropriate or too brief a course of antibiotic therapy in cases of streptococcal or *Corynebacterium* abscesses may lead to intractable pneumonia. Radiographs are good prognostic aids in those situations. Iatrogenic immunosuppression from prolonged corticosteroid or other anti-inflammatory therapy promotes opportunistic bacterial infection.

Immunodeficient foals, such as Arabians with combined immunodeficiency, do not respond to treatment of pneumonia. Adenovirus, *Aspergillus* and *Pneumocystis carinii* have been isolated from such foals. It is uneconomical to prolong the life of a foal with combined immunodeficiency; however, immunodeficiency stemming from malnutrition or iatrogenic causes offers a better prognosis if management changes are instituted.

Additional causes of poor therapeutic results include poor stall ventilation, heavy parasite burden, stress from handling during treatment, and exposure of affected foals to sick or carrier animals. Environmental causes should be suspected if a foal with acute pneumonia initially responds to therapy with an appropriate antibiotic but relapses with a fever, sibilant rhonchi and minimal pulmonary changes on radiography. Reduction of sibilant rhonchi after a test dose of atropine indicates a reaction to environmental irritants. Hay should not be fed and dust should be controlled by watering; short-term use of corticosteroids may also be beneficial. Nonresponding pneumonia related to coccidioidomycosis or histoplasmosis is rare in foals and generally restricted to enzootic areas.

Control: The ideal environment is a large clean pasture with plenty of sunshine and consistent temperatures. Drastic changes in temperature should be avoided. The extreme daytime heat and nighttime cold of desert climates may account for the high incidence of pneumonia in those areas.

Overfeeding of foals should be avoided. Good endoparasite control programs reduce the burden of parasites, which irritate the lungs during larval migration and reduce host resistance to disease. Pastures should not be overcrowded, dusty run-in shed floors should be watered, and stables or barns should be kept clean and well ventilated.

Such procedures as breeding the mare, separation of the mare and foal, deworming, vaccination, or transportation of the mare and foal should be minimized to reduce stress of the foal. Quiet, early training of the foal reduces stress of the foal when it is subsequently exposed to new environments.

References

1. Anon. J Eq Med Surg **2** (1978) 400, 428.
2. Knight, HD. Proc Ann Mtg Am Coll Vet Int Med, 1978. p 120.
3. Woolcock, JB *et al.* Res Vet Sci **28** (1980) 87.
4. Mansmann, RA *et al.* Proc 17th Ann Mtg Am Assoc Eq Pract, 1971. p 143.
5. Mansmann, RA. Vet Clin No Am **5** (1975) 87.
6. Hughes, WT. N Engl J Med **297** (1977) 1381.

Acute Lower Respiratory Tract Disease in Adult Horses

Acute lower respiratory tract disease in adult (older than a yearling) horses includes pneumonitis, pneumonia, pleuritis and pulmonary edema. They can be progressive and more than one condition can occur in an animal. Typical signs include fever, anorexia, hyperpnea, and occasionally cough and nasal discharge.

Pneumonitis

Cause: Although viral infections of the respiratory tract are typically confined to the upper airway, viral pneumonitis may descend to the lungs in some cases. Myxoviruses, herpesviruses and other types of viruses may be involved. The viruses can destroy the mucociliary blanket and alter the bactericidal capability of macrophages.[1]

Clinical Signs: Viral pneumonitis should be suspected if dry rhonchi are auscultated throughout the lungs of a horse with fever, anorexia and hyperpnea.

Treatment: Antipyretic administration encourages resumption of eating and should be on an alternate-day basis so the body temperature can be monitored. A fever that persists longer than 5 days is a sign of secondary bacterial pneumonia. Because of the possibility of altered respiratory tract defense mechanisms by viral infection, broad-spectrum antibiotics should be administered to prevent secondary bacterial infection. Stress should be minimized and exercise curtailed for at least 3 weeks. Hand-walking may be beneficial.

Control: A dust-free, sanitary environment is ideal to minimize mechanical irritation of the respiratory tract. An adequate vaccination program against respiratory diseases is important since viral pneumonitis typically affects unvaccinated horses.

Pneumonia

Cause: Bacterial pneumonia is usually secondary to a primary viral infection when affected horses are stressed by shipping, inclement weather, malnutrition or strenuous exercise. Pneumonia may also result from inhalation of dirt during a race, smoke inhalation, inadvertent infusion of anthelmintics into the lungs, and aspiration of food secondary to laryngeal or pharyngeal paralysis from various causes, including chronic lead poisoning.

Clinical Signs: Affected horses typically have a mucopurulent nasal discharge and a fever of 38.3-39.4 ·C (101-103 F). Anorexia is not as marked as in viral pneumonitis. Thoracic auscultation reveals mild, sibilant rhonchi to severe, moist rales.

Diagnosis: Diagnosis is based upon clinical signs. Transtracheal aspiration should be performed for culture and sensitivity testing of any organisms involved. Gram-negative bacteria are often isolated from horses with aspiration pneumonia. About 50% of bacteria isolated from horses with pneumonia are resistant to penicillin.[3] Serial CBCs should be performed to monitor the response to therapy.

Treatment: Treatment is dictated by culture and sensitivity test results. Corticosteroids may be administered with antibiotics in cases of smoke inhalation and aspiration pneumonia characterized by severe fluid accumulation in the lungs. Treatment for pneumonia should be continued 7 days after remission of signs.

Pleuritis

Pleuritis is an inflammation of the lining of the thoracic cavity. Clinical signs include mild

Table 1. Characteristics of Abnormal Pleural Fluid[14]

Condition (no. of horses)	Gross Appearance	Specific Gravity	Protein (g/dl)	WBC[a] (/mm³)	RBC (/mm³)	Volume (L)	Bacterial Culture[b]
ACUTE							
Primary pleuritis, including postviral pleuritis (5)	Serous, yellow to cloudy, sanguineous	1.0110-1.0216	1.3-5.5	4900-350,000	10,000-230,000	<0.5-3	Neg
Pulmonary abscess, pneumonia or both (8)	Cloudy, yellow to cloudy, reddish brown	1.0172-1.0206	3.7-4.9	15,600-115,000	0-870,000	6-35	5 of 7 pos
Lympho-sarcoma (2)	Sanguineous to serosanguineous	1.0120-1.0127	1.6-1.9	14,000-32,000	40,000-950,000	20-50	Neg
CHRONIC							
Primary pleuritis (11)	Cloudy, yellow	1.0184-1.0275	4.1-7.8	14,500-200,000	0-42,000	2-40	3 of 10 Pos
Pulmonary abscess, pneumonia or both (5)	Cloudy, yellow to serosanguineous	1.0166-1.0203	3.5-4.8	8100-71,000	2000-90,000	<1-10	1 of 4 Pos
Pulmonary granulomas (2)	Sanguineous, reddish brown	1.0173 (1)	3.6 (1)	39,700 (1)	590,000 (1)	3-5	Neg
Lymphosarcoma (2)	Serosanguineous	1.0142 (1)	2.5 (1)	.4100 (1)	60,000 (1)	4-30	Neg
Coccidioidomy-cosis (1)	Cloudy, pale yellow	1.0117	1.5	8400	6000	1	Neg
Equine infectious anemia (1)	Cloudy, yellow	ND	ND	ND	ND	6	Neg

a—Mainly neutrophils except in cases of lymphosarcoma, in which lymphocytes predominated.
b—Number of positive per number tested since cultures not obtained on all samples.
ND—Not determined.

fever, hyperpnea and decreased appetite. Coughing and nasal discharge may not be present. Thoracic auscultation in the first 24-48 hours of the disease may reveal no abnormalities; however, stiffness and thoracic splinting are evident at that time. After 48 hours auscultation generally reveals reduced or absent respiratory sounds in the ventral 25-75% of the thorax. Thoracentesis should be performed to determine the presence and character of fluid.

Acute Pleuropneumonia: This rapidly progressive type of pleuritis is usually related to stress, such as shipping or racing, and may be associated with a ruptured abscess or gangrenous pneumonia usually of the right apical lung lobe. Young racing Thoroughbreds and Standardbreds are commonly affected.

Clinical signs include tachycardia, prolonged capillary refill time and leukopenia. Thoracentesis produces a foul-smelling effusion containing anaerobic, aerobic and gram-negative bacteria. Affected animals should be treated for endotoxic shock and pneumonia with IV fluids, corticosteroids, the appropriate antibiotics and

intensive supportive care. Few affected horses survive despite treatment.

Acute Pleuritis: Acute pleuritis has an onset of 2-3 days and may be secondary to pneumonitis. Early diagnosis and initiation of treatment are critical in assuring recovery.

Thoracic auscultation early in the disease may be unremarkable but decreased respiratory sounds become evident in the ventral thorax after the first day. Other clinical signs include fever, thoracic splinting, and apparent colic or front-leg lameness, such as laminitis or shoulder lameness. Thoracentesis early in the disease typically produces small amounts of fluid with slightly increased WBC numbers and protein content (Table 1). As the disease progresses, the WBC count in aspirated fluid increases. The fluid is typically sterile and not odoriferous.

Treatment involves drainage of thoracic fluid every other day using a sterile teat cannula and suction at a negative pressure of 2-6 lb/inch^2. A one-way Heimlich valve can also be installed for continuous drainage. Asepsis is

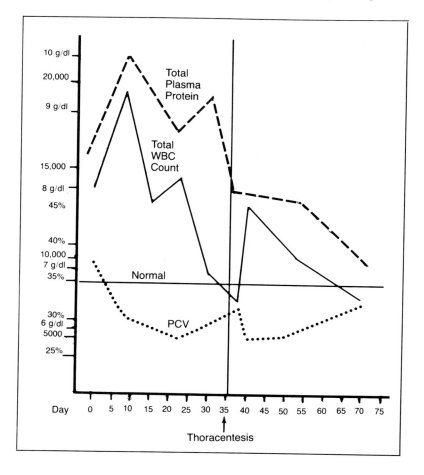

Fig 32. Blood values of a 2-year-old Thoroughbred stallion with a fluctuating fever for 6 weeks prior to treatment. A thoracic abscess, later drained by thoracentesis, caused hyperproteinemia and progressive anemia.

critical in placement of the drain to avoid thoracic contamination. Drainage should continue until less than 500 ml are obtained per aspiration. Removal of large amounts (> 20 L) of fluid at one time may cause hypovolemic shock. Penicillin or kanamycin should be administered for 10-14 days. The prognosis is poor if the WBC count remains high, the total plasma protein level remains above 8.5 g/dl, and the PCV is subnormal (Fig 32).

Chronic Pleuritis: Chronic pleuritis occurs in some horses not completely cured of acute pleuropneumonia or pleuritis. Such animals may develop generalized, extensive fibrin deposits on the visceral pleura, which is honeycombed with pockets of effusion. Although these animals may temporarily respond to antibiotic therapy, the prognosis for recovery is poor. In other horses the pleural effusion resolves after administration of high levels of antibiotics; however, abscesses may remain in the pleura or lungs after such treatment. Single, large abscesses can be located by radiography and/or auscultation, and drained by thoracentesis. The medial wall of the abscess prevents significant pneumothorax during drainage. Thoracic surgery and thoracic abscess drainage have been described.[4,5]

Some horses with chronic pleuritis have no history of pleural or other respiratory tract disease. Such animals may have chronic weight loss and fluid in the ventral thorax upon auscultation and thoracentesis. Chronic pleural effusion has been associated with lymphoma, equine infectious anemia and coccidioidomycosis (Table 2); however, many cases have no identifiable cause.[6,7] The prognosis for recovery from chronic pleuritis is poor.

Thoracic Wounds: Any penetrating thoracic wound can cause pleuritis. Such wounds should be treated as acute pleuritis with high levels of broad-spectrum antibiotics. A simple treatment for pneumothorax has been described.[8] After the wound was sutured, a chest tube was placed, with the external end in a bucket of water. Air could exit but not re-enter the tube.

Pulmonary Edema

Although pulmonary edema can occur in cases of anaphylaxis, it is most commonly associated with aspiration pneumonia. Auscultation reveals dull respiratory sounds throughout the lung fields because of sound reduction by interstitial and alveolar fluid accumulation. Transtracheal aspiration can be used to help determine the cause, and to obtain fluid samples for bacteriologic and cytologic examination.

Large doses of penicillin or kanamycin should be administered until culture and sensitivity test results are obtained. Corticosteroids (*eg,* prednisolone at 1 mg/lb) should be used for only 1-3 days because of their immunosuppressive effects. Diuretics help remove some alveolar fluid. Aminophylline can be used on a long-term basis to dilate airways and remove edema fluid through its mild diuretic action. Although nebulization therapy with 50% alcohol may be beneficial, the stress associated with administration of such therapy may undermine the beneficial effects.

Smoke Inhalation

The case history of 20 horses that survived a stable fire exemplifies the effects of smoke inhalation.[9] Rectal temperature was elevated to 38.9-40 C (102-104 F) 1-7 days after the fire. Hyperpnea paralleled the febrile course. The most severely affected horses had respiratory alkalosis. A spontaneous cough developed in most horses a week after the fire but resolved within a month. Fine rales and sibilant rhonchi were auscultated in half the horses the first week, but all were normal within a month. Al-

Table 2. Precipitins in Serum of Normal Horses and Horses with Heaves[15]

	Heaves (9)*	Controls (9)*		Heaves (9)*	Controls (9)
Alternaria	0/1**	1/0	Pullularia	0/0	0/0
Aspergillus clavatus	0/0	0/2	Rhizopus	0/0	0/0
Aspergillus fumigatus	0/1	1/0	Trichoderma	0/0	0/1
Candida	1/1	0/2	Moldy hay	2/2	5/1
Cephalosporium	6/3	7/2	Micropolyspora faeni	0/0	0/1
Fusarium	2/3	2/2	Thermactinomyces vulgaris	6/2	7/0
Hormodendrum	0/0	0/1	Housedust extract	3/1	4/2
Mucor	0/0	0/0	Chicken serum	1/1	2/0
Penicillum	1/0	0/1	Pigeon serum	1/1	2/1
			Saline	0/0	0/0

*   Number of horses
** Faint reactions/strong reactions

though secondary pneumonia can occur in humans 14-21 days after smoke inhalation, none of these horses developed pneumonia.[10]

Severely affected horses were treated with IV prednisolone and IM penicillin until 7 days after clinical signs were normal. Aminophylline was administered beginning on the third day after the fire. Severely affected horses received ultrasonic humidification in a plastic-enclosed stall 12 hours daily for 2 weeks.

Although some observers have noted a chronic cough or chronic obstructive lung disease in horses subsequent to smoke inhalation, such was not the case here.[11-13] However, 50% of the horses did not train or race up to their previous ability and 3 horses had marked exercise intolerance. The degree of decreased performance paralleled the length of exposure to smoke.

References

1. Reed, SE and Boyde, A. Infect Immun **6(7)** (1972) 68.
2. Holmes, JA *et al*. Report of the Selby Smelter Commission. Bull 98. US Govt Printing Office, 1915.
3. Mansmann, RA *et al*. Proc Am Assoc Eq Pract, 1971. p 143.
4. Fowler, ME *et al*. Am J Vet Res **24** (1963) 766.
5. Callahan, PT and Knight, HD. JAVMA **174** (1979) 1231.
6. Smith, BP. JAVMA **170** (1977) 208.
7. DeMartini, JL and Riddle, WE. JAVMA **155** (1969) 149.
8. Thompson, JV. VM/SAC **72** (1977) 250.
9. Mansmann, RA, Ohio State Univ: Unpublished data, 1973.
10. Pruitt, BA *et al*. J Thor Card Surg **59** (1970) 7.
11. Churchill, E, Chesapeake City, MD: Personal communication, 1973.
12. O'Dea, J, Genesco, NY: Personal communication, 1973.
13. Evans, L, Univ Penn: Personal communication, 1973.
14. Smith, BP. JAVMA **170** (1977) (in legend of Table 1).
15. Reed, CE, Univ Wisc: Unpublished data, 1970.

Chronic Respiratory Disease

Many names have been given to chronic respiratory disease in horses, including "broken wind," "heaves" and chronic alveolar emphysema. Although such terms connote a grave prognosis to owners, many affected horses can return to normal if treated properly.

Animals 6 years of age and older are typically affected. Many horses are affected seasonally and the history usually includes confinement in an enclosed, poorly ventilated stable. The owner may notice that the respiratory disease began with an upper respiratory infection and pro-

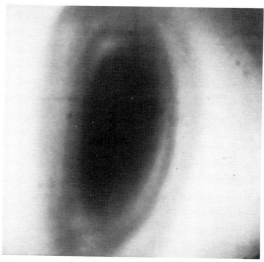

Fig 33. Endoscopic view of laterally flattened trachea ("scabbard trachea") in a 17-year-old pony with chronic progressive respiratory distress.

gressively became more significant. Clinical signs include chronic cough and dyspnea that increases with exercise. Fever, nasal discharge and hereditary predisposition are usually not part of the syndrome.

Rhinolaryngoscopic examination and evaluation of tracheal symmetry aid differentiation of chronic respiratory disease from chronic pharyngitis, congenital malformations or severe tracheal trauma, such as "scabbard trachea" in ponies, all of which may cause chronic cough and exercise intolerance (Fig 33). Affected horses should be methodically examined so a diagnosis, prognosis and treatment can be given (Fig 34).

Horses with chronic respiratory disease may be divided into 2 categories by physical examination. Mildly affected horses have no apparent weight loss. Respiratory rate and pattern are normal, but a moist cough and mucous sounds in the first divisions of bronchi may be present.

Severely affected horses have weight loss, continuous or intermittent dyspnea, flared nostrils, slightly elevated respiratory rate, and a prolonged, double expiratory phase. Prolonged expiration is associated with the presence of a "heave line," hypertrophy of the external abdominal oblique muscles from forced expiration because of decreased elastic recoil of the lungs. Sibilant rhonchi, which may resemble the sound of crinkling cellophane, are heard in the lung periphery. A deep, dry cough can be elicited by occluding the nostrils for 30 seconds

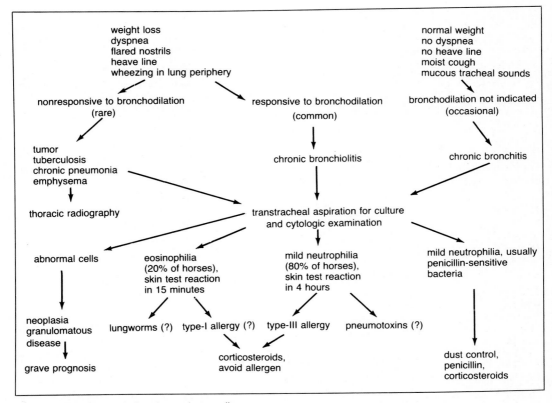

Fig 34. Management of chronic respiratory disease.

and allowing the horse to take a deep breath. Sputum may occasionally be coughed up, but nasal discharge is not typical.

Blood for a CBC should be drawn prior to exercising the horse during the examination to avoid the effects of stress on the hemogram.

Further subdivision of affected horses is achieved by pulmonary function testing or bronchodilation. In a few equine hospitals, pulmonary function testing can be performed on standing animals before and after bronchodilation. When pulmonary function testing is not available, the clinician may assess pulmonary function by comparing respiratory sounds before and after administration of bronchodilators, such as isoproterenol (0.2 mg in 6 ml sterile saline/450 kg body weight) or atropine (0.01 mg/lb). These drugs cause relaxation of pulmonary smooth muscle and cessation of the sibilant rhonchi immediately and their effects last about 30 minutes.

The use of bronchodilators in horses with mucous sounds, primarily in the trachea, and of normal weight is not helpful since the main portions of the lungs are unaffected. Pathologic changes are limited to the trachea and first divisions of bronchi, and are generally categorized as increased mucus production and not by smooth muscle contraction. These horses are said to have chronic bronchitis.

Horses with sibilant rhonchi in the lung periphery that disappear upon administration of bronchodilators have reversible obstructive pathologic changes, as seen in the typical case of "heaves."

Horses with sibilant rhonchi in the lung periphery that do not disappear upon administration of bronchodilators have irreversible changes of the peribronchiolar area, such as emphysema, or space-occupying lesions that compress the bronchial tree, such as a tumor or granuloma.

Transtracheal aspiration should be performed to obtain samples for cytologic examination and culture after pulmonary function testing or bronchodilation.

The following specific conditions should be considered after assessment of the horse's history, clinical signs, pulmonary function and tracheal washings.

Chronic Bronchitis

Cause: The disease is caused by constant irritation of the respiratory tree, usually by a very dusty environment. If the irritation continues, superimposition of a chronic streptococcal infection is common.[1]

Clinical Signs: Horses with chronic bronchitis are generally of normal weight and may have some exercise intolerance or a moist cough on exercise but do not have major dyspneic episodes. The fundamental pathologic change in chronic bronchitis in humans is hypertrophy of mucus-secreting goblet cells and tracheobronchial glands. Mucous rales are easily heard over the trachea, decreasing over the mid-lung portion of the primary bronchus. Because the periphery of the lung sounds normal, bronchodilation does not significantly change the auscultatory findings. A CBC and cytologic examination of easily obtained heavy mucus from transtracheal aspirates reveal mild neutrophilic leukocytosis.

Treatment: The condition is usually alleviated by controlling environmental dust or replacing moldy hay. Penicillin therapy for 2-4 weeks is also of benefit.

Chronic Bronchiolitis

Chronic bronchiolitis is the condition responsible for the "heavey" horse. Although the terms "pursiveness," "broken wind" and emphysema have been applied to this condition, they are very misleading in that chronic bronchiolitis involves neither permanent respiratory damage nor emphysema. Terms more specific than chronic bronchiolitis are unwarranted until more investigation properly categorizes the condition.[5]

Cause: Factors that may contribute to the primary mechanisms of chronic bronchiolitis or aggravate established cases include allergy, infection, irritants and toxins. The disease appears to be acquired and has no hereditary predisposition. Affected horses are typically quartered in dusty environments and have clinical signs during periods of reduced ventilation, as in a poorly ventilated stable in the winter. Because chronic bronchiolitis is the most common chronic respiratory disease in horses, further discussion is warranted.

In regard to allergy, no one specific antigen or type of immunologic disease has been identified as a general cause for chronic bronchiolitis. A few attempts have been made to create experimental models of allergic respiratory disease in horses. Histamine injected IV produced a response similar to that in horses with acute respiratory distress.[7] Bovine serum albumin given by nebulization caused clinical and histopathologic findings similar to chronic bronchiolitis. Nebulized ascarid antigen caused immediate respiratory hyperventilation.[2]

Horses appear to have homocytotropic antibodies similar to those in other animals, as demonstrated by Prausnitz-Küstner passive transfer of bovine serum albumin and ascarid extract.[2] How these reactions relate to clinical disease is still unknown.

There are 4 types of immunologic disease: type-I immediate hypersensitivity mediated by IgE, type-II autoimmune reactions, type-III Arthus reactions caused by specific circulating IgG, and type-IV delayed hypersensitivity reactions mediated by specific lymphocytes. Types I and II have been most implicated in chronic bronchiolitis.

Of 6 studies of 138 horses severely affected by obstructive lung disease, in only one study involving 14 horses was there a clear implication of type-I allergy as a general mechanism for heaves.[2,9-13] Using intradermal testing, there were far more delayed reactions (4 hours), noted primarily to mold antigens, than immediate reactions. The distinction between control and diseased horses was not absolute since some controls had large numbers of positive reactions and diseased horses had few reactions. For this reason, survey skin testing is not useful in the diagnosis of this disease.

In the hypersensitivity pneumonitides in humans, which have been more commonly related to the type-III immunologic reaction, precipitin reactions have been used to isolate the specific antigen involved. This is usually a disease acquired by inhalation of a specific antigen over a period, increasing the circulating specific IgG serum, which then produces the positive precipitin test. Precipitins to the molds *Micropolyspora faeni* and *Aspergillus fumigatus* were observed more frequently in diseased horses than controls, but there was no clear distinction.[13] Table 2 illustrates the precipitating reaction in horses with chronic respiratory disease and in normal horses. The survey results in Table 2 indicate that no specific etiologic agent can be determined by survey serum precipitin testing. Testing for precipitins in bronchial secretions rather than in serum may be more diagnostic.[15]

To definitively study the role of allergy in chronic respiratory disease, specific cases should be studied to define the type of immunologic mechanism and specific antigens involved. In Europe, *Micropolyspora faeni* has been implicated as one cause of farmer's lung in humans and as a cause for type-III allergic obstructive lung disease in horses.[13,16] By the use of skin testing, precipitating antibody, and inhalational challenge, 2 horses were determined to have an acquired type-III obstructive lung disease related to exposure to chickens.[17]

Viral, bacterial and parasitic infections are important in chronic respiratory disease. Influenza virus destroys respiratory tract epithelium, which takes at least 3 weeks to heal. If affected horses are exercised prior to healing, the respiratory tract becomes susceptible to secondary bacterial infection and hypersensitive to pollutants, dust and other allergens.[20] In a Swiss survey of 270 horses with chronic pulmonary disease, 47% continued to cough after remission of acute influenza.[6] The role of chronic viral infections in development of chronic respiratory disease remains unclear.

Bacteria can be the primary cause of chronic pneumonia in foals and occasionally in older horses. More often, however, bacteria are secondary invaders of the damaged respiratory tract epithelium. For this reason, culture and sensitivity testing is indicated in nonresponsive chronic respiratory disease. Penicillin-sensitive organisms are the most common type isolated from horses with chronic bronchitis and bronchiolitis.[1]

The interpretation of bacterial or fungal culture results must be related to the clinical condition of the animal and the environment in which the culture was taken. For example, potentially pathogenic bacteria may be isolated from the lungs of normal horses if the sampling was performed in an equine hospital. Fungi may be cultured from samples obtained from normal horses stabled in old, dusty barns.[21] Antibiotic therapy is indicated if pure cultures of pathogens, such as *Streptococcus zooepidemicus,* are isolated.

Migrating ascarid larvae are an important cause of lung disease in foals. Lungworms are another cause of chronic respiratory disease (see below). In general, parasite control programs improve a horse's condition and decrease its susceptibility to disease.

Control of environmental irritants is important in preventing respiratory disease. Bedding and feed should be as dust-free as possible. Stall walls may be coated with marine varnish and a fungicide, and floors sprayed with trisodium phosphate to reduce fungal contamination. Stable air may be dehumidified with hanging sacks of $CaCl_2$ or through the use of forced-air filtration.

Bedding material, such as straw, peanut hulls and fine wood shavings, cause considerable dust accumulation. A recommended bedding material is large wood chips sprayed with mineral oil at 1 gal/100 ft^2 stall area.

Dust control when feeding horses with chronic obstructive lung disease is also important. Hay should be eliminated from the diet. Beet pulp or alfalfa cubes or pellets may be fed free-choice or intermittently during the day to provide dietary bulk. Feeding of dust-free grain is also recommended.

The evaluation of apparently clinically normal horses that perform poorly is difficult. Older race horses may have normal upper respiratory tracts but decreased exercise tolerance. Hemoptysis may also occur. Maintenance of a dust-free environment for such animals helps them perform better.

The role of air-borne irritants, as in smog, on horses at urban racing centers has yet to be evaluated. However, acute (1 hour) and chronic (6 months) inhalation of sulfuric acid mist impaired bronchial mucociliary clearance.[22,23] Sulfate is a major component of the ambient aerosol in many urban areas. An inefficient mucociliary system may result in prolonged retention of inhaled particles, rendering the lung more susceptible to disease.

Acute pulmonary emphysema in cattle has been related to ingestion of tryptophan and subsequent appearance of the metabolite 3-methylindole. Oral administration of 3-methylindole at 0.2 g/kg body weight in horses caused bronchiolar cell proliferation, infiltration by neutrophils and eosinophils, and lamina propria thickening in small airways.[3] Acute pulmonary edema in horses feeding on pasture lush in *Perilla frutescens* may be a pneumotoxicity induced by *Perilla* ketone, a substance different from 3-methylindole but possibly acting on the lung in a similar way.[25] More research is required to document this interesting relationship of 3-methylindole to chronic bronchiolitis in horses.

Hereditary predisposition and seasonal variation have been long recognized in type-I atopic asthmatic disease in humans. However, the reports of chronic respiratory disease in horses suggest no hereditary predisposition. An inherited form of emphysema in children is related to a deficiency of serum alpha-1 antitrypsin. With the lack of antitrypsin activity, the proteolytic enzymes from inflammation may destroy pulmonary parenchyma. Although no horses with chronic respiratory disease have been shown to lack serum alpha-1 antitrypsin, in a study of 52 horses and ponies with chronic respiratory disease, there was an increased frequency of the electrophoretically slower Pr antitrypsin alleles, which are the homologue of human alpha-1 antitrypsin.[18] Because of both the mixed breeding and lack of correlation with low serum trypsin inhibitory capacity, the significance of this observation was difficult to assess.[19]

Clinical Signs: Affected animals have weight loss, dyspnea, a dry, deep cough and sibilant rhonchi in the lung periphery. They respond to IV administration of bronchodilators by loss of sibilant rhonchi on auscultation. A CBC and cytologic examination of tracheal aspirates may reveal mild neutrophilia and occasionally eosinophilia.

The most common and diffuse histopathologic change is mononuclear peribronchiolitis.[2-4] Mucosal-cell metaplasia, if present, may occasionally lead to bronchiolitis obliterans in small airways. Some interstitial fibrosis may also be present. Any emphysema is generally located paraseptally along the apical and anterior diaphragmatic lung lobe borders and is of little clinical significance (Fig 35).

In the past, horses with chronic bronchiolitis have been given a poor prognosis for recovery. However, with the use of corticosteroids, strict avoidance of offending antigens, such as moldy hay, and reduction of environmental irritants, such as dust, many horses can be greatly benefited. Use of oral prednisolone at 0.25 mg/lb body weight SID for 7 days and then on alternate days is recommended. Antihistamines are generally ineffective.

Lungworm Infection

A condition that can mimic chronic bronchiolitis and that may be more prevalent than previously thought is infection with the lungworm, *Dictyocaulus arnfieldi,* which causes a chronic cough, sibilant rhonchi and, occasionally, increased respiratory rate. Fever is generally not seen in lungworm infection. A CBC and examination of a transtracheal aspirate may reveal eosinophilia.[26]

Lungworm infection in horses has been related to contact with burros or donkeys, which have a 25-100% infection rate. However, a review of Russian literature revealed reports of an infection rate of 70% in horses without contact with burros or donkeys.[26]

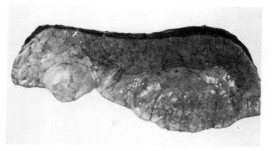

Fig 35. Section of an apical lung lobe affected by paraseptal emphysema. This can be observed in normal horses and those with chronic bronchiolitis, and represents only a minute portion of the entire lung.

When 3 forms of therapy for lungworm infection were compared, 2 doses of oral thiabendazole at 440 mg/kg body weight given 24 hours apart were superior to treatment with diethylcarbamazine or levamisole.[27] Since levamisole has been reported as a treatment for chronic respiratory disease, lungworms may play a more important role in some cases of chronic respiratory disease than previously recognized.

Neoplasia

A survey of 207 cases of chronic respiratory disease revealed a 0.6% incidence of pulmonary neoplasia.[6] An unusual tumor, the granular-cell tumor (myoblastoma), was found in 11 horses. A 14-year-old Thoroughbred broodmare had weight loss and reduced air sounds on one side of the thorax. Lateral radiographs revealed a large mass within the pulmonary field. Pulmonary function studies indicated pulmonary hypertension without evidence of generalized obstructive pulmonary disease. At necropsy, many large, firm, yellow-white nodules were observed in the right lung and confirmed as a granular-cell tumor histologically.[29] Thoracentesis may aid diagnosis (Table 1).

Chronic Granulomatous Pneumonia

This type of pneumonia may be secondary to aspiration of significant amounts of foreign material or related to infection by a specific organism, such as *Mycobacterium.* Horses with chronic pneumonia have weight loss, sibilant rhonchi and tachypnea, rather than typical double expiratory phase breathing. Radiographs and thoracentesis may aid diagnosis of chronic pneumonia (Table 1). Treatment is nearly always unsuccessful.

Nine horses of various breeds, ranging in age from 2½ to 20 years, had weight loss, increased respiratory rates and exercise intolerance associated with silicate granulomatous pneu-

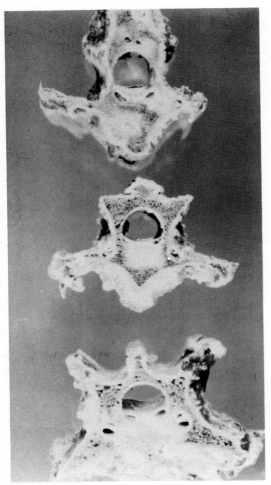

Fig 36. Vertebral osteoporosis and osteolysis in a horse with tuberculosis.

monia.[30] Granulomas consisted primarily of large, foamy macrophages, with occasional associated lymphocytes and plasma cells. The degree of fibrosis varied but was most severe in horses with large, confluent lesions. Refractile particles 1 μ in diameter and smaller were discernible within macrophages, which were occasionally birefringent. These particles were identified as cristobalite, a fibrogenic and cytotoxic type of silica, using energy dispersive x-ray analysis and x-ray diffraction. The high concentration of cristobalite was found in the soil in the environment of affected horses.

Tuberculosis

Tuberculosis is rare in horses and generally manifested as weight loss and stiffness of the neck. Bronchodilators are ineffective because of the large degree of granuloma formation.

Because *Mycobacterium* often causes cervical osteolysis and osteoporosis, cervical vertebral radiographs may be useful for diagnosis (Fig 36).[31] The results of tuberculin testing are very unpredictable in horses. Despite the rarity of the disease in horses, many are tuberculin-positive and have no history of prior exposure to *Mycobacterium* spp.[32]

Chronic Mycoses

Chronic fungal pulmonary infections are rare in American horses (see Chapter 10). Coccidioidomycosis, histoplasmosis, cryptococcosis and aspergillosis may cause chronic pulmonary disease and cachexia. Treatment is usually unrewarding. The most common fungal infection is coccidioidomycosis.[33-36] Affected horses were from 3½ to 15 years of age and had chronic weight loss. Pulmonary lesions ranged from pinpoint to 3-cm abscesses, with pleural effusion in some cases (Table 1). Peritoneal effusion and splenic and hepatic lesions have also been observed.

Emphysema

Emphysema is an unnatural distension or rupture of alveoli from excessive expiratory effort. Although small areas of permanent alveolar wall destruction occur paraseptally in the apical and anterior diaphragmatic lobes in horses with chronic bronchiolitis, severe emphysema as observed in humans is rare in horses. Clinically normal horses may have some paraseptal pulmonary emphysema.

References

1. Mansmann, RA *et al.* Proc 17th Ann Mtg Am Assoc Eq Pract, 1971. p 143.
2. Mansmann, RA. Doctoral thesis, Univ Calif, 1972.
3. Breeze, R. Proc Ann Mtg Am Coll Vet Int Med, 1978. p 105.
4. Thullbeck, WM and Lowell, FC. Am Rev Resp Dis **94** (1967) 82.
5. Edge, J *et al.* Br J Dis Chest **60** (1966) 10.
6. Gerber, H. Eq Vet J **5** (1973) 26.
7. Andberg, WG *et al.* JAVMA **98** (1941) 285.
8. Eyre, P. Vet Rec **90** (1972) 36.
9. Lowell, FL. J Allergy **35** (1964) 322.
10. Sertic, V. Vet Arch **38** (1968) 1.
11. Eyre, P. Vet Rec **91** (1972) 134.
12. Halliwell, REW *et al.* JAVMA **174** (1979) 277.
13. Lawson, GHK *et al.* Eq Vet J **11** (1979) 159, 172.
14. Reed, CE, Univ Wisc: Unpublished data, 1970.
15. Warren, CPW and Tse, KS. Am Rev Resp Dis **109** (1974) 672.
16. Pauli, B *et al.* Path Microbiol **38** (1972) 200.
17. Mansmann, RA *et al.* JAVMA **166** (1975) 673.
18. Breeze, RG *et al.* Vet Rec **100** (1977) 146.
19. Matthews, AG. Eq Vet J **11** (1979) 177.
20. Robinson, NE and Sorenson, PR. JAVMA **172** (1978) 299.

21. Mansmann, RA and Strouss, AS. JAVMA **169** (1976) 631.

22. Schlesinger, RB *et al*. Am Indust Hyg Assoc J **39** (1978) 275.

23. Schlesinger, RB *et al*. J Environ Path Tox **2** (1979) 1351.

24. Lindley, WH. Mod Vet Pract **59** (1978) 64.

25. Breeze, R *et al*. Mod Vet Pract **59** (1978) 301.

26. Mackay, RJ and Urquhart, KA. Eq Vet J **11** (1979) 110.

27. Round, MD. Vet Řec **99** (1976) 393.

28. Calverley, AH. Proc 23rd Ann Mtg Am Assoc Eq Pract, 1977. p 363.

29. Nickels, FA *et al*. Mod Vet Pract **61** (1980) 593.

30. Schwartz, LW *et al*. Chest. *In press,* 1981.

31. Nielsen, SW and Sprating, FR. Br Vet J **124** (1968) 503.

32. Francis, J: Tuberculosis in Animals and Man. Cassell, London, 1958.

33. Zontine, WJ. JAVMA **132** (1958) 490.

34. Maddy, KT. Vet Med **54** (1959) 233.

35. Crane, WS. Vet Med **57** (1962) 1073.

36. DeMartini, JC and Riddle, WE. JAVMA **135** (1968) 149.

EPISTAXIS IN RACE HORSES
by G.L. Ferraro

The veterinarian presented with epistaxis in a patient will be dealing with disease somewhere within the respiratory system or its related structures. Epistaxis is not always true nasal bleeding but rather only a sign of hemorrhage in some area that drains to the nasal passages. The source of that hemorrhage must be determined before a diagnosis can be made or treatment rendered.

The source of bleeding can be discovered by acquiring an adequate history and by thorough examination of the head and respiratory tract. In investigating the history, one should determine the duration of bleeding, the quantity and character of the blood seen at the nares, and whether the epistaxis is exercise-related. One should ascertain the age and activity of the patient, and determine if any other disease exists concurrently. The clinician should determine if the animal suffers from epistaxis only or if hemorrhage has occurred in other areas of the body, which would indicate generalized disease or toxicity.

Having completed the history, the veterinarian should then conduct the examination with the idea of locating the area of hemorrhage. The 3 major areas likely to be a source of hemorrhage are the nasal and sinus cavities, the guttural pouches and the lung.

Nasal and Sinus Cavity Hemorrhage

Hemorrhage originating from the nasal or sinus cavities can occur in any age horse but is probably more common in older horses due to a higher incidence of nasal tumors or polyps in those animals. The most consistent observation in these patients is that epistaxis is unrelated to exercise. In fact, the usual history is that epistaxis occurs intermittently in the stall or paddock. Hemorrhage may follow physical activity but physical exertion is not necessary to elicit epistaxis; epistaxis need not be related to fatigue during exercise. Hemorrhage from the nasal or sinus cavities is generally characterized by only small quantities of blood. In cases related to sinus infections, the blood may be mixed with catarrhal or purulent exudate (Fig C7).

When examining a horse for evidence of nasal or sinus bleeding, one should always percuss and auscultate the sinus for evidence of dullness. The nasal turbinates and openings of the maxillary sinuses should be examined using a fiberoptic endoscope. Any light source placed in the nasal cavity of the animal in a darkened room should be easily visible through the facial bones and sinus cavities. A variation in light transmission from one side to the other may indicate disease of the sinus cavity. Radiographs of the head and sinuses are indicated if nasal or sinus disease is suspected. The cheek teeth of any animal with sinus disease should also be examined since many cases are related to tooth abscesses or dental cysts.

Guttural Pouch Hemorrhage

Hemorrhage originating from the guttural pouches most frequently occurs in areas with severe winters, where animals are housed indoors for long periods and chronic guttural pouch disease is prevalent. It is more common in older horses but should be considered as a source of hemorrhage in all animals. Bleeding from this area is usually caused by mycotic infections, which erode the major arteries in close proximity to the guttural pouch. Affected animals usually have a history of a few incidents of epistaxis, characterized by large volumes of fresh blood gushing from the nares. These animals are gravely ill and should be treated immediately. In fact, in many cases the first incident of bleeding causes death. Therefore, early diagnosis of epistaxis is important.

Diagnosis of bleeding of guttural pouch origin is made by examining the guttural pouches with a flexible fiberoptic endoscope. Often the blood is evident at the openings of the pouches into the pharynx; in any case, the pouches themselves should be examined. Tranquilization of these animals prior to examination is indicated since arousal of the animal and subsequently elevated peripheral blood pressure may elicit a hemorrhagic incident.

The only effective treatment for animals with severe mycotic erosions of the major arteries near the guttural pouch is ligation of the endangered vessels.[1]

Pulmonary Hemorrhage

Pulmonary hemorrhage is almost always exercise-induced and is, therefore, most common in race horses.[2] Epistaxis in race horses was once thought to be of nasal origin, as from irritation of diseased or edematous nasal turbinates by increased airflow. Horses often hemorrhage from only one nostril and do not bleed until they return to the stall and lower their heads. These signs, together with the fact that venous blood often flowed in a stream at the floor of the nostril, seemed to indicate that the source of hemorrhage was in the head.

It was assumed that, as in humans, any blood from the lungs had to be expelled by coughing and was always frothy because it was mixed with air and tracheal secretions. However, it was subsequently demonstrated that, because a horse's lungs are ventral to the head, blood pools in the major bronchi, and rolls down the trachea and out the nares when the animal lowers its head.[3] Unilateral bleeding occurs when pooled blood takes the path of least resistance through one nostril. A recent study determined that over 95% of racing Thoroughbreds that hemorrhage as a result of exercise do so from the lung.[2] Pulmonary bleeding does not appear as frothy blood and is not generally coughed up. Further, less than 10% of animals with pulmonary hemorrhage show any evidence of bleeding from the nares.[2]

In determining if pulmonary hemorrhage has occurred, it is absolutely essential that the upper respiratory tract, including the trachea, be examined with a fiberoptic endoscope 30-60 minutes after a workout or race (Figs C8, C9).

Pulmonary hemorrhage should be suspected in animals with sudden, unexpected fatigue during a race. Such animals suddenly quit running during competition or seem to flatten out and tire toward the end of a race. They often seem to choke when they are pulled to a stop by the rider, or may seem excessively winded immediately after stopping and evidence a rather anxious, startled expression. Upon returning to the stable, these animals generally swallow excessively and may take more time than normal to cool out and relax after a workout. Although some clinicians feel that excessive coughing is an indication of pulmonary hemorrhage, recent studies have proven this to be an unreliable sign.[2] Horses frequently cough excessively after a race due to inhalation of dirt and debris from the race track, especially muddy or sloppy tracks. Animals may also experience substantial pulmonary bleeding and not cough at all. In fact, while evidence of hemorrhage in the respiratory tree can be demonstrated in as many as 40-50% of racing animals, not all animals show clinical signs and, in some, performance is not impaired.[2]

The current management of pulmonary hemorrhage is generally preventive in nature and usually consists of daily administration of ascorbic acid, rutin and vitamin K in the ration, although the value of such therapy is open to question. A more effective preventive measure is administration of furosemide, estrogens or a combination of both within a few hours of competition. An average of 250 mg (150-400 mg) furosemide is generally administered 2½-4 hours before a race. Estrogens are usually used in conjunction with furosemide and are generally given about an hour before competition. While the mechanism of action of these drugs to prevent pulmonary hemorrhage is not fully understood, they are generally accepted as effective.

Treatment of severe pulmonary hemorrhage, once it occurs, is generally ineffective. Animals with mild to moderate hemorrhage after exercise may not need any therapy. Moderate to severe cases are best treated with supportive therapy and antishock medication. In cases of rupture of the visceral pleura, with bleeding into the thoracic cavity, death is the usual result regardless of therapy. The amount of blood at the nostril does not necessarily indicate the severity of the incident.[2] Many animals experience severe pulmonary hemorrhage and show no evidence of blood at the nostril. Therefore, vital signs must be monitored when attempting to determine severity.

Any underlying chronic pulmonary disease should be treated as needed. Thoracic radiographs should be obtained, if possible, to determine the condition of the lungs. Animals with uncontrollable pulmonary hemorrhage should be removed from training and be given an extended period of rest and therapy.

References

1. Cook, WR. Eq Vet J 6 (1974) 45.
2. Pascoe, J et al. Am J Vet Res 42 (1981).
3. Cook, WR. Vet Rec 78 (1966) 396.

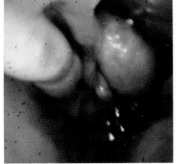

C1

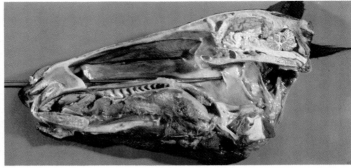

C2

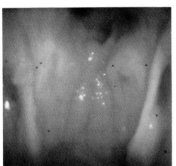

C3

Fig C1. Progressive ethmoidal hematoma.

Fig C2. Sagittal section of the head illustrating introduction of a bent-tipped catheter into the guttural pouch.

Fig C3. Endoscopic view of purulent exudate draining from the guttural pouch.

Fig C4. Endoscopic view of diphtheria of the guttural pouch. Note the nerves beside the necrotic plaque.

Fig C5. Endoscopic view of a catheter inserted into the guttural pouch. The dark material is dilute povidone iodine solution and the light material is pus.

Fig C6. Subepiglottal cyst.

Fig C7. Blood exiting the maxillary opening in the nasal passage.

Fig C8. Blood from the lower respiratory tract is evident on the epiglottis.

Fig C9. Blood from pulmonary hemorrhage is evident in the trachea.

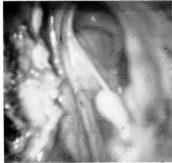

C4

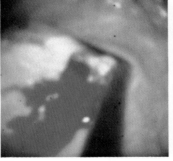

C5

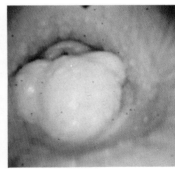

C6

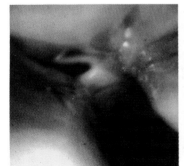

C7

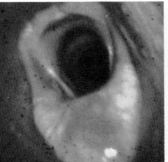

C8

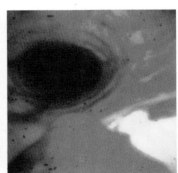

C9

Fig C10. Grade-I pharyngeal lymphoid hyperplasia. A few white follicles scattered over the dorsal wall of the pharynx is normal. Several larger pink follicles may also be present. (Courtesy of J Eq Med Surg)

Fig C11. Grade-II pharyngeal lymphoid hyperplasia. Numerous white and pink follicles cover the dorsal wall of the pharynx, extending to or slightly beyond the openings to the guttural pouches. (Courtesy of J Eq Med Surg)

Fig C12. Grade-III pharyngeal lymphoid hyperplasia. Many large red follicles cover the dorsal wall of the pharynx and extend onto the lateral walls to the epiglottis. Left laryngeal hemiplegia is also present. (Courtesy of J Eq Med Surg)

Fig C13. Grade-IV pharyngeal lymphoid hyperplasia. Many large red follicles, lying close together, arise from all areas of the mucosa. The follicles may extend onto the epiglottis, aryepiglottic folds and into the guttural pouches. Large aggregates of lymphoid follicles may resemble a polyp. (Courtesy of J Eq Med Surg)

Fig C14. Endoscopic view of dorsal displacement of the soft palate. The epiglottis is not visible nor is its outline apparent.

Fig C15. The soft palate bulges into the nasopharynx rostral to the epiglottis. This configuration is best appreciated as the endoscope is introduced or withdrawn.

Fig C16. The left arytenoid cartilage does not abduct to the same extent as the right. At rest the arytenoid cartilage lies in a median position. This condition may be corrected by laryngeal sacculectomy alone.

Fig C17. The left arytenoid cartilage has moved mediad into the laryngeal airway, causing obstruction. This endoscopic view demonstrates advanced laryngeal paralysis. Laryngoplasty, in addition to laryngeal sacculectomy, provides the best repair.

Fig C18. The epiglottis is entrapped in the aryepiglottic folds. The shape of the epiglottis can be appreciated but the normal vasculature and serrated margins are not apparent.

Fig C19. The epiglottis is hypoplastic and lacks the normal cartilage substance. It appears flaccid and has no obvious serrated margins or normal dorsal vascular pattern. Other forms of epiglottic hypoplasia are characterized only by an undersized epiglottis.

Fig C20. Chondritis of the right arytenoid cartilage. The cartilage is grossly misshapen and deformed. The airway is severely compromised and a small secondary granulomatous lesion is seen on the airway surface of the left arytenoid cartilage.

Fig C21. Tracheal stenosis as a result of previous tracheotomy. The lumen is narrowed by a scar.

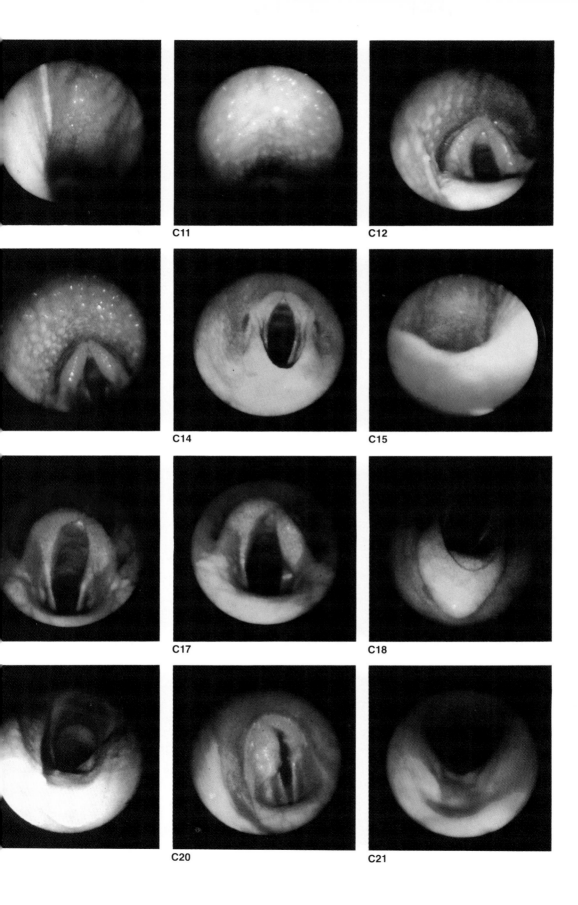

C11

C12

C14

C15

C17

C18

C20

C21

16

The Skin

by W.C. McMullan

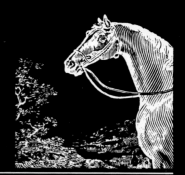

Structure and Function

Epidermis and Dermis

In terms of bulk, the skin is the largest organ of the body. This epithelial-connective tissue covering consists of 2 layers: the epidermis, a keratinized stratified squamous epithelium that serves as the protective horny layer of the skin, and the dermis, an intricately woven feltwork of collagen, elastic and reticular connective tissue fibers. Hair follicles, sweat and sebaceous glands, blood and lymph vessels, and nerves are embedded at various levels throughout the dermis, which nourishes the epidermis.[1]

Vitamin A is necessary for the normal development and maintenance of the horny layer, but excessive vitamin A causes abnormally rapid cell degeneration, altering the skin toward a mucous type of epithelium. Corticosteroids counteract the influence of excessive vitamin A but inhibit the metabolism of mucopolysaccharides and the formation of normal keratin. Cystine and methionine are important keratin precursors, and their use and uptake are inhibited by excessive vitamin A.[2] Vitamin A deficiency causes hyperkeratinization.

The skin has many functions. It acts as a barrier to microorganisms and is nearly waterproof, allowing relatively fluid body tissues to exist in a dry or excessively saline environment. Skin pigmentation protects against solar radiation and vitamin synthesis occurs within the skin in response to solar radiation. Receptors in the skin detect tactile, heat, cold and pain sensations. The evaporation of sweat from the skin surface provides temperature regulation.[2]

Skin Glands

The skin glands consist of sweat glands and sebaceous glands. Sweat glands are derived from the epidermis and infundibulum of hair follicles formed into a coiled secretory portion within the dermis. The straight ducts of these glands penetrate the epidermis of the hair follicle just before it opens onto the skin surface.[2] Sweat glands are present in almost all parts of the skin but are largest and most numerous at the lateral wing of the nostril, flank, mammary glands and free part of the penis.[3] They perform a thermoregulatory function and secrete under the influence of epinephrine. The adrenal medulla in response to impulses from the thermoregulatory center in the hypothalamus releases epinephrine into the circulation.[1] Sweat is strongly alkaline and contains serum proteins, urea (causing foam), ammonia, uric acid, phosphates and other materials normally found in urine (Na and Cl). When sweat dries, a salt deposit remains.[4]

Sebaceous glands are almost always associated with hair follicles and open into the upper part of the follicle (the infundibulum). Their secretory product, sebum, is composed of cellular debris and has a high lipid content, contributing to the water repellency and bactericidal and fungicidal properties of the skin. Other important functions of sebum are to provide luster to the coat and to serve as an identifying pheromone or olfactant signal. The secretion of sebum is continuous and regulated by various factors. Physiologic levels of estrogen have little influence, but high doses inhibit sebum secretion. Testosterone causes enlargement of sebaceous glands. Large doses of progesterone in laboratory animals caused glandular enlargement, but physiologic doses in women did not. Hypophysectomy alone produces a reduction in size and activity only partially reversed by either progesterone or testosterone alone. Thus, secretions of the hypophysis other than gonadotropins also exert an influence upon sebaceous glands.[1,2]

Pigmentation

Of several pigments related to skin color, the most important is a dark, reddish-brown pigment, melanin, produced by melanocytes within the basal layer of the epidermis and in the dermis. Melanin is synthesized from tyrosine by a copper-containing enzyme, tyrosinase, which catalyzes the oxidation of tyrosine to dihydroxyphenylalanine (dopa) and to dopa quinone. Tyrosinase also catalyzes dopa to form hallachrome and then 5, 6-dihydroxyindole, which is spontaneously oxidized to melanin. Carbon monoxide, cyanide ions, hydrogen sulfide and many compounds containing organic sulfur affect melanin formation by physiologically inhibiting enzyme activity through inactivating the copper component of tyrosinase by forming weakly dissociable complexes with copper. Within the resting melanocyte, the concentration of sulfhydryl compounds maintains an equilibrium with the concentration of tyrosinase so that modifications of either factor may alter melanin formation.

In albinism, there is a lack of melanin formation by melanocytes due to a congenital lack of tyrosinase even though sufficient numbers of melanocytes are present.

Melanin formation is influenced by many factors, including hormones produced by the hypophysis, thyroid, adrenals and gonads, and ultraviolet radiation.[2]

Hair

Hair is a flexible, keratinized structure produced by a hair follicle. The visible portion is the shaft and the part within the follicle is the root. A hair follicle is an epidermal invagination and, in the horse, all follicles are primary, ie, of large diameter rooted deeply in the dermis, and usually associated with sebaceous and sweat glands and an erector pili muscle. Each follicle has only one hair. The root has a terminal, hollow knob, the hair bulb, attached to a dermal papilla. The shaft is composed of an outermost cuticle, a cortex of densely packed keratinized cells and a medulla of loose cuboidal or flattened cells. The pattern of the cuticular cell surface, together with the cellular arrangement of the medulla, is characteristic for each species of animal and can be used for medicolegal purposes.

In the epidermis, the process of keratinization is continuous, but in the hair follicle it is intermittent, allowing for the seasonal changes in haircoat. Following a period of hair growth, during which the hair reaches its maximum length, the matrix cells cease mitotic activity and the follicle enters a resting phase. Following the resting phase, mitotic activity and keratinization start again and a new hair is formed. As the new hair grows, the root of the old hair gradually moves toward the surface, where it is eventually shed.[5]

External temperature has some effect on spring shedding, but probably more important is an increasing photoperiod. Mares placed under indoor lights on December 11 were shedding in Michigan before February 1, about 60 days earlier than control mares.[6]

Various hormones are also important in determining the hair growth cycle. Steroids of the adrenal cortex and sex glands prolong the resting stage. Thyroid hormone shortens the resting stage and inhibition of thyroxine production by propylthiouracil lengthens it.[2]

Permeability

Cutaneous permeability is thought to be limited by a superficial barrier between the stratum corneum and the outermost layers of epidermis. This barrier is particularly effective in preventing passage of water and some water-soluble substances, such as electrolytes. Substances unable to penetrate the superficial barrier may be absorbed in varying quantities through the more permeable cells of the sebaceous gland, sebaceous duct and follicular epithelium. Once past the barrier, there is no significant deterrent to further penetration of the remaining layers of the epidermis and dermis and into the general circulation via lymph vessels and capillaries.

Factors that increase absorption are seasonal temperature increases, hyperemia, trauma, irritant chemicals, keratolytic agents, solvents and persistent hydration of the stratum corneum (outermost epidermal layer).

Water and electrolyte absorption or penetration is thought to occur to some extent, but lipid-soluble substances are absorbed through the skin fairly rapidly and completely. Compounds soluble in both lipids and water are absorbed almost as rapidly as by the oral or parenteral routes.

Phenol (lipid-soluble) caused death in humans following application of carbolic acid to large areas of the skin. Other lipid-soluble substances that penetrate the skin with ease are estrogenic hormones, testosterone, progesterone and vitamins A, D and K. The best penetration of the skin is obtained by the use of vehicles containing water, propylene glycol, wetting agents and solubilizers.[7]

Examination

History

A complete history is vital in making a diagnosis of skin disease. Some of the more important questions are:

1. When and on which part(s) of the body did lesions first appear? Most insect dermatoses appear in late spring and affect specific parts of the body.
2. Are other animals or humans involved? Allergic dermatitis seldom involves more than 1-2 animals in a herd. Dermatophilosis, dermatomycoses and mange may spread from horse to humans.
3. Is the patient in a stall or at pasture? Horses in stalls are much less likely to have dermatophilosis; pastured horses are candidates for photosensitization or muzzle dermatitis due to irritant weeds.
4. Is the animal off feed or losing weight, indicating a problem in some other body system? In some cases (lymphoma, amyloidosis, hirsutism due to pituitary tumor, seborrhea), the skin is an indicator of the internal disorder.
5. Is pruritus evident? Of granulomatous diseases, phycomycosis is very pruritic, habronemiasis is moderately so, while sarcoid and squamous-cell carcinoma are not.
6. How old is the animal? *Culicoides* allergy is seldom if ever seen in yearlings, whereas dermatomycosis is commonly seen in young animals.
7. Has the animal had any previous treatment and, if so, what was the response? Horses with habronemiasis have a favorable response to systemic trichlorfon administration, but those with phycomycosis do not.
8. Have there been any additions to the herd? Dermatomycosis, viral papular dermatitis and coital vesicular exanthema frequently appear within 2 weeks of an infected new arrival.
9. Questions on diet, bedding, daily routine, nearby agricultural or industrial activi-

ties, resident insect population, sexual status, breed, color, duration of the problem, possible mineral deficiencies or excesses in the soil or water should be asked routinely.

Description of Lesions

An accurate visual description of the lesion(s) is helpful as a matter of good records, in discussion of a case and in searching for a diagnosis. The presence of certain lesions may lead to an etiologic agent. The following terms are descriptive and useful:

Acne: A chronic inflammatory condition of the pilosebaceous structures. The primary lesion is a comedo (blackhead), a plugged hair follicle(s) that progresses to a papule, pustule or nodule.

Alopecia: Loss of hair.

Excoriation: A superficial loss of epidermis usually caused by rubbing or other physical damage; an abrasion.

Hyperkeratosis: An increased thickness of the horny layer of the epidermis.

Nodule: A small, circumscribed solid elevation that usually extends into the deeper dermis, 0.5-2.5 cm in diameter; a large papule.

Papilloma: A neoplastic growth of surface epithelium supported on cores of papillae or vascularized connective tissue; a wart.

Papule: A small, solid elevation up to 0.5 cm in diameter; the typical skin eruption in allergic conditions.

Parakeratosis: A condition of abnormal cornification with excess scaling.

Pruritus: Itching.

Pustule: A small, circumscribed elevation of the skin filled with pus.

Scale: An accumulation of fragments of the horny layer; also called scurf or dandruff.

Seborrhea: Excessive scaling due to rapid epidermal proliferation.

Urticaria: A pruritic condition characterized by wheals; also called hives.

Vesicle: A small eruption of the skin filled with serous fluid; a blister; a large vesicle is called a bulla.

Vitiligo: An acquired condition characterized by depigmentation of the skin; also called leukoderma.

Wheal: A sharply circumscribed raised lesion caused by edema of the dermis.

Lesion Distribution

The lesions of many skin diseases are found primarily in certain areas of the body. A high percentage of squamous-cell carcinomas are located at a mucocutaneous junction. The nodules of *Hypoderma* are commonly found in the saddle area and seldom on the legs. The lesions of sporotrichosis characteristically follow the lymphatic distribution in an ascending chain. In linear keratosis, the lesions form a line. A symmetric pattern suggests an endocrine or some other internal etiology. Knowledge of specific locations common to certain diseases helps in the differential diagnosis.

Physical Examination

Observe the horse at a distance and close-up to examine every square inch of skin. Record your general impression of the haircoat as to gloss and areas of alopecia, and hair condition as to dry, oily, brittle, etc.

Describe the primary lesion(s) present as crusts, nodules, papules, pustules, scale, wheals, vesicles or other. Record their location, distribution and shape. The description and location of secondary lesions, such as depigmentation, excoriation, fistulae, hyperkeratosis, necrosis, seborrhea and ulcers, should be recorded.

Observe closely for external parasites. Many owners cannot conceive how a little gnat can aggravate a horse. A hand magnifying lens is helpful when looking for lice as well as in close examination of lesions.

The character of the skin should be recorded as to thickness, sensitivity, pruritus, pliability and odor, if present.

Laboratory Aids

Laboratory test selection is determined by physical examination results. The most valuable laboratory aids and what many consider standard procedure for skin cases are biopsy, skin scrapings and culture.

Biopsy: Biopsies are indicated in isolated lesions, such as papules and nodules, all neoplastic or suspected neoplastic masses, all persistent ulcerations, any case that is apparently unusual or quite serious, and in a disease that is not responding to rational therapy.[8,9] The indications for biopsy are many and contraindications few. Postbiopsy hemorrhage must be considered in patients with bleeding tendencies, a comparatively rare situation. Secondary sepsis may be a factor in debilitated horses or those receiving immunosuppressive drugs. Scar formation is not a problem with the "punch" technic.

Choosing the best site for biopsy greatly increases the information returned. Selection of biopsy site is guided by the following general rules:

(1) In generalized dermatosis, select a typical lesion not subjected to trauma nor encrusted, and not modified by treatment.

(2) Avoid scarred lesions.

(3) Remove small vesicles or bullae intact.

(4) Biopsy of ulcerative lesions should always include normal skin, the leading edge and the area of ulceration. Either a large sample by excision or multiple punches are required.

(5) When using a biopsy punch, do not include normal tissue if the entire lesion cannot be excised.

(6) If there is more than one stage of development in the disease process, ie, nodules and pustules, multiple biopsies should be taken.

Most biopsies can be performed under local anesthesia. Lidocaine HCl should be injected SC and not intralesionally. Circumferential local anesthesia may be necessary when a large sample is to be excised. Preparation of the site varies according to the type of lesion. A nodule, for example, is given a routine surgical preparation with omission of vigorous scrubbing that might alter microscopic appearance. Do not use iodine preparations to clean the skin because they often interfere with histologic staining. Loose crusts may be removed mechanically and included with the underlying sample. With excisional biopsies, normal surgical preparation is performed on the skin surrounding the lesion. In some cases, the lesion may be soaked with an antiseptic gauze pack before punch biopsy.

The Keyes cutaneous punch (V. Mueller, Chicago), an instrument similar to a cookie cutter, has a circular cutting edge and a handle. Inexpensive disposable punches are also available (Baker Laboratories, Miami). The sizes applicable for the horse are 4-6 mm in diameter. The punch is drilled with a rotary motion into the subcutis, including the entire depth of the lesion. The specimen is then atraumatically lifted out with a skin hook or needle. The excessive use of forceps has ruined many biopsies. The base of the sample and subcutaneous attachment usually must be snipped with scissors or cut with a scalpel blade. If there is excessive bleeding or if minimal scarring is desired, a single suture can be placed. Routine wound care and tetanus immunization should follow.

The biopsy should be blotted on absorbent paper to remove excess blood and placed in 10% buffered formalin immediately. The volume of formalin should be about 20 times that of the sample. If formalin is not available, the sample should be wrapped in gauze soaked in physiologic saline. If an excisional biopsy was performed, place the tissue on or between blotter paper before putting in formalin to prevent curling. If the temperature is below freezing, keep the specimen in formalin at room temperature for 4 hours before mailing so that ice crystals do not disrupt tissue architecture.

The sample bottle of formalin should have a wide mouth, a screw top and adequate identification. A detailed history and gross description aid pathologic interpretation.

A large and deep sample may be obtained with an elliptical excision by a scalpel blade. Small nodules or tumors are frequently handled this way, affording treatment and diagnosis simultaneously.

Skin Scraping: Select a typical lesion of recent origin, *ie*, one not altered by treatment or excoriation. The safest instrument for scraping is a bone curette, but a less expensive similar tool can be fashioned by a blacksmith to provide a strong, reasonably sharp, rounded edge. A scalpel blade and handle are satisfactory if used with care. Scrape at the margin and toward the center, both superficially and into the upper dermis. A drop of mineral oil at the chosen site helps trap material on the blade for easy transfer to a microscope slide. Material is scraped into a small plastic container and then sprinkled on a slide moistened with a drop or 2 of water or mineral oil. A coverslip or another slide is placed on top and the preparation is examined microscopically.

In searching for demodectic mites, it is helpful to squeeze a fold of skin to express mites from the hair follicle or sebaceous glands. Sarcoptic mites are frequently found under active crusts. Since equine mange mites are extremely difficult to find, it is often necessary to place the collected material in a small beaker and add 10% KOH. Stir and heat gently, but do not boil. This mixture is added to a saturated sugar solution in a centrifuge tube and spun until the mites and ova float to the surface. A drop or 2 of surface fluid is examined on a slide under a coverslip.[10] Alternatively, at least 5-10 scrapings should be examined directly before any confidence is attributed to a negative diagnosis.

Scrapings for dermatophytes are more useful when put on culture medium, but practitioners with training in dermatophyte identification report success with direct microscopic examination. The skin is wetted with water or saline and the scraping placed on a slide with a few drops of 10% KOH. The slide is allowed to stand for 30 minutes or heated gently (avoid boiling) for 15-20 seconds over a flame. A DMSO-KOH solution allows examination of the preparation for the presence of hyphae and/or spores on hair shafts within one minute without heating.[19] Broken hairs plucked from the periphery of a lesion are also examined by this technic.

Culture: Bacterial cultures are usually taken only when there are definite signs of infection, such as pustules or purulent tracts. Large pustules are aspirated with a sterile needle and syringe or lanced and touched with a sterile swab. The sample should be placed in a transport medium if more than 2 hours will transpire before inoculation onto agar plates for identification and sensitivity testing.

A draining tract should be washed lightly with bland soap and water. Pressure is applied to the area and a sterile swab applied to the fresh discharge.

Fungal Cultures: Fungal culture is the most reliable method for diagnosis of dermatomycosis. If the suspected site is grossly contaminated with dirt and manure, gentle washing with a bland soap, followed by rinsing and drying, is necessary. About 10 peripheral hairs (not mats) and scraped keratin (not large crusts) are placed on a culture medium with a color indicator, such as DTM (L.A. Mosher, Atlanta) or Fungassay (Pitman-Moore). Good contact should be made but the material should not be buried. The cap of the vial should be loose to allow air entry. Incubation at room temperature is satisfactory for most dermatophytes. If desired, a second tube may be incubated at 37 C. The sample should be identified, dated and examined daily.

A positive dermatophyte culture is indicated by a color change from amber to a dark cherry red. Dermatophytes use protein in the medium and produce alkaline metabolites that turn the medium red. Saprophytes use carbohydrates and produce acid metabolites that cause no color change. Saprophytes later use protein and may cause a color change after 7 days or more.[10] The color change should be coincident with early colony growth. A dermatophyte col-

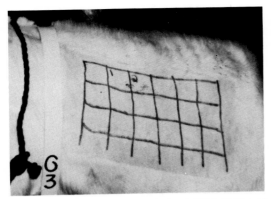

Fig 1. In allergy testing, 0.1 ml of a 1:1000 dilution of antigen is injected intradermally into a square marked on the neck. The size of the bleb is measured at 30 minutes, 4 hours and 24 hours.

ony is fluffy and cream or white. Most saprophyte colonies are grey, green or black. Heavy saprophytic growth can cause false-positive red color reaction on the medium.

Identification as to genus and species is done by harvesting the colony with a loop and placing a sample on a slide for a lactophenol cotton blue stain. Another technic is to make a flag of acetate tape on an applicator stick and touch the sticky side to the surface of the colony. The tape is then pressed, sticky side down, on a slide with a drop of lactophenol cotton blue stain. Microscopic examination is made to determine the shape and architecture of the macroconidia characteristic for most fungi.

Cytologic Examination: Cytologic examination of the skin is accomplished by needle aspiration, tissue imprints, tissue scrapings and smears of exudates.[11] Tumors, draining tracts, deep fungal infections or any lesion that contains an exudate can be examined.

Needle aspiration is used to differentiate inflammatory, hemorrhagic and neoplastic processes or to establish a specific type of tumor. It is used as an alternative to surgical biopsy.[8]

The site is surgically prepared and a sterile 20-ga needle attached to a sterile 10-ml syringe is inserted into the tissue. A vacuum is maintained while the needle is moved back and forth several times. Vacuum should be released before the needle is withdrawn from the skin. The aspirate is contained within the needle. Most aspirates coagulate, so the contents of the needle should be rapidly expressed onto a slide and a smear made, as with a blood smear.[11] Any large particles present should be crushed and smeared between 2 slides.

Tissue imprints are best made by touching the excised surface of a lesion to a slide after first blotting with a paper towel to remove excess serum or exudate. A lesion may be cleaned and touched with a slide to transfer cells for examination, but the surface may not be representative of deeper disease.

Smears are also made by scraping a lesion with a scalpel blade or by spreading exudate on a slide as for blood smears. In dermatophilosis, if the lesions are chronic and insufficient exudate is present under a mat of hairs, some of the crust can be minced or crushed in a few drops of water before making the smear. An air-dried smear is then routinely stained with Wright's or new methylene blue prior to cytologic evaluation by a pathologist.

In suspected allergic dermatitis, a biopsy seldom provides information about the etiology. Other diagnostic methods applicable are:

(1) Provocative exposure. The horse is moved to an "inert" isolation area and maintained until free of signs. Materials from the previous environment are then added singly and the horse observed for reappearance of signs.

(2) Environmental control. One element, such as bedding or hay, is removed singly and the horse observed for improvement, indicating the allergenic substance.

(3) Intradermal testing. Presently, the value of intradermal testing in horses is controversial; however, with improved antigens and standardized technics, it appears to have potential in working with equine allergy. The horse must not have received any immunosuppressive medication for the past 5-7 days or up to 30 days in the case of long-acting corticosteroids. The lateral aspect of the neck is clipped with a #40 blade. The area is washed with surgical soap, rinsed, swabbed with alcohol and marked into 2.5-cm or larger squares, the number depending on the number of test antigens (Fig 1). Tuberculin syringes with ⅜-inch, 26-ga needles are numbered and loaded with 0.1 ml of 1:1000 aqueous test antigens. One syringe is also loaded with 0.1 ml of a positive control, histamine, and one with a negative control, sterile diluent, both supplied by the antigen manufacturer. All injections are made intradermally with the bevel of the needle up. No air should be injected. The wheals produced are then measured at 30 minutes, 60 minutes, and again at 4, 24 and 48 hours. The response is graded as negative if the bleb is less than 5 mm greater than the negative control. Positive reactions are graded as 1+ through 4+ if the

bleb measures 5, 10, 15 or 20 mm greater than the negative control. If the horse does not show a 2+ or 3+ at the histamine square, immunosuppression should be suspected.

Anaphylactic reaction to administration of test antigens has been reported in heavey horses and extreme exacerbation of pruritus in horses with dermatitis.[12] Therefore, a 1:10,000 dilution is used by some veterinarians. If in 15 minutes no side effects are noted, testing is continued. All reactions at 1:10,000 are considered positive and the negatives at 1:10,000 are repeated at 1:1000. At the present time, no antigens are commercially produced specifically for horses, but human antigens seem satisfactory.

Laboratory tests helpful in special cases, such as possible hormonal conditions or immunologic diseases, include:

(1) Thyroid: serum samples for radioimmunoassay (RIA) T_3 and T_4, cholesterol, thyroid stimulation with TSH and biopsy. Thyroid scan is available at some universities.

(2) Adrenal: CBC, serum cortisol levels before and after ACTH stimulation, cholesterol, alkaline phosphatase, glucose, RIA T_3 and T_4, and creatinine clearance ratio for Na and K.

(3) Sex hormones: CBC, serum RIA T_3 and T_4, RIA levels for sex hormones are available at some laboratories.

(4) Immune system: CBC, antinuclear antibody, LE preparation, intradermal PHA, lymph node or skin biopsy, electrophoresis and/or immunoelectrophoresis, immunofluorescence.

A diagnostic tool that should not be forgotten is response to therapy. For example, if corticosteroid therapy does not relieve pruritus, chances are good the problem is not allergy. Recheck for sarcoptic mange in such cases.

Diseases Characterized by Granulomatous Reaction

Regardless of the cause of granulomatous lesions, the loops of newly formed capillaries and fibroblasts (granulation tissue) are a response to chronic inflammatory foci. The etiologic agent may be parasitic, bacterial, fungal, viral, traumatic or carcinogenic. The diseases are listed more or less in order of prevalence, with some variation as to locality.

Exuberant Granulation Tissue

Exuberant granulation tissue ("proud flesh") is a common sequela to untreated or mistreated wounds below the hock and carpus. It is covered in detail under wound management

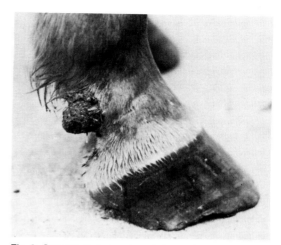

Fig 2. Sarcoid that developed 4 months after a wire cut.

but is mentioned here because of importance in the differential diagnosis of this group. It is not pruritic and responds well to surgery and reasonable aftercare.

Sarcoid

Equine sarcoid is a locally aggressive, nonmalignant fibroblastic tumor of equine skin and the most common tumor of the horse.[13] It occurs most frequently on the head, legs and ventral abdomen of horses, donkeys and mules (Fig 2). About a third of affected animals have multiple lesions. There is apparently no predilection for sex, age, breed, color or season of the year. Metastasis to internal organs has not been reported nor has invasion of blood vessels or lymphatics. Approximately one-half of sarcoids recur within 3 years after surgical re-

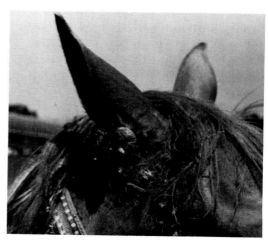

Fig 3. A fibroblastic, verrucous sarcoid.

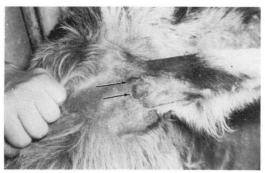

Fig 4. Occult sarcoids resembling a nodular lesion (arrows).

moval, most of these within 6 months and some before the incision heals.[14]

Cause: The cause is thought to be a virus. Bovine papilloma virus has been considered a possible cause, but current opinion leans toward a different viral agent and/or an atypical response to trauma and wound treatment.[15,16]

Gross Lesions: Sarcoids are seldom, if ever, pruritic, but may vary considerably in appearance. They are either verrucous (warty), fibroblastic ("proud flesh"-like) or less often a mixture of the 2 types (Figs C1,3). They are either pedunculated or sessile. The warty type is rarely larger than 6 cm in diameter and may remain static for years. Larger sarcoids often have a papillomatous or cauliflowered appearance. If they are traumatized and/or infected, they may change to the fibroblastic type. Occasionally, an "occult" sarcoid is encountered that is only slightly raised, with little disruption of the skin and easily confused with nodules due to a local inflammatory reaction. These are most common about the head, especially the ears and eyelids (Fig 4).

There is usually a history of a wound 3-6 months previously, but sarcoids may occur spontaneously. It is also thought they can be transferred to the lips and eyelids by biting or rubbing and by contamination of bridles, halters, etc. In one report of familial tendency, all the offspring of one mare developed sarcoids by 24 months of age, while unrelated horses in the herd were unaffected.[17]

Diagnosis: Since the gross appearance may resemble other conditions, such as papillomas, granulation tissue, phycomycosis, habronemiasis, squamous-cell carcinoma, neurofibroma, melanoma and fibrosarcoma, histologic examination of biopsy specimens is necessary for diagnosis. (Exception: static, flat hairless sarcoids are best left untreated.)

In submitting skin samples for analysis, include both normal and abnormal tissue and incise sufficiently deep to include the entire dermis and parts of the subcutis. Fix half the specimen in 10% formalin and send the other half in a refrigerated plastic bag for culture if necessary.

Treatment: Evaluation of any method of treatment is difficult because individual tumors may fluctuate in size with time and even completely regress, only to reappear later. Warty lesions may be present for years before progressing to aggressive fibroblastic growths. Early single lesions have a much more favorable prognosis than do multiple lesions.

Bovine wart or autogenous vaccines have not been more than 50% successful at best and often less.[18,19]

Freezing and thawing with dry ice or liquid nitrogen has been rated as 66-80% effective.[14,20,21] Under regional nerve blocks, thermocouple needles (Frigitronics, Shelton, CT) are placed at the base of the tumor, which is frozen by a direct spray of liquid nitrogen to -30 C as measured by thermocouples. After thawing, the tumor is frozen again to -30 C (see Cryosurgery). A less expensive "thermos" type unit adequate for general use is available (Town Mfg, San Antonio). A description of a do-it-yourself kit has been published.[22]

For many years prior to the development of cryotherapy, surgical excision followed by extensive electrocautery of the base of the tumor was considered the best technic.[14,19,23] Postsurgical irradiation is also recommended. Cobalt 60 or cesium implant needles are placed at the base of the excised lesion.[24]

A 5-fluorouracil ointment (Efudex:Hoffman-LaRoche) has been used successfully as a topical treatment.[25] It is a human cancer drug, an antimetabolite that irritates normal skin. Petrolatum is applied to normal skin and 5-fluorouracil is applied daily to the tumor base (after excision) for long periods, usually 30-90 days or until the lesion heals. Healing is delayed considerably by this drug, but its value in preventing recurrence of the tumor warrants its use.

Podophyllum (Merck) is an irritant cathartic manufactured in powder form. It is mixed in equal parts with tincture of benzoin to help retain it on the sarcoid. The drug should not contact healthy tissue because it causes cellulitis. The treatment procedure is simple and can be done by the client, with periodic progress

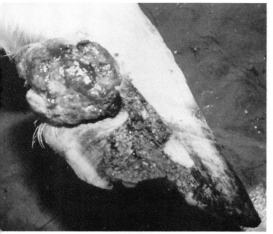

Fig C1. A granulomatous sarcoid.

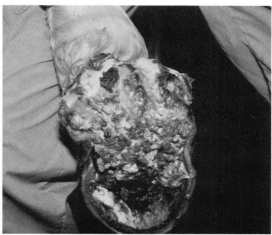

Fig C2. Phycomycosis subsequent to a wire cut.

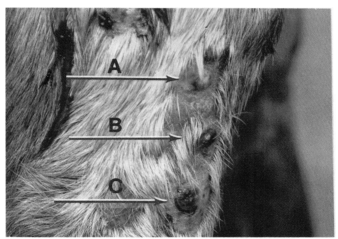

Fig C3. Nodules (A), pustules (B) and ulcers (C) in sporotrichosis.
(Courtesy of Dr C.H. Bridges)

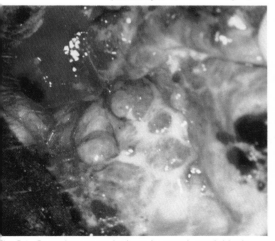

Fig C4. Granulomatous lesions in nasal amyloidosis. Air flow was completely obstructed in one nostril and reduced 50% in the other.

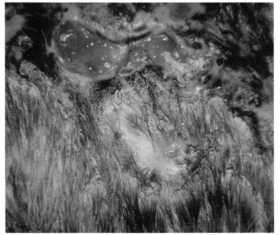

Fig C5. Severe ulcerative lesion caused by *C pseudotuberculosis* infection (saddle acne, contagious acne).

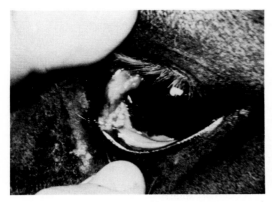

Fig 5. Ocular habronemiasis. Gritty calcifications embedded in the conjunctiva must be removed before healing can occur.

checks by the veterinarian.[26] The medication is applied daily to the lesion with a cotton-tipped applicator until a firm black scab forms. Treatment is then discontinued until the scab loosens, which usually takes 3-4 days. At this time, the scab is wiped away and daily treatment is repeated until another black scab forms. The growth reduces in size with each treatment.

The duration of treatment depends on the size of the tumor. The more active the tumor, the more rapidly it responds. Treatment is discontinued when the tumor disappears. The area must be watched carefully and treatment started again if abnormal tissue reappears.

It is important to warn the client of the likelihood of recurrence and the duration of treatment necessary.

Immunotherapy has been used in the treatment of sarcoids. Regression of sarcoids has followed within 1-6 months when slivers of sarcoid approximately 5 x 10 mm were surgically transplanted SC at the neck. New sarcoids developed at the transplant site, but these regressed along with the other lesions.[27] This technic is used to advantage when the sarcoid is anatomically dangerous to treat otherwise. Cryonecrosis of the transplants prior to implantation decreases the likelihood of new sarcoids at the site.

Spontaneous regression of nontreated multiple sarcoids after cryotherapy of other sarcoids has been reported, suggesting that cryotherapy may enhance the immune response of a host to neoplasia.[21] It has been postulated that this is a result of exposing the defense systems to the lipoprotein complexes released when tumor cells break up during cryonecrosis.[28]

Immunotherapy using BCG (bacillus Calmette-Guerin) is another method of treatment for sarcoids.[29,30] The BCG was originally isolated from a virulent strain of *Mycobacterium bovis*, requiring 13 years and 231 sequential passages in culture medium.[31] It has since been found to be a potent reticuloendothelial stimulant and nonspecific immunostimulant that enhances the immune response to a wide variety of antigens, including tumor-specific antigens.[32] It has been used for treatment of human acute lymphocytic leukemia and malignant melanoma.[33]

The best technic for use in horses has not been determined, but one involves multiple injections of lesions at 1- or 2-week intervals. All cases reported have been periocular sarcoids. To prevent anaphylaxis, the administration of antiprostaglandins and corticosteroids before each BCG injection is advised.

Habronemiasis

Habronemiasis ("summer sore") is caused by *Habronema* larvae deposited in skin wounds and moist places like the eye, sheath and penis (Figs 5-7). The house fly, *Musca domestica*, and stable fly, *Stomoxys calcitrans*, are the usual vectors. An infected wound may granulate slowly only to suddenly enlarge and become prominent with exuberant granulation tissue. This rapidly growing reddish-brown tissue protrudes above the normal skin, and is quite hemorrhagic and covered with a greasy, coagulated exudate. There is usually a serosanguineous drainage from the lesion. Severe pruritis

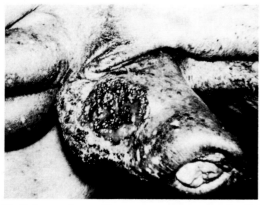

Fig 6. A necrotic, pruritic summmer sore on the sheath.

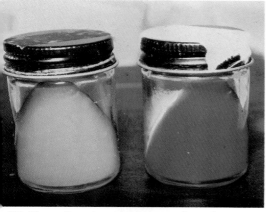

Fig C6. The yellow dermatophyte medium changes to red upon growth of a pathogenic fungus.

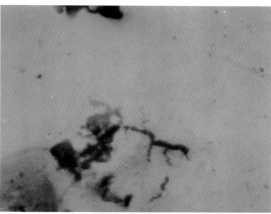

Fig C7. *Dermatophilus congolensis* in a stained smear.

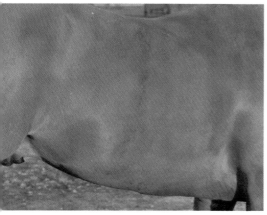

Fig C8. Linear crusting and alopecia in linear keratosis.

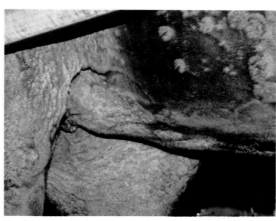

Fig C9. Circular lesions in pemphigus foliaceous resemble those of a dermatophyte infection.

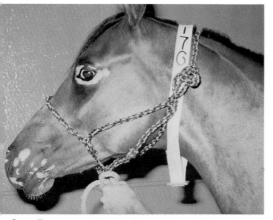

Fig C10. Pronounced leukoderma in an 18-month-old Arabian stallion with Arabian fading syndrome.

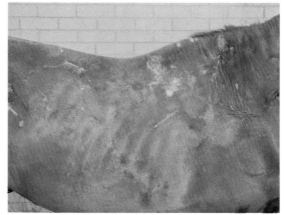

Fig C11. Thin, loosely attached skin that tears easily in a horse with hyperelastosis cutis. (Courtesy of Dr G. Grote)

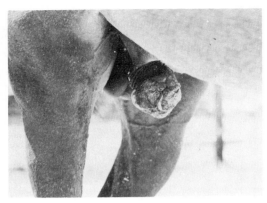

Fig 7. Summer sore on the glans penis.

is a common sign. Initially the sores are irregular in shape, but as they grow and extend, they gradually assume a circular contour (Fig 8). Areas of caseation, calcification, fibrosis and necrosis may be intermingled in the same lesion (Fig 5). These calcified granules are highly suggestive of habronemiasis, but must be differentiated from the calcified "leech" of phycomycosis. Occasionally the 2 conditions may exist simultaneously.

As the name "summer sore" implies, the condition appears when the ambient temperature remains above 70 F and fly vectors become numerous. Strangely enough, extensive wounds seldom become infected, perhaps because of the

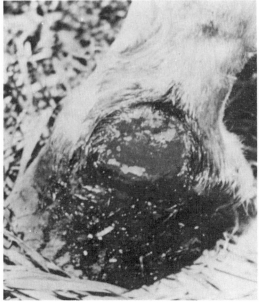

Fig 8. Summer sore that developed after a wire cut. Note the circular contour.

treatment received as compared with minor wounds. Lesions may heal with the coming of cold weather only to break out again the next summer. Certain horses seem to be more susceptible and have lesions year after year.

Although a history of a wound is usual, infective larvae may penetrate unbroken skin to cause typical lesions.[34] The bite of the fly itself is considered enough of a wound to initiate an infection.

Life Cycle: The larvae are passed in the feces and invade or are ingested by fly maggots. The larvae reach the infected stage in the pupa of the fly. Thus, if an infected fly is swallowed by the horse or deposits the larvae on the mouth or lips of the horse, development into adult *Habronema* takes place in the stomach. The adults live in nodular lesions of the stomach wall. If the fly deposits the larvae on a wound, cutaneous habronemiasis may result.

Larvae may reach the lungs, presumably by the blood and lymphatics or by migration from the mouth and down the trachea. A grey fibrous capsule forms around the larvae initially. As the nodules age they are surrounded by a thicker fibrous wall and the contents become caseous and then calcified. Usually no respiratory signs are noticed.[35]

Larvae deposited in the eye may produce a granular conjunctivitis, most noticeable at the medial canthus, involving the third eyelid. The lesion is at first red and later yellowish due to caseation and calcification. The conjunctival mucosa may bear many small yellowish flecks of necrotic superficial tissue that resemble grains of sand. Frequently a circular lesion ranging from a few millimeters up to 2 cm is apparent 1-2 cm from the medial canthus, toward the nose over the nasolacrimal duct. Larvae apparently migrate into the lacrimal puncta and the lacrimal sac before penetrating the tissues.

Chronic abscesses in the pectoral region of California horses are thought to be caused by *Corynebacterium pseudotuberculosis* possibly liberated by infected *Habronema* larvae.[36]

Diagnosis: The history and gross appearance of habronemiasis are very characteristic; however, the lesion is confused most easily with pyogranuloma, proud flesh, phycomycosis and sarcoid. A biopsy from a caseous area of the lesion and one from a more granulative area should be put in formalin for histopathologic examination. Occasionally a larva may be found if some exudate is squeezed onto a slide and examined microscopically.

The larvae are readily recognized by their large size (2.5-3 mm x 60 μ) and by the small spiny process on their tails. Generally only a few larvae are present in the average lesion, so their absence in a particular biopsy sample does not rule out habronemiasis.

A toxic action has been postulated for the necrosis and marked hypervascular granulation, but it is likely that a local hypersensitivity reaction from repeated reinfection is the basic cause.[34] The eosinophilia, which may reach 15-20%, and regression of the lesions during the winter when the intermediate hosts cease their activity support this idea. It has also been suggested that the presence of mature *Habronema* in the stomach may induce a state of general hypersensitivity.[34] Animals affected by summer sores are almost always heavily parasitized by the adult worms.

Treatment: One of the earliest treatments of habronemiasis was application of glycerin. By osmotic pressure, it floods the sore with serum, stimulates cellular function and promotes epithelial regeneration. It has been used in combination with 5 parts phenol, 10 parts oil of tar and 85 parts glycerin to prevent attraction of flies.[37]

Chromic acid (10%) applied 2-3 times to the lesion reportedly kills the larvae and also causes the formation of a thick crust to help prevent reinfection.[35]

Organophosphates have been used PO and IV. Ronnel powder has been given by stomach tube every 2 weeks at 45 g/1000 lb or at 8 mg/lb/day on the feed for 2-4 weeks.[36,38] Trichlorfon (Combot:Haver-Lockhart) has been given IV at 25 mg/kg body weight in a liter of 5% dextrose or saline.[39] The solution is preferably autoclaved before use and administered with a 2½-inch, 16-ga needle to avoid perivascular injection. The IV treatment may be repeated as often as once a week but is usually repeated at 2-week intervals. Precautions ordinarily observed with organophosphate use should be followed. Be sure the animal has not been dewormed or sprayed with organophosphates within the last 2 weeks. The use of organophosphates is not without some risk. Over the last 10 years, only one horse out of about 500 died after treatment and it died from a ruptured aneurysm. Several horses have shown mild signs, such as restlessness and pawing, and several had colic. Since the pretreatment use of atropine has been discontinued, no cases of flatulent colic have been observed nor have any moderate or severe organophosphate reactions. In many cases only one IV treatment is necessary.

The use of systemic corticosteroids minimizes reaction to the larvae. Trichlorfon is used in combination with an antibacterial agent, such as nitrofurazone, and a penetrant, such as DMSO. A mixture of 4.5 g trichlorfon and 4-8 oz nitrofurazone dressing is added to 1 oz DMSO to make a thick paste. This mixture is packed on the lesion under a bandage.

Satisfactory results have been obtained with Williams' ointment made as follows: 3 oz 24% ronnel in a small quantity of mineral oil are mixed with approximately ¾ lb heated petrolatum topical ointment and into this mixture is stirred 3 oz thiabendazole powder. This is applied daily or put under a bandage, which is changed every 2-3 days.[40] Three other similar recipes are:

3 oz 24% ronnel
1 oz mineral oil
¾ lb vaseline
3 oz thiabendazole
1½ oz tannic acid
1 oz nitrofurazone powder

3 oz DMSO
15 ml dexamethasone
40 ml nitrofurazone solution
1 oz trichlorfon powder

1 oz fenthion
½ lb nitrofurazone ointment
10 mg triamcinolone acetonide powder

Ocular habronemiasis is treated with 2 drops fenthion topically each day, plus a topical corticosteroid-antibiotic ophthalmic ointment in conjunction with IV treatment.

Injection of organophosphates directly into the lesion has proven successful. A shoulder lesion 5 cm in diameter was injected intralesionally and SC with 10 ml fenthion (Spotton:Cutter); improvement was noted in 10 days. One out of 6 horses developed cellulitis after injection of 2 lesions close to the medial canthus, but all showed rapid improvement.

Ten horses with recent lesions responded to the use of a feed grade of diethylcarbamazine at 1 oz/900 lb/day for 7 days. The treatment is repeated as indicated if reinfection occurs before healing is complete. The drug is almost completely nontoxic. Diethylcarbamazine liquid or tablets can be used at 2-6 mg/lb daily for 7-14 days. Diethylcarbamazine was not effec-

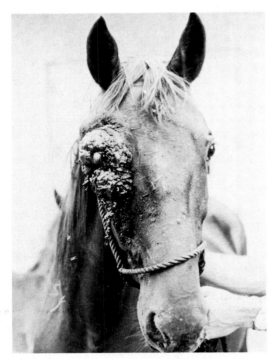

Fig 9. Advanced squamous-cell carcinoma.

tive the next season if a horse developed a lesion in the same location. Presumably the fibrous tissue does not allow enough circulation and drug to contact the larvae.

If lesion size is not prohibitive, cryosurgical treatment appears promising.[41] Very large lesions are best treated surgically and medically. In any of the aforementioned treatments, once the larvae are killed, the problem of granula-

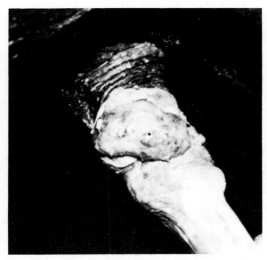

Fig 10. Squamous-cell carcinoma of the penis.

tion tissue and infection must be dealt with by the usual manner, *ie*, excision, pressure bandages, corticosteroid ointments, copper sulfate, etc. When possible, bandaging helps prevent reinfection and seems to decrease healing time.

Treatment for gastric adult *Habronema* infestation reduces recurrence but should not be done within 2 weeks of use of any other organophosphate medication. The use of dichlorvos (Equigard:Squibb), levamisole-piperazine (American Cyanamid) or carbon disulfide is recommended and all horses on the premises should be treated.[42] Predosing with 8 qt 2% $NaHCO_3$ may increase anthelmintic efficacy by dissolving some of the mucus plug at the opening of the *Habronema* nodule.[35]

Squamous-Cell Carcinoma

Squamous-cell carcinoma is a malignant epidermoid tumor that may occur anywhere but has a predilection for areas close to body openings, such as the eyelids, lips, nose, vulva, prepuce and penis, particularly on unpigmented skin (Figs 9,10). In one survey, 30 of 32 squamous-cell carcinomas were situated at a mucocutaneous junction.[43] The lesion may begin as a superficial, slightly indurated nodule covered with apparently normal skin. In the course of several weeks or months, scaling, ulceration and granulomatous reaction develop. Carcinomas are not pruritic unless complicated by habronemiasis or phycomycosis. In some cases, squamous-cell carcinoma may be initially papillomatous, with a verrucous surface often covered by a yellow purulent exudate. They bleed easily and have a broad base with an ulcerated surface that extends into the underlying tissue. Tumor growth produces a mound-like, crusty lesion and finally infiltration of surrounding tissue. The cut surface is pink or pink-grey. Those involving the glans penis are often cauliflower-like and slow to metastasize. Diagnosis is based upon histologic examination of biopsy specimens.

Treatment: Radical surgical excision and/or radiation therapy is commonly employed. In the eye region, 500 R are delivered to the tumor and the surrounding tissue every other day for a total of 5 doses.[7] As a forerunner to cryotherapy, good results were reported using CO_2 snow to produce a local temperature of -20 F.[44]

Cryosurgery alone or in combination with cesium needle implants produces the best results (see Cryosurgery). Cesium needles are implanted close to the tumor and left in place 5-7 days.

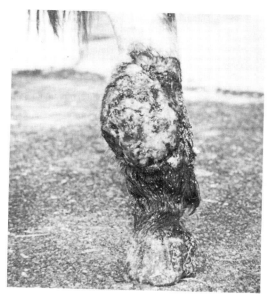

Fig 11. Pyogranuloma that developed subsequent to trauma.

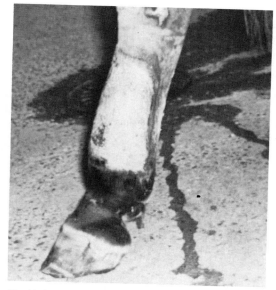

Fig 12. Leg in Figure 11 after surgical removal of the pyogranuloma and skin grafting.

Pyogranuloma

Pyogranuloma describes the granulomatous response of wounds attempting to heal in the face of significant bacterial infections. Such granulation returns rapidly after surgical removal and is difficult to control by routine measures. In some cases, enormous masses of granulation tissue intermingle with fibrous tissue in varying stages of maturity. This has been termed botryomycosis, but most often is a staphylococcal granuloma (Fig 11). An uncomplicated pyogranuloma is not particularly pruritic. Many times the amount of granulation is only moderate but wound healing is very slow.

Diagnosis: Diagnosis is by histologic examination of biopsy specimens.

Treatment: Treatment is successful when appropriate, intensive antibiotic therapy is instituted along with routine treatment for "proud flesh" (Fig 12).

Phycomycosis

Phycomycosis is usually a localized subcutaneous fungal infection caused by several fungi in the class Phycomycetes and characterized by exuberant granulation tissue, pruritus and necrotic draining tracts. *Hyphomyces destruens* and *Entomophthora coronata* are the most commonly recognized etiologic agents, although *Mucor pusillus* and *Basidiobolus ranarum* have been isolated from localized lesions of the leg and lung of 2 horses and the eye of another.[45,46]

In the early 1890's a disease of horses in Florida was reported that the horsemen of the area called "leeches" because they thought the elongated masses of necrotic tissue within the chronic granulomatous lesions were parasitic leeches (*Hirudinea*) that entered the tissues as horses stood in water.[45] In Texas, it also is known as the "Gulf Coast fungus" since most cases occur in low prairie land along the Gulf of Mexico.

Entomophthora coronata produces lesions similar to those of *Hyphomyces destruens*, but has a predilection for skin around the nostrils and nasal cavity mucosa. These mycoses were confused with cutaneous habronemiasis for many years because of the intense local eosinophilia and the presence of necrotic blood vessels that simulated degenerating larvae.

Clinical Signs: In Australia, the incidence of phycomycosis is related to winter seasons and is seen more in young horses. Most affected horses have one or more masses of exuberant granulation tissue on various parts of the body for weeks or months. Simultaneous involvement of opposite limbs is not unusual. The lesions usually develop at the site of an injury, such as a wire cut (Figs 13, C2). They are occasionally first recognized as focal swellings with serum exuding from small sinuses in the skin. Although the lesions occur most fre-

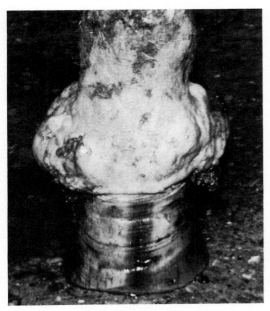

Fig 13. Phycomycosis of 30 days' duration. The lesion was very proliferative and had many fistulous tracts containing "leeches."

quently from the hock or knee to the hoof, they are not uncommon on the abdomen, neck and lips or skin surrounding the nostril. The mucosa of the nasal cavity, lips, trachea or stomach may be affected occasionally. Lesions of several weeks' duration usually contain necrotic sinuses and gritty, grey-white branching masses of hyphae and surrounding reactive tissue commonly called "leeches" (Fig 14).

Horses bite or lick the lesions when possible as though there were intense pruritus, and may destroy portions of the granulating tissue. Lameness develops as lesions on the legs enlarge and involve functional structures. Lesions in the nasal cavity or nostril cause respiratory embarrassment or, in later stages, may extend to the upper lip and affect prehension of food. Lesions expand peripherally in all directions. Those about the fetlock may encircle it and extend dorsad and ventrad to the hoof. Those on the ventral abdomen form an expanding, saucer-shaped mass up to 10-12 inches in diameter. Overlying and adjacent skin is destroyed by the inflammatory reaction and self-mutilation.

Systemic infection is manifested by signs referable to affected organs or may be found incidentally at necropsy of an animal with a peripheral lesion.[47] Cutaneous phycomycoses seldom produce significant clinical lesions by metastasis, but they may spread to regional lymph nodes and lungs.[48,49]

Transmission to humans or other horses has not been reported. However, contaminated bandages and soil contaminated naturally or by wound discharge are possible sources of infection. The fungus evidently must be in a non-host growth phase to be infective.

Lesions: The lesions are granulomatous, fistulated and/or ulcerated and characterized by the presence of yellow-grey necrotic masses or cores of tissue (also known as roots, leeches or kunkers).[50] The superficial surface of the granulation tissue frequently is hemorrhagic due to trauma inflicted by the horse. In more advanced lesions, small sinuses drain pus from the deeper foci of infection and hard, yellow, irregular plugs of necrotic tissue may be expressed. These frequently are found on a bandage when it is removed. Dense, mature, white fibrous tissue with many channels make up the matrix of the lesion. Pieces of creamy-white, necrotic tissue from fulminant lesions frequently branch and are easily dislodged to reveal a rough, uneven and at times jagged, coral-like surface.[50] Tendons and bones ordinarily are not invaded, but tendon sheaths may be.

Histologically, eosinophils are extremely numerous, especially in superficial parts of the lesions and throughout the sinuses. Fungi are found within the necrotic tissue.

Metastasis does not occur in *Entomophthora coronata* infections.

Diagnosis: A rapidly expanding granulomatous, highly pruritic, draining lesion originating from an originally insignificant wound is highly suggestive of phycomycosis. The presence of large, irregular, usually elongated grey to yellow masses of hard necrotic tissue (leeches) in sinuses permeating granulation tissue is sufficient for field diagnosis. Early and slowly progressing lesions may have minute foci of necrosis with less purulent exudate and may be confused with invasive squamous-cell carcinoma or cutaneous habronemiasis. In cutaneous habronemiasis, the yellow foci of necrosis and inflammation are seldom larger than a grain of rice and tend to regress spontaneously during cold weather. Hyphae may sometimes be found in necrotic tissue by microscopic examination of sediment left after treatment with 10-20% KOH or NaOH. Care must be taken not to confuse persistent, branching elastic fibers with fungal hyphae.

Histologic examination of deep biopsy samples is necessary in many cases.

Treatment: Because the fungus most frequently is embedded in hard, dense masses of necrotic tissue that permeate exuberant granulation tissue, radical surgical extirpation of all foci of infection is essential for effective treatment. Recurrence is frequent following excision of the lesions, however, and surgery should be repeated as soon as new foci are noted. These are recognized as dark hemorrhagic patches 1-5 mm in diameter in the granulation bed.

Of 10 horses with moderate to severe phycomycosis, 8 were treated successfully using radical surgery followed by IV, topical and intralesional therapy with amphotericin B (Fungizone:Squibb).[49] Depending on the severity of the lesion(s), amphotericin B at 150 mg/1000 lb is given daily and increased by 50 mg every third day until a maximum of 350-400 mg/day are given. The daily dose is reconstituted as per manufacturer's directions, added to 1 L 5% dextrose and carefully given IV with a 16-ga, 5-cm needle to prevent perivascular injection. Treatment of severe lesions should be continued for up to 30 days.

At the 350-mg dose level, alternate-day treatment is probably sufficient. Large lesions (>25 cm²) require larger doses and longer treatment. Treatment may be discontinued when drainage stops, granulation tissue takes on a healthy appearance with no fistulous tracts, and epithelization begins. General physical condition and rectal temperature should be monitored daily. The BUN and PCV values should be monitored weekly. If the horse becomes depressed and anorectic or if BUN levels become abnormally elevated, systemic therapy should be temporarily discontinued.

The main drawback to systemic use of amphotericin B is expense. The cost of the drug and diluent alone for a 450-kg horse for 30 days is about $700 (1979 prices).

Six pregnant mares treated systemically with amphotericin B had 5 normal foals and one stillborn foal with arthrogryposis. However, histologic examination of the deformed fetus did not establish amphotericin B as the cause of the abnormality.[51]

Local treatment of subcutaneous phycomycosis has been successful. As much affected tissue as possible is surgically removed and the surgical site is treated by topical application of a gauze dressing soaked in amphotericin B solution (50 mg amphotericin B in 10 ml 5% dex-

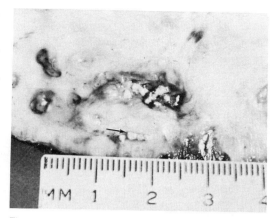

Fig 14. "Leeches" (arrow) in phycomycosis of the nasal mucosa.

trose), gauze dressing soaked in amphotericin B solution plus DMSO, or injection of amphotericin B into the base of the lesion. Surgery may be repeated for small necrotic tracts.

Compared with IV administration of amphotericin B, advantages of local application include less drug expense, treatment of the horse by the owner under supervision of a veterinarian, no phlebitis, and less chance of kidney damage. Disadvantages are poor results when used to treat large lesions, local tissue necrosis from extravenous injection of the solution, and lack of deep penetration of the drug in therapeutic amounts when applied topically.

Mycetoma

Mycetoma (maduromycosis) refers to a group of tumefactions or mycotic granulomas caused by a variety of fungi belonging to the classes Ascomycetes, Deuteromycetes and Actinomycetes. The common diagnostic feature is the presence of granules in exudate and lesions.[52] The fungi occur in the tissues as microcolonies in granules composed of large, segmented mycelial filaments and usually chlamydospores or other spores. The disease is a chronic debilitating process that does not respond to medical treatment.[53]

The fungi cause progressive, invasive subcutaneous and submucosal granulomas and often cause osteomyelitis.[52] The clinical appearance varies from a large granulomatous, cutaneous or subcutaneous mass to multiple cutaneous and subcutaneous nodules 10-25 mm in diameter, some of which rupture and drain (Fig 15).[53-55] A helpful diagnostic feature of mycetoma is dark brown specks scattered through the pink granulation tissue seen upon

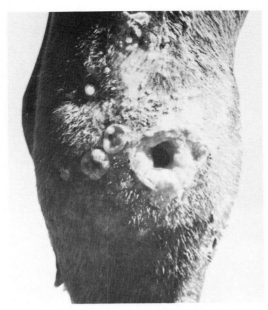

Fig 15. Mycetoma of the hock. Note the multiple draining tracts lined with granulation tissue.

close examination of a cut surface. The lesion looks as though someone sprinkled pepper on it. The specks and granules (microcolonies) are up to 1.5 mm in diameter. Fungal organisms isolated include *Helminthosporium* spp, *Curvularia spicifera* and *Hormodendrum* spp (chromoblastomycosis). Most of these are saprophytes of soil or plants.

Diagnosis is by histopathologic examination of biopsy specimens and cultural identification on Sabouraud's agar.

Rhinosporidiosis

Rhinosporidiosis is a chronic infection of the nasal, vaginal and ocular mucosae by the fungus *Rhinosporidium seeberi* and characterized by the formation of sessile or pedunculated polyps (Fig 16). These consist of granulation tissue through which the fungal sporangia are scattered. Only the nasal form has been observed in animals; dissemination apparently does not occur. The disease is seldom fatal and is evident clinically only by respiratory obstruction and chronic rhinitis. Humans, cattle, horses and mules are affected.[56]

A 12-year-old gelding with no regular contact with other horses had mildly noisy breathing, especially upon inspiration. Inspection of the nasal cavity revealed 4 nearly spherical protrusions attached by narrow pedicles to the mucosa of one nostril, and 2 similar lesions in the other. All growths were located toward the central portion of the nasal cavity and within 2½ inches of the external nares. The largest growth was about 1¼ inches in diameter and the smallest about ½ inch. The growths were mottled red, well-vascularized and covered with a thin, glistening membrane. Surgical removal of the lesion and a small portion of the mucosa resulted in healing within a few weeks.

Scattered through the growth and constituting approximately one-third of its bulk were large numbers of *Rhinosporidium seeberi*. Numerous large sporangia, approximately 200-300μ in diameter and containing 300-500 small endospores, were present.[57] A second case was later reported on a farm 5 miles from the above horse.[58]

The return of polyps 2 years after removal has been reported.[59]

Diagnosis of rhinosporidiosis is by histopathologic examination of biopsy specimens since the organism is very difficult, if not impossible, to culture.[60]

Diseases Characterized by Nodules

A nodule is a small (5-25 mm), circumscribed solid elevation that usually extends deeply into the dermis. Etiologic agents include parasites, fungi, viruses and neoplasia. Many nodules are of undetermined etiology. Observation as to number, location, alopecia, scab formation, pruritus and palpation for pain help differentiate the type of nodules, but of paramount importance is histopathologic examination.

Treatment of nodules is surgical if only a few are present or by systemic or intralesional administration of corticosteroids. The safest systemic corticosteroid in terms of possible adrenal suppression and drug-induced laminitis is oral prednisone or prednisolone at 1-1.5 mg/kg each morning for 10-14 days, followed by 10-14 days

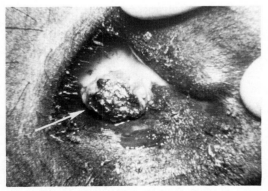

Fig 16. An intranasal polyp of granulation tissue (arrow), characteristic of rhinosporidiosis.

of alternate-day therapy at the same dosage or by daily administration at 0.75 mg/kg. Oral triamcinolone acetonide powder at 10 mg/454 kg each morning for 4 days, then every other day for 7 additional days, may alternatively be used. If the nodules are regressing but not completely, administration of triamcinolone acetonide may be continued at 3 doses/week. Signs of drug-induced hyperadrenalism, such as polydipsia, polyuria and loss of muscle mass over the loins, are not observed with these dosage schedules.

For intralesional therapy, a Luer-Lok syringe is used to create adequate pressure and a ⅜-inch, 23-ga needle to inject 4 mg triamcinolone acetonide into and under the nodule. No more than 20 mg triamcinolone should be used at one time. Treatment may be repeated in 10 days if necessary.

The following listing of nodular diseases is roughly in order of prevalence.

External Parasitic Nodules

Nodules due to bites from external parasites are common during warm months. Most regress spontaneously but may be replaced by new ones. The most frequent offenders are the mosquito and stable fly (dog fly).

Stable flies may explode to swarm numbers in wet summers. Affected horses have areas of raised hair up to 4 mm in diameter. After parting the hair, a small area of edema with a minute central scab is evident. Horses are affected mainly on the back, neck, chest and legs (Fig 17). In young horses, particularly imported horses, parasitic nodules cause severe edema and pain to the extent of self-mutilation of affected areas by biting. Mosquito bites are similar but have no central scab and subside in 3-4 days without treatment.[61]

Control of house and stable flies on farms is made easier by good sanitation, ie, proper collection and disposal of manure, waste feed and other fly-breeding media. Treatment of manure piles and bedding with a larvicide reduces multiplication and fly numbers. However, insecticides are usually also needed.

Surface or residual sprays usually provide effective control of flies in stables, barns and other farm buildings. Organophosphates are the most effective sprays now available for fly control. Those recommended for residual treatments include carbaryl 0.5%, ciodrin 0.15-2.0%, coumaphos 0.125% (Co-Ral), diazinon, dioxathion 0.15-0.6% (Delnav), dichlorvos 1.0%, dimethoate (Cygon), fenthion, malathion 0.5%,

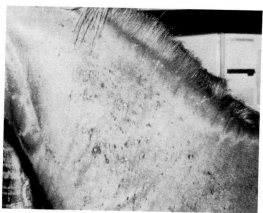

Fig 17. Nodular reaction and alopecia from stable fly bites.

mexthoxychlor 0.5%, rabon, ravap, ronnel 0.25%, ruelene, toxaphene 0.5%, and pyrethrins and synergist (0.05-1.0%).

Researchers may have an answer for stable fly control. Fiberglass panels termed "attractant toxicant devices" emit an invisible ultraviolet light highly attractive to stable flies. When they make contact, they pick up a small but lethal amount of a pesticide called permethrin. Tests of the panels near Fort Walton Beach, Florida, indicate reductions in stable fly populations by 98%.[62]

Another promising method of control is the fly predator system.[63] These natural enemies of pest flies are tiny beneficial insects no larger than the period at the end of this sentence. The female finds pest fly pupae in manure and lays eggs on it. Fly predator eggs hatch quickly and use the pest fly, caught in an inactive stage in the middle of its metamorphosis, as a food source. One female fly predator can destroy up to several hundred pest fly pupae. Pest fly reduction ranged from 83-93% within 30 days.

Another method under study is the sterile male release technic (as for screw worms).[64]

Mosquitoes are controlled in several ways. Since the larvae develop in water, elimination of breeding places by drainage, filling and elimination of receptacles, such as tin cans, buckets and auto tires, is helpful. Stagnant water can be sprayed with #2 fuel oil or residual organophosphate sprays.[65] For protection of the horse, repellents should be applied at times of greatest mosquito activity. Most commercial preparations are similar and none lasts more than a few hours. Diethyltoluamide (DEET) works well against mosquitoes.[66]

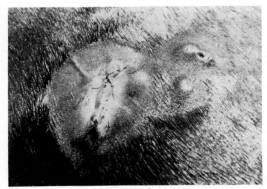

Fig 18. Nodular necrobiosis of the saddle area. Biopsy site is on the left.

Chemically treated wide-mesh (0.635 cm) netting of 100% knotted cotton (McLaughlin Goomly King, Minneapolis) provided 99% protection against mosquitoes for over 100 days.[67]

Clock-operated mist systems that dispense nonresidual sprays at a regular prescribed rate offer an excellent means of insect control even under extreme conditions, such as in poultry houses. A small unit suitable for a box stall costs about $25 and the spray bomb, which lasts about a month, costs $4-5. Pipeline systems offer more economical control.

Nodules may also be caused by ticks, black widow spiders, horse flies, deer flies and other

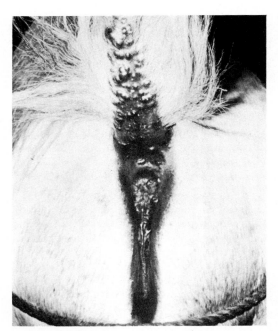

Fig 19. Melanomas of the tail and perianal region of a grey mare.

arthropods. The nocturnal black widow causes hot, edematous and painful swellings, especially on the head and neck of stabled horses.[68] Corticosteroid treatment affords quick relief.

Thin-skinned horses often are markedly sensitive to any of the instars of *Boophilus microplus*. This is mainly a reaction to foreign protein with small areas of raised hair and skin swelling as the ticks bury their mouth parts in the skin until engorged or a molt occurs.[69] The lesions are most numerous on the lower parts of the legs and on the muzzle.

Nodular Necrobiosis

Nodular necrobiosis (collagen granuloma) is thought to be a hypersensitivity reaction. It is more common during the summer. The nodules on the sides of the neck, withers and back are from 5-50 mm in diameter and are neither pruritic nor painful (Fig 18). The hair is seldom affected. The primary histologic change consists of one to several foci of necrobiosis (collagen degeneration) in which the collagen fibers have an amorphous, granular appearance. In older lesions, some foci become mineralized and there is a tremendous infiltration of eosinophils. Other names applied to this disease are eosinophilic granuloma and eosinophilic dermatitis. *Hypoderma* nodules are similar but frequently have a breathing pore.[9]

Melanoma

Melanoma is a common equine tumor, especially of older grey horses. Approximately 80% of greys over 15 years of age have melanotic growths.[70] The nodules are generally found at the perineum, vulva and undersurface of the root of the tail, but also on the male genitalia, limbs, neck and ears (Fig 19).[13] While melanomas are very rare in horses under 6 years old, congenital malignant melanoma has been reported in a foal.[71] Melanomas may be hard or soft, solitary or multiple, and dark brown to black. They vary in size from 10 to 20 mm but may be larger (Fig 20). The course of the disease is prolonged even though metastasis to local lymph nodes occurs early.[72] Melanomas remain benign for 10-20 years on the skin; however, the disease is rapidly fatal once vital organs are involved.

Treatment for early solitary nodules is surgical excision or cyronecrosis. Treatment in advanced cases has seldom been attempted.

In humans the most dramatic and definitive demonstration of the antitumor activity of BCG has been the regression of multiple intradermal metastases of malignant melanoma after intralesional injection of viable BCG. Lesions injected with BCG regressed in 58% of cases vs 14% in noninjected lesions, indicating a systemic response to tumor-associated antigens.[32] Apparent visceral metastases did not respond and long-term survivors had disease limited to the skin, subcutaneous tissue and regional lymph nodes. This technic has been used in horses (see Sarcoid).

Cutaneous Mastocytoma

Cutaneous mastocytoma (mastocytosis) is a nodular disease of unknown etiology. Tissue changes appear more hyperplastic than neoplastic. Localized aggregates of mast cells occur in certain conditions, such as chronic inflammation, parasitic infestation and human urticaria pigmentosa. In one case of disseminated mast cell tumors, a viral etiology was suggested.[73] An antigen-antibody reaction is another possibility.[70]

The most common form is a single 2- to 20-cm cutaneous nodule on the head, neck or distal extremities (Fig 21). The surface of the nodules may be normal in those lesions restricted to the dermis and hairless or ulcerated in more superficial lesions. The incidence is 5:1 males vs females, with an age range of 1 day to 15 years. Lesions in a newborn foal appeared and regressed in 30-day cycles until, at one year, the colt had only a few regressing nodules left.[74] Heavily mineralized limb lesions may resemble tumoral calcinosis radiographically.[9]

Total excision biopsy is the best method of diagnosis and treatment. Microscopic examination reveals variably sized aggregates of well-differentiated mast cells and foci of necrosis, many of which are partly mineralized.

The nodules are apparently self-limiting and reportedly do not metastasize. Only a small percentage recur after removal. Intralesional corticosteroids may be useful when surgery is not desirable.

Occult Sarcoid (see Sarcoid)
Hypoderma Nodules

Hypoderma spp nodules are of variable incidence, depending on the section of the country. A 1939 survey of the northeastern US showed 27% of 79 horses to be infested.[75] In a few small herds in Montana, a 40-60% incidence was reported.[76] High-risk horses are young and poorly conditioned, and share the range with cattle.

In the hottest part of the summer, adult warble flies attach their eggs to horse hairs. After hatching, the larvae penetrate the skin and migrate to the dorsum, especially around the

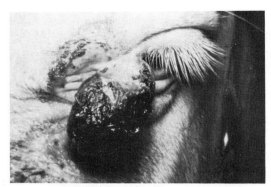

Fig 20. Large melanoma at the medial canthus.

withers, back and neck, during the fall and winter. Most larvae develop a breathing hole in the skin, which aids their identification. Grubs in horses are usually smaller (2-3 mm x 1-1.5 mm) than in cattle. Many fail to develop completely and are killed by host tissues and absorbed, but a few become mineralized and create a permanent nodule. Usually only 1-2 grubs are present, but occasionally 4-5 and rarely more than 10 occur. A few larvae may drop to the ground and burrow into the soil to emerge as a fly in about a month, the total cycle being 2-3 weeks shorter than in cattle. In the US, a life cycle in equine hosts is rarely completed. Another difference between equine and bovine species is that *Hypoderma* larvae in equidae are more likely to migrate to the brain and cause acute neurologic disease, with or without concurrent skin nodules.[77] Sudden onset of muscular weakness or localized paralysis that proceeds to profound loss of motor control,

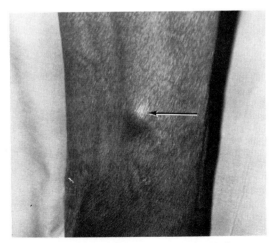

Fig 21. Cutaneous mastocytoma (arrow) on the craniomedial aspect of the foreleg. This stallion also had 2 tumors over tendons on the rear legs.

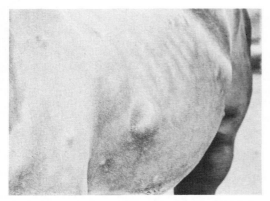

Fig 22. A very large nodule and many of the usual size in cutaneous lymphoma.

convulsions and death within 1-7 days is the usual clinical picture.

One or 2 lesions can be treated simply by enlarging the breathing hole with a scalpel blade and removing the larva with a hemostat. Early treatment of suspected *Hypoderma* spp nodules by intralesional injection of 4 mg triamcinolone acetonide and 0.5 ml fenthion may kill the developing grub and minimize local reaction.

In areas of high incidence, pour-on insecticides (13.4% cruformate *eg*, ruelene applied at 30 ml/45 kg) prevent the development of cattle grubs.[76] Treatment should be done at the time of year recommended for treatment of cattle.

Lymphoma

Lymphoma (lymphosarcoma) is a term used to designate primary tumors of the lymphoid system and includes sarcomatous and leukemic states. All affected horses in one review had at least one sarcomatous mass but all were not leukemic.[78] Of 26 affected horses, 14 were leukemic and 6 of the 14 had WBC counts over 30,000/mm[3]. Large subcutaneous nodules are present in about 10% of all cases surveyed. The age range was 2 months to 23 years and 75% of affected horses were over 6 years old. Males outnumbered females 2 to 1. Lymph node involvement was present peripherally in 50%, in the abdomen of 33% and in the thorax of 20%.[79] The liver, spleen and kidney are commonly involved.

Clinical signs vary widely with the degree of involvement. The most consistent signs are capillary fragility, pleural and pericardial effusion, ascites and ventral edema. The usual history is chronic illness, poor growth and intermittent colic.[80]

Cutaneous lesions include alopecia, sores over the bridge of the nose, subcutaneous nodu-

lar swellings over the neck, shoulder, forelegs and perineum, and ulcerations of the vulva and cervix (Fig 22).[81-84]

Treatment has been unsuccessful.

Sporotrichosis

Sporotrichosis is a chronic sporadic infection, primarily of the skin and subcutaneous tissues, although visceral and skeletal involvement sometimes occur. The disease is caused by *Sporotrichum schenckii*, a dimorphic aerobic fungus that is usually saprophytic. It is cigar-shaped in the yeast phase and gram-positive. The fungus exists on various plants and the infection is an occupational disease of horticulturists. Infection in animals and humans is usually introduced through cutaneous wounds by plant barbs or thorns. Humans, horses, mules, mice, dogs, cows, cats, rats and domestic fowl are susceptible.[85]

Clinical Signs: The lesions are hard subcutaneous nodules that develop along the lymphatics of the front and/or rear limbs, especially on the medial surface. Nodules are most numerous at the thigh or the upper foreleg and chest, are raised above the surface of the skin and vary in size from 1-5 cm (Fig C3). They eventually ulcerate and discharge a small amount of thick pus. There is no tendency of the nodules to coalesce, although they may appear connected by the lymphatics, which may be conspicuously thickened. Lymph nodes are not usually involved. Small nodules are usually solid, while larger ones often contain a purulent core. Rupture of the latter results in a crateriform ulcer (Fig C3). Occasionally a horse may have moveable subcutaneous nodules that do not ulcerate and do not involve the lymphatics. Usually only one horse in a herd is infected.[86]

Diagnosis: Nodules, pustules and ulcers along the lymphatics suggest sporotrichosis but should be differentiated from ulcerative lymphangitis caused by *Cornynebacterium pseudotuberculosis,* which is more often found at the fetlock, epizootic lymphangitis caused by *Cryptococcus neoformans,* which is more often found at the hock with ulcers that coalesce and involve lymph nodes, and the cutaneous form of glanders, which is evidently not present in the US.[87]

Diagnosis is rarely made by demonstrating the yeast phase in tissue sections. The mycelial phase may be demonstrated after inoculation on Sabouraud's agar at 20 C. Black colonies typical of the mold phase of *S schenckii* are evident. There is a characteristic triad arrangement of spores borne on slender conidiophores.[88] The organism may grow well on a maltose medium.[87] Culture at 37 C may cause the organism to revert to the yeast phase.[89]

Smears of the purulent material stained with Giemsa stain may reveal a few gram-positive ovoid or coccoid bodies. The organism occurs in much larger numbers in the tissues and pus of inoculated rats or hamsters and is correspondingly easier to find.[57]

Treatment: Iodides given IV, iodine locally and organic iodide PO usually give good results if continued for a long period. A 125-ml dose of 20% NaI is given IV and repeated 24 hours later, followed by 1 oz organic iodide in the feed daily for 30-60 days or until cured. The dosage and treatment schedule may be varied up to the point of producing iodism.

Use of griseofulvin at 10 g daily for 2 weeks, followed by 5 g daily until disappearance of lesions, has been effective when iodine treatment failed.[90]

Fibroma

A fibroma is a benign connective tissue tumor that may be hard or soft. Hard fibromas develop slowly and occur most frequently on regions subject to repeated impact or pressure, such as the head, saddle or harness regions. They vary in size from 1-8 cm and are not usually sensitive. They move with the skin and have a smooth or lobular surface.

Soft fibromas vary in size from 1-10 cm or larger and are usually circular, with a smooth or lobulated surface. They are usually located on the neck or tail and are attached to and move with the skin. The course may be acute or chronic.[91]

Treatment by surgical removal is usually quite successful but may be unnecessary except for cosmetic purposes.

Aberrant Parasitic Larvae

Aberrant larvae of several parasites may cause a nodular reaction due to host attempts to wall off migration. Specific identification is usually impossible in biopsy specimens, but those listed on histopathology reports include *Habronema, Hypoderma* and *Gasterophilus.* Onchocercamata, frequently associated with *Onchocerca* dermatitis in humans, are quite rare or nonexistent in horses.

Nodules suspected of being caused by aberrant larvae are treated as outlined previously.

Protein Bumps

"Protein bumps" is a condition rarely authenticated but suspected to be caused by over-

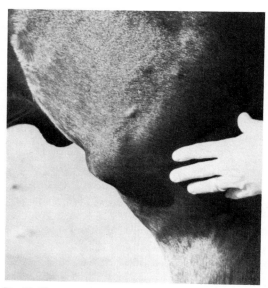

Fig 23. Tumoral calcinosis of the lateral aspect of the stifle.

feeding of grains, especially those of high protein content. Small itchy lumps, mainly on the thorax, but sometimes also on the neck and back, are reported in sales yearlings. Response to corticosteroids is rapid.[92] Change to a more moderate ration also is effective.

Mycetoma

Nodules due to early mycetoma have been described.

Tumoral Calcinosis

Tumoral calcinosis (calcinosis circumscripta) in 14 horses had the characteristic feature of a large (3-12 cm), dense subcutaneous nodule located at the lateral aspect of the gaskin, adjacent to the femorotibial articulation (Fig 23).[93,94] In no instance did history indicate trauma or injection reactions. Radiographic examination indicated that the nodules were oval masses irregularly infiltrated with radiopaque deposits of material with a density similar to that of cortical bone. At least 2 of these were intimately associated with the joint capsule, making surgical removal difficult. The calcified masses were enclosed by a dense fibrous capsule from which many internal trabeculae arose.

The etiology of tumoral calcinosis is unknown but is thought to be the effect of noxious influences, such as prolonged and repeated trauma.[95]

Surgical removal is recommended only in lame horses or those in which cosmetic surgery is warranted.

Unilateral Papular Dermatitis

Unilateral papular dermatitis presents a striking clinical picture characterized by multiple (30-300) nodules 5-15 mm in diameter on one side of the body only. Most nodules occur on the lateral thorax but may extend to the lateral aspects of the shoulder, neck and abdomen. Lesions develop in the spring and early summer and are nonpruritic. Spontaneous regression in 2-8 weeks is common. Horses in contact with an affected animal remain unaffected.

The etiology is unknown but the unilateral nature suggests peripheral nerve involvement somewhat similar to *Herpes zoster* infections in humans. Treatment is not necessary, but corticosteroids seem to shorten the course of the disease.[9]

Viral Papular Dermatitis

The initial skin lesions of viral papular dermatitis are numerous firm, concentric "BB" shot-sized papules, although some may be nodules up to 25 mm. The papules are not pustular, vesicular, painful or pruritic. Within 7 days, the papular lesions become covered with scabs that later drop off, leaving circumscribed, desquamated and hairless areas. Stages of the disease may overlap in the same animal, with new papules appearing while others heal. The body temperature remains normal.

In the original report, 17 of 22 horses in a barn were affected, the majority being 3-year-olds.[96] The incubation time was 6-8 days and the course of disease was 10-42 days, with an average of 24 days. Numerous examination for mites, fungi and larvae were negative. Growth appeared on the chorioallantoic membrane of embryos injected with a macerated scab lesion and a virus was isolated that caused the disease in experimental horses. Elevated temperatures were noted in the 2 experimental mares (ages 13 and 19 years) on days 6 and 7 postinoculation, 24 hours before 20 or so papules were observed, none of which were at the site of inoculation.

In Australian horses, the disease is clinically identical and appears annually when yearlings are brought to training establishments.[97] Because lesions appear initially around the girth region, harnesses, rugs and grooming gear are considered important transmitters of the disease. This highly contagious disease seriously interferes with training programs. In 2 other reports, the virus was found to be immunologically related to vaccinia and cowpox viruses.[98] Using electron microscopy, virions were seen in biopsy scabs and skin scrapings that were morphologically similar to vaccinia virus.[99]

While this disease is rarely reported, the clinical picture is easily passed off as a "fungus." The course of disease elapses during treatment for fungal infection, convincing all concerned that it was such. It is probably more common at tracks and breaking farms than is realized.

Amyloidosis

Any continual immunologic, chronic infectious or inflammatory stimulation of the reticuloendothelial system may result in amyloidosis, which is the deposition of amyloid glycoprotein fibers in parenchymatous organs. In the horse, the spleen and liver are chiefly involved, with the kidney and adrenals involved less often.[100] Two "atypical" types occur in the horse. Local "tumor-like" amyloidosis is characterized by nodular deposits in the mucosa of the upper respiratory tract and regional lymph nodes (Fig C4). The cutaneous form is characterized by multiple cutaneous and subcutaneous firm, painless nodules 0.5-10 cm or larger in diameter, especially on the head, neck and pectoral region. These may regress spontaneously or in conjunction with corticosteroid therapy, resembling urticaria, only to return and assume a chronic progressive nature.[9]

The lesions are produced by the deposition of amyloid fibers, the major protein component of which is derived from the elevated immunoglobulin levels associated with persistent antigenic stimulation. Frequently both atypical forms are seen in one horse and, in most cases, no visceral lesions are present. In one cutaneous case, electron microscopy revealed nodule composition of granulation tissue and numerous reticuloendothelial cells that contained amyloid in their cytoplasm.[101]

Diagnosis is established upon histopathologic examination of specially stained biopsy specimens.

No successful treatment is known, but affected horses may remain useful for a long time unless respiratory embarrassment is severe.

Disease Characterized by Pustules and Ulcers

Sporotrichosis (see above)
Corynebacterium Infection

Corynebacterium pseudotuberculosis causes cutaneous pyogenic reactions in several locations and forms on the horse. Ulcerative lymphangitis, caused by *C pseudotuberculosis,* becomes clinically apparent with the development of subcutaneous nodules most common at the rear fetlocks. The affected limb is usually very edematous (Fig 24). Some nodules ulcerate and discharge a creamy, green-tinged pus. The resulting ulcers are slow to heal and rarely spread to regional lymph nodes to cause systemic infection.[87] Culture of the discharge and sensitivity testing provide a diagnosis and indicate the most effective antibiotic to be used in conjunction with local treatment with povidone iodine washes and topical antibiotics. Advanced cases usually do not respond to treatment.

Another form of *C pseudotuberculosis* infection is sometimes called contagious acne.[102] Painful papules develop into pustules and then into furuncles in areas of the skin in contact with harness or tack. Infection is thought to result from contact of contaminated grooming equipment and tack with previously traumatized skin. Infection is more common in summer. Some lesions coalesce to develop crateriform ulcers that are less responsive to antibiotics and may require surgical removal, with healing by second intention (Fig C5).

A third form to be considered later is *Corynebacterium* "chest abscesses."

Epizootic Lymphangitis

Epizootic lymphangitis is a rare subacute or chronic disease of horses and mules caused by *Histoplasma farciminosum.* It is usually a primary wound infection followed by metastasis to regional lymphatics. While lymphatic involvement is common, the disease may also be evident as suppurative wounds, conjunctivitis, keratitis, ulceration of the nasal mucosa, sinusitis and pneumonia. Transmission from one horse to another may occur through direct contact, contaminated equipment and biting flies.[45] Spread of infection among horses is usually rapid.

The incubation period ranges from several weeks to as long as 6 months. Ulcerated cutaneous lesions usually appear on the rear legs but may also develop on the neck, lips and harness regions. The ulcers develop significant reddish granulations and discharge grey-yellow pus mixed with lymph or blood. As the disease progresses, infection spreads to adjacent lymph vessels, which become swollen and develop nodules. The nodules change into fluctuant furuncles and rupture into ulcers. Sometimes the ulcers coalesce into large ulcerative areas. When animals suffering from epi-

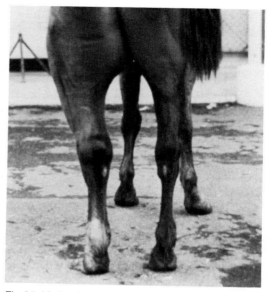

Fig 24. Limb edema caused by infection with *C pseudotuberculosis.*

zootic lymphangitis are kept confined in a closed stable, a characteristic moldy odor may be noted.[91]

Exudate, secretions or tissue from a lesion should be examined microscopically or cultured for confirmation of the diagnosis.

Amphotericin B therapy gives favorable results in humans and experimental animals. Systemic iodides plus surgical excision may be of benefit. Careful disinfection, isolation and fly control limit spread of the disease.

Staphylococcal Folliculitis

Staphylococcal folliculitis is probably the most common of dermal pustules, especially so-called "summer scab" or "summer rash." Many of the pustules extend into the dermis and subcutis to produce a profound inflammatory process, furunculosis. Lesions are most common in the saddle and harness areas but occur almost anywhere. Early inflammation produces a papule that soon progresses into a very small, painful pustule. When the pustules rupture, the exudate causes matting of hair and crusts, and the lesion is easily visible. Papules can be detected by careful palpation. Circular, scaly areas of alopecia are the end stage of the disease. The course of disease may be as short as 2 weeks with treatment or, if untreated, may last all summer.

Excessive sweating and friction from tack are important in allowing *Staphylococcus aureus* to become established. Less trouble is seen

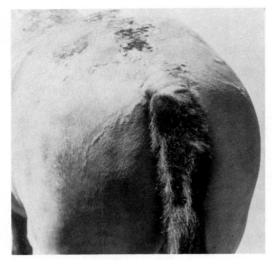

Fig 25. Lumbosacral lesions and "rat-tail" in severe *Culicoides* allergy.

in well-groomed horses that are bathed after workouts.[103]

A diagnosis is fairly obvious upon close clinical examination but culture of lesions is advisable since staphylococcal and *Corynebacterium* pustular dermatitis are virtually indistinguishable from folliculitis caused by dermatophytes or *Dermatophilus congolensis*.

Treatment with IM procaine penicillin at 10,000 IU/lb BID for 7 days and daily baths with povidone iodine scrub is usually effective.

Disease Characterized by Pruritus and Alopecia

Culicoides Dermatitis

The most common cause of pruritic alopecia is an allergic dermatitis caused by hypersensitivity to the bite of any of several species of

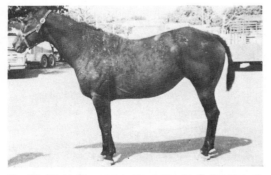

Fig 26. "Rat-tail" and sparse mane in *Culicoides* allergy.

biting gnats of the genus *Culicoides*. The name "Queensland itch" has been given to this disease since it is very common in that section of Australia. Similar if not identical syndromes are called "sweet itch" in England and Ireland, and "kasen" in Japan. The pathogenesis of Queensland itch was established in 1954 when *Culicoides robertsi* was determined as the etiologic agent.[104] *Culicoides pulicaris* is believed to be the most important species in England.[105] This and several other forms of seasonal allergic dermatitis are often termed "summer itch" or "summer eczema."

Culicoides gnats are also referred to as biting midges, "punkies," "no-see-ums" and other colloquial terms. They are improperly called sand flies, which is more accurately used in referring to members of the genus *Phlebotomus*.

Culicoides gnats are of such minute size, generally 1-3 mm long, that most horse owners have difficulty comprehending how the gnats cause such terrible itching. They are readily recognized by the large dark spots on the costal border of the wings, which are folded flat over the abdomen when at rest, with the thorax humped over the head (Fig 27).[35,116]

The bite of *Culicoides* is accompanied by immediate intense sharp pain and irritation, followed by development of red wheals. The intense irritation reportedly lasts for 1-3 weeks.[117] Because of their immense numbers, *Culicoides* gnats may have been responsible for the lack of early development of the southern areas along the Atlantic seaboard.[64]

Culicoides larvae have been found in mud, sand and debris at the edges of ponds, springs, creeks, the margins of practically any small body of still or slowly running fresh, brackish or salt water, compost piles, rotting leaf mold, peaty soils, manure and any other wet vegetable matter.[117] Adult gnats are most active when there is little or no breeze and when temperatures are over 50 F. They seldom fly more than 2 miles but may be passively transported by high winds.

Culicoides variipennis was the most common of 34 species of biting flies attacking horses in 3 southwestern states, accounting for 29.8% of the total of 4767 females identified during a survey. *Psorophora columbiae,* in the mosquito family, was second at 28.4%. *C variipennis* is found throughout most of the US, with seasonal activity in the north and year-round activity in the extreme south, except during the worst cold spells. In the southwest, activity is much greater in the morning. The favored feeding sites are the bare and short-haired areas high on the inside rear flanks between the leg and udder on mares.[118] This area frequently has circular patches of depigmentation 5-25 mm in diameter.

Clinical Signs: Signs appear with the advent of warm weather and subside only when cool weather leads into winter. Horses of all ages are affected, but cases in animals less than 3 years old are uncommon and usually not severe. Since this is an allergy, only a small portion of a herd is affected.

In the early stages of the disease, small papules with erect hair may be seen by the careful observer at the favored feeding sites of the gnat along the ears, poll, mane, withers, tail head and ventral abdomen. Severely affected animals may have lesions on the neck and lumbosacral areas (Fig 25). In a few days severe pruritus of the sites causes frequent rubbing. Broken hairs, scattered areas of alopecia, fresh excoriations and scabs on healed abrasions are evident. Rubbing of the tail head leaves a stubble of hair about 1-1.5 cm long on the upper portion of the tail, giving rise to the name "rat-tail." Lesions heal and hair grows back the first winter. However, the papules and pruritis return with the warm weather.

Some horses rub the mane almost completely out and, after several seasons, much of it fails to grow back (Fig 26). The skin over the withers by then is thickened and wrinkled. *Culicoides pulicaris* bites at the mane and tail 96% of the time.[105] The predominant area of involvement is probably related to the biting sites of particular species involved.

Diagnosis of Queensland itch is strongly suggested by the season, location and character of lesions, few horses affected, course of disease, and recurrence the next season. Diagnosis is confirmed by intradermal testing with *Culicoides* antigens. Unfortunately, none is commercially available. An effective antigen has been made by grinding the entire insects with a mortar and pestle, adding a small volume of saline to produce a homogenate and then adding enough saline to produce a final concentration of 1:100. The suspension is then passed through graded millipore filters of decreasing pore size, the final pore size being 0.22 μ.[106] Testing is done as previously described (see Examination). A normal horse and the suspect animal should both be tested. Biopsies of affected horses only confirm an allergic dermatitis without identifying the allergen. Eo-

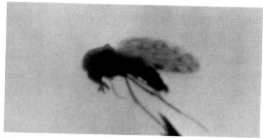

Fig 27. *Culicoides variipennis,* with its mottled wings, is one of the main causes of "summer itch."

sinophilia is a common finding in hemograms but is not diagnostic.

Treatment: An attempt should be made to protect allergic horses from *Culicoides* gnats. Stabling is helpful. Where species of gnats attack at dawn and dusk, horses may be turned out to graze only during the day.[107,108] However, worldwide the genus *Culicoides* numbers 1000 species of biting gnats, some of which bite at all hours of the day and night.[109] Therefore, constant stabling is recommended when the biting habits of the species involved are unknown. Screening the stalls is most helpful provided the screens are special 32 x 32 mesh. *Culicoides* gnats are small enough to pass through conventional 14- and 16-mesh mosquito screens. Painting the screens with 6% malathion in ethanol gives further protection.[107]

Time-operated spray-mist insecticide systems are helpful if the stall is not too exposed. Repellents, while effective against *Culicoides* for only a matter of hours, should at least be used at dawn, dusk and whenever the horse is out of the stall. Undiluted butoxypolypropylene glycol 800 prevented biting for 4-10 hours.[110] A light-weight stable sheet altered to cover the bites may also help if the patient tolerates wearing such. Insect control measures are best started in advance of the season. Any lotion or oily preparations that provide at least a mechanical barrier to gnats are beneficial.

Larvicidal treatment of water in breeding areas would be a logical solution were it not of such environmental concern. Alteration of larval habitat by diking, draining or flooding reduces populations but is seldom practical.

Despite diligent efforts to protect horses, gnats often gain access to horses and long-term, low-level corticosteroid administration is necessary. While repository products are used by some at 3- to 4-week intervals, oral treatment is safer when considering long-term use. Triamcinolone acetonide in oral doses of

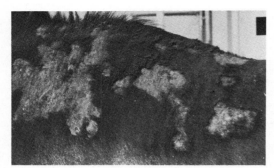

Fig 28. Alopecia on the withers from *Onchocerca cervicalis* infestation.

10 mg can be given daily for 4 days, followed by alternate-day 10-mg doses for 4 doses. Treatment twice a week can then be tried. The goal is to maintain the horse on the lowest dosage possible. When pruritus is very severe, the initial dose may be raised to 20 mg. Corticosteroids suppress the adrenal gland less if administered at the time of day when natural output of cortisol is highest, ie, between 4 AM and 10 AM.[111] The termination of corticosteroid treatment during cool weather should be gradual over 2-3 weeks, rather than abrupt, to allow adrenal function to resume normally.

Prednisone or prednisolone, although perhaps not quite as effective, is thought to be safer than triamcinolone for long-term administration. The lowest possible daily dose that prevents itching must be determined for individual horses and that dose is then doubled and given every other morning for the duration. The maintenance dose for the average horse is 250-500 mg every other morning. As with any chronic corticosteroid administration, the owner should be alerted to signs of iatrogenic Cushing's syndrome, such as thin skin, poor coat, loss of muscle mass (especially gluteal and intercostal), chronic laminitis, polydipsia, hirsutism (long, wavy hair), and docility.[112] If any of these are noted, the dosage should be reduced by one-third to one-half and the CBC and glucose, Na and K levels monitored.

At the end of the gnat season, a decreasing dosage often is not necessary with the use of prednisone or prednisolone. Signs associated with iatrogenic Addison's disease (hypoadrenalism) are weakness, debilitation, poor coat, weight loss, hypoglycemia, diarrhea and dehydration.[111] A diagnosis of hypoadrenalism is supported by a less than doubled serum cortisol level at 6 hours postinjection of 200 IU ACTH given IM.

Treatment of hypoadrenalism requires continued corticosteroid use on a decreasing schedule and ACTH. The following regimen has been suggested: [112]

Day 1:   10 mg dexamethasone
Day 2:   5 mg dexamethasone
Day 3: 2.5 mg dexamethasone and 80 IU ACTH
Day 4: 2.5 mg dexamethasone and 40 IU ACTH
Day 5: 2.5 mg dexamethasone and 40 IU ACTH

Hyposensitization by weekly injections with allergen of increasing concentration has been attempted in horses but is still experimental. Repeated doses of allergen stimulate production of IgG-blocking antibodies that interfere with insect allergen-IgE reaction. In humans and dogs, IgE coats tissue mast cells. When allergens reach those coated mast cells, the reaction causes mast cell degranulation and subsequent release of histamine, slow-reacting substance of anaphylaxis (SRSA), bradykinin and proteolytic enzymes. These active substances induce cellular changes that result in clinical skin disease.[113] Equine IgE has recently been identified and linked to chronic obstructive pulmonary disease.[114] In humans, insect allergy is mediated by IgE.[115]

Another treatment related to IgE and mast cell release of active compounds involves the use of diethylcarbamazine. While the drug is well known for its filaricidal properties, it is also an effective SRSA blocker at higher dosages. Diethylcarbamazine has been used with some success in the treatment of equine allergic dermatitis when given orally at 6.6 mg/kg BID, usually mixed in the grain ration.

Onchocerciasis

In humans, *Onchocerca volvulus* is one of the top causes of blindness in the world.[119] Other symptoms in humans are pruritus, subcutaneous nodules, and atrophy, mottled depigmentation, flaccidity and premature wrinkling of the skin.

The disease in horses is somewhat controversial. The presence of microfilariae in the skin and eyes of horses is well documented.[120-124] However, since many infected horses show few or no skin lesions, the pathogenicity of *Onchocerca cervicalis* in horses is doubted by some.[125] In humans, the most significant pathologic skin changes are caused by dead microfilariae and associated immune reactions, which may vary among hosts.[126] The number of microfilariae present, as well as the number that die, at any one time also affects the pathologic changes of onchocerciasis.

Clinical Signs: The initial lesions consist of thinning hair, especially about the face, neck, chest, withers and ventral midline, and mild to severe pruritus (Fig 28).[127,128] More advanced cases exhibit scaly alopecia and occasional abraded lesions that are seldom moist. The abrasions heal rapidly but recur frequently. Neck lesions are usually close to the mane and at the withers, and are 5-15 mm in diameter with some confluence of lesions. Thinning hair to near total alopecia is common on the face and especially around the eyes and ears. Thinning hair or alopecia on the ventral midline is diffuse in contrast to the well-delineated, narrow strip caused by horn flies. When itching is severe and the problem is compounded by biting insects, the entire area may be thickened with many minute, moist lesions. Some owners report the horse lies down and attempts to drag or rub its belly on the ground. Some horses straddle and rub stumps or similar objects.

Most affected horses are over 4 years of age. The youngest observed was a 2-year-old with lesions on the head and crest only.

Intracutaneous nodules are rare. Dry, scaly seborrhea is a frequent concurrent condition. Large flakes are found on the mane and tail, and small dandruff-like particles are visible over most of the body. Rubbing of the tail is seldom seen in onchocerciasis.

Onchocercal depigmentation in horses has been reported.[122,129] An 8-year-old stallion had several white circular patches of hair up to 2 cm in diameter over the withers and rib cage, and large zones of depigmentation of the scrotum, all of which appeared in the previous 5 months (Fig 29). Examination of skin biopsies from a circular white lesion on the withers, normal skin 2.5 cm from this lesion, and depigmented scrotal skin revealed 1423, 35 and 5150 microfilariae, respectively.

Diagnosis: Thinning of the hair and scaly lesions on the withers, neck, head and ventral midline, with mild to moderate pruritus, suggest onchocerciasis. Finding microfilariae in skin biopsies or deep scrapings is necessary for confirmation.

The biopsy site should be clipped and surgically scrubbed before it is infiltrated SC with 2-3 ml lidocaine. The sample is removed with a # 6 biopsy punch and placed in 5 ml physiologic saline and incubated at 37 C (98.6 F). More microfilariae are usually found in the

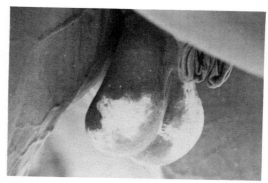

Fig 29. Scrotal depigmentation from heavy concentrations of *Onchocerca* microfilariae.

half of the sample that is minced with scissors; the other half is placed in formalin for histopathologic examination. Some active microfilariae may be observed as early as 10 minutes later, lashing about in an eel-like motion.

Onchocerca cervicalis is a whitish, thread-like nematode. Males are 6-7 cm long and 70-100 μ thick. Females are up to 30 cm long and 400 μ thick.[34] Microfilariae are 200-400 μ long and 4-5 μ in diameter, and have a very short tail (Fig 30). They seldom occur in blood. The life cycle begins when microfilariae are ingested by the biting midge *Culicoides* spp. Development to the infective larval stage takes about 25 days, at which time they are transmitted to the horse by the bite of an infected midge. The infective larvae subsequently develop into adults. Microfilariae are produced by newly matured adults and migrate to the skin in 4-5 months in humans infected with *Onchocerca volvulus*.

Treatment: Of the many drugs evaluated as a filaricide in humans, diethylcarbamazine has given the best results.[130,131] Other effective

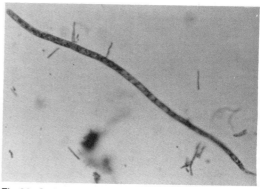

Fig 30. Stained *Onchocerca* microfilaria.

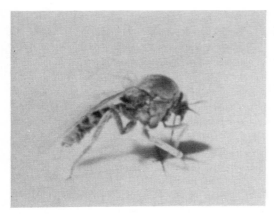

Fig 31. The black fly, *Simulium*. Note the humped thorax and transparent wings.

drugs are trichlorfon (7.5-10 mg/kg) and metriphonate (15 mg/kg).[132,133]

Diethylcarbamazine is stable and of very low toxicity. It kills virtually all microfilariae in the skin and eyes of humans, and considerable local reaction occurs around the dying parasites. Although microfilariae disappear rapidly from the skin, they usually reappear 1-3 months after treatment ceases. The action of this drug on adult worms is slight. Killing microfilariae obviously does not effect a total cure, but adulticidal drugs are usually too toxic to be used routinely. Topical treatment of human eyes with diethylcarbamazine caused disappearance of microfilariae from the aqueous humor after 48 hours.[134]

Diethylcarbamazine is an effective microfilaricide for horses at 2 mg/lb PO for a minimum of 5 consecutive days.[122] Many horses require treatment for 21 days or prophylactically throughout the summer.[124] In many instances, it is advisable to administer corticosteroids to control increased pruritus during the first few days of treatment, especially when ocular lesions are present. Acute eye lesions should be treated symptomatically and diethylcarbamazine treatment delayed until inflammation subsides.[124]

The severity of reaction to treatment is thought to be proportional to the number of microfilariae in the skin rather than the dose and is presumably caused by the liberation of antigens from microfilarial destruction in a sensitized individual.[130] This reaction is so specific in humans that it is frequently referred to as a diagnostic test called the Mazzotti test.[135] The same increased pruritus occurs in horses during the first few days of treatment.

Levamisole has been used as a filaricide in horses with good results.[136] It is given orally mixed with Karo syrup or in capsules at 5 mg/lb/day for 7-10 days. Some horses develop edema in areas with concentrations of microfilariae, such as the face and ventral abdomen. These side effects can be minimized by concurrent corticosteroid therapy. Other less frequent side effects include excessive sweating and mild colic. Injectable levamisole should not be used since severe cellulitis, seizures and death have occurred from its use. Oral treatment may have to be repeated in 2-3 months.

Until an effective drug is found to kill adult *Onchocerca* residing in the ligamentum nuchae, the problem will continue. A drug called Compound E, a combination of an aresenical and a benzimidazole, has been tested in dogs and cattle and appears promising.[137,138]

Control of this disease is impossible unless the horse is protected against bites of the vector, *Culicoides* spp.

Black-Fly Dermatitis

Black flies rank second only to the mosquito as annoying pests.[64] Their anesthetic bite is usually not perceived at the time, but subsequent swelling and itching may persist for weeks. In India, they are affectionately known as "dam-dims."[116]

These members of the family Simuliidae are black or grey and are 1-5 mm long (the house fly and stable fly are 6-7 mm). The thorax is humped over the head and the piercing proboscis is short (Fig 31). The long antennae, which have 11 segments, protrude like the horns of a cow. The wings are broad and not spotted. They have no scales and are not hairy, except for bristles on the thick cranial veins. The body is covered with short golden or silvery hairs.[35] There are 60 species over the US and Canada.

Unlike mosquitoes, black flies breed on grass and other plants along swiftly running, well-aerated water. An exception is the southern buffalo gnat, *Cnephia pecuarum,* which breeds in slow streams.[103] Some species have adapted to still water, while others breed only near waterfalls. The life cycle is complete in 2 months and 3-6 generations are produced annually. The life span varies from a few days to a few weeks. They are most active morning and evening, resting during the hot part of the day on the underside of leaves near the ground, and usually feed on the nectar of flowers. The adult *Simulium* never enters houses in search of a blood meal. Only 2 of more than 50 species of black flies in North America cause severe losses of farm animals. The southern buffalo gnat is an annual spring pest in the lower Mississippi Valley and, in outbreak years, thousands of mules and cattle have been killed in Louisiana, Arkansas and Mississippi. Flooding of the lower Mississippi and its large southern tributaries appears to increase black fly numbers and annual spring outbreaks sometimes occur for 2 or 3 years following a major overflow. *Simulium arcticum* killed many cattle in Saskatchewan during 1913-1919 and 1944-1946[103] Swarms of *S columbaczense* on the shores of the River Danube in 1923 killed 20,000 horses, cattle, sheep, goats and pigs, as well as wild animals.[35]

Clinical Signs: Animals pastured in fields surrounded by hedges or woods are most often attacked. Dark-colored animals are particularly affected. The udder, scrotum, prepuce, inner surface of the thighs and upper forelimbs, mandibular lymph nodes, inside the ears, ventral abdomen, cranial thorax and body orifices are favored sites (Fig 32).[7,139]

Since black flies only live 2-3 weeks, clinical signs may subside until a new batch of flies hatch. Black fly dermatitis is more common in late spring and early summer, but is seen briefly following heavy rains and flooding during a mild winter.

Lesions take the form of hyperemic, hemorrhagic, edematous swellings associated with excoriations caused by scratching and rubbing. In addition to the painful bite, a heat-stable, alcohol- and ether-soluble toxin secreted by the insect causes cardiorespiratory problems. The toxin causes increased capillary permeability, with a consequent great loss of fluid from the circulatory system into the tissue spaces and body cavities.[103] General signs appear only when large numbers of the flies attack an animal and may be evident immediately or within a few hours of insect attack.

Affected animals are depressed, listless, weak and unsteady, and may lie down. The body temperature is normal or subnormal; fever occurs only in advanced or terminal cases. Respiration is rapid and accompanied by groaning. The pulse is weak and accelerated and, in advanced cases, cardiac palpitation is striking. When excessive swelling of the nasal or pharyngeal mucosae occurs as a result of bites, the animal may die suddenly of suffocation. Cold, edematous swellings sometimes develop on the neck, thorax and ventral abdomen. The appetite diminishes or is lost altogether. Pregnant

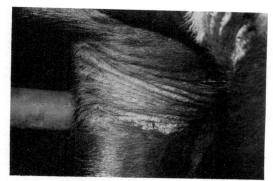

Fig 32. Foreleg lesions from bites of *Simulium*.

animals may abort. In very severe cases, paresis and paralysis develop, followed by death within 5-30 hours.[7] Petechiae are characteristic on the body parts mentioned. On the ventral abdomen, blood-encrusted areas of different sizes are common.

The females of some species of black flies have a special affinity for feeding on the inside of the ears, causing horses to shake their head and rub a lot. Scabs and bloody crusts are seen on the internal pinna (Fig 33). The condition commonly known as "ear fungus" or papillary acanthoma may be the result of this chronic irritation. After healing has taken place and the tenderness is gone, one to several grey or white plaques 1-20 mm in diameter can be found. Heavy keratin crusts overlie a pink, nonulcerated base. The plaques are not sensitive and constitute no problem for the horse but may annoy the owner since the lesions persist for the life of the horse.

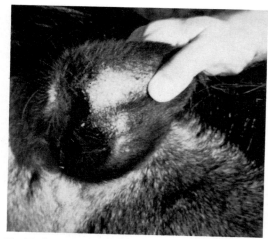

Fig 33. Crusts and small scabs on the inner aspect of the pinna from bites of *Simulium*.

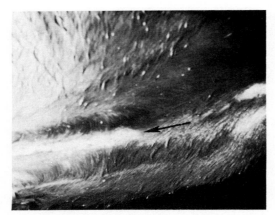

Fig 34. Hairless depigmented strip (arrow) on the linea alba from horn fly bites.

Treatment: Treatment of black-fly dermatitis is much the same as that for any other dermatitis caused by biting insects. Systemic corticosteroids offer relief until fly populations are controlled. Larvicidal treatment of streams is effective but ecologically unacceptable in most areas. Fly repellents must be applied to horses 2-3 times a day. On the ears, petroleum jelly is an effective mechanical barrier.[140]

Insecticides effective for other flies in the stable area are of some benefit. Stabling during daylight hours is beneficial. Complete control is difficult since adult flies may fly 15-20 km in a day.[141]

Stable-Fly Dermatitis

The stable fly, *Stomoxys calcitrans,* is about the size of the common house fly (6-7 mm), but is much more bothersome to horses. Horses and mules have reportedly lost 10-15% of their body weight during massive outbreaks of stable flies. In a 1912 Texas outbreak, 300 cattle, horses and mules were killed.[142]

During wet summers, stable fly population may reach plague proportions, especially in areas where manure disposal is inefficient. Injuries occur in horses galloping to evade fly bite. Affected horses have wheals up to 4 mm in diameter, with erect hair. If the hair is parted, a small area of edema with a minute central scab is evident. Lesions are most common on the back, chest, neck and especially the legs. Horses may stand in water to avoid bites until their joints are swollen and stiff.[143] In young or unexposed horses, the bites may be painful enough to cause self-mutilation.[92]

Since female stable flies lay eggs in manure and decaying straw or hay, especially if contaminated with urine, proper stall hygiene is important in fly control.[35] Insecticides and repellents are helpful. Stabling is beneficial since stable flies prefer a fairly strong light and are not usually seen in dark stables, except in autumn or rainy weather.[35] Along the Gulf Coast, where they are also called dog flies and beach flies, a sterile male release program has been successful experimentally.[64] Fly attractant panels treated with permethrin, as previously described, appear most promising.

Horn-Fly Dermatitis

The horn fly, *Haematobia irritans* in the US and *Lyperosia irritans* in many other parts of the world is mainly a pest of cattle.[35] It is morphologically very similar to the stable fly but only about half the size (about 4 mm). When large numbers of horn flies are present, an easily noticed feature is that their heads are all pointed toward the ground when feeding.

Lesions are caused when clusters of flies bite horses for their blood meal, which produces pruritus of varying degrees. A few days later, sharply defined areas of alopecia and scaling are noted on the sides of the neck and on the ventral abdomen (ventral midline dermatitis). Lesions on the ventral abdomen may reach 20-25 cm in diameter, while those on the neck are seldom more than 5 cm. Excoriation occurs if pruritus is severe. The ventral midline form of horn-fly dermatitis is sharply demarcated, while ventral lesions of onchocerciasis and/or *Culicoides* infestation are more diffuse (Fig 34).

Treatment with an antibiotic-corticosteroid ointment may be needed in severe cases, but insecticides and repellents usually suffice. Since horn flies spend most of their time on the host, control is easier than with stable flies.

Lice Infestation

Infestation by lice (pediculosis) is most common during the winter and early spring when horses have long, heavy coats. Both the biting louse, *Bovicola equi* and the sucking louse, *Haematopinus asini,* cause skin irritation. Affected horses rub and bite at their neck, flanks and tail head and may rub their jaw on fence rails. A rough coat with varying degrees of alopecia and self-inflicted lesions is typical.

Transmission through a herd is by direct contact primarily, but may be by tack and grooming equipment.

Diagnosis is by examination of the skin and parted hairs, with a hand lens if necessary.

Two treatments with water-based insecticide sprays or powders 2 weeks apart usually eradicate lice.[103]

Rhabditic Dermatitis

Pelodera (Rhabditis) strongyloides dermatitis is characterized by pruritic alopecia, papules and pustules, primarily on those areas in prolonged contact with contaminated bedding. Lesions are usually seen on the ventral aspect of the abdomen and thighs. Self-inflicted bite wounds may be present.[144]

The free-living causative nematode is ordinarily found in decaying organic material or moist soil.[145]

A horse with pruritic, pustular alopecia in the areas mentioned and confined in a filthy stall should be examined by taking scrapings for microscopic examination.

Correction of the unsanitary stabling situation may result in spontaneous recovery. If not, or in severe cases, bathing with selenium sulfide, followed by topical application of thiabendazole solution (Omnizole:Merck), has been successful.[145]

Chigger Infestation

Infestation with chiggers (trombiculosis) is uncommon, but has been reported in horses with mange-like lesions scattered over the body, especially on head, neck and legs. Scabs occurred in some areas and easily removed tufts of hair in others. Papules with erect hairs were also evident. Close examination revealed orange clusters of mites, *Euschoengastia latchmani*.[146] The reddish larvae of trombiculid mites (harvest mites) accumulate in small groups on the legs and abdomen, causing swelling and intense irritation.

Treatment with 5% lime sulfur washes and removal or insecticide treatment of infected bedding are effective.[61]

Trombicula autumnalis, the heel bug, is found in grass, hay and fodder. The mites prefer the mane, tail and feathers of the fetlock.[147]

Sarcoptic Mange

Although mange is comparatively rare in horses in the US, sarcoptic mange is probably the most common type. It is a purulent dermatitis caused by *Sarcoptes equi* and easily transmitted from one host to another, including horses, sheep, dogs, pigs, camels, rabbits and humans.[148]

The disease commences with an intense pruritus (characteristic of all mange) and the development of alopecic small patches. Papules are often seen on the neck, shoulders and head, gradually progressing to the entire body in untreated cases. Small vesicles are formed over and around the burrowing mites and the ser-

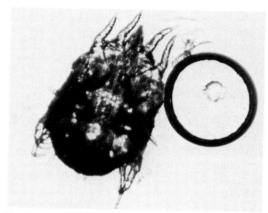

Fig 35. *Psoroptes* mite taken from the ear of a horse. The circular structure on the right is an air bubble.

ous discharge forms small, dry scabs. In chronic cases, rubbing and secondary infection cause thickened and wrinkled skin.[143]

Some horses exhibit an "itch reflex." When scratched over the withers, they tuck the nose close to the chest and make smacking noises with marked movement of the lips.[147] Pruritus is greatly increased when the body surface is warmer, as with exercise or blanketing.

Deep skin scrapings are necessary to recover this species of mite.

Psoroptic Mange

Psoroptic mange, which is caused by *Psoroptes equi*, is highly contagious and host-specific among horses (Fig 35). Infection is more easily transmitted at higher temperatures (above 25 C or 77 F). Horses with long, thick, dirty coats are more susceptible.[7]

Lesions are usually first noticed at the base of the mane, on the head under the foretop, at the base of the tail, or on any part of the body thickly covered with hair. The first sign is rubbed or broken hairs, followed by an eruption of small vesicles and papules. The vesicles rupture and serum collects in the hair to form crusts and scabs. The scabs are usually more moist than in sarcoptic mange.[143]

Psoroptic mites prefer skin folds, the throat and areas covered by long hair. They feed on lymph and serum but do not burrow deeply as do sarcoptic mites. With destruction of sebaceous glands, the skin becomes dry and cracked, and sweating may be diminished. Hematologic examination usually reveals eosinophilia.

Several horses in India infested with psoroptic mange had severe blood-red lesions mostly over the dorsum from the neck to the tail. Hair loss and pruritus were extensive and scabs were easily detached when the animals were brushed. Fresh lesions bled easily.[149]

Psoroptes mites also invade the ear canal, causing head-shaking, rubbing and droopy ears, but no lesions elsewhere on the body.

Chorioptic Mange

Chorioptic mange is caused by *Chorioptes equi* and is also known as foot or leg mange because the lesions are usually found on the lower limb around the foot and fetlock. Lesions occasionally extend up to the thigh and abdomen. The hindlegs are often affected and cause the horse to stomp and bite.[143] Chorioptic mange is most severe in winter and subsides almost to the point of recovery in summer.[103]

The mites live on the skin surface and do not penetrate. One case involved only the tail.[150]

Demodectic Mange

Demodectic mange is caused by *Demodex equi* and is comparatively rare in horses. A 7-month-old colt had lesions on the cranial part of the body, forelimbs and head. Alopecic patches were covered with large, bran-like scales.[151] In another case, the head, eyelids, neck, withers and hindquarters were involved. Other cases involved lesions starting at the neck and withers, and spreading to the back, forelimbs and head.[152] The coat was thin, with denuded areas and dry, scaly, roughened skin. Demodicosis may occur in an unusual pseudonodular form with sebaceous cysts that become suppurated. In thick-skinned or relatively resistant horses, the infection is limited to local folliculitis, with hypersecretion of the sebaceous glands.[153]

As in dogs, *Demodex* mites may be found on normal skin. Demodectic mange may be of the pustular or squamous form in the horse, the squamous form resembling that of the dog.[154]

Diagnosis: Demonstration of the mites in skin scrapings from the edge of a lesion, including adjoining apparently normal skin, is necessary for diagnosis. To make a scraping, grasp the skin between the thumb and forefinger and squeeze to evacuate the superficial skin glands. Pull up a fold of skin, the crest of which should be scraped until lymph or serum seeps out. Mineral oil is usually placed on the skin to collect scrapings, but 10% KOH may be better.[155]

Since finding mites in scrapings is difficult, several methods should be employed to ensure success: direct microscopic examination of a wet preparation cleared in 10% KOH; microscopic examination of centrifuged sediment of material macerated in cold 10% KOH for 24 hours; and flotation fluid (saturated sugar or saline) is added to the centrifuge tube containing the sediment produced by maceration and centrifugation. The material is mixed and allowed to stand for 12-24 hours. The surface film is transferred by a flat-ended glass rod to a clean, grease-free slide and a cover slip added. Examination of the material, free of the majority of epidermal and other debris, facilitates identification of mites.[155]

Another technic for handling skin scrapings is to place the debris in a small tube or beaker, add 10% KOH, stir and heat gently. Add the mixture to a saturated sugar solution in centrifuge tubes and spin until the mites and ova float to the surface. Examine a drop or 2 of the surface solution on a slide under a coverslip.[10]

Corridors containing female mites and eggs may be seen in the epidermis of biopsy sections on histologic examination and thereby afford a diagnosis when scrapings are negative.

The diagnostic procedures may at first appear somewhat superfluous. However, in one case in Minnesota, only 9 of 42 scrapings were positive and a total of only 12 mites were observed.[151] One or 2 routine scrapings would likely have been inadequate.

Treatment: In addition to general supportive therapy, such as good nutrition and hygiene, bathing and application of an effective miticide are the usual treatment. In recent years, chlorinated hydrocarbons, especially 0.01-0.03% lindane (gamma benzene hexachloride), have been used.[156] Benzyl benzoate is often added to the lindane preparation. Also recommended are diazinon and fenchlorphos applied 2 or more times at 10- to 14-day intervals.

In several cases of psoroptic mange, good results were obtained by bathing with soap, water and NaHCO$_3$, followed by the application of a 1% water emulsion of malathion to the dried horse with a brush. This was repeated every 3 days for 8 applications. No mites were found after the fifth treatment.[149]

Since mange can be spread by contaminated equipment and stables, disinfection with 2-3% cresol USP for 2-3 hours is also important. The mites are also susceptible to temperatures above 70 C (158 F) for an hour.

Dioxathion 1% (Navadel:Delmar) in cottonseed oil or lindane 1% in cottonseed oil is effective for otic *Psoroptes*.[157]

Ear-Tick Infestation

Several species of ticks (spinose ear tick, *Otobius megnini*; tropical horse tick, *Dermacentor nitens*) live deep in the ears and are not dislodged by dipping, dusting or spraying. Alopecia is limited to the area of the ear and may be inconspicuous. Ear-tick infestation may also cause ataxia and other neurologic signs.

Under proper restraint, horses may be effectively treated for ear ticks with 1 part lindane (25% emulsifiable concentrate or wettable powder), 12 parts cottonseed oil, and 12 parts pure pine oil. Add the cottonseed oil to the pure pine oil and mix. Add the lindane and mix thoroughly. Apply deep in the ear canal with a spring-bottom oil can. To prevent injury to the ear, cut off the spout to a 2-inch length. Slip over the oiler spout a 2½-inch length of flexible rubber tubing of ⅜-inch inside diameter. The tubing should extend ½ inch beyond the edge of the spout. After application, massage the ear to diffuse the mixture. This remedy dissolves ear wax, kills ticks and protects against reinfestation for at least 3 weeks.[68] Malathion, coumaphos and ronnel are also effective.[143] The use of 1% dioxathion in cottonseed oil has been recommended in Florida, where piroplasmosis is a problem.[157]

Diseases Characterized by Nonpruritic Alopecia

Dermatophytosis (Ringworm)

Dermatophytosis is a superficial fungal infection of the skin, hair and/or hooves, caused mainly by dermatophytes of the genera *Microsporum* and *Trichophyton*. Synonyms for this disease are ringworm, dermatomycosis and girth itch.

Cause: Five dermatophytes cause over 95% of equine cases. *Trichophyton equinum* is by far the most common.[9,158] The incidence of the other 4, *Trichophyton mentagrophytes, Trichophyton verrucosum, Microsporum gypseum* and *Microsporum canis*, is variable, depending on exposure to infected cattle (*T verrucosum*), humans or dogs (*M canis*), or geographic location.

Epizootiology: Natural infection results from direct contact with infected animals or humans. Indirect infection may be acquired from infected grooming equipment, tack, blankets or clothing. Ringworm in horses also has been transmitted by infected rats. Warm, damp, dirty, overcrowded, poorly ventilated stables encourage mycotic infection. Conversely, sufficient sun and fresh air attenuate the growth of dermatophytes.

Young, thin-skinned horses are particularly prone to ringworm. The incubation period after natural infection is generally a week to a month. When conditions are particularly favorable, the incubation period may be shortened to 4-6 days. Minor trauma of the skin is a prerequisite for the introduction of infective spores into the horny layer or hair follicles.

Animals treated excessively with antibiotics may lose their previous resistance to fungal infection. Dietary inadequacies also predispose animals to ringworm infection.

The ringworm fungus lives only in devitalized, superkeratinized skin and does not penetrate the deeper, living skin layers unless there is conversion to a yeast phase. It is most abundant in hair follicles. The fungus causes dermatitis and alopecia. When the hair shafts themselves are penetrated, they become brittle and break or split, leaving short stumps. Dermatophytic lesions spread in a characteristic circular fashion. Peripheral regions are the youngest, while there may be healing in the center, even without treatment.[159]

In an English study of ringworm incidence, specimens were examined during an 11-year period from 976 horses on 908 premises.[160] Ringworm was diagnosed in 303 animals from 251 premises at a rate of 31.1%. *Trichophyton equinum* and *Microsporum equinum (canis)* were primarily isolated. There was a marked seasonal distribution, with 70.5% of the outbreaks occurring between early September and the end of January. During this time, 47% of all specimens were positive for ringworm.[160] *Dermatophilus congolensis* infection in 92 horses on 70 premises (9.4%), cutaneous filariasis in 3 horses, and mite or lice infestation in 10 horses (1%) were also diagnosed. One US survey revealed that most infections occurred in the summer and fall, while another reported infections as more prevalent during colder months.[161,162]

Clinical Signs: In general, a similar clinical picture is produced by all equine ringworm agents, with minor variations in the severity of lesions, contagiousness of the infections, and the manner of hair invasion.

The clinical features of typical dermatophytosis include multiple foci of scaling and crusting, alopecia, variable pruritus, and peripheral spread (Fig 36). The lesions may initially resemble fly bites, but in a day or 2 the hair falls out and a scaly, crusty alopecia appears.[9] Lesions may expand for 4-8 weeks and then regress as the horse develops an immune response.

A description of an epizootic in French artillery horses deserves repeating: "The animals

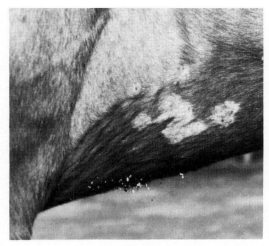

Fig 36. Early "girth itch" lesions from *Trichophyton*.

presented a number of ringworm plaques. Isolated lesions were scattered over the hindquarters and shoulders, others were grouped together on the posterior part of the saddle area and some were confluent. The isolated lesions first appeared as swellings and were perceptible by touch before they could be seen. Some days later, the plaques became visible because the hairs were matted and disordered in these areas. At this time the hair came out easily. Slight traction detached most of the infected hairs in a single block, the remainder being held at their base by a scaly crust. The skin in the area was at first moist and had a rosy and greyish cast. Soon afterwards, the plaque itself became dry, becoming powdery or granular and dark slate-grey in color. The lesions enlarged through the loss of peripheral hairs. They were most numerous in the saddle and girth area and formed large patches by their confluence."[163]

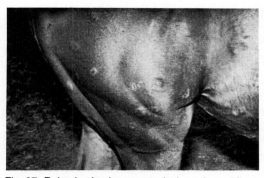

Fig 37. Raised, circular, crusty lesions from *Microsporum gypseum* infection.

Lesions may occur elsewhere, including the pasterns, where it may be erroneously called "scratches" or "grease heel."

Trichophyton equinum is highly resistant to destruction and remained viable for 18 months when kept in a dry test tube.[91] Therefore, hair samples may be mailed to a laboratory for diagnosis. In one survey, *T equinum* was found on the left girth region 9:1 over the right side.[164] Early lesions may be evident only as broken hairs rather than bare areas.

Microsporum gypseum normally inhabits soil and as such is inoculated into insect bites when horses roll in the soil.[165] Circular, raised lesions with heavy crusts and matted hair are typical (Fig 37). More inflammation and exudation is evident than with other dermatophyte infections and lesions are more likely to be on the legs or thorax than at the girth area.[158] Infection by *M gypseum* seems to be more common in summer and fall.

Although many dermatophytes are less contagious than commonly believed, *Microsporum canis* is the most likely dermatophyte to be highly contagious.[7,60]

Lesions caused by *Trichophyton mentagrophytes* are located mostly on the head, neck, at the base of the tail and on the extremities.[91] It is contagious to humans.

Diagnosis: A KOH preparation is a rapid method that is useful only after one has considerable practice and experience in its interpretation. The equipment necessary is 10% KOH, microscope slides and coverslips, an alcohol or Bunsen burner, thumb forceps and a scalpel handle and blade. Hair from early lesions are deposited on a slide. Several drops of 10% KOH are applied, a coverslip added and the slide gently heated for 15-20 seconds. The preparation should not be boiled. Alternatively, it may be allowed to stand for 20-30 minutes at room temperature.

An excellent result is obtained if the mount is placed on the microscope lamp for gentle heating. The preparation is ready for examination in 15-20 minutes and the structures are better preserved. A fungal stain is made by adding 7.3 g KOH to 73 ml Parker's permanent blue-black ink. The solution should be centrifuged to remove impurities.[9]

Mycotic infection, especially on glabrous skin, is identified by the presence of branching mycelia. Hair shafts should be examined at low and high power for spores. Ectothrix spores, in a sheath or chain outside the hair shaft, occur in *Microsporum* and *Trichophyton* infections.

Although some professional mycologists can diagnose 70% of fungal infections by the direct microscopic method, it is doubtful if a clinician with less special training could do so. In a study of 132 horses, 9 were positive on microscopic examination and 31 were positive on culture.[166]

With the use of fungal culture media, proper preparation of the lesion and correct inoculation of the medium are very important if confusing results are to be avoided. The following guidelines reduce the chance for error:

1. Pick the site for culture carefully. Look for frayed, broken or distorted hairs. The periphery of the lesion is usually the best place for sample collection.

2. Clean the hair at the site gently with water and dry with an absorptive material to decrease the amount of saprophytic fungal and bacterial contamination. This step may be omitted if the horse is well groomed.

3. Using a hemostat or thumb forceps, remove only a small portion of hair and scales from the lesion. Large amounts of hair and crust often are overgrown with contaminants, so avoid gathering excess material.

4. Press the sample onto the medium, but do not bury it.

5. Replace the culture container cap, but make certain that it remains loose on the jar for air exchange. A tightly closed lid inhibits culture growth and interferes with indicator color change.

6. Label the sample with the date, owner's name, and lesion site if more than one sample is collected.

7. Incubate at room temperature (22.2-30 C or 72-86 F) in a dark environment. In a few cases, incubation of a second sample at 37 C is rewarding.

8. All cultures should be observed daily for indicator color change and colony growth.

Trichophyton equinum requires niacin for growth and *T verrucosum* requires thiamin and inositol. Commercial indicator media do not supply this need. However, one can easily overcome this problem by applying 2 drops of injectable B-complex to the slant before applying the hair sample.[167]

Culturing lesions that have undergone treatment with antifungal agents is not very successful. Antifungal medication interferes with fungal culture growth and may produce false-negative results.

Indicator media are 98.6% accurate in the detection of human dermatophytes.[168] Experiments at the veterinary dermatology labora-

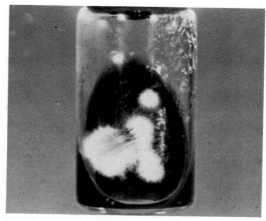

Fig 38. White, fluffy colonies on the cherry-red dermatophyte medium 6 days after inoculation.

tory of Purdue University resulted in approximately the same accuracy of diagnosis in dogs and cats.[169] A positive culture should change the color of the medium from amber to cherry red before extensive colony growth is present, usually in less than 10 days, sometimes as early as 4-7 days (Fig C6). Positive cultures have light cream or white fluffy colonies (Fig 38). Saprophyte colonies are usually brown, grey, green or yellow.[170]

A Wood's light may also be used in the diagnosis of ringworm caused by *M canis*. A Wood's light consists of ultraviolet light filtered through nickel oxide. A positive response to Wood's light examination is a bright yellow-green to green-blue color not unlike that seen by shining the light on the numerals of a fluorescent watch face. It is very important to note that medication, dirt, petrolatum and scales may fluoresce and give false-positive reactions.

Fungal fluorescence is rare in horses. *Microsporum canis* is the only major dermatophyte to produce this phenomenon.

Treatment: Most cases of dermatophytosis regress spontaneously in 2-3 months unless the horse is immunodeficient. To reduce chances for spread and to shorten the course of the disease, topical and/or systemic treatments are usually employed. If possible, all lesions and a 2.5-cm area surrounding the lesion should be clipped closely. (The clippers must be disinfected before subsequent use.) The entire horse is bathed with povidone iodine shampoo and the lather is allowed to stay on 15 minutes. After the animal is rinsed, a solution of captan (1-2 oz 50% powder to 1 gal water) is applied to the lesions with a brush and is sponged on the

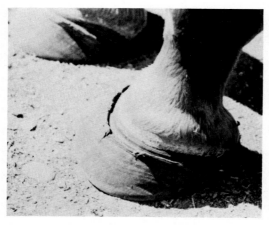

Fig 39. Cracked hooves in selenium toxicosis. (Courtesy of Veterinary Practice Publishing Co.)

rest of the body. The solution is allowed to dry on the horse. This should be repeated daily for a week, then 2-3 times a week until the lesions are healed. The application of 5% lime sulfur solution also gives good results.[61]

Various commercial keratolytic preparations that contain salicylic acid or undecylenic acid help destroy fungi. Thiabendazole has antifungal properties and can be used as a 4% solution in saline. It is not irritating to conjunctivae.[171] Efficacy is improved if applied repeatedly in 90% DMSO.

Most small animal antifungal preparations can be used but are often too expensive for use in horses because of the number and size of lesions. If economy is critical, sodium hypochlorite in a 6% solution can be used on the horse and for disinfection.[172]

Local treatment of lesions with iodine is an old effective treatment but staining associated with its use may be undesirable. Systemic therapy with griseofulvin is used in stubborn cases but it is somewhat expensive. The proper dosage of griseofulvin for a horse has not been established. Most veterinarians use 2.5 mg/lb/day PO or 17.5 g by stomach tube once a week. The latter schedule may be of doubtful value since, in humans, griseofulvin is detected in the outer layers of skin within hours after administration and quickly disappears after administration of the drug is discontinued.[9] In view of the increased dosage of griseofulvin necessary for dogs, 2.5 mg/lb may be woefully inadequate. Response to griseofulvin at low dosages or during short-term treatment (1-2 weeks) may actually be due to acquired immunity. Griseofulvin should be given for 30-60 days if required. Griseofulvin should not be used in pregnant mares. Topical therapy and clipping are usually necessary despite griseofulvin therapy.

In addition to the use of therapeutic agents, environmental factors, such as overcrowding and filth, should be corrected. Disinfection of equipment, pens and feed bunks is vital in reducing spread. Povidone iodine, 6% sodium hypochlorite, 3% cresol, 5% lime sulfur, benzalconium chloride, 3% captan, and lime (1%)-copper sulfate (1.5%) are just a few of many effective preparations for disinfection of premises.

Prevention of ringworm by vaccination may be possible in the near future. A vaccine against T verrucosum has already been tested in Russia on 1.4 million young calves and was 96% effective. Two IM injections were given 10 days apart.[173]

Patchy Shedding

Patchy shedding in the spring alarms owners but is of little consequence. For unknown reasons, some horses shed large patches that leave alopecic areas as large as 20 cm. The skin is absolutely normal in appearance and negative on fungal culture. There is no pruritus. New hair appears in about 3 weeks when the rest of the coat sheds normally. This seasonal alopecia is often diagnosed and treated as a fungal infection. A similar alopecia sometimes occurs a few days after a very high fever during respiratory disease.

Mercury Poisoning

Mercury poisoning due to ingestion of mercury-treated seed grain caused complete loss of hair from the body first and finally from the mane and tail. There was no abnormality of the hooves and only slightly scaly skin. Daily doses of 4 g potassium iodide for 14 days, coupled with stabling and blanketing, resulted in new hair growth in several months.[61]

Selenium Poisoning

Selenium (Se) toxicosis was first recorded in the US in 1860.[174] The acute disease is caused by consumption of large amounts of plants that require Se for metabolism. Signs of acute Se intoxication reflect involvement of the CNS, GI tract, cardiovascular system and respiratory system. Death may occur in 3-72 hours.[175]

Subacute Se toxicosis causes "blind staggers" from liver damage and subsequent effect on the brain. Chronic Se toxicosis ("alkali disease") causes thinning of the mane and tail ("bobtail disease") and transverse cracks in the hooves (Fig 39). In some horses, rear limb and, later, front limb lameness is the first sign. Great pain is evident upon palpation of the coronary band. In about 14 days, a break in the coronary band may be noticed. The crack may grow out completely or the hoof may be shed.[174] In some cases, body hair as well as mane and tail hair is lost. Serum sorbitol dehydrogenase and alkaline phosphatase levels are elevated due to liver damage.

Selenium intoxication may occur in as short as 3 weeks after an animal is placed on high-Se soil. Seleniferous soils and vegetation are found in the western US from North Dakota to southwestern Texas and west to the Pacific Ocean. Montana, Wyoming, Nebraska, North and South Dakota, and Colorado are states in which selenosis is a serious problem.[176] Water usually is not a source of Se intoxication except in isolated instances; water in most such areas is unpalatable.[176] However, chronic poisoning by Se salts in water containing 0.5-2 ppm Se has been reported.[177]

Chronic Se intoxication may result from consumption of cereals or grass grown in seleniferous areas or from plants that accumulate Se. Seleniferous soils should be suspected if plants of the species *Astragalus* (milk vetch), *Xylorhiza* (woody aster), *Oonopsis* (goldenweed) and *Stanleya* (prince's plume) are present.[176]

Selenium intoxication seems to be worse in dry years. Only parts of a farm or pasture may be dangerous.

Diagnosis: While loss of mane and tail hair in lame horses with a transverse separation and transverse corrugations of the hooves is highly suggestive of Se toxicosis, a definitive diagnosis must be reached by testing for abnormal amounts of Se in the blood (1-4 ppm), hair (5 ppm) or hooves (8-20 ppm).[174,177] Hair samples must be from hairs that grew after Se intake; therefore, the ends of long hairs are of little value.[174] The tolerance limit of dietary Se is considered to be 5 ppm.[177] The third phalanx is normal radiographically.

The disease has been produced experimentally by feeding an 826-lb gelding 72 lb *Morinda reticulata* (Indian mulberry) over a 56-day period. Analysis showed the 72 lb contained 7.3 g Se. Selenium levels in the mane, tail, hoof and liver were 12 ppm, 6 ppm, 6-8 ppm and 2.6 ppm, respectively.[178]

Treatment: Good nursing is an important part of treatment for Se intoxication. Deep bedding for recumbent horses, phenylbutazone to relieve pain, and removal of the patient from the Se source are imperative. Increased dietary protein is beneficial.[174] Drinking water containing 5 ppm inorganic arsenic is recommended and salt containing 40 ppm arsenic is also useful to prevent toxicity. Dietary arsanilic acid at 50-100 ppm has been used prophylactically in calves and pigs. Adult horses have been treated for toxicity with 4-5 g naphthalene PO for 5 days and another 5-day treatment after a 5-day interval.[177]

Disease Characterized by Mats or Clumps of Hair

Any dermatophytosis causes lesions of this category before the development of alopecia; *Microsporum gypseum* infection is an especially good example.

Dermatophilosis

Dermatophilosis (streptothricosis) is an acute or chronic exudative dermatitis, primarily of horses, cattle, sheep, goats and rarely humans, caused by *Dermatophilus congolensis*, an actinomycete (not a fungus). It is also known as "rain scald."[179] Dermatophilosis is more common during the fall and winter, and almost always follows periods of exposure to prolonged overcast and rainy weather, especially when rainfall levels are well above average.[180-184] Water-soaked skin is more easily abraded and probably more susceptible to infection. Concurrent attack by ectoparasites, especially stable and house flies, constitutes sufficient trauma.[185] Abrasion of the skin is necessary to produce the disease.[186] Dermatophilosis may be spread by using contaminated clippers or by wetting the

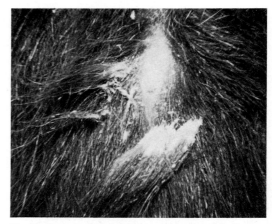

Fig 40. Typical clump of hair easily epilated in *D congolensis* infection.

CHAPTER 16

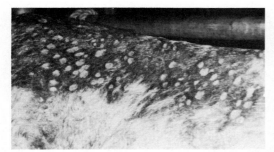

Fig 41. "Rain scald" (dermatophilosis) on the back, after mat removal.

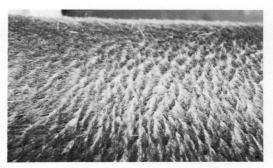

Fig 42. "Paint-brush" effect in diffuse dermatophilosis.

lesions, which results in the release of infective zoospores.[9]

Clinical Signs: The term "rain scald" relates to the predisposing rainy weather, after which focal lesions appear (Fig 40). Lesions are frequently found on the dorsum (rump, loin, saddle area) and may give the impression that large drops have scalded the skin, causing an exudate that mats the hair together in the form of plaques. Such plaques are usually less than 2 cm in diameter but may coalesce to cover much larger areas. They may be tender to the touch in the acute stage but are not pruritic. Removal of a matted tuft of hair reveals a moist, pink, bleeding lesion. The concave undersurface of the scab is wet with varying amounts of yellow to green pus or grey gelatinous exudate. There may be no exudate on the

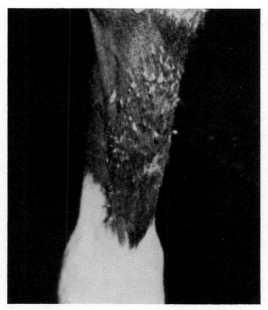

Fig 43. Clumping of hair caused by folliculitis in *D congolensis* infection.

underside of scabs on old lesions. Removal of scabs from older lesions reveals a smooth or scaly alopecia (Fig 41). Pain is often exhibited when crusts are removed early in the disease. Developing lesions not yet visible may be palpated by rubbing the palm over the coat.

A diffuse form of dermatophilosis in the croup and/or loin area results in hundreds of clusters of matted hairs that produce a paint-brush effect (Fig 42).

Various forms of dermatophilosis affect the legs (Fig 43). In one report on a condition called "aphis," white-faced, stocking-legged horses were first affected on the unpigmented areas of the skin.[186] After 3-4 days, there was a gradual spread to pigmented areas. Involvement of all 4 legs in a foal stabled in a muddy lot has been reported.[182] The lesions were described as a moist exudative dermatitis extending as high as the shoulder and gaskin, into the flank and along the ventral abdomen. There was thickening and wrinkling of the flank skin and generalized erythema of all affected skin. In another outbreak, the principal areas involved were the caudal pastern region, coronet, bulb of the heel and dorsal face of the rear cannon. The front cannons were not affected. Fetlock edema was also noted. Mares grazing on flooded creek and river flats had foot lesions; mares on stony hillside paddocks did not. Infection of the rear cannons only was thought to be caused by mud and cinders thrown by the front feet while running.[183] The pastern dermatitis is similar, if not identical, to early "scratches."

Diagnosis: Tufts of hair, matted at their base to form a scab with a concave undersurface and exudate coating, are fairly diagnostic. Similar lesions are observed with *M gypseum* infection.

Diagnosis should be made by laboratory examination. Smears from pus or from material of the inner scab surface of the scab crushed on a slide are good sources for isolating and identifying the causative organism. The crushed material should be diluted with sterile water and air-dried, heat-dried or fixed with methyl alcohol for 30 seconds, then stained with undiluted Giemsa or gram stain for 10 minutes. Under oil immersion, the organism appears as branching filaments dividing both transversely and longitudinally to form pockets of up to 8 coccoid cells. Demonstration of the characteristic filaments in stained smears is diagnostic (Fig C7). Parallel rows of coccoid bodies in one filament is adequate for diagnosis. Old lesions may show fragmentation of the filaments into tetrad, diplococcal and chain-like groups of gram-positive cocci. Occasionally individual motile cocci appear. Preparations from the inner surface of freshly collected scabs in acute cases often contain the organism in pure culture. In chronic cases, cultural examination is usually unsatisfactory because of the high degree of contamination.

Cultures on blood agar contain rough brown colonies that resemble drops of applesauce.[86] *Dermatophilus* does not grow on Sabouraud's medium or phenol red indicator media.[187,188] Brain-heart infusion agar is recommended for culture.

Treatment: More important than the drug used is the removal of infected, "ripe" scabs. However, if scab removal is very painful, systemic antibiotics and iodine shampoos should be used for several days prior to attempts at scab removal. *Dermatophilus* persists in the scab for as long as 42 months.[189]

Of equal importance is keeping the patient dry and protected from biting insects. *In vitro*, the organism is sensitive to griseofulvin, penicillin, dihydrostreptomycin, chlortetracycline, oxytetracycline and chloramphenicol. Other preparations, such as 1% gentian violet in alcohol, 5% salicylic acid and alcohol, Iodex ointment, tincture of iodine, 1-3% copper sulfate solution, copper naphthalene, quaternary ammonium compounds and 5% lime sulfur dip, have been used; however, evaluation of treatment is difficult since some horses recover spontaneously.

In an extensive outbreak in Australia, a topical aqueous solution of 0.25% chloramphenicol worked best. If deep fissures were present on the legs, the chloramphenicol was mixed in cod liver oil.[182]

The most popular antibiotic treatment is IM procaine penicillin at 22,000 IU/kg and dihydrostreptomycin at 11 mg/kg BID for 5-7 days.

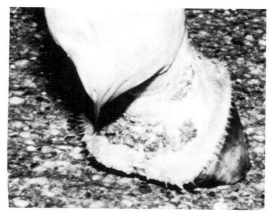

Fig 44. "Scratches" caused by *Staphylococcus aureus* infection.

Scratches

Scratches ("grease heel," "mud fever," "cracked heels") is a seborrheic dermatitis of the caudal heel and pastern seen most often in breeds with long hair in those areas under muddy or unsanitary conditions or when rough stubble in pastures traumatizes the heels and pasterns. Grit particles on some track surfaces cause the initial irritation, allowing a variety of organisms to gain entry and establish an infection. "Heelbug" mite infestation is another inciting factor. However, the disease may occur in the absence of these predisposing factors. Pain, swelling, alopecia, exuding serum and eventually ulceration usually begin at the heel. Serum exudate ("grease") mats the erect hairs (Fig 44). Some horses may be lame or

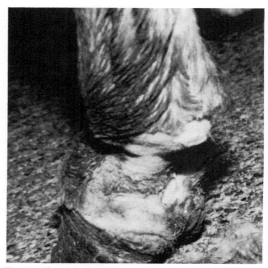

Fig 45. "Cracked heels," a severe form of scratches.

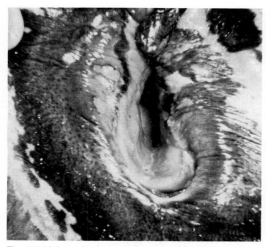

Fig 46. Vulvar depigmentation and ulcerations of the vaginal mucosa in coital vesicular exanthema.

have a stringhalt-type gait. In chronic cases, the skin may crack and have a foul odor (Fig 45). Occasionally, vegetative granulomatous growths ("grapes") appear from hypertrophy of the dermal papillae.[103]

Treatment: A mild soap and warm water are used to soak scabs and mats, which are removed by clipping after rinsing and drying. Astringents, such as McKillip's powder (Med-Tech), or mild astringent lotions, such as white lotion (zinc and lead sulfate) or calamine lotion, are applied in cases of serum transudation. A thiabendazole-DMSO paste or sulfapyridine cream has also been used successfully in such cases. Use of antibiotic-corticosteroid ointment under a bandage is recommended if the skin is irritated. Systemic sulfapyridine or antibiotics are beneficial in complicated cases.

Granulomatous masses or "grapes" should be removed by surgery and/or electrocautery. Early development of such masses may be controlled with the application of corticosteroid-antibiotic ointments.

The recurrence of scratches may be prevented by keeping heel and pastern hair short and by application of an antibiotic udder ointment prior to exercise.

Ringworm

Microsporum gypseum infection may closely resemble the focal form of dermatophilosis. Stained smears and dermatophyte culture may be necessary to differentiate them. *Microsporum gypseum* infection has been described (see Dermatophytosis).

Staphylococcal Folliculitis (see above)

Disease Characterized by Vesicles

Equine Coital Exanthema

Equine coital exanthema is a contagious disease of the male and female genitalia caused by a herpesvirus (probably type 3). It is most commonly spread at breeding but may be spread by biting insects, contaminated grooming equipment or inhalation of fomites.[190]

Infection with the herpesvirus does not result in clinical disease in every case. The virus may persist in affected horses over long periods. Immune carriers may have no clinical signs.[191]

Clinical Signs: Signs in the mare may appear as early as 7 days after coitus and consist of a purulent discharge and scab formation on the labia.[192] Shallow erosions with hyperemic bases are revealed when the scab is rubbed off (Fig 46). The erosions fill with exudate and heal rapidly, leaving a white scar for 3-4 weeks.[193]

Some mares initially have small vesicles 1-3 mm in diameter on the vulvar and vaginal mucosae. The vesicles become pustular and progress to small ulcers. The vulva becomes swollen and itchy, the buttocks are stained by a whitish discharge, urination is frequent, and switching of the tail is common. Signs subside after a few days to leave nonpigmented spots that persist for several weeks.[194] One infected mare had a single lesion at the same site on the vulva on 2 occasions about 30 weeks apart.[190] Intrauterine inoculation of a pregnant mare with equine herpesvirus type 3 produced small raised lesions on the clitoris. A 6- to 7-month fetus was aborted and had disseminated focal cutaneous lesions 0.1-1 cm in diameter.[195]

In the stallion, lesions may vary from only a few hemorrhagic 1- to 3-mm erosions to progressive lesions on the penile shaft and glans as described for the mare. Fertility in one stallion was only 30%.[191]

Diagnosis: Proof of exposure and/or subclinical infection is established by serum-neutralization testing. Rising titers on serial samples indicate active infection. Serum-neutralizing antibodies are present by the time lesions are fully developed. Virus isolation from vaginal swabs and vulvar skin scrapings permits a more definitive diagnosis. The virus has not been recovered from semen. Similar but more superficial erosions resulting in white plaques have been produced by the equine rhinopneumonitis virus.[192]

Treatment: Treatment is usually not necessary since the lesions heal rapidly with enforced sexual rest for 21-30 days. Both sexes may remain inapparent carriers. The disease may reappear the next season or may not be apparent for several years or ever again.

Vesicular Stomatitis

Two similar but serologically distinct viruses produce macules, vesicles and erosions that appear successively on the buccal mucosa or on the skin at the coronet. Cattle, hogs, several wild species and humans are also affected by these viruses. Wooded pastures with streams and wetland favor the spread of the disease. During a 30-year period, 90% of the reported cases occurred in August and September. Rather than direct contact, vector transmission, perhaps by mosquitoes, stable flies, horn flies and tropical sand flies, may be involved in dissemination of vesicular stomatitis.

Clinical Signs: Following a 1- to 3-day incubation period, salivation, slight depression and polydipsia occur. Vesicles on the tongue usually coalesce before rupturing; the resulting erosion may cover half the tongue. The wound is deep, raw and bleeding and has shreds of dead epithelium at the margin.

Vesicles at the coronary band are painful enough to cause lameness. Separation of the hoof wall may occasionally cause sloughing of the entire hoof. Both foot and mouth lesions may be observed in a single animal.

Diagnosis: The clinical signs are highly suggestive of vesicular stomatitis and are confirmed by virus isolation. A bit of epithelium, saliva or vesicular fluid from an infected horse can be used to inoculate a mouse or chicken embryo, which is observed for effects of the viruses. Fluid from lesions can be used as an antigen source for a complement-fixation test, the results of which are available in hours.

Serologic testing is also used. Within 10-14 days after infection, neutralizing and complement-fixing antibodies may be detected in the blood. The titer of both increases for 2-4 weeks and persists at a high level.

Treatment: Treatment is mainly supportive unless there is secondary infection that necessitates antibiotic therapy. Recovery is usually prompt and complete. Stabling and insect eradication drastically reduce infection.

The virus has been inactivated in the laboratory by treatment with 1% formalin for 15 minutes. A longer period or heavier treatment is suggested in the field since the virus resists physical and chemical agents longer in the presence of body substances and fluids.[196]

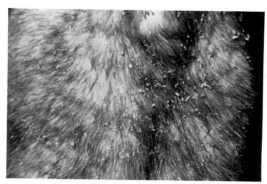

Fig 47. Severe scaling on the chest in idiopathic seborrhea.

Mercury Poisoning

Mercury poisoning was seen years ago when mercurial compounds were used as antiseptics, laxatives and skin preparations. Clinical signs generally appear several days after exposure in the form of vesicles and pustules that progress to crusted pruritic lesions (see Chapter 7).

Disease Characterized by Scaling and Crustiness

Many of the conditions previously described cause scaling and crustiness, especially dermatophytosis. The following diseases should also be considered:

Seborrhea

Seborrhea is really a sign caused by hyperkeratinization and/or hyperproduction of sebum and is not a disease *per se.* However, seborrhea is most often observed as a reflection of various internal disorders, the diagnosis of which may be difficult. Fortunately, generalized seborrhea is relatively rare.

Clinical Signs: Early or mild cases are characterized by scaling and epidermal flakes in a generalized, symmetric pattern, with little involvement of the extremities (Fig 47). Some horses have seborrheic scaling of the mane and tail only. Pruritus is absent. The signs are somewhat worse in winter.

In severe cases, the scale accumulates and is held together by sebum to form heavy crusts, sometimes 1-1.5 cm thick. Considerable loss of condition is usually evident despite a good appetite. In some areas, the crusts may peel off to leave areas of alopecia up to 10 x 20 cm in size. Pruritus is absent or mild. Hyperkeratosis is frequently seen in chronic cases (Fig 48).

Diagnosis: An attempt should be made to discover the basic underlying cause of sebor-

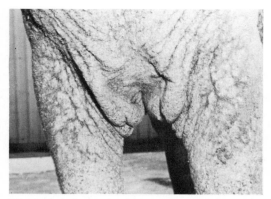

Fig 48. Hyperkeratosis and severe crusting in chronic seborrhea.

rhea. Serum evaluation for radioimmunoassay T_3 and T_4 levels may reveal hypothyroidism (T_3<60 µ/dl, T_4<1.5 µ/dl). A liver profile (sorbitol dehydrogenase, alkaline phosphatase, serum electrophoresis, BSP clearance, biopsy) may incriminate chronic hepatitis. Malabsorption may be diagnosed by absorption tests for glucose, xylose and fatty acids (see Chapter 13). Serum sex hormone analysis is also indicated. However, few reports are available since hormone assay has only recently become available.

Temporary seborrhea sometimes occurs during convalescence from febrile illnesses. Vitamin A deficiency can theoretically produce seborrhea but is rare unless horses are fed exclusively on poor-quality, old hay or some very unusual diet. Examination for dermatophytes and ectoparasites should also be performed.

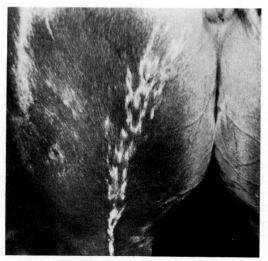

Fig 50. Generalized scaling in pemphigus foliaceous.

Undoubtedly there are other causes yet to be elucidated. Autoimmune seborrhea is confirmed by immunofluorescent tests of skin biopsies.

Treatment: If a specific diagnosis has been established, therapy should be directed accordingly. Regular use of sulfur-based keratolytic shampoos is beneficial. Sulfur promotes exfoliation and has keratolytic properties. Other keratolytics include selenium sulfide, salicylic acid, coal tar derivatives and polythionates.[70] For systemic treatment a saturated solution of sodium thiosulfate is given in the feed at 1 tsp TID for a week and repeated after 2 weeks off medication. Response to nonspecific treatment is generally poor to fair.

Linear Keratosis

Linear keratosis is readily apparent because of the nature of the lesion(s), which consist of one or more on linear areas of alopecia and keratinous crusting on the lateral aspect of the neck, shoulder or thorax (Fig C8). No exact etiology has been determined. In one case, the ventral progression of lesions suggested larval migration. Lesions appear most commonly in Quarter Horses 1-5 years old.[19]

Clinical Signs: The hyperkeratotic lesions consist of one or more linear areas of alopecia and keratinous crusting, 3-5 mm wide and 5-50 cm long, on the lateral neck or thorax and occasionally in other locations (Fig 49). Inflammation is minimal and there is no pruritus. The lesions may persist indefinitely.

Treatment: Keratolytic preparations (coal tar and sulfur ointments and shampoo, salicylic acid, undecylenic acid) are of temporary benefit if used regularly. A larvicidal dose of thiabendazole (440 mg/kg orally for 2 consecutive days) may be of benefit in early cases.

Pemphigus Foliaceus

Pemphigus foliaceus, an autoimmune disease in which autoantibodies are formed to the intercellular cement, result in cell separation (acantholysis) just deep to the stratum corneum.

Clinical Signs: Generalized scaling and crusting are the most outstanding signs, which are preceded by undetected vesicle formation and rupture (Fig 50). Depression is present in 80% of cases. Lesions are usually first apparent about the head and upper neck. Limb edema is common and more prominent over the joints. Edema of the male genitalia also occurs. Many horses are intermittently febrile and pruritic. Stertorous, rapid respiration was observed in 2 cases. Signs persist for the life of the horse.

Over half the cases reported have been in the Appaloosa breed.[197]

Diagnosis: Pemphigus foliaceus is easily confused with dermatophytosis and other autoimmune skin diseases (Fig C9). The disease is diagnosed by a punch biopsy that includes the edge of a lesion and some normal skin. If a vesicle is to be sampled, complete excisional biopsy causes less distortion than does a punch biopsy.

The sample should immediately be placed in Michel's fixative for transport. A quick-frozen sample is adequate but must not thaw prior to processing at the laboratory for direct immunofluorescent testing. Immunofluorescent study reveals subcorneal deposition of IgG in the intercellular spaces.[198] Routine histopathologic studies are also indicated.

Treatment: Long-term corticosteroid therapy is presently the only method of control. Oral prednisolone at 1-2 mg/lb daily is the dosage for the first 7 days. The continuing dosage should be reduced to 0.5-1mg/lb or the least possible dosage that controls the disease. After 2-3 months of treatment, gradual withdrawal from corticosteroids may be attempted; however, most horses require medication indefinitely. If chronic corticosteroid therapy becomes life-threatening, combination therapy with low doses of corticosteroids with another immunosuppressant, such as cyclophosphamide, may be attempted as in humans and dogs.

Disease Characterized by Depigmentation of Skin and/or Hair

Onchocerciasis

Depigmentation of the skin and hair from onchocerciasis has already been described.

Parasitic Dermatitis

Depigmentation of the skin of the upper inner thighs may occur from infestations of *Culicoides* gnats and *Onchocerca*.

Physical or Chemical Agents

Physical or chemical agents frequently damage melanophores, with resultant depigmentation. Sorrel horses commonly regrow white hair at the site of skin wounds, saddle galls and spur marks.[199] White hair may also occur at the site of a nerve block when the local anesthetic contains epinephrine. White hair from cryogenic treatment is useful for identification (freeze branding). Phenol compounds and many other chemicals, as well as radiation, cause depigmentation.[200] Black rubber bits and feed

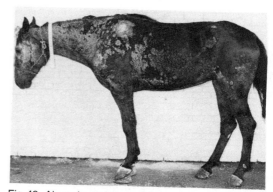

Fig 49. Alopecia, crusting and scarring in linear keratosis.

buckets have been associated with depigmentation about the mouth.

Arabian Fading Syndrome

This condition, also known as "pinky syndrome," is an idiopathic, nonpruritic, nontraumatic and noninflammatory depigmentation seen in Arabians and occasionally in other breeds. A similar condition in humans is termed vitiligo. Varying amounts of skin pigment are lost around the eyes, muzzle and, in some cases, the anus (Fig C10).

Depigmentation has been observed in weanlings, yearlings, and horses as old as 23; most affected horses are young. (Depigmentation in old horses may be a separate pathologic entity.) Any color of horse may be affected but it is most common in greys. There is no sex predilection. Depigmentation more commonly appears in mares during pregnancy or just after foaling. In a few mares it is present only when they are pregnant. Offspring from affected parents are more likely to be affected, although one severely affected stallion has never sired an affected offspring. It more commonly appears when the horse is stabled rather than pastured. The general health of the affected horse is almost always excellent.

The etiology of the Arabian fading syndrome is unknown. Judging from the variety of information related by trainers, breeders and veterinarians, a multiple etiology is likely. An increased incidence in certain family lines suggests a genetic predisposition. A similar condition in Belgian Tervuren dogs is thought to have some degree of heritability.[201] Loss of pigment only during pregnancy may be related to endocrine disorders since melanin formation is influenced by hormones produced by the hypophysis, thyroid, adrenal gland and gonads. A nutritional basis for depigmentation is sup-

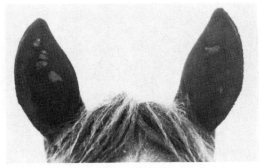

Fig 51. Raised, depigmented lesions on the inner aspect of the pinna in papillary acanthoma.

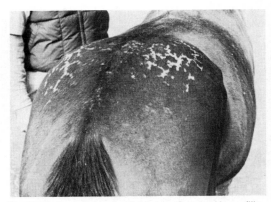

Fig 52. Reticulated leukotrichia in a Quarter Horse filly.

ported by the fact that many horses regain pigmentation while on commercial or specially formulated vitamin-mineral supplements.[202]

Vitiligo in humans is often associated with thyroid disease, pernicious anemia, adrenocortical insufficiency, melanoma and scleroderma. Strong support for an autoimmune or neural etiology is reported.[201,203,204]

Repigmentation in horses varies from none to complete. Some animals regain pigmentation when turned out to pasture or moved to a different section of the country. Dietary supplementation has been the most successful treatment. Feeding of a commercial vitamin-mineral supplement (Clovite:Ft. Dodge) was discontinued in the case of a recovered 23-year-old stallion and depigmentation was noticed again in 6 days; reinstitution of vitamin-mineral supplementation resulted in complete repigmentation. Feeding of the same supplement helped many other horses but has not helped horses on some farms. Other horses have regained pigment while fed sea water, iodine or fishmeal. The incidence of this decreased by 90% on one farm after soil testing, hair analysis and formulation of a special feed supplement.[202]

Papillary Acanthoma

Papillary acanthoma (aural plaques, "ear fungus") is a raised, depigmented area on the inner pinna. The condition is thought to be a chronic irritation from bites of the black fly (Fig 51). Histologically, however, the lesion is identical to verruca plana, a wart-like disease of humans.[197]

Reticulated Leukotrichia

Reticulated leukotrichia is characterized initially by a crusting, nonpainful dermatitis on the dorsum, between the withers and the tail, in young Quarter Horses. Hair is lost and regrows white and in a cross-hatched, reticulated patern (Fig 52). The skin does not lose pigmentation. The cause is unknown; since it has been seen almost exclusively in Quarter Horses, there may be a hereditary influence. No successful treatment has been reported.

Coital Vesicular Exanthema

Depigmentation associated with this disease appears on the vulva of affected mares (see Disease Characterized by Vesicles).

Warts

Depigmentation has been observed following the shedding of warts on the muzzle.

Copper Deficiency

The pigment melanin is synthesized from tyrosine by the enzyme tyrosinase, which contains Cu. Therefore, Cu is essential to maintain the color of skin and hair. Physiologic inhibitors of this enzyme are carbon monoxide, cyanide ions, hydrogen sulfide and many compounds containing organic sulfur.[2]

Copper deficiency occurs most often when its absorption or use is prevented. Cattle and sheep downwind from industries emitting sulfur dioxide have lost haircoat pigment but

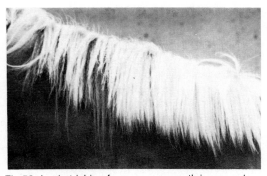

Fig 53. Leukotrichia of new mane growth in secondary copper deficiency.

have regained color when moved. Cadmium emission from a zinc plant was responsible for a secondary Cu deficiency in ruminants.[205] A similar case of secondary Cu deficiency occurred in a horse (Fig 53). Zinc, molybdenum, ferrous sulfide, calcium carbonate and ascorbic acid all have depressing effects on Cu metabolism.[206] Inhibition of Cu function may occur in a matter of hours; such changes are reflected in pigmentation of the haircoat.

Disease Characterized by Wheals

Wheals or urticaria may arise from ingestion of specific foods, administration of medication, a sequel to infection or toxic hepatitis, inhalation of chemicals or pollens, parasitism, as a reaction to insect stings, and as an idiopathic disease. Such factors cause pronounced local edema in the corium secondary to increased capillary permeability and diminished resorption of serum by the lymphatics. Pruritus may be present.

Foods frequently causing reactions include potatoes and their by-products, distillery wastes, malt, coconut cake, beer, pulp, buckwheat, clover, lucerne, St. Johnswort, glucose, wheat, oats, tonics, barley, bran and chicory.[7] Medications typically involved are antibiotics, hormones, insecticides, biologics, phenothiazine, acepromazine, phenylbutazone and procaine. Wheals usually develop in a bilaterally symmetric pattern minutes to hours after use of an offending drug. The lesions usually subside in several hours. Serum sickness, however, may occur many days after administration.

Infectious urticaria has occurred in cases of strangles, contagious equine pleuropneumonia, dourine and horsepox.

Edematous plaques with flat tops and steep sides appear and often disappear rapidly. They occur on the lateral aspects of the neck, shoulders and thorax, or occasionally all over the body and upper limbs. Some affected animals may also have edema around the vulva, anus or prepuce.[207] Lesions on the head and dorsum are often associated with drug reactions (Fig 54). In the early stages, wheals are 0.5-3 cm in diameter. They may become very large when several lesions coalesce.

Treatment with antihistamines and/or corticosteroids is usually very effective. In severe cases accompanied by respiratory or cardiac distress, parenteral administration of epinephrine and/or a tracheotomy may be necessary.

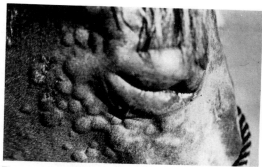

Fig 54. Wheals caused by the administration of drugs.

Amyloidosis

Wheals that respond initially to treatment with corticosteroids or that regress spontaneously but return and develop into nodules are a sign of amyloidosis.

Ticks

Some horses are allergic to the larvae of the common cattle tick, *Boophilus microplus*, and develop wheals at the site of attachment. The lower legs or muzzle are usually affected but it occasionally occurs on any part of the body. The lesions are intensely irritating.[70]

Allergy to *Amblyomma americanum* was diagnosed in a horse having seizures. Wheals

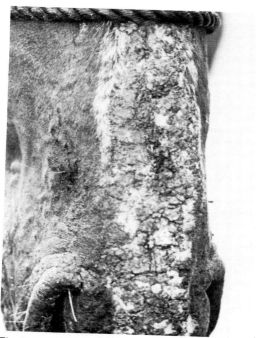

Fig 55. Photosensitization involving only nonpigmented skin.

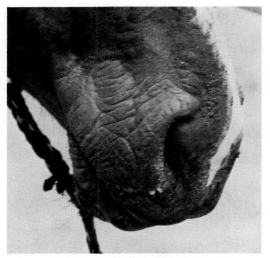

Fig 56. Thickened, hard skin on the muzzle from contact with *Helenium microcephalum*.

were proven to be a response to the female ticks. Other horses were not affected.[208]

Disease Characterized by Local Inflammation

Photosensitization

Primary photosensitization is caused by ingestion of photodynamic plants like buckwheat, St. Johnswort, oats, clover, vetch and alfalfa. The absorbed photosensitizing pigment causes inflammatory exanthema of the unpigmented skin when the horse is exposed to sunlight. Edema, erythema, necrosis, and cracking and peeling of the skin occur (Fig 55). In severe cases, vesicles form and the skin is swollen and tender, with a weeping surface. Lesions are most common on the face and distal extremities. Treatment involves removal of the offending plants and keeping the horse out of the sun. Application of topical antibiotic-corticosteroid ointments soothes cracked skin.

Photosensitization after treatment with phenothiazine may not be primary but may be due to failure of a damaged liver to excrete or detoxify the photodynamic metabolite, phenothiazine sulfoxide.[209] Other photosensitizing drugs include tetracyclines, chlorothiazides and sulfonamides.[210]

Horses that do not respond to dietary change and shade, and those that lose weight and have congested and/or icteric mucous membranes and CNS signs are candidates for hepatogenous photosensitization. The photodynamic agent

in such cases is phylloerythrin, a porphyrin derivative of chlorophyll that is formed in the intestine by bacteria. Some phylloerythrin is absorbed from the intestine and enters the portal circulation. In normal animals, phylloerythrin is effectively removed by the liver and excreted in the bile. In hepatic failure, however, phylloerythrin excretion is significantly reduced so that phylloerythrin enters the peripheral circulation and reaches the skin. In the superficial layers of skin, phylloerythrin absorbs ultraviolet radiation of the sun. Energy from the activated phylloerythrin molecule is then transferred to adjacent cells, causing necrosis and chronic inflammation. Only unpigmented areas of skin are damaged in hepatic photosensitivity.[211]

Leguminous plants and those containing pyrrolizidine alkaloids, *eg*, *Amsinckia intermedia* (teaweed), *Senecio* (ragwort) and *Crotolaria* (rattlebox), are frequent offenders when acute hepatic necrosis or chronic cirrhosis is present. These plants may be eaten in pasture or present as contaminants of hay.

Treatment of photosensitivity secondary to hepatic insufficiency is often unsuccessful but includes sedation with tranquilizers and chloral hydrate if CNS signs are present, administration of laxatives to prevent intestinal stasis, administration of 10 g neomycin orally QID to reduce intestinal bacterial numbers, slow IV infusion of 5% glucose if the horse is hypoglycemic, administration of 100 mg thiamin daily, and administration of 30 g choline daily PO. The value of corticosteroid therapy is debatable.

Contact Dermatitis

Contact of the skin with various plants, chemicals and medications causes local inflammatory reactions, ranging from wheal formation to eczematous dermatitis, with desquamation to hyperkeratosis.

Helenium microcephalum (small-headed sneezeweed), when overly abundant due to exceptional summer rains, caused conjunctivitis and chronic inflammatory dermatitis of the muzzle and eyelids in a band of pastured broodmares (Fig 56). Mowing the pasture eliminated the problem. A similar case of dermatitis of the muzzle and head was caused by the prickly spider flower, *Cleome gynandra*. *Urtica urens* and *U dioica* (stinging nettle) produce wheals in thin-skinned horses during summer months.

Chemicals and drugs that cause dermatitis when applied topically include carbolic acid, mercury compounds, mustard oil, crude oil, diesel fuel, turpentine, cattle screw-worm bomb, various blisters used in lameness treatment, leather preservatives and benzalkonium chloride. The last has caused alopecia after being applied to the skin prior to an injection. Minor irritation is manifested as erythema in white areas of the skin, while severe irritation appears as vesicles or large blisters. Acute, blistering dermatitis of the legs occurred in horses working in grain fields badly contaminated with *Euphorbia* sp (spurge).

Disease Characterized by Abnormal Sweating

Anhidrosis

Anhidrosis ("drycoat," "nonsweater") is an increasing problem of considerable economic importance to the racing industry in hot, humid climates. An incidence as high as 20% was reported on Louisiana tracks in 1979.[212] For many years this problem was seen only in Thoroughbreds shipped south for racing; however, the disorder is now seen in other breeds and native southern horses.

Clinical Signs: Affected horses appear normal for 1-2 months after shipping but then do not sweat immediately on exercise ("delayed sweats"). The onset of anhidrosis is often preceded by profuse sweating and excessive "blowing." Depending on the degree of anhidrosis, affected horses may have a temperature of 37.8-38.9 C (100-102 F) at rest, and up to 40-42.2 C (104-108 F) after exercise. Such animals require twice as long to cool out as a normal "free-sweater." The respiratory rate is up to 150/minute. The term "blower" stems from the labored respiration and exaggerated dilation of the nostrils. Many affected animals are initially treated for shipping fever. In partially affected animals, decreased sweating may be evident under the mane, on the ventral aspect of the neck and between the thighs. Horses affected for several months have a dull, rough, scurfy haircoat, and alopecia of the face and body friction areas. Performance decreases as the disease becomes more severe. Forced exercise has caused death in affected animals.[213]

Cause: The exact cause of anhidrosis is unknown. Hypothyroidism, electrolyte imbalance, hypoadrenalism have been suspected but not confirmed as causes. The most plausible concept suggests anhidrosis as a consequence of prolonged stimulation of the sweat glands by epinephrine, which is secreted as a response to a hot, moist climate. The sweat glands adapt to the increased blood level of epinephrine and eventually become insensitive to it. Supporting this theory is the finding that affected horses have higher blood epinephrine levels than normal horses and IV injection of epinephrine precipitates or aggravates anhidrosis.[214]

Diagnosis: Anhidrosis is diagnosed on the basis of history and signs. The diagnosis is confirmed by demonstrating a lack of sweating in response to intradermal injection of epinephrine in the skin under the mane or over the dorsal ribcage. A 25-ga needle is used to inject 0.1 ml epinephrine at dilutions of 1:1000, 1:10,000, 1:100,000 and 1:1,000,000. Normal horses sweat in a matter of minutes after injection of epinephrine in any dilution. Horses with anhidrosis sweat only after injection of epinephrine at the 1:1000 dilution or do not sweat at all.[215] Laboratory tests that may detect the underlying cause and indicate a course of therapy include radioimmunoassay of serum T_3-T_4 levels, creatinine clearance ratio for Na, Cl and K, and ACTH-stimulation test.

Treatment: The most logical treatment is to move the horse to a cooler, more arid climate. When this is not feasible, an air-conditioned stall with low humidity is the best solution. Reported medical treatments include administration of 15 g iodinated casein (Protomone: AgriTech) daily PO, 1000-3000 IU vitamin E daily PO, 1-2 L NaCl daily IV, 1-2 oz NaCl daily PO, 100-400 units ACTH IM, and 100-200 mEq KCl diluted in 1-2 L saline IV.[216,217]

Hyperhidrosis

Hyperhidrosis or excessive sweating occurs after administration of various drugs, such as epinephrine, acetylcholine, prostaglandin F_2alpha and promazine, in response to severe pain, and after transection of sympathetic innervation (in which case sweating is localized to the area supplied by the transected nerve). Trauma, focal infection or neoplasia in the region of the cervical vagosympathetic trunk may lead to a temporary or permanent Horner's syndrome. Due to the proximity of the cranial cervical ganglion and pre- and postganglionic sympathetic fiber to the caudal aspect of the guttural pouch, guttural pouch infections or careless IV injections may cause hyperhidrosis.[218]

Disease Characterized by Fragility and Hyperelasticity

Hyperelastosis Cutis

This unusual disease is easily recognized because affected animals have skin that is loosely

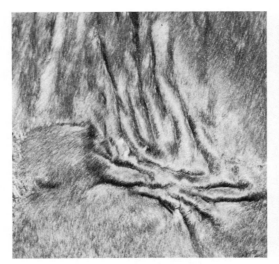

Fig 57. "Wrinkles of velvet" in hyperelastosis cutis.

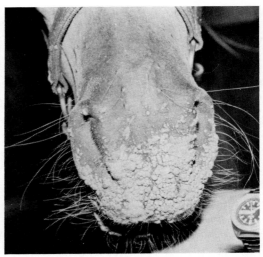

Fig 58. Viral papillomatosis in a yearling.

attached to the subcutis, and easily traumatized. The most common sites affected are the
back and adjoining thoracic wall (Fig C11). The
size of the lesions varies from 2-8 cm. The skin
has a velvety feel and may be pulled 5-10 cm
away from the body, returning to its former position when released (Fig 57). The lesions are
sharply demarcated and depressed 1-2 mm below the normal surface. Pain may or may not
be present. Areas may tear open from what
would normally be insignificant tension, such
as innocuous bites or abrasion by the feet of a
stallion breeding a mare.[219] Such wounds hold
sutures poorly and are extremely slow to heal,
resulting in extensive scars. Although the condition may be present at birth, owners generally do not notice anything unusual until 6-12
months of age. General health is good.

A similar condition in humans (Ehlers-Dan-
los syndrome) is characterized by dysplasia of
connective tissue, decreased numbers of colla-

gen fibers, and a relative or actual increase in
numbers of elastic fibers. It is an autosomal
dominant trait in humans, dogs and mink. Two
affected horses had the same grandsire and 2
other affected horses were full brothers.[220] All
4 were Quarter Horses.

Diagnosis is based on history and signs. Biopsy of lesions has not been informative in several cases. Treatment involves basic wound
care. Affected horses should not be bred.

Miscellaneous Skin Diseases

Warts (Viral Papillomatosis)

Warts are caused by a virus and most often
appear on the muzzle and lips of horses less
than 2 years of age. Occasionally they may be
present on the ears, eyelids or lower limbs.
Warts vary in size from 0.5-20 mm. When first
noticed, the few warts present are slightly
raised, flat, smooth and flesh-colored (Fig 58).
In a short time, they proliferate in number and
size, becoming rougher in texture, grey and
horny. They remain for 3-6 months and regress
spontaneously.[92]

Natural immunity develops with the passage of time and the warts disappear spontaneously. If the warts must be removed within
a matter of weeks, *eg*, before a sale, cryosurgery is the treatment of choice. Chemical cautery with trifluoroacetic acid is also safe and
effective. A solution of 25 g anhydrous trifluoroacetic acid, 3 g water and 20 g glacial acetic
acid is carefully applied to affected tissue only.
Adjacent tissue should be protected with petrolatum. Second and third applications are

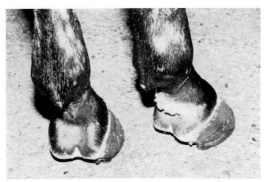

Fig 59. Keloid on the right pastern after a wire cut.

made on the fourth and seventh days after the initial treatment. The resulting scab sloughs within 2 weeks.[221] Salicylic acid 25% with podophyllin cream or crude castor oil has also been used to cauterize warts.[92]

Wart oils for daily application over long periods of time are also available. These contain castor oil and/or oil of thuja and are of questionable value.

Potassium or sodium iodide may be used PO at 8 g daily for 10-14 days. Arsenic preparations have also been used orally. Vitamin A injection into the wart tissue has provided good results. Procaine has been used successfully IV or by infiltration.[222] Efficacy claimed for some treatments may be due to natural immunity.

Therapy with autogenous vaccine is moderately to highly effective.[223] Injection of 5-10 ml autogenous wart vaccine, as a single SC dose on each of 4 occasions at weekly intervals, was of value.[207] Since the virus is species-specific, cattle wart vaccine is not effective.

Removal of a few warts for vaccine production has resulted in disappearance of the remaining ones. This same phenomenon has also occurred when only a few warts are treated by cryosurgery. Rarely, depigmentation occurs when warts drop off, especially if they have been treated.

Keloid

A keloid is considered by some to be a type of hard fibroma that develops from apparently normal tissue. Usually they grow out of scars on the limbs, especially on the lower joints (Fig 59). These hard, raised lesions develop gradually and have a keratinized surface.

Unfortunately, keloids often recur following surgical removal. Podophyllum or fluorouracil, as used in sarcoid treatment, can be used. Scarification, followed by the application of a mixture of 1 g ichthammol, 1 g pyrogallol and 10 g collodion, has been recommended.[4]

Hirsutism

A long, sometimes curly, shaggy, unseasonal haircoat occurs in older horses with pituitary tumor (Fig 60). Retention of long winter hair occurs in horses with chronic illness and/or dietary deficiency.

Curly Coat

In Percheron horses, a condition called "curly coat" is due to simple recessive inheritance. It has also been seen in Missouri Fox Trotting horses, small Bashkin horses, in which it is a breed characteristic, and other breeds (Fig 61).

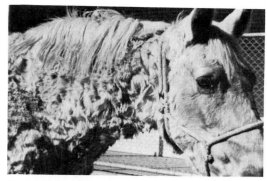

Fig 60. Long, shaggy coat during the summer on a horse with a pituitary tumor.

It may occur only on the mane and tail or may affect the whole body. Rather than normal, round hair shafts, the hair shafts of horses with curly coat are somewhat flattened.[224]

Epitheliogenesis Imperfecta

This rare congenital disease of foals is of possible hereditary origin and is characterized by the complete absence of all layers of epithelium in various parts of the body. It has affected the limbs of 3 foals, the head of one foal and the tongue of one foal. In an unreported case, both front limbs of a pinto foal were entirely devoid of epithelium from the carpus distad. The right hindleg had no epithelium over the fetlock and pastern. These affected limbs had no hooves, leaving sensitive laminae exposed to the environment. The foal was unable to stand long enough to nurse.[225]

Pigeon Breast

Corynebacterium pseudotuberculosis, in addition to causing ulcerative lymphangitis, con-

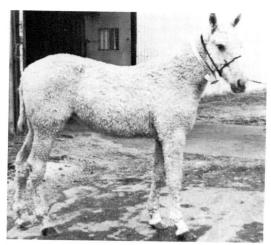

Fig 61. "Curly coat" on a Missouri Fox Trotter.

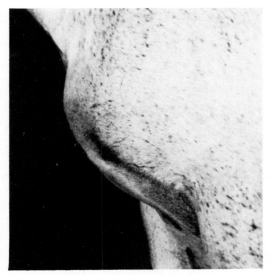

Fig 62. Large, firm pectoral abscess (pigeon breast) from *C pseudotuberculosis* infection.

tagious acne and abortion, periodically causes large (10 x 10 x 20 cm), deep, slowly developing, thick-walled abscesses (dry-land distemper, Colorado strangles, chest abscesses). The abscesses form primarily in the pectoral area, but occasionally occur in the axillary area, ventral abdomen or on the limbs (Fig 62). There is no age or sex predilection. Most cases have occurred in California and Texas in the late summer and early fall.[226-228] Several horses on one farm have been infected.

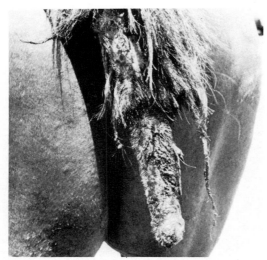

Fig 63. Severe staphylococcal pyoderma of the tail.

The fact that most horses had previously been treated or were being treated for cutaneous habronemiasis at the time of abscess formation leads to the suspicion that migrating *Habronema* larvae carry the bacteria into the tissues.[226] General health is good except for the unusual case in which generalized infection becomes apparent due to abortion and/or numerous small, nodular abscesses scattered all over the body.[227]

Administration of antibiotics delays rupture of the abscess and prolongs the disease. Poultices should be applied to encourage maturing of the abscess. Aspiration of the contents of the swelling with a long, large-bore needle (4-inch, 12-ga) can be performed to determine when the abscess should be lanced. A large volume of thick, creamy exudate containing *C pseudotuberculosis* in pure culture is typical.

Temporal Teratoma

A temporal teratoma (ear fistula, conchal sinus) is a soft, circular swelling, 2-4 cm in diameter, located rostroventral to the base of the ear. The wall of the cyst resembles thickened human skin and may contain sebaceous material and/or hair follicles. The cyst may drain at the edge of the pinna.[229] A cyst containing dental fragments of various stages of development may be completely covered by normal hair and skin (dentigerous cyst). Drainage from such a cyst may scald the area, resulting in hair loss. The dental fragments are sometimes attached to the temporal bone.[230]Surgical resection of the cyst is the best treatment.

Hepatodermatitis

Waste motor oil applied for dust control in an arena adjoining a riding stable produced a generalized ulcerative dermatitis. There was extensive hair loss, especially on the mane and tail, but also on the nose, face, legs and ventral abdomen. The fumes of the oil were hepatotoxic and caused secondary ulcerative dermatitis.[231]

Staphylococcal Tail Pyoderma

Staphylococcus spp invade skin abrasions produced by tail-rubbing, insect bites, psoroptic mange, pinworms or other causes. Small pustules subsequently form on the dorsal surface of the tail. Pruritus leads to self-mutilation, which results in a severe chronic disease that responds poorly to treatment (Fig 63). Discharge from rupture of the pustules mats the long tail hairs. Pustules heal and rupture in an unending process.

Treatment includes administration of large doses of an appropriate antibiotic, as determined by culture and sensitivity, for 14-21 days. Sublesional injection of antibiotic may also be beneficial. Clipping, washing and application of antibiotic soaks are helpful. Prevention of self-mutilation by rubbing is very important. Autogenous bacterin therapy is worth trying.

Despite intensive treatment, only 25% of affected animals have responded.

References

1. Bal, HS, in Dukes' Physiology of Domestic Animals. 9th ed. Comstock, Ithaca, 1977.

2. Breazile, JE: Textbook of Veterinary Physiology. Lea & Febiger, Philadelphia, 1971.

3. Getty, R: Sisson & Grossman's Anatomy of Domestic Animals. 5th ed. WB Saunders, Philadelphia, 1975.

4. Dellman, HD: Veterinary Histology. Lea & Febiger, Philadelphia, 1971.

5. Calhoun and Stinson, in Dellman: Textbook of Veterinary Histology. Lea & Febiger, Philadelphia, 1976.

6. Oxender, WE et al. Am J Vet Res 38 (1977) 203.

7. Kral, FA and Schwartzman, RM: Veterinary and Comparative Dermatology. JB Lippincott, Philadelphia, 1964.

8. Allen, SK and McKeever, PJ. Vet Clin No Am 4 (1974) 269.

9. Stannard, AA. Proc 22nd Ann Mtg Am Assoc Eq Pract, 1976.

10. Muller, GH and Kirk, RW: Small Animal Dermatology. 2nd ed. WB Saunders, Philadelphia, 1976.

11. Duncan, JR and Prasse, KW. Vet Clin No Am 6 (1976) 637.

12. Saunders, L, Canonsburg, PA: Personal communication, 1980.

13. Sundberg, JP et al. JAVMA 170 (1977) 150.

14. Ragland, WL et al. Eq Vet J 2 (1970) 2.

15. Ragland, WL et al. Eq Vet J 2 (1970) 168.

16. England, JJ et al. Am J Vet Res 34 (1973) 1601.

17. James, VS. Southwest Vet 21 (1968) 235.

18. Page, EH et al. JAVMA 150 (1967) 177.

19. Wheat, JD. Mod Vet Pract 45 (1964) 62.

20. Joyce, JR. VM/SAC 70 (1975) 200.

21. Lane, JG. Eq Vet J 9 (1977) 127.

22. Farris, HE et al. VM/SAC 70 (1975) 299.

23. Adams, OR: Lameness of Horses. 2nd ed. Lea & Febiger, Philadelphia, 1966.

24. Lewis, RE. Proc 10th Ann Mtg Am Assoc Eq Pract, 1964. p 199.

25. Roberts, WD. VM/SAC 65 (1970) 67.

26. Metcalf, JW. Proc 17th Ann Mtg Am Assoc Eq Pract, 1971. p 45.

27. Voss, JL. Am J Vet Res 30 (1969) 183.

28. Holden, HB. J Laryng 86 (1972) 821.

29. Wyman, M et al. JAVMA 171 (1977) 449.

30. Murphy, JM et al. JAVMA 174 (1979) 269.

31. Guèrin, C: The History of BCG. Little, Brown and Co, Boston, 1957.

32. Bast, RC et al. N Eng J Med 290 (1974) 1413.

33. Morton, DL et al. Ann Int Med 74 (1971) 787.

34. Soulsby, EJL: Textbook of Veterinary Clinical Parasitology. FA Davis, Philadelphia, 1976.

35. Soulsby, EJL: Helminths, Arthropods, and Protozoa of Domesticated Animals (Monnig). 6th ed. Williams & Wilkins, Baltimore, 1968.

36. Reid, CH. VM/SAC 60 (1965) 233.

37. Underwood, JR. Vet Bull US Army 30 (1936) 16.

38. Wheat, JD. Vet Med 56 (1961) 477.

39. Boyd, CL and Bullard, TL. JAVMA 153 (1968) 324.

40. Brown, DS. Proc 14th Ann Mtg Am Assoc Eq Pract, 1968. p 187.

41. Migiola, S et al. VM/SAC 73 (1978) 1073.

42. Drudge, JH et al. Am J Vet Res 35 (1974) 67.

43. Bridges, CH. Proc 9th Ann Mtg Am Assoc Eq Pract, 1968.

44. Epstein, AA. Arch Klin Chir 175 (1933) 344.

45. Bridges, in Catcott: Equine Medicine and Surgery. 2nd ed. American Veterinary Publications, Santa Barbara, 1972.

46. Connoli, MD: Equine phycomycosis. Aust Vet J 49 (1973) 214.

47. Austin, RJ. Can Vet J 17 (1976) 86.

48. Murray, DR et al. JAVMA 72 (1978) 834.

49. McMullan, WC et al. JAVMA 170 (1977) 1293.

50. Hutchins, DR and Johnston, KG. Aust Vet J 48 (1972) 269.

51. Joyce, JR and McMullan, WC. J Eq Med Surg 1 (1977) 256.

52. Johnson, GR et al. Can Vet J 16 (1975) 341.

53. Bridges, CH. Am J Path 33 (1957) 411.

54. Schiefer, B and Mehnert, B. Berl Munch tierarzt Wschr 78 (1965) 230.

55. Brown, RJ et al. Mod Vet Pract 53 (1972) 47.

56. Saunders, LZ. Cornell Vet 38 (1948) 213.

57. Smith, HA and Franksons, MC. Southwest Vet 16 (1961) 22.

58. Smith, HA and Franksons, MC. Southwest Vet 17 (1963) 58.

59. Myers, DD, et al. JAVMA 145 (1964) 345.

60. Jungerman, PF and Schwartzman, RM: Veterinary Medical Mycology. Lea & Febiger, Philadelphia, 1972.

61. Pascoe, RR. Aust Vet J 49 (1973) 37.

62. Anim Nutr and Health. (October, 1978) 6.

63. Appaloosa News. (July, 1978) 65.

64. Newsom, HD. Ann Rev Ent 22 (1977) 333.

65. Little, VA: General and Applied Entomology. 2nd ed. Harper and Row, New York, 1963.

66. Schreck, CE et al. J Med Ent 13 (1976) 115.

67. Grothaus, RH et al. Am J Trop Med Hyg 23 (1974) 533.

68. McDuffie, WC. Agr Res Survey. Washington, DC, 1969.

69. Rick, RF. Aust Vet J 30 (1954) 142.

70. Stannard, in Catcott: Equine Medicine and Surgery. 2nd ed. American Veterinary Publications, Santa Barbara, 1972.

71. Hamilton, DP and Byerly, CS. JAVMA **164** (1974) 1040.

72. Jubb, KVF and Kennedy, PC: Pathology of Domestic Animals. Academic Press, New York, 1970.

73. Altra, K and Clark, L. Path Vet **7** (1970) 43.

74. Prasse, KW *et al*. JAVMA **166** (1975) 68.

75. Baker, DW and Monlux, WS. J Parasit, Suppl **25** (1939) 16.

76. Scharff, DK. VM/SAC **68** (1973) 791.

77. Hadlow, WJ, *et al*. Cornell Vet **67** (1977) 272.

78. Newfeld, JL. Can Vet J **14** (1973) 149.

79. Newfeld, JL. Can Vet J **14** (1973) 129.

80. Kirk, MD. VM/SAC **66** (1971) 448.

81. Gupta, BN *et al*. Cornell Vet (1972) 205.

82. Gillis, MF. VM/SAC **60** (1965) 609.

83. Theilen, GH and Fowler, ME. JAVMA **140** (1962) 923.

84. Ward, JM and Whitlock, RH. VM/SAC **62** (1967) 1003.

85. Fishburn, FJ and Kelley, DC. JAVMA **151** (1967) 45.

86. Ditchfield, in Bone: Equine Medicine and Surgery. 1st ed. American Veterinary Publications, Santa Barbara, 1963.

87. Jones, TC and Maurer, FD. Bull US Army Med Dept 74 (1944) 63.

88. Koehne, G *et al*. JAVMA **159** (1971) 892.

89. Kirkham, WW and Moore, RW. Southwest Vet **7** (1954) 354.

90. Davis, HH and Worthington, WE. JAVMA **145** (1964) 692.

91. Kral, F: Compendium of Veterinary Dermatology. Pfizer Laboratories, New York, 1959.

92. Pascoe, RR. Aust Vet J **49** (1973) 37.

93. Dodd, DC and Raker, CW. JAVMA **157** (1970) 968.

94. Hutchins, DR. Aust Vet J **48** (1972) 200.

95. Thompson, SW *et al*. Cornell Vet **49** (1958) 265.

96. McIntyre, RW. Am J Vet Res **10** (1949) 229.

97. Hutchins, DR. N Zeal Vet J **8** (1960) 85.

98. Kaminjolo, JS *et al*. Zbl Vet **21B** (1974) 592.

99. Kaminjolo, JS *et al*. Zbl Vet **21B** (1974) 202.

100. Jakob, W. Vet Path **8** (1971) 292.

101. Stunzi, F *et al*. Vet Path **12** (1975) 405.

102. Knight, in Catcott: Equine Medicine and Surgery. 2nd ed. American Veterinary Publications, Santa Barbara, 1972.

103. Scott, DW and Manning, TO. Eq Pract **2** (1980) 11.

104. Rick, RF. Aust J Agr Res **5** (1954) 109.

105. Mellor, PS and McCoig, J. Vet Rec **95** (1974) 411.

106. Baker, KP and Quinn, PJ. Eq Vet J **10** (1978) 243.

107. Linley, JR and Davies, JB. J Econ Ent **64** (1971) 264.

108. Nelson, RL and Bellamy, RE. J Med Ent **8** (1971) 283.

109. Braverman, Y and Galun, R. Refuah Vet **30** (1973) 62.

110. Granett, P *et al*. J Econ Ent **42** (1949) 281.

111. Gribble, in Catcott: Equine Medicine and Surgery. 2nd ed. American Veterinary Publications, Santa Barbara, 1972.

112. Coffman, JR and Frey, RA. Proc 19th Ann Mtg Am Assoc Eq Pract, 1973.

113. Halliwell, REW. J Sm Anim Pract **12** (1971) 431.

114. Halliwell, REW. Proc Am Coll Vet Int Med, 1976. p 33.

115. Sobatka, AK *et al*. Fed Proc **35** (1976) 673.

116. Roy, DN and Brown, AWA: Entomology. 3rd ed. Bangalore Print, Bangalore, India, 1970.

117. Weinburgh, HB and Pratt, HD: *Culicoides*: Public Health Importance, Biology, Survey and Control. US Public Health Service, Comm Dis Center, Atlanta, 1962.

118. Jones, RH *et al*. J Med Ent **14** (1977) 441.

119. Stoll, RN. J Parasit **33** (1947) 1.

120. Rabalais, FC *et al*. Am J Vet Res **35** (1974) 125.

121. Mellor, PS. J Helminth **47** (1973) 97.

122. McMullan, WC. Southwest Vet **25** (1972) 179.

123. Alicata, JE. No Am Vet **17** (1936) 39.

124. Cello, RM. Eq Vet J **3** (1971) 148.

125. Mellor, PS. J Helminth **47** (1973) 111.

126. WHO Expert Committee on Onchocerciasis. WHO Tech Rep Ser 335 (1966) 13.

127. Dikmans, G. Cornell Vet **38** (1948) 3.

128. Underwood, JR. Vet Bull US Army 30 (1936) 227.

129. Thomas, AD. J So Afr Vet Assoc **34** (1963) 17.

130. Hawking, F. Trans Royal Soc Trop Med Hyg **52** (1958) 109.

131. WHO Expert Committee on Onchocerciasis. WHO Tech Rep Ser 335 (1966) 33.

132. Salazar, MM and Gonzalez, RD. Salud Publ Mex **10** (1968) 663.

133. Salazar, MM *et al*. J Tropenmed Parasit **21** (1970) 213.

134. Ben-Siru *et al*. Am J Ophth **70** (1970) 741.

135. Mastrandrea, G and Sanguigni, S. Arch Ital Sci Med Trop Parasit **49** (1968) 195.

136. Stannard, AA. Proc Western States Vet Conf, 1979.

137. Friedheim, EAA. Bull WHO 50 (1974) 572.

138. Denham, DA and Mellor, P. J Helminth **50** (1976) 49.

139. Ruhm, W. Vet Med Rev **1** (1969) 31.

140. Appaloosa News. (Oct, 1976) 87.

141. Thompson, BH. Ann Trop Med Parasit **70** (1976) 343.

142. Sterlman, CD. Ann Rev Ent **21** (1976) 155.

143. Batte, in Catcott: Equine Medicine and Surgery. 2nd ed. American Veterinary Publications, Santa Barbara, 1972.

144. Dozsa, J. Mod Vet Pract **47** (1966) 45.

145. Farrington, DO *et al*. VM/SAC **71** (1976) 1199-1202.

146. Brennan, JM and Yunker, CE. J Parasit **50** (1964) 311.

147. Hayes, MH: Veterinary Notes for Horse Owners. Hayes Areo, New York, 1974.

148. Schwartzman, in Orkin: Scabies and Pediculosis. JB Lippincott, Philadelphia, 1977.

149. Patid, K *et al*. Indian Vet J **44** (1967) 65.

150. Mehls, HJ. Berl Munch tierarztl Wschr **1** (1952) 9.

151. Besch, ED and Griffiths, HJ. JAVMA **128** (1956) 82.

152. Koutz, FR. Speculum **17** (1963) 21.

153. Euzeby, J. Rev Med Vet **121** (1970) 981.

154. Gibbons, in Catcott: Progress in Equine Practice. American Veterinary Publications, Santa Barbara, 1970.

155. Thomsett, LR. Eq Vet J **1** (1968) 91.

156. Wood, JC. Vet Rec **24** (1968) 218.

157. Tropical Horse Tick Eradication in Florida. USDA-ARS Equine Piroplasmosis Progress Report. (April, 1971) 8.

158. Pascoe, RR. Aust Vet J **52** (1976) 419.

159. Kral, in Bone: Equine Medicine and Surgery. 1st ed. American Veterinary Publications, Santa Barbara, 1963.

160. Pepin, GA and Austwick, RK. Vet Rec **208** (1968) 208.

161. Kaplan, W. Arch Derm **96** (1967) 404.

162. Kester, WO. Quarter Horse J **14** (1961) 43.

163. George, LK et al. Am J Vet Res **18** (1957) 798.

164. Pascoe, RR. Aust Vet J **52** (1976) 420.

165. Pascoe, RR and Connoli, MD. Aust Vet J **50** (1974) 380.

166. Bohm, KE et al. Berl Munch tierarztl Wsch **81** (1968) 397.

167. Simpson, RB, College Station, TX: Personal communication, 1972.

168. Taplin, D et al. Arch Derm **99** (1969) 203.

169. Blakemore, JC. VM/SAC **66** (1971) 357.

170. Carroll, HF. JAVMA **165** (1974) 192.

171. Robinson, HJ et al. Tex Rep Biol Med **27** Suppl **2** (1969) 537.

172. Experimental Reports of Equine Health Laboratory. Racing Assoc **10** (1973) 41.

173. Suskisov, AK et al. Izdatil'stvo Kolos (1972) 189.

174. Crinion, RAP and O'Connor, JP. Irish Vet J **32** (1978) 81.

175. Fowler, in Catcott: Equine Medicine and Surgery. 2nd ed. American Veterinary Publications, Santa Barbara, 1972.

176. Rosenfeld, I and Beath, OA: Selenium, Academic Press, New York, 1964.

177. Hultine, JD et al. Eq Pract **1** (1979) 60.

178. Knott, SG and McCray, CWR. Aust Vet J **35** (1959) 161.

179. Scarnell, J. Vet Rec **72** (1961) 795.

180. Searcy, GP and Hulland, TJ. Can Vet J **9** (1968) 7.

181. Kaplan, W and Johnston, WJ. JAVMA **149** (1966) 1162.

182. Pascoe, RR. Aust Vet J **47** (1971) 112.

183. Pascoe, RR. Aust Vet J **48** (1972) 32.

184. Smith, JB et al. Cornell Vet **51** (1961) 334.

185. Richard, JL and Pier, AC. Am J Vet Res **27** (1966) 419.

186. Edgar, G and Keast, JC. Aust Vet J **16** (1940) 120.

187. DiSalvo, AF et al. VM/SAC **64** (1969) 502.

188. Ford, RB et al. VM/SAC **69** (1974) 1557.

189. Lloyd, DH and Sellers, KC: Dermatophilus Infections in Animals and Man. Academic Press, New York, 1976.

190. Burrows, R and Goodridge, D. Proc 4th Int Conf Eq Infect Dis, 1978. p 159.

191. Thein, P. Proc 4th Int Conf Eq Inf Dis, 1978. p 36.

192. Gibbs, EPJ and Roberts, MC. Eq Vet J **4** (1972) 74.

193. Bryans, JT and Allen, GP. Proc 3rd Int Conf Eq Infect Dis, 1972. p 322.

194. Lieux, in Catcott: Equine Medicine and Surgery. 2nd ed. American Veterinary Publications, Santa Barbara, 1972.

195. Gleeson, LJ et al. Aust Vet J **52** (1976) 349.

196. Hansen, in Catcott: Equine Medicine and Surgery. 2nd ed. American Veterinary Publications, Santa Barbara, 1972.

197. Stannard, AA. Proc Ann Mtg Am Acad Vet Derm, 1980.

198. Halliwell, REW and Goldschmidt, MH. JAAHA **13** (1977) 431.

199. Meifer, WC, Dtsch tierarztl Wschr **73** (1966) 85.

200. Kahn, G. Geriatrics **26** (1971) 106.

201. JAVMA **173** (1978) 390.

202. McMullan, WC. College Station, TX: Unpublished data, 1980.

203. Hentz, KC et al. N Eng J Med **297** (1977) 634.

204. Morohashi, S et al. Arch Derm **113** (1977) 755.

205. Hennig, A et al. Trace Element Metabolism in Animals. 2nd ed. Univ Park Press, Baltimore, 1974.

206. Underwood, EJ: Trace Elements in Human and Animal Nutrition. 3rd ed. Academic Press, New York, 1971.

207. Thomsett, LR. J Vet Postgrad Clin Study **1** (1979) 15.

208. Tritschler, LR. VM/SAC **60** (1965) 219.

209. Clare, NT. Aust Vet J **23** (1947) 344.

210. Berry, J, and Merriam, JG. VM/SAC **65** (1970) 251.

211. Tennant, B et al. Vet Clin No Am **3** (1973) 279.

212. Beadle, R. student chapter SAVMA Ed Symp, Louisiana State Univ, 1980.

213. Correa, JF and Caldesin, GG. JAVMA **149** (1966) 1556.

214. Evans, CL et al. Vet Rec **69** (1957) 1.

215. Evans, CL. Br Vet J **22** (1966) 117.

216. Currie, AK and Seager, SWJ. Proc 22nd Ann Mtg Am Assoc Eq Pract, 1976. p 249.

217. Marsh, JH. Vet Rec **73** (1961) 1124.

218. Smith, JS and Mayhew, IG. Cornell Vet **67** (1977) 529.

219. Lerner, DJ and McCracken, MD. J Eq Med Surg **2** (1978) 350.

220. McMullan, WC, College Station, TX: Unpublished data, 1979.

221. Erlich, J. J Mod Med **40** (1972) 12.

222. Scientific Papers, Vet School, Sofia, Bulgaria **1** (1960) 143.

223. Quinn, AH. Vet Med (1963) 207.

224. Chalkley, L: Equine Genetics and Selection Procedures. Equine Research Pubns, Dallas, 1978.

225. Schumacher, J. Graduate paper, Texas A & M Univ, 1979.

226. Reid, CH. VM/SAC **60** (1965) 233.

227. Liu, IKM et al. JAVMA **170** (1977) 1086.

228. Mayfield, MA and Martin, MT. Southwest Vet **32** (1979) 133.

229. Mason, BJE. Vet Rec **95** (1974) 226.

230. Baker, in Catcott: Equine Medicine and Surgery. 2nd ed. American Veterinary Publications, Santa Barbara, 1972.

231. Case, AA and Coffman, JR. Vet Clin No Am **3** (1973) 273.

SKIN GRAFTING PROCEDURES
by D.V. Hanselka

Wounds of horses, particularly those of the distal limbs, have plagued owners and veterinarians for ages. Wounds that fail to respond to orthodox treatment may respond to skin grafting. This technic is often the only treatment by which successful covering of the lesions with skin can be accomplished.[1] A uniform epithelial covering develops in a shorter time on successfully grafted lesions than on those allowed to heal naturally.[2-4]

Classification of Grafts

Transplants may be classified according to the donor-recipient relationship of the tissues, *ie*, as homografts, heterografts or autografts. A homotransplant is one made from one animal to another of the same species. Homografts often stimulate a destructive immune response in the recipient. In these animals, the whole transplant is usually rejected and gradually replaced by scar tissue. Under specific circumstances, homografts survive for long periods.

A heterograft is one made between animals of different species. Heterografts are decidedly inferior to homografts because they evoke an even greater immunologic response in the recipient than do homografts.

An autograft is one made to a new site in the same animal. A rejection response is not stimulated in the host with autotransplantation.[1-3,5-7] Autografts may be categorized as free grafts and pedicle grafts. A free graft consists of an isolated piece of tissue which, at the time of transplantation, is completely devoid of vascular and nervous connections. A pedicle graft remains connected to the donor site for a time by a pedicle containing blood vessels. When a new blood supply has developed, the pedicle is usually divided.[5,7]

Grafts classified according to thickness may be either full thickness (epidermis and all of the dermis) or split thickness. Split-thickness grafts may be thin (Thiersch's graft), intermediate or thick.[8]

Autografts are most successful since the graft and host are antigenically identical.

Considerations for Skin Grafts

Autogenous transplantation of skin is the most useful method for resurfacing large skin defects and promoting wound healing after conventional therapy has failed.[9] A decision to use a skin graft should be made after consideration of the value of the animal, cosmetic effect desired, and location, duration and size of the wound.[11,12]

Before attempting a grafting procedure, the overall condition of the animal should be evaluated. Debilitated individuals with chronic disease have a greater tendency toward infection and graft rejection. Local factors, such as the nature of the tissue lost and condition of the recipient bed, should also be considered.[13] The skin selected for donor tissue should match the recipient bed's adjacent integument as closely as possible.

Several skin grafting procedures used in human surgery have been successfully applied to horses.[1-4,9-12,14-19] However, adequate restraint, effective bandaging and the increased possibility of contamination are major obstacles encountered. The surgeon must use judgment in selection of the grafting technic that will work best under the circumstances in each individual case.

Factors Affecting Graft Acceptance

Graft acceptance is defined as establishment of an arterial and venous network within a graft.[20] Conditions necessary for graft acceptance include a recipient bed that is free of infection, a richly vascularized graft bed, hemostasis of the recipient bed, proper preparation of the granulation bed, proper suture tension for the graft, adequate immobilization, and sufficient contact between the graft and recipient bed to permit serum imbibition and prompt revascularization of the graft.[8,21]

The growth phase of a successful skin graft may be divided into the period before revascularization, the phase of revascularization, and the phase of organic union. During the first phase, the graft, anchored by fibrin formed from coagulating plasma, is nourished by interchange of fluids between the transplant and its bed. The phase of revascularization may begin within 24 hours after grafting. Development of anastomotic vessels is usually complete by the tenth day. As the third stage begins, there is a firm fibrous union between the graft and its bed. The processes of contraction, pigmentation and reinnervation occur during this period and may require up to 18 months for completion.[7]

The main factors responsible for loss of a skin graft are accumulation of blood and/or serum beneath the graft, improper immobilization of the graft and its bed, bacterial infection, and an unacceptable recipient bed.[8,22] A seroma may form under a graft that stretches across concavities and is not held against the bed by a pressure bandage.[22] Such a graft only revascularizes after contact is made with the bed. If excessive hemorrhage persists when a recipient bed is being prepared to receive a graft, it may be wise to apply a nonadherent pressure pad to the bed and wait several days before grafting. Other precautionary measures to control bleeding include gentle pressure on the bed with saline-soaked gauze sponges, clamping and ligation of vessels, cauterization, use of topical epinephrine (1:10,000) or topical thrombin, use of a tourniquet, and meshing the graft.[5,8,10,22,23] If a hematoma or seroma develops, it should be carefully expressed by gentle pressure, flushed with saline, or swabbed with a cotton-tipped applicator after several sutures have been removed at the most dependent portion of the graft.[22] A pressure bandage is maintained until adequate adherence is obtained.

Infection in the bed slows cell migration into the wound and subsequently delays revascularization of the graft. Bacterial elements not only cause cell death in the graft and recipient bed but also destroy the fibrin film that holds the graft to its bed.[24] In addition to antimicrobial agents used to control infection, mechanical cleansing of the wound can be accomplished by debridement of unhealthy granulation tissue. The signs of postgrafting infection include an odor and redness around the graft margin between the second and fourth postoperative days.[8] An unsuccessful graft appears necrotic and bleached. Extensive exudates may actually float the graft off its bed.

Lack of immobilization does not allow revascularization of the graft from its recipient bed. Until the graft adheres firmly to the bed and vascular connections are established, movement between the graft and its bed breaks down the developing vascular connections.[25] The area that presents the worst immobilization problem is the cranial tarsal region.

Skin graft losses are also observed from unacceptable recipient beds. A graft will not "take" on any of the body's epithelial surfaces. Fat, tendon, cortical bone, heavily irradiated tissues, long-standing granulation tissue, and the exposed surfaces of chronic ulcers are poor recipient beds for skin grafts.[8] An unlevel, irregular graft bed may cause the graft to be lost. Smooth, convex, immobile recipient beds provide the best graft bed contact.[13]

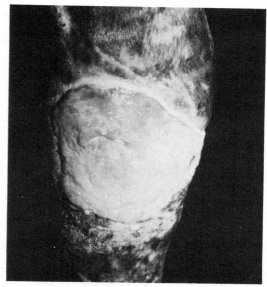

Fig 64. A healthy granulation bed on the cranial tarsal region, an excellent recipient site for a skin graft.

Preparation of the Recipient Bed

When a good blood supply is present, in 7-10 days open wounds develop a granulation tissue covering that serves as a mechanical barrier to invading microorganisms.[25] The time necessary to fill the void to skin level with granulation tissue may vary between 10 and 35 days, depending upon the amount of tissue lost. When necessary, several procedures may be used to stimulate granulation tissue growth, including application of hydrotherapy, wet saline bandages, dilute cresol bandages, and dilute povidone iodine dressings. Most water-soluble antimicrobial ointments used under bandages are mildly stimulating to the granulation tissue bed.

Healthy granulation tissue is firm, flat and red (Fig 64). Epithelialization around the bed's margins is a general indication that it will accept a graft. Chronic granulation beds are usually greyish red, edematous, covered with a tenacious exudate, more fibrotic and less vascular.[8] These should be radically excised several days prior to grafting to allow a new granulation bed to form. The excision should include 2-4 mm of the peripheral epithelium. The undesirable granulation tissue may be shaved off with a straight razor or scalpel blade.[5] This may be accomplished using a tranquilizer and twitch as restraint since granulation tissue has no innervation; a general anesthetic may be necessary if the nature of the animal dictates. After removing chronic

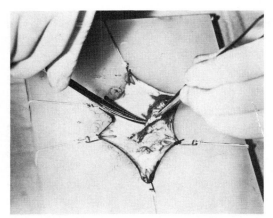

Fig 65. Full-thickness donor skin, placed with the hair side down on a polypropylene board, is held in place by 3 elastic skin hooks. Fat and fascia are trimmed away.

granulation tissue, a compression dressing with antimicrobial ointment is applied. This permits hemostasis and growth of a fresh, healthy recipient bed within 2 days in most cases.

Other factors that complicate the growth of a skin graft include habronemiasis, sarcoids and other neoplasia, phycomycosis, bone sequestration, joint and/or tendon sheath effusion, and foreign bodies. Any complication should be corrected prior to surgery.

The appropriate time for grafting is best determined by the appearance of the granulation bed. It should be free of exudate and should appear firm, flat and red, with evidence of epithelialization of the wound edges.[8]

Donor Sites

Horses have a tremendous reservoir of skin that can be used in skin grafting procedures. The considerations for selection of a donor site for a full-thickness graft include the looseness and abundance of the skin, and the color, thickness and texture of the hair as they relate to the recipient area.[24] Although similar criteria should be evaluated for a split-thickness graft, an additional concern arises: the postsurgical appearance of the donor site. Since a portion of the hair follicles are removed from the donor site during harvest of the graft, the final result is a sparser hair growth in this area, which may be cosmetically unacceptable.

Types of Skin Grafts

The 5 types of skin grafts to be considered are the free full-thickness graft, the free split-thickness graft, the mesh graft, the pinch graft, and the punch graft. Since the postsurgical care of grafted lesions is very similar for all of the technics, it will be discussed after the technics have been described.

Free Full-Thickness Grafts

A free full-thickness graft (Wolfe's graft) is composed of the epidermis and the entire thickness of the dermis. It closely mimics normal skin in color, texture, elasticity and hair growth. Such grafts undergo minimal contraction postsurgically, tolerate friction well, and maintain functional glandular components.[8-22]

Free full-thickness grafts require optimum conditions, *ie,* immobilization, a good blood supply, and minimal infection, for acceptance since they revascularize much more slowly than split-thickness grafts.[21]

This graft is indicated in situations in which the best cosmetic effect is desired. Its use should also be considered for areas over pressure points and flexion surfaces.[8]

Technic: This grafting procedure is usually performed aseptically, with the animal under general anesthesia. The donor tissue for the free full-thickness graft is taken from the cranial pectoral region since there is usually an abundant amount of loose skin in this area. The skin surface is surgically prepared and draped, as are the recipient bed and surrounding skin for a distance of 8-12 cm. The recipient bed should then be prepared for the grafting procedure. Any exuberant granulation tissue should be trimmed to skin level with a straight razor, followed by the application of sterile gauze sponges and gentle pressure to control hemorrhage. If the wound is not exuberant, brisk rubbing with a gauze sponge will suffice.

Once the bed is ready, a tracing of the outline of the wound is made with a piece of sterile towel, disposable drape, piece of developed x-ray film, or sheet of nylon. The pattern is placed on the donor area so the direction of hair growth on the graft is the same as that of hair growth surrounding the recipient area.[25] The donor skin is removed with a #15 scalpel, being careful to avoid any undue pressure and tension since this can distort the skin and result in a misshapen graft.[5] The donor site is usually closed by undermining the surrounding skin and closing the defect with deeply and superficially placed sutures. It may be wise to convert the defect to an elliptical shape for ease of closure. Do not harvest a piece of skin too large to permit suturing of the wound. It may be better to harvest several pieces and splice them on the recipient bed.

The donor skin is placed with the hairy side down on a polypropylene board (Surgical Plastic Block:Cyanamid) or piece of sterile vinyl tile and and held in place by 3 elastic skin hooks. All fat and fascia are trimmed from the donor tissue with rat-toothed thumb forceps and curved scissors (Fig 65). Dissection may seem tedious but is relatively easy with equine skin as compared with that for other domestic species. Appearance of the bases of the hair follicles signals that all fat has been removed.[9]

The graft should be kept moist at all times by placing it immediately on the recipient bed or using saline-moistened gauze sponges to sandwich the donor skin.

The graft is placed on the recipient bed and anchored in place by a few sutures at key points. This is necessary to evenly distribute the pliable skin over the entire defect. The remaining graft edges are sutured to the wound margin using 3-0 chromic catgut or braided nylon (Surgilon:Cyanamid) on a swaged reverse-cutting needle in a simple-interrupted pattern. The sutures are placed approximately 4-5 mm apart. Before tying the last sutures, all blood clots should be removed from beneath the graft (Fig 66).

Immediately after placing a graft on its bed, it appears greyish-white.[21] During the first 3-5 days after grafting, it appears bluish-grey; by postoperative day 8, the tissue takes on a reddish-blue color. It becomes more normal in appearance over the next 2 weeks.[26]

Skin that is severed from its blood supply is subject to degeneration of both the dermis and epidermis. The most viable elements of the skin are the hair follicles and sebaceous glands, which are the last structures to disappear in a sloughing graft. Sloughing of the epidermis is common. In thicker grafts, areas of necrosis and ulceration in the dermis easily become infected. Such areas may be located over a blood clot in the underlying bed.[27]

Blue, pink and red are generally considered favorable colors for a graft, whereas a white or black appearance of some duration is an unfavorable sign. A lack of drainage, firm adherence to the bed, and pink coloration indicate graft acceptance.

The surgeon should not panic when a graft takes on an adverse appearance. When a graft fails, epithelialization from the wound margins is stimulated. Consequently, a surprising amount of regeneration can occur under a dark, hard, nonviable piece of grafted skin.[25]

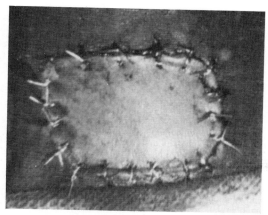

Fig 66. Sheet graft immediately after being sutured in place.

Free Split-Thickness Grafts

This graft is composed of the epidermis and a variable quantity of the dermis. It may be thin, intermediate or thick, depending upon the amount of dermis included. The thicker the dermis, the closer the properties approach those of a full-thickness graft.[22]

The split-thickness graft is indicated in repair of extremely large defects. The percentage of "takes" is better than that of a free full-thickness graft because revascularization occurs faster.

Technic: This procedure is performed aseptically, with the animal under general anesthesia. The donor areas used most frequently are the sternal region caudal to the elbow, the ventral abdomen, and the lateral thigh. A liberal area in the donor region is surgically prepared and draped, as is the recipient bed and its surrounding skin for a distance of 8-12 cm.

A split-thickness graft may be harvested with a grafting knife (Weck, Aloe Medical), a drum-type dermatome (Mueller, Bard-Parker), or electric and pneumatic dermatomes (Zimmer, Stryker, Mueller). The action of each instrument is that of a sharp blade moving back and forth to cut a piece of skin whose thickness is controlled by a calibrated setting.[8] The donor area must be flat, held under tension, and immobile.[13] Skin-graft knives have been developed for freehand cutting; several types have modifications to control the cutting depth on the knife. Once the donor area is held taut by tongue depressors or some other flat instrument, the surgeon lays the knife against the skin and angles it at about 15-20°. The blade is moved back and forth with short strokes about 5 cm behind the instrument that is creating

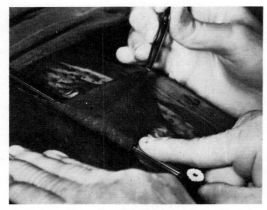

Fig 67. Split-thickness graft being harvestd with a Ferris-Smith skin graft knife.

tension (Fig 67). If the graft sticks to the blade, the blade can be lubricated with sterile mineral oil. The shims and rollers on some knives may be used to control the depth of the cut or the surgeon may judge the depth by sight. The surgeon can determine how thick the graft is soon after the cut is begun and adjustments can be made accordingly. A very thin graft is somewhat translucent; thicker grafts become increasingly opaque.[8,22]

Freehand cutting has been performed with an unmodified Schick injector razor to cut split-thickness grafts 0.012-0.014 inches thick and 1.25 inches wide.[28] A similar technic uses a Gillette safety razor modified by filing out the central strut of the safety guard.[29]

Drum-type, electric and pneumatic dermatomes are precision instruments designed to cut a graft of more uniform thickness than the freehand knives and eliminate some of the

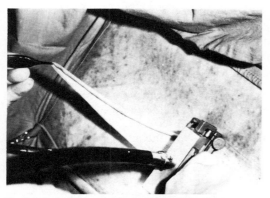

Fig 68. Split-thickness graft being harvested with a Stryker skin graft dermatome.

clumsiness of freehand cutting (Fig 68). However, they are considerably more expensive than the freehand instruments.[22] It is advisable to practice the harvesting technic of choice on a cadaver prior to one's initial grafting procedure since it may be difficult to obtain a good split-thickness graft with any of the above-mentioned instruments.

Once the donor skin has been harvested, care is taken to prevent drying of the graft. It is placed on the recipient bed with the proper direction of hair growth and attached in a similar manner as that described for the free full-thickness graft. The graft should not be stretched excessively in the suturing process. Overlapping graft edges may be trimmed to match the wound margin or allowed to necrose and slough. All blood clots must be removed prior to placement of the final sutures.

When a split-thickness graft is removed from the donor site, the epidermis is taken with it. Healing occurs by epithelium spreading over the denuded area from the cut surfaces of the hair follicles, sebaceous glands and sweat glands that remain in the dermis. Healing of the donor site occurs under a scab, usually in 2-4 weeks.

Mesh Grafts

A mesh graft (expansion graft) is a full-thickness or split-thickness skin graft in which multiple tiny slits have been cut to allow the graft to be stretched or expanded in 2 directions to many times its original size.[21,30] Indications for this grafting technic include coverage of large skin defects when there are inadequate donor sites, application of a graft to a somewhat less than ideal recipient bed, ie, one in which exudate, blood or serum is present, and reconstruction of irregular surfaces that are difficult to immobilize.[10-12,31]

Technic: This procedure is performed aseptically, with the animal under general anesthesia. The donor and recipient sites are surgically prepared and draped. A split-thickness graft may be harvested from the sternal region in a manner similar to that described for a free split-thickness graft. If a full-thickness graft is desired, it may be taken from the cranial pectoral region as an elliptical piece of skin, the size depending upon the defect to be covered. The resulting wound is closed with the suture pattern of choice. The long axis of the graft should be about one-third longer than the long axis of the wound and one-third to one-half the width of the defect to be covered. It may be necessary to harvest several pieces of skin and splice them together after expansion on ex-tremely large lesions.[11]

The donor skin is placed hairy side down on a polypropylene board and held in place by 3 elastic skin hooks. A piece of hard rubber cut-ting board or vinyl tile can be satisfactorily substituted for the polypropylene board. All fat and fascia are trimmed from the donor tissue with a rat-toothed thumb forceps and curved scissors. The graft should be moistened with sterile saline solution to prevent dehydration. Numerous incisions 1.0-1.5 cm long are made in the donor skin with a #11 scalpel blade. The cuts should be made in parallel rows about 2-5 mm apart. The incisions of each row should ex-tend beyond those adjacent to it. This produces a lattice network of the skin and allows it to be stretched into any desired shape (Fig 69).[11]

The size of the graft can also be expanded with a special mesh-grafting dermatome (Padgett), which cuts slits in the graft. The in-strument may be used to expand split-thick-ness or full-thickness grafts after fat and fascia have been removed. The dermatome is com-prised of a solid aluminum base, into which multiple parallel rows of cutting edges are mounted. The skin for transplantation is care-fully placed hairy side up on the mesh derma-tome so that all wrinkles are eliminated. To perforate the skin, a Teflon roller is passed across the graft in the direction of the blades, using moderate pressure. A graft with an ex-pansion ratio of 3:1 is produced that may be used to graft an area 3 times larger than the size of the graft before it was meshed (Fig 70).[10]

Before placing the expanded graft on the re-cipient bed, any excess granulation tissue should be excised to skin level. If the tissue is not exuberant, it is necessary only to freshen the site by rubbing it briskly with a gauze sponge. Hemorrhage can be controlled by ap-plying gentle pressure with gauze sponges.[3]

The cosmetic effect is improved when the cuts in the graft are placed parallel to the skin tension lines; the direction of hair growth on the graft should match that of hair growth of the surrounding area.[8,11] Since the main reason for using an expansion graft is to cover a large area with a small graft, the graft should be placed so the mesh can be expanded to cover the wound. This type of skin graft heals faster, is thicker and resembles more closely the sur-rounding skin if it is not expanded to its full extent when placed on the bed.[3]

The mesh is held in place with simple-inter-rupted sutures placed at the periphery of the

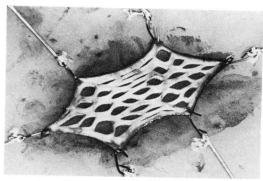

Fig 69. Full-thickness graft, stretched on a polypropy-lene board, has been meshed with a #11 scalpel blade to allow expansion. The staggered incisions are made in parallel rows.

graft, using 2-0 medium chromic catgut or non-absorbable material. On large wounds, the meshed skin is sutured to the underlying bed in a random fashion over the entire lesion with an interrupted suture pattern (Fig 71).

The diamond-shaped areas in the meshed skin heal by epithelialization, which is rapid since there is a 9-fold increase in the number of borders from which it can occur.[24] If grafting is successful, wounds usually heal in 12-18 days.[12] Initially a cosmetically undesirable diamond pattern is obvious, especially where the meshed donor skin was stretched to its maximal ex-tent. As the graft matures, however, it tends to assume more of the characteristics of a stan-dard split-thickness graft. Hair growth covers any residual mesh pattern (Fig 72).[10]

Pinch Grafts

A pinch graft is a type of seed graft in which small pieces of skin are placed in or on a gran-

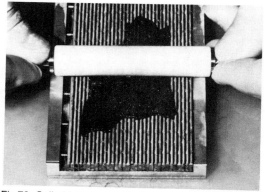

Fig 70. Split-thickness graft being expanded on a Padg-ett mesh dermatome.

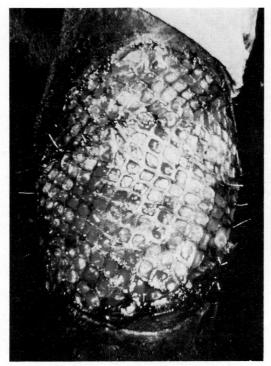

Fig 71. Mesh graft on a cranial tarsal recipient bed immediately after surgery.

ulating bed, with some regular spacing between the pieces of skin.[5]

This technic is indicated to repair large granulating wounds, to reconstruct contaminated and infected wounds, and to cover large wounds that cannot be well immobilized.[4,16,32]

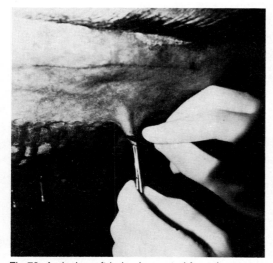

Fig 73. A pinch graft being harvested from the ventrolateral aspect of the thorax.

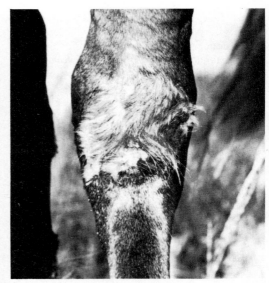

Fig 72. Split-thickness mesh graft on the cranial tarsal region 8 months postoperatively.

Although immobilization is of prime importance in any graft, this type of graft is not affected to a great extent by a small amount of movement because the lesion is covered by many small grafts embedded in the granulation bed itself. This nonsuture grafting technic does not require any special equipment.

Technic: The procedure may be performed with the horse standing and adequately restrained or recumbent and under general anesthesia. The donor and recipient sites are surgically prepared. Surgical drapes are used if the animal is under general anesthesia. The recommended sites for harvesting pinch grafts are the thorax, ventral abdomen, and lateral aspects of the neck and thigh. Generally the grafts should be taken from areas in which a slight cosmetic defect will not be noticed. Each graft may be harvested by first tenting the skin with a hypodermic needle, a curved suture needle or fine-toothed forceps. The skin is cut at right angles to the tent with a scalpel to produce a small piece of skin that is 2-4 mm in diameter, full thickness in the center and thinner at the edges (Fig 73).[4] These grafts are placed on a saline-moistened gauze sponge until transferred to the recipient bed. The donor sites may be left to heal as open wounds or may be sutured.

Pinch grafts may be embedded in the granulation tissue in 2 ways. First, the bits of skin may be thrust into the granulation tissue with forceps, the blunt end of a needle or probe and left below the surface of the bed.[4] Small pockets, 0.5-1.0 cm apart in every direction, may also be cut with a scalpel blade in the granulation tissue almost parallel to the wound surface, with the openings upward. The pinches of skin are placed in these pockets, which are 2-4 mm deep (Fig 74).[14] The latter technic has worked better. Grafts "floated" out of the pocket by hemorrhage can be held in place with forceps or digital pressure applied on the outside of the pocket. When placing pinch grafts in a standing horse, one should always work from the ventral area of the wound dorsad to prevent hemorrhage from obstructing the surgical field.

These grafts heal by the spreading of epithelial cells from the edges of each graft over the granulation tissue until the epithelial zones coalesce with each other and the wound margin.[5] By the sixth day, the granulation tissue over the pinch is gone and the graft appears as a small greyish-white spot.[33] Usually by the third or fourth week the epithelial tissue has coalesced over the entire wound if there is a good percentage of "takes."

Punch Grafts

The punch graft, also a type of seed graft, involves placement of small cylinders of full-thickness skin into previously created receptacle sites in the recipient bed.[9] This technic has been used extensively in hair transplantation in men.

The indications for this technic are similiar to those for the pinch graft except that this method cannot be used in areas that cannot be bandaged. This is an economical nonsuture grafting technic that allows a certain amount of mobility of the recipient bed.

Technic: The procedure is performed with the animal standing and adequately restrained or recumbent and under general anesthesia. The donor and recipient sites are surgically prepared. The recommended sites for obtaining punch grafts are the thorax, lateral aspect of the neck, and cranial pectoral region. The surgeon may harvest the individual grafts directly from the neck and thorax or remove an elliptical piece of skin from the cranial pectoral area, close the wound edges with simple-interrupted sutures, and harvest the grafts from the excised skin. The latter technic should be used if many punch grafts are needed. The donor skin is placed hairy side down on a polypropylene board or piece of vinyl tile and held in place by elastic skin hooks. All fat and fascia are trimmed from the donor tissue and a 7-mm

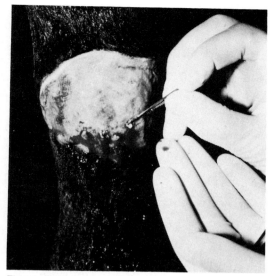

Fig 74. The pinch grafts are carefully tucked into the recipient "envelopes" with a #11 scalpel blade.

skin biopsy punch (Aloe Medical) is used to produce the small uniform cylinders of skin. This is done by placing the cutting edge of the punch on the stretched skin and, with firm pressure and a twisting motion of the hand, removing a small circular piece of skin (Fig 75). This is repeated until a sufficient number of free grafts are produced. The grafts are placed temporarily on a gauze sponge kept moist with sterile saline.[9]

If individual grafts are harvested, the same pressing, twisting action with a 7-mm skin biopsy punch is used until the entire thickness of skin is penetrated. The grafts, clinging to the body by subcutaneous fat and fascia, are then gently lifted with fine-tooth forceps and separated with curved scissors, cutting as close to the dermis as possible. These small cylindric

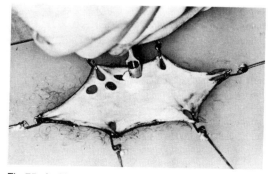

Fig 75. A skin punch is used to produce small circular plugs of skin after fat and fascia have been removed.

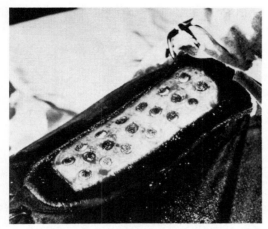

Fig 76. Punch grafts in their recipient bed immediately after surgery.

openings may be allowed to heal as open wounds or closed with one suture each.

The recipient sites for the skin punches are prepared as follows. Any excessive granulation tissue is sharply excised to skin level. The recipient beds for the small circular grafts are produced with a 5-mm skin biopsy punch. The cutting edge of the punch is placed on the gran-

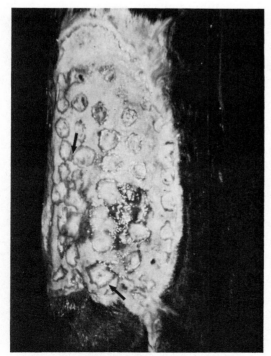

Fig 77. Lesion 21 days after punch graft surgery. Arrows denote the dark rings of epithelial tissue surrounding the grafted plugs.

ulation surface and, with slight pressure and a rotating movement, a circular plug of tissue removed. The depth of the recipient bed should correspond to the thickness of the skin transplant. These are spaced about 1.0 cm from each other in every direction. Clots that have formed in the recipient areas are teased out with a dry, sterile gauze sponge. The donor grafts are then placed into the recipient beds.[9]

On initial examination of the area after bandage removal 5-8 days after surgery, many of the grafts have sloughed their epidermal layers. The transplants appear as small, whitish-grey islands. Two weeks postoperatively, each grafted plug of skin is encircled by a dark red ring of epithelial cells, which gradually spreads until it coalesces with its neighboring grafts at about 3-4 weeks. By 6 weeks hair can usually be seen on the grafts, which have now taken on a greyish appearance. At 7-8 weeks pigmentation is progressing, while contraction of the lesion continues at a rapid rate (Figs 76-78).[9]

The cosmetic effect is considerably better than that obtained by the usual healing process. Although hair is present, it does not take on a smooth appearance but remains rough because the direction of hair growth has not been aligned with that of the grafted pieces of skin or that of the skin surrounding the lesion.[9]

Postoperative Care

Proper bandaging of the graft site is a very important step in obtaining a successful graft. The dressing should be nonadherent and provide protection, immobilization and adequate pressure.[25]

After the graft has been adequately secured on the recipient bed, an aqueous antibiotic powder (Neosporin:Wellcome) and a bandage are applied. The transplant is first covered with a nonadherent Telfa pad held firmly in place by an Elastikon adhesive bandage. Additional protection is afforded by a rubber foam pad (Reston Foam Pad:3-M) placed over the initial bandage and held by more elastic adhesive bandage material. A modified Robert-Jones bandage may be substituted for the foam pad bandage if additional protection and/or partial immobilization is desired. In areas of great mobility, a cast or a splint may be necessary to restrict movement of the grafted region. When the bandage is applied, care should be exercised to prevent excessive pressure on the graft itself, which would interfere with blood flow and result in ischemic necrosis.[24] The bandage is changed on the fourth postoperative day. At this time the graft is examined, cleansed carefully with saline-soaked gauze sponges, and rebandaged as previously described. An antibiotic ointment is used on the graft instead of the powder. The bandage is changed every 2-3 days after the initial examination until the wound is healed or completely epithelialized.

The donor site is treated according to the type of harvest. The defect created by harvesting full-thickness skin is usually closed by suturing, and healing is by primary intention. Split-thickness defects are allowed to heal by secondary intention. A scab is used as a natural bandage in this case; insects should be controlled accordingly. Use of postoperative systemic antibiotics is optional, but tetanus prophylaxis is essential.

Sliding Skin Flaps

Sliding skin flaps are useful in closing wounds that require considerable suture tension, such as those created by tumor or scar removal. A skin flap consists of skin and superficial fascia, with its arteries and veins. It is attached to the body at all times during transfer and its survival depends upon the efficiency of its circulation. If the blood supply is inadequate at the outset, nothing can save the flap. Assuming there is an adequate blood supply, the most common cause of trouble after transfer is development of tension. In designing a flap, the transfer must not create tension severe enough to lead to necrosis. The design of a skin flap should, therefore, consider the provision of an adequate blood supply, avoidance of excessive tension during and after transfer, and minimization of infection.[25]

Flaps are classified as local, in which the tissue transferred is in the vicinity of the defect, and distant, in which the transferred tissue is some distance from the defect.[25] Distant flaps are seldom used in large animals.

Wound repair by a local flap is usually preferable to use of a free skin graft. Flaps are more durable and can withstand the trauma to which they are subjected by the animal.[34] Local flaps also provide the best cosmetic effect because of the similarity in texture, thickness, color and hair type of the skin immediately adjacent to the wound.[6] The use of skin flaps on the distal extremities of horses is very limited since there is a scarcity of redundant skin in this region.

Flap construction should always be planned prior to the actual surgical procedure, with the animal in a normal standing position.[8] Flaps should be designed slightly larger than the de-

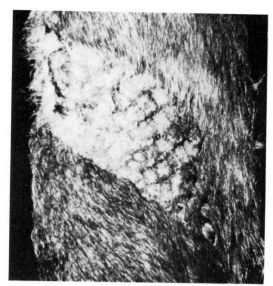

Fig 78. Lesion 6 months after punch graft surgery. Pigmentation, hair growth and wound contraction are complete.

fect to compensate for skin contraction.[35] It is also advisable to design a flap with slightly rounded corners if possible since sharp corners are subject to ischemic necrosis.[6]

The surgeon must keep in mind the direction of hair growth when placing flaps or free grafts. One must be certain that the hair growth of the flap in its final position will correspond to that of the surrounding area.[35]

The length:width ratio of a flap depends primarily upon the type of flap and area of the body involved. An acceptable ratio ranges from 1:1 to 3:1[36] The length:width ratio may be increased when large blood vessels pass into the base along its axis, the flap is located in an area of greater vascularity, or final placement of the flap has been "delayed."[8] A skin flap may be delayed to improve its vascularity or to condition the tissues to ischemia, allowing it to survive on less blood flow than normally needed.[37] This in turn helps ensure survival when the flap is transferred to its recipient bed. Delaying may be accomplished by incising the skin and subcutaneous tissue along 3 sides of the flap. This cuts off all blood supply to the flap except for that entering the pedicle and the deep surface of the flap. The wound is resutured and allowed to heal. In 7-10 days the flap is reincised and transferred.[8]

Once the flap has been designed, the recipient bed must be prepared. The site should be a healthy, fresh wound or a healthy granulating

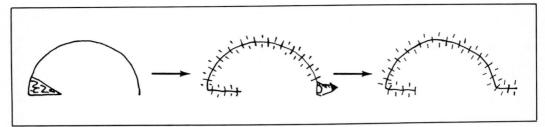

Fig 79. Rotation flap technic.[22]

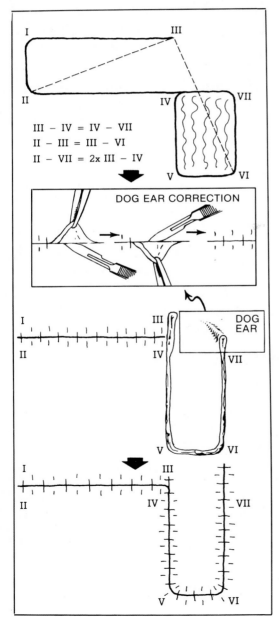

III – IV = IV – VII
II – III = III – VI
II – VII = 2x III – IV

DOG EAR CORRECTION

DOG EAR

Fig 80. Transposition flap technic, with "dog ear" correction.[25]

surface.[35] If a granulation bed exists, excess tissue should be removed so the normal skin around the lesion apposes well with the skin of the flap.

Hemostasis is important during the transfer procedure. Hematomas create tension, embarrass circulation and prevent early union of the flap with the recipient bed.[38]

Placement of a few vertical mattress tension sutures at strategic positions, to bring the flap's edges into apposition with the wound edges of the recipient site, prevents undue tension on the primary skin sutures. The remaining simple-interrupted sutures of fine nylon or silk are placed between the tension sutures.[26]

Bandages are usually placed over the grafted area to provide gentle pressure and protect the area from contamination and trauma. In certain areas of the body it may be necessary to resort to a stent or tie-over pressure bandage.

Because infection can cause loss of a flap, asepsis should be observed during the surgical transfer. The appropriate systemic antibiotics should be given for 5-7 days thereafter and tetanus prophylaxis also administered. Bandages and dressings are usually changed every 2-3 days for 14 days, at which time the skin sutures are removed.

Rotation Flaps

A rotation flap is a semicircular flap of skin and its subcutaneous tissue that rotates about a pivot point into the defect to be closed. The donor site is usually closed by suturing. The skin incision made to create a rotation flap should be 4 times longer than the space through which the skin is to be rotated. A dog ear is usually created as a result of skin flap rotation and is corrected as described in the section on the transposition flap technic (Fig 79).[22]

Transposition Flaps

A transposition flap is basically a rectangular piece of skin and its subcutaneous tissue turned on a pivot point to reach the adjacent wound to be closed. The defect is on a different axis from that of the flap, usually at a right angle to the axis of the flap.[22] This type of flap becomes shorter in effective length the further it is rotated and is used when the recipient area is adjacent to an area covered by loose skin.[39]

To design a flap that will transpose at a 90° angle with no tension, one edge of the defect should be incorporated into one edge of the flap, the width of the base of the flap should be at least equal to the width of the defect, and the edge of the flap that incorporates the edge of the defect should be at least twice as long as the base of the flap.[39] A flap designed according to these criteria has a sizable "dog ear," which must be removed from the area of abundant skin at the base of the flap. If removal of this skin will result in narrowing the base of the flap and jeopardizing its blood supply, it is better to remove the dog ear after the flap's circulation has been re-established. A dog ear is corrected by holding the excess skin to one side and extending the original incision just beyond the redundant pucker of skin. This triangular flap of skin is held up and removed by continuing the original incision to the end of the previously extended skin incision (Fig 80).[40]

Advancement Flaps

An advancement flap is a flap of skin mobilized by undermining and advanced into a defect without any rotation or lateral movement.[39] This graft is effective in defects around which the skin is loose and abundant.

To help equalize the length between the sides of the flap and the adjacent wound margins, triangles (Burow's triangles) may be excised lateral to the base of the flap.[39] This

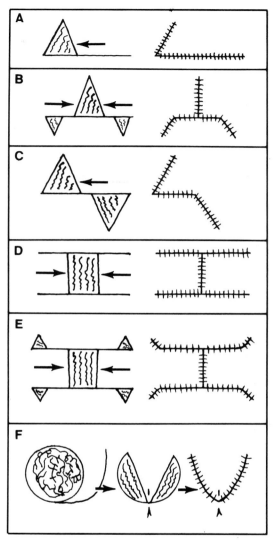

Fig 81. Single pedicle advancement flap technics used to close square, triangular and circular defects.[40]

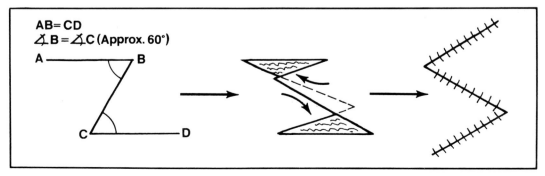

AB=CD
∠B=∠C (Approx. 60°)

Fig 82. Z-plasty technic.[25]

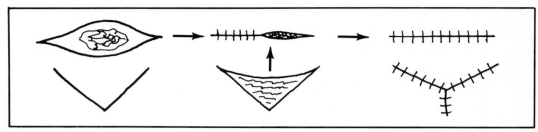

Fig 83. V-Y-plasty technic.[25]

overcomes the problem of tension created in the flap-advancement procedure. Many variations of advancement flaps have been designed to close square, rectangular, triangular and circular lesions (Fig 81).

Tension-Relieving Flaps

Several procedures have been developed to relieve tension created by scar contracture. These technics are referred to by letters of the alphabet the incisions resemble.

Z-Plasty: Probably the most commonly used tension-relieving flap is the Z-plasty, which involves transposition of 2 interdigitating triangular flaps.[27] It consists of a central limb and 2 arms positioned in the shape of the letter Z. The arms of the Z are equal in length to the central limb and are at an angle that varies from 30° to 90°.[8] By interchanging the 2 triangular flaps, the length of the original line can be increased 25-75%, depending upon the angle size. The wider the angle, the greater the increase in length (Fig 82).[22] This technic is used for excision of linear scars requiring relief of tension along their longitudinal axis.

V-Y Plasty: This flap is indicated to advance skin to cover a lesion. The procedure provides a small amount of tension relief when the apex of the V-Y flap is placed on the tension axis.[40]

A V-shaped incision is made in the skin, after which the skin on each side of the V is advanced. The closure changes the V to a Y, with the relief of tension and the amount of advancement of the flap proportional to the length of the leg that converts the V to a Y.[6] The V-Y plasty is helpful in correction of scars of the palpebrum and as a relaxing procedure for elliptical defects (Fig 83).[40]

W-Plasty: The W-plasty technic is used to revise a straight or curved scar, using a zigzag incision pattern without rotating the tissue.[41,42] It works best on a skin-level linear scar that crosses the lines of skin tension.

The W-plasty involves the surgical creation of a series of triangular flaps on each side of the scar in a design that allows the flaps to interdigitate perfectly when the wound is closed.[41,42] The limbs of the triangular flaps, which are about 6.5 mm long, are made alternately on each side of the scar until the entire length of the scar has been incised. The flaps created are isoceles triangles, each about 6 mm at its base and 6.5 mm high, with 2 65° angles and 1 50° angle.[43] The ends of a W-plasty use Ammon's triangles to prevent dog ear formation when the zigzag incision is closed (Fig 84).[41,42]

After removal of the scar, the flaps are undermined and apposed with a continuous intradermal suture to assure good interdigitation. Final apposition of the skin edges is with simple-interrupted sutures placed at the tip of each flap.[41]

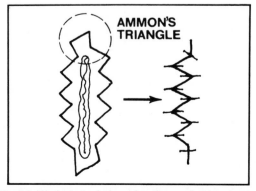

Fig 84. W-plasty technic, using Ammon's triangles to prevent "dog ears" at the ends of the W-plasty.[25]

References

1. Neal, PA. Vet Rec **73** (1961) 1399.
2. Boyd, CL. JAVMA **151** (1967) 1618.
3. Boyd, CL. Southwest Vet **20** (1967) 265.
4. Hogle, R *et al*. JAVMA **135** (1959) 165.
5. Brown, JB and McDowell, F: Skin Grafting. 3rd ed. JB Lippincott, Philadelphia, 1958.
6. Epstein, E: Skin Surgery. 1st ed. Lea & Febiger, Philadelphia, 1956.
7. Woodruff, MF: The Transplantation of Tissues and Organs. 1st ed. Charles C Thomas, Springfield, IL, 1960.

8. Grabb, WC and Smith, JW: Plastic Surgery: A Concise Guide to Clinical Practice. 2nd ed. Little, Brown and Co, Boston, 1973.

9. Boyd, CL and Hanselka, DV. JAVMA 158 (1971) 82.

10. Hanselka, DV. JAVMA 164 (1974) 35.

11. Hanselka, DV. Proc 21st Ann Mtg Am Assoc Eq Pract, 1975. p 191.

12. Hanselka, DV and Boyd, CL. JAAHA 12 (1976) 650.

13. Padgett, EC and Stephenson, KL: Plastic and Reconstructive Surgery. Charles C Thomas, Springfield, IL, 1948.

14. Mackay-Smith, MP and Marks, D. JAVMA 152 (1968) 1633.

15. Meagher, DM and Adams, OR. Eq Vet J 11 (1970) 239.

16. Neal, PA. Vet Rec 70 (1958) 401.

17. Obel, AN. Nord Vet Med 10 (1951) 869.

18. Sherinberg, YI. Veterinariya 33 (1956) 52.

19. Woolsey, JH and Shaffer, MH. JAVMA 121 (1952) 173.

20. Peacock, EE and Van Winkle, W: Wound Repair. 2nd ed. WB Saunders, Philadelphia, 1976.

21. Converse et al, in Converse: Reconstructive Plastic Surgery: Principles and Procedures in Correction, Reconstruction and Transplantation. 2nd ed. WB Saunders, Philadelphia, 1977.

22. McGregor, IA: Fundamental Techniques of Plastic Surgery. 6th ed. Churchill Livingston, Edinburgh, 1972.

23. Stark, RB: Plastic Surgery. Harper & Row, New York, 1962.

24. Cawley and Archibald, in Archibald: Canine Surgery. 2nd ed. American Veterinary Publications, Santa Barbara, 1974.

25. Swaim, SF: Surgery of Traumatized Skin: Management and Reconstruction in the Dog and Cat. 1st ed. WB Saunders, Philadelphia, 1980.

26. Pullen, in Bojrab: Current Techniques in Small Animal Surgery. 1st ed. Lea & Febiger, Philadelphia, 1975.

27. Converse, in Epstein: Skin Surgery. 2nd ed. Lea & Febiger, Philadelphia, 1962.

28. Snow, JW. Plastic Reconstr Surg 41 (1968) 184.

29. Shoul, MI. Am J Surg 112 (1966) 959.

30. Tanner, JC et al. Plast Reconstr Surg 34 (1964) 287.

31. MacMillan, BG. Surg Clin No Am 50 (1970) 1347.

32. Ross, GE. JAVMA 153 (1968) 1759.

33. Hoffer, RE and Alexander, JW. JAAHA 12 (1976) 644.

34. Spreull, JS. JAAHA 4 (1968) 71.

35. Krahwinkel, DJ and Howard, DR. AAHA Sci Proc 2 (1975) 439.

36. Johnston, D. AAHA Sci Proc 2 (1975) 383.

37. Myers, in Grabb and Myers: Skin Flaps. Little, Brown and Co, Boston, 1975.

38. Millard, in Cooper: Craft of Surgery. 2nd ed. Little, Brown and Co, Boston, 1971.

39. Grabb, in Grabb and Myers: Skin Flaps. Little, Brown and Co, Boston, 1975.

40. Stashak, TS. JAVMA 170 (1977) 143.

41. Borges, AF: Elective Incisions and Scar Revision. Little, Brown and Co, Boston, 1973.

42. Kirk, MD. VM/SAC 71 (1976) 801.

43. Borges, AF. Br J Plast Surg 12 (1959) 29.

WOUNDS AND THEIR MANAGEMENT
by D.V. Hanselka

Wound management demands a great deal of time of any veterinarian involved in general equine practice. Horses panic in many situations and make violent attempts to free themselves from any entanglement. Loud and unusual noises, such as thunderstorms, sonic booms, low-flying aircraft and gunshots, often cause horses to run blindly through fences and into solid objects, with total disregard for their well-being. Barbed wire is most commonly responsible for wounds, although many other objects can be incriminated.[1]

Successful wound management involves prevention and/or control of infection in contaminated wounds, elimination of sepsis in infected wounds, and promotion of healing as quickly as possible.[1] The treatment of wounds, especially of those below the knee and hock, can be extremely frustrating to both owner and veterinarian. Lesions of the lower limbs frequently fail to respond properly because of minimal soft tissue, poor circulation, inadequate drainage, increased exposure to contamination and infection, and excessive movement. The treatment selected depends upon the value, use and temperament of the animal, type of wound and its location, geographic location, facilities available, client demands, and veterinarian's preference.[2,3]

Types of Wounds

Open Wounds

Wounds may be classified as open or closed, depending on the degree of penetration of the skin. Open wounds are those in which the entire thickness of skin has been separated.[4,5] Open wounds may be classified as follows.

Incisions: These are wounds produced by sharp objects, intentionally with a scalpel during surgery, or accidentally by glass, sheet metal and similar objects. The skin edges are cleanly cut, with very little tissue damage. Hemorrhage is not severe unless a large vessel has been interrupted; a minimal amount of pain is present. The chief danger from incised wounds inflicted accidentally is damage to underlying blood vessels, nerves, muscles, tendons and abdominal or thoracic viscera.[1,5]

Lacerations: These wounds are probably the most common. They are usually produced by angular objects, such as barbed wire, and by animal bites. Lacerations are characterized by irregular skin edges and extensive damage to underlying tissue. Unless large vessels are opened, hemorrhage is usually not profuse because the vessels are often torn, resulting in marked vascular constriction. Severe pain is associated with the severe bruising of tissues. The chances for infection and tissue necrosis are great. When tissue has been torn away, the laceration is termed an avulsion.[1,5]

Punctures: These wounds are produced by sharp objects and are characterized by small, superficial perforations of variable depth. Punctures may produce serious complications and are commonly caused by nails, splinters, bites, goring and pitchforks. Dirt, manure and other debris often are carried into the depths of the wound. Joint cavities, tendon sheaths, and the abdominal and thoracic cavities may be invaded by the penetrating objects. Punctures may be characterized as penetrating into a body cavity, perforating a body cavity and back out, or a stab that goes into deep tissue only.[1,5]

Closed Wounds

Closed or subcutaneous wounds are those in which the skin has not been broken through all of its layers.[4,5] Closed wounds can be classified as follows.

Abrasions: An abrasion results from a friction injury to the superficial surface of the skin or mucous membrane and causes oozing of serum and minimal hemorrhage. These wounds are very sensitive and heal more slowly than would be anticipated. Usual causes include falls on gravel, rope burns, and scraping of the legs on the tailgate. They may lead to complications, such as habronemiasis, excessive fibrosis and keloid formation.[1,5]

Contusions: These wounds are characterized by loss of continuity without actual division of the skin. The trauma, usually a fall or kick, ruptures subcutaneous or deep blood vessels but leaves the skin intact. Contusions are categorized as first, second or third degree. A first-degree contusion consists of slight hemorrhage into and under the skin, producing discoloration but very little hematoma formation. A second-degree contusion is a subcutaneous hematoma, which will probably be absorbed if small. If it is large, the contusion may lead to scar formation and a possible blemish. It may also form a seroma after the blood cells of the clot have been absorbed. There is some danger of abscess formation from hematogenous origin. A third-degree contusion is a hematoma so extensive that the tissue is damaged beyond

repair. Although the skin is not broken from the original blow, thrombosis of the underlying blood vessels results in necrosis and sloughing of superficial tissues.[1,5] An excellent example is a skin slough observed on the withers, resulting from an ill-fitting saddle ("saddle sore").

Burns

Burns, which involve coagulation of tissue proteins, are caused by exposure of the skin to excessive heat or corrosive substances. Freezing, in which tissue fluids are frozen, may be considered a type of burn.[6]

Thermal burns have been classified according to the severity and the type of lesion produced. First-degree burns involve damage to the epithelium, transient erythema and subsequent desquamation. Second-degree burns consist of damage to the entire epithelium and varying depths of the dermis, accompanied by vesicle formation. Third-degree burns are characterized by complete destruction of the full thickness of the skin, variable amounts of damage to subcutaneous tissues, subsequent ulceration and sloughing. More recently, burns have been described as superficial, partial thickness or full thickness, as they relate to depth of the damage to the skin.

Tissue Repair

The skin is the largest and most exposed organ of the body. Consequently it is very susceptible to trauma. Skin defects not only result from accidental injury, but also from the surgical removal of pathologic conditions involving this organ.[7] Tissue damage may result from physical, chemical and/or biologic insults.[4] The many types of wounds of the skin and underlying tissues are all associated with certain anatomic, physiologic, pathologic and microbiologic factors. Although all of these factors affect wound healing, the basics of the process remain the same, ie, cell migration to bridge the gap, cell multiplication to replace the lost cells and, finally, cell maturation so that the tissue can function again.[4,6]

The sequence of events in the healing of a wound can be divided into the inflammatory, debridement, repair and maturation stages.[7] It is important to remember that these stages or phases of tissue repair tend to overlap and should be considered a continuous sequence of events proceeding in an orderly manner. Some of the processes of healing may continue for years after the physical integrity of the affected tissue has been re-established.[6]

Inflammatory Stage

The inflammatory phase of healing is basically a vascular and cellular response that disposes of microorganisms, foreign material and devitalized tissue. The mechanisms responsible for tissue repair are also initiated.[8,9]

Following a full-thickness skin injury, the normal elasticity and external muscular tension tend to enlarge the defect. As a result, the shape of the defect may have little resemblance to the size and shape of the skin segment removed.[10] Immediately after injury the small vessels constrict and vascular occlusion tends to limit hemorrhage at the wound site.[11] Blood flows into the gap, providing fibrinogen and other clotting components. As the clot forms, enzymatic activity provides an intricate network of interconnected fibrin strands, which provides a framework for further healing.[11]

Normally the clot contracts and dehydrates to form a protective scab.[9,11] If there is excessive hemorrhage, this blood must be clotted, organized and removed by absorption before healing can proceed.

Active vasodilation, with increased blood flow to the injured area, follows the initial vascular constriction. Capillary and venule permeability increases, plasma-like fluids rich in enzymes, proteins, antibodies and complement arrive in the tissue by diapedesis and active movement, and WBC escape from the affected vessels and congregate around the injured tissue.[8,9,11] The duration and intensity of this stage vary according to the degree of local tissue damage.

Debridement Stage

Within 6-12 hours after injury, neutrophils and monocytes migrate to the affected tissue. Neutrophils, which are short-lived as compared with mononuclear cells, are necessary to clean up infected wounds since healing does not progress until infection is controlled. This is accomplished through ingestion of organisms by phagocytosis. The neutrophils, in turn, die and degenerate, releasing enzymes that attack extracellular debris.[11]

Monocytes become macrophages when they enter the wound. They then phagocytize dead tissue and debris, which are partially digested. Mononuclear cells may also coalesce to form multinucleate giant cells or evolve into epithelioid cells and histiocytes. Macrophages attract fibroblasts into the injured site and promote collagen synthesis.[11]

Tissue fluids, combined with WBC and necrotic tissue, make up the inflammatory exudate. In time this exudate takes on the appearance of pus. The enzymes associated with pus interfere with epithelialization and fibroplasia. Healing can be hindered by insufficient drainage of an infected wound.[8,11]

Repair Stage

Repair starts soon after injury and proceeds as rapidly as blood clots, necrotic debris and other barriers are removed from the wound. Fibroblast proliferation, capillary infiltration, and epithelial proliferation and migration are involved in wound repair.[9]

Fibroblasts, which originate from undifferentiated mesenchymal cells in nearby connective tissue, move into the wound by advancing along fibers within the fibrin clot that forms soon after injury. They also move along capillaries that are growing into the wound. These cells slide along a cytoplasmic extension of their wall (ruffled membrane). As they encounter other fibroblasts, movement ceases and the cells stick together (contact inhibition). This aggregation of cells eventually fills the defect created by lost tissue. Fibroblasts usually appear in the wound about the third day and continue to multiply for 14-21 days.[11]

In small incisions, the fibrin strands of the clot are oriented vertically. Consequently the fibroblasts migrate vertically, producing a similar arrangement to new collagen fibers that they produce. Where there is tissue loss, the elasticity of the skin places tension on the clot that is adherent to the wound margins. The fibrin strands are subsequently oriented toward the edge of the wound. Entering fibroblasts are guided along these fibrils toward the center of the defect.[11]

After fibroblasts have entered a wound, they secrete protein-polysaccharides and various glycoproteins that make up the wound's ground substance. The mucopolysaccharides of this substance surround the fibroblasts and affect the aggregation and orientation of collagen.[9] Collagen is synthesized by the fibroblasts from hydroxyproline and hydroxylysine beginning about the fourth or fifth day. The small collagen bundles gradually aggregate and enlarge to form a dense collagenous scar that binds the edges of the severed tissues together. As the collagen content of the wound increases, the level of glycoproteins and mucopolysaccharides decreases due to the diminishing number of synthesizing fibroblasts. Collagen content in a wound is also controlled by collagenase, which is liberated from proliferating epithelial cells and fibroblasts that have come in contact with the new epithelial cells.[11]

The repair phase may last several weeks to many months. There is an early rise in tensile strength as collagen is produced and deposited in the wound. A slower increase in tensile strength takes place over a long period, resulting from maturation and remodeling of the collagen. The strength of scar tissue never reaches that of normal skin.[12] Research indicates that a healed skin wound in a rat is only 80% as strong as comparable unwounded skin.[13]

A major component of connective tissue is elastin. This fibrous element is not replaced when removed through injury, which explains the lack of elasticity of scar tissue.[11]

Capillary proliferation and infiltration play a major role in fibroblastic replication and synthetic activity. Oxygen is necessary for cell migration, cell multiplication and protein synthesis.[11] Following trauma, the center of the wound is most deficient of O_2. This lack of O_2 tension may be partially responsible for the branching and ingrowth of new blood vessels from the periphery of the wound.[12] Bright-red granular tissue appears in an open wound 3-6 days after injury as a result of proliferation of capillary loops. These loops originate from the endothelial cells of cut capillaries and grow into the wound immediately behind the fibroblasts at a rate of about 1 mm/day. Granulation tissue is red, firm, flat and nonexuberant as it grows to cover the entire wound. As granulation tissue develops, the simple blood channels differentiate progressively into arterioles, capillaries and venules.[11,12] Granulation tissue is extremely resistant to infection and allows the epithelium to migrate across its surface. Wound contraction is probably initiated in this tissue.[9] Exuberant granulation tissue ("proud flesh") is common in horses, especially with wounds below mid-radius and mid-tibia. Excessive granulation tissue develops when collagen fiber deposition has exceeded new capillary formation.[11] Although proud flesh may form, wound healing may progress in spite of its presence, but usually at a much slower pace.

A system of lymphatics is produced in the wound, basically in the same manner as blood vessels. Lymphatic endothelial cells that arise from previously damaged lymphatics migrate into the granulating tissue and undergo mitotic activity, resulting in lymphatic channels.[7]

Epithelial proliferation and migration begin very soon after injury. The marginal basal cells enlarge, flatten and extend superficially and deep over the exposed dermis. Excess cells migrate out over the defect to replace the epithelial cell deficit.[11] Coverage of an incision can occur in 12-24 hours.[12] However, in an open wound that penetrates the entire dermis, a granulation bed must form before epithelial migration can occur.[14] There is usually a period of 4-5 days before the epithelium begins to migrate from the wound margins across the developing granulation tissue. In preparation for migration across the wound surface, there is a tremendous buildup of peripheral epidermal cells (reservoir of cells). Epithelial migration proceeds in a manner similar to that described for fibroblasts. The epithelial cells slide across the granulating surface until they are surrounded by similar cells (contact inhibition).[15] If a scab is present, the epithelial cells secrete collagenase, which dissolves the base of the scab so it can be shed.[11] As the epithelium thickens, the cells become more columnar and mitosis is increased. The epithelium becomes layered and acquires some of the structural features of the adjacent epidermis. Migration is rapid at first but, as the line of cells from the wound margin extends, the epithelium becomes a single layer and its progress slows tremendously. Days, weeks or even months may pass before epithelialization is complete.[12] In some large wounds, epithelialization may not be sufficient to cover the wound.

Maturation Stage

During the early stages of wound healing, collagen synthesis adds to the ultimate strength of the wound. As collagen content stabilizes, various tissue collagenases remove nonfunctional and unnecessary collagen fibers; functionally oriented fibers are preserved. In the course of tissue maturation and remodeling, wound strength is achieved as a result of increased intermolecular and intramolecular cross-linkage of collagen fibers and a change in the physical weave of the fibers. The fibrils increase slightly in thickness and compactness and group into bundles.[11] Scar tissue of a healed wound is initially quite vascular, cellular and pink. As the scar matures and contracts, the vessels and cells become fewer and the scar becomes white and flattened.[14]

Wound contraction is a reduction in size of an open wound as the result of centripetal movement of the full-thickness skin that surrounds the lesion.[11] Granulation tissue contains fibroblasts (myofibroblasts) that develop characteristics typical of smooth muscle, including contractile ability. This allows the skin margins to be pulled centripetally so that the area to be covered by epithelialization is reduced.[11] In areas where skin is loosely attached to underlying structures, closure of the wound can be completed by wound contraction, leaving minimal scar tissue. Where contraction cannot reach the ultimate conclusion, a wider scar is left.[9] Wound contraction is a natural phenomenon that greatly facilitates management of large skin defects. The beneficial effects of wound contraction greatly outweigh the ill effects.[12]

Factors Affecting Wound Healing

Many elements and conditions enhance or inhibit wound healing. These factors must be carefully considered by the surgeon so that appropriate decisions can be made in managing the wound.

Condition of the Patient

The physical condition of the animal definitely affects wound healing. Dehydration, endocrine imbalances, and diseases of the heart, kidney and liver can alter wound healing.[14] Hypoproteinemia and chronic anemia have a deleterious effect on wound healing.[12,14] The age of the animal may affect healing; older individuals usually have decreased fibroplasia and cell proliferation and an increased susceptibility to infection.[14]

Infection

Bacterial infection can interfere with wound healing in several ways. Bacterial invasion of the injured site may lead to exudation that mechanically separates the wound surfaces. Ulcers, abscesses, fistulas or sinuses may form from bacterial contamination. Bacteria also produce necrotizing toxins or enzymes that destroy tissues. These include hyaluronidase, which favors the spread of infection, collagenase, which destroys and inhibits collagen production, fibrinolysins, which destroy developing fibrin, coagulases, which produce vascular thrombosis, and hemolysins, which destroy hemoglobin.[14]

Contaminated wounds may become infected when large amounts of necrotic tissue or certain types of foreign bodies are present, and in interference of local tissue defenses, as in burns or immunosuppression. When organism numbers reach a concentration of 1×10^6/g tissue, the wound is considered infected. The lower the initial number of bacteria, the longer it takes to reach the point of infection.[11] Not only the number of bacteria but also the environment within the wound determines if the wound becomes infected.

Movement

Movement of the wound edges tends to delay, if not totally disrupt, the healing process. This results from rupture of new capillaries and disturbance of the growth pattern of new fibers, often causing deposition of excess collagen fibers.[7] Wound edges should be immobilized with sutures and/or bandages if feasible.

Foreign Bodies

If a foreign body in the depths of the wound promotes infection or causes irritation, the wound usually does not heal until the material is removed. As long as a draining tract remains open to the body surface, little harm is done except that the wound does not heal. If the tract seals over, a deep-seated abscess may result.[12]

The most common foreign bodies encountered in equine wounds are grass, straw, wood, iron scraps and gravel. Included in the list of foreign bodies are sequestra of bone. A bone sequestrum usually results from trauma to the periosteum and cortex, which causes vascular impairment and ventual necrosis of the affected bone. Talcum powder and other insoluble powders may lead to granuloma formation.

A few materials are basically inert and cause little or no tissue response, such as carbon fibers and certain suture material, such as stainless steel. Lead bullets, shell fragments and birdshot cause little tissue reaction.

Sharp objects, such as broken hypodermic needles and slivers of glass, may not cause any appreciable tissue reaction. However, they may migrate through tissues, as a result of muscle movement, and penetrate vital organs.

Drugs

Certain drugs can have a detrimental effect upon tissue repair. Anti-inflammatory drugs, such as phenylbutazone, corticosteroids and ACTH, reportedly affect the healing process. However, it is unlikely that physiologic levels or therapeutic doses of these compounds adversely affect the quality of wound healing.[11]

Because topical antimicrobial powders and ointments may impede healing due to their irritant nature, the veterinarian should carefully select a topical powder or ointment to use in wound therapy.

Cytotoxic drugs usually interfere with cell proliferation, which is detrimental to wound healing. Long-term application of thiotepa and fluorouracil may completely prevent healing.[11]

Hematomas and Seromas

Collections of blood or serum within a wound can retard healing by mechanically separating the tissue edges. The fluid can also exert enough pressure to interfere with the vascular supply to the surrounding tissues. Serosanguineous fluid also provides an excellent medium for bacterial growth and abscessation.[14]

Neoplasia

Wounds or surgical incisions made in neoplastic tissue may not heal due to proliferation of tumor cells.[14] The neoplasms most commonly encountered in horses are sarcoids, squamous-cell carcinomas and melanomas. For this reason, it is advisable to biopsy nonhealing wounds.

Parasitism

Due to the environment in which horses live, open wounds are very susceptible to infestation by parasites. The irritation created by the presence of these parasites usually delays healing. The most frequent infestation that presents some difficulty in treatment is habronemiasis ("summer sores"). During fly season, the larvae of *Habronema* are deposited in the open wound. Through their migration and subsequent irritation, the wound fails to heal. Other parasites that disturb wound healing include maggots, screwworms and other flies.

Mycosis

Phycomycosis, which has been reported in Florida and Texas, is caused by a fungus, *Hyphomyces destruens*. Open wounds are usually contaminated by wading in ponds, rice canals and swampy areas. The extreme irritation in the wound causes the animal to mutilate the granulating area. Chronic granulomatous disease is recognized by the yellowish-white necrotic cores ("leeches") that form in the depths of the wound.[16]

Trauma

Prolonged trauma to a wound can delay healing indefinitely. The tendency of horses to chew or rub healing wounds must be anticipated and appropriate precautions taken, including use of a neck cradle, bib, cross-tie, heavy bandage, cast, or various repellents, such as cayenne pepper, on a bandage.

The surgeon should prevent excessive intraoperative trauma by handling tissues carefully, preventing dehydration of tissues, and limiting exposure of tissues.[14]

MANAGEMENT OF SKIN INJURY

Therapy for Contaminated and Infected Wounds

Most self-inflicted wounds should be considered contaminated due to the circumstances under which they occur. They are also often needlessly contaminated by overzealous owners attempting to provide first aid. When dealing with open wounds, the veterinarian should instruct the client on proper care of the wound prior to transport of the animal to the clinic or arrival of the veterinarian at the farm. Instructions should simply be to do nothing more than apply a large, clean occlusive dressing of cotton and gauze or an improvised bandage of clean cloth held firmly in place. Disposable diapers are ideal for small wounds. Such a bandage helps protect the wound, prevents further contamination, and helps stem profuse hemorrhage. Antiseptics, ointments and powders should not be applied to wounds since they increase the possibility of additional contamination and chemical irritation to the tissues. Ointments make cleansing and debriding difficult if the wound is to be sutured.[12]

It is often difficult to decide whether to suture a wound or allow it to heal by granulation. Factors that influence the treatment of lacerations include the type and location of the wound, temperament and use of the horse, economics, demands of the client, facilities available, and the veterinarian's preference.[2]

Equine wounds are generally extremely traumatic because of the severe bruising and tearing of tissue that occur as a result of the horse's size and explosive nature. Lacerations of the lower leg most often cause severe scarring and sometimes disability if allowed to heal poorly. Wound repair tends to be poor in this region because of the minimum of soft tissue, poor circulation, inadequate drainage, increased opportunity for contamination and infection, and excessive movement.[2] These conditions promote development of exuberant granulation tissue, which delays or prevents healing. Surgical intervention, if feasible, promotes "optimum healing of these wounds with maximum preservation of tissue and maximum return of function in a minimum of time with a minimum of scar tissue."[2]

After the health and nutritional status of the animal has been evaluated and the wound is thoroughly examined, a decision on surgical intervention should be made. If surgery is elected, one must attempt to prevent or stop infection in contaminated wounds, eliminate sepsis in infected wounds, immobilize the wound, support the site, and protect the area from additional contamination.[2]

A series of organized steps necessary in achieving first-intention healing include restraint of the animal, preparation, cleansing and debridement of the wound, placement of drains if necessary, wound closure, protection and support of the closed wound, and postoperative care of the animal.[2]

Restraint

The choice of restraint is dictated by the situation. Most wounds can be sutured with the horse standing, using sedation and local anesthesia. However, there are circumstances in which general anesthesia should be used, such as for severe lacerations in inaccessible regions of the body and for intractable animals.

Anesthesia of wounds in standing horses may be achieved by specific nerve blocks or infiltration of the area with a local anesthetic, preferably one that does not contain a vasoconstrictor. Vasoconstrictors may cause necrosis of the skin in thin-skinned animals and may interfere with healing near the wound edge. The anesthetic agent should be infiltrated around the wound but not near the free edges of a laceration. This minimizes postoperative swelling and allows easier visualization of the tissues during surgery. If it is necessary to anesthetize the area from within the wound, care should be exercised in cleansing the wound prior to infiltration to minimize the hazard of forcing contaminants into deeper tissues.

Preparation of the Site

Protection of the wound is important while the surrounding area is being prepared. One of the most popular methods for protecting the wound is packing it with saline-moistened sterile gauze sponges.[14] Another widely used technic is to fill the wound with a sterile, water-soluble lubricant, such as K-Y jelly (Johnson & Johnson). Once the wound is prepared, the lubricating jelly is washed from the wound, along with any hair or soap adhered to it. Small lacerations may be temporarily closed with towel forceps, Michel wound clips or a

continuous suture.[14] However, these technics inhibit removal of hair from the very edge of the wound.

The hair around the wound is clipped with a #40 blade from an area ample enough to allow adequate aseptic preparation of the site. Use of suction with the clippers helps remove loose hair particles. The wound edge is further prepared by shaving with a straight-edge razor or a large scalpel blade.

After clipping and shaving are complete, any gauze sponges used to pack the wound are removed and replaced with fresh sponges. The peripheral skin is then scrubbed with a mild surgical soap as for aseptic surgery.

Cleansing the Wound

Following preparation of the wound periphery, attention is focused on cleansing the wounded tissue itself and preparing it for primary closure. Most agree that soaps and detergents are somewhat irritating to damaged tissue. Surgical scrub solutions are a mixture of surface-active detergents and antiseptic agents. The bacteria are destroyed by the antiseptic compound and the detergent reduces the surface tension between the wound and debris to facilitate removal of contaminants. However, the detergents in surgical scrubs are mildly toxic to tissues, especially muscles, tendons and blood vessels, and inhibit their defense systems, thereby potentiating bacterial infection. Some feel that even though soaps are toxic to cells, their action on contaminants overrides their adverse effects on tissues.[17] If one chooses to scrub the wound with an antiseptic detergent, the wound should be thoroughly rinsed with physiologic saline or a water-antibiotic mixture to prevent trapping any of the detergent in the depths of the wound.

Washing a wound with tap water effectively removes bacteria and tissue debris lying unattached on the surface. After use of tap water, one should freely irrigate with sterile saline or sterile water.[11] Addition of antibiotics to the irrigating solution is an efficient way to treat contaminated wounds. The combination of penicillin-streptomycin and water is 5 times more effective than water alone.[18]

Physiologic saline solution is an effective wound lavaging agent.[14] It does not cause appreciable tissue damage and is more effective in contaminated wounds when combined with antibiotics.

Care should be exercised when selecting an antiseptic agent to cleanse a contaminated wound.

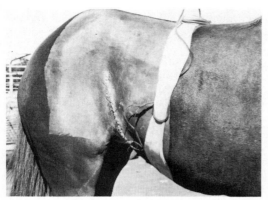

Fig 85. Plastic accordion-type reservoir used for vacuum drain, positioned on the lumbar area to relieve fluid accumulation from a laparotomy site.

It should be remembered that any antiseptic strong enough to kill bacteria is also strong enough to kill tissue cells.[11] Dilute solutions of povidone iodine have been used for cleansing wounds.[2,17,19] Povidone iodine (Betadine:Purdue Frederick) controls wound sepsis, has a broad antimicrobial spectrum of activity without bac-

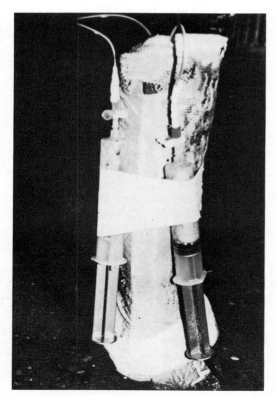

Fig 86. Vacuum drains, constructed from large plastic syringes, are secured to a cast after tendon surgery.

terial resistance, is effective in blood, pus, serum and necrotic debris, and causes minimal tissue reaction.[19] Another popular antiseptic is 0.05% chlorhexidine (Nolvasan:Fort Dodge) solution, which has many properties similar to povidone iodine compounds.[20]

Hydrogen peroxide is a good cleansing agent because of its mechanical foaming action, which lifts debris and clotted blood from the wound.[20] However, damage to the microvascular system of the wound has been observed after use of 3% hydrogen peroxide in distilled water.[21]

Irrigating the wound appears to have a distinct advantage over simply pouring an antiseptic solution into the wound to decrease the incidence of infection. Irrigation or lavage not only floats away debris and particles of tissues but also removes, dilutes or reduces the number of bacteria within the wound.[22] A disadvantage is the possibility of spreading infection to deeper tissues.[14] Lavage may be accomplished with a rubber bulb-type syringe, a large syringe with a small hypodermic needle, or a Water Pik (Teledyne Aquatic). The last device provides a pulsating, high-pressure stream of water for lavage. The Water Pik is 3 times more effective than a bulb syringe in removing tissue fragments and 7 times more effective in removing bacteria from a wound.[18] Increasing the volume of irrigating solution also decreases the incidence of infection.[23]

When cleansing a wound by any method, it is imperative that tissues be handled gently to prevent additional trauma. Overzealous scrubbing can be detrimental to wound healing.

Wound Debridement

After the wound has been thoroughly cleansed, it is ready for debridement. Adhering to the principles of aseptic technic, the surgeon should drape the wound if feasible. Self-adhering plastic drapes are best suited for standing animals. The surgeon should be gloved at this point in the procedure. The debridement technic varies according to the type of wound and its location. Wound debridement basically involves removal of devitalized, contaminated and necrotic tissue.[20] During surgical debridement all incisions should be made by sharp dissection, using a scalpel or scissors in conjunction with rat-toothed forceps.[18] Layered debridement involves removal of tissue beginning at the surface and progressing to the depths of the wound.[24] This facilitates removal of all edematous, devitalized, contaminated tissue and entrapped microscopic debris, leaving a freshly uncovered surface with a good vascular supply. Care should be exercised in avoiding vital structures, such as nerves, large vessels and joint capsules. A 3-mm strip should be removed from badly damaged skin edges without evidence of capillary oozing.[22] The skin edges may be scraped to freshen them if there is not ample tissue present to permit removal.[2] When testing a skin flap for viability, a sharp line of color demarcation that indicates adequate circulation on one side and abnormal circulation on the other is the most important clinical observation.[20] Jagged wound edges should be straightened by excision to facilitate good closure.[17] To accomplish good apposition of the skin edges without excessive tension, it may be necessary to undermine them to allow sliding of the skin.[2]

During surgical debridement, the objectives to be considered include removal of all foreign bodies, provision of adequate hemostasis, restoration of normal structure, if possible, use of adequate lavage during debridement, and drainage of deadspace and deep pockets.[14,22,24] One should avoid excessive tearing and prolonged pressure on tissue, as well as extensive exploration that breaks down natural fascial barriers to the spread of infection.[12,14]

Placement of Drains

A drain placed in the depths of a wound may be beneficial in the presence of massive contamination, excessive deadspace, foreign material and incomplete debridement.[25] Drains should be soft, pliable and nonirritating, and should not weaken in the presence of tissue fluids. The most common types used are fenestrated or unfenestrated thin latex rubber tubing (Penrose) and rubber or plastic tube drains.[18] Closed-suction or negative-pressure drains may be used in aseptic surgical wounds that are sutured for primary closure but in which large amounts of deadspace are still present. These drains greatly decrease the possibility of ascending infection. Commercial drains (Bel-O-Vac:Aloe Medical) are also available (Fig 85). One may also be constructed from a short piece of polyethylene tubing and a 60-ml syringe with a needle adapter (Fig 86).

If a drain is necessary, it should be placed in the wound after debridement and prior to wound closure. One end of the drain should be fixed at the site to be drained with a skin suture independent of the wound edge sutures. The other end of the tube should pass ventrad by the shortest route to the outside. At the

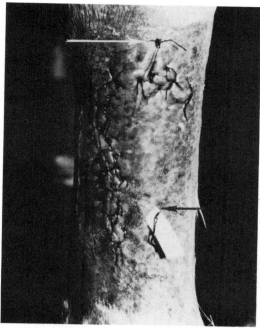

Fig 87. Penrose drain (black arrow) exiting through a separate skin opening. A single ligature (white arrow) must be cut to remove the drain.

point of exteriorization, a separate stab wound large enough to provide adequate drainage is created for exit of the drain (Fig 87). The drain must not emerge through the distal end of the suture line, which would be jeopardized by exiting fluids and sepsis. The drain should be anchored where it exits the skin to prevent it from being pulled out or slipping back into the wound.[25]

An alternate technic involves placement of a drain with each end emerging from a stab incision at opposite ends of the wound, with each end anchored by a suture. A modification of this type of double-ended drain is the seton, in which the ends of the tubing emerging from the wound are tied together outside the wound.[7]

Lavage fluids or antibacterial solutions may be flushed into the wound from the protruding end of the tube after careful cleansing of the site. If possible, the wound and drain tube should be bandaged. This allows evaluation of the amount of drainage, minimizes ascending infection along the drain, and prevents premature removal of the drain by the animal. Drains should be removed when there is little or no drainage, usually 3-5 days postoperatively. However, one must use good judgment so that drains are not removed prematurely.

Disadvantages associated with use of drains include possible ascent of infection around a drain, encroachment of rigid drains on adjacent structures, foreign body reaction if left in place too long, and loss of the drain.[14,25] Another factor considered to be a disadvantage is the false sense of security that may tempt the surgeon to close a wound that is better left open to heal by granulation.

Control of Hemorrhage

Hemostasis, in both surgically created and accidental wounds, is essential for optimum healing. Hemorrhage from a fresh wound must be evaluated carefully. If excessive, it may be necessary to apply direct pressure to the wound with a sterile pressure bandage to preserve life or prevent serious blood loss. Most wounds stop bleeding after a pressure bandage has been in place for 15-20 minutes. Large vessels that persist in hemorrhaging during lavage and debridement should be carefully clamped with mosquito hemostats and ligated with fine catgut. Overzealous use of large crushing forceps and electrocoagulation tends to increase the local inflammatory response as a result of the destruction of tissue. Excessive swabbing with gauze sponges disrupts the small clots over the ends of the smaller vessels, thus perpetuating bleeding. Prior to wound repair, consideration should be given to replacement of blood volume with whole blood in animals that have suffered severe blood loss. Most injured large animals do not require blood transfusions.[26]

Primary Wound Closure

Whether the wound is created surgically under aseptic conditions or accidentally under less than aseptic circumstances, the mechanics of wound closure are basically the same. A wound should not be closed until all tissues are healthy since premature apposition is likely to result in wound breakdown and persistent infection.[27] Wound closure soon after occurrence is referred to as primary closure. This technic uses first-intention healing, which may be defined as "the uncomplicated healing process of a clean incision that has been readily closed and that requires minimal epithelialization and formation of granulation tissue."[4]

Accidental wounds of several days' duration may sometimes be cleaned, debrided and sutured to complete the healing process by first intention. This is known as delayed primary closure.

Wound closure varies according to the surgeon's preference and the type of wound. Yet the same basic principles must be followed if first-intention healing is to be achieved. Once the wound has been properly cleansed and debrided, and hemorrhage controlled, a staged closure is undertaken. Every effort should be made to obliterate deadspace with deep absorbable sutures of appropriate size in a simple-interrupted pattern. The absorbable suture material recommended for use in a contaminated wound is polyglycolic acid (Dexon: Cyanamid) since this material is not affected by inflammation and enzymes as are catgut and collagen. Polyglycolic acid also has intrinsic bacteriostatic properties.[28] If primary closure cannot be accomplished to one's satisfaction, adequate drainage should be established with Penrose drains. It is important to remember that correct tension of the suture and proper apposition of the tissue are paramount in this technic. Proper tension of the suture may be defined as that amount necessary to bring the tissues into apposition sufficient to prevent gaping. Sutures placed too loosely create deadspace for serum accumulation; those placed too tightly cause necrosis of the tissue entrapped by the suture.

Buried absorbable sutures are basically foreign bodies and stimulate an inflammatory response. Therefore, only the least number of sutures necessary should be used to achieve proper tissue apposition. Since one of the objectives of sutures is to give temporary strength to the wound, in addition to hemostasis and obliteration of deadspace, it is important that deep sutures be placed in fibrous tissue, such as the muscle sheath and fascia.[11] The holding power of the tissue in which sutures are placed has a greater effect in determining the strength of the temporary tissue union than the strength of the suture material itself.[29]

Subcutaneous tissues are apposed with 00 or 000 absorbable material placed in a simple-continuous pattern to provide adequate freedom to suture the skin edges.

The skin edges should be apposed without undue tension. Irregular skin wounds may require some effort on the part of the surgeon to properly distribute the skin throughout the length of the wound. Many suture materials and suture patterns are available, each with its advantages and disadvantages. However, the surgeon's technic is of more importance than the choice of suture material or pattern.[14] A good surgeon can usually achieve satisfactory results with any type of suture material and pattern.[11]

It is generally best to use a nonabsorbable, noncapillary suture material with as small a diameter as needed to provide the necessary tensile strength for the temporary union. Those available include polypropylene, nylon, stainless steel, Dacron, silk and cotton, the last 2 of which are the least desirable. Many synthetic nonabsorbable sutures have a low coefficient of friction and thus require at least 4 single throws or a surgeon's throw, followed by a square knot, for adequate security.

The aim in closing wounds is to appose the skin edges accurately, with no overlapping. This is accomplished by passing the needle through the skin perpendicular to the skin's surface on both sides of the wound. The sutures should be placed squarely across the wound and should take equal bites into both sides of the wound. The distance between the needle puncture site and the wound edge generally should equal the thickness of the skin. The distance between sutures varies but generally should be equal to twice the skin's thickness.[30] Another guide to spacing sutures is to place as many sutures as close together as necessary for satisfactory coaptation of the wound edges.[7] Proper suture tension is as important in skin sutures as it is in buried sutures. Sutures tied too tightly can lead to excessive exudation, tissue necrosis, wound disruption, delayed healing and excessive scarring. Loose sutures allow gaps to form, entry for further contamination and greater scar formation. As a rule of thumb, sutures should be tied so they just approximate the skin edges.[7]

Selection of a proper suture pattern may sometimes determine the eventual outcome of a sutured wound. The simple-interrupted suture pattern is by far the most versatile and dependable pattern available. Others, such as the vertical mattress, horizontal mattress and continuous-interlock patterns, may be used alone or in combination. A common combination is the vertical mattress pattern with alternate simple-interrupted sutures (Fig 88).

Wounds in horses commonly cannot be closed without excessive tension placed on the sutures because of skin loss or wound edge retraction. Relaxing (relief) incisions or tension sutures may be used in such cases to alleviate much of the tension on the primary suture line. Tension sutures are usually placed a sufficient distance from the skin edges to minimize the chances for strangulation and margin necrosis.[7] The tendency for sutures to cut through tissue may be reduced by using bolsters or

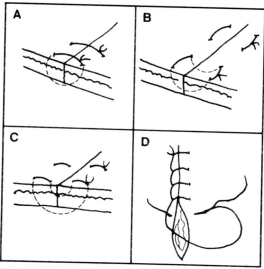

Fig 88. Commonly used skin suture patterns. A. Simple interrupted. B. Horizontal mattress. C. Vertical mattress. D. Continuous interlock.

stents under the sutures before they are tied. Bolsters, which distribute suture pressure over a large surface area, may be purchased or constructed from old IV rubber tubing, coat buttons or gauze. Patterns used to distribute tension include the simple interrupted, horizontal mattress, vertical mattress, far-near-near-far, and stent. A simple-interrupted suture may be used as a tension suture by alternating wide and narrow bites of tissue taken when placing the sutures. When horizontal mattress sutures are used for tension relief, they are placed well away from the skin edges and simple-interrupted sutures used to approximate the skin edges.

Horizontal mattress sutures have a greater tendency to interfere with circulation in the skin edge than do vertical mattress sutures. This potential disadvantage may lead one to choose the latter for tension relief. The vertical mattress pattern is placed in the same fashion as its horizontal counterpart and is used in conjunction with the simple-interrupted pattern to close the skin edges. The far-near-near-far pattern is a combination of tension and approximating sutures, which works well in wounds with widely separated skin edges. This suture is placed in the order of its name, with the "far" component supplying the tension and the "near" component apposing the skin edges. Excessive tightening of the suture should be avoided to prevent suture line inversion (Fig 89). Stent sutures help obliterate deadspace and serve as

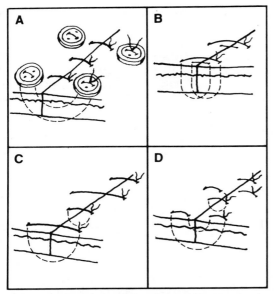

Fig 89. Commonly used retention suture patterns. A. Vertical mattress, using buttons. B. Far-near-near-far. C. Simple interrupted (wide bites), with alternating simple-interrupted sutures with normal bites. D. Vertical mattress, with alternating simple interrupted.

effective tension sutures.[31] Prior to closure of the deep tissues and skin edges, an appropriate number of large, simple-interrupted sutures are preplaced and left untied along the length of the wound. After the wound edges have been apposed with a simple-interrupted pattern, a gauze roll is laid on the surface line and over-tied with the free ends of the sutures. This multipurpose suture acts as a self-retaining bandage that exerts even pressure between the wound edges and underlying tissues (Fig 90).

Other means for cutaneous closure that have not been universally accepted by veterinarians include the use of tissue adhesives, adhesive tape, and metal clips.[7,32]

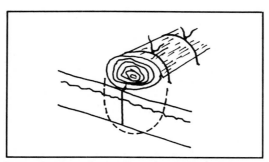

Fig 90. A stent or tie-over gauze bandage secured over the suture line in an area that cannot be bandaged.

Many theories exist on the subject of suture removal times. One should remove sutures when the wound is sufficiently healed and removal is judged to be safe. However, this depends upon the surgeon's experience and judgement, and many wound-related factors, such as the tension on the wound and location of the wound. No specific time can be set for suture removal that applies to all cases. As a general guideline, suture-supported wounds that have healed by first intention have usually gained sufficient strength by 10-14 days postoperatively to allow safe removal of sutures.[4]

Delayed Wound Closure

Delayed primary closure of wounds is a very useful technic. Many horses are presented with fresh lacerations that are badly contaminated and have severe tissue damage that results in extensive necrosis and swelling. Other animals have been injured several days before medical attention is requested. Most of these cases, barring severe skin and/or tissue loss, respond very well to this procedure.

In delayed primary closure, the wound is converted to one resembling a clean laceration through surgical removal of infected and devitalized tissue. The wound is initially treated the same as that for primary closure by thorough cleansing, lavage and debridement. However, it is not sutured until later. The laceration is kept under a medicated bandage and systemic antibiotic therapy given for 3-5 days, after which time primary closure with sutures is accomplished if the tissue appears healthy and there is minimal exudation. Additional time is allowed if moderate exudation exists and more debridement is necessary.

When closure is performed later than 5 days after injury, it is referred to as secondary closure. After this time, fibrocollagenous tissue is forming rapidly and the wound has lost much of its pliability. Once granulation tissue has been created, the skin edges adhere to the underlying tissue and apposition is possible only by excising much of the fleshy bed. A narrow rim of the skin at the wound margin is also excised. Primary closure is then accomplished.

After delayed primary or secondary closure, a firm, well-padded, partially immobilizing bandage is applied. For lacerations in highly mobile areas, a cast may be necessary to provide strict immobilization for 10-12 days. Delayed closure provides the opportunity to observe the progression of healing and allows any redebridement that may be necessary. Wound closure can then be performed when all tissues of the laceration are ready for closure.[7]

Protection of the Closed Wound

The bandage plays a very important role in wound healing in animals. The bandage provides immobilization, obliterates deadspace, protects the wound from contamination and trauma, and minimizes postoperative edema and hemorrhage. Bandages of various kinds are quite easily applied to the extremities of horses but are more difficult to apply to the head and trunk. Correct application of a pressure bandage is a critical maneuver. If applied too tightly, restricted circulation may result in retardation of healing and possible skin necrosis and sloughing. This is especially true for elastic-tape bandages that are used alone or in conjunction with other materials. Extreme caution must be exercised when applying these tapes to a horse's leg. If applied too loosely, the bandage does not obliterate deadspace or prevent edema and may slip away from the wound, thereby allowing access to contamination and additional trauma. A firm, well-padded partially immobilizing bandage is one that extends well above and below the wounded area.

The style of the bandage and type of bandage material used varies with the preference of the surgeon and location of the wound. Many kinds of material are available for bandaging, from a simple combination of sheet cotton and gauze to the more sophisticated military field bandage (LilyWhite), elastic adhesive (Elastikon: Johnson & Johnson), and self-adhering tapes (Vetrap:3-M). A good bandage material frequently recommended to clients is the disposable baby diaper. Also readily available is the elastic, nonadhering tape (Ace:American Hospital Supply), which can be used in conjunction with other bandage material.

Whatever bandage is ultimately chosen, the sutured wound itself must be covered initially with a sterile, nonadherent pad (eg, Telfa:Kendall). This, in turn, is usually held in place by circumferential wrapping with some type of soft, rolled bandage material (eg, Kling:Johnson & Johnson). A bandage is then placed over this primary bandage. This method allows minimal disturbance of the sutured wound during bandage changes.

The stent or tie-over bandage allows pressure to be maintained over areas, that would not easily accept a conventional bandage, such as the elbow, head and gaskin. The tie-over sutures should be tied with a release knot so the gauze stent may be easily removed and replaced upon examination of the wound.

When bandaging the proximal portion of the leg, a bandage should be applied to the distal portion first to support or maintain the position of the proximal bandage and to prevent edema of the distal extremity.[4] A many-tailed or spider bandage allows for motion of the carpus or hock without bandage slippage.[26]

In addition to providing pressure, a bandage also provides immobilization. This feature is very important in attaining rapid, uneventful healing of wounds located near joints. It may be necessary to increase the immobilization by incorporating more padding (modified Robert-Jones bandage) into the bandage. Splints made from PVC pipe, wood, aluminum and other rigid materials may be applied over a bandage to improve immobilization. If total immobilization is necessary, a cast (plaster of Paris, fiberglass, polyurethane) may be applied to the limb for 10-14 days. This is especially indicated for lacerations of the bulb of the heel, fetlock and carpus/tarsus.

Bandages must be evaluated frequently and changed as needed. An excessively moist wound, especially one with a drain, may need daily bandage changes. As healing progresses, exudation usually decreases and the interval between bandage changes increases to every 3-5 days. Bandages should be changed if they become soaked with urine or rain since a wet bandage provides a favorable medium for bacterial growth.[7]

Excessive pressure or other problems may cause the horse to constantly chew or rub at the bandage. This should be critically evaluated without hesitation. Often there is no problem with the bandage but the chewing is related to boredom or pruritus associated with healing. Nevertheless, the surgeon must devise some method to prevent destruction of the bandage and mutilation of the wound. Restrictive measures include use of a bib, neck cradle or muzzle, application of a cast, and application of offensive substances, such as hot sauce, to the bandage. Bandages should only be changed when needed.[2]

Postoperative Care

Topical Antibiotic Therapy: The use of topical antibiotic therapy in wounds can be beneficial. Although topically applied antibiotics are advantageous, they are not a replacement for the proper surgical care of wounds, which always includes debridement.[14] Antibiotics used topically should be in aqueous solution. Antibiotic powders generally should not be used in wounds because many contain filler substances and tend to cake on the surface of a wound, protecting the underlying bacteria. When applied in large amounts they can act as a foreign body. Hydrophilic antibiotic ointments, placed into wounds prior to closure, make wound lavage and debridement difficult. Ointments on sutured skin edges keep the area moist and may slow the healing process. Wounds sutured for primary closure should be allowed to remain dry under the protection of a bandage.

Systemic Antibiotic Therapy: Systemic antibiotic therapy should be initiated for all major injuries. Antibiotics are best selected based on results of culture and sensitivity tests. If this is not possible, penicillin is the drug of choice for most aerobic and anaerobic gram-positive infections. Ampicillin has activity against both gram-positive and gram-negative bacteria, including *E coli* and *Proteus* spp.[7] Samples from wounds in critical areas, such as joints, tendon sheaths and the thoracic cavity, should be obtained for culture. Systemic antibiotics should be administered for at least 3-5 days after all clinical signs of infection have subsided.

Prophylaxis against tetanus should be considered for all wounds in horses. Tetanus antitoxin and/or tetanus toxoid may be administered, depending upon the animal's prior protection against this disease.

The use of analgesics should be considered for animals in a great deal of pain as a result of a wound. The use of nonsteroidal anti-inflammatory drugs may be indicated in horses that have sustained excessive bruising and exhibit considerable edema. Use of corticosteroids is contraindicated due to their effects on lysosomes and fibroblastic activity.[2]

Often the nutrition of the animal is overlooked. It is important that this element be evaluated to ensure that ample protein, trace minerals and vitamins are provided since these are essential for tissue repair.

During the convalescent period, the animal should be confined in a dry, well-bedded box stall to restrict movement.

OPEN WOUND MANAGEMENT

Many wounds in horses should not be closed so that healing can take place by second intention. This method of healing should be considered for all extensive lacerations that cannot be properly immobilized, with wounds exhibiting excessive avulsion, and in any wound requiring a great amount of suture tension for closure (Fig 91). Heavily infected wounds also respond better if allowed to heal as an open wound. Economics may also dictate that the wound heal by granulation.

Healing by second intention is achieved by aiding the normal healing process. There are no magic drugs that accelerate wound healing but there are acceptable methods that assist, rather than interfere with, the processes of tissue repair. An open wound that is handled properly usually heals rather well and is quite compatible with function. Wound contraction plays an important role in minimizing the size of the resultant scar or blemish. Horses, more than other species, must have proper care in the treatment of open wounds. Mismanagement results in exuberant granulation tissue, excessive scarring, blemishing and sometimes unsoundness. Wounds distal to the carpus/tarsus are especially sensitive and require careful treatment to prevent complications.[5]

Another drawback in second-intention healing is the increased time required for healing as compared with that of primary closure, and the poor quality of tissue covering the healed wound. Healing by second intention involves formation of granulation tissue, wound contraction and epithelialization. In many areas, especially the distal extremity, a lack of redundant skin results in inability of the granulation bed to contract. For this reason, it relies upon epithelialization to provide an intact surface. This covering is inelastic, poorly attached and not very durable. The result is a wound covering that is easily abraded, exposing the underlying scar tissue and leading to secondary infection and more scar formation.[11]

When presented with a wound that cannot be closed, the same protocol should be followed as that previously described for first-intention therapy except for closure of the wound: restraint and anesthesia, preparation, cleansing and debridement of the wound, control of hemorrhage, placement of drains if necessary, protection of the wound, medication, and care of the animal.

Initial Care of Open Wounds

One of the objectives in open wound healing is to assist the normal reparative processes in closing the raw surfaces. Wounds close naturally if the factors that complicate healing, especially infection, do not overwhelm normal tissue repair.

Any required emergency care, such as controlling hemorrhage with ligation and/or pressure, treating shock, and preventing additional trauma to the injured tissue, should be administered initially. The animal should be properly restrained and provided with adequate analgesia to the injured site. The distal portion of the wound usually requires very little local anesthesia because it is detached from its nerve supply. The proximal portion should be anesthetized by infiltration of a local anesthetic without epinephrine or through a regional nerve block.

The hair is then removed with a pair of clippers, straight-edge razor or a #21 scalpel blade from a liberal area surrounding the wound. The skin edges of the wound must be free of hair since it may provide sufficient irritation to produce exuberant granulation tissue.[5]

Once the edges of the wound have been prepared, the lacerated tissues are thoroughly cleansed with normal physiologic saline solution, to which an aqueous antibiotic solution has been added. If antiseptic soaps, such as the povidone iodine scrubs are used, they should be thoroughly rinsed from the wound with normal saline or tap water since they are somewhat irritating. Mild povidone iodine and chlorhexidine solutions may also be used to rinse and cleanse the wound. Hydrogen peroxide (3%) provides cleansing by its mechanical foaming action; however, it may damage the microvascular system of the wound.[21]

Irrigating the wound with a bulb-type syringe or a Water Pik may have an advantage over simply pouring an antiseptic solution into a wound. Caution should be exercised not to drive debris into deep tissues.[14]

A very important procedure directed toward eliminating development of infection is thorough debridement. It must be done carefully and completely. All dirt, hair, loose bone fragments and tissues obviously torn from their blood supply should be removed from the wound by sharp dissection.

When surgical debridement cannot be carried out, enzymatic agents may be used to accomplish debridement of nonviable or questionable tissue. Enzymatic debridement aids repair of open wounds even though it may take longer than surgical debridement.[11,18] Several types of enzymes are commercially available, including fibrinolysin-desoxyribonuclease (Elase:Parke-Davis), trypsin (Granulex:Dow Hickam, Trypzyme:Burns-Biotec), chymotryp-

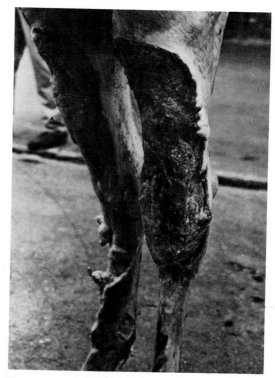

Fig 91. Large granulating wounds in the tibiotarsal region of a colt.

sin-trypsin (Kymar:Burns-Biotec), and sutilains (Travase:Flint).

Large blood vessels that continue to bleed during cleansing and debridement should be ligated with fine catgut. However, the preservation of the blood supply to injured tissues is paramount if maximal healing is to be attained. Maintaining blood flow through the damaged area is more effective in preventing infection than is application of medication.[4]

If pockets in the wound will allow exudation to accumulate, ventral drainage should be established with a latex rubber drain. Drainage is especially important in wounds that cannot be properly bandaged, such as those in the pectoral area.

After a wound has been thoroughly cleansed and properly debrided, a protective pressure bandage with proper topical medication should be applied if possible. Initial medication under the bandage should consist of a nonirritating, water-soluble antibiotic ointment. Mastitis preparations and nitrofurazone (Furacin: Norden) are often used. Injectable aqueous antibiotics may be applied topically or injected into the tissues around the wound.[5] It is important to remember that topical medication of the wound with antiseptics (ointments or solutions) is of limited value when used for the control of infection. There are no antiseptics that do not have some adverse effect on the immature, cellular repair process when used in a concentration sufficient to control sepsis. Antibiotics remain as the most beneficial agents in controlling pathogenic bacteria.[4]

Once the wound has been properly medicated, a firm, well-padded, partially immobilizing bandage is applied. A bandage may prevent secondary contamination, keep wound edges in near apposition, and limit self-mutilation. Edema is minimized and protection from insect irritation is afforded by a bandage. Wounds distal to the carpus/tarsus tend to develop exuberant granulation tissue; pressure supplied by a bandage usually retards this overgrowth. Wounds on the distal extremity should be kept bandaged until nearly healed. The partial immobilization supplied by the bandage allows healing to progress at a faster pace. A cast should be used if total immobilization is necessary, as in lacerations across the bulb of the heel, pastern region and joint surfaces. The cast should be left in place for 10-14 days unless earlier removal is warranted.

When bandaging the proximal part of the leg, a bandage should be applied to the distal part of the leg to maintain the position of the proximal bandage and prevent edema of the distal extremity.[4]

The need for changing a bandage is determined by the condition of the wound. An excessively moist lesion is not compatible with optimal healing. Bandages should be changed often enough to preclude accumulation of exudate and subsequent irritation of the wounded tissue. As healing progresses, exudation usually decreases and the time interval between bandage changes is increased to 3-5 days.

Care should be exercised when changing a bandage so as not to disturb the new epithelial and granulating growth. Contamination should always be avoided during a bandage change. The results of a wound healed under a properly applied pressure bandage are more cosmetic, more stable and less likely to form keloids than those healed under a scab.

The previous discussion on bandaging has applied principally to wounds distal to the mid-radial/mid-tibial regions. Lacerations located proximal to these points do not lend themselves to application of a bandage very easily. Development of exuberant granulation proximal to the mid-radial/mid-tibial areas is generally not a problem. Wounds in these areas heal quite adequately without the aid of a bandage through contraction and epithelialization. Nevertheless, the area should be kept reasonably clean and protected from additional trauma if maximal healing is to be achieved. Dirt, bedding and insects can complicate unbandaged lacerations. Complications can be minimized by more frequent cleansing, use of clean bedding or a grassy paddock, and application of insecticides around the wound periphery. Insect repellants put into the injured tissues greatly retard healing. Self-mutilation, which is a problem especially during summer months, may be reduced through the use of a bib, neck cradle or cross-tie.

The exudate from an open wound is toxic to normal skin when it is allowed to drain down and accumulate. To reduce this reaction, the exudate is cleansed from the skin daily and a coating of petrolatum ointment is applied to the skin as a protectant.[4]

Systemic antibiotic therapy should be considered for all major injuries, especially in wounds that are severely contaminated and adequate debridement cannot be accomplished, cannot be kept free of secondary contamination, and penetrate a joint or body cavity.[4] Penicillin is preferred unless culture and sensitivity tests indicate otherwise. Therapy should continue for at least 5-7 days. Tetanus prophylaxis with antitoxin and/or toxoid should be administered for all wounds.

The care of the animal as a whole should be reviewed. If healing is to progress satisfactorily, adequate nutrition should be provided. Parasitism, bad teeth and other chronic diseases may delay wound healing. The horse should be kept reasonably confined in a clean, dry area, such as a box stall or paddock.

Management of Granulation Tissue

In second-intention wound healing, the raw surfaces are closed by tissue growth from within. Deeper defects created by loss of tissue are closed first by replacement with fibrocollagenous proliferation (granulation tissue) before final closure of the surface (epithelialization) can take place. The proliferative phase of healing is greatly prolonged in second-intention healing when compared with that in first-intention repair. Many factors determine the ultimate healing time of an open wound, including size and location of the wound, as well as the complicating factors previously described. Our main goal should be to decrease this period as much as possible without jeopardizing tissue repair. Procedures that assist rather than interfere with healing include stimulation, suppression and removal of granulation tissue.

Stimulation of Granulation Tissue

If the granulating process can be stimulated, the defect in the depths of a large wound fill more rapidly. All agents that stimulate production of granulation tissue are irritating to the wound. One should choose a substance that is mild and relatively harmless to the wound and surrounding tissues.

Water: Water or moisture is the most common agent used to stimulate granulation tissue. Horses in areas of high humidity tend to form more granulation tissue than animals maintained in a dry environment.

Stimulation may be achieved by applying a wet bandage over the wound or by spraying the wound with tap water from a hose with a shower head attachment (Fig 92). While the wound is being gently stimulated, it is also being cleansed.

Ointments: Hydrophilic antibiotic ointments are mildly stimulating because they maintain a moist environment within the wound. These compounds should not contain any insoluble substances that may be trapped in the granulation bed and eventually act as foreign bodies.

Scarlet Oil: This topical preparation has been used for many years on wounds that cannot be bandaged. The scarlet red and the bland oil base gently stimulate the granulation process, while the balsam of Peru deodorizes the wound.[4] This product also basically produces a moist environment for the wound.

Creosol Solution: This substance (Kreso Dip:Parke-Davis), when used in a 1% solution, is slightly more irritating and subsequently more stimulating than water alone. It is generally applied to the wound by wetting the bandage. This product not only stimulates the granulation bed but also has a broad antimicrobial spectrum.

Suppression of Granulation Tissue

A granulation bed eventually reaches a point when growth must be slowed or stopped, especially in a wound on the distal extremity. This can be accomplished by several methods.

Pressure: The pressure bandage is probably the most useful method to suppress granulation growth, especially on the extremities.

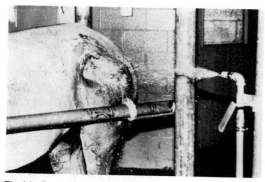

Fig 92. Shower head attached to a pipe stand is used to irrigate a large wound in the hip area.

Corticosteroids: Corticosteroids applied topically in conjunction with an antibiotic ointment suppress growth of granulation tissue by inhibiting lysosomal and fibroblastic activity. They do not adversely affect epithelialization.

Scab: A scab is basically a natural bandage. A lesion not subjected to repeated injury heals satisfactorily under a scab. The scab must be firmly attached to be an integral part of the healing process.[4] All tissue defects and gaps should be filled with granulation tissue to skin-level before induction of "scabbing" should be considered. In larger wounds a scab is not easily maintained.

A scab may be produced in several ways. The surface of a small wound without a tissue defect usually dries and forms its own scab as soon as topical medication is stopped. Application of a corticosteroid or DMSO ointment or solution usually allows the surface of the bed to dry. The use of irritants, such as 7% iodine, 10% formalin, 2% picric acid and gentian violet-tannic acid mixtures, on the surface of a wound destroys the most superficial layer of granulation tissue, with the dried layer then becoming a scab.[4] A favorite scabbing agent is a mixture of equal parts of 7% tincture of iodine and 10% formalin, painted on the wound surface 3-4 times at 2-hour intervals. Another preparation used to promote development of a scab is "bloodwax," which consists of equine RBC, zinc sulfate, water and DMSO mixed into a wax-like paste and applied to an open wound with a tongue depressor.[33]

Removal of Granulation Tissue

Wounds with excessive granulation tissue are very common in horses, primarily because of improper treatment. Removal of this exuberant flesh may be accomplished by several means.

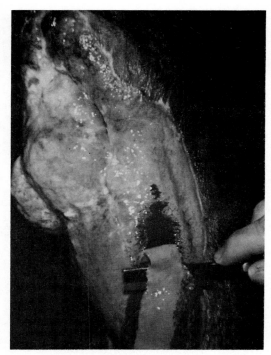

Fig 93. Exuberant granulation tissue being removed with a straight razor. A pressure bandage is used to control hemorrhage.

Surgical Removal: This is by far the best way to remove large amounts of excess tissue. The tissue should be excised to the level of the surrounding skin and a pressure bandage applied to control profuse capillary bleeding (Fig 93). Anesthesia of the wound itself is not needed since it does not have a nerve supply.[4] However, tranquilization and use of a twitch may be necessary while working on the extremities of some animals. The bandage may be changed the following day or the wound left open to be scabbed.

Chemical Cautery: Chemical cautery involves use of very irritating caustic agents, such as copper sulfate, zinc sulfate, antimony trichloride and alum. These escharotics destroy varying thicknesses (1/8" to 3/16") of the superficial granulation tissue, thereby removing excess flesh. Repeated daily applications of these agents to the wound surface under a bandage eventually remove the tissue down to skin level. These caustics are severely irritating and repeated use may create a nonhealing wound, more exuberant granulation tissue, or excessive fibrosis of the healed wound, causing a permanent blemish. They usually hinder healing more than they help it. This group of prod-

ucts has been the most misused by horse owners in wound therapy. Owners should be advised that if it takes more than one application of a caustic agent to remove the exuberant tissue, surgical removal is recommended.

The granulation bed can be easily managed, no matter how large or small it is. There are times when one needs to suppress as well as stimulate granulation tissue within the same wound. This can be easily accomplished by using a combination of the methods previously described. It should be remembered that the granulation bed should always have a pink, healthy appearance as it grows to fill the void in the wound.

Epithelialization and Contraction

After the raw surfaces and defects have been filled with fibrocollagenous proliferation, most wounds close naturally by epithelialization and contraction.[4] In an open wound that fully penetrates the dermal layer, a layer of granulation tissue must form before the wound can epithelialize.[14] Usually there is a latent period of 4-5 days before epithelial cells begin to migrate from the wound margins across the developing granulation tissue. The migration of epithelial cells is rapid at first but soon slows. Epithelial proliferation and migration occur most efficiently when the granulation bed is level with the surrounding skin edges.

Occasionally, the skin edge of the wound becomes inverted. The position of this edge is not conducive to maximum epithelial cell proliferation and migration. It should be trimmed and the granulation bed freshened adjacent to the skin edge.

In some large wounds, epithelialization may take weeks to months to completely cover the granulation bed. Others may not have sufficient epithelial growth to cover the wound entirely; skin grafting may be necessary to ultimately heal these wounds.

Wound contraction is an important factor in the healing of open wounds. This natural phenomenon is the reduction in size of an open wound as the result of centripetal movement of the whole-thickness skin surrounding the lesion.[7] While granulation tissue is forming and epithelialization is occurring, the granulation bed contracts, pulling the skin margins centripetally so the area to be covered by epithelialization is greatly reduced.[11,12,14] Contraction, which begins shortly after injury and may continue for weeks, is always more apparent and dramatic when the wound is located in an area of loosely attached or redundant skin, such as the shoulder or cranial pectoral region. In these regions, wound closure is essentially completed by wound contraction, with very little epithelialization being necessary. The subsequent scar is minimal and the appearance acceptable. In areas where contraction cannot occur satisfactorily to reduce the size of the wound, such as the distal legs, a wider, more fragile scar is left (Fig 94).[12]

Epithelialization and contraction occasionally cease before the lesion is healed, especially in larger wounds. The phenomenon has been referred to as "regeneration fatigue."[1] This failure to heal is often the result of repeated trauma from caustic drugs, infection, movement, self-mutilation and foreign bodies. Several methods are available to stimulate completion of healing after the underlying cause has been eliminated.

Freshening the Granulation Bed: Trimming (freshening) the granulation bed and its peripheral skin edge with a scalpel blade stimulates the wound even though the granulation tissue is not exuberant. Most of these wounds have a very pale, smooth, relatively avascular (mature) bed that is no longer responsive.

Biologic Dressings: Biologic dressings have been used to stimulate a favorable response in slow-healing wounds. These "temporary skin bandages" are allografts (equine cadaver skin) or xenografts (bovine cartilage and porcine skin). Equine cadaver skin has been used as a protective bandage to enhance healing of chronic lesions.[34] The use of bovine cartilage, prepared from calf tracheas and ears, has produced a significant effect upon the healing of many chronic wounds. The cartilage can be applied topically as a powder (Lescarden:Balassa) or as whole bovine ear cartilage sutured over the wound.[35,36] Several theories have been proposed on how cartilage accelerates wound healing.[37] The use of pigskin as a biologic dressing has accelerated the rate of healing in painful, slow-healing leg wounds in horses. The commercially available porcine skin dressing (Burn Treatment Skin Bank, Phoenix, AZ) provided a more complete and normal granulation and epithelialization than other methods of treatment.[38]

Insulin: The application of protamine zinc insulin topically stimulates wound healing and acts as a debriding agent.[39] Insulin increases protein synthesis and conditions the cell membranes of epithelial, fat and muscle cells so that glucose can enter the cell.[39,40] In-

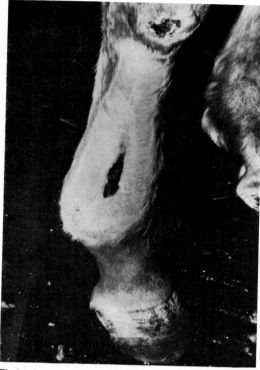

Fig 94. Large metacarpal wound healed by granulation-epithelialization in an area lacking redundant peripheral skin. Note the extensive scarring.

sulin is apparently more effective in treatment of chronic and infected wounds than in fresh and noninfected lesions.[7] The most effective concentration of insulin is 30 units protamine zinc insulin per 1 g nitrofurazone base.[39] However, other concentrations have been used effectively, from 10 units protamine zinc insulin per 1 g base to 30 units of insulin per 28 g nitrofurazone ointment base.[7]

Vitamin and Mineral Supplementation: Certain vitamins and trace minerals are essential to wound healing. The need for supplementation is especially necessary in debilitated, undernourished horses. Vitamin A is essential for epithelial health.[41] It also acts as an antagonist against the anti-inflammatory effects of corticosteroids.[11]

Vitamin C is necessary for epithelial regeneration and synthesis of collagen.[11,41] A deficiency of vitamin C delays healing. Following major stress such as surgery and burns, the human body loses ascorbic acid in varying amounts.[42] Animals similarly may also lose vital levels of ascorbic acid after trauma and may require supplementation.[7]

Wounds in Zn-deficient animals heal poorly. Characteristically there are problems with epithelialization and tensile strength in the wound.[12]

All horses should receive a well-balanced ration during convalescence to ensure optimal healing.

Skin Graft: Wounds occasionally fail to heal completely, regardless of the technic used. This is especially true of large wounds on the distal limbs of horses. The only recourse the surgeon may have is the use of free or pedicle skin grafts. Skin grafting technics are discussed elsewhere in this chapter.

TREATMENT OF PUNCTURE WOUNDS

A puncture wound is dangerous since it may lead to malignant edema, tetanus or extensive cellulitis. Perforations of the skin are often overlooked because they are covered by hair. Bacteria and/or foreign bodies may be carried deep into the tissues beneath the skin and produce swelling, tenderness or exudation. Puncture wounds create an especially favorable environment for multiplication of anaerobic bacteria.

The wound site should first be cleansed by clipping a liberal area and scrubbing the skin with an appropriate surgical soap. The wound should be irrigated with a sterile saline-antibiotic mixture or a mild povidone iodine solution. The tract should always be gently explored with a flexible probe, hemostat or gloved finger, depending upon its size and depth.[26] If the opening is too small to accommodate the finger, it may be wise to enlarge the perforation so that digital palpation can be accomplished.[6]

Ventral drainage should be established if pocketing of the wound permits accumulation of discharges. With the animal properly restrained, the skin is anesthetized and incised at a point below the estimated location of the deep pocket. The stab incision, which is extended into the cavity, is enlarged sufficiently to permit passage of a latex rubber tube, which is then passed out to the exterior by way of the original puncture wound. The 2 ends of the tube can be sutured or tied together to form a seton.

Suturing is contraindicated in all puncture wounds. Punctures invariably close very rapidly, causing bacteria to be trapped by this prompt healing process.[6] It is desirable to maintain drainage, allowing the wound to heal from within.

The wound should be lavaged daily with an appropriate antimicrobial solution until it is obviously healing properly. In the presence of an active cellulitis, local treatment should be supplemented with systemic antibiotics. Tetanus prophylaxis with antitoxin and/or toxoid is always warranted.

The presence of a chronic draining sinus is often due to a foreign body in the puncture wound.[5] Foreign bodies may range from small wooden splinters to bits of metal or bone (Fig 95). Foreign material may be discovered through use of a probe, radiography and surgical exploration. Since wood and other soft materials may not be revealed by conventional radiography, radiopaque material, such as 2% aqueous iodine or a commercial preparation (Hypaque: Winthrop), may be injected to outline the tract and foreign body. The draining sinus may be a great distance from the foreign object, especially in soft tissues that allow the foreign body to migrate. The foreign body and its accompanying tissue tract must be removed before healing can be completed.

TREATMENT OF ABSCESSES

A diffuse, painful inflammation of the subcutaneous connective tissues (cellulitis) develops in the early stages of trauma and/or contamination of soft tissues. If severe enough, this cellulitis may lead to marked toxemia or septicemia.[6] Systemic antimicrobial therapy is usually indicated, along with the conventional care previously described. An abscess may form as a sequel to the cellulitic reaction if pathogenic bacteria become entrapped in the subcutaneous tissues. The collection of purulent exudate in these tissues leads to development of a pus-filled cavity. It is wise to wait until the abscess has matured or "come to a head" before an attempt is made to lance it. Maturation of an abscess may be stimulated by applying hot packs or mild rubefacients. In some locations it may be necessary to aspirate the fluctuant mass to distinguish it from a hernia.[6]

Once the abscess is ready for invasion, the skin should be adequately cleansed and injected with local anesthetic if necessary. Using appropriate chemical and physical restraint, the abscess is incised at the most ventral point of the cavity to provide optimum drainage. A large enough opening should be made to ensure that the cavity is completely eliminated prior to healing of the skin incision.[6] Once the pus has been evacuated, the cavity may be flushed with an antibiotic solution or chemically cauterized with an iodine solution such as Lugol's. This is accomplished by swabbing the space with iodine-soaked gauze sponges or packing the cavity for 24 hours with iodine-soaked rolled gauze. The cavity should be lavaged daily with water to remove superficial exudates until the wound is nearly healed. Appropriate insect control should also be carried out.

TREATMENT OF ABRASIONS

An abrasion, which is a partial-thickness friction injury to the skin, is treated by gentle cleansing with surgical soap and rinsing with normal saline or water. Dried hair, grit and other debris imbedded in the skin should be carefully removed. A moist antiseptic dressing should be applied, usually in the form of an ointment. In small wounds, application of the ointment may be discontinued after several days and the lesion allowed to dry and form a scab. Local therapy of more severe wounds with emollient ointments should be continued to keep the scab soft as the lesion heals. If infection develops under the scab, the scab should be removed, the surface cleansed and antibiotic ointment reapplied. Abrasions that continue to "weep" serum may be treated with a mild astringent.[5]

Severe abrasions, especially rope burns in the pastern region, may be complicated by excessive fibrosis and keloid formation.[1,5]

TREATMENT OF CONTUSIONS

Most first-degree contusions heal without consequence. Contusions of the second and third degree generally require therapy. Immediate care of second-degree contusions consists of application of cold packs or cold hydrotherapy to the affected area to stop hemorrhage and limit the extent of the hematoma. Topical use of DMSO may help limit seroma and/or hematoma formation.[5]

Hematomas and seromas, which occur most commonly in the cranial pectoral and ventral abdominal areas, must be properly diagnosed when the horse is presented some time after injury. They must be differentiated from an abscess, hernia or neoplasm. On palpation, a hematoma or seroma may feel like an indurated, well-encapsulated mass or fluctuant enlargement.[26] Aseptic aspiration should be used to evaluate the contents, especially for hematomas over the abdominal wall that must be distinguished from a hernia.

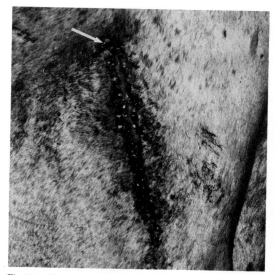

Fig 95. Chronic draining sinus near the point of the shoulder. A large sliver of wood was removed from the sinus and the wound healed.

In addition to the initial therapy described, most hematomas or seromas require either aspiration or surgical drainage. Hematomas with a volume of less than 50 ml usually are absorbed spontaneously. Whether aspiration is performed for diagnosis or treatment, it should be done aseptically. Tranquilization and/or physical restraint is adequate. Once the area has been surgically prepared, a sterile 16-ga hypodermic needle of adequate length is inserted into the hematoma. The fluid is drained as thoroughly as possible in an attempt to obtain union of the skin with the subcutaneous tissue. It is usually difficult, if not impossible, to apply a pressure bandage due to the location of the lesion. An exception to this is the hygroma, which is basically a seroma on the cranial aspect of the carpus, caused by repeated trauma.

If the hematoma is to be opened surgically, it should be performed 7-10 days after occurrence to allow sufficient organization of the clot and to minimize postsurgical hemorrhage from the ruptured vessels. A local anesthetic may be used to infiltrate the proposed line of incision after sufficient chemical and/or physical restraint is achieved. After the skin is prepared, a liberal incision is extended to the most ventral portion of the swelling. Care must be exercised to preserve any vital structures, such as large vessels, nerves or tendon sheaths, in the path of the incision. An incised seroma empties immediately by gravity, whereas a hematoma usually requires a gloved finger or hand to remove the blood clot. Fresh hemorrhage may be controlled through ligation or pressure from sterile gauze packed tightly into the cavity. This pack, which is removed in 36-48 hours, may be saturated with a 5% Lugol's solution to destroy the surface lining. Following pack removal, the cavity should be lavaged with a mild povidone iodine solution to remove exudates. Swabbing with Lugol's solution may be continued until secretion has ceased. Warm hydrotherapy to the area may speed resolution. Flushing with antiseptic solutions is discontinued as healing progresses and the amount of fluid discharge decreases.[26] Systemic antibiotics are given if indicated and tetanus prophylaxis is always given.

In third-degree contusions, a localized area of skin usually undergoes necrosis and eventually sloughs. Basic therapy should include debridement of all necrotic tissue, gentle cleansing of the wound, and prevention of infection by local application of an antibiotic ointment and administration of systemic antibiotics, if necessary. A healed "saddle sore" may necessitate use of a special blanket or pad. Large wounds on the withers may require a skin graft durable enough to withstand subsequent saddle pressure.

A specialized form of the third-degree contusion is the decubital ulcer or "pressure sore," created by the crushing of the skin between the body weight and the surface upon which the animal is lying.[6] Common sites for these ulcers in recumbent horses are the shoulder and hip. Repeated cleansing and application of emollient dressings are recommended for those sores. Padding should be provided in the form of a mattress or deep bedding. The animal should be turned regularly from one side to the other. A body sling may be used if warranted and if the animal will tolerate it.

EMERGENCY CARE OF SPECIAL WOUNDS

Wounds in certain regions of the body may initially require special care because of possible complications. Although the detailed therapy of the various complications is covered in their respective systems within this text, basic emergency care will be mentioned here.

Head and Neck

Lacerations of the eyelids are rather common in horses. Torn eyelids should be sutured as soon as possible to re-establish normal contact with the cornea and to prevent drying of the cornea. Badly torn eyelids often heal usually well when promptly sutured. Reconstructive surgery may be necessary for large defects.[1]

Ear lacerations are also common. If not sutured, these wounds usually heal as a split in the free margin of the ear. The surgeon may choose to suture this wound as a fresh laceration or allow healing to occur and suture it at a later date after freshening the edges. The raw edges of the cartilage may be sutured prior to suturing the skin; an alternative technic involves suturing only the skin. Protective bandages and/or splints should be used.[43]

Large vessels severed in the cervical region require immediate aid to prevent severe or fatal blood loss. Pressure compresses (cotton, gauze, cloth) temporarily control bleeding until the vessel is ligated. Large vessels should be ligated dorsal and ventral to the wound. When the carotid artery is involved, the vagosympathetic trunk should not be included in the ligatures.[1]

Lacerations of the trachea may cause extensive subcutaneous emphysema. This may be minimized by performing a tracheostomy ventral to the wound. Usually the entrapped air is of no concern and is eventually absorbed. Tracheal stenosis may result if damage to the cartilage is severe.[1]

Laceration of the esophagus presents several problems. A serious complication to a lacerated esophagus is saliva and ingesta invading the cervical tissues, causing severe cellulitis. This infection may gravitate into the thoracic cavity, causing devastating pleuritis. Swelling from the cervical infection may interfere with respiration and venous return from the jugular vein. Therapy includes parenteral antibiotics, incision of the inflamed area to allow drainage of the entrapped fluids, and conventional care previously described for acute cellulitis. Suturing the esophagus may be attempted in the early stages if feasible. Frequently the edges are devitalized, friable and edematous, allowing the sutures to tear out easily. In these cases provisions must be made to provide adequate water and food to the animal parenterally or through an indwelling stomach tube installed ventral to the cervical wound.[44] The most common complication of esophageal invasion is development of an esophageal fistula, through which saliva constantly exudes.

Thorax

Penetrating thoracic wounds are serious. They may result in aspiration of air into the pleural cavity, causing complete collapse of the lungs. Penetrating wounds demand immediate systemic antimicrobial therapy and complete closure, temporarily through bandage compresses or permanently with sutures. The pending infection must be controlled and pneumothorax corrected.[1]

Abdomen

As in the thorax, penetrating wounds of the abdomen may cause serious complications. The most common complications of abdominal invasion are peritonitis and intestinal herniation. Immediate care must be provided to protect any exposed viscera. Anesthesia should be induced at once and the defect repaired if possible. Placement of peritoneal drains may be warranted and massive systemic antibiotic therapy instituted. Appropriate treatment should be administered if shock is present or imminent.[1]

Joints and Tendon Sheaths

Invaded joints and tendon sheaths, characterized by discharge of straw-colored, oily fluid, require prompt therapy if function is to be restored.[1] Severe contamination from the laceration often causes extensive infectious arthritis and tenosynovitis if not properly treated. Fresh wounds should be protected from additional contamination and treated as soon as possible. Therapy may include joint or sheath lavage, capsule or sheath suturing, systemic antimicrobial treatment and supportive bandages or casts.

Axilla

Wounds in the cranial pectoral region and axilla are common in horses. Wounds of the axillary space characteristically develop extensive subcutaneous emphysema because of the suction-like movement of the parts. When complications do not exist, the axillary wounds heal readily with routine treatment. Any subcutaneous air is generally absorbed after some time.[1] Gaseous cellulitis, as a result of a clostridial infection, must be considered as a cause of crepitous enlargement.

THERAPY FOR BURNS

Burns in large animals are uncommon but devastating when they do occur. Not only is the skin involved, but often many other systems suffer damage, especially the cardiovascular system, liver, kidneys and respiratory tract. Depending upon the magnitude of the burn, there can be a tremendous fluid and electrolyte shift. Most animals with burns over more than 50% of their body surface die because of water and electrolyte shifts.[45]

Burned patients should be carefully evaluated to determine the extent of the injury. An estimate of the percentage of body surface affected may be calculated by dividing the total body surface area ($S = 0.1$ x weight in kg x $\frac{2}{3}$, where S is expressed in m^2) into the measured area of burned skin and multiplying by 100.[45] The burned area can be determined with the aid of a metric ruler or tape. If the involved area is less than 15% of the total surface area and consists basically of first- and second-degree burns, minimal supportive therapy will be required. Patients burned over an area greater than 15% or with third-degree burns will require intensive fluid replacement, which should be initiated immediately by indwelling IV catheter. The most rapid loss and translocation of fluids and electrolytes occur during the first few hours after injury.[45] Lactated Ringer's solution is the fluid of choice until electrolyte values are obtained and dictate otherwise.[46] The hydration and electrolyte levels should be monitored at regular intervals so that needs can be adjusted accordingly.

Analgesics are essential to control pain in severely burned animals. Systemic antibiotics should be administered since these animals are extremely vulnerable to infection. Corticosteroids may be warranted if shock or pulmonary edema is present. Tetanus prophylaxis should also be administered. One of the most important aspects in the treatment of shock from burns is careful and frequent evaluation of the animal's progress.[45]

Previous discussion has been limited to the initial emergency and systemic therapy for burned animals. Although these are very important, local management of the burn should receive its share of attention. The main goals in local treatment are prevention of infection, promotion of rapid healing, minimization of scar formation, and prevention of self-mutilation of the wound.[45] Whether the burn is caused by heat, cold or corrosive substances, topical management is essentially the same as that for other open wounds.

References

1. Boyd and Britton, in Catcott: Equine Medicine and Surgery. 2nd ed. American Veterinary Publications, Santa Barbara, 1972.
2. Beeman, M. Proc 19th Ann Mtg Am Assoc Eq Pract, 1973. p 163.
3. Hanselka, DV. Proc 21st Ann Mtg Am Assoc Eq Pract, 1975. p 191.
4. Heinze, in Oehme and Prier: Textbook of Large Animal Surgery. 1st ed. Williams & Wilkins, Baltimore, 1974.

5. Adams, OR: Lameness in Horses. 3rd ed. Lea & Febiger, Philadelphia, 1974.

6. Greenough and Johnson, in Oehme and Prier: Textbook of Large Animal Surgery. 1st ed. Williams & Wilkins, Baltimore, 1974.

7. Swaim, SF: Surgery of Traumatized Skin. 1st ed. WB Saunders, Philadelphia, 1980.

8. Bryant, WM. Clin Symp 29 (1977) 2.

9. Johnston, DE. J Am Anim Hosp Assoc 13 (1977) 186.

10. Peacock, in Schwartz: Principles of Surgery. McGraw-Hill, New York, 1969.

11. Peacock, EE and Van Winkle, W: Wound Repair. 2nd ed. WB Saunders, Philadelphia, 1976.

12. Johnston, DE. Arch Am Coll Vet Surg 3 (1974) 30.

13. Levenson, SM et al. Ann Surg 161 (1965) 293.

14. Archibald and Blakely, in Archibald: Canine Surgery. 2nd ed. American Veterinary Publications, Santa Barbara, 1974.

15. Epstein, in Epstein: Skin Surgery. 4th ed. Charles C Thomas, Springfield, IL 1977.

16. Bridges, in Catcott: Equine Medicine & Surgery. 2nd ed. American Veterinary Publications, Santa Barbara, 1972.

17. Lipowitz, AJ. JAAHA 12 (1976) 813.

18. Jennings, PB. Arch Am Coll Vet Surg 4 (1975) 43.

19. Dedo, DD et al. Trans Am Acad Ophth Otolar 84 (1977) 68.

20. Altemeier, WA and MacMillan, BG. Ann NY Acad Sci 150 (1968) 966.

21. Branemark, PI et al. J Bone Jt Surg 49A (1967) 48.

22. Committee on Trauma, Am Coll Surg: Early Care of the Injured Patient. 2nd ed. WB Saunders, Philadelphia, 1976.

23. Singleton, AO and Julian, J. Ann Surg 151 (1960) 912.

24. Hoover, NW and Ivins, JC. Arch Surg 79 (1959) 701.

25. Postlethwait, in Sabiston: Textbook of Surgery. 11th ed. WB Saunders, Philadelphia, 1973.

26. Johnson et al, in Oehme and Prier: Textbook of Large Animal Surgery. 1st ed. Williams & Wilkins, Baltimore, 1974.

27. Brown, PW. Clin Orth 96 (1973) 42.

28. Furneaux, RW. Canine Pract 2 (3) (1975) 22.

29. Howes, EL. Surg 7 (1940) 24.

30. Irwin, DHG. J Sm Anim Pract 7 (1966) 593.

31. Smithcors, JF. Mod Vet Pract 47 (1976) 401.

32. Grabb and Smith, in Grabb and Smith: Plastic Surgery. Little, Brown & Co, Boston, 1968.

33. Roberts, WD. Proc 14th Ann Mtg Am Assoc Eq Pract, 1978. p 192.

34. Roberts, WD. Proc 10th Ann Mtg Am Assoc Eq Pract, 1964. p 243.

35. Prudden, JF and Allen, J. J Am Med Assoc 192 (1965) 352.

36. Roberts, WD. VM/SAC 61 (1966) 961.

37. Prudden, JF et al. Surg Gyn Obstet 128 (1969) 1321.

38. Marden, DT. VM/SAC 69 (1974) 771.

39. Belfield, WO et al. VM/SAC 5 (1970) 455.

40. Rosenthal, SP. Arch Surg 96 (1968) 35.

41. Lewis, JR: The Surgery of Scars. McGraw-Hill Book Co, New York, 1963.

42. Schwartz, PL. J Am Diet Assoc 56 (1970) 497.

43. Titus, in Oehme and Prier: Textbook of Large Animal Surgery. 1st ed. Williams & Wilkins, Baltimore, 1974.

44. Hofmeyer, in Oehme and Prier: Textbook of Large Animal Surgery. 1st ed. Williams & Wilkins, Baltimore, 1974.

45. Davis, in Swaim: Surgery of Traumatized Skin. 1st ed. WB Saunders, Philadelphia, 1980.

46. Fox, CL. Ann NY Acad Sci 150 (1968) 823.

CRYOSURGERY
by J.R. Joyce

Cryosurgery is the destruction of tissue by controlled freezing. Since the mid-1970's, cryosurgery has become popular in veterinary medicine to treat superficial tumors and some inflammatory diseases that do not respond well to conventional therapy. In equine medicine, cryosurgery has been used to treat sarcoids, squamous-cell carcinomas, cutaneous habronemiasis, exuberant granulation tissue, papillomas and melanomas, as well as for partial and total neurectomies.[1-11]

There are several advantages of cryosurgery over conventional surgery. The mechanics of cryosurgery are easy to master. The procedure usually takes a minimum of time to perform and can often be performed with only regional anesthesia. Cryosurgery is generally safe for both the surgeon and the patient. Minimal pain is associated with the freezing process. Hemorrhage is generally nonexistent or minimal, and tumor cells are not disseminated by the surgical procedure. There is evidence of increased immune response to some types of neoplasms following cryonecrosis.[12] Postoperative care is usually minimal and cryosurgical scars are usually small.

There are several disadvantages to cryosurgery. Following freezing, moderate to severe edema develops around the lesion. Large tissue masses undergoing necrosis after freezing have a bad odor and attract flies until the necrotic tissue sloughs. White hair may grow over the site or around the resulting scar. Vital normal tissue can be accidentally destroyed by inexperienced operators. Finally, sophisticated cryosurgical instrumentation is expensive.

Cryosurgical Equipment

A variety of cryosurgical equipment is available from less than $100 for a home-made unit or solid probe to several thousand dollars for large, sophisticated units.[5,9] Each unit has advantages and disadvantages. The various types of cryosurgical equipment available should be studied to select a unit that fits one's particular requirements. Discussions with users of a particular unit can provide useful information.

Various cryogens are used in cryosurgery. Liquid nitrogen (boiling point -195.6 C) and nitrous oxide (boiling point -98 C) are the most popular; however, CO_2 and freon are also used. Each has advantages and disadvantages that vary in different circumstances.

Although not always necessary, especially as one gains experience and confidence, a pyrometer (tissue thermometer) is extremely helpful to monitor the temperature of the ice ball and surrounding tissue. Its use permits much more accurate control of the area destroyed and results in a higher percentage of successful treatments. The pyrometer also helps prevent excessive freezing and damage to tendons, ligaments and other vital anatomic structures. However, the surgeon should keep in mind that sometimes the temperature being recorded may not be a true reflection of the extent of the freeze. If the thermocouple of the pyrometer is placed against large blood vessels, it records the warmer temperature of the flowing blood. Occasionally a thermocouple malfunctions. Use of 2 thermocouples reduces the chances of error and serious harm to the patient.

Cryonecrosis

Tissue destruction by cryosurgery results from direct cellular damage and anoxia (infarction) due to damage to small blood vessels. Some knowledge of these mechanisms enables one to better understand and perform cryosurgery successfully.[12-14] Cellular destruction is related to size and location of ice crystal formation, toxic electrolyte concentrations, cell dehydration and denaturation of all membrane lipid-proteins.

Freezing damages cells of capillaries and arterioles. Vasodilation occurs after a brief period of vasoconstriction. Thrombosis then creates an area of infarction, with a sharp line of demarcation between damaged and viable tissue. Large vessels are more resistant to the effects of cryosurgery due to the quantity of warm blood flowing through them.

Most cryosurgeons adhere to the following guidelines to ensure maximum lethal effects upon tissue to be removed: The tissue to be destroyed should be frozen rapidly for optimal formation of intracellular ice crystals. The area should be frozen to a minimum of -20 to -30 C and should extend several millimeters into healthy tissue if possible. Thawing of the frozen tissue should be slow and unassisted to expose the cells to lethal salt concentrations that result from the freezing process, and to allow intracellular ice crystals to form larger, more damaging crystals.

When possible, a double or triple freeze-thaw cycle should be used. This ensures maximum cell death by speeding the rate of freezing with subsequent freezes, thereby increasing the direct effects of cellular destruction and thrombus formation in the microcirculation of the unwanted tissue. A few cryosurgeons recommend a single freeze-thaw cycle when minimum tissue destruction and scarring are desired, as in the adnexa of the eye.

Application of the Cryogen

Cryogens are applied to unwanted tissue by contact probes or direct spray.

Circulating contact probes are available in a variety of sizes and shapes. The cryogen circulates through the tip of the probe and is vented safely away from the patient. This prevents splattering of the cryogen on adjacent tissue and allows somewhat better control of the area to be frozen. However, probes generally do not freeze as large an area as the spray apparatus. To compensate for this lower freezing power, the surgeon may treat several overlapping areas, or remove the bulk of the lesion surgically and freeze the base. On deep tumors, a core or cores of tissue can be surgically removed from the mass and the contact probe inserted into the holes to allow faster, deeper freezing.

Solid cryoprobes (cotton-tipped applicators or solid metal probes) are less expensive than circulating contact probes and can be used successfully on small, superficial lesions. The probes are prechilled by immersion in the liquid cryogen and are then applied to the unwanted tissue. A water-soluble lubricant jelly can be applied to the tissue to ensure that the chilled probe maintains firm contact.[15]

Spray application allows direct application of the cryogen to the unwanted tissue. The cryogen is under pressure and the amount applied is controlled by valve or spray tips with different-sized apertures. Spray application allows larger and deeper areas to be frozen than with contact probes. Healthy tissue must be protected from excess cryogen. Not clipping the hair over surrounding healthy tissue is one method of protection. Dry hair helps insulate tissue from the effects of freezing. Other insulators that can be used are styrofoam, foam rubber and petroleum jelly. Styrofoam cups are

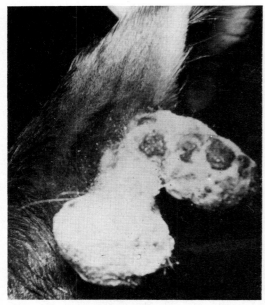 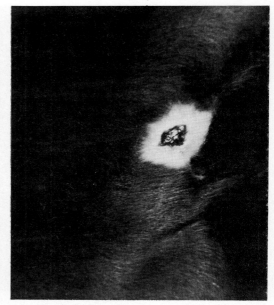

Fig 96. Aural sarcoid immediately after (left) and 3 weeks after (right) cryosurgery.

inexpensive and easily cut to various shapes. A thick layer of petroleum jelly gives good protection, especially over dry hair. Metal or plastic spray "cones" are available to direct and contain the cryogen spray. This not only protects surrounding tissue, but speeds the freezing process.

On extremely large tumors, the bulk of the mass can be removed and the tumor base frozen. Overlapping the areas frozen allows freezing of relatively large areas.

Controlling Necrosis

The ice ball must be carefully monitored to avoid excessive tissue damage. Manual palpation, visual examination, clinical experience and use of a pyrometer aid the cryosurgeon in determining the amount of tissue to be destroyed. Thermocouples placed just below the unwanted tissue allow accurate delineation of the area to be frozen. However, use of the pyrometer can have a few drawbacks. One must be aware that artificially high readings may be obtained if a thermocouple is against a large blood vessel. Also, the temperature at the thermocouple can "bottom out" below the optimal -20 to -30 C when a large ice ball is produced or with very rapid heat loss. Palpation and visual examination are valuable methods of assessing the area frozen, especially as one develops clinical experience with cryotherapy. In difficult cases, several layers of unwanted tissue can be removed over a period of weeks.

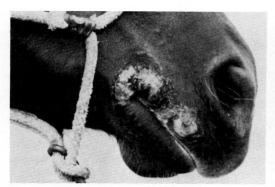 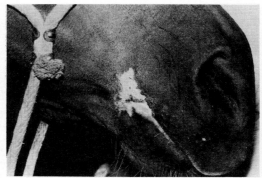

Fig 97. Labial sarcoid before (left) and 6 months after 2 cryosurgical treatments at an 8-week interval (right).

Aftercare

Aftercare is usually minimal. Cryotherapy often causes considerable local edema that usually resolves in several days. The thawed tissue may ooze a serosanguineous fluid and take on a reddish-black color the following day. A separation develops between necrotic and viable tissue in 7-14 days. A small amount of pus may be evident at this demarcation. The necrotic tissue may be dry and hard, and remains in place to function as a bandage or scab. With small areas of necrosis, complete healing may take place under this scab. The scab can be removed if it is loose or irritating to the animal. As with any other large area of tissue necrosis, there is an odor and fly problem.

Hemostasis following cryosurgery is excellent provided no vessels have been severed during biopsy or by reducing the size of tumor with a scalpel. Vessels severed just before or during cryosurgery may bleed profusely upon thawing.

Healing is generally without complications and antibiotics are not usually administered. The time for complete healing varies from 3-4 weeks for superficial cryolesions up to 2-3 cm to 2-3 months for large, deep lesions. Scarring is minimal in proportion to the tissue destroyed. White hair may regrow around the scar edges. Although healing and granulation proceed rapidly, formation of exuberant granulation tissue is minimal following cryosurgery.

Cryosurgery may stimulate the formation of antibodies to certain types of neoplastic cells left *in situ*.[11,13] Rupture of cell membranes by the freeze-thaw process may allow antigens to be released into the systemic circulation.[12,16] In several horses, pea-sized pieces of equine sarcoid harvested from the patient were treated with a double freeze-thaw cycle and implanted sc. Sarcoid tissue that could not be removed or treated due to its extent and/or location subsequently regressed.[17]

Examples of successful cryosurgery are illustrated in Figures 96 and 97.

Anesthesia

Although cryosurgery desensitizes nerves as freezing progresses, anesthesia prior to treatment is usually necessary. Many tumors can be frozen using only xylazine sedation or xylazine sedation in combination with regional anesthesia. The choice of anesthetic remains the clinical judgement of the veterinarian and is based on the size and location of the tumor, disposition of the patient, facilities available, and expertise of the cryosurgeon.

References

1. Joyce, JR. JAVMA **168** (1976) 226.
2. Farris, HE *et al.* VM/SAC **71** (1976) 325.
3. Joyce, JR. VM/SAC **70** (1975) 200.
4. Krahwinkel, DJ *et al.* JAVMA **169** (1976) 201.
5. Farris, HE *et al.* VM/SAC **70** (1975) 299.
6. Farris, HE and Fraunfelder, FT. JAVMA **168** (1976) 213.
7. Hilbert, J *et al.* JAVMA **170** (1977) 1305.
8. Migioia, S. VM/SAC **73** (1978) 1073.
9. Twidale, JD. Proc 23rd Ann Mtg Am Assoc Eq Pract, 1977. p 317.
10. Animal Nutrition and Health. (March, 1978) 9. (Abstr).
11. Tate, LP. Proc 23rd Ann Mtg Am Assoc Eq Pract, 1977. p 321.
12. Greiner, TP *et al.* Vet Clin No Am **5** (1975) 565.
13. Bojrab, MJ. Norden News (Spring, 1978) 16.
14. Goldstein, RS: Handbook of Veterinary Cryosurgery. Spembly, Santa Clara, CA, 1977.
15. Farrell, KR. VM/SAC **73** (1978) 1377.
16. Withrow, SJ *et al.* JAAHA **11** (1975) 271.
17. Joyce, JR, Texas A&M Univ: Unpublished data, 1980.

17

The Endocrine System

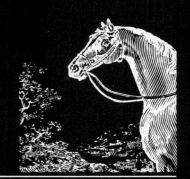

THE PITUITARY GLAND
by D.A. Deem and R.H. Whitlock

Anatomy and Physiology

The hypophysis cerebri or pituitary gland is located in the sella turcica of the cranial vault. It is composed of 2 main sections, the adenohypophysis and neurohypophysis, which differ in their origin, structure and function. The adenohypophysis forms from an evagination of the roof of the pharynx (Rathke's pouch) that extends dorsad during embryogenesis and contacts an outpouching of the floor of the third ventricle, which becomes the neurohypophysis. The gland normally weighs 1-3 g, and measures 2 x 2 x 0.5 cm.

The adenohypophysis consists of the pars tuberalis, pars distalis and pars intermedia. The distal and intermediate parts are fused, and the pars intermedia is particularly well developed and completely surrounds the neurohypophysis.[1] The pars tuberalis functions primarily as a scaffolding for blood vessels to the pars distalis and hypophyseal portal system. The pars intermedia is the source of melanophore-stimulating hormone (MSH) or intermedin, the function of which in mammals is not known. The intermediate lobe produces adrenocorticotropic hormone (ACTH). This and other experimental evidence points to a similar, if not identical, cytologic source of MSH and ACTH. Cells secreting ACTH may be in a different secretory stage from those that elaborate MSH.[2]

The pars distalis is the functionally most active portion of the adenohypophysis. It is responsible for elaboration of ACTH, thyroid-stimulating hormone (TSH), somatotrophic or growth hormone (STH), follicle-stimulating hormone (FSH), luteinizing hormone (LH) and prolactin. The cytologic source of these hormones is controversial. The previous classification of pituitary cells as acidophils, basophils and chromophobes does not explain the independent secretion of 6 known hormones and other peptides, the physiologic significance of which is unknown. There is enormous species variability and it is most logical to classify pituitary cell types on the basis of the hormone secreted. Histochemical, immunofluorescent and electronmicroscopic evaluations have supported the concept that each major hormone is secreted by a distinct cell type. Prolactin and STH arise from acidophilic cells, and TSH, FSH and LH arise from basophilic cells. The source of ACTH is controversial. Some authors feel it is secreted by basophilic cells, which also can secrete MSH.[3] These cells are present in the pars distalis and pars intermedia, and the relative distribution and predominant secretory product vary among species. Relatively agranular cells, called chromophobe cells, were originally believed to be the source of ACTH.[4] However, these cells are now believed to represent undifferentiated precursors of the secretory cells or those that have temporarily been depleted of granules and are in a resting state.[3]

Somatotropic Hormone

The primary role of STH is to stimulate an increase in body size. Epiphyseal plates of long bones are uniquely sensitive to STH. Cartilage proliferation and skeletal growth are promoted through somatomedin, a polypeptide released from the liver in response to STH, in synergism with thyroxine.[5] Along with ACTH, STH mobilizes fat and causes increased levels of ketone bodies in the blood. Glucose use in muscle and adipose tissue is inhibited by STH, resulting in hyperglycemia. The mechanism of control of STH synthesis and release is not definitively known; however, hypoglycemia, exercise, certain types of excitement and administration of amino acids (particularly arginine) stimulate STH secretion.[3]

Blockade of hypothalamic and adrenergic receptors with drugs, such as phentolamine, decreases STH response to provocative stimuli. An inhibitory peptide for STH release has been isolated from porcine hypothalamic extracts, and the existence of a releasing factor has been suggested.[6] After inactivation of the inhibitory factor with normal serum, highly active fractions of somatotropic hormone-releasing factor are demonstrable. The balance of these controls remains to be elucidated.

Prolactin

Prolactin initiates and maintains lactation.[3] After the mammary gland has been prepared by estrogens, progestins, corticosteroids and insulin, prolactin causes milk secretion. Both STH and ACTH are necessary and synergistic with the action of prolactin on mammary growth and secretion. Increased prolactin levels are observed at proestrus, parturition and after suckling. The role of the hormone in males is unknown. Interference with dopaminergic mechanisms in the hypothalamus by certain drugs induces lactation and hyperprolactinemia in women.[3] This is presumably due to interference with the normal secretion of a prolactin-inhibitory factor. Catecholamine content is correlated with prolactin-inhibitory activity of hypothalamic extracts.[7] However, material devoid of catecholamines exhibits prolactin-inhibitory activity, and gamma amino benzoic acid may be the definitive prolactin-inhibitory factor.[8] The hypothalamus may also contain prolactin-releasing factors. Thyrotropin-releasing hormone (TRH) is a potent stimulus for prolactin secretion in some species.[4,6] Equine prolactin has been isolated from equine pituitary glands.[9]

Follicle-Stimulating and Luteinizing Hormones

Follicle-stimulating hormone (FSH) and luteinizing hormone (LH) have primary action on the gonads and are therefore called gonadotropins (see Chapter 23). The 2 hormones are synergistic in their actions; however, FSH is primarily responsible for ovarian follicular development and testicular gametogenesis, and LH (also called interstitial cell-stimulating hormone) promotes luteinization in the ovary and secretion by the Leydig cells in the testes. Secretion of gonadotropins is regulated by the hypothalamus through luteinizing hormone-releasing hormone (LHRH). No hypothalamic releasing factor for FSH has been isolated, so it is assumed LHRH also causes FSH release. Many environmental stimuli, such as odors and light, act through the hypophysiotropic releasing mechanism. Sex steroids act by feedback inhibition on the pituitary and hypothalamus to modify gonadotropin release.

Thyroid-Stimulating Hormone

Thyroid-stimulating hormone (TSH) or thyrotropin has morphologic and functional effects on the thyroid gland. The height of the alveolar epithelium in the thyroid is increased and colloid becomes depleted by TSH administration. It increases all aspects of thyroid physiology, including iodine trapping, organic binding, thyroglobulin synthesis, iodotyrosine and iodothyronine formation, thyroglobulin proteolysis, and thyroxine (T_4) and tri-iodothyronine (T_3) release. The TSH acts at a specific site on the thyroid cell membrane.[10] The secretion of TSH is determined partially by the level of hypothalamic thyrotropin-releasing hormone (TRH) and partially by the level of circulating thyroid hormones. The TRH is thought to delicately adjust TSH secretion, since the pituitary possesses some degree of autonomy.[11] Serum TSH levels in humans increase rapidly within 10 minutes of TRH injection. Administration of TSH prior to TRH blocks TSH release, suggesting the formation of an inhibitor to TRH action.[10] Negative feedback acts primarily at the pituitary level and free thyroxine (T_4) is believed to be the primary physiologic regulator of TSH secretion.[12,13] Secretion of TSH is stimulated by exposure to cold via a hypothalamic release of TRH.[11] During cold adaptation, the rate of thyroxine secretion increases by two-thirds.[14] Release of TSH is suppressed by glucocorticoid administration, suggesting modulation by adrenocortical function.[10]

Adrenocorticotropic Hormone

Corticotropin (ACTH) binds with specific surface receptors of adrenocortical cells and, in the presence of Ca, activates adenyl cyclase and increases the intracellular concentration of cyclic AMP. Key enzymes are phosphorylated, resulting in increased steroidogenesis and secretion. Although ACTH stimulates aldosterone production, its primary action is on the secretion of glucocorticoids by the zona fasciculata. Extra-adrenal effects of ACTH cause fat mobilization, enhanced ketogenesis, increased content of glycogen in muscle, hypoglycemia, and decreased blood amino acid concentrations.[4] Pituitary secretion of ACTH is under dual control. Circulating cortisol inhibits ACTH secretion by action on pituitary corticotropic cells and also possibly on the hypothalamus. Secretion of ACTH also occurs in response to hypothalamic release of corticotropin-releasing factor (CRF) in response to stress, such as pain, anxiety, hypoglycemia, exercise, circadian rhythm and other neurogenic stimuli. Using plasma cortisol levels as an indicator, profound hypoglycemia (<20 mg/dl) is required to stimulate ACTH release.[15] Although high plasma levels of cortisol and administration of corticosteroids diminish ACTH release, this negative feedback system is of secondary importance in stressful situations, in which ACTH release occurs despite elevated plasma cortisol levels.

Melanophore-Stimulating Hormone

The pigment granules of melanocytes of certain fish and amphibians are dispersed by MSH. In higher animals, the functional significance of MSH is unknown. The pituitary of all species contains 2 melanocyte-stimulating peptides. In lower animals, hypothalamic control of MSH secretion is exerted by a melanophore-stimulating, hormone-inhibiting factor. In humans, MSH shares the same feedback inhibition by cortisol as does ACTH.[3] Serum levels of MSH are elevated in Addison's disease (adrenocortical atrophy) and decreased after glucocorticoid administration.

Oxytocin and Vasopressin

The neurohypophysis is the distal component of a neurosecretory system that includes 2 pairs of nuclei in the hypothalamus (the supraoptic and paraventricular nuclei) and the neurohypophyseal tract, which carries axons from these nuclei to terminate there. The axons make up the neural stalk and contain the biologically active neurosecretory octapeptides, oxytocin and vasopressin. The exact mechanism by which neurohypophyseal hormones are released is not clear, but a wide variety of stimuli is involved. Nerve impulses originating in the hypothalamus are conducted along the axons of the pituitary stalk, resulting in depolarization of neurosecretory terminals and release of the hormones.[3]

Oxytocin and vasopressin share many physiologic actions, but oxytocin is primarily concerned with reproduction. Oxytocin exerts a stimulatory effect on the myometrium when it

is under estrogenic influence during late gestation and the follicular phase of estrus.[4] Cervical stretching results in oxytocin release. Oxytocin also stimulates contraction of myoepithelial cells surrounding milk alveoli, causing mild ejection or letdown. The suckling stimulus acts via a neural afferent path to the hypothalamic nuclei, resulting in oxytocin release from the neurohypophysis. Oxytocin may be involved in prolactin release since its injection prolongs lactation in female rats from which the young have been removed.[4]

Because the major physiologic role of vasopressin relates to its antidiuretic activity, it is called antidiuretic hormone (ADH). The target organ is the kidney, in which ADH makes the distal tubule and collecting duct permeable to water. The osmotic gradient between the dilute urine formed by Na and Cl absorption in the loop of Henle and hypertonic interstitium results in water resorption and antidiuresis. Vasopressin may disrupt the permeability of tubular membranes by affecting cell protein or intercellular cement substance. The intracellular mediator of ADH is cyclic AMP, which is formed when membrane-bound adenyl cyclase is activated.

Dehydration is the usual stimulus for release of ADH. Osmoreceptor cells within the supraoptic nucleus of the anterior hypothalamus react to increased extracellular osmolarity and release ADH. Plasma vasopressin levels in rats rise sharply when plasma osmolarity is increased.[16] Dilution of the plasma or body fluids suppresses the release of ADH, resulting in profuse diuresis and excretion of hypotonic urine. Therefore, a negative-feedback system, including the kidney and CNS, preserves the total solute concentration of body fluids. There is a close anatomic and physiologic relationship between the thirst and ADH centers in the hypothalamus. The combination of ADH release and the thirst mechanism ensures the normal osmotic concentration of body fluids. Stimulation in the rostromedial portion of the hypothalamus in goats causes polydipsia and diuresis. Whether there exist 2 separate, overlapping centers or a single one with nervous connections is yet to be established. A reduction in effective plasma volume, as in hemorrhage, shock or decreased cardiac output, stimulates ADH release, even in the presence of hypotonic body fluids. Under homeostatic conditions, plasma osmolarity and blood volume are the major physiologic controls.[16] Minor factors control vasopressin release in some situations. Pain and emotional states that result in neural stimuli may cause antidiuresis. Many pharmacologic agents, such as acetylcholine, morphine and barbiturates, cause ADH release.[3] Alcohol inhibits ADH release by blocking normal releasing stimuli. Absence of glucocorticoids may increase ADH release and the renin-angiotensin mechanism may affect secretion of ADH.[17] The contribution of these minor mechanisms is poorly understood.

Vasopressin can cause smooth muscle contraction when present in quantities greater than necessary for maximal diuresis. A generalized increase in vascular resistance occurs and can cause a rise in blood pressure in anesthetized animals. The mechanism of action on smooth muscle is unknown, but ADH and its analogs have been used to control bleeding from gastric and esophageal varices in humans.[18] Vasopressin can cause a rise in plasma cortisol levels in humans, either through the release of hypothalamic corticotropin-releasing factor or by mimicking its action on the pituitary. This is used to help differentiate Cushing's disease from Cushing's syndrome due to adrenocortical carcinoma.[19,20]

Diseases of the Pituitary Gland

Hypopituitarism

Cause: Primary hypopituitarism may result from pituitary destruction by nonsecretory pituitary tumors, metastatic neoplasia, cysts, infarction, and a number of infiltrative and granulomatous processes.[21] Atrophy of the gland is usually the result of local pressure by cysts or tumors of the gland or adjacent areas of the brain. The basophils are more pressure-sensitive than acidophils, but a large degree of atrophy must occur before clinical signs are seen. Acquired cysts are common in horses but do not produce an obvious functional deficit.[1]

Necrosis of the hypophysis occurs rarely as a result of local inflammation, sinus thrombosis or ischemia. The last sometimes occurs in the adenohypophysis in extreme anemia. Inflammation of the neurohypophysis is common and usually associated with meningitis or encephalitis. The adenohypophysis is remarkably resistant to inflammation. Destructive, suppurative inflammations can involve both portions of the gland. Embolism from other sites of infection and local extension from otitis media or retropharyngeal inflammation are the usual routes. Parasitic inflammations are occasionally seen.

Clinical Signs: Hypopituitarism is manifested in various ways because of the lack of hypophyseal hormones. In humans, gonadotropin deficiency causes gonadal atrophy and loss of body hair. Signs of adrenal insufficiency and hypothyroidism usually occur. Dwarfism and failure of growth result if hypopituitarism develops before puberty. Moderate normocytic normochromic anemia may be observed.[3] Adenohypophyseal insufficiency has not been observed in horses but would be expected secondary to massive destruction of the gland by inflammation or neoplasia. Although isolated pituitary hormone deficiencies occur in humans, they have not been observed in horses.

Diagnosis: Diagnosis of insufficiency of the adenohypophysis is based on low blood levels of cortisol, thyroxine and the pituitary gonadotropins. Stimulation tests with the tropic hormones should produce a positive response unless the target organs have atrophied.[3]

Treatment: Therapy consists of replacing adrenal, thyroid and gonadal hormones. Prognosis depends upon the cause of the pituitary deficiency. The prognosis is grave since most cases in horses are secondary to an expanding neoplasm.

Diabetes Insipidus

Cause: Neurohypophyseal insufficiency is commonly associated with adenohypophyseal insufficiency and is manifested by failure to conserve water because of a lack of ADH. Although common in humans and dogs, diabetes insipidus has not been documented in horses. The polydipsia and polyuria that frequently accompany tumors of the pars intermedia in horses have been ascribed to ADH insufficiency through destruction of the neurohypophysis by the expanding tumor.[22] However, other factors may be involved (see below) and ADH therapy does not result in concentration of the urine.

Clinical Signs: Clinical signs of diabetes insipidus are pronounced polydipsia and polyuria. Deprivation of water results in rapid dehydration, weight loss, profound thirst and extracellular hypertonicity. In affected dogs and humans, the urine specific gravity is usually 1.001-1.005.[3,16] Plasma osmolality rises because of inability to concentrate urine.

Diagnosis: Induction of dehydration by water restriction should be a maximal stimulation for ADH release and consequently increased urine specific gravity. If the animal still produces urine with a specific gravity of 1.005 or less after water deprivation, true diabetes insipidus should be suspected. The diagnosis can be confirmed by demonstrating that the kidneys respond to exogenous ADH. The ADH-response test is performed in dogs by injection of 2-10 pressor units vasopressin tannate in oil, following bladder evacuation and recording of urine specific gravity.[16] Urine specimens are collected 8, 12, 16 and 20 hours postinjection and should exhibit maximal concentrations. Fluid should be limited during this period for best evaluation of concentrating ability.

The most difficult condition from which to differentiate diabetes insipidus is psychogenic polydipsia, in which urine specific gravity may be consistently less than 1.005. This primary psychic polydipsia results in water diuresis. A distinctive feature of primary polydipsia is that plasma osmolarity tends to be decreased to low normal or less.[23] The urine is concentrated after moderate water deprivation for several days.

Polyuria may occur during K depletion or hypercalcemia, both of which impair renal concentration mechanisms.[24] However, the urine is usually not persistently hypotonic because only maximal concentration is impaired.

Hyperadrenocorticism can also produce polyuria and polydipsia. The urine specific gravity is usually greater than 1.005. It is thought that cortisol increases glomerular filtration, thereby initiating diuresis. Alternatively, ADH synthesis, release or action on the kidney may be blocked by cortisol.[25,26] Compression of the posterior pituitary gland, hypothalamus or hypothalamic stalk by an ACTH-producing anterior pituitary tumor is another possible mechanism.[26,27] However, exogenous ADH does not cause urine concentration.

Polyuria is a common manifestation of chronic renal failure; however, urine specific gravity is usually fixed near that of plasma (1.008-1.012). The polydipsia and polyuria are not nearly as pronounced as in diabetes insipidus.

Treatment: Treatment of diabetes insipidus requires IM injection of vasopressin at a dosage and frequency determined for the individual. A dosage of 0.22 pressor units/kg relieves signs in canine patients for 24-60 hours.[16] The oral hypoglycemic agent, chlorpropamide, as well as the hypolipidemic agent, clofibrate, reduce polyuria in some human patients with diabetes insipidus.[26] These are used in patients with some residual capacity to release ADH because they stimulate ADH release and potentiate its effect on renal tubule cells.[21] Thiazide diuretics, especially hydrochlorothiazide, is useful in treating human patients with nephrogenic diabetes insipidus. They produce Na depletion, causing a fall in glomerular filtration rate and enhanced absorption of fluid in the proximal portion of the nephron.[26] The value of these drugs for use in animals has been disputed.[16,23] There are no reports of successful therapy of polyuric syndromes with any of these agents in horses.

Prognosis depends upon the cause of ADH insufficiency. Primary and metastatic intracranial neoplasms are the most common causes in dogs.[27] The prognosis is grave if other signs of neurologic dysfunction accompany or quickly follow signs of diabetes insipidus. Diabetes insipidus may also occur subsequent to traumatic or inflammatory destruction of the neurohypophysis. Some cases of reduced vasopressin secretion have no known cause (idiopathic diabetes insipidus). Familial diabetes insipidus has not been observed in domestic animals.

Hyperpituitarism

Hypertrophy of the pituitary gland occurs during pregnancy and is associated with an increased size and number of acidophils. Nodular hyperplasia is common in older horses. The hyperplastic nodules in the pars distalis are usually microscopic.

Pituitary Neoplasia

Neoplasia is the most common type of pituitary disease in horses. The tumors are derived from cells of the pars intermedia, and only infrequently is the pars distalis affected.[28] Since most equine pituitary adenomas arise in the pars intermedia, this discussion pertains to these. Older horses are affected, with females more so than males. The tumors expand mainly toward the hypothalamus. Even in very large tumors, remnants of the normal gland can be found and signs of adenohypophyseal deficiency are not clearly demonstrated.[1] Diabetes insipidus and hypothalamic dysfunction may occur due to compression.[1,22]

Clinical Signs: The clinical syndrome associated with tumors of the pars intermedia in horses is characterized by weight loss, muscle wasting, lethargy, ravenous appetite, and varying degrees of polyuria and polydipsia.[28,29] Some affected horses develop hirsutism; the hair over the trunk and extremities may grow to 10-12 cm and become wavy. The pattern varies, but usually the long hair is bilaterally

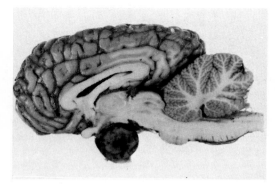

Fig 1. Pituitary adenoma in the pars intermedia.

symmetric.[22,30-32] The skin is often greasy or dry and scaly. Superficial skin infections, such as streptothricosis, are common.[29] Some affected animals sweat excessively.[30] Muscle wasting gives the animals a sway-backed appearance, with bony prominences and a pendulous abdomen. Chronic infectious processes commonly occur, such as abscesses, sinusitis and fistulous tracts; these, as well as wounds and surgical incisions, are slow to heal.

The most consistent laboratory findings are insulin-resistant hyperglycemia (often >200 mg/dl) and glycosuria.[22,33-35] Intravenous glucose-tolerance tests, using glucose at 0.5-1 g/kg body weight, usually reveal elevations of blood glucose levels for up to 3 hours;[33,34] however, results are variable and should be interpreted cautiously. Blood glucose levels in normal horses are said to return to preinjection levels within 120 minutes.[34,35] Ponies fasted for 72 hours prior to testing had elevated blood glucose levels for up to 6 hours.[36] Dietary factors may also significantly influence glucose tolerance; animals accustomed to grain have a greater glucose tolerance. Because of the apparent great individual variation in normal animals, glucose-tolerance testing may not be a useful diagnostic tool for horses with pituitary adenomas.

The leukogram may reveal a relative neutrophilia, lymphopenia and eosinopenia.[29] Total eosinophil counts usually reveal no eosinophils. Unless there is a systemic infection, the total WBC count is within normal limits. A mild, normochromic normocytic anemia is common. Lipemia and hypercholesterolemia may be observed.

Polydipsia and polyuria may be striking; some affected horses drink up to 80 L water daily and produce large volumes of dilute urine. Glycosuria is present in horses with hyper-

glycemia. Ketonuria often reflects progressive weight loss.

Plasma cortisol levels may be elevated or normal, but plasma MSH levels are consistently elevated.[29] Many affected horses do not exhibit a diurnal variation in blood cortisol levels as seen in normal horses.[15,37,38]

Diagnosis: Although the characteristic clinical signs aid diagnosis, not all affected animals exhibit striking hirsutism, muscle wasting, polyuria and polydipsia. Parasitism, inadequate diet, poor dentition, chronic infections, and chronic renal and liver disease must be ruled out. Other endocrine disorders may cause similar clinical signs. For example, hyperhidrosis and hyperglycemia are also observed in cases of pheochromocytoma.[39]

Necropsy Findings: Adenomas of the pars intermedia cause symmetric pituitary enlargement. The adjacent adenohypophysis is often compressed, remaining only as a rim of tissue on the rostral margin of the mass (Fig 1). The overlying hypothalamus is compressed if the tumor is very large. The neurohypophysis is frequently grossly obliterated. The tumors are often nodular and may be cystic, but hemorrhage and necrosis are rare, even in very large neoplasms. They vary in color from yellow to grey-white or pink. Adrenal gland enlargement is common and the cortex:medulla ratio is usually greatly increased.[35] The pancreas is grossly normal. The liver and kidney are often pale, and the liver may be slightly enlarged. Pneumonia, abscesses and evidence of bacteremia are common.[22,33-35]

Adenomas of the pars intermedia do not have a distinct capsule, but are sharply delineated from the compressed anterior lobe parenchyma. Fine septa of connective tissue, containing numerous capillaries, subdivide the tumor into nodules. The tumor cells are arranged in cords and nests along these septa, and the histologic pattern is similar to that of the pars intermedia of normal horses. Numerous secretory granules are present in the tumor cell cytoplasm. The cells vary from cuboidal to spindle-shaped. They seem to have differing staining characteristics and have been described as chromophobic, eosinophilic and basophilic.[22,33-35]

The neural lobe is most commonly infiltrated with neoplastic tissue, which results in replacement by fibrous astrocytes and hemosiderophages. This is in striking contrast to the pars distalis, which is compressed but not invaded. If the tumor enlarges sufficiently to compress the hypothalamus, there is a marked loss of nerve bodies and increased glial cell numbers.[28]

Hepatic parenchymal cells are often swollen and contain increased glycogen; fatty infiltration is prominent in the centrolobular region. There may be moderate portal infiltration with lymphocytes and plasma cells. The kidney may have similar degenerative changes.

Findings vary, but there seems to be no obvious pancreatic degeneration that would support insulin deficiency (diabetes mellitus). The fact that insulin does not correct the persistent hyperglycemia speaks against beta-cell deficiency or dysfunction as a primary abnormality despite many reports to the contrary.[33-35]

Treatment: The long-term prognosis for affected horses is poor regardless of treatment. The progression of clinical signs depends upon how quickly the tumor enlarges and presumably how actively it secretes its corticotropic product. Septicemia, encephalitis and pneumonia are usually the immediate cause of death. Affected animals commonly become severely wasted and debilitated before death. Many become blind from compression of the optic nerve. The adrenocorticolytic agent, O, p'-DDD (Lysodren:Calbio), has been used experimentally in horses but has proven impractical due to highly variable results and prohibitive expense. This drug and others may provide a temporary benefit to animals with slowly enlarging adenomas. Although feasible, bilateral adrenalectomy is not performed in horses.

References

1. Jubb, KVF and Kennedy, PC: Pathology of Domestic Animals. 2nd ed. Academic Press, New York, 1970.
2. Orth, DN and Nicholson, WE. Ann NY Acad Sci **297** (1978) 47.
3. Williams, R. Textbook of Endocrinology. 5th ed. WB Saunders, Philadelphia, 1974.
4. Dickson, in Swenson: Duke's Physiology of Domestic Animals. 9th ed. Cornell Univ Press, Ithaca, 1977.
5. Irvine, CHG and Evans, MJ. J Repro Fert Suppl **23** (1975) 709.
6. Boyd, AE et al. Endocrin **103** (1978) 1075.
7. Schaar, CJ and Clemens, JA. Endocrin **95** (1974) 1202.
8. Schally, AV et al. Endocrin **100** (1977) 68.
9. Chen, CL et al. Am J Vet Res **40** (1979) 1303.
10. Hershman, JM and Pittman, JA. N Engl J Med **285** (1971) 997.
11. Reichlin, in Martini and Ganong: Neuroendocrinology. Academic Press, New York, 1966.
12. Cryer, PE: Diagnostic Endocrinology. Oxford Univ Press, New York, 1976.
13. Wahner, HW and Gorman, CA. N Engl J Med **284** (1971) 225.
14. Irvine, CHG. J Endocr **39** (1967) 313.
15. James, VHT et al. J Endocr **48** (1970) 319.
16. Bovee, KC. Vet Clin No Am **7** (1977) 603.
17. Agus, ZS and Goldberg, M. J Clin Invest **50** (1971) 1478.
18. Merigan, TC et al. N Engl J Med **266** (1962) 134.
19. Bethge, H et al. Acta Endocr **60** (1969) 47.
20. Coslovsky, R et al. Acta Endocr **75** (1974) 125.
21. Hays, RM. N Engl J Med **295** (1976) 659.
22. Loeb, WF et al. Cornell Vet **56** (1966) 623.
23. Joles and Mulnix, in Kirk: Current Veterinary Therapy VI. WB Saunders, Philadelphia, 1977.
24. Schrier, in Beeson et al. Cecil Textbook of Medicine. 15th ed. WB Saunders, Philadelphia, 1979.
25. Owens, JM and Drueker, WD. Vet Clin No Am **7** (1977) 583.
26. Streeten et al, in Thorn et al: Harrison's Principles of Internal Medicine. 8th ed. McGraw-Hill, New York, 1977.
27. Madewell, BR et al. JAAHA **11** (1975) 497.
28. Capen, in Moulton: Tumors in Domestic Animals. 2nd ed. Univ Calif Press, Berkeley, 1978.
29. Gribble, in Catcott: Equine Medicine and Surgery. 2nd ed. American Veterinary Publications, Santa Barbara, 1972.
30. Backstrom, G. Nord Vet Med **15** (1963) 778.
31. Ericksson, K et al. Nord Vet med **15** (1963) 778.
32. Holscher, MA et al. VM/SAC **73** (1978) 1197.
33. Baker, JR and Ritchie, HE. Eq Vet J **6** (1974) 7.
34. King, JM et al. Cornell Vet **52** (1962) 133.
35. Tasker, JB et al. JAVMA **149** (1966) 393.
36. Argenzio, RA and Hintz, HF. J Anim Sci **30** (1970) 514.
37. Bottoms, GD et al. Am J Vet Res **33** (1972) 785.
38. Zokolovick, A et al. J Endocr **35** (1966) 249.
39. Evans, LH et al. JAVMA **159** (1971) 209.

THE THYROID GLAND
by F.A. Kallfelz

Anatomy and Physiology

The thyroid gland of the horse is composed of 2 lobes located on the ventrolateral surfaces of the trachea, just caudal to the larynx. Each lobe is about 5.0 cm x 2.7 cm x 1.5-2.0 cm. In adult horses, a band of connective tissue, the isthmus, connects the 2 lobes across the ventral surface of the neck. The isthmus in foals generally contains functional thyroid tissue.[1]

The thyroid gland is composed of roughly spherical follicles of variable size. The follicles consist of an outer single layer of cuboidal epithelium enclosing a cavity. The apical ends of the cells face the central cavity and the bases are attached to a thin basement membrane. Inside the outer sphere of cells is a homogeneous gel-like substance, the follicular colloid. The colloid contains thyroglobulin, a glycoprotein that includes several iodinated amino acids, including the active thyroid hormones, thyroxine and triiodothyronine.

The space between follicles contains a network of blood vessels and connective tissue, in which are clumps of parafollicular cells or C-cells, which secrete the hormone calcitonin. Occasionally, C-cells are seen in follicles, but the apical borders do not contact the colloid.

The principal function of the follicular portion of the thyroid gland is secretion of thyroid hormone. The thyroid follicular cells trap inorganic iodide by an active transport process. Iodide is then oxidized to elemental iodine and incorporated into mono- and diiodotyrosine. This formation of iodinated amino acids takes place in the thyroglobulin molecules within the lumen of the follicle. These iodinated amino acids then undergo coupling reactions to form iodothyrines, including triiodothyronine (T_3) and tetraiodothyronine or thyroxine (T_4). The active thyroid hormones are released to the circulation after hydrolysis of thyroglobulin.

Thyroid hormone secretion is mediated directly by TSH elaborated by the pars distalis of the adenohypophysis. As stated previously, this hormone enhances all aspects of thyroid hormone production. Secretion of TSH is stimulated partially by low serum levels of thyroid hormones and partially by the level of TRH in the blood of the hypothalamic hypophyseal portal system. The level of TRH is also affected by the level of circulating thyroid hormones.

Upon release to the circulation, T_4 and T_3 become bound to plasma proteins, including thyroxine-binding globulin, prealbumin and albumin. Thyroxine is almost completely bound to these proteins, with less than 0.1% being found free in the circulation. Somewhat more T_3 is found in the free form.[2] It is generally assumed that the free thyroid hormone is the physiologically active fraction.[3]

Considerable argument still exists as to the identification of the most active thyroid hormone. Since T_3 is biologically more potent than T_4 and is formed from deiodination of T_4 at the tissue level, many feel that T_3 is the active form of the hormone.[4,5] However, the circulating levels of T_3 are in the 100 ng/dl range in most species, while those of T_4 are 1-8 μg/dl. Therefore, the circulating level of T_4 is 20-50 times that of T_3, which balances the increased potency of T_3. Also, some studies in humans have suggested that euthyroidism requires normal levels of both T_4 and T_3.[2]

Measurements of the levels of circulating thyroid hormones indicate that normal levels of thyroxine are in the range of 2.5 μg/dl using a competitive protein-binding procedure;[6,7] normal levels are only 1.6 μg/dl using radioimmunoassay procedures.[8] More recent measurements using radioimmunoassay procedures in adult horses suggest normal levels of total serum thyroxine of 2.21 μg/dl ± 0.15 μg/dl and of total serum triiodothyronine of 45 ng/dl ± 6 ng/dl based on about 80 observations.[9] Analysis revealed no significant difference in hormone levels by breed, sex or use.

The principal physiologic role of thyroid hormones is to increase the metabolic activities of body tissues, ie, increase the basal metabolic rate. The precise role of thyroactive substances at the cellular level appears to be stimulating synthesis of enzymes that cause increased size, number and function of mitochondria, although some tissues, such as brain, spleen and testes, do not increase their metabolic activity in response to thyroid hormones. When thyroid dysfunction occurs, clinical abnormalities are seen in the skin, hematopoietic and reproductive systems. Alterations are also seen in maturation of young animals and in basal metabolic rate and lipid metabolism in adults.

Diseases of the Thyroid Gland

Hypothyroidism

The literature suggests that hypothyroidism may be responsible for such conditions as laminitis, infertility, anhidrosis, alopecia, anemia and osteodystrophy in horses. Such reports are based on the observation that many such conditions appear to respond to treatment with thyroid hormones. However, documented cases of clinical hypothyroidism are rare.

Hypothyroidism has also been associated with myopathy in race horses.[10] This conclusion was based on low levels of circulating thyroxine and on histopathologic examination of the gland. However, decreased levels of circulating thyroid hormone in normal, trained race horses has also been reported.[11] Also, the histologic findings described are not incompatible with a normal, resting thyroid gland. The TSH responses in these horses were normal. Therefore, the diagnosis of hypothyroidism in horses with myopathy is open to question.

Cause: From a theoretic standpoint, hypothyroidism is the clinical manifestation of a deficiency of circulating thyroid hormone. This deficiency may be due to primary disease of the

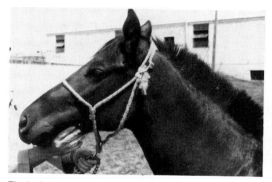 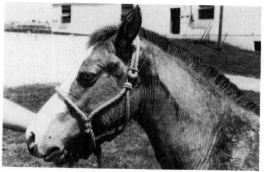

Fig 2. A. Normal female at approximately 2 years of age. Note normal haircoat, sharp angular features and alert appearance. B. Thyroidectomized 2-year-old female 5 months after thyroidectomy. Note coarse, dry haircoat, wrinkled skin, thickened facial features and dull appearance. (Courtesy of Cornell Vet)

gland, either hereditary or acquired, secondary to disease of the pituitary or hypothalamus, resulting in a decrease in TSH level, to unavailability of precursors needed for elaboration of thyroid hormone, specifically iodine, or to antithyroid or goiterogenic substances that inhibit synthesis or release of thyroid hormone.

Clinical Signs: Since few reports of documented cases of clinical hypothyroidism are available, the expected range of clinical signs must be based on the results of experimental trials. The long-term effects of thyroidectomy in horses have been investigated in a trial lasting more than a year.[12] The animals used in this study were thyroidectomized at about 1.5 years of age and observed for 61 weeks after ablation. Several changes were noted in the thyroidectomized animals. Hypothyroid young horses were generally small, lethargic and slow-moving. The haircoat was coarse, rough and dull, and shed 4-6 weeks late as compared with controls (Fig 2). These horses were sensitive to cold and would shiver continually when exercised in a chilling wind or cold rain.

Rectal temperatures were consistently and significantly lower in thyroidectomized horses than in control horses. However, since the difference was only about 1° F, this might be difficult to evaluate in a clinical situation. The PCV of thyroidectomized horses was also significantly lower than those of controls; it was frequently below 30% in thyroidectomized animals and always above 30% in controls. Serum cholesterol values were elevated in some affected animals. Another manifestation of hypothyroidism in young, growing animals was slowing of bone growth to the point of stunting, and a failure of closure of the epiphyseal plates.

Of 3 thyroidectomized mares, 2 became pregnant and delivered normal foals. Semen evaluation of thyroidectomized stallions revealed no abnormalities, although the hypothyroid state may have affected libido and general animation.[13]

Total serum thyroxine values in control animals were consistently 1.4-3.0 μg/dl, while those of thyroidectomized animals fell to undetectible levels.

The signs of hypothyroidism observed in this study, therefore, included lethargy, sensitivity to cold, low-grade anemia, dry haircoat, and decreased rectal temperature. Laminitis or skeletal disease was not observed in this study. Previous reports of altered reproductive performance were not verified. Also, no signs of constipation or steatorrhea were observed.

Diagnosis: Observance of the above-mentioned signs should make one suspect hypothyroidism as the cause. Based on the data on serum thyroid hormone concentrations, serum thyroxine values below 0.5 μg/dl and triiodothyronine levels below 0.1 ng/ml are consistent with this diagnosis.

The TSH-response test, a technic widely used in small animal medicine, has been used to further evaluate thyroid function in horses.[9,14] A blood sample is drawn for T_4 and/or T_3 evaluation. Immediately thereafter, 20 IU TSH are given IM and a second sample is drawn 12 hours later for evaluation. Increases in hormone level to 2-5 times baseline values are observed in normal horses. A diagnosis of primary hypothyroidism is reasonable if the level of thyroid hormone in the second sample is less than doubled. A response to TSH might also be expected in secondary hypothyroidism, but the increase is not as large as that seen in normal animals. A diagnosis of hypothyroidism is warranted when typical signs of hypothyroidism are accompanied by very low values of circulating thyroid hormone. A thyroid biopsy is necessary to confirm the diagnosis.

When such a diagnosis is made, it is imperative that the cause of the problem be investigated. The diet should be carefully evaluated to ensure that it does not contain deficient or excessive amounts of iodine. High dietary iodine levels cause hypothyroidism in several species, including horses.[15] While ration levels of 0.5 ppm (7-10 mg/day) are normal, intakes of 50-500 mg resulted in goiter and other signs of hypothyroidism in newborn foals and horses. The diet should also be evaluated for the presence of ingredients containing antithyroid compounds, such as linseed, raw soybean, and members of the family Brassicaceae, including cabbage, turnips and kale. If nutritional factors might explain the clinical signs, elimination of those factors from the ration should result in alleviation of clinical signs. If nutritional factors are not involved, primary or secondary hypothyroidism is probably the cause.

Treatment: Treatment of primary or secondary hypothyroidism is accomplished by feeding iodinated casein (Protomone:Agri-Tech), which contains significant quantities of thyroactive substances. Preliminary data suggest that a daily oral dose of 5 g iodinated casein restores normal levels of serum thyroxine and results in elimination of clinical signs of hypothyroidism. This could also be accomplished by the use of thyroxine but would be much more expensive. A blood sample should be obtained for thyroxine determination 1-2 weeks after initiating iodinated casein feeding. If the serum thyroxine level is low, the dose of iodinated casein should be increased. If the level of thyroxine is above 5 μg/dl during therapy, the dose should be reduced. The owner should be informed that therapy is required indefinitely once a diagnosis is made.

Hyperthyroidism

Although hyperfunction of the thyroid is common in humans, hyperthyroidism in animals is apparently quite rare. A few cases of hyperthyroidism in dogs have been ascribed to functional tumors of the gland.[16] Hyperthyroidism has also been associated with functional thyroid adenomas in aged cats.[17] This is now diagnosed regularly and is treated by thyroidectomy or by radioiodine therapy.

There are very few reports of hyperthyroidism in horses. One report associates nervousness, hyperexcitability and sweating with laboratory evidence of increased thyroid function.[18] The syndrome has been suspected in other high-strung, unmanageable horses. In at least one case, thyroidectomy resulted in a change in demeanor of a high-strung horse; the owner was able to train and ride the animal after surgery, whereas this was impossible preoperatively.[12]

Neoplasia

Thyroid neoplasia is apparently common in horses. In an early study of the thyroid glands of 100 horses, 37% contained adenomas. This finding was most common in aged horses; the average age of the horses in this group was 18 years.[19] In another study of thyroid glands of 59 horses of various ages, one thyroid adenoma was found in an aged mare.[20] In a study from India, thyroid adenoma was the most common tumor in aged horses.[21] In this study of 69 horses with neoplasia, 30% had thyroid adenomas; 87% of affected horses were 16 years of age or older.

Adenoma of the thyroid gland is a common finding during necropsy of aged horses. Occasionally an owner presents a horse because of a visible goiter, usually not associated with clinical signs. Rarely these goiters become large enough to impinge on the trachea or esophagus, resulting in dyspnea or dysphagia. Enlarged thyroid glands are almost always adenomatous, well encapsulated and easily removable by surgery. They are apparently nonfunctional and do not cause clinical signs or biochemical evidence of hyperthyroidism.

Nutritional Hypercalcitoninism

As previously mentioned, interspersed among the follicles of the thyroid gland are clumps of parafollicular or C-cells. These cell types are vestiges of the ultimobranchial glands of lower animals. In the early 1960's the existence of a hormone with an effect opposite to that of parathyroid hormone was demonstrated. Because of its effect of lowering the blood Ca level, it was called "calcitonin." While it was first thought that this hormone was secreted by the parathyroid gland, it was subsequently shown that the source was the parafollicular cells of the thyroid gland.

Calcitonin reduces the blood Ca level by decreasing the activity of osteoclasts, thus diminishing the outflow of Ca from bone to the blood pool. This decreased osteoclastic activity, if sustained, could result in a diminution of bone remodeling, which could have clinical significance, particularly in growing animals in which bone remodeling is important for normal growth and skeletal development.

It has since been hypothesized that high-Ca diets may result in nutritional hypercalcitoninism in some species, including dogs and cattle. This syndrome has been identified only in growing animals and is characterized by grossly deformed bones, with morphologic and histologic evidence of osteopetrosis.

Almost no evidence has been published regarding this syndrome in horses. In one study involving the feeding of high-Ca diets to horses, no clinical abnormalities were observed over 17 months.[22] However, Ca kinetic evaluation showed that bone resorption was inhibited by high levels of dietary Ca. Also, histologic results indicated an increased amount of lamellar as compared to osteonic bone, suggesting decreased bone remodeling.

High levels of dietary Ca may be associated with lesions of the epiphyseal plate in heavily fed, rapidly growing horses. This condition, termed "epiphysitis" by some, has been thought to be due to feeding rations high in P and marginal in Ca. In some cases, therefore, this condition may be secondary to high levels of dietary Ca and, hence, possibly a form of nutritional hypercalcitoninism.

THE PARATHYROID GLANDS

Anatomy and Physiology

The horse has 2 pairs of parathyroid glands. The external or cranial pair is frequently found on the dorsomedial edge of each thyroid lobe. They are 1.0-1.3 cm long and are generally a reddish-yellow color. The external parathyroid glands may, however, be found either cranial or caudal to the thyroid glands, as well as imbedded in the connective tissue around the trachea. The internal or caudal parathyroid glands are found within the parenchyma of the thyroid gland lobes, generally on the medial surface. Since the external parathyroid glands are most often not connected to the thyroid glands, thyroidectomy in horses can be performed without danger of hypocalcemic tetany, a common sequela to thyroidectomy in such species as the dog and cat.

Microscopically, the parathyroid gland is made up of intertwined cords of cells, with cap-

illaries located among the cords of cells. The cords are made up mainly of chief cells, with a much smaller number of oxyphil cells. The primary function of the chief cells is secretion of parathyroid hormone. The function of the oxyphil cells is unknown.

Parathyroid hormone (PTH) secretion is controlled through a feedback mechanism by the ionic Ca concentration in the extracellular fluid. Small decreases (on the order of 0.1 mg/dl) in serum Ca concentration result in a prompt increase in circulating PTH levels. On the other hand, slight increases in serum Ca levels cause a reduction in serum PTH levels. Therefore, PTH elevates blood Ca levels by activation of bone resorptive mechanisms, releasing Ca into the circulation, increasing tubular P excretion and Ca resorption in the kidney, and enhancing intestinal Ca absorption by increasing production of the active form of vitamin D. Under normal conditions, PTH, calcitonin and vitamin D metabolites interact in the maintenance of Ca homeostasis.

Diseases of the Parathyroid Glands

Dysfunction of the parathyroid glands can be due to primary or secondary causes. Primary diseases result in hyperfunction or hypofunction. Primary overproduction of PTH is generally a result of neoplasia of the parathyroid glands, while hypofunction is due to atrophy or destruction of the glandular tissue.

Nutritional Secondary Hyperparathyroidism

Cause: Primary dysfunction of the parathyroid glands in horses has not been reported. However, altered parathyroid function can be induced by other (secondary) problems. The most common condition of this nature seen in horses is nutritional secondary hyperparathyroidism, due to feeding diets high in P and low in Ca. Diets high in grain or grain products and low in legumes are frequently associated with this problem.[23] In this condition, high levels of dietary P inhibit intestinal absorption of the minimal amounts of dietary Ca. High levels of serum P cause the ion product of Ca and P in the plasma to exceed normal, with a resulting decrease in ionized Ca level. The lowered level of serum Ca stimulates PTH secretion, causing bone resorption and returning the plasma Ca level to normal. Because of the continuous lack of dietary Ca, the hyperparathyroidism persists, resulting in excessive loss of bone tissue. This is replaced by fibrous connective tissue, hence the term "fibrous osteodystrophy."

Clinical Signs: The clinical signs of nutritional secondary hyperparathyroidism result from bone lesions and are most prominent in those bones with significant amounts of trabecular as opposed to lamellar bone, *eg*, the cancellous bone of the skull, ribs and long-bone metaphyses.[23] As bone is replaced by fibrous tissue, the bones increase in size. The term "bighead" has been used to describe the enlarged maxillae and mandible seen in this condition.[24] Affected horses often have a shifting-leg lameness and enlarged carpi, fetlocks and hocks ("epiphysitis").

Diagnosis: The diagnosis is often based on the clinical signs, in combination with a good history of the animal's diet. While serum P and alkaline phosphatase levels may be elevated and serum Ca levels may be slightly decreased, the results of single evaluations may be of little value in individual animals. If the condition is suspected, the ration should be evaluated and changed if the Ca:P ratio is abnormal. A Ca:P ratio of about 1.2:1 is normal, while in some cases it may be as low as 1:5 or less. Calcium carbonate and legume hay are good sources of additional Ca. Bone meal or dicalcium phosphate should not be used since they contain high levels of P. While the bone lesions are theoretically reversible, many factors affect the rapidity and completeness of the reparative process. Thus, a guarded to fair prognosis for complete recovery is warranted.

Renal Secondary Hyperparathyroidism

Another common form of secondary hyperparathyroidism is renal secondary hyperparathyroidism, which in many species occurs in part as a result of P retention from chronic renal failure. This condition has not been observed in horses, probably because horses with chronic renal failure generally develop hypercalcemia and hypophosphatemia, although the reason for this is unknown.[25]

Pseudohyperparathyroidism

Pseudohyperparathyroidism is due to production of compounds with parathyroid hormone activity by tissues other than the parathyroid glands. Such tumors as lymphosarcoma and perianal adenoma have resulted in pseudohyperparathyroidism in some species; however, this condition has not been observed in horses.

References

1. Venzke, in Getty: Sisson and Grossman's Anatomy of The Domestic Animals. 5th ed. WB Saunders, Philadelphia, 1975.

2. Chopra, IJ *et al.* J Clin Endocr Metab **36** (1973) 1050.

3. Clark, F and Horn, DB. J. Clin Endocr **25** (1965) 39.

4. Gross, J *et al.* Lancet 2 (1952) 1044.

5. Pitt-Rivers, R *et al.* J Clin Endocr Metab **15** (1955) 161.

6. Kallfelz, FA and Lowe, JE. JAVMA **156** (1970) 1888.

7. Hightower, D *et al.* JAVMA **159** (1971) 449.

8. Thomas, CL and Adams, JC. Am J Vet Res **39** (1978) 1239.

9. Davidson, H *et al*, Cornell Univ: Unpublished data, 1981.

10. Waldron-Mease, E. Eq Pract **3** (1979) 124.

11. Irvine, CHG. Am J Vet Res **28** (1967) 1687.

12. Lowe, JE *et al.* Cornell Vet **64** (1974) 276.

13. Lowe, JE *et al.* J Repro Fert Suppl **23** (1975) 81.

14. Kallfelz, FA. Vet Clin No Am **7** (1977) 497.

15. Baker, HJ and Lindsey, JR. JAVMA **153** (1968) 1618.

16. Rijnberk, A. Tijdschr Diergeneesk **91** (1966) 789.

17. Holzworth, J *et al.* JAVMA **176** (1980) 345.

18. De Martin, BW. Rev Fac Med Vet Zootec, Univ S Paulo **10** (1973) 35.

19. Schlottauer, CF. JAVMA **78** (1931) 211.

20. Dimock, WW *et al.* JAVMA **104** (1944) 313.

21. Damodaran, S and Ramachandran, PV. Indian Vet J **52** (1975) 531.

22. Whitlock, RH *et al.* Proc 16th Ann Mtg Am Assoc Eq Pract, 1970. p 127.

23. Krook, L and Lowe, JL. Path Vet 1 Suppl 1 (1964) 1.

24. Sturgess, GW and Crawford, H. Admin Report on Osteitis Fibrosa to Govt Vet Surg, Ceylon, 1927.

25. Tennant, B *et al.* Proc Soc Biol Med **167** (1981) 365.

THE ENDOCRINE PANCREAS
by J.J. McClure

Anatomy and Physiology

The pancreas originates very early in embryologic development from the epithelium of the primitive gut. From common progenitor cells, the endocrine and exocrine portions of the pancreas develop into distinct anatomic and functional parts that play specialized roles in digestion and metabolism. The exocrine pancreas participates in digestion by the production of digestive enzymes. The endocrine pancreas plays a key role in the disposition of absorbed dietary nutrients and maintenance of homeostasis of those nutrients by storage and mobilization.

The endocrine pancreas is organized into millions of pancreatic islets (islets of Langerhans), 100-200μ in diameter, dispersed throughout the parenchyma of the exocrine pancreas. Each islet consists of a labyrinth of anastomosing capillaries, with islet cells interspersed among the vessels. This arrangement is conducive to rapid release of hormonal secretions into the bloodstream and transport of nutrients into the cells. Fenestrations in the endothelial cells of the capillaries permit rapid exchange of materials. Venous drainage is into the portal vein.[1]

The endocrine pancreas synthesizes a number of polypeptide hormones. Three functional secretory cell types have been identified in mammalian islets. Beta cells are the site of insulin production, "A" or alpha-2 cells are the source of glucagon, and "D," delta or alpha-1 cells, are the source of gastrin and somatostatin. In some species other hormones associated with the pancreas include thyrotropin-releasing factor and human pancreatic polypeptide.[2] Insulin is comprised of 2 polypeptide chains and joined by 2 disulfide bridges. Proinsulin synthesized in the rough endoplasmic reticulum of beta cells is a single polypeptide chain consisting of the A and B peptides joined together by a connecting C peptide. Following synthesis, proinsulin moves into the Golgi apparatus, where enzymes cleave off the C peptide, and packaging into secretory granules begins. Appropriate stimuli cause the secretory granules to migrate to the plasma membrane, where insulin, C peptide and some intact proinsulin are secreted by emiocytosis (exocytosis).[3]

The liver is the major site of inactivation of insulin; as much as 50% of active insulin is removed from the circulation with each passage of blood. Since insulin secreted into the portal circulation must initially pass the liver before reaching the peripheral circulation, blood levels may not reflect the actual secretory rate of this hormone.

Glucagon is a single polypeptide chain synthesized and secreted in a fashion similar to insulin. The half-life of this hormone in the peripheral circulation is about 10 minutes. The kidney is the major site of inactivation. Extrapancreatic sources of production of glucagon-like activity have been identified, including alpha-2 cells in the GI mucosa, which secrete enteroglucagon.[3]

Simplistically, insulin promotes the storage of dietary nutrients. Glucagon, in concert with a number of other counterinsulin hormones, including glucocorticoids, epinephrine and growth hormone, promotes mobilization of nutrients from storage forms. The antagonistic effects of insulin and the counterinsulin hormones play a major role in glucose homeostasis and serve to maintain blood glucose levels within remarkably narrow limits considering the variations in nutrient intake and metabolic needs from moment to moment.

The blood glucose level is the major factor controlling the secretion of insulin. Secretion is stimulated primarily by increases in blood glucose levels above a specific threshold value that generally approximates postprandial levels. Insulin secretion decreases as blood glucose levels drop in response to the effects of insulin.[4] Amino acids, particularly lysine, arginine and leucine, can also stimulate insulin release. Volatile fatty acids stimulate the release of insulin in ruminants, but they do not have this effect in horses.[5] Several hormones, including glucagon, ACTH, TSH, enteroglucagon, gastrin, secretin and cholecystokinin, augment the glucose-induced release of insulin but are not effective in the absence of glucose.[1]

Insulin stimulates the normally limited uptake of glucose into muscle and adipose tissue, and promotes glucose storage as protein, glycogen and triglycerides. These tissues then become an indirect source of glucose since they do not possess the enzymatic machinery to convert the storage form back to glucose and cannot release glucose directly into the circulation. They must release gluconeogenic substrates (amino acids, fatty acids, glycerol, pyruvate, lactate), which must travel to the liver to be converted to glucose (gluconeogenesis). Adrenocorticoids promote the release of these intermediates from muscle, growth hormone stimulates their release from adipose tissue, and insulin inhibits the release of these substrates from both tissues.

The liver differs from muscle and adipose tissue in that glucose diffuses freely into and out of hepatic cells, and enzymatic machinery allows for reconversion of gluconeogenic substrates and storage forms back to glucose. The effect of insulin on the liver is to increase the storage of glucose as glycogen and lipids, and to inhibit gluconeogenesis, thus decreasing the need for substrates from the peripheral tissues. Quantitatively, the liver is a much more significant site of glucose metabolism because it is exposed to insulin levels often 3-10 times those in the peripheral circulation; absorbed glucose first reaches the liver via the portal vein prior to its delivery to peripheral tissues. Therefore, the liver, under the influence of insulin, serves as the first and major site of disposition for absorbed glucose, rather than the peripheral tissues.

In addition to lipogenesis in adipose tissues and the liver, insulin inhibits a hormonally sensitive lipase in adipose tissue, which in turn decreases lipolysis and limits the amount of ketogenic and gluconeogenic substrates presented to the liver. A major effect of insulin in hepatic fat metabolism is inhibition of the rate of beta-oxidation of fatty acids, the process by which ketone bodies are produced. These effects occur with lower levels of insulin than are required for an effect on glucose metabolism. For this reason, insulin is considered a potent antiketogenic agent.

Although the major effects of insulin on protein metabolism are usually associated with muscle, there is evidence that protein synthesis is stimulated in other tissues as well and the effect of insulin on growth is a general one involving almost all tissues. Insulin increases body protein stores by increased uptake of amino acids, increased protein synthesis, decreased protein catabolism, and decreased oxidation of amino acids.

Insulin has a hypokalemic action due to stimulation of uptake of K by muscle and liver. This effect is demonstrated in the absence of changes in glucose metabolism. Insulin also has an antinatriuretic effect that results in conservation of Na by the kidney.

As one of the counterinsulin hormones, the net effect of glucagon secretion is to increase blood glucose levels by promoting mobilization of glucose from the liver by glycogenolysis and gluconeogenesis. This action is presumably mediated through a membrane-bound adenyl cyclase system on the hepatic cell membranes. Glucagon does not exert its hyperglycemic effect by altering peripheral use of glucose, nor does it exert a major effect directly on protein or lipid metabolism, although it may augment ketone production by the liver. Glucagon is secreted at a relatively constant, low rate except under extreme situations, such as acute hypoglycemia, prolonged exercise, hypercorticism, and stimulation of the ventromedial hypothalamus or adrenergic nervous system. Its physiologic role appears to be maintenance of a constant minimum glucose output from the liver in the face of fluctuations in insulin activity and dietary intake. The ingestion of glucose tends to result in higher blood glucose levels than does IV administration of similar quantities of glucose. This effect has been attributed to the stimulation of enteroglucagon production by the presence of the ingested carbohydrates.

Although not of pancreatic origin, other counterinsulin hormones deserve comment in the context of their interaction with insulin and their role in regulation of blood glucose. Adrenocorticoids, as stated earlier, promote the breakdown of protein in peripheral tissues, primarily muscle, and thus promote gluconeogenesis and glycogen synthesis by providing increased amino acid substrates to the liver. In addition, they reduce the effectiveness of insulin by blocking its action on muscles and adipose tissue. Hypercorticism has also been associated with increased glucagon secretion.

Epinephrine increases blood glucose levels by a number of mechanisms, including inhibition of insulin secretion and stimulation of glucagon secretion. In addition, it decreases glucose uptake by muscle and stimulates glycogen breakdown in muscle and liver. Glycogenolysis in the liver results in a direct increase in blood glucose levels, while in muscle it results in increased release of lactate, which can be used as substrate in gluconeogenesis by the liver. Epinephrine-induced lipolysis also results in increased availability of substrate for glucose production.

The major insulin-antagonizing effect of pituitary growth hormone is the result of altered peripheral glucose uptake and use. Growth hormone stimulates lipolysis and promotes the uptake of free fatty acids into muscle while reducing the effectiveness of insulin in glucose transport. At the same time it inhibits glycogen breakdown and promotes protein synthesis in muscle, thus forcing the body to depend on fat as a source of energy rather than carbohydrate or protein. These antagonistic actions of growth hormone require the presence of insulin. The anti-insulin effect of growth hormone is countered by its ability to stimulate insulin secretion which, except in extreme cases, prevents the development of hyperglycemia. Acute administration of growth hormone causes a transient insulin-like response, including a drop in blood glucose levels, which is quite unlike the effects of prolonged or continuous administration. The effects of growth hormone are thought to be mediated by a family of secondary substances, called somatomedians, elaborated under the control of growth hormone. Those that have been characterized have nonsuppressible insulin-like activity because their activity is unaffected by anti-insulin antibody. Whether they account for the signs associated with acute growth hormone administration and what their role is in mediating the other effects of growth hormone are not yet defined.[3]

Diseases of the Endocrine Pancreas

Clinical endocrine disorders may be associated with altered secretion rates or altered target tissue response to specific hormones. Diseases associated with hyperfunction of the endocrine pancreas, such as seen with insulin- or glucagon-secreting neoplasms, have not been observed in horses, and only rarely has hypofunction of the endocrine pancreas been observed.[6-11]

Diabetes Mellitus

Diabetes mellitus is not a single disease entity but rather a clinical syndrome that may be produced in a number of different experimental and natural situations. The common feature is a lack of insulin effect due to an absolute deficiency of circulating insulin or to hormonal or tissue factors that modify its activity. Based on etiology, the syndrome of diabetes mellitus can be classified as: primary (spontaneous, essential, idiopathic, genetic, hereditary) diabetes, which in humans is further subdivided according to the age of onset and/or severity into juvenile and adult diabetes types; pancreatic diabetes, which is secondary to direct destruction of the pancreatic islets by chronic inflammation, neoplasia or surgical removal; endocrine diabetes, which develops secondary to endocrinopathies, such as hyperpituitarism, hyperadrenalism and hyperthyroidism; and iatrogenic diabetes, which is associated with administration of drugs, such as corticosteroids and certain thiazide diuretics.[12]

Primary or spontaneous diabetes mellitus, which occurs in humans and dogs, has not been observed in horses. Diabetes mellitus has occurred secondary to chronic pancreatitis and to suspected endocrinopathies associated with pituitary tumors.[7-11] The use of the term diabetes mellitus to refer to secondary types of the syndrome may be inappropriate, but it is useful from a clinical standpoint in that it defines a group of physical and laboratory findings which, when present, aid differential diagnosis.

Clinical Signs: The predominant clinical signs associated with diabetic syndromes include emaciation despite normal or increased food intake, polydipsia, polyuria, hyperglycemia, glycosuria, ketonuria and lipemia. Altered glucose tolerance may be demonstrated by IV or oral glucose-tolerance tests.

Diagnosis: Diabetes mellitus is diagnosed by glucose-tolerance tests. The theory of glucose-tolerance testing is that normal animals can remove a glucose load from their blood within a specified period of time. Those unable to do so are said to have a "reduced glucose tolerance."

In the IV glucose-tolerance test, glucose is administered IV as a 50% solution at 0.5-1 g/kg body weight. Blood glucose levels are determined prior to injection and at 30-minute intervals for 3½-4 hours after injection. Blood glucose levels normally peak immediately, then gradually return to normal within 1½ hours. However, because several factors, including fasting and roughage rations, may prolong this time to as long as 3½ hours in normal horses, results should be interpreted cautiously.[5,13,14] Persistence of elevated glucose levels beyond 3 hours has occurred in diabetic horses.

The oral glucose-tolerance test is used to assess glucose absorption from the small intestine and to evaluate pancreatic endocrine function. The test is conducted after a 12-hour overnight fast. Glucose is administered as a 20% aqueous solution via nasogastric tube at 1 g glucose/kg body weight. Blood glucose levels are determined prior to administration and at 30-minute intervals for 2 hours, then hourly for the next 4 hours. Blood glucose levels normally double within 2 hours and return to resting levels within 6 hours. The initial rise provides information concerning the absorptive capacity of the small intestine for glucose. Assuming adequate absorption occurs, the subsequent decline in blood glucose levels is an insulin-mediated response to the hyperglycemia and is an indication of glucose tolerance.[15]

Differential diagnoses include chronic pancreatitis, hyperpituitarism associated with neoplasia, primary adrenocortical hyperfunction (Cushing's disease), and pheochromocytoma. The last 3 conditions may be associated with additional clinical signs and some specific diagnostic tests are available to differentiate these conditions (see Adrenal and Pituitary Diseases). Hyperglycemia associated with these conditions tends to be insulin-resistant.[16] The suspected mechanism of increased blood glucose levels in these conditions is related to alterations in sensitivity of peripheral tissue to insulin rather than to an absolute decrease in insulin levels. Therefore, an insulin-tolerance test may assist in establishing a diagnosis and determining the feasibility (if not the practicality) of insulin therapy.

No standardized approach to insulin-tolerance testing has emerged. Both rapid-acting (regular, crystalline, zinc) and long-acting (protamine zinc) insulin preparations have been used in a wide variety of dosages in fasted and fed horses. Regular insulin decreases blood glucose levels within an hour, whereas the maximum effect of protamine zinc insulin is within 12 hours.[7,8,17] Initial IV dosages of regular insulin should probably not exceed 0.1-0.3 u/kg body weight and even this dosage can produce insulin shock in some normal ponies.[16,17] Fasted animals are more resistant to the hypoglycemic effect of insulin than are fed animals. This makes fed animals more prone to insulin shock. Conversely, fasting may give an erroneous impression of the presence of insulin resistance associated with disease. Since fasting may aggravate the altered metabolic state of a diabetic animal, the test should be conducted on fed animals.[16] Response is measured by monitoring blood glucose levels prior to administration and at 30-minute intervals for 2 hours after administration. If a decline in blood glucose levels occurs, the magnitude of the decrease can be used to determine the dosage of insulin to obtain the desired effect on blood glucose levels. If there is no response, the test can be repeated on subsequent days using higher insulin doses.

Signs of insulin or hypoglycemic shock include muscular tremors, incoordination, increased pulse and respiratory rates, sweating, hyperirritability and nystagmus. Mild cases may be reversed by oral administration of sugar or Karo syrup. In more severe cases, IV administration of glucose results in prompt recovery.[7,16,17]

Treatment: Successful management of a case of diabetes mellitus associated with chronic pancreatitis in a pony, with protamine zinc insulin, has been reported.[7] Stabilization of blood glucose levels and improvement in clinical condition were eventually attained with a dosage of 0.5 u/kg body weight administered IM at 12-hour intervals. The pony was fed hay and grain 4 times daily. Insulin shock was a frequent complication but was adequately managed by glucose administration. Discontinuation of insulin therapy after 6 weeks resulted in rapid deterioration in clinical condition.

Prognosis: The prognosis in diabetes mellitus ultimately depends on the primary disease with which it is associated. The prognosis is poor in those areas associated with neoplasia of other endocrine organs.

References

1. Greep, RO and Astwood, EB: Handbook of Physiology. American Physiological Society, Washington, DC, 1972.
2. Track, NS. Can Med Assoc J **122** (1980) 287.
3. Felig, in Bondy and Rosenberg: Metabolic control and disease. 8th ed. WB Saunders, Philadelphia, 1980.
4. Evans, JW. J So Afr Vet Assoc **54** (1974) 317.
5. Argenzio, RA and Hintz, HF. J Anim Sci **30** (1970) 514.
6. Jubb, KVF and Kennedy, PC: Pathology of Domestic Animals. 2nd ed. Academic Press, New York, 1970.
7. Jeffrey, JR. JAVMA **153** (1968) 1168.
8. Tasker, JB *et al:* JAVMA **149** (1966) 393.
9. Baker, JR and Ritchie, HE. Eq Vet J **6** (1974) 7.
10. King, JM *et al.* Cornell Vet **52** (1962) 133.
11. Loeb, WF *et al.* Cornell Vet **56** (1966) 623.
12. Steinke and Soeldner, in Thorn *et al:* Harrison's Principles of Internal Medicine. 8th ed. McGraw-Hill, New York, 1977.
13. Robie, SM *et al.* Am J Vet Res **36** (1975) 1705.
14. Coffman, J. VM/SAC **74** (1979) 719.
15. Roberts, MC and Hill, FWG. Eq Vet J **5** (1973) 171.
16. Gribble, in Catcott: Equine Medicine and Surgery. 2nd ed. American Veterinary Publications, Santa Barbara, 1972.
17. Argenzio, RA and Hintz, HF. J Nutr **101** (1971) 723.

THE ADRENAL GLAND
by J.E. Palmer, R.H. Whitlock and D.A. Deem

The adrenal glands consist of 2 anatomically distinct parts, the cortex and the medulla. Despite the close anatomic relationship of these areas, they apparently function independently. However, this view may not be entirely correct since medullary hormones may influence cortical activity through the hypothalamic-pituitary axis and the cortex produces substances that are important in medullary hormone production, at least in the fetus.[1]

The Adrenal Cortex

The 3 layers of the adrenal cortex produce different classes of corticosteroids. The outer zona glomerulosa produces the mineralocorticoid aldosterone, which helps regulate Na and K balance and is under the control of the renin-angiotensin system. The central zona fasciculata forms the bulk of the cortex and is the site of glucocorticoid production. Glucocorticoids help regulate carbohydrate and fat metabolism, and are under the influence of adrenocorticotropic hormone (ACTH). The inner zona reticularis produces cortical androgens, estrogens and progesterones, which are also released in response to ACTH stimulation.[1]

Secretion of glucocorticoids is under the direct control of ACTH secreted from the anterior pituitary gland. Since glucocorticoids are not stored in the cortex, ACTH regulates their rate of production, which then becomes their rate of secretion.[2] The rate of release of ACTH from the pituitary gland is influenced by a number of factors, including exercise, stress, ambient temperature, light and hypoglycemia.[2] The depth and duration of hypoglycemia are important factors; however, only severe hypoglycemia (< 20 mg/dl) causes an effective release of ACTH.[3] The most important control of ACTH secretion is the feedback inhibition of cortisol.

Cortisol and corticosterone are the principal glucocorticoids of horses.[2-5] As with other diurnal animals (eg, humans, monkeys, dogs, cats), there is a circadian rhythm of adrenal activity.[3-5] The peak secretion of cortisol and corticosterone occurs at about 10 AM, with a low point 6-12 hours later. This daily rhythm probably reflects the variation in ACTH secretion secondary to the light-dark cycle.[5] Because of this cyclic variation and the marked day-to-day variation in normal animals, a single measurement of plasma concentration of corticosteroids should be viewed with caution. Because the half-life of plasma cortisol is short (80 minutes), cortisol levels may fluctuate rapidly.[3]

Surgery, exercise and severe hypoglycemia (<20 mg/dl) increase plasma cortisol levels in horses.[3] The common factor in these situations is probably stress, which apparently increases ACTH secretion and modifies the feedback mechanism so that a high plasma cortisol level is maintained. During exercise, an increased metabolic rate causes decreased plasma cortisol levels and stress causes increased cortisol output. Moderate exercise produces a 30% increase in plasma cortisol levels.[3] Venipuncture, if done with the usual minimal amount of stress, does not affect the plasma cortisol level.[3] Anesthesia with acetylpromazine, thiopental and halothane also does not affect plasma cortisol levels, although other agents have been found to do so in humans.[3] Age, sex and stage of pregnancy do not affect plasma corticosterone levels in horses.[4] However, administration of small doses of dexamethasone decreases plasma cortisol levels for 72 hours.[3,4]

Corticosteroids have a variety of physiologic and pharmacologic activities. These hormones initiate their actions at the cellular level by first binding with a cytoplasmic receptor. The complex migrates to the nucleus and initiates messenger RNA production, which in turn is responsible for protein synthesis.[2,7,8] Corticosteroids influence protein, fat and carbohydrate metabolism, water and electrolyte balance, and renal, nervous, cardiovascular and skeletal system function. They also cause catabolism of peripheral protein, and an increase in blood amino acid levels and amino acid use by the liver.[2,7,8] Corticosteroids stimulate gluconeogenesis, liver glycogen deposition and decreased peripheral use of glucose, resulting in elevated blood glucose levels.[2,7,8] They also increase blood fatty acid levels and facilitate lipid use. They have a "permissive" effect on sympathomimetic amine lipolysis and interact with other metabolic hormones, such as glucagon and growth hormone.[7,8]

Mineralocorticoids cause Na resorption, and K and H excretion by the kidney, salivary gland, sweat glands, exocrine pancreas and GI mucosa.[2,7] Musculoskeletal weakness occurs with a lack of mineralocorticoids.[7]

Glucocorticoids at physiologic levels also have specific effects on the hemogram. There is an increase in circulating neutrophils due to an increase in the rate of entry into circulation from the bone marrow and a decrease in margination. There is also a decrease in the number of circulating lymphocytes, eosinophils, monocytes and basophils. Lymphopenia is probably due to redistribution rather than destruction.[7] Eosinopenia may not occur in all horses; it has only been reproduced experimentally with the use of long-acting ACTH or prolonged, severe hypoglycemia and not by other stimuli that cause a marked increase in plasma cortisol levels.[3]

Glucocorticoids dramatically block the immune response, which, along with other anti-inflammatory properties, is the basis of their popularity as therapeutic agents. However, the basis for their interference with immune function is not understood. They have no effect on circulating antibody titers and the dramatic lympholysis observed in rodents may not occur in other species. In fact, interference with cell-mediated reactions is probably related to interference with the inflammatory response since there is normal development of cell-mediated immunity.[7]

The anti-inflammatory properties of glucocorticoids have long been known and exploited therapeutically. They suppress local heat, swelling, erythema and pain. They inhibit the edema, fibrin deposition, capillary dilation, WBC migration, phagocytic activity and other phenomena associated with acute inflammation. They also suppress capillary and fibro-blast proliferation, deposition of collagen and cicatrization in the late stages of inflammation. The effect of glucocorticoids is local and their mechanism of action was thought to be lysosomal stabilization. However, it now appears that the anti-inflammatory effect is probably due to the summation of multiple, discrete effects on different aspects of the inflammatory response. Whatever their mechanism of action, glucocorticoids decrease the body's response to the disease but do not interfere with the underlying cause. The disease remains and may progress without causing the signs commonly used to monitor its progression or evaluate the efficacy of therapy.

Another important pharmacologic effect of glucocorticoids is their ability to produce premature parturition in some species. However, parturition could not be induced in ponies by one large dose of dexamethasone (0.1 mg/kg) 96-144 hours before normal parturition.[9]

Adrenocortical Function Tests

Thorn Test

The Thorn test involves the suppression of circulating eosinophils by ACTH administration and has been used as a screening test for adrenal function.[10] Absolute eosinophil counts are easily performed and inexpensive. This is not a quantitative test and small amounts of circulating corticosteroids cause maximal suppression.[4,11] However, this does not seem to be true in horses. In fact, although many stimuli increase plasma cortisol levels, only long-acting ACTH consistently causes a pronounced decrease in eosinophil count.[3] The Thorn test is not a sensitive indicator of adrenal function in horses and should not be used in place of plasma cortisol determinations.

Resting Plasma Cortisol and Corticosteroid Levels

Cortisol and corticosterone are the major circulating corticosteroids in horses. Their measurement is important in determining adrenocortical function. Competitive protein-binding analysis, chromatographic technics, automated fluorometric methods, and radioimmunoassay have all been used to measure glucocorticoid levels in horses.[3,4,12] Each method has a slightly different range of normal values. For this reason, normal values must be established by each laboratory using the available technic before the significance of a result can be determined. Normal equine plasma cortisol levels, as determined by radioimmunoassay, are 43.3 ± 9.13

ng/ml. Care must be taken in interpreting single blood values due to the diurnal variations and day-to-day fluctuation in individuals. Although venipuncture has no effect on plasma cortisol levels, excessive excitement during blood-taking, and the stress of shipping or hospitalization may cause erroneous results.[3] Concurrent diseases may also affect results. Plasma corticosteroid levels are increased in acute states, such as shock, colic or fractures, and are decreased in chronic debilitating diseases.[11]

ACTH-Stimulation Test

The ACTH-stimulation test determines if a low resting plasma corticosteroid level is due to primary failure of the adrenal gland or a secondary failure due to a lack of ACTH stimulation. The test is performed by injecting ACTH gel at 1 IU/kg IM after obtaining a sample for determination of the plasma cortisol level. The peak plasma corticosteroid level in normal horses occurs 8 hours after injection. However, levels determined 2-10 hours after injection are greater than the normal resting range.[11] The normal 8-hour peak is 2-3 times the resting value.[3,4,11] Other doses of ACTH have been used (10-500 IU).[3,4,11-14] Intravenous administration of 100 IU synthetic aqueous ACTH doubles the plasma corticosteroid level in 2 hours.[13]

Less than a doubling of the resting value by 8 hours reflects an unresponsive adrenal gland and possible adrenal disease. However, care should be used in interpreting the results of the test since an atrophied gland may not adequately respond to a single ACTH injection. If atrophy, secondary to a chronic lack of circulating ACTH, is suspected, the horse should be treated with ACTH at 0.5 IU/kg twice daily for 4 days and the test repeated.[13]

The ACTH-stimulation test has also been used to better define high plasma cortisol levels. If an abnormally high resting plasma cortisol level is the result of an ACTH-secreting tumor, there may be some further increase in the plasma cortisol level after ACTH administration. However, if the abnormally high plasma cortisol level is due to an adrenal tumor, there should be no change in the level after ACTH administration.

Dexamethasone-Suppression Test

The dexamethasone-suppression test is used to help define the reason for an elevated plasma cortisol level. After a blood sample is obtained for resting plasma cortisol determination, 10 mg dexamethasone (22 μg/kg) are given IM. The plasma cortisol level should be at least a quarter of normal by 13 hours after the injection.[4] The decrease begins within an hour of injection and may continue for 48 hours.[4] During the initial 2½ hours, the plasma cortisol level decreases by half.[3] However, the kinetics have not been well defined.

Elevated plasma cortisol levels occur in normal horses under stress, horses with ACTH-secreting pituitary tumors (Cushing's disease), and horses with cortisol-secreting adrenal tumors (Cushing's syndrome). If the horse is normal, administration of dexamethasone should significantly suppress the plasma cortisol level. If the horse has an ACTH-producing pituitary tumor, the plasma cortisol level may decrease slightly or remain unchanged after dexamethasone administration.[4,14,15] The test is invalidated by the administration of ACTH within the preceding 48 hours.

Combined Dexamethasone-Suppression ACTH-Stimulation Test

A combined dexamethasone-suppression ACTH-stimulation test has been used in horses.[12] After taking a blood sample for resting plasma cortisol determination, 10 mg dexamethasone are given IM. Three hours later, a second blood sample is taken and 100 IU synthetic ACTH are injected IV. The final blood sample is taken 5 hours after beginning the test.[12] The 3-hour blood sample should have a decreased or nearly undetectible level of cortisol and the 5-hour sample should contain 1.5-2.5 times the cortisol in the resting sample. The major advantage of the test is the simultaneous evaluation of both pituitary and adrenal gland competence.

Determination of Urine Steroids and Metabolites

Steroid and steroid metabolite determinations on 24-hour urine samples have been used to measure adrenal function in other species. The 17-ketosteroids and 17-ketogenic steroids can be measured by the Zimmerman reaction and 17-hydroxycorticosteroids by the Porter-Silber reaction to quantitate corticosteroid production.[8] These technics have not been used in horses because of the difficulty in collecting 24-hour urine samples. There is also some indication that dietary substances of herbivores interfere with the 17-ketosteroid determination.[16]

Diseases of the Adrenal Cortex

Hyperadrenocorticism

Cause: Hyperadrenocorticism (Cushing's syndrome) has 3 causes. First, excessive ACTH secretion from the pituitary gland overstimu-lates the adrenal glands, resulting in increased cortisol secretion and secondary hyperadrenocorticism. This is most often caused by a beta-cell adenoma in the pars intermedia of the pituitary gland. Second, adrenocortical tumors can secrete cortisol, resulting in primary hyperadrenocorticism. These tumors usually are not ACTH-responsive. Adrenal tumors, although not rare, are an uncommon cause of Cushing's syndrome in horses.[3] Third, some nonpituitary tumors may secrete ACTH, resulting in excessive cortisol production. Such tumors have not been observed in horses. Nodular hyperplasia of the adrenal cortex can also be associated with abnormally high blood corticosteroid levels and signs similar to Cushing's syndrome.[1] Although nodular hyperplasia is common in older horses, the relationship with adrenal function has not been explored.[17]

Clinical Signs: The signs of primary hyperadrenocorticism include weight loss, muscle wasting, poor haircoat, chronic infection, polydipsia, polyuria, low urine specific gravity, acid urine, glycosuria, increased PCV, neutrophilic leukocytosis with lymphopenia and eosinopenia, normal or high plasma Na levels, hypokalemia and hyperglycemia. If the condition involves a functioning adrenal tumor, a sublumbar mass may be palpated rectally and there may be other organ involvement due to metastasis. Development of signs depends in part on whether both glucocorticoids and mineralocorticoids are produced. It is unusual for all of these signs to occur in one animal.

Diagnosis: Adrenocortical hyperfunction can only be definitively diagnosed by detecting increased plasma corticosteroid levels or abnormal function. Although increased plasma corticosteroid levels in the absence of other physiologic stimuli are expected, plasma cortisol levels may be normal in secondary adrenocortical hyperfunction. Adrenal function tests are useful in attempts to define the lesion causing increased function.

Lack of suppression of plasma cortisol levels by dexamethasone administration suggests a functional adrenal tumor or a dexamethasone-insensitive ACTH-producing tumor. Lack of increased plasma cortisol levels after ACTH stimulation suggests a nonresponsive functional adrenal tumor, although some adrenal tumors may be responsive and some cases of secondary adrenocortical hyperplasia may not be responsive. In general, functional adrenal tumors do not respond to the normal feedback mechanisms.

The only reported case of primary adrenocortical hyperfunction in a horse involved an 8-year-old Standardbred mare with an adrenocortical adenocarcinoma.[18] Clinical signs included weight loss, anorexia, polyuria, polydipsia, a large sublumbar mass, increased PCV, neutrophilic leukocytosis with lymphopenia, low urine specific gravity, acid urine, hyponatremia and hypokalemia. Plasma corticosteroid levels were not determined. A 14-year-old horse that may have had a functional adrenocortical adenoma had convulsions, a normal to high blood glucose level, and excessive fat deposits similar to those seen in Cushing's disease in humans.[19] Unfortunately, no blood corticosteroid assays were performed.

Iatrogenic Cushing's Syndrome

With the widespread use of synthetic corticosteroids in equine medicine, iatrogenic Cushing's disease is inevitable. However, with the exception of a few minor side effects, untoward effects of long-term glucocorticoid therapy are not often reported. The real problem seems to be adrenocortical atrophy secondary to long-term treatment, resulting in the "turning-out syndrome" when the administration of corticosteroids is discontinued (see below).

Chronic Hypoadrenocorticism

Cause: Chronic primary adrenocortical hypofunction (Addison's disease) occurs in humans when 9.0% of the adrenal cortex is unresponsive; however, there is a report of an undocumented case of Addison's disease in a horse with unilateral adrenal tumors.[20] The opposite adrenal gland was normal. Destruction of the adrenal tissue due to expanding nonfunctional tumors, vascular disease, amyloidosis, granulomatous disease (tuberculosis or mycotic infection), toxins and withdrawal after prolonged iatrogenic administration of corticosteroids have all been associated with Addison's disease in other species.[14]

Clinical Signs: The signs of chronic primary adrenocortical insufficiency include weakness, poor exercise tolerance, depression, weight loss, hypoglycemia, anemia, hypotension, polydipsia, polyuria, increased salt intake, hyponatremia, hypochloremia, hyperkalemia, GI signs and hypoglycemic convulsions. If the insufficiency is secondary to a tumor, a sublumbar mass may be detected on deep rectal palpation. All of these signs are not necessarily present in any one individual. The presenting signs depend on the plasma cortisol levels. Since the resting plasma cortisol level may be normal, it is best to document the insufficiency with an ACTH-stimulation test.

The only reported case of primary adrenocortical hypofunction in a horse occurred in a 10-year-old Standardbred stallion.[20] The animal had convulsions that responded to IV glucose therapy, as well as profuse sweating, polydipsia, polyuria, increased salt intake, a large, painful sublumbar mass, hyponatremia, hypochloremia, hyperkalemia and hypoglycemia. Hypoglycemic convulsions are probably rare in adrenocortical hypofunction in horses since the degree of hypoglycemia needed before clinical signs appear is severe (<8 mg/dl when induced with insulin).[3] However, the rate of decrease of blood glucose levels is probably as important as the severity of hypoglycemia.[20] Necropsy revealed a large adrenocortical adenoma. Unfortunately, no plasma cortisol determinations were performed.

Treatment: Treatment of chronic adrenocortical insufficiency should be individualized to the patient's particular corticosteroid and/or mineralocorticoid deficiency and the cause of the deficiency. Rest and hormone replacement therapy are of utmost importance. In cases of glucocorticoid deficiency, dexamethasone (2-5 mg) or hydrocortisone (60-150 mg) may be given once a day.[14] If mineralocorticoids are deficient, desoxycorticosterone may be used. In cases of adrenal atrophy secondary to iatrogenic Cushing's disease, ACTH (40-80 IU daily) should be used.[19]

Acute Hypoadrenocorticism

Acute adrenocortical hypofunction (Addisonian crisis) is a rapidly fatal disease if not treated. An Addisonian crisis may be precipitated by bacterial infection or infarction of the adrenal cortex, or by stressful conditions encountered by a patient with marginal adrenal function. Resultant hypotension causes acute renal failure, oliguria, cyanosis, muscle weakness and prostration. There may be hyponatremia, hyperkalemia and eosinophilia. Corticosteroid replacement, fluids, antibiotics and other symptomatic therapy are usually initiated in an attempt to save the patient's life before a definitive diagnosis is reached with laboratory analysis.

Turning-Out Syndrome

The "turning-out syndrome" or "steroid letdown syndrome" occurs when horses are taken off the race track and turned out after the racing season. Despite good nutrition and parasite control, affected horses appear unthrifty, lose weight and have a poor haircoat. They are dull, depressed, mildly anemic, easily fatigued, and subject to mild abdominal pain.[2,11,21,22] This syndrome usually only occurs in a few horses of a group. Because of the similarity of these signs with those in humans with Addison's disease and the widespread use of glucocorticoids at race tracks, it has been widely assumed that this syndrome results from iatrogenically induced adrenal insufficiency.[2,21,22] However, this has not been documented with plasma cortisol determinations or adrenal function tests. If it is hypoadrenalism from adrenal suppression secondary to prolonged iatrogenic corticosteroid administration, one would expect low or normal resting plasma cortisol levels and a decreased response to ACTH stimulation. This syndrome has been treated successfully with rest and ACTH (2 doses of 400 IU each given IM 48 hours apart).[3,22] Clinical improvement occurs within several days but the full effect is not for 30 days.[21]

There is no doubt that exogenous corticosteroids can cause adrenal atrophy. However, the dosage and period of administration required are not known. The route of administration and agent used are probably important in determining the time required to produce significant atrophy. A dose of 20 mg dexamethasone given IM daily for 10 days causes a significant decrease in plasma corticosteroid levels and a decreased response to ACTH stimulation, with peak plasma corticosteroid levels one-third that of control horses.[11] If adrenal insufficiency is diagnosed by a decreased response to ACTH stimulation and exogenous corticosteroids are the suspected cause, the test should be repeated in 14 days to allow possible return of normal function of the gland.[12]

The Adrenal Medulla

The adrenal medulla, along with sympathetic ganglia, originates from the primitive neural crest. It has been thought of as a modified sympathetic ganglion in which the postganglionic cells have become secretory (chromaffin) cells containing fine granules of epinephrine or norepinephrine. Epinephrine is the predominant adrenomedullary hormone in horses.[14] There may be extra-adrenal cells, known as organs of Zuckerkandl, associated with paravertebral and visceral sympathetic ganglia.[1,14,17] Pheochromocytomas arising from the organs of Zuckerkandl are clinically indistinguishable from adrenomedullary tumors.

Adrenomedullary stimulation results in an increased blood pressure, heart rate and respiratory rate. It also causes hyperthermia, hyperhidrosis, nervousness, mydriasis, neutrophilia, hypoptyalism and decreased GI motility. Glycogenolysis and lipolysis also result in hyperglycemia and glycosuria. Weight loss occurs in protracted cases. These adrenergic actions are mediated by epinephrine and norepinephrine released from the adrenal medulla.[14] Very little research has been done on equine adrenal physiology.

Adrenomedullary Tests

Hormone Assays

Epinephrine and norepinephrine have short plasma half-lives. They are oxidized and excreted in the urine as metanephrine, normetanephrine and vanilmandelic acid.[14,23] Levels of these hormones and metabolites in the blood and urine can be measured but normal values have not been established.

Adrenomedullary Function Tests

Diagnosis of a pheochromocytoma in humans has been based on the response to administration of certain blocking agents, such as phentolamine (Regitine:Ciba), or certain stimulating agents, such as tyramine, histamine and glucagon.[23,24] However, such tests are not safe without intensive monitoring of the patient because of the possibility of over-response to either type of agent. There are no reports on the use of such tests in horses.

Adrenomedullary Disease

Neoplasia

Although medullary hyperplasia is not an uncommon necropsy finding, it has not been reported to cause disease in horses. However, functional tumors are occasionally found. Usually these are small benign pheochromocytomas arising from chromaffin (secretory) cells. Other tumors that may occur include malignant pheochromocytomas, neurofibromas, ganglioneuroblastomas and neuroblastomas.[7,17] Malignant pheochromocytomas may extend via the adrenal vein into the caudal vena cava to cause thrombosis and metastasis.[1,17]

Early signs of a functional pheochromocytoma may be paroxysmal in nature because the release of excessive amounts of hormone may not be constant. An important clinical sign that occurs in humans and may occur in horses is hypertension. Other clinical signs include increased heart rate, respiratory rate and temperature, sweating, dry mouth, GI atony, dilated pupils, nervousness, hyperglycemia and glycosuria.[14] Ante mortem diagnosis may be made on the basis of clinical signs, blood chemistry determinations and hormone assay. However, due to the periodic nature of tumor functional activity, blood chemistry determinations and hormone assays must be performed when clinical signs are evident. It may be possible to alleviate signs, such as hypertension, by the use of a blocking agent to confirm the diagnosis. Differential diagnoses include abdominal pain, sympathomimetic drug intoxication, primary or secondary hyperadrenocorticism, diabetes mellitus, pancreatic alpha-cell tumor, and hyperthyroidism. Definitive diagnosis can only be made with hormone assays. Postmortem recognition of the tumor is aided by a positive reaction to chromaffin staining.

A pheochromocytoma in a 15-year-old mare caused excessive sweating, polydipsia, polyuria, periodic anorexia, depression and apprehension, weight loss and laminitis.[24] The mare had glycosuria and hyperglycemia, and the results of an insulin-tolerance test were negative and a glucose-tolerance test were abnormal. A second case occurred in a 25-year-old pregnant mare with a 2-day history of episodic excitement, tremors, and profuse sweating.[25] The mare had dilated light-responsive pupils, tachycardia, tachypnea, fever and profound hyperglycemia.

References

1. Appleby, EC and Sohrabi, I. Vet Rec **102** (1978) 76.
2. Tobin, T. J Eq Med Surg **3** (1979) 10.
3. James, VHT *et al.* J Endocr **48** (1970) 319.
4. Hoffsis, GF *et al.* Am J Vet Res **21** (1970) 1379.
5. Bottoms, GD *et al.* JAVMA **33** (1972) 785.
6. Zolovick, A *et al.* J Endocr **25** (1966) 249.
7. Hayes and Larner, in Goodman and Gilman: The Pharmacological Basis of Therapeutics. 5th ed. Macmillan, New York, 1975.
8. Williams *et al,* in Thorn *et al:* Harrison's Principles of Internal Medicine. 8th ed. McGraw-Hill, New York, 1977.
9. Drost, M. JAVMA **160** (1972) 321.
10. Thorn, GW *et al.* J Am Med Assoc **137** (1948) 1005.
11. Hoffsis, GF and Murdick, PW. JAVMA **157** (1970) 1590.
12. Eiler, H *et al.* Am J Vet Res **41** (1980) 430.
13. Eiler, H *et al.* Am J Vet Res **40** (1979) 724.
14. Gribble, in Catcott: Equine Medicine and Surgery. 2nd ed. American Veterinary Publications, Santa Barbara, 1972.
15. Eiler, H *et al.* Am J Vet Res **40** (1979) 727.
16. Holtz, AH. Acta Endocr **26** (1957) 75.
17. Jubb, KVF and Kennedy, PC: Pathology of Domestic Animals. 2nd ed. Academic Press, New York, 1970.
18. Raker, CW and Fegley, H. JAVMA **147** (1965) 848.
19. Kral, F. JAVMA **133** (1951) 235.
20. Evans, LE *et al.* JAVMA **152** (1968) 1778.
21. Kirk, MD. VM/SAC **69** (1974) 1383.
22. Solomon, JA. Blood Horse **85** (1963) 714.
23. Hickler and Thorn, in Thorn *et al:* Harrison's Principles of Internal Medicine. 8th ed. McGraw-Hill, New York, 1977.
24. Evans, LH *et al.* JAVMA **159** (1971) 209.
25. Buckingham, JDE. Can Vet J **11** (1970) 205.

18

The Urinary System

by R.P. Hackett, J.T. Vaughan and B.C. Tennant

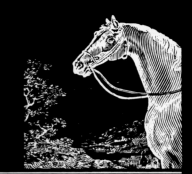

The urinary system, which consists of the kidneys, ureters, urinary bladder and urethra, is responsible for maintenance of water and electrolyte homeostasis, and for excretion of many of the products of metabolism. The kidney also has certain endocrine functions, including production of erythropoietin, the polypeptide hormone responsible for regulation of erythrogenesis, synthesis and release of renin, production of angiotensin, which functions in the regulation of the cardiovascular system, and production of 1,25-dihydroxycholecalciferol, the active, polar metabolite of vitamin D_3. Diseases of the renal parenchyma may be associated with disturbance in many or all of these regulatory and excretory functions. Diseases of the lower urinary tract are characterized primarily by disturbances in normal urinary flow.

In many cases, diseases of the kidney or the lower urinary tract are suspected because of such signs as dysuria, polyuria and hematuria. Laboratory abnormalities indicative of renal or urinary tract disease may be discovered in some cases during routine examination for other problems.

Signs of Urinary Tract Disease

Dysuria, simply defined, is abnormal urination. Straining or pain associated with urination, stranguria, occurs in association with cystitis, cystic calculi and urethritis, and is manifested by frequent passage of small quantities of urine, pollakiuria. Grunting during or at the end of urination and remaining in the crouched posture are signs of painful urination. Differentiation of painful urination from other types of abdominal pain, eg, intestinal obstruction, usually depends on signs that localize the problem to the lower urinary tract.

Polyuria is the passage of unusually large volumes of urine and may occur in normal horses ingesting excessive salt or certain rations, eg, alfalfa hay. Some horses may inexplicably drink large volumes of water and become polyuric. Polyuria is a characteristic sign in horses with adenoma of the intermediate lobe of the pituitary gland (see Chapter 17). Affected horses may be hyperglycemic, and polyuria is caused by osmotic forces associated with excessive renal loss of glucose. In others, glycosuria is absent and polyuria appears to be related to disturbances in hypothalamic or posterior pituitary function.

During convalescence after acute tubular nephrosis, a period of spontaneous diuresis may be associated with polyuria. In chronic renal disease, the inability to concentrate urine may result in polydipsia and obligatory polyuria, but many horses with advanced renal failure are presented with oliguria or reduced urine volume. Oliguria also may be a sign of prerenal defects (shock, dehydration) or acute nephropathy, eg, oxalate nephrosis, or other causes of acute tubular necrosis.

Anuria, the complete absence of urination, is a very unusual sign in horses. Even in the most severe renal disease, small quantities of urine are produced, and anuria should never be ascribed to primary renal failure until patency of the urethra has been established. Rarely, cystic calculi may completely obstruct the urethra and result in anuria associated with rapid enlargement of the bladder with characteristic signs of dysuria.

Hematuria, the presence of blood in the urine, may be recognized by the appearance of the voided specimen (gross hematuria) or by identification of increased numbers of RBC microscopically (microscopic hematuria). It is necessary to differentiate hematuria from hemoglobinuria caused by intravascular hemolysis. This often requires laboratory examination of the urine or blood except when frank clots of blood are present.

When hematuria is most conspicuous at the beginning of urination or when blood is observed flowing directly from the urethra, the origin of the hemorrhage is most likely the lower urinary tract. Hematuria most obvious at the end of the urinary stream suggests hemorrhage originating from the bladder. Renal hemorrhage is characteristically associated with blood present throughout the urinary stream; however, when significant hemorrhage occurs from the renal pelvis (granuloma, renal-cell carcinoma), blood with clots may be most obvious at the termination of urination.

Edema of the extremities and the ventral abdomen occur frequently in horses with advanced renal failure. In most cases, protein-losing nephropathy is present and edema is due, in part, to hypoalbuminemia. Such horses typically are oliguric and expansion of extracellular volume appears related to salt and water intolerance.

Physical Examination of the Urinary Tract

The external urethral orifice may be examined in mares by digital palpation or by direct visualization with a vaginal speculum. The bladder of the mare is easily catheterized with a standard metal mare catheter. The lumen of the bladder in the mare may be examined with a fiberoptic endoscope. In the male, it is almost always necessary to tranquilize the animal to relax the retractor muscles of the penis so the glans penis can be examined or the urinary bladder catheterized. The external urethral process protrudes from the fossa glandis; dorsal to the urethra is the urethral sinus, which is a diverticulum of the fossa. The diverticulum sometimes becomes impacted with caseous sebaceous and epithelial cell debris (smegma), requiring removal of the material. Catheterization of the male after thorough washing of the penis is accomplished with a flexible rubber catheter.

In adult horses the urinary bladder can be palpated per rectum, and in mares it also may be palpated per vagina. Its position in the caudal abdomen or the pelvic canal depends on the volume of urine present. When completely contracted and empty, the bladder is about the size of a human fist and is located on the ventral wall of the pelvic cavity caudal to the pelvic inlet. With increased urine volume, the bladder extends craniad along the ventral abdominal wall. The normal capacity of the bladder is about 4 L.

The left kidney is located medial to the spleen and ventral to the psoas muscles. The caudal pole of the left kidney can be palpated per rectum in most horses as a smooth, firm structure located at about the level of the third lumbar vertebra. The kidney is surrounded by renal fascia, and in well-conditioned horses, perirenal fat, located beneath this fascia, may create the false impression of enlargement. In acute nephrosis, the kidneys may be enlarged several times their normal size and are palpable more caudad and ventrad than normal. The kidneys may be remarkably decreased in size in horses with advanced chronic glomerulonephritis. The right kidney is located caudal to the liver. Its caudal pole can almost never be palpated in normal horses and can be reached only when there is significant enlargement.

If possible, it is useful to observe urination as part of the examination of horses with disease of the urinary tract. Horses normally urinate in the standing position. It is unusual for a recumbent horse to urinate, and retention of urine is a frequent complication in paralyzed horses, even in the absence of bladder paralysis. Catheterization is often required to prevent discomfort or damage to the bladder caused by overdistension.

Both males and females spread the hindlimbs in preparation for urination. They then lower the rump and press forward, exerting pressure by contraction of the abdominal musculature. Normal horses sometimes emit a grunt or groan during urination. Males usually extend the penis from the sheath, but some older geldings urinate within the sheath. Adult horses urinate 4-6 times per day and produce urine volumes ranging from 4 L to 15 L per day, depending on water intake and the diet.

The first signs of urinary tract disease may be evidence of pain or abnormal posture during urination. When it is necessary to overcome increased resistance to urine flow, as with cystic calculi, straining typically precedes and accompanies the passage of urine. If the obstruction to flow cannot be overcome, only a small volume of urine is passed and the effort is repeated. Inflammation of the urethral mucosa is characterized by straining or discomfort after urination. The volume of urine in such cases may be normal, and there is a gradual reduction of straining after urine has been passed. Straining and frequent attempts to urinate may also be signs of intestinal obstruction. It is usually possible to differentiate such cases from those with primary diseases of the urinary tract based on other clinical signs that usually accompany intestinal obstruction.

Laboratory Evaluation

Urinalysis: Urinalysis, if properly performed, usually indicates the presence of urinary tract disease and provides information regarding the type of disease present. Equine urine varies in color from light yellow to amber. Upon standing, the urine may become much darker, assuming a coffee color, which is due to the oxidation of various urochromogens present in normal urine. Equine urine may be clear but, unlike that of most other species, it can also be very turbid. This normal cloudy appearance is particularly obvious in horses receiving large quantitites of Ca in the diet and is caused by $CaCO_3$ crystalluria. Cloudiness combined with the normally high mucus content of equine urine is sometimes mistaken for pyuria. Before this diagnosis can even be considered, however, it is essential to examine the urinary sediment microscopically.

Like other herbivores, horses normally excrete alkaline urine, with a pH of 7.5-8.5. The urine may be acidic in fasting or anorectic horses and, in horses receiving high-grain diets, the urine pH also may fall below 7.

The specific gravity of equine urine ranges from 1.020 to 1.050. The capacity to concentrate urine decreases in most diseases of the kidney, often at an early stage and before azotemia develops. Specific gravity varies with water intake, and a low specific gravity is clinically significant only when measured after a period of water deprivation. Restriction of water intake, however, is contraindicated in horses in which azotemia is present or suspected because the loss of renal concentrating capacity in such individuals can result in severe dehydration and further deterioration in renal function.

In normal mammals, the urine contains small amounts or protein consisting of serum proteins derived primarily from the glomerular filtrate and other proteins secreted by the renal tubules and the remainder of the urinary tract. The concentration of urinary protein, however, is less than that detected by the usual tests for urinary protein, and persistent proteinuria detected by such tests is abnormal. The commercially available "dipsticks" are formulated for use in acidic urine. In the normally alkaline urine of horses, a false-positive protein reaction (trace to 1+) is often observed. The standard sulfosalicylic acid test for urinary protein, however, is characteristically negative in normal horses. The concentration of urinary protein varies with urine volume. In very dilute urine, a spuriously low protein reaction may be observed. Strong protein reactions may be detected in foals during the first 1-2 days of life, during which a variety of small milk proteins are absorbed by the intestine and filtered by the glomeruli.

The differentiation of hematuria from hemoglobinuria, based on identification of abnormal numbers of RBC in the urine, is usually not possible on the basis of inspection of the urine specimen unless frank clots are present. When examination of urine is delayed or when the urine is extremely dilute, spontaneous disruption of RBC may occur, but RBC ghosts remain in the sediment.

Several chemical reagents, the most common being orthotoluidine, are available for detection of small quantities of blood or heme pigments. This test, however, does not distinguish between hematuria, hemoglobinuria and myoglobinuria. In large amounts, myoglobin may produce a port wine-colored urine indistinguishable from that due to other heme pigments. On the basis of clinical signs and other hematologic and biochemical tests, one can often differentiate diseases associated with myoglobinuria from those associated with either hematuria or hemoglobinuria. In severe intravascular hemolysis, frank hemoglobinemia is frequently present, while in myolytic disease, it is very unusual to detect myoglobinemia, except during the very earliest stages. Myoglobin or hemoglobin in urine may be differentiated in the laboratory by spectrophotometry or electrophoresis.

Glucose appears in the urine of horses when the plasma concentration exceeds the renal threshold of 160-180 mg/dl. The threshold level may be exceeded temporarily during excitement or exertion. Hyperglycemia is also a characteristic of certain endocrinopathies, such as Cushing's syndrome, caused by adenoma of the intermediate lobe of the pituitary. Diabetes mellitus is, however, rare in horses. Dipstick tests for urinary glucose usually are based on the glucose oxidase reaction and are therefore specific for the glucose molecule. Ketonuria is very unusual in horses, even in such conditions as starvation that, in other species, are characterized by increased ketone body excretion.

Examination of urine sediment is an essential part of urinalysis. A few epithelial cells, RBC and WBC may be present in normal urine. The concentration of cells varies in normal urine, depending on the rate of urine flow. However, in both upper and lower urinary tract diseases, the number of these cells is often increased significantly. Interestingly, some horses with cystic calculi have virtually no increase in the number of WBC or RBC in the urine.

Casts are cylindric molds of the tubular lumina and are formed by precipitation of protein and, in some cases, clumps of cells. When present in urine, casts are an indication of renal parenchymal disease. In alkaline urine, casts are either not formed or rapidly disintegrate. Therefore, it is very unusual to observe hyaline or cellular casts in equine urine. Even in severe renal disease, they are seen only when the urine is acidic.

Serum Biochemistry: The blood urea nitrogen (BUN) and serum creatinine levels are the most widely used indicators of the amount of nitrogenous wastes retained in renal failure. Creatinine and urea nitrogen are excreted primarily by glomerular filtration. Increases in both usually are not observed until there is a loss in function of more than 75% of the nephrons. Therefore, significant renal disease can be present without evidence of azotemia. Normal values are 10-25 mg/dl for BUN and 1.0-1.5 mg/dl for creatinine. Increases in noncreatinine chromogens, such as bilirubin, occur frequently in horses and may interfere with creatinine level determination, resulting in spurious elevation in the reported serum creatinine concentration.

Both acute and chronic renal failure are characteristically associated with moderate hyponatremia, hyperkalemia and metabolic acidosis. In acute tubular nephrosis, there may be moderate hypocalcemia and hyperphosphatemia; however, in end-stage glomerulonephritis with oliguria, hypercalcemia and hypophosphatemia have been reported. These latter changes are common in horses but very unusual in other domestic species, and are believed to be related to a unique role of the equine kidney in Ca homeostasis.

DISEASES OF THE KIDNEY

Acute Renal Failure

Cause: Acute renal failure in horses is characterized by acute and usually rapid deterioration in renal function and has multiple etiologies. Prerenal causes of acute renal failure impair renal perfusion and include hypovolemia due to severe dehydration or blood loss, and circulatory insufficiency, as from shock or congestive heart failure. Prerenal azotemia refers specifically to hemodynamic changes believed to be reversible.

Postrenal forms of azotemia are the result of physical disruption in urine flow, such as that caused by obstruction of the neck of the bladder or urethra due to urinary calculi, and spontaneous rupture of the urinary bladder. Both are characterized by oliguria or anuria. Typically, obstruction of the urethra causes anuria and colic. Spontaneous rupture of the bladder is also associated with dysuria and oliguria, and progressive abdominal distension typically accompanies progressive azotemia.

Acute tubular necrosis is the most common renal cause of acute azotemia. When renal ischemia associated with prerenal vascular disturbance is severe or sufficiently prolonged, degeneration of renal tubular epithelial cells occurs. Necrosis of renal tubular cells also may be associated with hemoglobinuria or myoglobinuria, the ingestion of nephrotoxins, such as soluble oxalate salts present in poisonous plants or in the diet, or the administration of nephrotoxic drugs, such as certain sulfonamides or aminoglycosides. In the case of prerenal factors (severe dehydration or shock), the etiology may be readily apparent. In horses with hemoglobinuria or myoglobinuria, renal insufficiency can be anticipated. In other cases of acute renal tubular necrosis, however, the cause cannot be established and it must be assumed that the cause is an environmental or dietary toxin.

Clinical Signs: Like other forms of acute renal failure, acute tubular necrosis is initially characterized by oliguria. The primary cause of oliguria in this form of kidney disease is still not completely understood, but reduced glomerular filtration rate is an important factor. The reduced glomerular filtration rate is probably related to reduced blood flow secondary to afferent arteriolar vasoconstriction, which is thought to be related to disruption in the renin-angiotensin regulatory system.

Because of tubular damage in acute renal failure, the urine is not concentrated and the specific gravity characteristically may be less than 1.020. Proteinuria and microscopic hematuria are also characteristic. In most cases, the swollen kidneys can be appreciated by rectal examination, and tenderness of the perirenal area is recognized during palpation.

Treatment: The best clinical approach is to avoid the renal circulatory insufficiency that leads to acute tubular necrosis and avoid exposure to nephrotoxic substances. In potential cases of hemoglobinuric or myoglobinuric nephrosis, saline diuresis and furosemide therapy are indicated. When renal insufficiency exists or is suspected, aminoglycoside antibiotics should be used cautiously.

During the initial oliguric phase of acute tubular necrosis, fluid therapy should be administered but should not exceed the needs of the patient. Horses with acute renal failure often are intolerant of Na and water, and rapidly gain weight and become edematous if excessive parenteral fluids are administered. It is necessary to monitor the serum electrolytes, particularly K, the serum level of which is often increased during the oliguric phase. Hyperkalemia may be effectively treated with isotonic (1/6 molar) $NaHCO_3$ solution administered IV.

In horses recovering from acute tubular necrosis, oliguria is characteristically followed by a diuretic phase that may last several weeks. Food intake increases significantly but polydipsia, polyuria and low urine specific gravity persist because of continued tubular dysfunction and the inability to concentrate urine. As with the oliguric phase, it is worthwhile, if possible, to weigh the horse at frequent intervals to detect rapid loss of fluids.

Recovery from acute tubular necrosis is determined by the nature and severity of the underlying cause. Persistence of oliguria is an unfavorable prognostic sign, while oliguria followed by diuresis is generally considered favorable. Acute oxalate nephropathy has a mortality rate of greater than 50%. In cases of hemoglobinuric or myoglobinuric nephrosis in which the hematologic or muscular diseases are satisfactorily resolved, the prognosis is more favorable, with mortality due to renal failure less then 20%

Chronic Renal Failure

Although chronic diseases of the equine kidney have been recognized for many years, the collective experience of practicing veterinarians suggests that clinical illness associated with primary renal failure is unusual. The frequency of clinical renal failure in horses is clearly less than that observed in some other domestic species, such as dogs, but the uremic syndrome in horses is not rare and accounts for a small but significant number of patients with histories of protracted weight loss and peripheral edema.

Cause: Most reports of equine renal disease are descriptions of pathologic lesions and provide little useful information regarding clinical manifestations or morbidity and mortality rates associated with such diseases. Glomerulonephritis appears to be the most frequent type of renal disease encountered clinically in horses.[1] Although reports of spontaneous glomerulonephritis are unusual, the frequency in horses used for antiserum production has been reported to be much higher.[2-6] The prevalence of subclinical glomerulonephritis appears to be much higher than would be anticipated, based on experience with clinical patients. In a survey of random equine necropsies, microscopic glomerular lesions were identified in over 40% of the horses examined.[7]

Chronic interstitial nephritis occurs less frequently than glomerulonephritis. The cause is unknown but in some cases has been attributed to pyelonephritis, presumably the result of ascending urinary tract infection.[1] Early descriptions of pyelonephritis due to *Corynebacterium renale* included cases in horses as well as cattle.[8] Oxalate nephrosis also has been described in horses with signs of renal insufficiency. In some cases it has been attributed to ingestion of plants containing high concentrations of soluble oxalate salts.[9] In others the cause of oxalate crystal deposition is unknown, but grain contaminated with oxalate-producing fungi may be involved.[10]

Occurrence: In a series of 9 uremic horses, the average age at admission was 12 years (range 5-19 years), with no unexpected breed or sex predisposition.[1] The duration of illness prior to admission averaged 3.5 months (range 1-7 months), with 8 of the 9 having histories of anorexia and weight loss during much of this period. Pica, characterized by an unusual appetite for soil or straw bedding, was in the histories of 4 cases. Polyuria and/or polydipsia were historical findings in only 3 of 9 cases.

Clinical Signs: Regardless of the nature of underlying renal lesions, clinical manifestations of chronic renal failure are similar. In the above series of cases, 8 or 9 horses were obviously cachectic at admission.[1] Lethargy and weakness were observed in most cases and in 7 of 9, there was conspicuous edema of the ventral abdomen and/or the distal extremities. Oliguria was observed in 5 of 9 cases and in 3 of 9, there were polyuria and polydipsia. Diarrhea was a terminal sign in 3 cases.

Rectal examination of the kidney often is useful. In horses with chronic interstitial nephritis and glomerulonephritis presented in advanced stages of uremia, the left kidney can be palpated and readily recognized as smaller than normal. In cases of oxalate nephropathy with a clinical course of only a few weeks, the left kidney is often much larger than normal.

Laboratory Findings: Anemia is a consistent finding in horses with chronic uremia. Frequently there is metabolic acidosis. The serum Na and Cl levels are normal or moderately reduced. Hyperkalemia associated with cardiac arrhythmias is characteristic. The BUN levels in clinical cases ranged from 75 mg/dl to almost 300 mg/dl, with correspondingly high serum creatinine values of 4-15 mg/dl.

The clinical and biochemical abnormalities associated with chronic renal failure in horses are similar to those observed in other species, with one notable exception. In uremic horses, hypercalcemia and hypophosphatemia are frequently but not always observed.[1,11-13] In other species, hypercalcemia is a highly unusual sequela of primary renal disease, and it is necessary, in cases of hypercalcemia associated with renal failure, to consider primary hyperparathyroidism and pseudohyperparathyroidism as differential diagnoses.[14,15] The latter condition has been associated with squamous-cell carcinoma of the stomach in a horse.[16]

Studies of normal Ca and P metabolism suggest that hypercalcemia in horses with renal disease is the direct result of renal failure. As the dietary intake of Ca increases, horses, unlike most other domestic species and humans, continue to absorb progressively more Ca from the intestine. The serum Ca level is maintained by increasing the excretion of Ca in the urine as $CaCO_3$. The equine kidney, therefore, appears to have a unique role in the control of serum Ca and Ca homeostasis.[17,18] The profound hypercalcemia observed after bilateral nephrectomy supports this view.[19] Much remains to be learned about the role of the kidney in Ca homeostasis in horses. However, when biochemical findings of azotemia are associated with hypercalcemia and hypophosphatemia, one must seriously consider primary renal disease as a differential diagnosis.

Several studies of normal renal electrolyte and water excretion in horses have been conducted.[20-23] Because of their diet, horses normally excrete much less Na and more K than omnivorous or carnivorous species. Creatinine excretion rates, adjusted for body weight, are lower in horses than in other species.[20] Unfortunately, most affected horses are presented in advanced states of uremia and quantitation of

functional deficits has not been possible. Renal function has recently been studied in clinical patients, and it is hoped that such studies will allow earlier recognition of renal insufficiency, with the hope of improved treatment.[24]

Treatment: When oliguria is present, the prognosis is very unfavorable. In such patients there is clear indication for protein restriction, but every effort should be made to provide adequate caloric intake. Salt restriction is indicated in most cases because of the peripheral edema, but the patient often limits its own water intake. Attempts to induce diuresis in oliguric patients by forced fluid intake, via nasogastric or IV administration, have been unsuccessful and in several cases have resulted in rapid deterioration and death.

References

1. Tennant, B *et al.* Proc 25th Ann Mtg Am Assoc Eq Pract, 1979. p 293.
2. Fincher, MG and Olafson, P. Cornell Vet **24** (1934) 356.
3. Frank, ER and Dunlap, GL. No Am Vet **16** (1935) 20.
4. Langham, RF and Hallman, ET. Am J Vet Res **1** (1940) 49.
5. Langham, RF and Hallman, ET. JAVMA **99** (1941) 471.
6. Schleifstein, J. Am J Path **15** (1939) 596.
7. Banks, KL and Henson, JB. Lab Invest **26** (1972) 708.
8. Boyd, WL and Bishop, LM. JAVMA **90** (1937) 154.
9. Steward, J and McCallum, JW. Vet Rec **56** (1944) 77.
10. Andrews, EJ. JAVMA **159** (1971) 49.
11. Brobst, DF *et al.* JAVMA **173** (1978) 1370.
12. Coffman, JR *et al* Proc 23rd Ann Mtg Am Assoc Eq Pract, 1977. p 161.
13. Brobst, DF *et al.* J Eq Med Surg **1** (1977) 171.
14. Finco, DR and Rowland, GN, JAVMA **173** (1978) 990.
15. Massry, SG *et al.* Arch Int Med **131** (1973) 828.
16. Meuten, DJ *et al.* Cornell Vet **68** (1978) 179.
17. Schryver, HF *et al.* J Nutr **100** (1970) 955.
18. Scvhryver, HF *et al.* Cornell Vet **64** (1974) 493.
19. Tennant, BC *et al.* Fed Proc **33** (1974) 670.
20. Knudsen, E. Acta Vet Scand **1** (1959) 52.
21. Tasker, JB. Cornell Vet **57** (1967) 649.
22. Rawlings, CA and Bisgard, GE. Am J Vet Res **36** (1975) 45.
23. Traver, DS *et al.* J Eq Med Surg **1** (1977) 378.
24. Traver, DS *et al.* Proc 22nd Ann Mtg Am Assoc Eq Pract, 1976. p 177.

DISEASES OF THE URINARY BLADDER

Cystitis

Cause: Cystitis, or inflammation of the urinary bladder, is uncommon in horses. It is rarely a primary disease and usually occurs secondary to diseases that result in incomplete emptying of the urinary bladder, such as urolithiasis or bladder paresis or paralysis.[1-3] Horses with cystic calculi almost invariably have coexistent cystitis.[1] Bladder paresis or paralysis associated with sorghum ingestion or other diseases results in urine retention, sediment accumulation and bacterial growth in the urinary bladder.[2] Less commonly, cystitis may be associated with chronic vaginitis or improper or prolonged urinary catheterization. Bacteria isolated from the urinary bladders of horses with cystitis include E coli, Staphylococcus sp, Corynebacterium sp, Pseudomonas aeruginosa and others.[2]

Clinical signs: Acute cystitis, an uncommon disease, is characterized by colic, straining and frequent passage of small amounts of urine.[4] Cystitis is usually chronic in duration. Clinical signs of chronic cystitis include frequent urination, straining, dribbling of urine, caking of skin with urine sediment, urine scalding and alopecia, vulvar "winking" in mares, and penile relaxation in males.[1-3] Urine may be more turbid than normal and may contain blood. Rear-limb incoordination may accompany cystitis in horses that have ingested sorghum.[2] Rectal examination is indicated to evaluate the bladder for calculi or urine sediment.

Diagnosis: The urinary bladder should be aseptically catheterized in animals with suspected cystitis to obtain a urine sample for urinalysis and bacterial culture and sensitivity tests. Bacteria, epithelial cells, mineral crystals, RBC and WBC may be evident upon microscopic evaluation.[1-3] Urine may be grossly blood tinged or positive for occult blood.[2,3]

Treatment: Successful treatment of cystitis depends upon elimination of the underlying cause and administration of systemic antibiotic therapy. Surgical removal of cystic calculi associated with cystitis is necessary.[1] Systemic antibiotic therapy is based on culture and sensitivity tests and is continued long after clinical signs of cystitis have disappeared.[3] Irrigation of the bladder with large volumes of sterile fluid to flush out urine sediment may be of value, but topical treatment of the bladder with antibiotics is rarely indicated.

Cystic Calculi (Urolithiasis)

Urinary calculi may form in any part of the equine urinary tract, but the most common site is the bladder.[5-9] There are no apparent sex or breed predispositions for calculus formation. Adult horses are most frequently affected.

Cause: Urinary calculi are precipitated urine solutes that have been deposited upon a nidus and bonded by a cementing agent. A cluster of desquamated epithelial cells or necrotic tissue ordinarily acts as the nidus for deposition of solute crystals. Factors that favor precipitation of solutes from urine are not well understood. Urine is a highly saturated solution with a large number of solutes, many in higher concentration than could occur in a simple solution. Urine colloids usually prevent precipitation of these highly concentrated solutes but in some circumstances the capacity of such colloids to prevent precipitation is exceeded.

Urine pH is a major factor affecting solute precipitation. An alkaline pH favors formation of both carbonate and mixed-phosphate calculi. The concentration of various urine solutes may also favor solute precipitation and is affected by diet and water intake or loss. Water deprivation or excessive water loss results in a urine concentration that favors solute precipitation. Consumption of feed or water with a high mineral content leads to a high urinary solute concentration and an increased tendency for crystal formation. As solutes precipitate, they are cemented upon the nidus to form a concretion or stone. The cementing agent is thought to be a mucoprotein, the quantity of which, in ruminants, increases with the ingestion of high-concentrate, low-roughage rations or with pelleted rations.[10]

A solitary calculus is usually formed in affected horses.[9] The calculi are composed of various forms of $CaCO_3$, predominantly calcite but also aragonite, vaterite and baterite.[11,12]

Clinical Signs: In horses of either sex, urinary calculi develop most frequently in the urinary bladder. Male horses infrequently may be affected with urethral calculi. Clinical signs of cystic calculi include straining to urinate, dribbling of urine, and frequent urination.[8,9] Less common signs include mild recurrent colic, loss of condition, stilted gait, urine scalding and soiling of the hair with urine salts.

Diagnosis: Urinalysis indicates concurrent cystitis, as evidenced by crystals, RBC, WBC and bacteria in the urine. A cystic calculus may occasionally be "felt" with a urinary catheter, but definitive diagnosis is by rectal palpation of the urinary bladder. The calculus can ordinarily be palpated as a hard oval mass near the neck of the bladder.

Treatment: Treatment of cystic calculi is through a variety of surgical approaches, including ischial urethrotomy and pararectal cystotomy (Gokel's operation) in males, urethral sphincterotomy in mares, and laparocystidotomy in either sex.

Ischial urethrotomy is indicated for removal of a small cystic calculus or a urethral calculus.[6,7,9] Preoperative evaluation should include urinalysis and bacterial culture and sensitivity tests of urine. Preoperative antibiotic therapy is recommended to control any existing bladder infection and to reduce the risk of postoperative infection. Surgery is performed on the standing horse, with local anesthesia preferably provided by epidural injection. The tail is secured overhead, the rectum is manually emptied, and the rear quarters are scrubbed and draped for aseptic surgery. If epidural anesthesia is inadequate, the operative site is anesthetized by local infiltration. The urethra is catheterized to facilitate its identification. An 8- to 10-cm vertical incision is made on the midline just ventral to the anus and over the ischial arch. Tension is applied to the soft tissues with the fingertips, and the incision is continued in depth between the retractor penis muscles, through the bulbospongiosus muscle, and into the lumen of the corpus spongiosum urethra, cutting down onto the surface of the catheter. Hemorrhage from sinusoidal spaces does not lend itself to ligation and must be controlled by packing or by careful suturing with fine catgut. Cautery is contraindicated unless done with caution since tissue damage delays healing and increases the risk of stricture. The incision can be lengthened as needed for access to calculi in the horizontal pelvic urethra and bladder craniad, or for access to urethral calculi distal to the arch. Only small, smooth calculi should be removed in this way. Rough stones are usually imbedded in the bladder mucosa and are difficult to remove through such limited exposure, even though broken down by a lithrotrite.

Upon removal of all calculi, the bladder is flushed clean of sand and blood. The urethral incision may be closed carefully with fine sutures of absorbable material, but usually the wound is allowed to heal by second intention, presumably to lessen the chances of stricture formation. If the latter method is used, care should be taken to obliterate any tissue pockets that would impede ventral drainage of urine and serum. Urination through the wound necessitates regular wound care. Epithelialization and granulation proceed rapidly and, within 2-3 weeks, the wound is healed sufficiently to discontinue treatment.

Postoperative medication should include antibiotics for 7-14 days and judicious use of urine acidifiers, such as ammonium chloride. Diuretics may be used until protein and occult blood disappear from the urine and the wound shows evidence of healing. Provision of abundant clean drinking water is essential. Some alteration of feed according to the mineral composition of the calculus may be necessary. For example, feeds containing less Ca or P than normal may be indicated.

Pararectal cystotomy (Gokel's operation) is used to remove a cystic calculus in males. Although not widely practiced in this country, the method has achieved a measure of acceptance in Europe. The patient is prepared in the same manner as for ischial urethrotomy. If epidural anesthesia alone is inadequate, a vertical line along the right side of the anus (for right-handed operators) in the space between the anus and the semimembranosus muscle may be infiltrated. A 10- to 15-cm sagittal incision is made through the skin, which has been tensed by tenaculum forceps placed across the anus. The forceps serve the added purpose of displacing and closing the anus to protect against contamination. The skin edges are retracted by stay sutures and the incision is deepened by blunt finger dissection through the pelvic fascia, along the right rectal wall to the neck of the bladder, exercising caution to stay in the retroperitoneal recess (rectogenital pouch). The bladder is evacuated by catheterization, to permit retrograde displacement of the calculus with the left hand, or the hand of an assistant, introduced into the rectum.

With the calculus so presented, an incision is made through the retroperitoneal portion of the bladder wall, using care to avoid the converging ampullae caudad and the ureters craniad. Blunt reflection of the peritoneum and pelvic fascia and partial retroflexion of the bladder wall allow direct visualization of the bladder for incision and closure. Good illumination and retraction by an assistant are essential to this phase of the operation. Removal of the calculus with forceps and subsequent closure of the incision are performed as described for laparocystidotomy. The pelvic fascia is closed with interrupted sutures of catgut and the skin with interrupted mattress sutures.

The major risks of pararectal cystotomy are peritonitis and pelvic abscessation. Constipation could be an added problem due to pelvic pain and swelling. Such complications may be prevented by the use of a light laxative diet, scrupulous wound care, analgesics, tranquilizers or sedatives, and continuous antibiotic therapy as required for healing and elimination of infection.[13-15]

Urethral sphincterotomy is used in mares to remove cystic calculi too large to be delivered through the intact urethra. The patient is prepared as for a standing aseptic gynecologic procedure, and straining is suppressed by epidural anesthesia and tranquilization. The rectum and bladder should be emptied. The vulva is retracted by forceps, sutures, blade retractors or by hand. Good illumination of the vestibule of the vagina is essential.

The calculus is displaced caudad by a hand in the vagina. Further traction on the calculus can be provided by forceps through the urethra, although use of forceps may be deferred until the urethra has been incised. The dorsal wall of the urethra is incised with a scalpel as it is stretched open over the underlying calculus. Care is used in calculus removal to minimize hemorrhage from the inflamed bladder mucosa. Once the calculus is removed and the bladder cleansed of sand and debris, the urethral incision is closed with simple-interrupted sutures of catgut or synthetic absorbable suture. An indwelling balloon catheter may be used for a few days to keep the bladder empty.

Preoperative and postoperative use of antibiotics should be based on bacterial culture and sensitivity test results. Any amendment of the diet and water depends on the mineral content of the calculus and etiologic factors. Acidification of the urine is a further consideration. Rigorous management of the associated cystitis is important if success is to be more than temporary. Chronic cystitis can be one of the most refractory and frustrating of all urologic problems.[9,13,16]

Laparocystidotomy is performed in male or female horses to remove a cystic calculus too large to be removed by any of the preceding methods. Since this is usually an elective procedure, time permits preoperative considerations designed to put the patient in the best condition for surgery. The appropriate antibacterials, as determined by culture and sensitivity tests, should be used preoperatively to control infectious cystitis and minimize the risk of postoperative peritonitis.

Surgery is performed with the horse in dorsal recumbency and under general anesthesia. The rectum is emptied manually and the bladder catheterized, and the site is prepared for aseptic surgery. A 16- to 18-cm longitudinal,

right paramedian incision is made midway between the midline (prepuce in the male) and the inguinal ring. Layers incised deep to the skin are the superficial and deep abdominal fascia, the rectus abdominis muscle within its superficial and deep layers of the aponeurotic sheath, the fatty fascia transversalis, and the peritoneum. The rich blood supply from external pudendal and superficial abdominal vessels necessitates good homeostasis to avoid postsurgical hematoma. Although some surgeons use an incision through the prepubic tendon caudal to the osseous symphysis pubis for greater access, it is preferable to end the incision at the prepubic tendon because of the large anastomotic branch of the deep femoral artery that traverses this structure.[13] Transection of this vessel causes considerable hemorrhage and access for ligature is limited because of its location in the substance of the heavy tendon. Moreover, adequate access to the urinary bladder does not depend on this small extension of the incision.

The laparotomy site is draped with a plastic fenestrated shroud. The bladder is located and retracted into the incision by slow, persistent traction until 2 stay sutures of umbilical tape can be placed in the apex bilateral to the urachal scar. The musculature of the bladder is slowly fatigued until stretching and relaxation occur. The bladder is carefully packed off to prevent contamination of the peritoneal cavity from spillage during subsequent operation. An incision is made in the apex or dorsal wall of the bladder, avoiding the ureters, until the calculus is located.

Rough calculi may be intimately attached to the mucosa, reminiscent of the bovine placental caruncle and uterine cotyledon. Removal or detachment is best accomplished by peeling the 2 surfaces apart. In this way, much hemorrhage from the bladder mucosa is avoided, as well as other possible complications. The bladder is cleansed of sand and debris with moist gauze sponges and copious saline lavage, and the effluent is aspirated to reduce the chance of contamination of the peritoneum. Control of hemorrhage prior to closure obviates the necessity of later removal of blood clots. If the bladder mucosa hemorrhages extensively, the bladder can be temporarily packed with warm saline gauze prior to closure, and parenteral agents, such as conjugated mare estrogens, may be given to hasten clotting.

The bladder is closed with 0 or 00 chromic catgut or synthetic absorbable sutures on tapered needles in 2 layers. The first row is a simple-continuous suture through all layers of the bladder. If the bladder wall is greatly thickened, only the mucosa is sutured. The second row is of interrupted Lembert sutures.[17] Alternatively, 2 layers of inverting sutures can be used. Indwelling balloon catheters may be used postoperatively, if necessary, to keep the bladder empty. The abdomen is closed in 4 layers. The deep sheath of the rectus abdominis muscle is apposed with continuous horizontal mattress sutures of #1 chromic catgut, with the peritoneum included or excluded. The superficial sheath of the rectus abdominis muscle (conjoined aponeuroses of the abdominal oblique muscles) is apposed by imbricating mattress sutures of monofilament nylon, polypropylene or dacron, #2 or larger. An alternative method uses simple-interrupted sutures of #2 polyglycolic acid. The third layer closes the superficial abdominal fascia with simple-interrupted sutures of #2 chromic catgut or polyglycolic acid suture. The skin is closed with continuous interlocking or interrupted mattress sutures of monofilament synthetic material, such as nylon or polypropylene, size #2.

Postoperative use of diuretics, urine acidifiers, abdominal drains, tension sutures, stent bandages and corsets is discretionary. The use of postoperative antibiotics is mandatory. Dietary management depends on the etiology and may entail reducing the source of the predominant mineral contained in the stone if the diet, such as feeds high in P, is incriminated. The long-range prognosis should be guarded since the individual may be predisposed to chronic cystitis and calculus formation.[9]

Paralysis of the Bladder*

Bladder Function: Urination is a function of sensory and motor pathways. As the volume of urine in the bladder increases, pressure receptors are stimulated and impulses are carried through branches of the sacral plexus over the sacral spinal nerves into the sacral segments of the spinal cord. This sensory information is then conducted up both sides of the spinal cord to the brainstem. From there, information on bladder pressure is conducted to the cerebellum and forward to the somesthetic cortex of the cerebrum.

Motor control of urination is regulated by an upper motor neuron system and a lower motor neuron system. The upper motor neuron sys-

tem probably begins in the motor cortex of the cerebral hemisphere, but the major center for micturition is in the reticular formation of the brainstem. Motor information is conducted over the reticulospinal tracts, primarily in the lateral funiculus of the spinal cord, which terminate in the grey matter of the sacral segments. These reticulospinal tracts have 2 major functions in the sacral segments. One is to facilitate the lower motor neuron (parasympathetic) system. The cell bodies of the lower motor neurons are located in the grey matter of the sacral segments, and the axons pass through the sacral spinal nerves into the sacral plexus, and through the pelvic nerve to innervate the detrusor muscle of the bladder. Facilitation of these neurons causes detrusor muscle contraction, which causes emptying of the bladder and opening of the neck of the bladder at the proximal urethra. The second function of the upper motor neuron system is to inhibit lower motor neuron (somatic efferent) function. The cell bodies of the lower motor neurons are in the ventral grey column of the sacral segments. The axons are conducted through the spinal nerves into the sacral plexus and out branches of the pudendal nerve to innervate the striated urethral muscle that surrounds the urethra. Inhibition of this lower motor neuron system causes relaxation of the urethralis muscle and therefore permits urine to be conducted through the urethra.

Causes and Clinical Signs: Bladder paralysis in horses occurs primarily in diseases that interfere with the lower motor neuron pathway in the sacral segments of the spinal cord and sacral spinal nerves, or the upper motor neuron pathway in the reticulospinal tracts of the white matter of the spinal cord. Lower motor neuron lesions cause complete atonia of the smooth muscle of the bladder and the urethralis muscle. Incontinence is prominent, and it is easy to evacuate the bladder by pressure.

In upper motor neuron paralysis, the urethralis muscle may actually be spastic. Although there may be no voluntary contraction of the bladder muscle, evacuation of the bladder by manual pressure is difficult because of hypertonicity of the urethralis muscle. Clinical evidence of paralysis of the bladder ordinarily occurs only in cases of severe upper motor neuron spinal cord disease.

Lower motor neuron disturbances most commonly associated with bladder paralysis include direct injury to the sacral segments of the spinal cord or the sacral nerves in either the

*by A. de Lahunta

vertebral canal or the pelvis ventral to the sacral vertebrae, protozoal myelitis localized in the grey matter of the sacral segments, and neuritis of the cauda equina, which profoundly affects the sacral nerves as well as the caudal nerves to the tail. In neuritis of the cauda equina, paralysis of the tail, anus, rectum and bladder are the most consistent clinical signs observed. One case of cryptococcal leptomeningitis was most severe in the area of the cauda equina and caused paresis of the tail, anus, rectum and bladder. Other causes of lower motor neuron-related bladder paralysis include abscesses of the sacral segments or sacral spinal nerves in the vertebral canal of young foals or, rarely, neoplasia at this site in older horses.

Upper motor neuron paralysis of the equine bladder is uncommon. The most common spinal cord diseases rarely cause complete paralysis of the pelvic limbs, in which one would expect paralysis of the bladder. Vertebral fractures and contusions of the spinal cord in young horses are the most common causes of severe paralysis of the pelvic limbs and are, of course, characterized by bladder paralysis.

There are 2 diseases of the horse in which a degree of paralysis of the bladder is present in association with weakness and ataxia of the pelvic limbs. Both usually involve the white matter of the spinal cord. The weakness and ataxia in horses compared with that in other species is not of the degree one would expect to associate with bladder dysfunction. One of these diseases is ischemic myelopathy, caused by EHV-1 (rhinopneumonitis).[18] Mildly affected horses have varying degrees of weakness and ataxia of the pelvic limbs, along with a very full bladder that is not evacuated normally; incontinence may sometimes occur. Some of these horses also have slight weakness of the tail, but anal function is usually normal. This syndrome has not been correlated with significant lesions in the sacral segments of the spinal cord and is not associated with the sensory deficits that usually accompany lower motor neuron paralysis from lesions of the sacral segments. Most spinal cord lesions in these horses are in the white matter. We do not know why this lesion produces bladder paralysis. It is common, however, and when there is any degree of bladder paralysis in horses with a sudden mild weakness and ataxia, a diagnosis of EHV-1 myelitis is suggested.

The other upper motor neuron disease in which there is a degree of bladder paralysis associated with weakness and ataxia of the pelvic limbs is that caused by sorghum or sudangrass poisoning.[19,20] Again, the lesions in the spinal cord are primarily in the white matter. They are degenerative, mild lesions that one would not necessarily expect to be associated with bladder paralysis. This syndrome differs from the other neurologic bladder problems in that there also is prominent cystitis, as is reported in sudangrass or sorghum poisoning. Any horse with bladder paralysis is susceptible to cystitis, but it is not commonly observed clinically except with this particular poisoning.

Treatment: Treatment of bladder paralysis is aimed at controlling cystitis with systemic antibiotics and keeping the bladder emptied by catheterization or manual expression. The practicality of such supportive care and the prognosis for recovery depend upon the cause.

Rupture of the Urinary Bladder

Rupture of the urinary bladder in mature horses is an unusual event ordinarily associated with parturition or urinary obstruction.[21,22] Rupture of the urinary bladder is more common in neonatal foals, with reported prevalences ranging from 0.2% to 2.5%.[23-26] The condition occurs primarily in male foals and is assumed to occur during parturition as extreme external pressure is applied to the distended bladder.[23-25] The bladder usually ruptures near its apex on the dorsal surface.

Clinical Signs: Affected foals represent a diagnostic challenge in the early stages of the disease. Parturition is typically unremarkable, and the foal appears normal after birth and suckles as expected. Depression may be noted by 24-48 hours after birth. The foal may relax its penis, strain and pass small amounts of urine. Complete anuria is not a characteristic observation. Straining and signs of mild colic may lead to confusion of this disease with meconium impaction. Foals straining from meconial impaction tend to hold their rear legs together, with the back arched and tail raised, whereas foals suffering from distension of the peritoneal cavity with urine extend their rear legs caudad, with the back and loins hollowed out and the head lifted.[23] Patients with a ruptured bladder have been observed to walk backward or crouch continually, usually with the tail elevated.[27] There is progressive lethargy, weakness, anorexia and, within 3-4 days of birth, conspicuous abdominal distension. Palpation and ballottement of the abdomen reveal fluid rather than gaseous distension.[1]

Diagnosis: Several methods are available to confirm a diagnosis of bladder rupture. The observation that the foal can urinate does not safely rule out bladder rupture nor does the ability to obtain urine upon catheterization of the urinary bladder.[28] Abdominocentesis typically yields a large volume of clear, yellow fluid, which may smell of ammonia when heated. Appearance of a dye, such as methylene blue or azosulfamide, in the peritoneal fluid after infusion into the bladder is considered diagnostic of bladder rupture.[1,28] Positive-contrast cystography is also a reliable diagnostic test for a ruptured urinary bladder.[29]

The BUN concentration is of limited diagnostic value since it may be normal or only slightly higher than normal in some cases.[28] A reliable laboratory test is comparison of the creatinine level in serum with that in the peritoneal fluid.[28] In bladder rupture, the concentration of creatinine in the peritoneal fluid is invariably higher than that of serum. Profound hyponatremia, hypochloremia and hypo-osmolality, coupled with an elevated serum K level, have been described as characteristic of bladder rupture in neonatal foals.[28]

Treatment: Surgical repair of a ruptured urinary bladder should be performed as soon as possible after the condition is diagnosed. Abdominocentesis to remove accumulated urine is indicated before induction of anesthesia to minimize respiratory and cardiovascular compromise in animals with marked abdominal distension. Replacement fluid and electrolyte therapy is initiated before surgery and is continued well into the postoperative period. Electrolyte abnormalities in this disease are typical and replacement with physiologic saline solution is indicated unless determined values dictate otherwise. The foal should be treated with broad-spectrum antibiotics before surgery and maintained on such treatment for a minimum of 5 days after surgery.

Because body heat is lost in the withdrawal of large quantities of fluid from the peritoneal cavity over a short period, use of a heating pad, an infrared lamp or hot-water bottles may be advisable if the ambient temperature is low.[26] Fluids should be readily available for IV infusion to maintain blood pressure. For these same reasons, the general anesthetic used should have the least possible depressant effect on vital functions. Despite frequent reference in the literature to the use of IV phenothiazine tranquilizers and barbiturate anesthetics, an-

esthesia in a depressed foal can be easily induced by the administration of halothane with a mask. After a shallow plane of anesthesia is induced, it can be maintained through an endotracheal tube, which permits assisted ventilation by hand-bagging or by machine and prevents aspiration pneumonia. Initial preparation of the ventral abdominal wall for aseptic surgery should be done prior to anesthesia if this is possible without undue struggling of the patient. Once anesthesia is induced, final preparation of the surgical site, including draping, should be accomplished without delay.

The preferred position for the procedure is dorsal recumbency, with the animal tilted toward the hindquarters. This relieves any fluid pressure on the diaphragm and facilitates drainage of the peritoneal cavity, once opened. The line of incision is midline in females. In males, a right paramedian incision is made beside the prepuce and extended caudad to the prepubic tendon. In males, the incision passes through the skin, superficial and deep abdominal fascia, rectus abdominis muscle and its sheath of aponeurotic fibers from the 2 oblique abdominal muscles and the transversus abdominis muscle, fatty fascia transversalis and peritoneum. Hemorrhage can be a problem in the paramedian incision and careful hemostasis should be exercised. Urine should be removed slowly from the peritoneal cavity by positioning and suction. Rapid removal precipitates hypotension caused by rapid filling of capillary beds previously compressed by abdominal fluid pressure. The newborn foal's elongated, fusiform bladder is easily identified and accessible. The rent is usually found on the dorsal surface at the urachal end.

The abdominal cavity should be thoroughly explored before the bladder is repaired. Special attention should be given to the urachus, umbilical vein and arteries, kidneys, ureters and pelvic urethra, which should be examined for abnormalities. The peritoneal cavity is cleansed, using additional lavage and suction. The bladder is identified and stay sutures are placed for its manipulation. A self-retaining abdominal retractor may be placed and the intestines packed craniad with saline-moistened towels or laparotomy pads to improve exposure. Both the dorsal and ventral surfaces of the bladder should be evaluated in all cases since tears in each location may occur. The edges of the tear are debrided as necessary and the rent is closed with 2 inverting layers of 00 chromic catgut or synthetic absorbable suture.

It is important to distinguish between a suture closure of a sharply incised wound, as in a cystotomy, and that of a tear resulting from extreme internal pressure. A weak closure may result from suture placement too close to the edge of the defect. When the muscle layers fail under tension, separation and shredding of the fibers may extend beyond the margins of the rent itself. This may account for the recurrence of perforations adjacent to the suture line during the first 24-48 hours after surgery. To avoid such complications, suture bites should be taken well back into healthy tissues, going deeply enough to provide strong supporting limbs of the suture line. Tapered, rather than cutting-edge, needles should be used.

Although the risk of laparotomy wound dehiscence and eventration is not as great in foals as in adults, the predisposition to umbilical hernias and the patient's weakened resistance dictate good suture technic in laparotomy wound closure. The peritoneum may be sutured or not. If suturing is elected, it is convenient to include the deep sheath of the rectus abdominis muscle in the same row, taking care to exclude the retroperitoneal fat. The superficial sheath of the rectus provides the principal internal support and should be sutured separately with a simple or an overlapping mattress pattern with #1 polyglycolic acid, chromic catgut, monofilament polypropylene or equivalent. The superficial fascia can be closed separately or in conjunction with the skin closure. The skin is sutured with 0 or #1 polypropylene or equivalent in interrupted mattress or continuous interlocking pattern.

Placement of abdominal drains is optional, applications of bandages and placement of an indwelling urinary catheter are advisable, and administration of antibiotics and tetanus immunization is mandatory. Any drains, bandages and catheters used must be kept clean. Bandages must be changed frequently enough to keep the incision dry. Drain ports must be kept under sterile, absorbent packs or exhausted into self-contained suction packs, necessitating use of sump drains rather than Penrose tubing. Catheter ends must be protected with one-way valves, eg, a split latex surgical glove finger, to prevent aspiration of air and contaminants. Drains and catheters usually can be removed in 3-4 days. Fluid and electrolyte balance are closely monitored and appropriate supportive care is given as necessary. The prognosis is favorable in cases that are promptly diagnosed and treated.

A novel approach through a urethral sphincterotomy (see Cystic Calculi) was used to repair a rent in the bladder of a postpartum mare. The lesion, located near the neck of the bladder, was diagnosed by cystoscopy. Under short-acting general anesthesia, a single layer of simple-continuous sutures of 0 chromic catgut was used to close the wound. Urine in the peritoneal cavity was drained by multiple abdominocentesis. Recovery was complicated by a period of incontinence and urine-pooling (vesicovaginal reflux), as well as adhesions of the pelvic viscera.[26]

Patent Urachus

Clinical Signs: In the prenatal foal, the urachus serves as a cord-like conduit between the urinary bladder and the allantoic cavity. In normal animals, the urachus closes at or soon after birth and persists as a mass of cicatricial tissue at the apex of the urinary bladder.[30] In affected foals, the urachus persists as a patent tubular connection between the urinary bladder and the umbilicus. Either sex may be affected. The hair around the umbilicus may be continually wet with urine, and urine passes from the umbilicus as drops in the resting foal or as a steady stream when the foal micturates. Associated omphalophlebitis, septicemia, joint ill or retrograde cystitis may occur.[1,8] One author has stated that patent urachus is invariably accompanied by umbilical infection; it is not known whether urachal patency is a cause or result of infection.[31]

Treatment: A patent urachus may close spontaneously but, in most cases, treatment is indicated to assure rapid, complete closure. Treatment with broad-spectrum antibiotics is recommended to control local umbilical infection or cystitis and to reduce the chance of hematogenous infection. Local treatment consists of repeated cauterization of the urachus to create sufficient inflammatory reaction within the urachus to suspend urine flow. A silver nitrate applicator or a cotton swab soaked in 90% phenol, Lugol's iodine solution or tincture of iodine is passed into the urachus for a distance of 3-4 cm twice daily for several days. The urachus should close by the conclusion of this course of treatment.

Surgical resection of the urachus is indicated in those cases that are unresponsive to conservative therapy. The foal is lightly anesthetized and the urinary bladder is evacuated by an indwelling urinary catheter. The foal is placed in dorsal recumbency and the urachus is swabbed with disinfectant solution or, in cases with umbilical infection, the urachus and umbilical vessels are excluded from the site with sutures. The ventral abdomen is prepared and draped for aseptic surgery. An elliptical incision, centered over the umbilicus, is made to include all layers of the abdominal wall and free the umbilicus from the body wall. If necessary, the linea alba can be incised in either direction to improve exposure. The umbilical vessels are doubly ligated and the urachus and urinary bladder are identified. In animals with a cord-like urachus and a distinct junction between the urachus and urinary bladder, simple double ligation of the urachus near its junction with the bladder is adequate. In cases with overt infection of the urachus or in cases with a subtle transition from urachus to urinary bladder, resection of a portion of the apex of the bladder is indicated. The bladder is delivered to the incision and stabilized with stay sutures. The site is carefully packed off with moistened laparotomy pads. The portion of the apex of the bladder that contains the urachus is cross-clamped with heavy forceps and is transected on the bladder side of the forceps. The urachus and attached umbilicus are discarded. The bladder defect is closed in 2 layers with 00 chromic gut or, preferably, synthetic absorbable suture. A Cushing layer, oversewn with a Lembert pattern, provides satisfactory closure. Use of nonabsorbable suture material should be avoided in closure of the urinary bladder, especially if the sutures may penetrate the bladder mucosa, because of the risk of calculus formation about these sutures.

The body wall is closed with heavy absorbable suture in a simple-interrupted or near-far-far-near pattern. Closure of the skin and subcutaneous tissues is routine. The foal is maintained on parenteral antibiotics for a minimum of 5 days after surgery. An indwelling urinary catheter is not necessary in most cases.[1,8]

Prolapse of the Urinary Bladder

Cause: Vesical prolapse is an uncommon event that occurs either as an eversion through the short, distensible urethra of the mare or as a prolapse through the disrupted vaginal wall. In either case, it is usually a complication of foaling. Relaxation of supporting pelvic muscles and ligaments, regional edema, distension of sphincters and increased irritability in the birth canal all predispose to straining and prolapse.[8] In one mare, increased intra-abdominal pressure caused by torsion of the left colon 6 days postpartum resulted in prolapse of the bladder.[32] Causes may be unrelated to parturition. Rarely, the tenesmus seen in rabies may result in prolapse.

Diagnosis: The diagnosis is self-evident upon identification of the prolapsed organ protruding from the vulva. If it is not everted, confirmation can be made by needle aspiration of urine. If the bladder is everted, the pink mucosa of the bladder and the twin papilliform openings of the ureters on the dorsal surface of the neck of the viscus are characteristic.

Treatment: Management must first be directed at control of straining. This requires epidural anesthesia with 5-10 ml 2% lidocaine or mepivacaine, depending upon the size of the mare, and general sedation or tranquilization. Contaminated surfaces must be cleansed, necrotic or abraded tissues debrided, hemorrhage controlled, and distension decompressed. The edematous bladder wall is then carefully massaged until the bladder can be replaced in the pelvic cavity. In cases of bladder eversion, if the urethra will not distend sufficiently to permit replacement, sphincterotomy may be required. The sphincterotomy defect is closed with synthetic absorbable or chromic catgut sutures after bladder replacement. Defects in the vaginal wall permit similar repair. One case of long duration required amputation of the bladder just distal to the ureteral openings.[6]

Complications include reprolapse when straining returns after anesthesia subsides. To avert this, the mare should be heavily tranquilized, with appropriate analgesics applied topically (lidocaine or Nupercaine gel or ointment) and given systemically (xylazine, phenylbutazone). Placement of an indwelling balloon catheter to maintain decompression of the bladder and to medicate the bladder may be advisable. In this event use of a one-way catheter valve is imperative. Use of urinary antibiotics is recommended to control urinary infections and lessen the likelihood of pelvic cellulitis. Tetanus immunization is mandatory.

References

1. Walker, DF and Vaughan, JT: Bovine and Equine Urogenital Surgery. Lea & Febiger, Philadelphia, 1980.
2. Adams, LG *et al*. JAVMA **155** (1969) 518.
3. Blood, DC and Henderson, JA: Veterinary Medicine. 5th ed. Lea & Febiger, Philadelphia, 1979.

4. Kajesekhar, M and Keshavamurthy, BS. Vet Rec **99** (1976) 214.

5. Jackson, OF. Vet Rec **91** (1972) 7.

6. Frank, ER: Veterinary Surgery. 7th ed. Burgess Publ, Minneapolis, 1964.

7. Wright, JG and Neal, PA. Vet Rec **72** (1960) 301.

8. Lundvall, in Oehme and Prier: Textbook of Large Animal Surgery. Williams & Wilkins, Baltimore, 1974.

9. Walker, DF and Vaughan, JT: Bovine and Equine Urogenital Surgery. Lea & Febiger, Philadelphia, 1980.

10. Blood, DC et al: Veterinary Medicine. 5th ed. Lea & Febiger, Philadelphia, 1979.

11. Grunberg, W. Zbl Vet Med **18A** (1971) 767.

12. Sutor, DJ and Wooley, SE. Res Vet Sci **11** (1970) 299.

13. Berge, E and Westhues, M: Veterinary Operative Surgery. Williams & Wilkins, Baltimore, 1965.

14. Pezzoli, G and Masetti, L. Atti Della Soc Ital Delle Sci Vet **23** (1969) 342.

15. Nickel, R et al: The Viscera of the Domestic Mammal. 2nd ed. Springer-Verlag, New York, 1973.

16. Firth, EJ. Eq Vet J **8** (1976) 99.

17. Grier, RL. Vet Clin No Am **5** (1975) 415.

18. de Lahunta, A: Veterinary Neuroanatomy and Clinical Neurology. WB Saunders, Philadelphia, 1977.

19. Adams, LG et al. JAVMA **155** (1969) 518.

20. Van Campen, KR. JAVMA **156** (1970) 629.

21. Firth, EC. JAVMA **169** (1976) 800.

22. White, KK. J Eq Med Surg **1** (1977) 250.

23. Du Plessis, JL. J So Afr Vet Assoc **29** (1958) 261.

24. Bain, AM. Aust Vet J **30** (1954) 9.

25. Rooney, JR. Vet Path **8** (1971) 445.

26. Pascoe, RR. Aust Vet J **47** (1971) 343.

27. Leader, GH. Vet Rec **64** (1952) 241.

28. Behr, MJ et al. JAVMA **178** (1981) 263.

29. Meynard, JA. J Sm Anim Pract **2** (1961) 131.

30. Ellenport, in Getty: Sisson & Grossman's Anatomy of the Domestic Animals. 5th ed. WB Saunders, Philadelphia, 1975.

31. Roberts, SJ: Veterinary Obstetrics and Genital Diseases. 2nd ed. Edwards Bros, Ann Arbor, MI, 1971.

32. Donaldson, RW. Vet Rec **92** (1973) 409.

DISEASES OF THE URETHRA

Urethral obstruction, urethral trauma and ejaculatory hemorrhage of urethral origin are diseases limited to males.

Urethral Obstruction

Urethral obstruction is uncommon but may arise from a variety of causes, including urethral calculi, smegma accumulation in the urethral sinus, neoplastic or granulomatous diseases of the penis or urethral process, and accumulation of mucus in the urethra of neonates. Signs of urethral obstruction include colic, straining, prolapse of the penis, dribbling of urine and dysuria.[1-3] Diagnosis is by physical examination and urinary catheterization.

Urethral calculi are rare compared with the prevalence of cystic calculi.[1] A urethral calculus usually lodges in the pelvic urethra proximal to the ischial arch or in the distal penile urethra. A catheter should be passed to determine the level of obstruction. Calculi in the penile urethra may be removed with a hemostat or dislodged with a urinary catheter. Surgical removal by urethrotomy directly over the calculus may be necessary. If a calculus in the penile urethra cannot be retrieved or if severe urethral necrosis or trauma occurs, a permanent subischial urethrotomy may be necessary. Calculi in the pelvic urethra are removed by ischial urethrotomy as described for removal of cystic calculi (see Cystic Calculi).[2]

Preputial smegma may accumulate in the urethral sinus and become sufficient in size to cause urethral obstruction, especially in older horses.[1,4] Such accumulations are commonly called "beans" and are easily removed manually. Lesions of the glans penis or urethral process, such as squamous-cell carcinoma or *Habronema* granuloma, may cause urethral obstruction.[2,3] These are treated by penis amputation, amputation of the urethral process, or topical organophosphates, as indicated. Urethral obstruction by a mucus plug may cause straining and distension of the urinary bladder in neonatal male foals.[1] Such plugs frequently may be dislodged by urethral catheterization.

Urethral Trauma

Blunt or sharp trauma may cause urethral obstruction or laceration. Partial or complete urethral obstruction, due to periurethral inflammatory reaction or hematoma, is associated with acute traumatic paraphimosis or blunt injury, usually a kick to the penis in the area where it crosses the ischial arch. Treatment in such cases is directed toward control of swelling around the urethra. Fresh, clean urethral lacerations should be sutured with absorbable sutures. Tissues superficial to the urethra are ordinarily left unsutured to prevent urine entrapment in the wound. Infected or badly traumatized urethral wounds are best left unsutured. If urethral continuity is lost, healing should be allowed to occur over an indwelling urinary catheter.[2] Urethral stricture may complicate any wound of the urethra. Amputation of the distal portion of the penis may be indicated in severe penile wounds involving the urethra.

Ejaculatory Hemorrhage

Ejaculatory hemorrhage (hemospermia) causes infertility in breeding stallions.[5,6] Such hemorrhage is commonly of urethral origin and usually caused by bacterial urethritis or urethral stricture. Diagnosis is based upon endoscopic evaluation of the urethra and urinary bladder, contrast urethrography, and biopsy and culture of urethral lesions.

References

1. Lundvall, in Oehme and Prier: Textbook of Large Animal Surgery. Williams & Wilkins, Baltimore, 1974.
2. Walker, DF and Vaughan, JT: Bovine and Equine Urogenital Surgery. Lea & Febiger, Philadelphia, 1980.
3. Stick, JA. VM/SAC **74** (1979) 1453.
4. Guard, WR: Surgical Principles and Techniques. Edwards Bros, Ann Arbor, MI 1953.
5. Voss, JL and Pickett, BW. J Repro Fert **23** (1975) 151.
6. Voss, JL and Wotowey, JL. Proc 18th Ann Mtg Am Assoc Eq Pract, 1972. p 103.

TUMORS OF THE URINARY TRACT

Renal Carcinoma

The most common neoplasm of the equine kidney is the renal-cell carcinoma. These tumors arise from dedifferentiation of cortical tubular epithelial cells and typically are quite large by the time a diagnosis is made. The presenting clinical signs vary, the most prominent of which may be massive ascites due to multiple tumor implants on the serosal surface of the abdominal organs, diaphragm and omentum. In other cases, tumor growth into the renal pelvis, with erosion of blood vessels, leads to frank hematuria. There is no evidence of dysuria and characteristically the greatest concentration of blood comes during the last part of the urine stream. In addition to RBC and protein, the urine contains numerous neutrophils, but tumor cells are difficult to identify.

The most important diagnostic feature in primary renal-cell carcinoma is the presence of an abdominal mass, which in some cases can be palpated in the paralumbar fossa. Tumor masses can be located during rectal examination in the sublumbar area caudal to the expected location of either the left or right kidney. Although solitary renal tumors have been removed from dogs, the advanced stage of development prior to clinical recognition precludes effective surgical treatment in most horses.

Transitional-Cell Carcinoma

Transitional-cell carcinoma of the bladder is very unusual in horses. The presenting history is typically one of progressive dysuria, with variable hematuria. Clinically the transitional-cell carcinoma can be confused with cystic calculi. With the latter, one or more concretions can be palpated by rectal examination. With transitional-cell carcinoma, the mass(es) has the consistency of firm tissue and metastases to regional pelvic lymph nodes may also be palpated.

19

The Muscular System

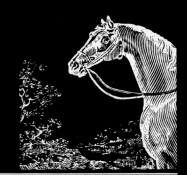

by E. Waldron-Mease, C.W. Raker and E.P. Hammel

As the name implies, the skeletal muscles of the body attach directly or indirectly to bone or cartilage and comprise the voluntary muscle system. Locomotion and maintenance of body posture depend in part on this huge mass of tissue. One must constantly refer to the nervous and skeletal systems when considering the normal function or disease of muscles. Although primary muscle disease in the horse is uncommon, when one encounters a muscular malfunction it is necessary to characterize the disease to differentiate among primary myopathy, neuromyopathy and a musculoskeletal problem.

Anatomy and Physiology

A brief review of the anatomy, biochemistry and physiology of skeletal muscle is necessary to establish a background for further discussion. Skeletal muscle is composed of long fibers (cells) that run essentially parallel to the long axis of the muscle. The whole muscle is covered by connective tissue fascia, which also branches centrally to divide the muscle into parallel bundles of fibers called fasciculi (Fig 1). These fasciculi are visible grossly and give the muscle its marbled appearance on cross section.

The muscle fiber (Fig 1c) is the cellular unit of the muscle. It is a long, multinucleated cell 10-100 μ in diameter that can be isolated under the dissecting microscope. Within each muscle fiber are numerous cylindric myofibrils (Fig 1d), each of which is composed of a highly ordered arrangement of myofilaments that are strands of contractile proteins (Fig 1e). The thick filaments are composed of many molecules of the protein myosin and the thin filaments are composed largely of molecules of actin, troponin and tropomyosin. Portions of myosin molecules protrude from the thick filaments to form cross bridges that probably in-

teract with surrounding thin filaments when contraction takes place.

Much is known about the structural conformation of skeletal muscle during contraction, but for this review it is sufficient to say that the interdigitating thick and thin filaments slide past each other. The cross bridges of the thick filaments are believed to alternately bind and release at successive sites along the thin filaments to cause movement of the filaments. When the thick and thin filaments overlap each other maximally, there is maximal shortening. Conversely, when the filaments are overlapped minimally, there is maximal lengthening. Each sarcomere or contractile unit, extending from Z line to Z line, actually shortens only a minute amount; however, when this is added to the shortening of the many sarcomeres that make up the length of the myofibril, the effect is profound. All the myofibrils of a fiber contract simultaneously. This causes the fiber to contract and, of course, the contractions of the fibers are what causes the whole muscle to contract.

When stained or specially illuminated, the muscle fiber appears to have striations extending across it. Figure 2 illustrates how these striations originate from the interdigitating pattern of the myofilaments. The most dense regions are where the thick and thin filaments actually overlap and the least dense regions are where there are only thin filaments. The alternating dense and light patterns along the myofibril correlate with those of adjacent myofibrils so that the patterns seem to extend from one side to the other and give the fiber its characteristic striated appearance.

A complex membrane called the sarcolemma surrounds the muscle fiber and contains the cytoplasm (sarcoplasm) of the cell (Fig 2). Beneath the sarcolemma lie flat cell nuclei. Throughout the sarcoplasm, among the myofibrils, are the mitochondria. These organelles

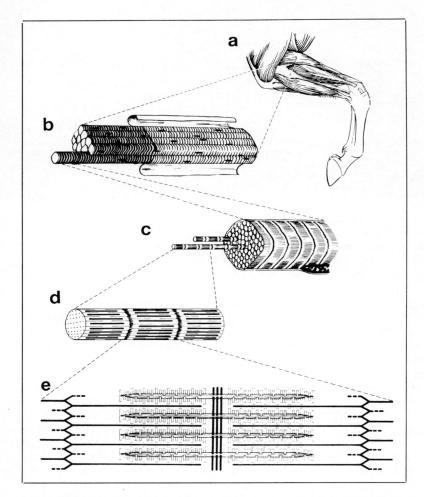

Fig 1. Schematic diagram of the microscopic structure of skeletal muscle: a, whole muscles covered with fascia; b, portion of a muscle fasciculus with fascia reflected to show muscle fibers and nuclei; c, portion of a muscle fiber with 2 isolated myofibrils; d, portion of a myofibril showing thick and thin filaments, and Z lines; e, detail of a sarcomere showing Z lines from which thin filaments originate. The cross bridges protrude from the thick filaments in a Lelical arrangement. In the region of overlap, each thick filament is surrounded by 6 thin filaments. (Drawing by KM Friedenberg)

are associated with metabolic reactions that involve molecular O_2, such as oxidative phosphorylation and Krebs cycle reactions.

The sarcoplasm contains the numerous ions and molecules necessary for energy production and contraction. Substances of major importance include Ca, K, Mg, Na, phosphocreatine and adenosine triphosphate (ATP). Also present are glycogen, the storage form of carbohydrate, and myoglobin, a pigmented respiratory protein. Enzymes are found in the mitochondria and sarcoplasm; certain of them can be of diagnostic significance.

Being selectively permeable to certain ions, the sarcolemma maintains a resting membrane potential and also propagates the action potential necessary for initiation of contraction. A transverse tubular system is continuous with the sarcolemma and conducts the action potential inward from the surface of the fiber. This conduction property of the tubular system allows excitation to spread rapidly to

all parts of the fiber, causing all the myofibrils within the fiber to contract at once.

The sarcoplasmic reticulum is a complex closed system of tubules surrounding the myofibrils. It consists of 2 confluent components, the longitudinal sarcotubules and the terminal cisternae. The terminal cisternae have intimate contact with the transverse tubules extending inward from the surface of the cell.

Chemical reactions must produce the energy the muscle converts into useful work during the contractile process. Although all details are not known, ATP is the basic fuel for contraction. As the ATP is metabolized, it must constantly be replaced and the rate of replacement must match or exceed the rate of use if contraction is to continue. This is accomplished by a number of different ATP-producing reactions available to the muscle. An extremely rapid mechanism operates when the compound phosphocreatine (PCr), which is present in muscle, transfers its phosphoryl group to adenosine diphosphate (ADP) and reforms ATP. This reaction is catalyzed by the enzyme creatine phosphokinase.

Stores of PCr are used within a few seconds during vigorous work and glycolytic metabolic reactions involving glycogen and glucose must occur quickly to supply additional ATP. Glycogen stored in the muscle is broken down and, after exhausting exercise, there is very little remaining in the muscle. There have been several reported cases in humans in which muscle weakness or rapid tiring has been associated with defects in the enzymes of the glycolytic pathway. In these cases muscle glycogen is not metabolized and there are abnormally high levels in the muscle.

In addition to ATP, glycolysis produces pyruvate that is either converted into lactate or enters the Krebs cycle. When glycolysis is proceeding rapidly and a limited amount of O_2 is available to the muscle, a high percentage of pyruvate is converted to lactate by a reaction catalyzed by lactate dehydrogenase. Although these reactions are fast, they are inefficient. The ATP yielded from the conversion of carbohydrate to lactate is small. If the demands for ATP are less and sufficient O_2 is available, most pyruvate enters the Krebs cycle and undergoes oxidative phosphorylation where high ATP yields are achieved for the amount of glucose initially metabolized. This aerobic metabolism makes the most efficient use of carbohydrate but is relatively slow. When muscle is at rest or doing minimal work, most energy is supplied by the oxidation of stored fats. Fat is metabolized by the Krebs cycle and oxidative phosphorylation, resulting in high yields of ATP.

Muscle fibers are innervated by motor neurons located in the ventral horn of the spinal cord grey matter. The nerve cell, axon and terminal branches, and related muscle fibers are considered a single motor unit. The number of fibers contained within a motor unit is related to the function of the muscle. Muscles involved in precise movements, such as eye muscles, have the fewest number of fibers per motor unit, whereas muscles concerned with gross movements have larger motor units. The fibers of one motor unit are usually scattered among the fibers of other motor units. However, the fibers of one unit function separately from those of a different unit. All fibers of one unit contract almost simultaneously in a twitch-like action, but the motor units within a muscle contract asynchronously. The result of this continuous shower of twitches at different fre-

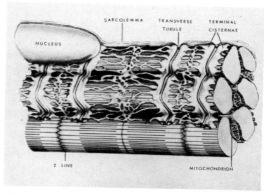

Fig 2. Schematic drawing of the internal structure of a skeletal muscle fiber. The transverse tubules course along the myofibrils at the level of the ends of the thick filaments. The sarcoplasmic reticulum ramifies over the myofibrils and the terminal cisternae are closely apposed to the transverse tubules. (Drawing by KM Friedenberg)

quencies is a smooth contraction of the whole muscle.

When an impulse travels down the motor neuron axon and arrives at the specialized neuromuscular junction, it causes the release of acetylcholine. Acetylcholine changes the membrane potential of the sarcolemma and excites an action potential. Inward spread of excitation along the transverse tubules results in the release of Ca from the terminal cisternae into the sarcoplasm. This increase of Ca ion concentration activates the contractile process by releasing inhibition of myosin-actin interaction.

The enzymatic ATPase activity of the myosin molecule is activated to split ATP and thereby release energy necessary for the sliding of filaments. When Ca is recaptured by the sarcotubules of the sarcoplasmic reticulum, ATPase is inactivated and the muscle fiber relaxes. Acetylcholine at the neuromuscular junction has in the meantime been broken down by acetylcholinesterase, removing primary excitation and allowing the sarcolemma and transverse tubules to repolarize. This repolarization is characterized by Ca removal from the sarcoplasm. The muscle fiber is now susceptible to another action potential and contraction.

Muscle cells, as other types of cells, respond to injury in a limited number of ways. The end result of insult to muscle, if sufficiently great, is grossly evident atrophy of the affected group(s). It is important to classify the underlying cause as this may determine to what degree muscle can be reasonably expected to return to normal form or function.

Local muscle atrophy caused by skeletal disease may be related only to disuse. Histologically, disused muscle fibers appear shrunken but otherwise normal. Return to full use and size is possible if the offending lesion and/or associated pain are alleviated. Permanent changes in disused muscles are more likely related to contracture of tendinous structures than to muscle dysfunction or damage.

Muscle atrophy secondary to loss of innervation has a prognosis directly related to recovery of nervous tissue function, which exerts considerable trophic effects on muscle in addition to initiation and integration of movement. Severance or other severe damage to a large nerve proximal to its entry into a muscle results in severe atrophy and loss of function. Damage to the facial nerve as it crosses the mandible or to the supraspinatus nerve ("sweeny") are well-known examples. Histologic findings of muscle in these extreme cases are quite similar to those of disuse atrophy. If nerve damage is not complete, the more classic histologic lesions of denervation may be evident, with well-circumscribed islands of normal muscle fibers interspersed with atrophied groups on cross section.

The repair process after denervation involves proliferation of remaining nerve endings to re-establish contact with adjacent denervated muscle fibers. This process has limited potential. Histologic examination reveals increased numbers of normal-sized muscle fiber groups. Histochemically these fibers are identical to unaffected, innervated muscle fibers. Hypertrophy of unaffected, innervated muscle fibers may also occur in time, restoring mass without increasing the actual number of muscle cells.

The prognosis for return to normal function depends primarily upon the original role of the muscle. Muscles requiring fine motor control, such as ocular muscles, are least likely to resume normal function if restoration of nervous function is less than complete. Damage to critical muscles of locomotion, such as the brachiocephalicus, and of motion and support, such as the adductor pectoral group, produces obvious gait deficits; prognosis is guarded to poor in such cases. Prognosis for use is best for muscles, such as the gluteals, in which a return to essentially normal function may occur even when the muscle group does not regain its original mass.

Direct insult of biochemical, mechanical or inflammatory origin may cause temporary disruption of muscle cell membrane and organelle functions, or may be of sufficient severity to cause rhabdomyolysis (muscle cell destruction). Histologic changes may range from slight pallor of cells to membrane rupture and/or loss of cross striation. Cellular response varies markedly from essentially no inflammatory response to varying degrees of round-cell, neutrophil or eosinophil infiltration.

Muscle cells repair themselves by increasing their metabolic activity, as do all cells. This phase is characterized histologically by increased basophilia of affected muscle cells on light microscopy, which is correlated with increased mitochondrial and sarcoplasmic reticulum activity. Muscle cell nuclei, which normally lie outside the sarcolemma, may move intracellularly, although in a series of postoperative and exercise-induced myopathies studied over a 2-year period this was not a prominent feature.

Muscle has very limited regenerative capacity. Cells may hypertrophy to double or triple their original diameter, and some fiber-splitting has been observed. Generally, massive muscle damage results in fibrous and/or fatty infiltration, and atrophy of the affected group.

Our knowledge of the basic properties of the muscular system far exceeds our ability to transfer this knowledge to the diagnosis and treatment of disease conditions. One slight malfunction in this complex structure and sequence of events is a potential cause of disease.

Examination of the Muscular System

Physical Examination

Examining the muscular system is difficult, and very little can be found about it in the veterinary literature. The human literature is replete with discussions of muscle diseases, but still little has been written about a systematic method for examining this system. The major problem is to characterize muscle lesions, in fact to decide whether they are muscle lesions at all, and to determine if they are myogenic or neurogenic in origin.

The initial examination should include an evaluation of the size, shape, tone, consistency, temperature and sensitivity of the muscles. An attempt should be made to determine the extent of the lesions, whether part of a muscle, a total muscle, a group of associated muscles, a whole limb or the total body musculature is involved. Whether the lesions are bilateral or unilateral is significant.

Muscle size is influenced by many factors. This tissue has the capacity to hypertrophy with exercise; individual muscle fibers increase in diameter due to an increase in the total number of myofibrils as well as in various nutrient and intermediary metabolic substances. The type of exercise is important in determining the degree of muscular hypertrophy. Contractions of maximal force, such as isometric exercise, even though sustained for only several seconds per day, are the most efficient for developing muscular strength. Repetitive, dynamic, forceful exercise, such as pulling weight, enhances both strength and muscle bulk. Relatively mild muscular activity, such as jogging or swimming, even though sustained for long periods of time, does very little to increase muscle size. This type of activity greatly enhances the endurance of muscles by increasing the efficiency of blood supply, O_2 utilization and rate of removing metabolic end products. Physiologic hypertrophy must be distinguished from pathologic states, such as myotonia, in which the muscles appear grossly hypertrophied but actually contain considerable fat and fibrous tissue (Fig 3).

A muscle decreases in size when it is not used or when used only for weak contractions. Neurogenic atrophy is the result of denervation, but nonneurogenic atrophy or wasting of muscle bulk may be due to decreased muscle use because of joint ankylosis, splinting or decreased weight-bearing due to pain. Some muscles, such as the gluteus medius, infraspinatus and supraspinatus, atrophy more rapidly than other muscles of the limbs. Studies in various species have shown that certain muscles are more susceptible or resistant than others to atrophy resulting from denervation. For example, the small muscles of the larynx atrophy quickly and become markedly shrunken within 2 weeks following section of the recurrent laryngeal nerve.[1]

In cases of muscle denervation, several clinical signs may be present. Voluntary muscle control is absent and the affected muscle group is flaccid. Muscle tone and tendon reflexes are diminished or absent. Fibrillations (spontaneous activity from single muscle fibers) begin to occur a few days after denervation. These fine contractions are not visible through the skin but are sometimes seen with reflected light on the surface of muscle. This activity continues for several months until fiber degeneration becomes extensive or reinnervation occurs. Spontaneous twitch contractions in motor

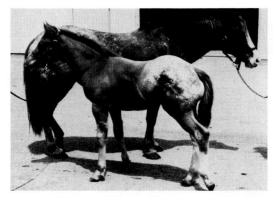

Fig 3. A 4-month-old filly with myotonia. Note the well-developed musculature of the hindquarters. (Courtesy of Dr W Moyer, Unionville, PA)

units are termed fasciculations. These are visible through the skin and are distinguishable from the smaller, more rapid contractions of fibrillation. Fasciculation indicates abnormal excitability in an intact motor unit. In muscle that has partially lost its motor innervation, this rhythmic twitching commonly occurs during mild contraction but ceases when the muscle is completely relaxed.

If reinnervation occurs during the first 3-4 months after denervation, recovery and full function of the muscle can be expected. If denervation persists for a longer period, the muscle fiber degeneration and replacement by fat and fibrous tissue will have progressed to such a degree that the muscle is unable to resume normal function. Fortunately, muscles usually function as a group and, despite some denervation, other muscles of the group may support the function of the denervated muscle and maintain overall function of a limb. When denervation and atrophy of the gluteus medius occur, the biceps femoris, semitendinosus and semimembranosus muscles can assume its action of extending the hip. A slight gait deficit usually results but the horse's usefulness may be relatively unaffected.

Attempts to delay or prevent muscle atrophy or wasting by direct electrical stimulation of the nerves and muscles have had varied success in human and veterinary medicine. It undoubtedly has greatest merit when nerve supply to a muscle is temporarily interrupted or when one is trying to minimize temporary muscle wasting due to confinement or splinting.[2]

The normal shape of a muscle may be altered due to atrophy of a local area, rupture of muscle fascia with prolapse of underlying fibers, rup-

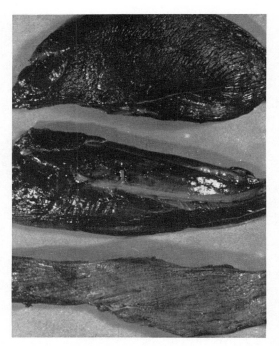

Fig 4. Normal skeletal muscle (top), moderately affected muscle, and severely affected muscle (bottom).

ture of the muscle fibers themselves, or rupture of the muscle tendon or its attachment. Atrophy of a portion of muscle may occur when the muscle is innervated by a number of nerves and the lesion causing the denervation is localized to one or a few of these nerves. Denervation atrophy of the gluteus medius is often most severe in the middle and caudal portions of the muscle, with the cranial portion being relatively unaffected grossly (Fig 4).

Myalgia is perceived in all voluntary and involuntary muscles. When muscles are pricked with a needle or cut with a sharp knife, the pain is slight; when the muscle is injected with an irritating substance or crushed, the pain is severe. One of the most common causes of muscle pain in humans is overexercise, particularly by those not used to strenuous exercise. The pain and soreness develop hours and even days after exercise. It is speculated that important contributing causes of this pain are overextension of muscles, with the resultant strain on muscle sheaths and tendons, and changes in intracellular and extracellular metabolites. Muscle pain is apparent in the early stages of equine influenza and other systemic infections. A defective blood supply to an area or limb may cause muscle pain but signs appear while the muscles are functioning and not while at rest.

The local [133]xenon-clearance method enables measurement of muscle blood flow during exercise. It involves injecting ^{133}Xe into muscles and measuring the isotope's clearance with scintillation detectors attached to the limb. In human patients with occlusive vascular diseases, this method has been useful in demonstrating abnormalities of blood flow.[3] There are no reports of using this technic in clinical veterinary medicine but it is being used experimentally and may eventually become a diagnostic procedure.

Laboratory Methods

Laboratory tests are often helpful in characterizing and classifying muscle lesions. These methods include determination of serum enzyme activity, biopsy and electromyography.

Serum Enzymes: The activity of several enzymes is increased in horses suffering myogenic disease or muscle trauma. Three have been found most useful: creatine phosphokinase (CPK), lactate dehydrogenase (LDH) and serum glutamate oxaloacetate transaminase (SGOT). Most research on the clinical significance of these enzymes has been done in cases of equine exertional myopathy and myopathies of nutritional origin.[4-6] Some general knowledge of the properties of these enzymes is necessary for their proper evaluation.

Enzymes may be of diagnostic value because of their specific chemical activity and their presence in specific tissues of the body. When a tissue is damaged or its metabolism altered so that increased amounts of enzymes leak from the tissue, tissue loss is reflected by increased serum levels of the enzymes. Several factors, such as the enzyme's location within the cell and constituent binding, affect the release rate of the enzyme from the cell. Mechanisms determining the rate of enzyme loss from serum are not known but destruction by the reticuloendothelial system, hepatic metabolism and renal excretion must be considered.

Some enzymes, such as LDH, are found in several tissues but tissue specificity can be assigned by studying the isoenzymes (isozymes). Lactate dehydrogenase is composed of at least 5 isozymes that are slightly different in physical properties, but all are capable of catalyzing the same chemical reaction. This slight property difference makes it possible to separate and identify the isozymes by technics such as electrophoresis (Fig 5). Tissues differ in their LDH_1 content, and skeletal muscle and liver, which are capable of anaerobic metabolism, contain high levels of LDH_5.[7]

Many recommendations have been made as to the best method for handling the blood sample to be assayed for enzyme activity. As RBC are high in LDH, it is important that there is no hemolysis in the sample. Studies of stability of different enzymes at room, refrigeration and freezer temperatures have resulted in varied conclusions. With horse blood very reliable results can be obtained for CPK, total LDH, LDH isozymes and SGOT by using the following procedure. The blood is collected carefully to avoid hemolysis. A firm clot is allowed to form within 1½-2 hours and then the sample is centrifuged. The serum is removed, frozen quickly and stored in a freezer until the assay can be performed, preferably within a week. Freezing serum does not alter its total enzyme or isozyme activity significantly. Samples with high activity can be grossly abused—left at room temperature for several days, thawed and refrozen several times, and stored for long periods—and they still reflect elevated levels clinically significant for substantiating a diagnosis of muscle damage. While improper handling of samples is discouraged, it sometimes is unavoidable in a clinical circumstance and it is helpful to know that an abused sample is not valueless.

A source of considerable confusion is the variety of different assay methods available for the same enzyme. One method may evaluate the enzyme activity in units unrelated to the units used in another method. Therefore, one must know the methods used when comparing data and the normal levels for that method.

Interpretation of serum enzyme levels in horses at rest must be done with caution and knowledge of enzyme kinetics and specificity, as well as familiarity with the animal's daily routine and stage of training. Elevated SGOT and serum CPK levels during the intensive end stages of training have been reported. One study on SGOT levels during training and competition revealed a return of SGOT levels to pretraining or lower than pretraining levels in horses that performed well or exceptionally well, respectively.[5] Horses with persistently high SGOT levels did not work well and developed clinical signs of rhabdomyolysis ("tying-up") in some instances. A resting serum CPK level of 600 IU/L in a hard-working horse with clinical signs of muscle pain and/or damage may be difficult to interpret without comparison with prior enzyme test results or serum CPK levels after exercise (see below).[5,8,9] Apparently inconsistent results for serum enzyme

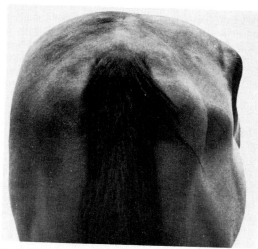

Fig 5. Muscle atrophy over the right hip 4 months after a severe attack of exertional myopathy with myoglobinuria. Even at this stage, the horse could jump well. There was significant improvement in the gross appearance of the area within a year of the episode.

levels, as obtained by various investigators, can be traced to differences in the intensity and duration of exercise and the use of varying sampling intervals.[8-10]

Acute muscle damage causes marked elevation in the serum activity of these enzymes, whereas in a slow progressive condition enzyme activity could be within the normal range. Myopathy of nutritional origin may be present for some time with no clinical signs and only mildly elevated serum enzyme activity. When exertion is suddenly required, the diseased muscle is unable to meet the stress and overt clinical signs and high serum enzyme levels occur.

Serum Electrolytes and Acid-Base Status: Elevated serum K and P levels occur with severe rhabdomyolysis because these ions are present in high concentrations in skeletal muscle. Altered serum Ca or Mg levels affect the electrical potential of the muscle cell membrane, causing hyperexcitability when serum levels are low and reduced excitability when serum levels are high.

Ammonia is normally produced by skeletal muscle as an end-product of purine metabolism. Plasma ammonia levels are normally elevated during and after exercise. In human sports medicine, the ratio of lactate to ammonia produced is used as an indirect measurement of relative anaerobic and aerobic activity.[11] This is a potentially useful tool for use in horses, although normal equine values have not been established. Blood for ammonia level determination must be collected in a heparinized tube and the plasma immediately separated and frozen.

A substitute for direct measurement of serum lacate is calculation of the anion gap using the following equation: anion gap = $([Na^+]$ + $[CO_2^-])$ + $([Cl^-]$ + $[CO_2^-])$. This method has the advantage of simple sample handling. Only 5 ml serum are required compared with the more cumbersome collection of blood into perchloric acid for lactate analysis. The calculated anion gap is expressed in mmol/L and represents the contribution to acid-base balance of all organic anions, such as lactate and pyruvate products of anaerobic metabolism.

Interpretation of serum electrolyte, enzyme and acid-base changes with exercise and/or disease requires an understanding of basic exercise physiology and establishment of normal control values. Transient rises in SGOT and serum CPK levels have been documented in horses during intensive training, but these levels usually return to normal as training continues.[5,8] A submaximal exercise test of 10 minutes at a trot has been used as an aid in interpretation of borderline serum CPK levels and to diagnose suspected myopathy cases.[10,12] Blood samples for CPK assay are collected before exercise, 5 minutes postexercise and 1 hour postexercise. Normal horses, both trained and untrained, have doubled or tripled serum CPK levels 5 minutes postexercise and have serum CPK levels equal to pre-exercise levels at 1 hour postexercise.[13] Many clinically normal horses with histories suggestive of myopathy have abnormal serum CPK curves when subjected to the submaximal exercise test. In most cases the test does not precipitate clinical signs. If desired, the anion gap and serum lactate and plasma ammonia levels can also be determined at the above 3 intervals. One horse with internal iliac thrombosis had a markedly increased anion gap (metabolic acidosis) following exercise.[10,12]

Biopsy: Microscopic examination of muscle can yield useful information if the specimens are carefully taken.[14] Excised tissue can be studied by light and electron microscopy. Various staining procedures differentiate structural components, and biochemical and histochemical technics are used to study the tissue's metabolism and to detect enzyme defects. The technics employed determine the best way for the tissue sample to be collected. For example, tissue must be frozen immediately when obtained for histochemical analysis. If possible, the pathologist who will examine the tissue sections should be consulted about the exact procedures to be followed.

Some general guidelines can be offered for obtaining useful muscle biopsies. The sample should be taken from a site of active disease, but severely diseased muscle is too friable and should be avoided. Ideally, both diseased and normal tissues are taken from the same muscle for comparison. The operation can be performed under local anesthesia, with care taken not to inject the anesthetic into the muscle. The incision should be long enough to obtain a piece of muscle approximately 2.0 cm by 0.7 cm by 0.7 cm. The fibers are dissected longitudinally with a sharp scalpel, carefully avoiding undue stretching, tearing or crushing of tissue. The specimen is fixed at rest length. One of the simplest ways of doing this is to lay a sterile applicator stick parallel to the fibers and tie the ends of the sample to the stick before excising the sample. The stick prevents the fibers from contracting when the ends of the sample beyond the ties are cut. It also prevents distortion when the tissue is placed in a fixative or is frozen. Muscle clamps are specifically manufactured for biopsy procedures, but they are expensive and unnecessary.

Various needles, forceps and drills have been devised for taking muscle samples but their use is generally not advised for critical evaluation of tissue morphology because the samples obtained are small and the fibers are often distorted.[15-19] Some authors believe that excellent samples can be obtained with a needle if care is taken in trimming and orienting the sample.[19] The advantages of a needle biopsy are obvious. The sample can be obtained quickly through a small stab incision with minimal trauma to the horse. Most owners, while extremely reluctant to allow open surgical biopsies, often agree to needle biopsies. The small amount of tissue obtained with a needle is not a great disadvantage for many of the biochemical assays done. Samples of 20-30 mg can be assayed with modern microtechnics.

Although postbiopsy complications are uncommon, dehiscence can be a problem if the biopsy specimen is removed from an area subjected to motion. Flushing the biopsy site with an antibiotic-saline solution is recommended when strict asepsis is not possible, as with standing biopsies. A 2-layer closure of the fascia and skin using horizontal mattress sutures of 0 catgut and 0 or #1 nonabsorbable material, respectively, has proven most effective.

Electromyography: This technic involves the observation and evaluation of the electrical activity of muscle. The basic electronic equipment required for this technic includes an oscilloscope and an audio amplifier. Electrical signals picked up from needle electrodes inserted into the muscle are amplified and displayed for visual observation as a function of time on the oscilloscope screen and for aural impression via the audio amplifier. Special needle electrodes are available in a wide variety of types from a number of manufacturers. Considerable thought should go into needle selection since size and configuration greatly alter the shape and magnitude of observed signals. Bare needles, such as 20-ga or larger hypodermic needles or scalp electrodes used in EEG recording, are generally unsuitable because of the large surface area from which they record.

Detailed evaluations of the electrical activity recorded in EMG studies require considerable experience. However, some basic and general observations can be made even by the inexperienced. To begin, muscle fibers are excitable tissue and electrical action potentials are part of their normal function. These action potentials are a part only of working muscle and should be absent in normal muscle that is completely at rest (unstimulated). Therefore, while electrical activity in muscle used to support a limb would be considered normal, such activity in an unloaded muscle or muscle in an anesthetized animal, should be considered a sign of disease. To be concise, electrical activity recorded from muscle in an anesthetized animal after needle electrode movement has ceased is pathologic. This is the simplest level of application of EMG studies and is often the most rewarding since it enables the investigator to localize and biopsy pathologic areas of muscle for detailed histologic evaluation.

In human medicine much detailed information is extracted from analyses of the waveforms of electrical activity observed in resting muscle or in muscle contracting at various tension levels. In veterinary EMG the level of sophistication in analysis of active muscle patterns does not permit any cogent observations at this time. However, without much difficulty one can learn to distinguish certain patterns of activity seen in resting diseased muscle. The most common form of pathologic activity is produced by muscle denervated for a week or longer. The pattern seen with denervation may include many kinds of wave forms but is best characterized by "fibrillation potentials." These are small potentials that are for the most part monophasic, *ie*, they are in one direction only on the oscilloscope screen. The magnitude of these potentials is about 200 μv or less, and they are of short duration (< 5 m Sec). These potentials are thought to arise from the firing of single muscle fibers with unstable membrane characteristics produced by denervation. Because they are random and monophasic, they are associated with the firing of individual hyperexcitable muscle fibers known to exist in denervation. To the ear, the randomness and single polarity of these potentials produce the impression of crackling and sizzling.

The fibrillation potential is the simplest of all waveforms. There are many more complex forms that may be seen on the oscilloscope screen. The motor unit, which may be seen in lightly anesthetized or awake animals, is much larger and more complex than the fibrillation potential. This potential is thought to arise from the quasisynchronous firing of all muscle fibers of a motor unit near the area of the active parts of the recording electrodes. These potentials are multiphasic. They change polarity several times within the waveform. This multipolarity is thought to be due to the algebraic summation of nearly synchronous firing of fibers located on both sides of the recording electrodes. They are further distinguished from fibrillation potentials by their characteristic rhythmicity, which is extremely regular. Perhaps the most easily recognized abnormal pattern of electrical activity is the myotonic pattern. This pattern is multiphasic like the motor unit but is much more rapid, perhaps because of the addition of several units firing all at once but in different phase. The amplitudes and frequencies of these units wax and wane to produce a characteristic "divebomber" pattern in the audio portion of the display. Its description is further detailed in the section on myotonia.

Histochemical Analysis: Histochemical analysis involves staining a sample of muscle for assay of specific enzyme activity. Muscle fibers are classified as slow-twitch (Group I) or fast-twitch (Group II) by the intensity of staining with oxidative enzymes such as ATPase, Na ATPase and NADH. Since histochemical typing may vary within the same muscle belly, the technic is theoretically useful for differentiating neurogenic and myopathic etiologies of dysfunction and/or atrophy, and in diagnosis of specific deficiency states.

If facilities are available, live muscle can be examined *in vitro* for response to chemical stimulation. Equine muscle defects documented by histochemical technics include malignant hyperthermia susceptibility and myotonia congenita.

Localized Myositis

Inflammation of skeletal muscle in the horse is most commonly caused by direct or indirect trauma. In the acute state, affected muscles are sensitive when palpated and there is increased heat, swelling and firmness. The signs usually are apparent for several days to several weeks. Chronic myositis can lead to muscle wasting and, therefore, may resemble atrophy from other causes. Muscle biopsy may help identify the character of the pathologic process.

Myositis is frequently secondary to an active degenerative disease of bones or joints. Such lesions of the thoracic, lumbar or sacral vertebrae (including their dorsal processes) or subluxation of the sacroiliac articulation may lead to secondary inflammation of back muscles. Frequently the primary lesion is in the bones or joints of one or both hindlegs. Lesions of the tarsus and stifle especially are likely to cause signs of myositis. There are cases in which inflammation of back muscles is apparently related to ill-fitting equipment, such as improperly adjusted hobbles, or to the horse's faulty manner of movement.

Inflammation of the longissimus dorsi, psoas and possibly the gluteal muscles may occur after strenuous work; it is most frequently observed in Standardbreds. Occasionally other types of horses, especially jumpers and hunters, may be similarly affected. Improperly fitted tack is a prime cause. Horses in dressage training frequently exhibit back soreness as training advances. The training schedule, conformational limitations, suitability of the rider, and tack must all be considered when formulating recommendations. A simple test for fit of tack is to place a piece of string along the dorsal midline between the saddle pad and the saddle, and to draw the string caudad with the rider's full weight in the seat. The string should pull out easily if the tack is properly adjusted.

Muscle soreness is reflected by a change in the gait of the hindlegs. Stride length may be shortened, the back may be slightly arched or stiff, and the hindlegs carried further forward than normal. Digital pressure applied to the back may cause the animal to drop its back excessively, tense the muscles and groan. This reaction must be differentiated from the normal vertebra prominens reflex resulting in dorsiflexion of the back.[20] The abdomen may appear tucked up and tense. Palpating the psoas muscles rectally can elicit evidence of pain.

Treatment: Therapy is designed to correct the primary cause, following which the muscle soreness usually disappears. Rest is often beneficial, especially if the myositis is primary or if the primary cause cannot be immediately determined. Administration of an anti-inflammatory agent, such as a corticosteroid, naproxen, meclofenamic acid or phenylbutazone, may alleviate the inflammation and associated pain.

Injection of corticosteroids directly into the affected area has been employed with varying success. Solutions of irritants, such as iodine, have also been directly injected. Use of irritant solutions results in varying degrees of relief but also results in extensive local tissue destruction, and should only be employed when sclerosis is deemed inevitable and when acceleration of the process could be beneficial.

Local therapy with hot packs, infrared light and massage increases local blood flow and aids in relaxation of muscle spasms when applied by competent operators. Persistent problems may indicate an underlying generalized condition and warrant further investigation.

Muscle Damage Related to Anesthesia

Malignant Hyperthermia

The advent of inhalant anesthetics and the relatively common occurrence of prolonged surgery have spawned a new type of surgical complication. Malignant hyperthermia is a syndrome classically characterized by the rapid onset of high fever and skeletal muscle rigidity associated with the administration of anesthetics and/or muscle relaxants.[21-23]

Cause: The exact cause of malignant hyperthermia is unknown but the syndrome has been characterized in humans as a pharmacogenetic defect of skeletal muscle metabolism. Administration of anesthetics and/or muscle relaxants, particularly succinylcholine and halothane, to susceptible animals causes accelerated release of Ca from the sarcoplasmic reticulum, which results in prolonged, uncontrolled contracture, increased O_2 consumption, depletion of ATP, and increased production of heat, lactate and CO_2. Muscle cell disintegration leads to release of myoglobin and massive amounts of K into the circulation. Subsequent sympathetic overstimulation and cardiac arrhythmias result in death.[22]

Clinical Signs: Although the classic syndrome involves fever and severe muscle contracture, some affected horses exhibit only postoperative muscle pain and swelling, elevated SGOT and serum CPK levels, myoglobinuria and varying degrees of electrolyte and acid-base imbalances. Muscle masses that bear the animal's weight during surgery tend to be severely affected; however, many animals are symmetrically affected or are affected in areas that do not bear weight during surgery.[24,25]

The syndrome has no apparent predisposition for sex, weight, age or condition of affected animals, although lean Thoroughbreds or Standardbreds may be more susceptible. Nutrition and stage of training may affect susceptibility; the significance of such factors warrants investigation. An individual or familial history of "tying-up" is extremely significant since susceptible horses often have clinical or subclinical exercise-related problems (see Primary Exertional Myopathy).

Diagnosis: Diagnosis of malignant hyperthermia is difficult in the absence of intraoperative or immediate postoperative temperature rise. In human patients an intraoperative temperature rise of 1° C or more is considered nearly pathognomonic for the syndrome. Definitive diagnosis is made only by biopsy and *in vitro* exposure of a muscle sample to varying concentrations of halothane and caffeine, which trigger contracture in susceptible samples.[22,26,27]

Pressure Myopathy

When pressure from prolonged recumbency is the cause of muscle damage, the muscles on the lower side of the animal are often more severely affected. Damage varies from tenderness to partial or complete paralysis. Edematous plaques often occur over affected areas. The muscle tenderness and plaques may be present in horses that can stand upon recovery from anesthesia.[28,29] Hypotension and decreased serum Ca levels have been reported in affected horses.[28-30] These factors, acting alone or in concert with others, may prove to be the cause of postoperative myopathy.

At necropsy, significant muscle lesions seem to reflect a lack of adequate perfusion, resulting in death of the affected muscle. The relaxation that occurs during a lengthy surgical procedure and the weight of the horse appear sufficient to prevent adequate perfusion of tissues in the areas under greatest pressure.

Treatment: The treatment of postoperative myopathy is aimed at relief of muscle pain and swelling, and correction of secondary and frequently life-threatening myoglobinuria, and electrolyte and acid-base imbalances.

Good nursing care is extremely important since the condition of recumbent horses can degenerate rapidly if adequate care is not provided. The stall floor should be kept clean, dry and well padded. Recumbent horses should be turned every few hours to prevent decubiti formation and allow perfusion of weight-bearing muscle masses. The animal's underside should be kept as clean and dry as possible to prevent scalding, and decubiti should be carefully dressed and padded. Perfusion in affected areas can be improved with the use of massage, infrared light and ultrasonic treatments. Bladder catheterization may be necessary to assure passage of urine.

The administration of anti-inflammatory agents helps combat associated inflammation. Muscular pain can be reduced through the use of morphine (100 mg given IM) or meperidine (0.5-1 g given IM). Muscle relaxants, such as methocarbamol (4-10 mg/kg body weight IV), help reduce muscle spasm and associated pain. Dantrolene sodium is a peripherally acting muscle relaxant that slows the release of Ca from the sarcoplasmic reticulum. The drug has prophylactic and therapeutic activity and can be used to prevent the development of malignant hyperthermia.[31] Dosages of 1 mg/kg body weight PO have been used to treat postoperative myopathy with good results.[24,26,31] Response to administration of the drug is strongly dependent upon the rapidity of administration to suspect animals. Dantrolene has not been approved for use in horses and its use in this situation must be considered experimental.

Fluid therapy should be tailored to maintenance of moderate diuresis, particularly when myoglobinuria is present. Myoglobin precipitation in the kidneys can be reduced by alkalinization of the urine and diuresis. Mild to moderate hyperkalemia is common initially but serum K levels may decrease rapidly as diuresis progresses. Metabolic acidosis is also common in horses with extensive tissue damage and should be treated empirically with $NaHCO_3$ at 1 mg/kg body weight IV until acid-base determinations are available.

The careful monitoring of horses affected by postoperative myopathy is critically important for the first 24-72 postoperative hours, during which fluxes in electrolyte and acid-base balance occur rapidly.

Prevention: Obtaining a thorough history is important to maximize the safety of all surgical patients. Any horse with a history of "tying-up" should be considered a high risk; testing for malignant hyperthermia should also be considered in such horses.

Provision of adequate padding of firm consistency (air, foam rubber or water) and attempts to reduce the duration of surgery greatly reduce surgery-related muscle damage. Since deep planes of anesthesia reduce peripheral circulation, only the depth of anesthesia necessary to perform the surgery should be used.

Fibrotic and Ossifying Myopathy

This condition has been reported in humans and horses.[32-34] It is initiated by trauma to or near a muscle that results in fibrosis during the reparative process. In some cases, bone is deposited in affected tissues. The condition should be differentiated from myositis ossificans progressiva, which is an inherited disorder of connective tissue characterized by progressive ossification within muscles. There is no effective treatment for the latter condition, which has been reported in humans and swine.[35,36]

Cause: Fibrotic and ossifying myositis is seen most frequently in Quarter Horses and stock horses. When used for cattle-cutting, calf-roping and similar events, such horses are subjected to sliding stops and quick turns in tight circles, which stress the semitendinosus muscles. "In a sliding stop the stifle and hock are extending while the large thigh muscles are contracting, jerking. Similarly, when the foot is caught in a halter, the thigh muscles contract against resistance in a jerking manner. The semitendinosus will be torn first, because of the insertion pattern of the three large thigh muscles at the stifle."[37] Since the semitendinosus inserts most distad on the tibia, ". . . a greater rotatory force is exerted on the semi-tendinosus than on the biceps or semimembranosus."

Clinical Signs: Signs reflect restricted normal function of traumatized muscle due to fibrotic and ossified tissue in the muscle and adhesions among surrounding muscles. In stock horses the lesions occur most frequently in one or both hindlegs, with unilateral involvement being more common. The condition also occurs in the forelegs. A characteristic abnormal gait is probably due to adhesions that form among the semitendinosus muscle and the adjacent semimembranosus and biceps femoris.

In an affected hindleg, the protraction (anterior) phase of the foot's flight is shortened, and when the foot is within a few inches of being placed on the ground it is suddenly pulled back 3-5 inches before making contact. With the shortened protraction phase of the foot's flight, the retraction (posterior) phase is lengthened. This abnormal gait is more evident when walking than when trotting.

Palpation over or near the insertion of the semitendinosus or other involved muscle usually reveals the tissue to be firmer than normal, occasionally with the consistency of bone.

Diagnosis: Radiographs of the area may be useful in diagnosis, particularly if ossified lesions are present.

Microscopically the fibrotic lesions consist of hyalinization of myocyte cytoplasm, loss of muscle striations, some pyknotic nuclei, and fibrosis.[38] As a rule, signs of active inflammation are absent except in the early stages.

Differential diagnosis must be made from lesions affecting surrounding joints. When the hindlegs are typically affected, the metatarsophalangeal, tarsal and stifle joints should be examined. Stringhalt and subluxation of the patella may occasionally produce similar signs. A case involving the gracilis muscle has been reported.[34] The accompanying signs were similar to cases in which the semitendinosus muscle was affected.

Treatment: In humans it has been recommended that local massage not be given, but that rest combined with bandaging may be beneficial.[33] The time required for recovery was approximately 6 weeks, and if the leg was used too soon the signs recurred. Radiotherapy was tried but its value was questionable.

The best method of treatment in horses with semitendinosus involvement appears to be excision of the affected portion of muscle and its tendon of insertion. Transection of the muscle near its insertion has been proposed as an alternate method of treatment, but in our experience this procedure seems to be less effective than excision.

Surgery may be attempted, with the horse standing, after inducing local anesthesia. Administration of a general anesthetic enables the surgery to be performed under better conditions, however, and is preferred.

Following preparation of the surgical site, a vertical incision 12-15 cm long is made through the skin over the semitendinosus muscle close to its insertion on the caudal surface of the stifle. With the leg in extension, the muscle is identified and all adhesions among juxtaposed muscles are separated and all newly deposited fibrous tissue removed. The distal end of the semitendinosus muscle is located and a 7- to 10-cm section is removed. At least 4 cm of the most distal segment should include the tendon of insertion. The incision is closed by approximating the edges of the incised muscle fascia with #1 chromic catgut sutures.

A Penrose drain is placed in the dead space created by removal of the muscle, tendon, fibrous tissue and retraction of the muscle after it is severed. The drain is brought to the outside through a stab incision in the skin distal to the original incision and secured with 1 or 2 sutures using a nonabsorbable material. The skin edges are approximated with a layer of subcuticular, interrupted horizontal mattress sutures of 00 chromic catgut. The final layer of sutures through the skin is a series of interrupted vertical or horizontal mattress sutures using nonabsorbable material.

If bone is present along with fibrous tissue, it is also removed. Ossified tissue usually is a plate or plaque of bone overlying the semitendinosus muscle; it can vary greatly in size.

Postoperative management consists of prophylaxis against tetanus and administration of a systemic antibiotic if deemed advisable. Exercise should be restricted for the first 7-10 days. The drain is removed when there is no longer evidence of drainage; this usually is about the fifth day. The skin sutures should not be removed for 10-14 days because these incisions tend to dehisce.

Clinical improvement usually is evident in 7-10 days and although all horses do not have complete regression of clinical signs after surgery, improvement is expected in all cases.

Myotonia
by G.C. Farnbach

Myotonia in skeletal muscle is characterized by a prolonged after-contraction, with difficulty in relaxation. The contraction may follow voluntary use of the muscle, direct percussion of the muscle, or stimulation mechanically, electrically or chemically.

In humans this disorder can occur alone, as in myotonia congenita, or as part of more complex disorders, such as myotonia dystrophica. The phenomenon has been well documented in goats, and herds of these animals are maintained for research of this condition.[39-41] The disorder has also been reported in dogs, cattle and horses.[42,43] Affected horses may have a variety of clinical signs and disease progressions.

Equine myopathies accompanied by myotonia are too poorly understood to adequately classify. These disorders can be compared to human muscular diseases only in a general way. In humans most myotonic myopathies display characteristic inheritance patterns. In the horse too few animals have been observed to make generalizations about inheritance; however, recently 2 offspring of one stallion were affected with myotonia and a third (the only untested offspring) had gait abnormalities characterized by stiffness. This suggests the possibility that a dominant pattern of inheritance might exist in at least one form of equine myotonia. On the other hand, a myotonic Thoroughbred mare bred to a myotonic Welsh pony twice produced normal offspring.

Cause: The biochemical defects responsible for the condition are not known explicitly but have been demonstrated to be inherent within the muscle rather than within the nervous system. Complete neuromuscular block by receptor inhibition or by depolarization fails to reduce the myotonic phenomenon.[43] In intracellular electrophysiologic studies, the repetitive discharge of individual muscle fibers has been eliminated by the disconnection of the transverse tubular system from the sarcolemma.[44] This work was done with biopsies from myotonic goats in which it is also known that, as in people with myotonia congenita, there is a marked deficiency in permeability to the chloride ion across the sarcolemma. It has been proposed that after an action potential, the accumulation of K in the long and tortuous transverse tubular system produces a degree of membrane depolarization. In muscle with normal chloride conductance the effect of this depolarization is minimized by chloride shunting. When low chloride conductance is present, depolarization becomes adequate to produce subsequent action potentials, resulting in the repetitive activity seen in myotonia. While this explanation appears reasonable and adequate for myotonia associated with decreased chloride conductance in the sarcolemma, membrane chloride conductance was not appreciably altered in 3 horses studied at the University of Pennsylvania and in some human patients with myotonic diseases. Therefore, some other mechanism must cause the observed repetitive electrical activity in these cases.

Clinical Signs: All equine cases of myotonia studied have varied in their severity but have had certain consistent characteristics. Clinical signs were first noticed when the animals were from 3 weeks to several months of age. Muscle abnormalities are most prominent in the hindquarters, where the animals appear extremely well muscled (Fig 3). The inability to walk in a fluid, smooth manner is most pronounced after a period of rest and becomes less prominent as exercise is continued. Muscular strength does not appear to be diminished.

Many affected animals exhibit complete stiffening and immobility when startled, and considerable difficulty in taking the first few steps when led from the stall. With percussion of affected muscles, there is an immediate visible and sustained contraction followed by slow relaxation. It may take more than a minute for the muscles to return to the resting state. These muscles always feel firm and tense, and never plastic as a normal relaxed muscle. Despite crippling disabilities in the hindquarters, affected animals may appear normal in the head, neck and forelimbs.

On EMG the affected muscles manifest the high-frequency continuous discharge pathognomonic for myotonia.[45] The audible signal is characterized by a shifting in frequency and amplitude similar to that of the old-fashioned divebomber. This characteristic pattern is produced by the repetitive firing of individual muscle fibers. As fiber excitability wanes, the frequency with which they self-excite decreases and the amplitude of each action potential diminishes to produce the characteristic features of the myotonic EMG.

Histologic evaluation of affected muscle reveals fibers with extreme variation in diameter with a range well beyond twice normal. The largest myofibers generally occur in groups, have extremely irregular borders and may be folded within themselves. There is centralization of nuclei, and degenerated and necrotic myofibers are frequently encountered. There is a noticeable paucity of inflammatory reaction in affected tissue. Electron microscopy reveals a variety of subcellular changes, including unusual accumulations of lipids and granules that appear to be glycogen. The spectrum of changes seen is similar to that seen in human muscular dystrophies.

Treatment and Prognosis: Drug therapy in horses has not been effective. In humans, the use of phenytoin, procainamide and quinine has been effective.[46] In equine cases these drugs might be tried if warranted, but the likelihood of success is remote.

Of 3 documented cases followed for several years at the University of Pennsylvania, 2 showed mild amelioration of signs with age. One has been used as a teaser stallion and another for breeding purposes. The mare used for breeding improved to the point that gait abnormalities become very subtle. Signs in the third animal worsened progressively and the musculature became grotesquely deformed by fibrous pseudohypertrophy. The gait also worsened and the mare moved about only with great difficulty. This animal had been the most severely affected one. On these limited data, there appears to be a spectrum of clinical courses that parallel the spectrum of signs and histologic findings.

Hypothyroid Myopathy

Hypothyroidism, particularly of a mild and secondary nature, is an insidious disorder that is difficult to diagnose. Horses in training have periods of suppressed thyroid function corresponding to periods of maximal stress. The demands of growth or the stress of infectious disease, transport or adverse weather conditions may further impair thyroid function.[47,48]

Clinical Signs: A common early manifestation of depressed thyroid function and hypothyroid myopathy is muscle cramping, with or without elevated SGOT and serum CPK levels.[49] Compromise of muscle function may be mild or marked. One affected horse had pseudomyotonia, dimpling of the muscles on percussion and stilted gait, but no EMG changes. Depressed appetite and weight loss are more common than weight gain. A decrease in endurance or performance is a common complaint. Nonresponsive, normocytic normochromic anemia may also be present.[50]

Diagnosis: Presumptive diagnosis of hypothyroidism is based upon the presence of decreased plasma T_4 levels on radioimmunoassay.[51] Plasma should be submitted to a qualified veterinary laboratory with established equine plasma T_4 values since technics used in human diagnostic laboratories are too insensitive for use on equine samples. The plasma should be immediately separated from blood cells and kept cool until tested.

Diagnosis of secondary hypothyroidism is supported by TSH-response test results.[51,52] Plasma T_4 levels are compared on samples taken before and after administration of TSH.

Preliminary studies indicate a transient rise to normal serum T_4 levels in hypothyroid horses given 5 IU thyroid-stimulating hormone (Thytropar: Armour). Serum T_4 levels return to subnormal in 12-24 hours. Horses with normal resting serum T_4 levels responded similarly but had smaller increases in serum T_4 levels after injection, followed by a return to normal levels.

Treatment: Horses suspected of having hypothyroidism induced by stress may benefit from daily administration of 3-7 g iodinated casein (Protomone: Agri-Tech) PO. Other forms of oral thyroid hormone replacement are not effective in horses. Weekly or biweekly monitoring of serum T_4 levels is critical for dosage adjustment.

Prevention: Growth, training, infection, adverse weather and other stress factors place heavy demands upon thyroid function. Recognition of these factors and astute observation of subtle, early signs aid early detection.[47,48,51]

Nutritional Myopathy
by D.C. Dodd

Nutritional myopathy (dystrophic myodegeneration, polymyositis, white muscle disease) occurs mainly in young, rapidly growing animals of all domestic species. It is characterized by noninflammatory degeneration of skeletal and cardiac muscle. Natural cases have been reported in Australia, New Zealand, the Netherlands, Great Britain and the US. The reported frequency in foals is very low compared with the known frequency in lambs, calves and pigs.[53-59] The cause of the muscular degeneration that is characteristic of this disease is a vitamin E-Se deficiency that may be either a primary dietary deficiency or a secondary one induced by various factors.

Cause and Pathogenesis: With regard to the cause, we must rely mainly on work done in other species. It seems clear, however, that white muscle disease (WMD) in foals is truly one of the protean manifestations of vitamin E-Se deficiency. The precise relationships and interactions between these 2 substances are not known but a primary or induced deficiency of either or both usually exists in nutritional myopathy. Vitamin E is known for its antioxidant activity and its intimate connection with the maintenance of cell membranes in general. One of the important functions of Se may be to permit or enhance the uptake of vitamin E from the lumen of the gut and from the blood to the tissues.

Brown pigmentation of adipose tissue is seen sometimes in vitamin E deficiency in the cat, rat, hamster, mouse and pig, but it occurs only when large amounts of long-chain polyunsaturated fats are in the diet. No specific information on this point is available for the horse, but it would seem reasonable to assume that the cause of the brown discoloration of fat is the same in this species as in the ones named.

It has been well established in various countries that WMD of lambs and calves occurs predominantly when the soil and pastures are low in Se or when the animals are grazing legumes. A succinoxidase inhibitor that interferes with vitamin E is present in some fresh leguminous pastures and hay, and it increases greatly if the hay gets damp.[60,61] It could be myopathogenic.

Clinical Signs: Foals usually are affected between birth and about 7 months of age. The clinical onset may be sudden or preceded by lethargy and a stilted stiff gait. The more acute form usually follows a period of increased muscular activity. Acutely ill foals usually have such severe and extensive muscle damage that they go down and are unable to rise. Death may follow within as short a period as 5 hours, probably from exhaustion and circulatory failure resulting in pulmonary congestion and edema. Rapid death can also be attributed directly to heart failure and pulmonary edema when the myocardium is extensively affected, as it is in some foals.

The less acute form is more common and is usually first apparent as gait abnormality, described variously as stiff, stilted or even incoordinated, and a stiff carriage of the head and neck. As there is no evidence of a neuropathy, it probably is incorrect to say that the gait is incoordinated. Any difficulty in using the legs can be attributed solely to muscular degeneration and foals that recover have no evidence of neurologic deficit. Because the extent and severity of muscular damage vary considerably, so do the associated clinical signs. Foals able to stand and move about, particularly those able to nurse, have a good chance of recovery. When the disease is progressive, the foal goes down after a variable period and death follows within a few days. Most affected foals have a dejected and lethargic attitude but some, even when recumbent, have been described as bright and alert.

In the early, more acute phase of this disease, many foals have painful subcutaneous swellings particularly prominent along the nuchal crest, ventral abdominal wall, and rump. The causes of these swellings are edema, hemorrhage, neutrophilic invasion and necrosis and calcification of the subcutaneous tissues and fat. The fat may have a peculiar yellow-brown discoloration and is usually flecked with 1- to 2-mm hemorrhages. As the disease progresses, the affected fat becomes much firmer and the pain subsides.

Some foals with difficulty in standing may nurse if assisted, but others have such extensive damage of the lingual and pharyngeal muscles that sucking and swallowing are difficult or impossible. Any difficulty in swallowing can lead to death from aspiration pneumonia. If this does not occur, lack of food soon results in death from starvation. The loss of condition may be masked by swelling of the subcutis and fat.

In 5 adult horses with nutritional myopathy subsequent to colic, clinical signs included edema of the head and neck, muscle stiffness and soreness, and tachycardia progressing to heart failure; myoglobinuria occurred in 4 of the 5 horses.[62]

Lesions and Chemical Changes: Extensive localized or generalized muscular damage causes liberation of large amounts of myoglobin that results in myoglobinuria and brown discoloration of the urine. This is likely to be noticed only in the early stages of acute cases. Also liberated from the damaged muscles are the enzymes GOT, LDH and CPK.

Although low serum Se and vitamin E levels are a good indication of nutritional myopathy, dependable normal values are unavailable.[62-64]

Gross lesions are bilaterally symmetric (unless prolonged unilateral recumbency precedes death) and include pallor of cervical, pectoral, pelvic and cardiac musculature (Fig 4).[62,65] Subcutaneous edema, especially of the neck and ventral body wall, usually is present. In the same areas the fat may be swollen and have a brown discoloration and hemorrhagic flecks. In the late stages of the disease, the fat becomes firmer and drier.

Microscopically there is noninflammatory myodegeneration with swelling, hyalinization, fragmentation, lysis, necrosis and mineralization of muscle fibers and proliferation of the satellite cell nuclei.[66] When subcutaneous and internal fat deposits are affected, the change is classified as a steatitis. Edema, focal hemorrhages and infiltration of fat with neutrophils, plus focal necrosis and mineralization, are present to various degrees. If the myocardium is affected, the changes are similar to those in skeletal muscle.

Treatment and Prevention: The minimum requirement of Se for horses is 2.4 μg/kg body weight daily when given parenterally or 10μg/kg when given orally.[64] To treat a foal with nutritional myopathy, 2 injections of 10-20 mg sodium selenite should be given a week apart.[66] At the same time, 1000 mg vitamin E are given orally for 3-5 days. Unless this treatment is given soon after the onset of clinical signs, it is unlikely to have the desired effect.

On farms where nutritional myopathy is known to occur, the condition can theoretically be prevented by injecting the dam with 20-30 mg Se a month before parturition or by injecting the foal with 10 mg Se at birth.

Analysis of 542 samples indicated that the serum Se status of suckling foals is low and remains low even at an age when suckling foals consume considerable quantities of grain and roughage. Orphan foals fed commercial milk replacers had more than twice as much serum Se as their nursing counterparts, indicating a possible inhibiting effect of mare's milk on dietary Se or a Se-dependent intestinal microflora of the suckling foal.[64]

Exertional Myopathy

Exertional myopathy refers to clinical signs secondary to exercise and referable to skeletal muscles. The terms "tying-up," "Monday morning disease," "azoturia" and "paralytic myoglobinuria," often used interchangeably, describe a group of signs rather than a single disease. Exertional myopathy may be primary, related to a defect in the skeletal muscle cell, or secondary, related to extrinsic factors that damage the muscle cell.

Secondary Exertional Myopathy

Myositis: As previously discussed, myositis is among the most common causes of secondary exertional myopathy. Signs may be as subtle as a shortened stride, reluctance to turn, refusal to jump, or reluctance to perform at speed ("sourness"). Pain on palpation or manipulation of the muscles, particularly if unilateral, aids in diagnosis. A thorough search for possible causes of myositis as well as a complete training history are essential for presumptive diagnosis.

Results of muscle-specific enzyme tests help confirm the diagnosis; however, samples taken after a single, isolated incident cannot differentiate between primary and secondary myopathy. Low-grade, localized pain should be further evaluated by thorough examination of the skeletal system. Administration of muscle relaxants and anti-inflammatory agents may help assess the contribution of myalgia (muscle pain) to the overall condition.

Obtaining a complete training history is critical when muscle pain is generalized or when large muscles, such as the femoral, gluteal and iliopsoas groups, are affected. Such horses may have signs of tying-up, including myoglobinuria, profuse sweating, reluctance to move, sawhorse stance, and general indications of distress, such as tachycardia, hyperventilation and low-grade fever. In the absence of myoglobinuria, cases of laminitis, pleuritis and colic may be mistaken for tying-up.

Serial SGOT determinations during stall rest and supportive care can be used to assess recovery (see Treatment). A complete diagnostic workup is indicated in horses with recurrent attacks or when there are no obvious problems with the exercise schedule, equipment and suitability of the horse to its work.

Hypothyroidism: Muscular manifestations of hypothyroidism may be mild or marked. Serum muscle-specific enzyme levels vary and spontaneous regression of signs may occur (see Hypothyroid Myopathy).

Nutritional Secondary Exertional Myopathy: Nutritional status is among the original suspected causes of secondary exertional myopathy. Carbohydrate loading, the ingestion of a high-carbohydrate diet during periods of rest and/or after a period of low-carbohydrate feeding, can produce increased muscle stores of glycogen.[67,68] Increased anaerobic metabolism and lactate production presumably account for a higher incidence of cramping with or without myoglobinuria.

Despite some success with inducing tying-up with high-carbohydrate diets, increases in muscle glycogen stores could not be detected histochemically. Neurohumoral factors may also be involved (see below). Some horses may have intrinsic deficiencies in carbohydrate metabolism (see Primary Exertional Myopathy).

Vitamin E-Se deficiency is a well-documented cause of muscular dystrophy in many species. These nutrients are critical to intracellular oxidative processes.[69] Many refractory cases of tying-up respond to vitamin E-Se supplementation.[70] One affected 13½-year-old Belgian mare had an inclusion-body myopathy reminiscent of similar nutritional dystrophies

in other species. A Canadian study of soil Se levels and serum vitamin E-Se levels revealed poor correlation between deficiency and clinical signs, suggesting a complex of causative factors.[71]

Skeletal muscle contains large amounts of K. Extracellular release of K is critical to local vasomotor control during exercise.[72] Depletion of body K may be caused by administration of diuretics, muscle damage, intense exercise, abnormal aldosterone secretion, and losses in sweat and urine in hot weather.[73] Detection of K depletion is difficult because serum K levels are maintained at the expense of intracellular stores until depletion is advanced.

Most equine diets contain adequate amounts of K. Free-choice feeding of K, as a salt or in solution with other electrolytes, may be advisable during periods of heavy training or following muscle damage. Fresh water should always be available. Mixing a K salt in feed is not advised. Potassium salts should be introduced in small quantities to determine tendencies of the horse to ingest potentially dangerous amounts.

Intermittent Claudication: Decreased blood supply to the muscles, from arterial thrombus formation by *Strongylus vulgaris* larvae, is frequently manifested as acute muscle pain and cramping during exercise. Early manifestations have not been described but probably include muscle pain. The iliac branches of the aorta are most severely affected. The affected limb(s) may feel cool and refill time of the saphenous vein is prolonged. Rectal palpation usually reveals decreased pulse pressure and/or thickening of affected arteries. One severely affected horse returned to galloping soundness after a 5-week program of 2 miles of walking prior to exercise.[74]

Although it has been suggested the condition is more common in stallions, the influences of management and gender are unknown. A fecal egg count may help determine if *Strongylus* infection is a cause of secondary myopathy.

Other Factors: Blustery and/or cold weather may predispose horses to secondary exertional myopathy. Myotonia is aggravated by cold; "cold myotonia" in humans is triggered by environmental conditions. Factors such as hormonal changes in response to cold, deleted exercise periods and decreased warm-up periods in cold weather should be investigated. The possible role of neurohumoral factors in secondary exertional myopathy is exemplified by the suggested higher incidence in fillies and clinical episodes after excitement.

Serum hormone levels are significantly altered in human athletes with exertional myopathy but have not been documented in horses.[75] Myopathy after administration of hormones has not been observed in horses.[76]

Primary Exertional Myopathy

Defects of glycogen metabolism (glycogen-storage diseases) occur in humans but have not been demonstrated in horses.[77-79] Defects in glycolytic or oxidative enzyme pathways may produce signs similar to those of tying-up.[80,81]

Malignant Hyperthermia: Susceptibility to malignant hyperthermia (see Postanesthetic Complications) has been documented in horses with exertional myopathy.[13] All affected animals were racing Standardbreds or Thoroughbreds. Their histories revealed rapid onset of severe myopathy at an early age or less dramatic, chronic debility and poor performance over a number of years, with some degree of muscle atrophy, primarily in the hindquarters. Animals in the latter group suffered isolated episodes of acute, severe signs of tying-up. Neither group responded well to drug therapy or manipulations of diet and training schedules, and none was exposed to inhalant anesthetics or succinylcholine.

Malignant hyperthermia is hereditary in humans and pigs but genetic transmission has not been proven in horses. A complicated pattern of inheritance could explain the wide range of clinical severity seen in horses.

Definitive diagnosis of malignant hyperthermia is by *in vitro* testing of live muscle strips for contracture in the presence of halothane and substances such as KCl and caffeine. Unfortunately, the procedure is time-consuming, costly and performed in only a few laboratories. Because a viable strip of muscle is required for testing, some animals must be shipped to facilities equipped for such testing. Diagnosis of malignant hyperthermia is aided by ruling out other causes of myopathy. Causes of severe, repeated episodes of tying-up, such as management, hormonal or dietary factors, should be evaluated. A familial history of tying-up or anesthesia-related complications is highly suspicious.

Treatment of malignant hyperthermia is described below.

Diagnosis of Exertional Myopathy

History: A thorough history is invaluable in determining the diagnosis, prognosis and rational therapy of suspected cases of exertional myopathy. A familial history of muscular problems, as well as information on past GI disorders, parasitism, laminitis or lameness, aids diagnosis. Duration, onset, severity and precipitating circumstances of the most recent attack should be noted. Laboratory test results from earlier episodes may be useful. Details on equipment, diet, training schedule, deworming programs and any drugs administered are also essential.

Clinical Signs: Signs of exertional myopathy occur during or after exercise. Occasionally signs of stiffness and pain are not noticed until several hours after a particularly strenuous workout. Such signs include a stilted gait, reluctance to move, generalized or localized (*eg,* over hindquarters) sweating, rigid stance similar to that in colic or laminitis, and anorexia (Fig 5). The pain and anxiety associated with exertional myopathy also commonly cause an elevated temperature, and elevated pulse and respiratory rates.

Palpation of muscles may elicit a painful response or exaggerated guarding. Assessment of the response to palpation depends on the operator's subjective judgement but is more obvious if an unusual response is unilateral. Dark, discolored urine (pigmenturia) from excretion of myoglobin is present in severe cases.

Laboratory Tests: Results of laboratory tests can confirm the diagnosis, determine the etiology, direct treatment and aid prognostication. The proliferation of commercial clinical pathology laboratories has provided practitioners with a wide range of diagnostic tests. Because "normal" values for various assays, especially enzyme activity, vary among laboratories, practitioners should submit samples from normal horses to establish "normal" values for laboratories to which samples are submitted.

Because serum enzyme, electrolyte and metabolite levels are heavily influenced by sample handling, the clinical pathology laboratory should be contacted for specific directions on obtaining and shipping a specimen. Delayed refrigeration or centrifugation and exposure to light can adversely affect serum assay results.

The most useful laboratory test in suspected cases of exertional myopathy is serum CPK level. Assay of serum LDH levels may also be helpful because that enzyme is less affected by improper sample handling (Fig 6). The SGOT level can be used to monitor recovery. Levels of SGOT rise slowly but remain elevated for days or weeks.

Serum creatinine levels should be determined in severe cases of exertional myopathy, with or without pigmenturia. Renal dysfunction from myoglobin precipitation in the renal tubules is rare but must be considered. Serum creatinine levels should be monitored throughout treatment.

Acid-base status and serum electrolyte levels should be evaluated in acute cases. Test results are often not available soon enough to influence initial therapy but can direct later treatment and assess the severity of the episode. Acidosis is common in exertional myopathy. Exercise or muscle damage results in release of intracellular K and severe muscle damage may result in life-threatening hyperkalemia. Renal clearance of excess K may be impaired by concurrent acidosis and myoglobin precipitation. Hypokalemia from excretion of K in the urine may be detected 24 hours after injury. The benefits of transfer of severely affected horses to facilities with on-site electrolyte and acid-base monitoring may outweigh the risks of shipment.

The severity of exertional myopathy can be difficult to interpret by clinical signs alone in some horses because of their temperament. Poor conformation and concurrent skeletal disease can also obscure muscular disease. In such cases, serial sampling before and after a controlled period of exercise may aid diagnosis. Horses may be trotted on a lunge line for 10 minutes.[12,13] Racing Thoroughbreds may be galloped 2 miles or made to run a mile in 1:15. Serum enzyme levels from affected horses should be compared with those of normal horses sampled in the same manner.

Blood samples should be obtained prior to exercise, and 5 and 60 minutes after exercise for CPK, SGOT, LDH, Na, K, Cl and CO_2 determinations. Fecal examination, rectal examination and serum T_4 determination should also be performed.

Discoloration of urine from pigmenturia may vary from a reddish tinge to dark brown. Pigmenturia primarily is caused by excretion of myoglobin, although hemoglobin may be present after exhaustive exercise. The simplest, but least sensitive, test to differentiate myoglobin from hemoglobin in urine is the benzidine-precipitation test.[82] More accurate methods involve electrophoresis and immunodiffusion.[50,82]

Although serum vitamin E and Se levels can be determined by some research laboratories, the assays are costly, complicated and difficult to interpret. A trial period of supplementation is a more practical method of diagnosing such deficiencies.

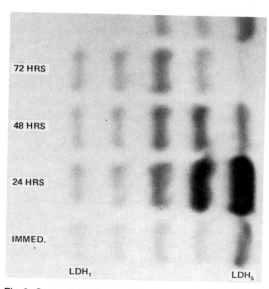

Fig 6. Serum LDH isoenzymes separated by electrophoresis. The bottom sample, obtained immediately after a moderate attack of exertional myopathy, revealed increased LDH_5 levels. The 24-hour sample had peak activity, and the 48-and 72-hour samples revealed a return toward normal levels and a slight shift to the isoenzyme distribution of myocardium.

Biopsy for microscopic and histochemical examination or special studies can be very useful. The laboratory should be contacted prior to biopsy for instructions on sampling.

Treatment of Exertional Myopathy

Treatment of exertional myopathy is aimed at relief of anxiety, muscle spasm and pain, and correction of complications, such as acidosis and renal dysfunction. Acutely affected animals should not be moved unnecessarily. The animal should be covered with a blanket that protects against chill but allows evaporation of sweat.

Tranquilizers are commonly used to calm affected animals and relieve some muscle spasm. A dose of 20-40 mg acepromazine is commonly given IV. Although the exact effect of acepromazine on equine muscle is not known, the vasodilator properties of the drug may be beneficial. Nonspecific analgesic/anti-inflammatory drugs may also be useful. Phenylbutazone (1-3 g IV), pentazocine (200-400 mg diluted, IV), morphine and meperidine have been used. Early administration of large doses of corticosteroids may also be beneficial.

The use of skeletal muscle relaxants is indicated when tranquilizers cannot provide relief. Methocarbamol is commonly used but is expensive and must be administered slowly to prevent excitement. A 450-kg horse should be given 2-9 g methocarbamol IV. Dantrolene sodium has been used with mixed results.[13,31] Administration is oral but IV doses parallel those in other species. Dantrolene is the only effective drug to treat malignant hyperthermia.

Fluid therapy is indicated in dehydrated animals or those with pigmenturia or abnormal blood chemistry values. Use of normal saline or dextrose in normal or half-strength saline is preferred, especially when serum K and lactate levels are not monitored. Mild diuresis produced by fluid administration minimizes myoglobin precipitation in the renal tubules. Acidosis is treated with $NaHCO_3$ given IV at 0.5-1 mg/kg body weight. All drugs should be administered cautiously until normal volumes of urine are produced.

The convalescent period in exertional myopathy is 2-5 days. Horses should not be exercised until clinical signs and blood chemistry abnormalities abate. Muscle spasms can be relieved by mixing 2-4 g naproxen granules (Equiproxen: Diamond) with the feed during convalescence. Continued use of analgesic/anti-inflammatory agents may be helpful. Electrolyte supplementation should be guided by test results.

Vitamin E-Se (E-SE: Burns-Biotec) injections are of questionable value, but a prophylactic regimen of 10 ml given IM twice in a 2-week interval, then monthly, may be beneficial. Vitamin E and Se may also be added to the feed.

Horses with low serum T_4 levels may benefit from thyroid hormone supplementation (see Hypothyroid Myopathy). Horses susceptible to malignant hyperthermia have been protected by small daily doses of dantrolene.

Prevention of Exertional Myopathy

Many cases of exertional myopathy can be prevented by good management, use of proper equipment and tailoring training schedules to individual horses. Horses with a familial history of myopathy should not be bred. Horses turned out daily are apparently not as often affected. Those with conformational defects that predispose to muscle strain benefit from massage and other topical therapy.

Horses responsive to vitamin E-Se supplementation may require supplementation indefinitely. Horses receiving thyroid hormone supplementation should be monitored to adjust dosage since this condition can correct itself spontaneously.

References

1. DeBuck, D and DeMoore, L. Nevraxe 5 (1903) 229.
2. Strong, CL: Horse Injuries. Faber & Faber, London, 1967.
3. Alpert, JS et al. Circ 39 (1968) 353.
4. Gerber, H. Eq Vet J 1 (1969) 1.
5. Cardinet, GH. Am J Vet Res 24 (1963) 980.
6. Freedland, RA and Kramer, JW. Adv Vet Sci Comp Med 14 (1970).
7. Coffman, JR et al. Proc 13th Ann Mtg Am Assoc Eq Pract, 1967. p 98.
8. Anderson, MG. Eq Vet J 7 (1975) 160.
9. Fowler, WM et al. J Appl Physiol 17 (1962) 943.
10. Bohmer, D. Proc 2nd Int Symp Biochem Exercise, 1973. p 229.
11. Poortman, JR. Proc 2nd Int Symp Biochem Exercise, 1973. p 212.
12. Waldron-Mease, E. J Eq Med Surg. In press, 1981.
13. Waldron-Mease, E. Proc 24th Ann Mtg Am Assoc Eq Pract, 1978. p 95.
14. Engel, WK. Pediatr Clin No Am 14 (1967) 963.
15. Bergstrom, J. Scand J Clin Lab Invest (Suppl 68, 1962).
16. Radner forceps. Stille-Werner, Stockholm.
17. Sabeh, G et al. J Lab Clin Med 65 (1965) 523.
18. Porro, RS et al. J Neuropath Exp Neur 28 (1969) 229.
19. Steinberg, S and Botelho, S. Science 137 (1962) 979.
20. Rooney, JR: Clinical Neurology of the Horse. KNA Press, Kennett Square, PA, 1971.
21. Lucke, JN et al. Br J Anaesth 48 (1976) 297.
22. Innes, RKR and Stromme, JH. Br J Anaesth 45 (1973) 185.
23. Waldron-Mease, E. JAVMA. In press, 1981.
24. Waldron-Mease, E. Proc 24th Ann Mtg Am Assoc Eq Pract, 1978. p 95.
25. Waldron-Mease, E. Vet Sci Comm 3 (1979) 45.
26. Rosenberg, H and Waldron-Mease, E. Abstr Ann Mtg Am Soc Anesth, 1977. p 333.
27. Moulds, RFW and Denborough, MA. Br Med J 2 (1974) 245.
28. White, KK and Short, CE. Proc 24th Ann Mtg Am Assoc Eq Pract, 1978. p 107.
29. Lindsay, W et al. Proc 24th Ann Mtg Am Assoc Eq Pract, 1978. p 115.
30. Johnson, BD et al. J Eq Med Surg 2 (1978) 109.
31. Pinder, RM et al. Drugs 13 (1977) 3.
32. Adams, OR: Lameness in Horses. 2nd ed. Lea & Febiger, Philadelphia, 1966.
33. Ellis, M and Frank, HG. J Trauma 6 (1966) 724.
34. Bishop, R. VM/SAC 67 (1972) 270.
35. Russell, RGG et al. Lancet (Jan 1, 1972) 10.
36. Seibold, HR and Davis, CL. Path Vet 4 (1967) 79.
37. Rooney, JR: Biomechanics of Lameness in Horses. Williams & Wilkins, Baltimore, 1969.
38. Adams, OR. JAVMA 139 (1961) 1089.
39. Brown, GL and Harvey, AM. Brain 62 (1939) 341.
40. Bryant, SH et al. Am J Vet Res 29 (1968) 2371.
41. Harvey, JC. Johns Hopkins Med J 125 (1969) 270.
42. Van Neikerk, IJM and Jaro, GG. So Afr Med J 44 (1970) 898.

43. Steinber, S and Botelho, S. Science **137** (1962) 1979.

44. Adrian, RH and Bryant, SH. J Physiol **240** (1974) 505.

45. Flora, GC. Postgrad Med **41** (1967) 148.

46. Rowland, in Cecil and Loeb: Textbook of Medicine. 13th ed. WB Saunders, Philadelphia, 1971.

47. Takagi, S *et al.* Exp Rep Eq Hlth Lab **11** (1974) 94.

48. Irvine, CHG. J Endocr **39** (1967) 313.

49. Takamori, M *et al.* Arch Neur **25** (1971) 535.

50. Waldron-Mease, E. J Eq Med Surg **2** (1978) 101.

51. Lowe, JE *et al.* Cornell Vet **64** (1974) 276.

52. Waldron-Mease, E. J Eq Med Surg. *In press*, 1981.

53. Gabbedy, BJ and Richards, RB. Aust Vet J **46** (1970) 111.

54. Hartley, WJ and Dodd, DC. N Zeal Vet J **5** (1957) 61.

55. Dodd, DC *et al.* N Zeal Vet J **5** (1957) 61.

56. Kroneman, J and Wensvoort, P. Neth J Vet Sci **1** (1968) 42.

57. Baker, JR. Vet Rec **82** (1968) 70.

58. Baker, JR. Vet Rec **84** (1969) 488.

59. Jones, RC and Reed, WO. JAVMA **113** (1948) 170.

60. Cartan, GH and Swingle, KF. Am J Vet Res **20** (1959) 235.

61. Roughan, PG. N Zeal J Agric Res **8** (1965) 607.

62. Owen, RR *et al.* JAVMA **171** (1977) 343.

63. Lindholm, A and Asheim, A. Acta Agric Scand **19** (1973) 40.

64. Stowe, HD. J Nutr **93** (1967) 60.

65. Wilson, TM *et al.* JAVMA **169** (1976) 213.

66. Mauro, A. J Biophys Biochem Cytol **9** (1961) 493.

67. Bergstrom, J *et al.* Acta Physiol Scand **71** (1967) 140.

68. Bergstrom, J *et al.* Nature **210** (1966) 309.

69. Bieri, JC. Fed Proc **22** (1963) 318.

70. Hill, HE. Mod Vet Pract **43** (1962) 66.

71. Owen, RR *et al.* JAVMA **171** (1977) 343.

72. Knochel, JP and Schlein, EM. J Clin Invest **51** (1972) 1750.

73. Knochel, JP *et al.* J Clin Invest **51** (1972) 242.

74. Fregin, FG and Waldron-Mease, E, Univ Penn: Unpublished data, 1980.

75. Hartley, LH *et al.* J Appl Physiol **11** (1972) 602.

76. Vignos, PJ and Greene, R. J Lab Clin Med **81** (1973) 365.

77. Layzer, RB *et al.* Arch Neur **17** (1967) 1.

78. Angelini, C *et al.* N Engl J Med **287** (1978) 948.

79. Pearson, CM *et al.* Am J Med **30** (1961) 502.

80. Whitaker, JN. Am J Med **63** (1977) 805.

81. Fishbein WN *et al.* Science **200** (1979) 545.

82. Boulton, FE *et al.* J Clin Path **24** (1971) 816.

20

The Skeletal System

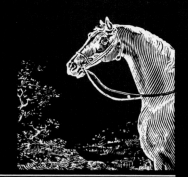

DIAGNOSIS OF SKELETAL DISEASE

The History
by B.D. Grant

The complete history should be obtained before the physical examination is begun. As with any other system, a systematic approach to obtaining the history should be followed so that important factors are not overlooked.

Age

The age of the animal is important when evaluating a horse for skeletal diseases. The incidence of degenerative conditions increases with age and the amount of use of an animal; such conditions include navicular disease and ringbone. Conversely, other conditions most commonly involve very young horses, including septic arthritis, osteochondrosis and angular deformities.

Sex

The sex of the animal does not usually play an important role in the definitive diagnosis of skeletal problems, but certainly one cannot expect to see in a female an acute hindleg lameness from a scrotal hernia nor in a male the limited hindleg extension and tail-switching associated with vaginitis. Young males may have more injuries because of their aggressive behavior than females of the same age. The sex of the animal also may influence the selection of treatment of various conditions.

Breed

The breed of the animal is important as there are breed predilections for some conditions, eg, the "bucked-shin" complex is rare in Standardbreds but common in Thoroughbreds and Quarter Horses. Navicular disease is rare in Arabians, especially compared with the prev-

alence in Quarter Horses. Carpal and fetlock injuries occur in race horses of all breeds but more often in racing Quarter Horses and Thoroughbreds because of their higher speed compared with Standardbreds.

Color

While not of great importance, the color of the patient can play a role in lameness. For example, a grey horse had a lameness confined to the elbow and shoulder. No external masses were noted, but necropsy revealed massive infiltration of the elbow and shoulder with a malignant melanoma.[1] The owner subsequently learned that the previous owner had had a number of skin lesions excised.

Light-skinned horses often have an increased inflammatory response to topical medication and irritants, especially when applied below the carpus.

Occupation

Because many injuries are related to a horse's use, it is important to determine the horse's present use, its past use, and its intended future use. For example, a hunter with a lip tattoo and suspected carpitis may have suffered a carpal osteochondral fracture during its racing career. Blemishes of the skeletal system that do not necessarily contribute to unsoundness are more important when one is dealing with show horses vs performance horses. For example, inflammation of the interosseous ligament in a racing Standardbred can cause a blemish and lameness early in its course, but its importance is reduced with time. In contrast, an obvious "splint" in a Quarter Horse used for a halter class would seriously affect the animal's relative value.

Duration

It is important to determine the occurrence and duration of signs involving the skeletal

945

system. Questions can be asked to determine if the problem was associated with one traumatic incident (fall), a specific activity (jumping, racing), or after breeding. Information regarding changes of feed, shoeing, or other stressful conditions that may predispose to laminitis should be obtained.

The duration of injury can often be roughly estimated by radiographic findings, by considering the rate of hoof-wall growth, and observing the degree of disuse muscle atrophy.

Response to Therapy

The determination of the animal's response to medical and surgical therapy is important in diagnosis and to avoid possible litigation. This is especially true with the widespread use of intra-articular corticosteroids, which may mask clinical signs.

The response to phenylbutazone is especially useful information since sole abscesses show little response to phenylbutazone, especially when compared with the dramatic response obtained in degenerative conditions, such as navicular disease or osteoarthritis.

Physical Examination
by J.H. Cannon

Diagnosis of equine lameness begins with a thorough and systematic physical examination. A working knowledge of anatomy of the limbs and a detailed knowledge of the normal variation of joints and their supporting structures are vital in evaluation of an injured leg. Such evaluation necessarily includes both visual and physical examinations. Visual examination is usually performed concurrently with the digital examination and includes detection of swelling, abnormal silhouettes, deformities and abnormal postures. Visual examination often leads the examiner to a suspicious area or structure, which can then be palpated.

Digital palpation detects heat and swelling or may elicit a painful response. Since evaluation of the painful response can be very subjective, extreme care must be taken to gain the horse's confidence during the examination; otherwise the horse may become overly apprehensive of the necessary manipulations. It may be advisable to bypass the leg in question or the obviously swollen joint to first examine normal structures to determine how the horse reacts to manipulation. If pain is elicited immediately in an examination, the horse becomes apprehensive during examination of

other areas; the resultant responses can be very confusing. By first examining normal structures, the degree of apprehension can be evaluated and compared with the response when the suspected areas are examined.

When manipulating an area of old inflammation, such as a splint, enlarged shin or bowed tendon, pressure applied should initially be moderate and slowly increased. Pain is often noted early but may decrease or disappear with continued manipulation.

The physical characteristics (heat, swelling, sensitivity to manipulation) of equine legs can change from day to day, morning to afternoon, and before or after exercise. Therefore, it may be necessary to evaluate these characteristics on several occasions to accurately determine the state of the structures in question.

Considering the anatomy and the variation of normal, a systematic approach to the physical examination is then employed. Each examiner uses a different system, but it is essential to be systematic and thorough. All areas are palpated and all manipulations are performed to eliminate or confirm suspected disease. One such system will be described.

Physical examination begins with the hoof. Because inflammation in the hoof commonly causes swelling proximal to the hoof, the examination should begin at the hoof to properly evaluate swelling in the remainder of the limb. Visual inspection detects rings, cracks, a dished wall, separated white line, etc. The coffin joint is palpated above the coronary band to detect excessive synovial fluid accumulation, and the strength of the pulse in the digital vessels is checked. Deep digital pressure over the bulbs of the heels, frog, toe and sole often elicits pain in diseased hooves, especially in thin-walled Thoroughbreds. Hoof testers are a valuable aid in locating a hoof lameness, but the diagnosis should not be made with this instrument alone. False-positive reactions are not uncommon with the hoof tester in Thoroughbreds. When hoof testers are used, the opposite hoof must always be evaluated to compare responses.

Palpation of the fetlock begins by determining the amount of synovial fluid in the joint and the amount of fluid in the digital tendon sheath. The joint is then flexed to evaluate the range of motion and to elicit a pain response. In a chronically inflamed joint, flexion may reveal a limited range of motion but may not cause lameness. Conversely, a stiff joint that is the cause of the lameness may not be painful upon flexion.

To localize pain from flexion of the fetlock, the joint should be flexed while applying pressure over the base of the sesamoid bones and distal sesamoidean ligaments, and again while applying pressure over the apex of the sesamoid bones. The pastern and its supporting structures are also examined at this time in both flexion and extension.

Moving proximad up the limb, the suspensory ligament and splint bones are thoroughly examined. Caution must be taken in evaluating pain on the palpation of the bifurcation of the suspensory ligament since many normal horses resent manipulation of this area.

The flexor tendons are evaluated in weight-bearing and nonweight-bearing stances. While the horse is standing, the texture and shape of the tendons are determined by palpation. In the nonweight-bearing state, the tendons can be separated and any soreness localized. The metacarpus is also examined in the weight-bearing and nonweight-bearing states. Digital pressure over the cranial surface of the third metacarpal bone is used to evaluate soreness. Young horses with previous shin soreness are very likely to "lie" to the examiner. To accurately determine the degree of soreness in such shins, pressure must be applied slowly over the areas in question. Manipulating other areas of the limb and metacarpus first is useful in gaining an apprehensive horse's confidence.

The carpus is the most difficult joint to evaluate in the lower forelimb. The degree of carpal lameness is often greater than the physical appearance would indicate. All areas of the carpus must be carefully palpated and manipulated to accurately evaluate these joints. Range of motion and pain on flexion are of limited diagnostic value since horses with severe carpal lameness often have complete range of motion and no pain on flexion. Only obvious carpal problems are detected by these 2 methods alone. Deep digital pressure over the articular edges and the synovial lining must be applied to elicit pain from these joints and to detect excessive synovial fluid accumulation. Pressure is applied while the carpus is flexed and the degree of flexion is varied to examine as much of the joint as possible.

The areas proximal to the carpus are also examined systematically. The elbow and shoulder are flexed and extended, abducted and adducted, and the joints and their supporting structures are thoroughly palpated. Physical examination of the areas proximal to the carpus is not as useful as in the lower leg since it is more difficult to adequately manipulate these areas.

During examination of the rear limb, the hoof, pastern, fetlock and metatarsus are examined as in the forelimb. It must be noted, however, that disease of the rear fetlock does not cause as much pain on flexion and palpation as does disease of a front fetlock. Particular care must be taken in evaluating heat and swelling in the rear fetlock.

Visual examination of the hock reveals any abnormal bony or soft tissue swelling. Since this is a complex joint, a thorough knowledge of normal structures and their appearance is important. The suspect joint should be compared with the opposite leg. The distal intertarsal joints, cunean bursa, tibiotarsal joint, tendon sheaths of the hock and plantar ligament should be palpated in a routine hock examination. Although not a specific test, the spavin test is a valuable aid in diagnosing hock lameness (see Chapter 1).

The size and limited mobility of the stifle joint are deterrents to adequate physical examination of this joint. The patella can be manipulated in the standing position and the patellar ligaments palpated. The joint capsules should be ballotted to detect excess fluid and to check for possible free-floating bodies.

The lumbar, ileosacral and gluteal areas are checked by deep digital pressure. These are also areas in which it is important to differentiate between an apprehensive response to palpation and a true pain response.

As outlined above, the physical examination is the first step in diagnosis of lameness. Areas of suspicion detected by a thorough physical examination can be further investigated by local anesthesia and radiography. Without correlating the physical examination, results of local anesthesia and radiography can be incomplete or confusing and lead to misdiagnosis.

Chapter 1 contains illustrations of the above palpation technics.

Diagnostic Anesthetic Injections
by R.P. Worthman

Diagnostic nerve blocks and anesthetic injections into synovial cavities may be used to help locate an obscure lesion causing lameness. Anesthetic may also be infiltrated around a bony enlargement to determine if it is the cause of lameness. Diagnostic nerve blocks are performed first on the most distal, discrete

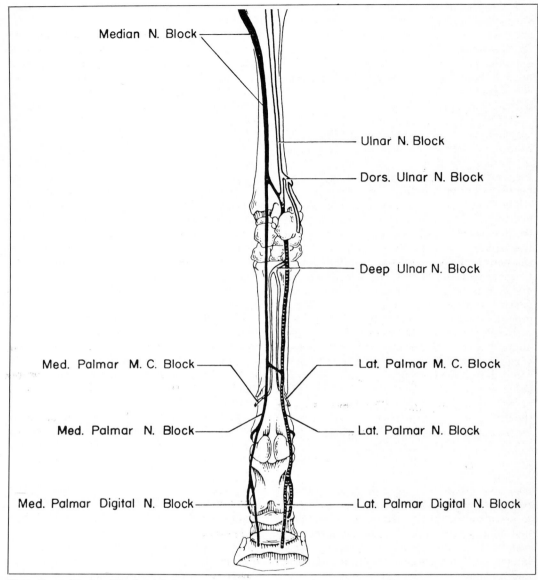

Median N. Block

Ulnar N. Block

Dors. Ulnar N. Block

Deep Ulnar N. Block

Med. Palmar M. C. Block — Lat. Palmar M. C. Block

Med. Palmar N. Block — Lat. Palmar N. Block

Med. Palmar Digital N. Block — Lat. Palmar Digital N. Block

Fig 1. Nerve blocks of the front limb.

branchings of nerve trunks and then progressively more proximal to locate a painful lesion.

Diagnostic nerve blocks and synovial injections should be used routinely only in obscure, chronic lamenesses that cannot be diagnosed by other means. The danger exists that a slight lesion (*eg*, hairline fracture) may be made a major one by the trauma resulting from the return to normal gait and weight bearing after pain is abolished by the anesthetic. Lameness caused not by pain but by mechanical factors (adhesions, exostoses, contractures) is not ameliorated by injection of an anesthetic.

The effects of a nerve block should be evident within 5-10 minutes, while synovial injections usually require at least 15 minutes to take effect. Remember that procaine has no topical effect and is of no value in anesthetizing synovial cavities. All injections should be made through aseptically prepared areas of skin and sterile equipment. Synovial fluid ordinarily does not flow freely from a needle smaller than 18 ga due to its viscosity.

Because diagnostic injection of nerves and joints in the front and rear limbs is similar, only the procedures for the front limbs are described below (Fig 1).

Medial and Lateral Palmar Digital Nerve Blocks

Interpretation: If the animal goes sound after blocking these 2 nerves, the lesion is in the more palmar portions of the hoof since the palmar digital nerves innervate the entire navicular bursa, the palmar portion of the coffin and pastern joint capsules, deep flexor tendon, digital cushion, palmar portion of the cartilage of the hoof, laminar corium and the corium of the bars, frog and sole. Skin desensitization in the bulbs of the heel may be incomplete due to variability of cutaneous nerve branches. If the palmar digital blocks have been performed properly, however, there is no response to application of hoof testers over the central third of the frog. Cutaneous desensitization in the dorsal coronary region indicates that dorsal digital branches have been included in the block, which may lead to misdiagnosis. Remember that the results of a specific neurectomy can hardly be expected to be better than the results obtained by blocking that nerve.

Technic: Using a 25-ga, ⅝-inch needle, no more than 1.5-2 ml anesthetic are deposited sc upon each of the 2 palmar digital nerves about midway between the fetlock and the coronet. A larger volume than this blocks dorsal branches of the palmar digital nerves, causing misleading results. The needle is inserted just dorsal to the superficial digital flexor tendon, where the often palpable digital vein, artery and palmar digital nerve course distad. The nerve is closely associated with the palmar aspect of the digital artery. At the midpastern level of the block, the artery and nerve emerge from beneath the ligament of the ergot, which can be made taut and palpable when the ergot is pushed proximad. Blocking more proximad than the ligament of the ergot increases the probability of including major dorsal branches in the block because of their closer proximity to the palmar digital nerve as one approaches the level of the fetlock.

Navicular Bursa Injection

Interpretation: If the animal goes sound after the palmar digital nerves are blocked, one may inject anesthetic into the navicular bursa, after the effect of the nerve blocks has worn off, to help localize the lesion to this specific structure within the hoof. This injection, however, anesthetizes not only the navicular bursa directly but also, by diffusion, the coffin joint capsule

and the digital tendon sheath. In addition, since a very slight misdirection of the needle causes deposition of anesthetic directly into the digital tendon sheath or the coffin joint instead of the navicular bursa, it may be prudent to omit this procedure. An injection made directly into the coffin joint is probably an easier and more reliable method to gain the information desired.

Technic: An 18-ga, 2-inch needle is inserted through the previously prepared and anesthetized skin of the bulbar fossa. The site is between the heels, just proximal to the coronary band. The needle is passed approximately parallel to the plane of the bearing surface of the hoof until bone is contacted. Up to 5 ml anesthetic may be injected into the bursa without resistance to its flow.

Coffin Joint Injection

Interpretation: Anesthetic injected into this joint anesthetizes not only the coffin joint capsule within 10 minutes but also, by diffusion, the navicular bursa after 10 minutes. By combining palmar digital nerve blocks with intra-articular injection of the coffin joint, involvement of the navicular bursa can be confirmed, more or less to the exclusion of other structures within the hoof. If the animal goes sound with palmar digital blocks, the lesion is located in the navicular bursa or in other structures within the palmar portion of the hoof. If the coffin joint is injected after sensation has returned from the nerve blocks and the animal again goes sound (after 10 minutes), the lesion most likely involves the navicular bursa.

Palmar digital blocks anesthetize the navicular bursa, together with many other structures within the hoof, but they do not desensitize the entire coffin joint, the dorsal portion of which is innervated by unblocked dorsal branches of the palmar digital nerves. To spare these dorsal branches, the palmar digital nerves should not be blocked proximal to the midpastern level and only a small volume of anesthetic should be used. Intra-articular injection of the coffin joint anesthetizes that joint directly, as well as the navicular bursa by diffusion, but not the other structures of the hoof, which are desensitized only by the nerve blocks. Therefore, when the animal goes sound after the nerve blocks and the coffin joint injection, other hoof structures are eliminated and navicular involvement is the most probable cause of the lameness. Few of the other digital structures are desensitized by both procedures.

Technic: A 20-ga, 2-inch needle is inserted 1.5 cm proximal to the coronary border of the hoof at either the medial or lateral border of the common extensor tendon. The needle is directed obliquely distad to pass deep to the tendon toward the extensor process. About 6-10 ml anesthetic are injected into the proximal dorsal pouch of the coffin joint capsule.

Ring Block at Midpastern

Interpretation: If the animal remains unsound after blocking the palmar digital nerves, a ring block at midpastern anesthetizes the entire digit distal to the level of the ring block. This includes both the coffin and pastern joints by blocking the palmar digital nerves, their dorsal branches and the terminal branches of the palmar metacarpal nerves.

Technic: The medial and lateral palmar digital nerves are blocked as previously described and additional anesthetic is injected SC around the entire circumference of the pastern at a level proximal to the pastern joint.

Pastern Joint Injection

Interpretation: If the animal goes sound after the ring block at midpastern, one must wait until sensation has returned to the digit before proceeding with injections into the coffin joint or the pastern joint. These injections determine the presence of intra-articular involvement of these joints, which were desensitized by the midpastern ring block but not by a palmar digital block alone.

Technic: Palpating dorsad from the distal collateral tubercles of the first phalanx along the articular line to the border of the common extensor tendon, which is 2 cm from the dorsal midline of the digit, a 20-ga, 2-inch needle is directed from this point dorsad and mediad (or laterad), deep to the extensor tendon, into the pastern joint capsule.

Low Medial and Lateral Palmar Nerve Blocks

Interpretation: If the animal remains unsound after the ring block at midpastern, these low palmar blocks anesthetize most structures distal to the fetlock. Although much of the fetlock joint capsule itself is anesthetized, it is not possible to completely desensitize this joint via medial and lateral palmar nerve blocks. In addition, cutaneous desensitization is incomplete on the dorsal aspect and sides of the proximal part of the digit. Blocking the medial and lateral palmar nerves at an even more distal level (at the swelling of the fetlock where the nerves are readily palpated) provides even more incomplete desensitization of the felock joint.

Technic: Using a 25-ga, ½-inch needle, 2-3 ml anesthetic are deposited over the medial and lateral palmar nerves 2-3 inches proximal to the fetlock joint, *ie,* at the same level as the distal ends of the splint bones. The nerves lie just dorsal to the medial and lateral edges of the deep digital flexor tendon in the groove between the tendon and the suspensory ligament. Normally at the level of the block the orientation of the palmar vessels and nerve is vein-artery-nerve, with the artery deep to the vein and nerve.

Ring Block Proximal to the Fetlock

Interpretation: If the lameness remains after blocking the medial and lateral palmar nerves, a ring block proximal to the fetlock anesthetizes most structures distal. Although largely desensitized, the fetlock joint retains some degree of sensitivity, however. This procedure blocks the 2 palmar nerves, the subcutaneous, terminal portions of the 2 palmar metacarpal nerves, and the cutaneous branches of the musculocutaneous and dorsal ulnar nerves.

The fetlock joint capsule is not anesthetized completely because the proximal palmar pouch of this joint receives some innervation more proximad from the palmar metacarpal nerves deep to the suspensory ligament. Some deeper fibers from the 2 palmar nerves proximal to the level of the infiltration may also help innervate the proximal palmar pouch of this joint capsule, as well as the proximal portion of the digital tendon sheath.

Technic: About 10 ml local anesthetic are injected SC in a ring at the level of the distal ends of the splint bones. Care should be used to infiltrate over the medial and lateral palmar nerves and at the distal ends of the splint bones to anesthetize the medial and lateral palmar metacarpal nerves.

Fetlock Joint Injection

Interpretation: If lameness decreases after the medial and lateral palmar nerves are blocked or subsequent to the ring block proximal to the fetlock, one may inject the fetlock joint to completely anesthetize the joint and detect an intra-articular lesion.

Technic: About 5 ml anesthetic are injected with a 20-ga, 1-inch needle into the proximal palmar pouch of the fetlock joint. Penetration of the pouch may be from the lateral or medial side of the joint, between the suspensory ligament and the third metacarpal bone just proximal to the level of the sesamoid bones.

Digital Tendon Sheath Injection

Interpretation: Involvement of the flexor tendons in the area of the digital tendon sheath can cause distension of the sheath with fluid, which must be differentiated from turgidity of the digital veins or swelling of the fetlock joint capsule (by its location caudal to the suspensory ligament instead of a distension proximal to it.)

If the animal remains only partially sound after injection of the fetlock joint and the digital tendon sheath is suspect, the sheath may be drained and injected with anesthetic. Such an injection eliminates the possibility that the proximal portion of the digital sheath has not been anesthetized by previous anesthetic procedures. Perhaps a more practical method of anesthetizing the entire digital tendon sheath is to block the medial and lateral palmar nerves at a more proximal level of the metacarpus.

Technic: The common synovial sheath for the superficial and deep digital flexor tendons may be entered by inserting a 20-ga, 1-inch needle between the suspensory ligament and the deep flexor tendon on either side of the appendage just proximal to the level of the sesamoid bones. The digital vessels and nerves at this site can be slid aside and spared from penetration by the needle.

High Medial and Lateral Palmar Nerve Blocks

Interpretation: This procedure may be performed instead of injecting the digital tendon sheath. In addition to the structures desensitized by the low palmar nerve blocks, these higher blocks primarily remove sensation from the superficial and deep flexor tendons in the metacarpal region, as well as from the entire digital tendon sheath.

Technic: The needle is inserted into the groove between the suspensory ligament and the deep flexor tendon in the proximal quarter of the metacarpus. Both the medial and lateral palmar nerves at this more proximal level lie deep to the heavy metacarpal deep fascia and are not palpable. The nerves may be blocked individually from both the medial and lateral approaches, or both nerves may be blocked from the lateral side by first blocking the lateral palmar nerve and then passing the needle through the space between the suspensory ligament and the deep flexor tendon toward the medial palmar nerve. Aspiration should be attempted before injection to ensure that the medial palmar vessels have not been entered. The

appearance of a bleb at either site indicates that the anesthetic has been deposited too superficially. Both palmar nerves in the proximal half of the metacarpus lie deep to the heavy metacarpal deep fascia.

Deep Branch of Lateral Palmar Nerve Block

Interpretation: If the animal remains lame, the deep branch, primarily composed of ulnar nerve fibers of the lateral palmar nerve, may be blocked. Branches of this deep branch innervate distal portions of the carpal joint, the suspensory and inferior check ligaments, and the proximal palmar pouch of the fetlock joint capsule before emerging at the distal ends of the splint bones as the 2 palmar metacarpal nerves.

Technic: With the carpus flexed, the needle is inserted from the palmar surface 3 cm distal to the accessory carpal bone. The needle passes into the palpable space between the lateral border of the flexor tendons and the distal ligament of the accessory carpal bone. Anesthetic solution should be injected into the space between the inferior check (accessory) ligament and the suspensory ligament.

Carpal Joint Injection

Interpretation: If the animal has remained lame up to this point (or even earlier *ie,* after the ring block proximal to the fetlock), one may wish to eliminate the carpal joint as the cause of lameness. The midcarpal joint cavity and the carpometacarpal cavity, with which it communicates, are injected first, then the radio-carpal joint is injected. These 2 injections of anesthetic solution complete the intra-articular examination of the 3 joints of the carpus for a lesion causing the lameness.

Technic: The midcarpal and carpometacarpal joint capsules communicate, so only the midcarpal joint need be injected. When the carpus is flexed, a "dimple" appears in the skin medial to the extensor carpi radialis tendon and superficial to the midcarpal joint space. Injection of 5 ml anesthetic through a 20-ga, 2-inch needle anesthetizes both joint capsules.

For radiocarpal joint injection, the carpus is flexed and the needle is inserted into the radiocarpal joint capsule at a second dimple located 3 cm proximal to the dimple penetrated by the needle used to inject the midcarpal joint cavity.

Ulnar and Median Nerve Blocks

Interpretation: Blocking the median and ulnar nerves removes sensation from the entire digit and, except for some areas of skin, from the metacarpus and carpus. It is still debated whether a branch of the deep radial nerve reaches the carpal joint by passing distad, deep to the extensor tendons.

Technic: For an ulnar nerve block, the needle is inserted in the palpable groove between the flexor carpi ulnaris and the ulnaris lateralis muscles about 10 cm proximal to the accessory carpal bone. The nerve is not palpable because it lies deep to the heavy antebrachial deep fascia. If a bleb appears at the time of injection, the tip of the needle is too superficial (subcutaneous rather than subfascial). Note that the ulnar nerve, artery and vein are immediately deep to the fascia and any anesthetic deposited more deeply than about ½ inch is lost within the flexor muscles.

Blocking the median nerve just distal to the elbow joint is contraindicated for diagnosis of lameness because of the probability of including muscular branches in the block. As an alternative procedure, the needle is inserted 10 cm proximal to the chestnut at the caudal border of the flexor carpi radialis muscle. The needle is directed toward the caudal aspect of the radius by following along the deep surface of the muscle. This leads toward the median artery, vein and nerve, the last being the most caudal. The vein is large, forcing the median nerve on its caudal aspect caudad. Should venous blood appear in the needle when blocking the median nerve, one can withdraw the tip of the needle from the lumen and deposit the anesthetic upon the nerve where it lies along the caudal aspect of the median vein.

Ring Block Proximal to the Carpus

Interpretation: The effects of blocking the median and ulnar nerves have been discussed above. The cutaneous sensation remaining in the carpus and metacarpus can be eliminated by a ring block proximal to the carpus. Subcutaneous infiltration blocks branches of the musculocutaneous, superficial radial, and caudal cutaneous antebrachial nerves, completing desensitization of all structures distal.

Technic: After the median and ulnar nerves have been blocked, additional anesthetic may be infiltrated SC in a ring proximal to the carpus. One or more of the previous procedures should have localized any painful lesion in the distal half of the front limb. If the animal remains lame at this point, one can inject the elbow and then the shoulder joint capsules, as well as the bicipital and infraspinous bursae to detect a painful lesion at any of these sites. However, before initiating this stage of the ex-

amination, one should consider the possibility that the lameness may be mechanical in nature and not subject to amelioration through nerve blocks. Another possibility, of course, is that the nerves intended to be blocked were partly or wholly missed due to faulty technic or, rarely, due to anatomic variation.

Elbow Joint Injection

The lateral ligament of the elbow joint, which connects the lateral epicondyle of the humerus with the lateral tuberosity of the radius, is palpated. An 18-ga, 2½-inch needle is inserted through the skin 1½ inches proximal and 1 inch cranial to the lateral tuberosity of the radius, directing it mediad and slightly caudad to a depth of 2 inches.

Shoulder Joint Injection

The caudal prominence of the lateral tubercle of the humerus, over which the infraspinatus tendon passes, is palpated. Cranial to the infraspinatus tendon lies the palpable cranial prominence of the lateral tubercle. A 16-ga, 3-inch needle is inserted through the skin in the notch between the 2 prominences of the lateral tubercle and is directed in a horizontal plane, caudomediad at a 45° angle, to a depth of about 3 inches.

Intertubercular (Bicipital) Bursa Injection

An 18-ga, 3-inch needle is inserted through the skin cranial to the proximal end of the deltoid tuberosity, and directed proximad and mediad between the biceps muscle and the humerus, toward the distal pouch of the bursa on the cranial aspect of the shoulder joint.

Infraspinatus Bursa Injection

The infraspinatus tendon is palpated where it crosses the lateral surface of the caudal part of the greater tubercle of the humerus. An 18-ga, 2-inch needle is inserted between the tendon and the tubercle from a cranial or caudal direction.

Radiographic Examination
by R.D. Sande

Radiographic examination for any purpose should be preceded by a thorough physical examination of the patient. Specific areas in question are determined from the clinical examination and these areas are then subjected to further study. Information provided by radiographic examination should satisfy qualitative and quantitative criteria. Properly performed radiographic examination, in conjunction with the physical examination, should confirm or support clinical findings. Negative radiographic findings should not be ignored since inability to demonstrate radiographic evidence of a disease does not preclude the clinical diagnosis.

Areas of Examination

Equine radiography has considerable limitations beyond those recognized in small animal and human patients. Anatomic areas amenable to radiographic examination include the limbs distal to the stifle and elbow, the skull and portions of the axial skeleton, including the cervical spine and tail. The thoracic and lumbar spine, thorax, abdomen, stifle, elbow, shoulder, coxofemoral articulations and pelvis provide a formidable diagnostic challenge, depending on the sophistication of the available radiographic facility.

Radiography of the equine limbs distal to the elbow and stifle should be performed with a rigid protocol designed to provide excellent visualization of soft tissue and skeletal structures. The radiographic examination must be performed in such a manner as to produce a profile of the entire area of interest. Properly performed, the examination should require a minimum of 4 exposures, including a dorsopalmar (or dorsoplantar), lateral, and 2 obliques that intersect the horizon or profile produced on the lateral projection. These obliques may be described as dorsopalmar (dorsoplantar) lateral-medial oblique (Fig 201) or palmar (plantar) dorsolateral-medial oblique, as defined by the direction and path of the primary beam from the x-ray tube to the film. Additional projections, including "skyline" (Fig 194) or flexed views, should be determined on the basis of the survey radiographic and physical examinations to ensure that the appropriate profile is projected onto the film.

Radiographic examination of the equine skull is perhaps the most rewarding of any performed in this species. Survey radiography of the equine skull is made difficult by skull size and variable densities encountered. As a result, thorough physical examination and exact localization of pathologic changes often precede the request for radiographic examination. Such a request is not made for discovery of a lesion but for confirmation and further definition. The physical examination findings predicate the protocol used to produce the best radiographic profile of the lesion.

The cervical and coccygeal areas of the spine are slightly more difficult to examine radiographically. Positioning of the patient is paramount to any radiographic study of the axial skeleton. Perfect lateral and ventrodorsal projections are necessary for most interpretations, excluding lateral radiography of the dens. Radiography of the spine, similar to that of the skull, is often preceded by physical and neurologic evaluation. Positive radiographic findings are frequent and negative examinations have little value.

Thoracic radiography may provide valuable information if extensive pathologic changes are present. Adequate visualization of thoracic changes is limited by the available diagnostic radiographic facility and size of the patient. Visualization of the dorsal and dorsocaudal segment of the thorax is usually adequate. Unfortunately, the cranial and ventral thorax is difficult to study. Right and left lateral projections should be routine for adequate visualization of each hemithorax.

Diagnostic radiographic examination of the abdomen, lumbar spine and thoracic spine is extremely difficult in most adult horses. Specialized radiographic facilities capable of generating high kilovoltage technics are necessary.

Radiographic examination of the equine pelvis, stifle, shoulder, and elbow is possible with most mobile and fixed radiographic units. Portable radiographic units may also prove inadequate for such studies.

Radiographic Equipment

Procedures involving the use of ionizing radiation should be performed only after careful consideration of the principle of "acceptable risk." More specifically, one should determine that the information that might be gained by the procedure is worth the risk to the patient and attendants. Failure to satisfy this criterion is cause for re-evaluation of the need for the procedure. Performance of a radiographic procedure should include efforts to reduce the hazards of exposure to ionizing radiation by the attendants and the patient.

Long-scale radiographic detail is achieved with technics using maximum KVp and minimum mAs. This type of technic allows visualization of a wide variation (long scale) of tissue densities. Adequate mAs is necessary to provide visual separation of individual tissue densities. In contrast, short-scale radiographic technics use high mAs and reduced KVp. With short-scale technics, more radiative interactions occur as a result of production of greater numbers of x-rays. While this may produce greater detail, it is limited to a narrow range of tissue densities and results in increased radiation exposure to the patient and attendants.

Radiographic technic is usually restricted by the quality and sophistication of the x-ray generator and tube. Equipment capable of producing high-mAs, high-KVp studies may be prohibitively expensive and is generally located at academic institutions. Mobile radiographic units are normally limited to less than 125 KVp and 200-300 mAs. This type of equipment is usually confined to use within a veterinary hospital and gives high-quality, safe radiography for an acceptable investment.

Portable diagnostic x-ray equipment is the most commonly used type for routine equine radiography. Unfortunately, portability is made possible at the expense of shielding and electronic sophistication. These units are best used for examination of the limb distal to the elbow and stifle, and portions of the skull.

Cassette, screen and film combinations are important factors in performing high-quality radiography. Rare-earth screens have proven especially valuable in equine radiography as they provide adequate radiographic detail using limited radiographic facilities. Use of rare-earth screens may reduce mAs requirements to one-eighth that required to produce an equivalent film with par-speed screens. Advantages include a significant reduction in radiation exposure to the patient and attendant, expanded capabilities and better use of x-ray equipment, shorter exposure times, and shorter scales of contrast, with better subject detail. The added expense involved in purchase of the screens is more than offset by savings in equipment investment and added radiation safety.

Proper collimation of the primary beam reduces scattered radiation, resulting in improved radiographic detail and reduced exposure to radiation. To further reduce loss of detail due to radiation scatter, a grid should be interposed between the patient and the film when tissue thickness exceeds 10 cm.

Protection from ionizing radiation is best accomplished by reducing the time of exposure, increasing the distance from the primary radiation source, and interposing a barrier. Lead aprons and gloves should be worn during all diagnostic procedures. These barriers are designed to protect against scattered radiation and should not be considered protective if worn in the primary beam.

Radiation-monitoring devices should be worn by attendants during radiographic procedures. The most popular device is a film badge that accurately measures total body exposure when used properly. The badge should be worn on the lapel, beneath the protective apron. When not in use, the badge should be stored safely out of the radiation zone and away from heat sources or direct sunlight.

Special Technics and Imaging Systems

Enhancement of subject contrast may provide additional diagnostic information. When one is unable to adequately visualize radiographic detail due to limitations of the equipment, a special procedure or contrast study may be performed. Special studies that have proven practical clinical application in equine radiography include contrast arthrography, upper GI contrast studies, sinography or fistulography, dacryorhinocystotography and localized selective or semiselective vascular studies. Myelography, angiocardiography and cerebral angiography have application but may require additional radiographic facilities. Any special study should be preceded by thorough physical and radiographic examination, a review of the technic to be performed and careful selection of the appropriate contrast agent.

Technologic advancements in imaging systems have made special imaging technics available and feasible in institutional and private veterinary practice. The application of xeroradiography in equine practice has become increasingly popular. This modality is useful in the radiographic study of equine lameness associated with pathologic changes in both soft and hard tissues (Fig 204).

Cinematography, Electrogoniometry, Thermography, and Dynamography
by M.H. Ratzlaff

Cinematography, electrogoniometry, thermography and dynamography have been used to evaluate the physiologic responses of horses to locomotor stress. Each method provides specific information that may aid in the diagnosis of lameness and the evaluation of surgical or medical treatments.

Cinematography

Cinematography involves the use of high-speed cameras to record the movements of horses moving at different gaits.[2-7] In its simplest form, one camera is used to photograph the horse moving at the selected gait and the films are empirically evaluated. A more precise method may be used in which the horse moves over a known distance while films are taken. In this method, anatomic landmarks on the limbs are identified and marked with small squares of tape or by other means. The horse is trotted over a level, known, marked distance. The high-speed camera is positioned perpendicular to the marked course and the field of view encompasses the entire course. The horse is photographed as it traverses the entire distance. The film speed should be at least 5 times the normal projection speed so that on film, the horse moves at least 5 times slower than normal. The analysis consists of plotting the position of each marked anatomic site for each frame until at least one full stride is completed. Using this method, the length of stride, stride rate, arcs of flight of the toe and joints, limb segment displacements, linear and angular velocities and accelerations, and the range of motion of each joint may be determined.

A third method employs 2 or more cameras. After the anatomic landmarks of the limbs are marked, one camera is positioned in front of the course and another at right angles to the course. A third camera may be placed directly behind the course. Analysis of films obtained by this method provides a 3-dimensional analysis of hoof and limb movements.

There are 2 main disadvantages of high-speed cinematography. First, the markers used to identify anatomic landmarks move with the skin, especially in the proximal regions of the appendages. Therefore, the accuracy of the measurements decreases significantly in the proximal parts of the limbs. Second, the analysis of slow-motion movies is delayed due to the time involved in processing the film. However, the advantages of cinematography far outweigh the disadvantages. Cinematography provides the greatest amount of information of all of the methods used to evaluate motion and usually supplements other technics. The development of computerized film analysis has permitted rapid, complete data analysis of locomotor patterns.

Electrogoniometry

Electrogoniometry provides for the continuous recording of joint motion and is accurate to within $\pm$ 1° of movement when properly performed.[6,8,9] Electrogoniometry may be used to determine the patterns of joint movement, specific points in the stride, range and amplitude of motion, angular velocities and accelerations, and the swing, support and total stride times.

Elgons (electrogoniometers), which function as electrical protractors, are calibrated and positioned over the center of rotation of the joints to be evaluated. The elgons are taped securely in place and the leads are attached to the saddle. The leads are connected to a control panel, which is connected to an oscillographic recorder. The elgon consists of a potentiometer mounted on a plastic or metal chassis. The signal generated by the potentiometer is amplified in the control panel and passes to the oscillographic recorder. The resulting goniograms may be analyzed directly or the data may be recorded on magnetic tape and analyzed by computer.

A second method, using radio telemetry, permits unrestricted movement of the horse. The leads from the elgons are connected to an FM transmitter, which may be mounted on the sulky or attached to the saddle. The signals generated by the potentiometers are amplified and transmitted to an FM receiver, demodulated and recorded on an oscillographic recorder or magnetic tape.

Several disadvantages are associated with electrogoniometry. First, errors are inherent in recordings of motion of the joints proximal to the carpus and tarsus. The elgons move with the skin and do not remain positioned over the center of rotation of the proximal joints. Second, unless telemetry is employed, the use of electrogoniometry normally is confined to the evaluation of joint motion at the walk and trot. The cable connecting the leads from the elgons to the control panel must be lengthy and elaborate for use on horses moving at faster gaits. Third, the interpretation of goniograms is difficult for the practitioner since electrogoniometry does not provide for direct visualization of movement.

Goniograms of the fetlock and carpus, as well as the positions of the limb at selected points in the stride, are illustrated in Figure 2. Flexion of the carpus begins during the second half of the support phase, continues through hoof lift and reaches its maximum during the first half of the swing phase. Carpal extension begins at this point and reaches its maximum shortly after hoof contact. Flexion of the fetlock also begins during the second half of the support phase, continues through hoof lift and reaches its maximum during the swing phase. Two points of maximum flexion, interrupted by a brief period of extension, occur during the

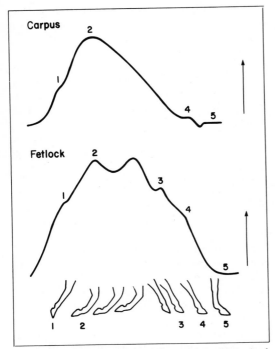

Fig 2. Typical goniograms of the carpus and fetlock of a trotting horse. The arrows indicate flexion, and the position of the limb during the stride is shown at the bottom. 1 = hoof lift, 2 = maximum flexion, 3 = flexion peak during extension of the fetlock, 4 = hoof contact, 5 = maximum support.

swing phase. Fetlock extension begins during the second half of the swing phase and reaches its maximum during the support phase. A brief period of flexion (point 3) occurs during extension at the point of maximum protraction of the limb. This is apparently due to the final positioning of the hoof by the actions of the digital extensor and flexor muscles prior to contact.

Electrogoniometry and cinematography were used to aid diagnosis of an obscure lameness of the right leg of a Thoroughbred hunter-jumper. Electrogoniometry was performed on the right and left carpal and fetlock joints. Side-view, slow-motion movies were also taken as the horse moved through a marked course. Movement of the right and left carpal joints was essentially normal; however, the right carpus had an increased amplitude due to an increased range of flexion ($+13°$) (Fig 3). The goniograms of the fetlock joints were flattened, apparently due to training. The right fetlock had a decreased amplitude due to decreased extension ($-7°$). Additionally, there was an abnormal period of flexion during the extension

phase immediately after hoof contact (point B). There was also a small amount of flexion prior to hoof lift (point A). The percent of the support time of the right limb was also slightly less than that of the left.

The arcs of the toe, fetlock and carpus of the right and left limbs are illustrated in Figure 4. At hoof contact, the right carpus and fetlock did not drop as far as those of the contralateral limb. During maximum weight-bearing, the loop formed by the fetlock joint was tighter than that of the left (point A) and the right carpus did not drop as far as the left (point B). At hoof lift, the right fetlock and carpus were higher than the left, and the arc of flight of the left toe was higher than that of the right (point C). The stride length of the right front was slightly shorter than that of the left.

The changes in movement of the right front limb indicated damage to the suspensory ligament. The pattern of movement and decreased range of extension of the right fetlock, and the abnormal changes immediately before hoof contact and hoof lift supported this conclusion. The changes observed on film analysis were consistent with those observed in the goniograms. During maximum weight-bearing, the fetlock and carpus did not drop as far as the left, which suggested pain at this point in the stride. Additionally, there was a decreased support time of the right limb. Subsequent clinical examination confirmed the diagnosis of suspensory desmitis in the mid-metacarpal area.

Thermography

Thermography is the graphic imaging of temperature gradients of the skin.[10-15] Different thermography patterns, due to temperature differences, indicate pathologic changes.

The basic instrumentation for medical thermography consists of an infrared scanner, which converts the radiated thermal energy (infrared rays) to electrical signals. A display unit converts and amplifies these signals into a thermal picture displayed on a video screen. The resulting thermogram may be black and white or color. Isotherm colors of known temperatures may be coded on the display screen. Therefore, color images may be used for the quantitative evaluation of the thermogram by comparing the color of these images to isotherm colors.

Thermographic examinations may be performed on all regions but is most frequently used as an aid in the diagnosis of lameness.

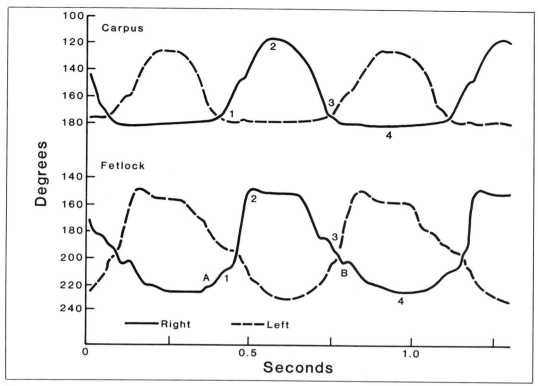

Fig 3. Goniograms of the carpal and fetlock joints of a Thoroughbred with an obscure lameness of the right limb. The right carpus showed increased flexion (2). The right fetlock joint had decreased extension (4) and abnormal flexion prior to hoof lift (A) and after hoof contact (B). 1 = hoof lift, 2 = maximum flexion, 3 = hoof contact, and 4 = maximum extension.

Most examinations use a temperature range of 10° C; temperature patterns are compared to isotherms of 1° C each on the color monitor. The infrared scanner is positioned perpendicular to the limbs, 6-8 ft from the horse. Dorsal, palmar/plantar, lateral and medial views are most commonly taken. Thermograms of both limbs are obtained for comparison.

The main advantage of thermography is the early detection of pathologic changes, often before clinical signs become apparent. Additionally, the equipment is not difficult to operate and is not harmful to the horse or operator. The major disadvantage of thermography is high initial cost of the equipment.[13]

On black and white thermograms, lighter areas indicate regions of higher infrared emissions due to increased surface temperatures, while darker areas are cooler (Fig 5). In normal horses, the highest temperatures are associated with the coronary band and coolest temperatures occur on the dorsolateral aspects of the fetlock joints.

Dynamography

Dynamography involves use of a force transducer to measure the amount and direction of the forces exerted by the foot upon the ground.[16,17] The force transducers in general use today consist of forceplates embedded in the ground. One type of force platform consists of a rigid metal surface plate suspended on a series of vertical and horizontal metal bars, on which strain gauges are mounted. Force exerted on the surface plate results in deformation of the metal bars. This deformation changes the electrical resistance of the strain gauges and the flow of current through the strain gauge circuit. These plates record the forces in vertical, cranial-caudal horizontal, and lateral-medial horizontal directions. The vertical forces result from the body weight during the support phase. Lateral and medial forces result from hoof impact, rotatory motion of the limb, and the direction of travel.

The force platform is calibrated, covered with a nonslip surface, and embedded in soil

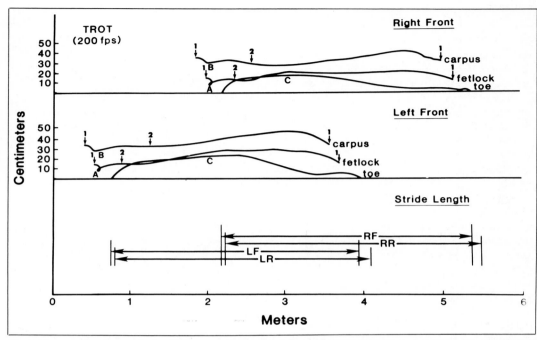

Fig 4. Slow-motion film analysis of the same horse as in Figure 3. The horse was moving at a trot and filmed at 200 frames/second. The arcs of flight of the right and left carpus, fetlock and toe are shown at the top and center. The length of stride of all four legs is shown at the bottom. At hoof contact (1), the right carpus and fetlock did not drop as far as those of the left leg, and the loop (A) formed by the right fetlock during the support phase was smaller than that of the left. The right carpus did not drop as far as the left during the support period (B). The arc of flight of the right toe was also lower than that of the left (C). The stride length of the right front leg was shorter than that of the left. 1 = hoof contact, 2 = hoof lift.

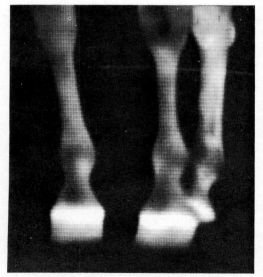

Fig 5. Thermogram of the forelimbs immediately after exercise. The lighter areas indicate regions of higher temperatures. (Courtesy of Dr R. Purohit)

with the surface plate level with the ground (Fig 6). The leads from the strain gauges are connected to amplifiers and a recorder. As the horse moves over the force platform, the amount and direction of the forces are recorded. A force-time pattern is obtained and peak forces can be measured. These forces are most commonly expressed as a percentage of body weight but may be expressed in Newtons.

The main disadvantage of the force platform is that horses tend to avoid striking the platform even when the surface is camouflaged. The major advantage of this technic is that locomotive forces are directly measured.

Bone Scintigraphy
by M.D. Devous, Sr. and J.L. Baum

Bone scintigraphy is an aspect of nuclear medicine that provides a sensitive and early means of detecting increased bone turnover and new bone formation. Most skeletal diseases, such as fractures, osteoarthritis, osteomyelitis, epiphyseal abnormalities and neoplasia, can be diagnosed and radiographic evaluations can be confirmed by scintigraphy. Certain injuries may take several days or may never become radiographically evident, while scintigraphic evidence of a bone abnormality is often visible 12-24 hours after injury. The progression or regression of skeletal disease can be accurately monitored through scintigraphy. Scintigraphic evidence of a healed fracture is based on the metabolic condition of the osseous tissue. Therefore, disappearance of a scintigraphic lesion is a clear indication of normal metabolic behavior. Interpretation of the state of healing under radiographic conditions is often more subjective. Scintigraphy can be used under all conditions in which lameness is not clearly identified by physical or radiographic examination. In many cases with radiographic evidence of a lesion, scintigraphy is used to determine the severity of the lesion and to monitor its progression or regression.

Bone scanning involves administration of a radiopharmaceutical. Once the radioactive material has concentrated in the organs of interest, the image is produced by detecting gamma radiation with a position-sensitive device. The result is a picture of the distribution of radioactive materials within the animal. It represents the physiologic or pathologic behavior of the target organ since the radioactivity distribution directly reflects the normal or abnormal abilities of the tissues to absorb the radiopharmaceutical. Radiographs depict structure via tissue densities, whereas scintigraphs depict pathologic changes via radiopharmaceutical distribution.

Instrumentation

The instrument used to measure radiopharmaceutical distribution is called a gamma camera. The gamma camera consists of a collimator (a lead shield with parallel holes), which focuses the gamma rays onto a radiation-sensitive crystal (sodium iodide) fitted with an array of photomultiplier tubes that detect the position of incoming gamma rays. Most cameras are equipped with a 10-inch crystal, which produces a circular field of view 10 inches in diameter. Diverging and converging collimators can be used to focus on smaller or larger areas of interest.

Radiopharmaceuticals

Most radiotracers accumulated by the skeleton do so by exchange with the inorganic components of hydroxyapatite, the principal mineral

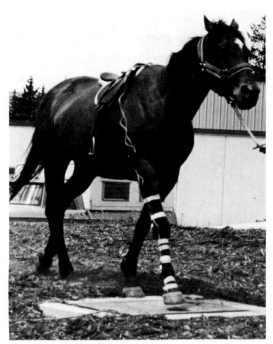

Fig 6. Three-directional force platform embedded in the ground. The right front hoof is about to strike the platform.

of the skeleton. In human and veterinary nuclear medicine, technetium 99M is the radioisotope of choice. The technetium 99M obtained from a generator is usually bound to pyrophosphate (PYP) or methylene diphosphonate (MDP). Both agents localize in the skeleton within 30 minutes of IV injection, and adequate clearance from the surrounding soft tissues for clear imaging occurs by 2 hours with MDP. Therefore, most bone imaging is conducted 2-5 hours after IV injection of the agent.

Scintigraphic Technic

Technetium 99M is obtained from the generator and mixed with sterilized MDP or PYP. The patient is given the material by IV injection and is placed in front of the camera for imaging 2 hours later.

Mild tranquilization permits imaging over periods of up to 2 minutes with very little motion and also eases positioning of the animal in front of the cameras. Some care must be taken in imaging the pelvic region to avoid overlap of bony structures with the bladder because of renal clearance of the radiopharmaceutical. Most images require 1-2 minutes for acquisition. Typically a forelimb is imaged from shoulder to hoof in 5 views. Rear limbs are im-

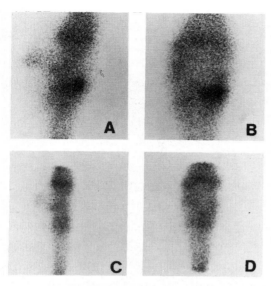

Fig 7. Lateral and cranial scintigraphs of the carpus. A fracture of the third carpal bone appears as a focal lesion in the craniomedial aspect of the distal row of carpal bones (A,B). The lesion was nearly healed after 6 months of rest (C,D).

owner suspected a splint lameness but the animal had a more severe lameness than generally found with splint problems. Radiographic evaluation suggested chronic inactive splints inconsistent with the degree of lameness. However, scintigraphic evaluation revealed a fractured third carpal bone (Fig 7).

There is great potential for the use of scintigraphy to diagnose lameness. The major stumbling blocks to be overcome before scintigraphy becomes practical in private practice are equipment costs and appropriate means of training and licensing. The former is almost within reason now. Typical used gamma cameras can be obtained for 2-5 times the cost of comparable radiographic equipment. The latter problem is just now being studied. The first residency program aimed specifically at nuclear medicine training allied with radiology training was recently initiated. Such training should be more common within a few years.

Arthroscopy
by C.W. McIlwraith

There are obvious limitations in the conventional methods of assessing diseased joints. For example, radiographs only demonstrate erosion of the articular cartilage when the erosion is advanced enough to cause narrowing of the joint space or subchondral bone changes. Also, although synovial fluid examination may demonstrate the presence of synovitis, the degree of pathologic change in the synovial membrane is difficult to assess.

Examination of the joint with an arthroscope enables evaluation of the nonosseous joint tissues, including the synovial membrane and its

aged from hip to hoof in 5-7 views, depending on the size of the animal. In general, clinical history restricts imaging procedures to a small area for 20-60 minutes. Lateral and cranial or caudal views are generally sufficient for complete identification and localization of abnormal bone activity. Unlike radiographs, in which structural detail is obtained by multiple views, hot spots on scintigraphic scans generally show up as long as perpendicular views of the area have been obtained.

An example of clinical use of scintigraphy involves a 4-year-old male Standardbred. The

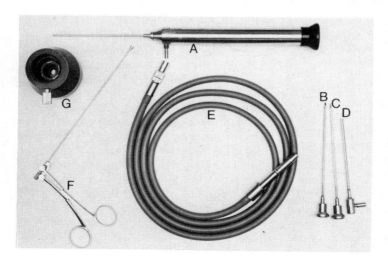

Fig 8. Equipment used in arthroscopy: arthroscope (A); sharp trocar (B); blunt obturator (C); insertion cannula (D); fiberoptic light guide (E); biopsy forceps (F); camera adapter (G). (Courtesy of JAVMA)

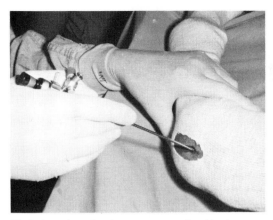

Fig 9. Insertion of arthroscope cannula with sharp trocar through fibrous joint capsule. The trocar is replaced with a blunt obturator before entering the joint.

associated villi, articular cartilage, intra-articular ligaments, and menisci. The technic has been widely used in humans.[18] The use of the arthroscope in equine clinical cases and research has been described.

Equipment

Several types of arthroscopes are available. A 2.2-mm diameter arthroscope (Dyonics) is illustrated in Figure 8. The 17° inclined-view model provides a 70° field of view and a magnification of 1-15 power, depending on the distance between the end of the arthroscope and the object. The arthroscope is illuminated by fiberoptic lighting via a 1.75-m flexible light guide. Other instrumentation includes an insertion cannula, a sharp trocar to penetrate the fibrous joint capsule, a blunt obturator to enter through the synovial membrane into the joint, and a pair of biopsy forceps (Fig 8).

Technic

General anesthesia and aseptic technic are used in all cases. Prior to insertion of the arthroscope, the joint may be distended by intra-articular injection of Ringer's solution to make insertion easier and safer. To insert the arthroscope, a stab incision is made with a #15 scalpel blade and the joint capsule penetrated with the insertion cannula containing a sharp trocar (Fig 9). The trocar is then exchanged for the blunt obturator and entry into the joint completed. If prior injection of Ringer's solution has not been performed, a synovial fluid sample may be aspirated at this stage. The joint is then flushed with Ringer's solution and the arthroscope inserted. Irrigating solution is flushed through the side cannula to remove

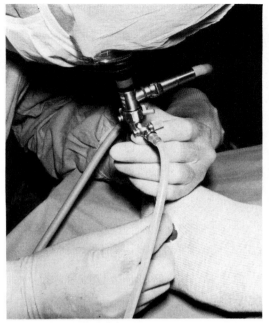

Fig 10. Visualization through a 2.5-mm Wolf arthroscope.

any debris or air bubbles and to distend the joint during visualization (Fig 10). Following visualization, a biopsy of the synovial membrane can be obtained by selecting the site, removing the arthroscope and inserting biopsy forceps through the cannula (Fig 11). At the completion of the procedure, the skin is closed with a single suture.

Arthroscopic findings should be documented by dictation, drawing, photography or a combination of all 3. Camera adapters are available for all name-brand single-lens reflex

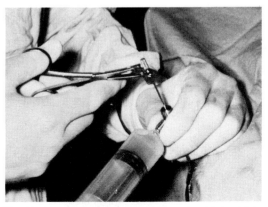

Fig 11. A synovial membrane biopsy is obtained following an arthroscopic examination.

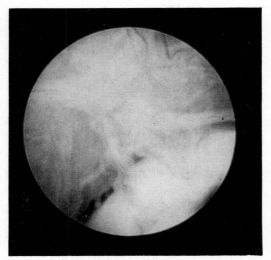

Fig 12. Synovial villi adjacent to lateral trochlear ridge of the talus in a normal tibiotarsal joint.

Examination of the fetlock joint is performed through the volar pouch. This limits the examination to the articular surfaces of the sesamoid bones, caudal distal metacarpus, and synovial membrane of the volar pouch.

Two entry sites are necessary for complete examination of the tibiotarsal joint. A craniomedial entry site allows visualization of the medial trochlear ridge of the talus and the synovial membrane of the medial tibiotarsal joint. A craniolateral entry is necessary for examination of the lateral trochlear ridge of the talus and the intermediate ridge of the distal tibia.

The femoropatellar joint of the stifle is examined by insertion of the arthroscope between the middle and lateral patellar ligaments distal to the patella. Complete examination of the femoropatellar articulation is difficult but it is generally possible to examine some areas of the trochlear ridges of the femur and the articulating surface of the patella. A technic for examination of the small, separate femorotibial joints has been described.[20] In that technic, the femorotibial joints are entered by an oblique approach from the opposite side.

The author has not performed arthroscopic examinations on the elbow, shoulder, hip or phalangeal joints.

General Arthroscopic Anatomy and Pathology

The structures of principal interest on arthroscopic examination of an equine joint are the synovial membrane and the articular cartilage, which are difficult to evaluate by standard clinical methods.

cameras for photographs. However, with conventional light sources and the small diameter arthroscopes, photographs are inferior to what is visualized. For good photographs, a light source with a flash generator is desirable.

The effectiveness of arthroscopic examination depends on how much of the joint can be visualized; this varies with different joints. The entire radiocarpal and intercarpal joints can be examined using entry sites lateral and medial to the extensor carpi radialis tendon. A single entry lateral to the tendon allows visualization of all but the lateral cul-de-sac and usually suffices for most clinical examinations.

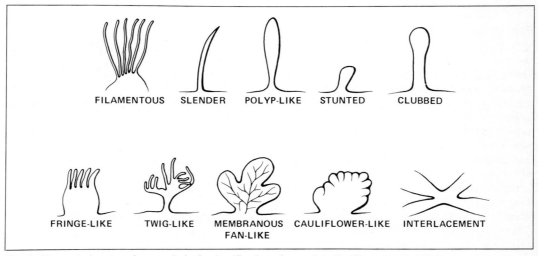

Fig 13. Suggested system for morphologic classification of synovial villi. (Courtesy of JAVMA)

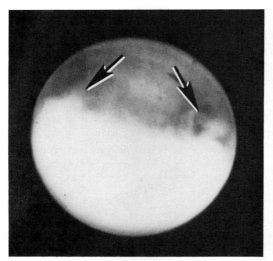

Fig 14. Arthroscopic view of superficial fibrillation of the articular cartilage of the trochlear ridge of the femur. Disrupted fibrils of articular cartilage are suspended in the irrigating solution (arrows).

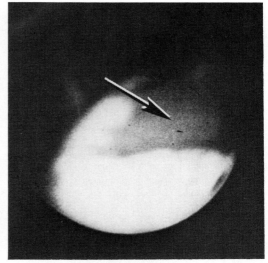

Fig 15. Arthroscopic view of erosion of the articular cartilage (arrow) on the proximal articular surface of the third carpal bone.

The morphology of the synovial villi is much more apparent with arthroscopy than with arthrotomy. With arthrotomy, villi tend to cling to the synovial membrane and cannot be seen distinctly. With arthroscopy, the villi stand out distinctly while suspended in the fluid medium (Fig 12). The magnification of the arthroscope also facilitates definition. A classification system for the morphologic characteristics of villi has been suggested (Fig 13).

In normal joints, villi are located in certain areas that must be recognized before one can interpret pathologic changes. The synovial membrane is nearly always inflamed in equine joint diseases. Hyperemia and petechiation of the synovial membrane and associated villi may be observed in acute synovitis. Small, hyperemic villi may form in locations where villi were previously absent. Membranous, fan-like and cauliflower-like villi have been observed in joints with synovitis but have never been seen in normal joints. Fusion of villi and formation of fibrinoid strands have also been observed in inflamed joints. In some cases of traumatic and degenerative arthritis, excess villous proliferation may be an indication for synovectomy.

Changes in the synovial membrane have been used to study the development of synovitis in the equine intercarpal joint.[19]

The potential usefulness of arthroscopy for the diagnosis of other soft tissue injuries in joints has been demonstrated.[21] In a prospec-

tive study of humans with injuries involving traumatic hemarthrosis but no or negligible instability on clinical examination, 72% of knees had disruption of the cranial cruciate ligament. Meniscal tears were also diagnosed in 62% of the knees. At our present stage of experience in horses, arthroscopic diagnosis of traumatic injury of the stifle is undeveloped but potentially useful.

The greatest clinical use of the arthroscope is in the assessment of articular cartilage when radiographic signs are equivocal or nonexistent. Arthroscopic examination allows the recognition of fibrillation and erosion of the articular cartilage (Figs 14, 15). Fibrillation may be more easily recognized by arthroscopy than by gross visualization due to a combination of factors. These factors include magnification and transillumination of collagen fibrils, as well as their suspension in the irrigation solution.

Severe erosion of the articular cartilage is generally obvious on arthroscopic visualization (Fig 15). Visualization of subtle defects in the articular cartilage may be improved by the addition of methylene blue to the irrigating solution but this is usually not necessary nor routinely practiced.

Specific Arthroscopic Anatomy and Pathology

A normal arthroscopic view of the medial half of the intercarpal joint includes the distal

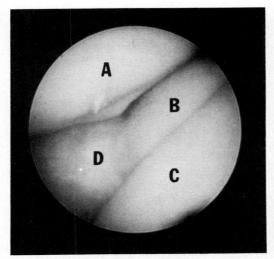

Fig 16. Arthroscopic view of the medial aspect of a normal intercarpal joint. Distal articular surface of the radial carpal bone (A); proximal articular surface of 2nd (B) and 3rd (C) carpal bones; synovial membrane (D).

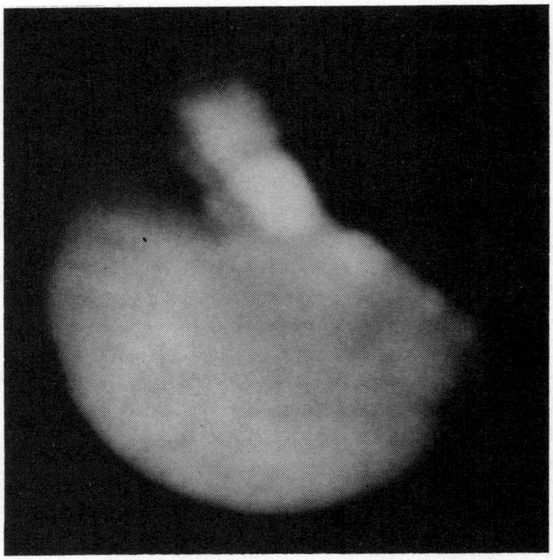

Fig 17. Arthroscopic view of a cartilage flap partially detached from the trochlear ridge of the talus in a case of degenerative joint disease. (Courtesy of JAVMA)

articular surface of the radial carpal bone, the proximal articular surface of the second and third carpal bones, the villous synovial membrane dorsomediad and the smooth synovial membrane of the medial cul-de-sac (Fig 16). Arthroscopic examination through this site generally allows identification of most pathologic states of the intercarpal joint. Intra-articular fractures can be identified by radiographs. However, in some cases, particularly in old fractures, the state of healing or condition of the articular surface is uncertain. These situations can be evaluated and a prognostic and therapeutic decision made using arthroscopy. The results of the examination may dictate the need for arthrotomy and removal of the chip, with or without curettage of some of the remaining articular cartilage. Alternatively, arthroscopy may reveal degeneration to the point where surgical intervention is not indicated. Such situations can be similarly evaluated in the radiocarpal joints.

Another clinical use of the arthroscope is illustrated by the case of the race horse with carpal soreness. Acute inflammation is present clinically but radiographic signs are equivocal. Using arthroscopy, observation of severe erosion dictates a poor prognosis and no surgical intervention (Fig 15). Localized lesions may serve as an indication for curettage of the articular cartilage, and synovitis with minimal cartilage degeneration is an indication for joint lavage.[22]

Joint lavage can be conveniently performed in conjunction with arthroscopy. The arthroscope cannula serves as an egress portal and a 10- or 12-ga needle is inserted in the medial aspect of the joint as an entry portal. The synovial membrane of the carpal joints undergo characteristic changes with inflammation. Small villi develop in the normally smooth medial areas and villi morphology changes in the villous areas.

The synovial membrane in the proximal recess of the fetlock joint has a characteristic lacy appearance. Fibrotic, thickened villi develop with inflammation in the joint. Cartilage degeneration may be detected on the articulating surface of the sesamoids and caudal distal metacarpus. Because one cannot evaluate the metacarpophalangeal or metatarsophalangeal articulations, the indications for arthroscopy of the fetlock are much less than in the carpal joints.

The synovial membrane of the tibiotarsal joint has a marked tendency for hypertrophy when inflamed. This situation is easily recognized by arthroscopy and appropriate treatment instituted. In degenerative joint disease of the tibiotarsal joint, craniocaudal radiographs may or may not reveal a decreased joint space. Using arthroscopy, the trochlear ridges of the talus can be visualized and the presence of fibrillation or erosion diagnosed (Fig 17). Degeneration of the articular cartilage in these cases is usually generalized and treatment generally not indicated.

Complete examination of the femoropatellar joint is not possible but enough articular surface of the patella and trochlear ridges of the femur can be visualized to confirm the presence of degeneration of the articular cartilage. The most significant clinical affliction in this area is osteochondritis dissecans, which can be diagnosed radiographically. However, radiographs are of little value in diagnosing patellar chondromalacia. In such cases, arthroscopy can confirm the presence or absence of fibrillation or erosion of articular cartilage. While the author has identified fibrillation in this area in a few clinical cases, the overall usefulness of arthroscopy in the stifle has not been assessed.

Limitations of Arthroscopy

Although the arthroscope is a useful clinical and research tool, it may not be destined for routine use in general equine practice. The arthroscope requires considerable experience before it can be used effectively and valid interpretations made. At least 50-100 examinations are required before one gains confidence in the technic. A thorough knowledge of arthroscopic anatomy and awareness of the pitfalls of overinterpretation are prerequisites. Magnification can make insignificant defects appear as major lesions. Relatively avascular projections of synovial membrane may be mistaken for loose bodies.

As previously mentioned, visualization of the entire joint is difficult in some instances. This is exacerbated by pathologic thickening and fibrosis in the fibrous joint capsule. Multiple entry sites and accessory instruments are used in humans to manipulate intra-articular structures and enhance visualization.[23]

Because available arthroscopes are rigid and delicate, the development of flexible arthroscopes to circumvent difficult obstructions could eliminate any need for multiple entry sites and may improve the examinations of the hock, stifle and fetlock in horses.

In humans, removal of loose bodies and shaving of chondromalacic cartilage is practiced under arthroscopic visualization, obviating the need for arthrotomy. One advantage is that such procedures can be performed under local analgesia in humans. Because of the necessity for general anesthesia in horses, these complex procedures have little advantage over simple arthrotomy and are more cumbersome. In the intercarpal joint, the size of the cannula used with the intra-articular shaver is too large to be practical.

The full potential of arthroscopy has yet to be evaluated. The arthroscope is a useful clinical and research tool in the carpal and tibiotarsal joints, has limited clinical but potentially good research value in the stifle, and is of limited clinical use in the fetlock. In specialty practices, the instrument can play an important role in the complete evaluation of traumatic and degenerative joint disease. However, because of some of the reasons outlined above, the technic is not destined for routine use.

Complications

Potential complications of arthroscopy are joint infection, hemarthrosis, iatrogenic damage to the articular cartilage, and breaking of the instrument within a joint. The author has encountered a few instances of iatrogenic damage to the cartilage and in no case was there significant damage. All of these cases occurred during learning of the technic. A review of 3714 arthroscopic examinations of human knees revealed no cases of infection, minor articular cartilage damage attributable to the instrument in 2% of the cases, 4 cases of subcutaneous emphysema from insufflation of gas, and 26 instances of bending or breaking of the instrument when negotiating the condyles.[24]

Synovial Fluid Analysis
by C.W. McIlwraith

Examination of the synovial fluid should be a routine procedure in the evaluation of arthritic conditions since it can provide valuable information in addition to that gained by clinical and radiographic examination. Although synovial fluid examination generally does not provide a specific diagnosis, it does give an indication of the degree of synovitis and metabolic degeneration within a joint.

An understanding of the basic nature of synovial fluid is necessary to appreciate the changes that occur in joint disease. Synovial fluid is a unique tissue fluid. Joint fluid is to a large degree a dialysate of plasma, to which is added hyaluronic acid.[25] The source of hyaluronic acid is generally believed to be the synovial membrane.[26] Studies of the structure of hyaluronate molecules indicate that each is a random coil with a moderate degree of stiffness. This particular constituent of synovial fluid provides most of its unusual properties such as viscosity.

In the past, hyaluronate has been regarded as the essential lubricant of articular cartilage. More recently it has been demonstrated that a lubricating glycoprotein is the essential component of the boundary lubricant system of articular cartilage;[27] not only does hyaluronic acid not lubricate cartilage but it appears to impede lubrication when tests are performed over an extended period.[28] The main role of hyaluronate is that of a boundary lubricant of the synovial membrane.[29]

The large asymmetric hyaluronic acid molecule in the synovial fluid itself influences the composition of the fluid.[30] Research data suggest that hyaluronate may obstruct some solute passage through the water surrounding the molecules. In this concept of excluded volume, the size and shape of the molecules play an important role. Small molecules are not excluded and large ones, such as fibrinogen, are excluded. The quantity and physical state of hyaluronate produced under pathologic conditions may well be the primary determinants of the nature of the remainder of the contents of the synovial fluid. Also, the hyaluronic acid in the perisynovial connective tissue may be of significance in the exclusion of certain plasma proteins from the synovial fluid.[31]

Because of its physiologic roles within the joint, hyaluronic acid has been used as a therapeutic agent.[32] However, as with its physiologic role, the exact mode of its therapeutic role is uncertain.

Synovial fluid may be considered as a tissue fluid that changes with disease. Joint injury is generally accompanied by synovitis. Most affected horses exhibit signs of increased production of synovial fluid with distention of the joint capsule. In more severe cases there is influx of fibrinogen and globular proteins into the synovial fluid, an increase in leukocyte numbers and a decrease in viscosity. Trauma is a major factor in initiating degenerative lesions in a joint and synovitis appears to be a common accompaniment to degenerative joint disease in horses.[34]

Both increased formation and decreased resorption of synovial fluid appear to contribute to the clinical phenomenon of effusion. Increased protein content increases the synovial fluid osmotic pressure and later acts as a barrier to fluid resorption. This effect is in addition to the change in permeability of inflamed synovial membrane.

Hyaluronic acid is depolymerized in untreated arthritis irrespective of etiology; this is considered the cause of reduced viscosity.[36] However, the viscosity of hyaluronic acid is apparently dependent on the length of the polysaccharide chain, the conformation of these chains, and interaction between adjacent chains and other molecules.[28] Therefore, the decrease in viscosity may not simply be depolymerization but could be due to an altered relationship with other molecules.

Most of the changes in synovial fluid in joint disease can be attributed to the associated synovitis. The degree of change is generally proportionate to the degree of pathologic change of the synovial membrane. Pathologic changes in articular cartilage are not reflected accurately in the character of synovial fluid. Signs of cartilage damage are limited to the change in joint fluid enzyme content and the presence of cartilage debris in a stain of the sediment.

Normal and abnormal values for equine synovial fluid parameters have been documented.[37,38] Most of these provide an indication of the relative amount of joint effusion or synovial membrane inflammation and so parallel the spectrum of inflammatory activity within the joint. Synovial fluid analysis alone generally does not provide a specific diagnosis. The exception to this is septic or infectious arthritis, although this is not always the case. However, the information on the intensity of metabolic derangement within the joint, coupled with other signs, often leads to a specific diagnosis.

Technic

Samples are collected using sterile needles and syringes. All sites for arthrocentesis should be clipped and aseptically prepared. The use of surgical gloves is recommended. Depending on the joint involved, infiltration of the sampling site with a local anesthetic may be appropriate. The fluid is aspirated in a syringe and transferred to both plain and EDTA vacuum tubes.

Characteristics of Synovial Fluid

The results of synovial fluid analysis are discussed below in general terms of the amount of inflammation present, but specific disease examples are given where appropriate. Grouping synovial fluid findings into disease entities is not recommended. While cases of osteochondritis dissecans and tarsal hydrarthrosis are characterized by mild and somewhat consistent changes, the changes in traumatic and infectious arthritis may vary widely.

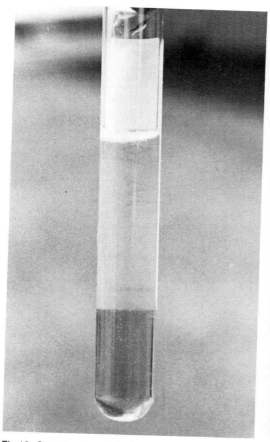

Fig 18. Sample of normal, clear synovial fluid. The label on the tube can be easily seen through the fluid.

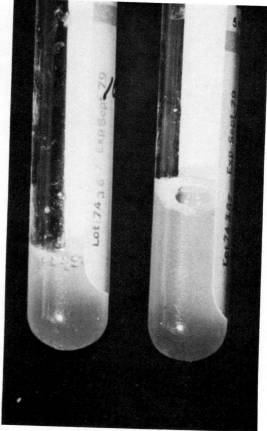

Fig 19. Opaque and discolored samples of synovial fluid from an infected joint.

Appearance: Synovial fluid appearance is evaluated by visual inspection at the time of collection. Normal synovial fluid is pale yellow, clear and free of flocculent material (Fig 18). Streaks of blood in the aspirate indicate hemorrhage during collection. Uniformly diffuse hemorrhage represents an acute traumatic condition, whereas dark yellow or pale amber samples (xanthochromia) represent previous hemorrhage and are most commonly associated with chronic traumatic arthritis. An opaque sample containing flocculent material reflects synovial membrane inflammation. Such change is variable and minimal in chronic degenerative joint disease and osteochondritis dissecans, and more marked in acute synovitis (traumatic or infectious). The intense inflammatory process in the synovial tissues in infectious arthritis is reflected by serofibrinous to markedly flocculent samples (Fig 19). The synovial fluid from infected joints is often bloody due to hemorrhage from the severely inflamed synovial membrane.

Volume: This is noted at the time of fluid aspiration. Attention must be paid to the particular joint when evaluating this parameter. Volume is increased in most cases of active synovitis. Decreased synovial fluid volume occurs in some cases of chronic degenerative joint disease and may be manifested as a "dry joint."[34] This situation can be associated with fibrotic synovial membrane. Synovial fluid volume is increased in cases of idiopathic synovial effusion, as in bog spavin. Volume increases in osteochondritis dissecans are variable. Marked synovial effusion is commonly seen in the femoropatellar joint with osteochondritis dissecans of the lateral trochlear ridge of the femur and is commonly the presenting clinical sign in osteochondritis dissecans of the tibiotarsal joint.[39] Synovial fluid volume is usually increased in cases of infectious arthritis.

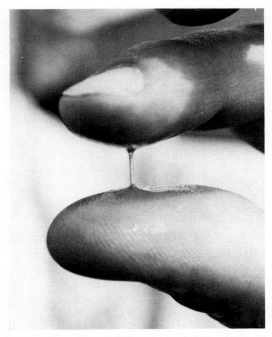

Fig 20. Evaluating the ability of synovial fluid to "string" as a simple test of viscosity. The length of the string was slightly decreased in this sample from a joint with osteochondritis dissecans.

Clot Formation: Normal synovial fluid does not clot. This property has long been attributed to a lack of fibrinogen but it is now known that other clotting factors are also absent in normal synovial fluid.[25] Clots do occur, however, in synovial fluid from diseased joints, and the size of the clot is roughly proportional to the severity of synovitis. In humans, clots have been graded by estimating the clot size in relation to the volume of fluid in the tube.[25]

Protein: The protein content and albumin:globulin ratio of synovial fluid can be determined accurately by the biuret method. For convenience, the author simply measures protein concentration using a refractometer. The different protein fractions in equine synovial fluid have been evaluated using paper electrophoresis following treatment of the sample with hyaluronidase.[38] Starch-gel electrophoresis has been described as superior to paper electrophoresis.[35]

Synovial fluid protein content is approximately 25-35° of the plasma protein concentration of the same animal. The normal value for horses is reported as 1.81 ± 0.26 g/d.[37] Synovial fluid, when compared with plasma, has a relatively increased albumin level.[33]

The total protein content of synovial fluid increases with joint inflammation. With increasing inflammation, the total synovial protein level approaches that of plasma and the various protein fractions appear in levels comparable to those of serum.[25] As the relative amount of albumin decreases, the amount of alpha-2 and gamma-globulins increase and fibrinogen is present. These changes are consistent with increased permeability of the synovial membrane associated with inflammation (possibly coupled with decreased steric hindrance from hyaluronic acid). However, the recognition of new protein components not present in normal serum, synovial fluid or plasma suggests that more than increased permeability is involved.[25]

Simple estimation of total protein concentration is sufficient for routine synovial fluid analysis; however, future research may show that electrophoretic examination has diagnostic value. One may be reasonably certain that synovial fluid is not normal when the total protein is above 2.5 g/d. A total protein level above 4 g/d indicates severe inflammation. Noninfectious inflammatory conditions generally cause total protein levels below this level. It should be emphasized that protein levels must be compared with normal values from the same joint if the increase is subtle. Significant differences in protein levels have been demonstrated between different joints in the horse and significant increases in protein levels have been demonstrated in horses in training.[38]

Viscosity: The viscosity of synovial fluid depends chiefly on its content of hyaluronate and is therefore a measure of the quantity and degree of polymerization of hyaluronate.[38] Normal values of relative viscosity of synovial fluid vary among laboratories. Within a laboratory the relative viscosity can reflect trends in the development and progression of an inflammatory state. Relative viscosity decreases with synovitis. The decrease may reflect dilution of hyaluronate by the effusion and depolymerization of hyaluronic acid, and is in proportion with the intensity of the inflammation. However, measurement of relative viscosity using a viscosimeter is tedious and not routinely used. The technic has been used to monitor the progression of an experimental synovitis in ponies.[40]

For practical field use a simple test for viscosity is to watch the fluid drip slowly drop by drop from the end of the syringe. With normal fluid, the drops usually string out as much as

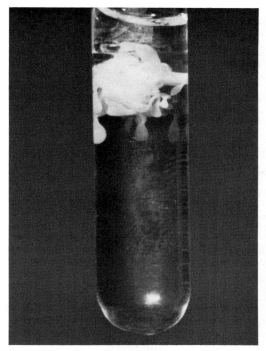

Fig 21. A "good" mucin clot. The precipitate is distinct and the remaining solution is clear.

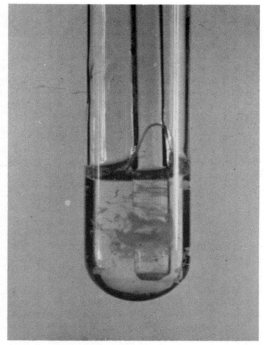

Fig 22. A "fair" mucin clot. Some disruption of the precipitate is evident.

2-3 inches before separating. Viscosity is low if the fluid drops from the syringe with the ease of water. Another test is to place a drop of synovial fluid on the thumb and touch it with the index finger. Separating the fingers then produces a string 1-2 inches long before it breaks if viscosity is normal (Fig 20). Decreased stringing occurs with decreased viscosity. Fluid from an infected joint does not string. These methods are of course subjective and only useful for detecting gross changes. A simple method of measuring relative viscosity using a WBC-diluting pipette has been developed.[41] The technic is reproducible with 2% accuracy and apparently adds little to the time required for routine synovial fluid analysis. This technic could be of value in monitoring clinical cases of arthritis and their response to therapy.

Because the viscosity of synovial fluid varies with shear rate, some authors have proposed the measurement of intrinsic viscosity of hyaluronate is more meaningful in evaluating the hyaluronate status of synovial fluids.[38] Intrinsic viscosity provides an estimate of the degree of polymerization of hyaluronic acid in synovial fluid. However, to measure intrinsic viscosity, the hyaluronic acid concentration must be determined; estimation of the latter is

fraught with problems. The measurement of relative viscosity is therefore thought to be the most useful parameter clinically and is certainly the most convenient.[42]

However, the significance of the relative viscosity findings should not be overemphasized and should not be considered a direct quantitative or qualitative estimate of the hyaluronic acid content. It is only an indicator of the relative amount of synovitis present and one's interpretation should be limited to this.

Mucinous Precipitate Quality: Evaluation of mucinous precipitate quality (MPQ) or the mucin clot is a simple test in which 0.5 ml synovial fluid is added to 2 ml 2% acetic acid and mixed rapidly with a glass rod. The mucin clot formed contains all the hyaluronate present in the synovial fluid. When the mucin clot is normal, a tight, ropy mass forms in a clear solution. Conventionally, this is called a "good" mucin (Fig 21). A softer mass with some shreds in solution constitutes a "fair" mucin (Fig 22). A "poor" result has shreds and small, soft masses in a turbid solution. Finally, some fluids may react to form only a few clumped flecks of mucin suspended in a cloudy solution. This is a "very poor" mucin test. In general, the more inflamed the joint, the worse the mucin clot.

Good to fair mucins are associated with traumatic and degenerative arthritides. Infected joints have poor to very poor mucin test results because bacterial enzymes, especially hyaluronidase, degrade mucin.

It has been reported that mucin clot tests should not be performed on synovial fluid samples containing EDTA because EDTA causes a decrease in synovial fluid viscosity by degradation of the hyaluronic acid component of mucin.[43] However, anticoagulant is needed to maintain the protein and hyaluronate of inflamed samples in solution. A suitable compromise is to use EDTA but perform the mucin clot test as soon as possible after sampling.

The results of MPQ generally parallel changes in relative viscosity. While it is recognized that synovial fluid protein is required for the formation of a mucin clot, little is known about how qualitative and quantitative changes in synovial fluid proteins, which occur in inflammatory joint disease, affect the results of MPQ. Although all the factors involved in the quality of the mucin clot are uncertain, the decrease in MPQ correlates well with the degree of joint inflammation. Therefore, MPQ is recommended as a routine part of synovial fluid analysis.

Cytologic Examination: Total WBC and RBC counts are performed on synovial fluid using hemocytometers. However, it is essential to use saline diluent and not the usual white-cell diluent containing acetic acid because the latter precipitates the hyaluronic acid-protein complex. If the volume of synovial fluid is very small, cell counts can be estimated by counting the white cells in a microscopic field of a smear and comparing this with a blood smear of known concentration. Smears for differential cell counts are made in the standard way as for peripheral blood but with minor modifications. If the WBC count is elevated, the smear may be made directly from the synovial fluid. Otherwise, the sample should be centrifuged and the sediment, resuspended in 0.5 ml supernatant, used to prepare a smear. The smears are air-dried and stained with Wright's stain or new methylene blue.

Erythrocytes are not considered normal constituents of synovial fluid. Their presence in small numbers is usually attributed to contamination of the sample at the time of arthrocentesis. Depending on the trauma to the vascular synovial membrane caused by arthrocentesis, the RBC count may vary greatly. Increased hyperemia in diseased synovial membrane may increase the tendency for bleeding. The normal value for RBC in equine synovia fluid is reported as 3791 ± 2373 cells/mm^3, with a range of 0-17,000.[37]

The WBC count of normal equine synovial fluid has been reported by different workers as 167 ± 21 cells/mm^3 and 87 cells/mm^3.[37,38] The percentage of neutrophils is generally less than 10%. Quantitative and qualitative changes in the WBC present in synovial fluid provide an indication of the magnitude of the inflammation of the synovial membrane. In most cases of infectious arthritis, cytologic examination provides a specific diagnosis. However, there is no specific cytologic pattern with the other diseases. Values characteristic of various diseases have been published but the author has encountered much wider ranges and is cautious about grouping types of effusion and matching them to diseases.[37] With this in mind, one may make some generalizations.

Idiopathic synovitis (bog spavin) and osteochondritis dissecans usually have synovial fluid WBC counts of fewer than 1000 cells/mm^3. These conditions have been classified as noninflammatory effusions but the use of the term is questionable. Histologic examination of the synovial membrane in osteochondritis dissecans has revealed inflammatory changes. The presence of effusion without inflammation has not yet been explained.

In traumatic arthritis and degenerative joint disease, the cell count may vary tremendously depending upon the amount of acute synovitis present. The cell count in degenerative joint disease is typically low in humans; however, synovitis seems to be more prominent in equine degenerative joint disease and, consequently, counts of 5000-10,000 cells/mm^3 may be encountered. In these more severe inflammatory effusions, the proportion of neutrophils is greatly increased.

Infectious arthritis causes the highest WBC counts in synovial fluid. In general, when the count is over 50,000/mm^3, infection is the prime suspect; counts over 100,000 are virtually pathognomonic. The synovial fluid WBC counts for infectious arthritis are reported as $105,775 \pm 25,525$ cells/mm^3 (range 59,250-178,000). Neutrophils are the predominant cell type. One may observe toxic changes in neutrophils but they are usually normal. Bacteria may be observed on synovial fluid smears in some instances.

It is not unusual for synovial fluid to contain cells and cell numbers typical of infectious arthritis and yet show a negative culture. This is common in joints of animals under antibiotic treatment but may occur in untreated animals. Treatment of an infected joint is an emergency and cytologic examination of synovial fluid provides a rapid diagnosis and is probably the best use for synovial fluid analysis. However, this does not diminish the significance or usefulness of a specific etiologic diagnosis if possible. Cultures from synovial membrane biopsies are useful in such cases.

More than a simple bacteriologic examination may be required for an etiologic diagnosis in some cases. *Chlamydia* and *Mycoplasma* have been associated with polyarthritic conditions in foals.[44,45]

Although infected joints typically have high WBC counts, some joints may not. The author has observed cases in which bacterial sequestration apparently occurred in the joint capsule. These cases "smouldered" and had nondiagnostic synovial fluid analyses. Degenerative joint disease finally resulted. The author has also encountered occasional cases of "latent" septic arthritis in which the synovial fluid analyses have been more typical of traumatic arthritis. Fortunately these cases are rare. In polyarthritis in foals, the count may sometimes be considerably less than 50,000 cells/mm^3.

As alluded to above, there is a "grey zone" between traumatic arthritis with a high WBC count in synovial fluid and infectious arthritis with a low WBC count. High WBC counts (up to 52,000 cells/mm^3) have been recorded in cases of traumatic arthritis in humans. Two cases of traumatic arthritis (52,000 WBC/mm^3, neutrophils 89%; 29,100 WBC/mm^3, neutrophils 74%) were differentiated from infectious arthritis by the presence of fat droplets in the synovial fluid.[46] The authors considered the synovial fluid leukocytosis secondary to lipid droplet phagocytosis. Intracellular and extracellular lipid globules in the synovial fluid and an upper fatty layer following centrifugation of hemorrhagic synovial fluid are indications of a traumatic etiology for arthritis.

One should be aware of the disparity that may exist between cellular changes observed in synovial fluid and synovial membrane. For example, while a nonseptic inflamed joint may have a preponderance of neutrophils in the synovial fluid, examination of the synovial membrane typically reveals an inflammatory infiltrate that is primarily lymphoid in nature. The presence of neutrophils in the synovial fluid in these cases has been related to the presence of strong chemotactic factors, which are products of activation of complement in the fluid.

Enzymes: In general, there is a close correlation between the levels of alkaline phosphatase, aspartate aminotransferase, (previously GOT) and lactic dehydrogenase (LDH) in synovial fluids and the clinical severity of joint disease.[37] The proportionate increase of enzyme activity with the degree of synovitis has been demonstrated experimentally in the equine intercarpal joint.[40] However, specific diagnoses cannot be made using enzyme levels.

Increased enzyme activities in joint fluid may result from one of several mechanisms including the release of enzymes from WBC, release of enzymes from necrotic or inflamed synovial tissue, or production and release of increased amounts of enzymes by altered synovial tissue.[47] A positive correlation observed between the number of WBC in the fluid and the height of the enzyme levels is indirect evidence for the first possibility.[47]

Recent work with LDH isoenzyme levels in equine synovial fluid indicates that it may be possible to differentiate between joint diseases with or without articular cartilage lesions.[48] The isoenzymes LDH$_4$ and LDH$_5$ were present in high amounts in articular cartilage, and increased levels of these isoenzymes were the most characteristic feature in synovial fluid from joints with arthrosis. More work is necessary to evaluate the clinical usefulness of this technic.

Gas-Liquid Chromatography: As discussed above, there is uncertainty in diagnosing some cases of infectious arthritis, and etiologic diagnoses are often never obtained from synovial fluid samples. Recently, gas-liquid chromatography to identify various fatty acids and their amount in the synovial fluid has been used to obtain a specific etiologic diagnosis of pyogenic arthritis in humans.[49] Some preliminary studies have been performed in horses and the potential usefulness of the technic in infectious arthritis diagnosis has been confirmed.[50] However, the establishment of control chromatography for the effusions due to each specific organism is necessary before specific diagnoses can be made. Consequently, it is not yet a routine diagnostic aid.

Other Technics: Relatively high levels of sulfate occur in the synovial fluid from humans with traumatic degenerative arthritis.[51] The source of the sulfate was not identified. The technic may be of potential value in horses.

Microscopic examination of metachromatically stained sediment (after centrifugation) for detection of cartilaginous debris has been described for horses;[37] however, the author has found the results of this technic inconsistent. The author has also abandoned the use of simultaneous measurement of serum and synovial fluid glucose levels because of inconsistency in samples from normal joints.

The author uses appearance, volume, protein level, gross viscosity estimation, mucin clot and cytologic examination routinely in synovial fluid examination. Generally, these parameters confirm the presence of an inflamed synovial membrane and provide an indication of the degree of pathologic change present. Infectious arthritis is usually specifically diagnosed by conventional synovial fluid examination.

Measurement of viscosity (laboratory method) and enzyme levels is indicated in certain cases. If the equipment is available, gas-liquid chromatography has potential value in obtaining a specific diagnosis. The presence and degree of articular cartilage damage is not generally demonstrated by synovial fluid analysis; LDH isoenzyme analysis may be potentially useful for this purpose. In the meantime, the development of a simple test that provides an indication of articular cartilage degeneration would be a welcome addition to tests currently used.

Synovial Membrane Biopsy
by C.W. McIlwraith

As discussed previously, synovitis is a prominent component in most instances of joint disease. Also, the changes in synovial fluid are generally a reflection of the pathologic changes in the synovial membrane. Therefore, histologic examination of the synovial membrane may be useful in evaluating a diseased joint and as an aid in differential diagnosis.

The diagnostic use of punch biopsy of synovial membrane and the histologic changes in rheumatoid arthritis, osteoarthritis, traumatic arthritis, gout and other common diseases in humans have been described.[52,54] Although the usefulness of such studies was generally agreed upon, each of the investigators noticed certain histologic changes common to a number of diseases and that accurate differential diagnosis could be difficult.

The histologic changes in the synovial membrane of horses with intra-articular fractures and osteochondrosis dissecans have been reported.[55] Synovial membrane biopsies obtained during arthroscopy have been used to evaluate the development of experimental synovitis in the equine intercarpal joint.[40]

The author has studied the changes in the synovial membrane in association with clinical joint disease and evaluated the potential usefulness of synovial membrane biopsies as a diagnostic indicator in the differential diagnosis of equine joint disease in a series of cases over 2 years. The samples were obtained by synovial membrane biopsy at arthroscopic examination or removed surgically at arthrotomy.

Twelve cases of intra-articular fractures and 6 cases of degenerative joint disease, involving signs of cartilage and/or bone pathologic changes but no chip fractures, were studied. Samples from animals with osteochondritis dissecans and villonodular synovitis were also examined. From this preliminary work it appears that the reaction of the synovial membrane in equine joint disease is rather nonspecific and the usefulness of synovial membrane biopsy in horses is limited. However, the technic is of value in assessing the progression of a joint problem and in the study of the pathogenesis of inflammatory and degenerative problems.

Synovial membrane changes in joints with intra-articular fractures were generally correlated with the length of time the chip had been present. Villous synovitis was present and vascular hyperemia in the subintima was prominent in joints with recent fractures. Endothelial cells were more prominent in these hyperemic capillaries. Amorphous eosinophilic material (presumed to be fibrin) was observed at the surface of the synovial membrane in these acute cases and polarization of synoviocytes, with the cytoplasm oriented toward the joint space, was associated with these areas. Subacute changes (2 weeks) were typified by subintimal edema and infiltration of the subintima with mononuclear cells (lymphocytes, plasma cells and, later, macrophages). Diffuse perivascular infiltration and lymphoid follicles have been observed. Hemorrhage may also be observed within the synovial membrane.

Other changes include perivascular fibrosis and a granulation response. Granulation tissue was observed in samples from joints 3 weeks or longer after intra-articular fracture. All the above findings were similar to those of other authores except that intimal hyperplasia was not observed in the present study.[55] However, the synoviocytes were hypertrophied.

Lesions of acute synovitis were observed in one case of degenerative joint disease. In this instance the changes included subintimal edema and hemorrhage, capillary congestion and a roughened intimal surface. The affected horse was still actively working despite the presence of fibrillation in both carpal joints. In the other 5 cases (all long-standing), varying degrees of chronic change were observed. A gradation was observed from fibrotic synovial membrane still containing congested vessels, to relatively avascular synovial membrane, to synovial membrane areas of hyalinization. The intima consisted of a single discontinuous layer of synoviocytes.

The author has consistently observed changes characteristic of acute synovitis in synovial membrane samples from race horses with acute carpitis. Degeneration of the articular cartilage and chronic fibrosis of the synovial membrane ensue with repeated exacerbation. The pathogenesis of these changes can only be conjectured but the biopsies provide a useful means of following some of the changes.

The synovial membrane changes accompanying osteochondritis dissecans are variable and nonspecific. The acute reactive changes of edema, congestion, surface fibrin deposition, subintimal hemorrhage and mononuclear cell infiltration have been observed in some samples, while other cases have been typified by the presence of osteochondral fragments buried in granulation tissue. Congested, edematous synovial membrane has been observed with subchondral cysts of the medial femoral condyle.

The synovial membrane changes are characteristic in infectious arthritis. In the early stages, congestion and edema with massive infiltration of neutrophils are observed. This is rapidly followed by overt destruction of the synovial membrane, and fibrin deposition.

Specimens of villonodular synovitis of the fetlock contain masses composed primarily of dense collagen, with sparse mononuclear cell infiltration; however, hemosiderin deposition has not been a feature of the samples examined. Other researchers have also reported this.[56] In humans, the lesions are typically brownish and villous. Histologically they consist of a stroma of connective tissue containing round and polyhedral cells, granules of hemosiderin and crystals of cholesterol.[57] The appearance of the lesions in horses suggests a concussive rather than a hemorrhagic pathogenesis.

The preliminary studies described above have not established a definitive role for synovial membrane biopsies in the differential diagnosis of equine joint disease but certainly demonstrate change in all types of disease and a means of studying disease progression.

References

1. Grant, BD and Lincoln, S VM/SAC **67** (1972) 995.
2. Fredricson, I and Drevemo, S. Eq Vet J **3** (1971) 137.
3. Fredricson, I et al. Eq Vet J **12** (1980) 54.
4. Nilsson, G et al. Acta Vet Scand, Suppl **44** (1973) 1.
5. Ratzlaff, M: Locomotion of the Horse (16 mm film). Michigan State Univ, 1976.
6. Ratzlaff, M. Proc 25th Ann Mtg Am Assoc Eq Pract, 1979. p 381.
7. Wentink, G. Anat Embry **152** (1978) 261.
8. Adrian, M et al. Am J Vet Res **38** (1977) 931.
9. Ratzlaff, M et al. Proc 3rd Int Symp Eq Med Control, 1980. p 397.
10. Delahanty, D and Georgi, J. JAVMA **147** (1965) 235.
11. Nelson, H and Osheim, D: Soring in Tennessee Walking Horses: Detection by Thermography. USDA-APHIS, Ames, IA, 1975.
12. Palmer, S. Am J Vet Res **42** (1981) 105.
13. Purohit, R and McCoy, M. Am J Vet Res **41** (1980) 1167.
14. Stromberg, B. J Am Vet Rad Soc **15** (1974) 94.
15. Vaden, M et al. Am J Vet Res **41** (1980) 1175.
16. Pratt, G and O'Connor, J. Am J Vet Res **37** (1976) 1251.
17. Ouddus, M et al. J Eq Med Surg **2** (1978) 233.
18. Johnson, LL: Comprehensive Arthroscopic Examination of the Knee. CV Mosby, St. Louis, 1977.
19. McIlwraith, CW and Fessler, JF. JAVMA **172** (1978) 263.
20. Nickels, FA: Radiographic and arthroscopic findings in the equine stifle. Master's thesis, Washington State Univ, 1976.
21. Noyes, FR. J Bone Jt Surg **62A** (1980) 687.
22. Norrie, RD. Proc 21st Ann Mtg Am Assoc Eq Pract, 1975. p 91.
23. Whipple, TL and Bassett, FH. J Bone Jt Surg **60A** (1978) 444.
24. Dick, W et al. Arch Ortho Traumat Surg **92** (1978) 69.
25. Cohen, in Cohen: Laboratory Diagnostic Procedures in the Rheumatic Diseases. Little, Brown and Co, Boston, 1967.
26. Roy, S and Ghadially, FN. J Path Bact **93** (1967) 555.
27. Radin, EL and Paul, IG. J Bone Jt Surg **54A** (1972) 607.
28. Swann, in Sokoloff: The Joints and Synovial Fluid. Academic Press, New York, 1978.
29. Radin, EL et al. Ann Rheum Dis **30** (1971) 322.
30. Ogston, AG and Phelps, CF. Biochem J **78** (1961) 827.
31. Nettelbladt, E et al. Acta Rheum Scand **9** (1963) 28.
32. Asheim, A and Lindblad, G. Acta Vet Scand **17** (1976) 379.

33. Marsh, FJ *et al*. Can J Comp Med **40** (1976) 202.

34. Raker, CW *et al*. Proc 12th Ann Mtg Am Assoc Eq Pract, 1967. p 229.

35. Fournier, G *et al*. Can Med Assoc J **100** (1969) 242.

36. Holt, PJL *et al*. Ann Rheum Dis **27** (1968) 264.

37. Van Pelt, RW. JAVMA **165** (1974) 91.

38. Persson, L. Acta Vet Scand Suppl **35** (1971) 1.

39. Moore, JN and McIlwraith, CW. Vet Rec **100** (1977) 133.

40. McIlwraith, CW *et al*. Am J Vet Res **40** (1979) 11.

41. Hasselbacher, P. Arth Rheum **19** (1976) 1358.

42. Levine, MG and Kling, DH. J Clin Invest **35** (1956) 1419.

43. Ogston, AG and Sherman, TF. Biochem J **72** (1959) 301.

44. McChesney, AE *et al*. JAVMA **165** (1974) 259.

45. Moorthy, ARS *et al*. Br Vet J **133** (1977) 320.

46. Graham, J and Goldman, JA. Arthr Rheum **21** (1978) 76.

47. West, M *et al*. J Lab Clin Invest **62** (1963) 175.

48. Rejno, S. Acta Vet Scand **17** (1976) 178.

49. Seifert, MN *et al*. Br Med J **2** (1978) 1402.

50. Brooks, JB *et al*, Cornell Univ: Unpublished data, 1979.

51. Chrisman, OD *et al*. J Bone Jt Surg **40A** (1958) 457.

52. Mikkelsen, WM *et al*. Arch Int Med **102** (1958) 977.

53. Rodnan, GP *et al*. Ann Int Med **53** (1960) 319.

54. Wilkinson, M and Jones, BS. Ann Rheum Dis **23** (1963) 100.

55. Johansson, HE and Rejno, S. Acta Vet Scand **17** (1976) 153.

56. Nickels, FA *et al*. JAVMA **168** (1976) 1043.

57. Cohen, in Hollander and McCarty: Arthritis and Allied Conditions. Lea & Febiger, Philadelphia, 1972.

BONE AND JOINT PATHOLOGY
by A.M. Gallina

Anatomy and Physiology

Bone

The skeleton is composed of living tissue capable of growth, modeling, remodeling and repair. Repair is the process by which fractures heal. Microfractures are likely to occur continuously and repair is probably an ongoing process. Modeling involves sculpting of bone and is probably influenced by distribution of skeletal load. Remodeling is the process associated with mineral homeostasis and redistribution of load through the skeleton. While minute-to-minute alterations of mineral balance do not involve the remodeling process, it is related to long-term homeostatic demands made on bone.

The organic osteoid matrix of bone consists of 90-95% collagen. Virtually all bone collagen is deposited in parallel lamellar bundles as seen by polarized or scanning electron microscopy. The deposition of collagen in bone must occur some days prior to its mineralization. The organic bone matrix yet to be mineralized is known as osteoid.

Proteoglycans are the major noncollagenous organic components of skeletal matrices but in lesser concentrations than in cartilage. The size and consistency of the hydrated molecule are responsible for many of the mechanical and physiochemical properties of cartilage. Giant molecules of protein-polysaccharides trapped between the collagen bundles also act as a molecular sieve, admitting small molecules but excluding large ones. The concentration of protein-polysaccharide in bone is much less than in cartilage and its role in osseous matrix is not clearly defined.

The bony skeleton is made rigid by the addition of mineral to the already deposited organic matrix. The solid mineral phase of mature bone mineral is a carbonate-containing analog of the mineral hydroxyapatite and characterized by mineral disorder. The mechanism of mineral deposition in the skeleton is not clear but organic components of bone play a role in the process.

The cells of the skeleton include osteoblasts, osteocytes, chondrocytes and osteoclasts. Osteoblasts are the cells responsible for the synthesis of bone matrix. Osteocytes represent osteoblasts that have been incorporated into the bone matrix. They are the most numerous bone cells and constitute the major portion of the bone cell syncytium. Chondrocytes are the mature cells of cartilage. They are larger and rounder than their precursor chondroblasts and characterized by numerous, interdigitating cytoplasmic processes. Osteoclasts are large, multinucleated cells responsible for most morphologically apparent resorption of bone and calcified cartilage. Although the precise mechanisms whereby these cells degrade bone and mineralized cartilage is not well defined, it certainly involves lysosomal activity.

Fetal formation and postnatal growth occur by endochondral bone formation and intramembranous growth. In endochondral bone formation, a cartilagenous model of the fully developed bone forms from primitive mesenchyma. The cartilagenous model undergoes calcification at its center, followed by the appearance of osteoblasts. The cartilagenous matrix is replaced by bone, except at the physis and articular surface. At the epiphyseal growth plate and metaphyseal juncture, vascular invasion of cartilage follows calcification of its matrix and death of chondrocytes. The calcified cartilage serves as scaffolding for the deposition of bone matrix and is resorbed at the same rate that the growth plate is expanded. This results in long-bone growth while the physis remains constant. Termination of growth occurs with cessation of interstitial expansion of the epiphyseal plate and its gradual obliteration.

Intramembranous bone growth, which predominates in the skull and facial bones, is almost entirely appositional. The bone first appears as many separate centers of ossification that enlarge and eventually fuse to form a single plate. Growth continues by formation of bone on the outer convex surface and resorption on the inner concave surface.

Remodeling implies bone resorption. Because remodeling proceeds at a more rapid pace in growing animals than in mature animals, pathologic effects are more severe or develop more rapidly in young animals. Various physiologic and pathologic stimuli increase or decrease the portion of bone undergoing remodeling; new foci are continually originating as others come to completion.

Remodeling foci are initiated by the appearance of osteoclasts, which resorb a quantity of bone to create a Howship's lacuna. The signals that activate and deactivate remodeling osteoclasts are unknown. Osteoclasts do not engulf bone but rather initiate enzymatic reactions that result in the breakdown of bone. Osteoclasis is, therefore, a surface phenomenon. Mature osteocytes are also responsible for bone resorption (osteolysis) within spicules of bone where osteocytes are entrapped.

With the disappearance of osteoclasts, a cluster of osteoblasts appears at the site of previous resorption. It is this focal coupling of bone resorption and formation that characterizes the remodeling process and distinguishes it from other skeletal activities. Since change in one of these activities results in a similar change in the other, the coupling of resorption and formation is most responsible for the difficulty of treating many osteopenic disorders.

Many factors influence bone growth, remodeling and maintenance. These may be divided into metabolic and nonmetabolic influences. The latter influences include genetics, gravity, work and environment, which are difficult to quantitate but are decisive factors. A diet with an adequate level of vitamins and minerals is of prime importance. Normal Ca metabolism also depends upon the intestinal tract and kid-

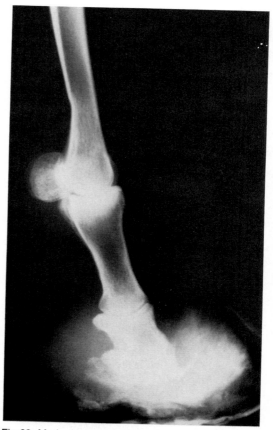

Fig 23. Marked osteoporosis as a result of disuse associated with chronic laminitis.

ney. Hormonal influences include growth hormone, parathormone and calcitonin.

Metabolic Bone Diseases: Metabolic bone diseases can be divided into those characterized by porosis, malacia and petrosis. Osteoporosis is a generalized atrophy of bone; little bone is present but the remaining bone is properly calcified. Osteoporosis is rare in domestic animals. The cause is not known but may follow defects in bone formation or excessive resorption during prolonged immobilization (Fig 23).

Osteomalacia is characterized by failure to mineralize osteoid into true bone. This disturbance in Ca and P balance is the predominant feature of rickets and osteomalacia (adult rickets). In these there is no defect in forming osteoid, but rather an excess production.

Fibrous osteodystrophy is a third disorder characterized by osteomalacia but differs from rickets or osteomalacia in that a marked increase of bone resorption is a constant feature. This results from prolonged and excessive stimulation of bone by parathormone, as in sec-

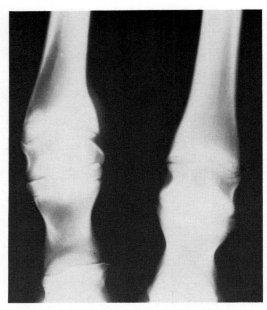

Fig 24. Radiographic appearance of nutritional osteodystrophy in a foal.

ondary hyperparathyroidism in response to hypocalcemia. Secondary hypothyroidism is not uncommon in animals with chronic renal disease or chronic nutritional imbalance, such as vitamin D deficiency, Ca deficiency or excess dietary P. Fibrous osteodystrophy starts as a simple osteomalacia that becomes altered due to increased bone resorption stimulated by parathormone. Rickets and osteomalacia may progress to fibrous osteodystrophy (Fig 24).

Osteopetrosis is characterized by an excess of calcified bone. It occurs infrequently in animals but has not been observed in horses.

Joints

Articulating joints are unions between 2 or more bones. Where motion is restricted, the bones are joined by fibrocartilage. A discontinuity exists between diarthrodial joints, which are composed of articular cartilage, the bone ends, a synovial lining, and surrounding ligaments and muscles.

Cartilage is firm, pliable, elastic tissue free of blood vessels, lymphatics and nerves. It is generally thickest at the periphery of concave surfaces and at the center of convex surfaces. Articular cartilage is bordered by subchondral bone. Bone and cartilage have no structural continuity but cartilage projections interdigitate and lock into the irregular surface of the bone. The junction between calcified and non-

calcified cartilage appears histologically as a basophilic line known as a tidemark.

Collagen in articular cartilage is distributed horizontally to resist forces acting on it. There is more collagen at the articular surface than in deeper portions. Collagen bundles in superficial cartilage are smaller in diameter and have a tighter weave than those in the body of cartilage. The collagen envelope is firmly attached at the articular margins and blends into the periosteum. In addition to its mechanical function, the dense collagenous layer retains proteoglycans while excluding harmful enzymes in the synovial fluid.

The distribution of proteoglycans varies from joint to joint and within a single joint. The articular surface contains much less proteoglycan than does deeper cartilage. Within many joints there are well-defined areas that are always softer than the surrounding cartilage and contain much less proteoglycans, probably related to loading patterns. Areas in a joint that are generally less loaded in normal use are usually chondromalacic.

Chondrocytes require very small amounts of O_2. The nutrition of articular cartilage in developing animals is derived from nutrients that diffuse from the blood supply of the perichondrium and vessels on the epiphyseal side of the epiphysis. In adults the nutrition of articular cartilage depends on the synovial fluid and hence on the vascular supply of synovium. Synovial fluid is composed of a vascular transudate from the synovial membrane and mucin from type-B synovial cells. Type-A synovial cells are much more numerous, produce degradative enzymes, and have phagocytic functions. Articular cartilage depends on a healthy synovial membrane and an adequate circulation of fluid through the joints for its nutrition.

References

1. Teitelbaum, SL and Bullough, PG. Am J Path **96** (1979) 283.
2. Heinze, CD and Lewis, RE. Proc 14th Ann Mtg Am Assoc Eq Pract, 1968. p 213.
3. Brown, MP and MacCallum, FJ. Vet Rec **98** (1976) 443.
4. Green, DA. Br Vet J **125** (1969) 539.
5. Ham and Cormack: Histology. JB Lippincott, Philadelphia, 1979.
6. Robbins and Cotran: Pathologic Basis of Disease. WB Saunders, Philadelphia, 1979.
7. Shively, JA and Van Sickle, DC. Am J Vet Res **38** (1977) 681.
8. Rankin, JS and Diesem, CD. JAVMA **169** (1976) 614.

Bone Diseases

Congenital Defects

Generalized anomalies are extremely rare in horses or not reported. "Contracted foals" is a generalized anomaly but appears to be a neuromuscular disease rather than a primary skeletal defect. This condition may include torticollis, scoliosis, distortion of the cranial bones and flexion contracture of the distal portions of the limbs. The etiology in most cases is unknown. Fetal ankylosis has been described in horses grazing on hybrid sudangrass. These plants, at a certain stage of their growth, may contain a toxic principle and the fetuses of mares in early gestation are also susceptible.

Localized developmental defects are relatively common. Most localized lesions occur in the vertebral column. The caudal vertebrae may fuse to the sacrum and the lateral facets of the lumbar vertebrae may fuse. Intervertebral joint and spinous process ankylosis has also been reported. Kyphosis, lordosis, scoliosis, hemivertebrae and "wobbles" are covered elsewhere in the chapter.

Appendicular anomalies are relatively uncommon. Polydactylism has been reported. Stifle anomalies are being recognized with increased frequency. Congenital absence of the patella and congenital patellar ectopia, with normal femorotibial articulations, are recorded. A more common condition is luxation of the patella secondary to hypoplasia of the femoral trochlea (Fig 25). The condition may be unilateral or bilateral and most cases involve hypoplasia of the lateral ridge of the femoral trochlea.

Rickets

It is difficult to find documented cases of classic rickets in horses. Under experimental conditions in which the Ca deficiency is neither severe nor prolonged, clinical rickets did not develop in young horses and ponies. The role that deficiencies of Ca, P and vitamin D play in the development of osteochondrosis dissecans and "epiphysitis" has not been elucidated.

Rickets is characterized by failure of adequate deposition of Ca in bones of growing animals. The primary cause is vitamin D deficiency. Dietary lack of Ca is a fundamental cause but seldom occurs. Dietary Ca levels may be adequate but absorption is impeded by excessive alkalinity of the intestine, escape of Ca in combination with fatty acids from unassimilated fats, and formation of insoluble com-

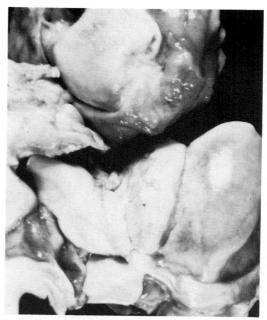

Fig 25. Hypoplasia of the lateral trochlea in a yearling with chronic gonitis.

plexes between Ca and oxalate or phytate. A severely unbalanced dietary Ca:P ratio and P deficiency can also cause rickets.

The gross lesions in rickets are enlargements of the ends of the long bones and of the costochondral junctions. The long bones may become permanently bent under the weight of the animal and other skeletal deformities may develop. At necropsy the enlarged costochondral articulations have been likened to a string of beads, the "rachitic rosary." The bones are abnormally soft and can often be cut with a knife. When a long bone is cut longitudinally, the epiphyseal plate is abnormally wide and irregular.

The principal microscopic changes are an increase in the zone of proliferating cartilage, disorderly arrangement of cartilage, disorderly penetration of cartilage by blood vessels, defective calcification and failure of normal degeneration of the cartilage, an excess of uncalcified osteoid in the metaphysis, and fibrosis of the marrow areas. Evidence of increased resorption is not a feature of rickets. Osteoclasts are fewer than one might expect.

Osteomalacia

Fibrous osteodystrophy ("bighead disease") is well documented in equidae. The cause of this disease is nutritional secondary hyper-

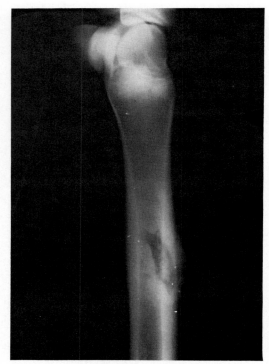

Fig 26. An involucrum in the rear cannon bone.

teolytic resorption, fibrous replacement and active osteoblasts producing osteoid, which fails to mineralize. All bones are affected, but the most striking changes occur in the facial bones and mandible. Metastatic calcification of soft tissues is a regular feature. The parathyroid gland is grossly enlarged.

Miscellaneous Nutritional Deficiencies

While vitamin D, Ca and P receive the most attention in relation to bone growth, other vitamins, minerals and protein are also essential for bone growth. Unfortunately, very little is known about the requirements in equidae; in some the minimal dietary requirements have not been established.

Young horses fed diets low in protein or lysine do not grow as rapidly as those on an adequate diet. Zinc deficiency also results in poor growth. Copper-responsive osteodysgenesis has been reported in foals. Iodine requirements for horses have not been determined but thyroidectomized horses had poor growth and delayed plate closure. These nutrients, in addition to Ca and P, may be involved in the development of "epiphysitis" and other musculoskeletal diseases.

Osteomyelitis

Factors other than the presence of bacteria in a bone are necessary to cause osteomyelitis. Many investigators postulate that venous thrombosis plays an important role in bone infection by causing stasis and plasma transudation. These factors favor localization of bacteria and furnish suitable culture for growth. Bacteria can reach bone by hematogenous spread from a distant focus of infection, from a source external to bone, from postoperative infection, post-traumatic wound infections and open fractures, or from an adjoining soft tissue infection (Fig 97).

There are no differences between cellular or humoral immune mechanisms of bone and those of other tissue. Acute inflammation results in production of exudate containing polymorphonuclear WBC and fibrin. When this occurs in bone, bacterial products, vascular ischemia and enzymes from degenerating neutrophils cause necrosis of marrow and possibly of trabecular bone. If the bacteria are of low virulence or there is high host resistance and the infection is overcome, the damaged bone regenerates and heals completely. If the infection persists and progresses, a problem peculiar to bone is encountered: a small volume of soft tissue space is surrounded by a rigid wall. Exudate can raise tissue pressure to force ex-

parathyroidism. Diets containing excess P result in an elevated plasma P level and a decreased plasma Ca level and stimulate parathormone secretion. Urinary P content is increased and urinary Ca level decreased, but parathormone is unable to establish Ca homeostasis because of the continuous excessive P intake. The disease has also occurred in pastured horses with a normal dietary intake of Ca and P. The cause was thought to be due to ingestion of plants containing oxalates. Experiments have demonstrated that oxalates inhibit Ca absorption in ponies.

Bony resorption and deposition of fibrous tissue is often exaggerated at skeletal sites of greatest mechanical stress. Flattening of the ribs may be apparent. The most classic changes are observed in the head. The lesions are initially observed at the lower and alveolar margins of the mandible, then in the facial bones. Teeth loosen and mastication becomes painful and difficult. Lameness occurs because of preferential resorption of outer cortical bone, resulting in focal periosteal avulsion and torn or detached tendons and ligaments. There may be obvious swelling of joints, bones may be bowed and spontaneous fractures occur.

Microscopically the lesions are those of fibrous osteodystrophy, with osteoclastic and os-

udate along the medullary canal and into the canals in cortical bone. The result depends on the thickness of the cortex and firmness of the attachment of its periosteum.

In young animals the metaphyseal cortex is thin and the periosteum is loosely bound to the underlying bone. Accumulating exudate more easily penetrates the cortex and elevates the periosteum, disrupting the periosteal vessels that supply the cortical bone. Without blood supply, the outer half of bone tends to die and sequestrate. Repair follows if the infection is brought under control. Formation of new bone (invelucrum) and fibrous tissue results from raising of the periosteum. Diaphyseal infections can be similar. Involucrum formation can be massive.

Adult periosteum is more firmly attached and the cortex is relatively thick. Infections tend to remain in the medullary canal and erode bone locally. Periosteal activity and new bone can also be seen but usually not the massive involucrum found in young animals (Fig 26). In addition to the bone changes listed previously, other tissues and systems may become involved. When the mandible is involved, the teeth are often shed and the mandible becomes distorted, interfering with mastication and prehension. Involvement of vertebral bodies may lead to secondary involvement of the meninges and paralysis.

Epiphysitis

The term "epiphysitis" is a misnomer because the condition is not an inflammatory process and involves the growth plate or physis rather than the epiphysis. Physeal dysplasia and dysplasia of the growth plate are more acceptable terms. This condition occurs in young horses and most commonly involves the distal extremities of the radius, tibia, third metacarpal/metatarsal bone, and the proximal aspect of the first phalanx. The condition is characterized by swelling at the level of the physis on the medial side. The physis may be wavy and uneven. Microscopically, the physeal cartilage appears crushed and thinned, and new bone is formed. A classification for the degree of physeal closure has been developed.

The cause of this syndrome is still unknown. Suggested causes include malnutrition, conformational defects, faulty hoof growth, fetal malpositioning, compression of the growth plate and toxicosis. The most acceptable hypothesis at this time appears to be the compression theory. However, the changes observed in "epiphysitis" also occur in clinically normal animals.

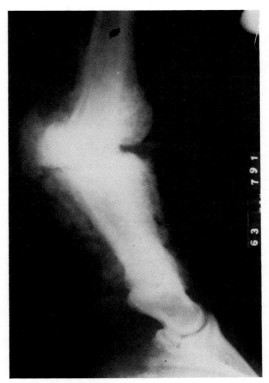

Fig 27. Hypertrophic pulmonary osteoarthropathy in the distal front limb of a horse with a granular-cell tumor of the lungs.

Hypertrophic Pulmonary Ostoarthropathy

Hypertrophic pulmonary osteoarthropathy, also known as Marie's disease, is a proliferative disease of long bones seen in association with chronic disease elsewhere in the body, usually in the thoracic cavity. Thoracic lesions in affected horses include neoplasms and pulmonary abscesses. The disease is characterized by bilateral, symmetric thickening and deformity of the limbs by new bone production. All limbs, from the femorotibial and shoulder joints to the phalanges, especially at the epiphysis, are involved. Joint surfaces are not involved, although there is periarticular proliferation and enlargement. The new bone is formed just under the periosteum, which is pushed outward. The irregular bony growths create a roughened surface (Fig 27). The combined effects of the osseous and pulmonary lesions are fatal.

Exostosis

Exostosis is the granulation tissue of bone in the form of a chronic proliferative inflammatory process. Horses are especially subject to

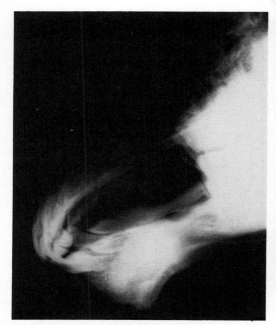

Fig 28. Osteoma of the mandible.

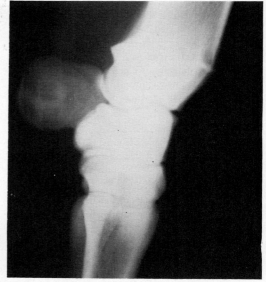

Fig 29. Solitary osteochondroma in the distal radius.

exostoses of the limb, ringbone and splints. An exostosis is comprised of compact bone but lacks the Haversian system arrangement observed in normal cortical bone. Islands of cartilage may be present. The junctions between the new exostotic bone and the old bone remain distinct.

Neoplasia

Primary bone tumors in equidae are rare. In a survey of equine tumors during a 5-year period, only 2 of 236 tumors were primary bone tumors and those were benign. A 10-year survey at Ohio State University listed 6 of 282 tumors arising from bone.

Osteosarcoma: This is the most common primary bone tumor of horses. The most common sites apparently are the mandible and maxilla. In one survey, the growths were observed in animals 1-7 years of age. Most equine tumors are combined sarcomas (compound), in which tumor cells produce not only osteoid but also malignant cartilage. These neoplasms present a challenge to pathologists because compound sarcomas may contain bone and osteoid, malignant cartilage, fibrosarcomatous-like areas, myxoid tissue and areas mimicking hemangiosarcoma. A definitive diagnosis can only be made by reviewing the clinical, radiographic and microscopic findings.

Osteoma: Osteomas are very rare and those reported have been restricted to the mandible and skull. Controversy still exists regarding the classification of these growths. One group considers these as hamartomas rather than true neoplasms. Fibrous dysplasia and exostosis cannot be microscopically differentiated from osteomas in many cases. The typical lesion is a benign, slow-growing mass composed of well-differentiated cancellous bone (Fig 28). Variation is seen in the amount of fibrous tissue present and in trabecular irregularity.

Chondrosarcoma: These rare tumors usually arise in flat bones but there is one report of long-bone involvement. Chondrosarcomas are characterized by formation of cartilage by tumor cells rather than bone. Endochondral ossification is common and must be distinguished from direct bone formation by tumor cells. If the latter occurs, the growth must be classified as an osteosarcoma.

Osteochondroma: Osteochondromas are benign bony projections covered with a cartilagenous cap on the external surface of a bone. Polyostotic and solitary osteochondromas occur in horses. The polyostotic form has been referred to as hereditary multiple exostosis. A single dominant autosomal gene is responsible. The lesions are generally congenital and tend to be bilaterally symmetric. Lesions on various parts of the body vary in size and shape. Those on flat bones continue to grow until the animal reaches maturity, while those on the leg do not.

Solitary lesions are usually on a limb and are located on the cortical surface of the metaphysis or distal end of the diaphysis (Fig 29). These irregular growths may be sessile, pedunculated, multiobulated, rounded, conical or spur-like. Osteochondromas are characterized by biphasic growth. Connective tissue and periosteum cover the cartilagenous cap. The cap resembles a physis and endochondral bone formation can be seen. Islands of cartilage sometimes occur in the cancellous bone base. Sarcomatous transformation in horses has not been reported.

References

1. Behrens, E et al. JAVMA 174 (1979) 266.
2. Cho, DY and Leipold, HW. Eq Vet J 9 (1977) 195.
3. Finocchio, EJ and Guffy, MM. JAVMA 156 (1970) 222.
4. Huston, R et al. J Eq Med Surg 1 (1977) 146.
5. Leathers, CW and Wagner, PC. J Vet Orthoped 1 (1979) 56.
6. Lerner, WJ and Riley, G. JAVMA 172 (1978) 274.
7. McGavin, MD and Leipold, HW. JAVMA 166 (1975) 63.
8. Prichard, JT and Voss, JL. JAVMA 150 (1967) 871.
9. Rooney, JR. Cornell Vet 56 (1966) 172.
10. Carbery, JT. N Zeal Vet J 26 (1978) 279.
11. Egan, DA and Murrin, MP. Irish Vet J 27 (1973) 61.
12. Grovendyk, S and Seawright, A. Aust Vet J 50 (1974) 131.
13. Hintz, HF and Schryver, HF. JAVMA 168 (1976) 39.
14. Joyce, JR et al. JAVMA 158 (1971) 2033.
15. Lowe, JE et al. Cornell Vet 64 (1974) 276.
16. Raker, CW. Cornell Vet 58 (1968) 15.
17. Coffman, JR. Mod Vet Pract 54 (1973) 53.
18. Vaughan, LC. Vet Rec 98 (1976) 165.
19. Campbell, JR. Eq Vet J 9 (1977) 116.
20. Ellis, DR. Vet Rec 98 (1976) 225.
21. Norden, CW. J Infect Dis 124 (1971) 565.
22. Jubb and Kennedy: Pathology of Domestic Animals. 2nd ed. Academic Press, New York, 1970.
23. Blood et al: Veterinary Medicine. Lea & Febiger, Philadelphia, 1979.
24. Alexander, JE et al. JAVMA 146 (1965) 703.
25. Cotchin, E. Eq Vet J 9 (1977) 16.
26. Jacobson: Comparative Pathology of Tumors of Bone. Charles C Thomas, Springfield, IL, 1971.
27. Kerr, KM and Alden, CL. Proc Ann Mtg Am Assoc Lab Diag, 1974. p 183.
28. Lee HA et al. Eq Med Surg 3 (1979) 113.
29. Moulton: Tumors in Domestic Animals. 2nd ed. Univ Calif Press, Berkeley, 1978.
30. Riddle, WE and Wheat, JD. JAVMA 158 (1971) 1674.
31. Shupe, JL et al. Am J Vet Res 40 (1979) 251.
32. Sundberg, JP et al. JAVMA 170 (1977) 150.

Joint Diseases

Degenerative Joint Disease

Degenerative joint disease is a common noninflammatory disease of moveable joints, especially those that bear weight. The disease is characterized by deterioration of articular cartilage and by formation of new bone in the subchondral areas and of the joint. Osteoarthrosis and osteoarthropathy are used synonymously with degenerative joint disease and are preferred over the term osteoarthritis, which implies a primary inflammatory process.

The etiology of this condition is not clear but most cases appear to be secondary to aging, severe trauma, chronic repeated low-grade trauma, joint instability, nutritional deficiencies or imbalances, abnormal loading (posture or limb deviation), or conformational defects.

The earliest changes observed on gross examination are that cartilage becomes opaque, less glossy and less elastic, with localized areas of softening. As the disease advances, the surfaces of the cartilage become frayed and begin to fibrillate. The cracks progress and penetrate deep into the cartilage. Eventually the articular surface becomes largely denuded of cartilage. The underlying bone becomes sclerotic from mechanical pressure and possible effects of synovial fluid, and resembles polished ivory. Spurs covered by cartilage (osteophytes) often form at joint margins and at insertions of ligaments and tendons. Osteocartilagenous bodies ("joint mice") form in advanced cases.

Histologically the areas of fibrillated cartilage are depleted of chondrocytes. Deep in the cartilage, large numbers of chondrocytes are grouped in clusters, with surrounding areas of attempted cartilage repair and regeneration. New bone appears beneath completely sclerotic cartilage.

The basic responses in the synovial membrane are proliferation of surface cells, increased vascularity, and fibrosis of subsynovial tissue. These changes are seen grossly as a thickening of the joint capsule and a granular surface.

Degenerative Arthropathy

Ringbone: Ringbone is a proliferative and degenerative arthropathy of the interphalangeal joints, usually of the forelimbs, thought to be caused by chronic mechanical stress. Erosion of the articular cartilages sometimes leads to fibrous or bony ankylosis, but the periarticular bony exostoses are more prominent than the intra-articular lesions.

Spavin: Spavin is a form of arthropathy that affects the cartilages of the second and third tarsal bones. In severe cases there may be fusion of the ends of the bones where apposing articular cartilages have eroded. Although the synovial membrane becomes hyperplastic, the periarticular lesions are minimal. Large irregular exostoses are formed in a few cases.

Osteochondrosis

Osteochondrosis is a disease that occurs during rapid growth. The most commonly affected site is the shoulder, with the primary lesion starting in the humeral head. Osteochondrosis may be unilateral or bilateral.

There is little agreement on the etiology and pathogenesis of the lesions. The principal change is cartilage degeneration but not inflammation of the synovium. Fissuring, fibrillation, microfractures, and separation of small fragments are among the early changes. The synovium becomes edematous and thickened but there is no significant increase in vascularization and infiltration by WBC is minimal. Pannus does not develop.

Subarticular bone is thickened because of compression or new bone formation. Marrow spaces are often filled with fibrous connective tissue and occasional nests of cartilage can be observed. In advanced cases, small islands of cartilage ossify to form periarticular osteophytes. Fragments of cartilage or calcific spurs may break off and become joint mice.

Infectious Arthritis

Infectious arthritis is a nonspecific term that refers to inflammation of the synovial membrane and articular cartilage due to invasion of an infectious agent. Organisms may enter a joint by hematogenous dissemination from a septicemic process, from an infection localized in other organs, by direct spread from an adjacent infection in soft tissue, or through a perforating injury. Any joint may be involved but larger joints are most frequently affected. Infection is usually limited to one joint but often affects several joints in neonates.

Infectious arthritis of hematogenous origin is usually characterized by initial synovitis, followed by changes in the articular cartilages and sometimes bone. The nature of the exudate in the joint depends on the infecting agent and may be serous, fibrinous, suppurative or a combination of these. The synovium becomes inflamed and edematous, with varying degrees of villous hypertrophy and fibrin deposition. Progressive infectious synovitis can result in pannus formation between articular surfaces, with erosion of articular cartilage, infection of subchondral bone and osteomyelitis. In the chronic state there is extensive granulation tissue formation, chronic synovitis and degenerative joint disease, with osteophyte formation. Ankylosis may occur. Suppurative arthritis destroys cartilage and bone and commonly there is rupture of the joint capsule.

Most cases of arthritis arise from perforation of the joint or by extension of an infection from surrounding soft tissue. However, specific infections can result in localization of infection in joints from bacteremia or septicemia. Navel or intrauterine infections by organisms such as *E coli*, *Streptococcus* and *Actinobacillus equuli* are important causes of polyarthritis in newborn foals. Polyarthritis due to *Chlamydia* also occurs in foals.

Villonodular Synovitis

Villonodular synovitis is not a form of arthritis but is an inflammation of the synovial membrane or tendon membranes. The cause is unknown. The metacarpophalangeal joints are most commonly affected. Bilateral involvement has been reported. The ages of affected animals is 2-18 years. A slightly higher incidence in males has been observed.

Intra-articular lesions are usually attached to the dorsal portion of the dorsal proximal pouch of the metacarpophalangeal joint by a broad stalk. The nodules are firm and greyish-white, and may be circumscribed or lobulated. Erosive bone lesions are typically associated with the mass; erosive lesions of the articular surfaces have been noted in some cases.

Microscopically the lesions consist of dense, well-collagenized stroma lined by synovial cells. Neovascularization is prominent and hyalin change in the stroma and osseous metaplasia are occasionally seen.

Giant-cell tumors of tendon sheaths may represent a form of villonodular synovitis. These growths represent inflammatory reparative granulomas and should not be classified as neoplasms. Microscopically these growths are comprised of a fibroblastic stroma, lipid-laden macrophages, hemosiderin pigment and numerous osteoclastic giant cells.

References

1. Barclay, WP *et al.* Cornell Vet **70** (1980) 72.
2. Mason, TA and MacLean, AA. Eq Vet J **9** (1977) 189.
3. McChesney, AE *et al.* JAVMA **165** (1974) 259.
4. Ragland, WL. Path Vet **5** (1968) 436.
5. Raker, CW *et al.* Proc 12th Ann Conf Am Assoc Eq Pract, 1967. p 229.
6. Rejno, S and Stromberg, B. Path Acta Rad Suppl **358** (1978) 139.
7. Schebitz, H. Proc 11th Ann Mtg Am Assoc Eq Pract, 1965. p 359.
8. Stromberg, B. Eq Vet J **11** (1979) 26.
9. Van Pelt, RW. JAVMA **155** (1969) 510.
10. Van Pelt, RW. JAVMA **158** (1971) 1658.

PRINCIPLES OF THERAPY
Orthopedic Surgery
by B.D. Grant

Immobilization

Immobilization of skeletal injuries reduces the chance of further injury. A simple form of immobilization is enforced stall rest. Enforced stall rest is usually of little benefit for short periods; rest for 1-6 months is often recommended. Good foot care, endoparasite control, and good stall ventilation, sanitation and lighting are critical. Feeding of a good-quality grass hay is recommended. The use of grain increases the chances of producing an overweight, overactive animal that places additional strain on the injured part. Removal of the animal from the stall every 2-3 weeks for progress checks should be avoided to prevent reinjury. Confined animals are also very susceptible to viral infections, especially if kept in a stable with a large transient horse population, and should be vaccinated regularly.

Crossties or overhead chains provide more immobilization to the injured part than stall rest. The use of these devices is usually limited to animals whose injuries would be made worse by attempts to lie down and rise, as in injuries of the pelvis and upper forearm. Animals less than a year of age do not respond well to crosstieing or overhead chains, and after 1-2 days simply lie down or attempt to leap out of their constraining devices.

Many types of slings are available for the immobilization of a horse with skeletal disease (see Chapter 8). The owner should understand that a sling can only be used successfully on a horse that can stand by itself. Application of a sling to an animal that cannot stand may result in further injury or even suffocation. Slings generally should not be used on adolescent animals.

Bandages are a common form of immobilization. An animal's foreleg may be bandaged in a flexed position to prevent weight-bearing. Young animals with fractures of the upper forearm tolerate this method very well for moderate periods.

Use of a Robert-Jones bandage is indicated for the immediate immobilization and protection of long-bone fractures below the elbow and hock (Fig 30). These bandages are also useful following surgery for osteochondral fractures. Several types of elastic adhesive bandages can be used directly over an incision or injured area. Elastic bandages should be applied carefully to avoid ischemia and pressure necrosis over bony prominences and flexor tendinitis.

The use of plaster resin-polymer or PVC tube casts is also an important form of immobilization for the treatment of long-bone fractures, wounds, osteomyelitis and exuberant granulation tissue. The use of casts is described in more detail in the section on fracture repair.

Surgery

Preoperative Management: The animal should be weighed when first admitted to the clinic for accurate dosage calculations. Recording of weight upon admission and discharge also plays an important role in considering the dietary intake of each animal. This is especially important when the owner's assessment of the quality of surgery is based on the appearance of the horse at discharge.

The preoperative use of antibiotics has always been controversial.[1] If antibiotics are to be used postoperaatively, the same antibiotic should be given in large doses preoperatively. Use of aminoglycoside antibiotics should be avoided to prevent potential interaction with the anesthetic agent. Tetracyclines also should not be used because of the association of these drugs with postoperative diarrhea.

Phenylbutazone can be administered 3-4 hours before surgery to reduce operative and postoperative pain, and to reduce the chance of postoperative myositis. All horses should be dewormed, if necessary, prior to surgery to reduce the occurrence of abdominal pain and/or diarrhea due to the increased activity of the parasites during anesthesia. Use of organophosphate anthelmintics should be avoided immediately before surgery.

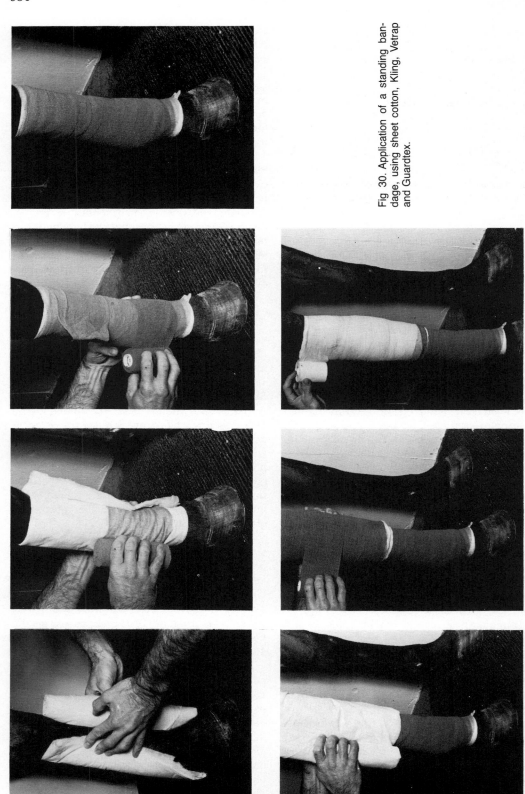

Fig 30. Application of a standing bandage, using sheet cotton, Kling, Vetrap and Guardtex.

Facilities: Orthopedic surgery should ideally be performed in a facility that allows a separate room for tabling and preparation of the patient. Only after the horse is anesthetized and fully shrouded, with the operative site prepared and the feet bandaged, should it be taken to the operating room. This room should only be available for aseptic procedures. The surgical room need not be elaborate but should have doors that can be tightly sealed to prevent the influx of barn dust, insects and casual observers. Proper lighting and the availability of resuscitative equipment are very important.

Some provisions for cauterization should be available although it may not be used routinely. Overuse of electrocautery in arthrotomies of the fetlock and carpal joints produces a characteristic circumscribed pale area at the incision edge that invariably leads to slow healing of the incision.

Tourniquets are commonly used in arthrotomies to reduce hemorrhage and improve visibility in the surgical field. The most common type of tourniquet used is a combination of an Esmarch bandage, followed by the application of a high-pressure, inflatable cuff (Fig 31). After 2 hours the tourniquet's effectiveness is decreased because of increased venous hemorrhage. Vessels and nerves may also be more difficult to identify when a tourniquet is used. For this reason, the surgeon must be very familiar with the anatomy of the area.

Surgical instruments should include stainless steel gouges, chisels, curettes, rongeurs, a bone file, osteotomes, mallets, hand-held and self-retaining retractors, a bowl, and some form of suction. Use of chrome-plated instruments should be avoided.

Anesthesia: Although surgery for osteochondral fractures can be done on a standing horse with the aid of sedation and local anesthetics, the most common practice is to have the animal under general anesthesia. The risks of general anesthesia are less than the risks of a poor-quality arthrotomy due to inadequate regional anesthesia, uncontrolled patient movements, injury to the operator and assistants, and postoperative infection.

Positioning: The surgeon should examine preoperative radiographs to confirm the correct location of the surgical site and to determine the best operative position. Although most arthrotomies are performed with the horse in lateral recumbency, some surgeons prefer dorsal recumbency, especially when multiple incisions are necessary. Dorsal posi-

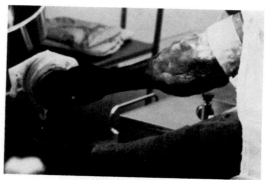

Fig 31. An inflatable cuff has been applied proximal to the carpus after the horse is positioned in lateral recumbency.

tioning allows good control of hemorrhage because the operative site is above the heart. However, there have been reports of unexplained deaths in animals recovering from anesthesia after surgery in dorsal recumbency.[2]

Site Preparation: The operative site is clipped, rinsed with an antiseptic solution, and bandaged with an antiseptic pack the day before surgery. At the time of surgery, sterile shrouds are applied to the entire animal. The antiseptic pack is removed, the area is shaved with a razor and the site is scrubbed routinely.[3] A moisture-proof drape is placed under the leg, and an adhesive drape over the operative site (Fig 32).

Arthrotomy Technic: The anatomic landmarks should be repeatedly palpated to assure the correct location of the skin incision. The skin and subcutaneous tissue are incised and retracted and entry into the joint capsule is heralded by the escape of synovial fluid. Insertion of fingers into the joint should be minimized to reduce the risk of septic arthritis.

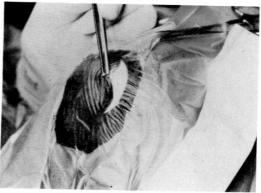

Fig 32. A curvilinear incision is made through a plastic drape and the skin on the craniomedial aspect of the carpus.

Ligatures of absorbable or .nonabsorbable material should be used to control hemorrhage to allow adequate visualization of the surgical field. Some surgeons feel the use of hemoclips, while effective, may cause clients and other veterinarians to attribute postoperative pain to the presence of these radiopaque bodies. The tourniquet should be released before the joint capsule is closed so that any large bleeders can be ligated before closure.

The joint capsule should be closed with nonabsorbable suture material, such as autoclaved Vetafil or Prolene, in a simple interrupted pattern for the synovium and a horizontal mattress pattern for the fibrous joint capsule. The closure is tested by injection into the joint of 6-8 m saline containing 1 million IU potassium penicillin. The subcutaneous tissue and skin are closed routinely. The incision is covered with antibiotic ointment and gauze pads held in place with adhesive tape. Standing elastic adhesive bandages are applied over this.

Recovery: The recovery room should be dimly lit, quiet, well padded and provided with O_2. While the horse is still recumbent, some clinicians examine and trim the feet, float the teeth and clean the penis of male horses. Antibiotics should be given when the horse is standing to minimize the possibility of an adverse drug reaction. The animal should be observed closely until fully recovered.

Postoperative Management: Antibiotics, if indicated, should be administered for at least 5 days. Phenylbutazone decreases enzyme activity in articular cartilage, and decreases postoperative swelling and pain. The drug can be given orally as boluses or as a phenylbutazone powder-molasses slurry at 4 g once daily for 5 days, then 2 g daily for 30 days. Administration of phenylbutazone should be discontinued if diarrhea develops.

An operated joint should be passively flexed 15-20 times daily for the first 2-3 postoperative weeks to reduce the formation of adhesions in the joint.[4] If moderate pain on passive flexion and/or swelling persist at 14 days postoperatively, 20 mg dexamethasone may be given IM every other day for 7 treatments. Ultrasound therapy, beginning on the fourteenth postoperative day, also reduces pain and swelling.

Intra-articular injections of corticosteroids, hyaluronic acid and orgotein have been used to reduce adhesion formation; however, only limited studies have been conducted on the efficacy of such treatments.

Bandages on the carpus should be changed on the third postoperative day, and those on the fetlock, tendons and splint bones are changed at 7 days. Bandages should be changed earlier in cases of swelling, excessive pain, hemorrhage, discharges, abnormal odors or fever. The bandage should then be changed every other day until suture removal at 12-14 days postoperatively. Application of a nonporous bandage over the standing cotton bandage provides support and reduces the chance of wound contamination (Fig 30).

Sutures are normally removed after 12 days, although some clinicians remove every other suture on day 12 and the remainder on day 14. The area should be surgically prepared and the horse properly restrained prior to suture removal. Postoperative radiographs should be obtained at the time of suture removal.

The horse can be hand-walked for 5 minutes daily beginning on postoperative day 10, and for increasingly longer periods during the following weeks. Galloping, either free in a paddock or under tack, should be avoided for at least 8 weeks. Swimming is an increasingly popular mode of postoperative exercise.

Postoperative Complications

Myositis: Postoperative myositis can result from poor positioning of the animal on the surgical table and inadequate padding. It is one of the most common causes of violent recovery from general anesthesia. The condition is described in detail in Chapter 19.

Diarrhea: Postoperative diarrhea occasionally occurs in horses subjected to general anesthesia. Proper anthelmintic and dietary therapy, as well as anti-inflammatory agents to reduce stress, should be a consideration before any surgery requiring general anesthesia. Chapter 13 contains details on the treatment of diarrhea.

Synovial Fistula: Fistula formation most commonly occurs after surgery on joints previously injected with corticosteroids or when a tendon sheath is inadvertently entered during joint surgery. Incomplete closure of the joint capsule and suture failure also lead to fistula formation.

A synovial fistula is diagnosed by evidence of synovial fluid emergence upon flexion of the limb or by contrast radiography. Conservative treatment is aimed at producing joint swelling and consequent closure of the fistula through the use of topical counterirritants, temporary bandage removal, and discontinuance of anti-inflammatory drug administration. Intra-articular injection of iodine-based contrast agents has benefitted some horses. Fistulas that fail to close after such treatment warrant surgical closure to prevent septic arthritis.

Seroma: The development of fluctuant accumulations of serosanguineous fluid is not unusual after joint surgery in which radical dissection was required or in which hemostasis was a problem. Seromas can be differentiated from a developing synovial fistula by aspiration; synovial fluid is typically a yellow, slippery tenacious fluid. Repeated aspiration should be avoided. Most seromas require only pressure bandages for resolution.

Wound Dehiscence: The failure of first-intention healing of an arthrotomy occurs most frequently in joints previously injected with corticosteroids. Vitamin A counteracts the inhibiting effect of corticosteroids on wound healing.[5] Therefore, postoperative care of an arthrotomy on a joint that has been previously injected with corticosteroids should consist of oral administration of vitamin A (5 million IU give PO) every other day for 7 treatments. Vitamin A should be administered parenterally (5 million IU given IM) if the animal is fed mineral oil. Loosely applied horizontal mattress sutures of heavy material prevents gross enlargement of the wound. Care should be taken to have the bandages changed daily in a clean environment to avoid as much contamination as possible.

Septic Arthritis: The development of septic arthritis following arthrotomy is the most serious complication possible as it frequently leads to humane destruction of the patient. Clinical signs include severe pain, fever, leukocytosis and lameness.

Dystrophic Calcification: Dystrophic calcification of soft tissues is most commonly associated with surgery requiring radical dissection, such as removal of fragments from slab fractures of the third carpal bone or P1 fractures. Dystrophic calcification is usually evident on radiographs obtained 2 weeks after surgery as soft tissue swelling and loss of clarity of the outlines of the carpal bones. The amount of physical impairment is not always related to the degree of radiographic change. Treatment includes systemic corticosteroids, ultrasound therapy, poultices, and limited exercise.

Compensatory Lameness: Compensatory lameness develops when an animal with a primary lameness shifts its weight onto the remaining sound limbs. Rotation of the third phalanx is the most common type in mature

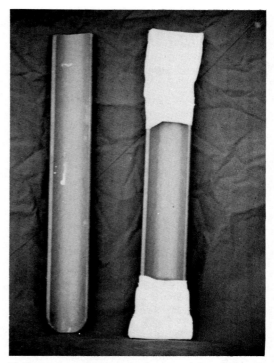

Fig 33. Splint made from plastic pipe cut along its length into thirds or quarters. The ends are rounded off and padded with felt.

horses, with a varus deformity most common in young horses. Preoperative and periodic postoperative radiographs of the weight-bearing limb should be made to detect such changes.

Suture Rejection: Suture rejection is uncommon and usually associated with nonabsorbable sutures. Swelling and a purulent discharge may be evident 2-12 months after surgery, but the animal may not be lame. Treatment requires removal of the offending suture(s).

External Coaptation
by A.S. Turner

Splints

Splints are useful in certain areas of equine orthopedics. They can be constructed out of wooden strips, thermoplastic material (Orthoplast:Johnson & Johnson, Thermoplastic:3 M), or from PVC pipe. Thermoplastic splints are conformed to the contours of the limb after softening by immersion in hot water. Plastic pipe is usually cut lengthways into thirds or quarters. The ends are usually rounded and padded to minimize trauma from sharp edges (Fig 33). Splints should not be the sole method of treatment for long-bone fractures in any size of horse because they do not have the strength and rigidity provided by a well-fitting plaster cast. They are useful for temporary immobilization of fractures below the carpus and the hock if the animal is to be referred for more elaborate treatment. Too much reliance must not be placed on splints as treatment; plaster casts are superior, even for temporary immobilization of a long-bone fracture.

Splints are sometimes useful in correcting certain angular limb deformities, especially in newborn foals, caused by ligamentous laxity. However, as with any external coaptation device, development of pressure sores must be minimized. If the splint must remain in place for more than a day, it should be periodically removed and replaced to help minimize pressure sores. A useful regimen is to splint the leg during the day and remove the splint during the night. Tetanus prophylaxis should be provided if pressure sores develop. The use of large amounts of padding, although beneficial from the standpoint of minimizing development of pressure sores, can be detrimental because it reduces the effectiveness of the splint. Plastic piping has a tendency to rotate around the limb if not applied correctly.

Modified Thomas Splints

There are still indications for the use of modified Thomas splints in horses, although with the advent of sophisticated internal fixation technics, they are used less and less. They are still used regularly in cattle because of economic limitations of treatment and their better tolerance of these devices.

Modified Thomas splints are almost always used as a method of immobilization in conjunction with internal fixation or casting. They are also useful for temporary immobilization of certain fractures when used with casts. These splints must not be relied on as a sole method of fracture stabilization. They limit motion in the limb, which is useful in certain tibial and radial fractures. If a cast is used with the splint, the cast generally can be made a little lighter than it otherwise would be.

The modified Thomas splint is a very awkward device for a horse to wear because the splint is always constructed longer than the leg. The animal usually drags the splint around the stall. Animals that lie with the affected limb down must be rolled over to enable them to rise, especially if the rear limb is in the splint. Excessive traction causes circulatory problems in the axilla and inguinal regions due to pressure from the ring of the splint.

The ring of the splint should be well padded to reduce the incidence of pressure sores. Usually a competent welder or blacksmith must be present for the construction and fitting of the splint. The hoof is generally wired to the distal end of the splint. Good nursing care and constant attention to the splint are essential or poor results can be expected. Pressure sores generally develop but, if managed carefully, are usually of minor significance when compared to the original problem.

Slings

A properly constructed sling is useful if the animal tolerates it. Unfortunately, only a small percentage of horses can manage themselves in a sling, despite the erroneous beliefs of many horse owners. Slings are usually used not as a sole method of fracture fixation but to reduce stress on a fracture site repaired by other means. They are also useful in horses that refuse to lie down to reduce stress on the sound limbs. A horse in a sling should be under constant supervision and must receive good general nursing care at all times.

Plaster Casts

A well-applied plaster cast is one of the most useful adjuncts in the treatment of certain equine limb injuries. They can be used for the management of certain soft tissue trauma as well as some fractures. Some fractures below the carpus and tarsus, and certain comminuted fractures of the sesamoids or phalanges can be managed solely with a well-made cast. Casts can also be used to stabilize fractures during transportation to a facility for internal fixation. Casts are frequently used to supplement internal fixation devices used in repair of some fractures, and they reduce the excessive force on the bones of the lower limb, especially in recovery from anesthesia. Luxations of various joints are generally treated solely with casts.

Lacerations of the lower limbs (including the heel and coronary band) are one of the most common indications for application of a cast. Clinicians are often reluctant to apply a cast over contaminated wounds of the lower limbs. However, the results obtained by cast application are superior to those obtained by pressure bandages. Pressure bandages, no matter how meticulously applied, do not immobilize the wound edges as effectively as a plaster cast. The old saying that a wound "needs air" should, for practical purposes, be ignored. Casts applied to contaminated wounds with copious exudation should be changed every 8-10 days rather than cutting a window in the cast. Windows severely weaken the cast and granulation tissue often grows through the window.

The joint above and the joint below the fracture should be immobilized by the cast. The cast should not end in the middle of a long bone because the fulcrum effect produces severe sores and places excessive pressure on the diaphysis. With very few exceptions, the cast should include the entire foot. If the foot is left exposed, the axial force of weight-bearing is transmitted up the leg, resulting in instability of the fracture site. It can also result in sores, especially at the coronary band. The foot may be left exposed when it is impossible to get the foot off the ground due to a painful injury and the horse is considered too much of an anesthetic risk to undergo cast application under general anesthetic.

A product suitable for cast application is the rapid-setting, resin-impregnated plaster Zoroc (Johnson & Johnson). This material is a combination of plaster resin and catalyst. Regular plaster of Paris has been used on equine limbs but is not recommended because it takes 3-4 hours to cure to a reasonable strength. A large heavy cast is required to withstand normal ambulation, and plaster casts lack strength.

The resin-impregnated plaster comes in 4- and 6-inch rolls sealed in foil packets. The material occasionally deteriorates when exposed to air or heat and becomes granular in texture; these rolls should be discarded because they do not bond well to adjacent layers, resulting in a weaker cast. The setting time for Zoroc is 5-8 minutes, although 20 minutes should pass before allowing the animal to stand on the cast. Tractable animals can have the cast applied while standing, but it is difficult to achieve a good fit if the cast is applied this way. Sometimes pain from the injury causes constant movement of the limb during cast application. A cast applied under these circumstances does not fit properly and can cause pressure sores.

General anesthesia is the best method of restraint for cast application. The animal is positioned in lateral recumbency, with the affected limb up. If a cast is to be applied in the field for temporary immobilization of a fracture, a temporary pressure bandage, such as the Robert-Jones bandage, should be applied during induction of anesthesia and replaced with the cast once the animal is anesthetized.

When the animal is anesthetized, the shoes should be removed and the feet trimmed prior to application of the cast. The foot of the limb

to be placed in the cast should also be trimmed because the heels can become quite contracted during confinement in a cast.

About 12 rolls of 4-inch Zoroc are used for a cast on the metacarpus or metatarsus of a 1000-lb (450-kg) horse. Heavier or fractious animals, or ones that may have a violent recovery from anesthesia need about 13-15 rolls of 4-inch Zoroc. About 12 rolls of 6-inch Zoroc are required for a 1000-lb adult horse. Materials required for cast application include 12-15 rolls of 4-inch Zoroc, various sizes of orthopedic stockinet (2-inch for foals, 3-inch for fractures below the carpus/tarsus in adults, 4-inch for full-limb casts), an aluminum walking bar (½-inch square), orthopedic felt (¼-inch thick), borax powder (optional), bandage scissors, one Backhaus towel clamp, rolled cotton or similar material, and tepid water. Materials required for removal are an oscillating saw, cast spreader, large screwdriver, and bandage scissors.

The material should be laid out in an orderly fashion prior to anesthetizing the animal so it is readily available (Fig 34). The felt used at the top of the cast should be cut to approximate length, the correct diameter stockinet located, and the walking bar shaped. Delays in application of the cast allow the plaster to cure in "shells," which greatly reduces its strength.

The water should not be too hot or the cast will set in "shells" rather than as one solid unit; use of cold water delays curing. The resin-impregnated plaster recommended in this technic should not be immersed as long as regular plaster of Paris. The plaster becomes too sloppy if held in the water until all the bubbles disappear. The end should be kept free and both hands should be used to immerse the roll. Im-

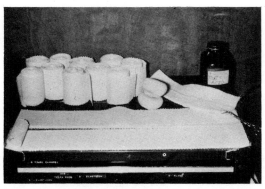

Fig 34. The cast material is arranged in an orderly fashion so the cast can be applied with minimal delay between each roll of plaster. This helps prevent the cast setting in "shells." The "splints" of plaster are also prepared.

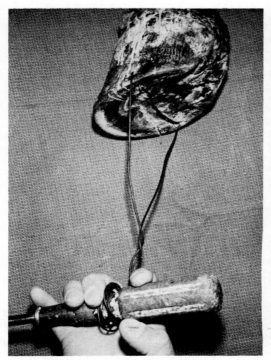 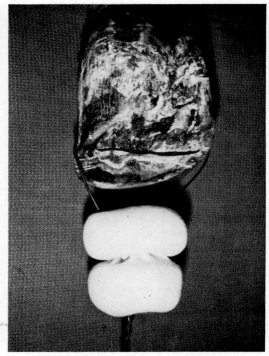

Fig 35. Baling wire is threaded through ⅛-inch holes in the hoof wall at a 45° angle to the sole. The wire is twisted and held by an assistant.

Fig 36. The stockinet is threaded over the wire.

mersion for only 2 seconds is generally all that is required for Zoroc; however, some clinicians prefer longer periods of immersion. Curing is indicated by a slight increase in temperature, due to an exothermic reaction. Such heat is usually of no consequence. Some cast products are limited in use by the excessive heat generated during curing, resulting in burns.

Prior to application of the cast, 2 rolls of 4-inch plaster are fashioned into "splints." One roll is folded back and forth on itself, in accordion fashion, to about the length of the cast plus 6 inches (15 cm). This enables the splint to fold over the toe region. For full-leg casts that extend to the top of the limb, 6-inch rolls are more economical. The splints are eventually placed on the dorsal and volar (or plantar) surfaces of the leg.

Incorporation of a walking bar into the cast is optional for small casts that come to the top of the metacarpus/metatarsus. A walking bar aids in transferring weight from the ground surface to the proximal end of the cast. It is therefore necessary to extend the bar beyond the weight-bearing surface of the foot. Although walking bars require additional time

and money, I recommend their use in all casts. Walking bars are also useful in full-leg casts because they provide the additional strength these casts need. The walking bar should be bent prior to anesthetizing the horse. The base of the walking bar should be about 1 inch (3 cm) wider than the widest part of the hoof across its weight-bearing surface.

Cast Application: Any wounds are debrided, sutured and treated as indicated. Sterile, non-adhering dressings are applied to wounds under the cast to prevent the stockinet from adhering to the wound. Specialist cotton can be used to protect the coronary band from abrasion and minimizes the chances of cutting the coronary band during cast removal.

Fractures are stabilized by closed reduction by attachment of baling wire to the hoof wall and traction applied by an assistant. Holes ⅛-inch in diameter are drilled in the hoof wall, directed at a 45° angle to the white line of the sole. Care must be taken not to penetrate the sensitive laminae. The drill holes are positioned depending on the degree of flexion or extension required in the fetlock, pastern and coffin joints. Holes should be drilled in the heel region for weight-bearing by the foot and in the toe region for extension of the foot. Wire is then threaded through both holes to form a U, twisted and held by an assistant (Fig 35). This technic is also used to reduce a fracture at the time of surgery. Restraint must be applied to the body of the animal if excessive traction is required to reduce a fracture. Patience is required to reduce equine long-bone fractures. Traction may be required for ½-1 hour. Most clinicians agree that muscle relaxants are worthless in that situation.

The leg is then dusted with borax powder to flatten the hair and to keep conditions in the cast relatively dry. The only significant padding applied under the cast is a double thickness of orthopedic stockinet. When more padding than this is applied, the weight of the animal soon compresses the padding and the cast becomes loose, resulting in abrasions. Some clinicians apply the cast directly over the hair. If wire has been used to stabilize the foot, the stockinet is threaded over the wire and rolled up the leg to a point about 10-15 cm proximal to the intended top of the cast (Fig 36). When rolling the stockinet proximal up the leg, care must be taken not to dislodge any dressings on the leg (Fig 37). A 4-inch (10-cm) wide strip of ¼-inch orthopedic felt is applied to the proximal end of the metacarpus/metatarsus to the top of the cast (Fig 38). In full-limb casts, the felt should be 6 inches (15 cm) wide and placed at the proximal end of the radius/tibia. In casts that extend proximal to the carpus and the hock, it is advisable to make a "doughnut" of felt and place it over the accessory carpal bone or medial malleolus of the tibia. A Backhaus towel clamp holds the felt in position. There should be no wrinkles in the stockinet.

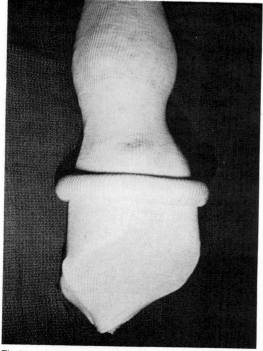

Fig 37. When rolling the stockinet up the leg, care must be taken not to dislodge any dressings.

Application of the first roll is critical. It should be closely applied without tightening, or circulatory embarrassment of the limb will result. The plaster should fit quite snugly under the fetlock joint. Each layer of material should be rubbed circularly until the fabric lines of the plaster disappear. This ensures that the cast sets up as a single unit. (Fig 39).

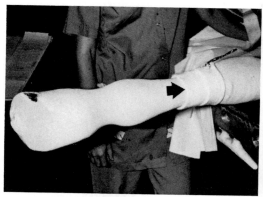

Fig 38. A 4-inch wide strip of ¼-inch orthopedic felt is applied to the top of the metacarpus/metatarsus (arrow).

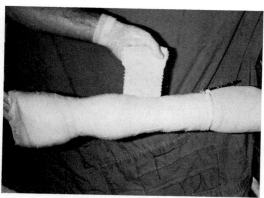

Fig 39. The first roll should be applied snugly without tightening. Excess stockinet can be cut from the toe region when 3-4 rolls of plaster have been applied.

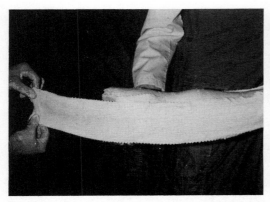

Fig 40. Previously prepared splints are applied to the cranial and caudal aspects of the cast and covered with another roll of plaster.

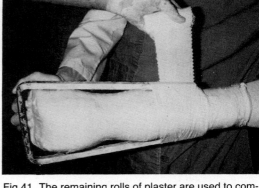

Fig 41. The remaining rolls of plaster are used to complete the cast by covering the walking bar. The plaster is twisted into a "rope" at the top of the cast to prevent the walking bar from breaking out of the top of the cast.

An assistant must support the limb at the carpus or tarsus and at the fetlock joint during the application of the cast or an angular deformity in the cast will result. One must be careful not to dimple the cast with the fingers. Such indentations result in abrasions.

When 3-4 rolls of plaster have been applied, the excess stockinet can be cut from the toe region. The wire applying traction to the foot should be left in place until the cast is nearly complete. Previously prepared splints are applied to the cranial and caudal aspect of the cast and are covered with another roll of plaster applied in the usual fashion (Fig 40).

The walking bar is held in position by an assistant, making sure it is correctly placed across the bottom of the foot. The bar is then covered with plaster; the toe is well covered since much wear occurs there (Figs 41, 42). The remaining rolls of plaster are used to complete the cast. At the top of the walking bar the plaster is twisted 360° to form a "rope" of cast material at the ends of the walking bar. If this is not done, the walking bar will break out of the top of the cast and will not transfer weight to the top of the cast.

Full-limb casts require larger-diameter stockinet to fit the muscle masses of the upper extremities. These larger casts should be reinforced in the area of the carpus and hock, which are the most common sites for breakage, with plaster applied in a figure-8 pattern. The rear limb should be placed in slight flexion to encourage the horse to adopt a more weight-bearing posture (Fig 43). Rear-limb casts are usually quite awkward. Prolonged struggling or falling with the cast behind the horse can lead to rupture of the peroneus tertius.

Combination Casts: A resin-impregnated cast to the proximal end of the radius/tibia can be so heavy for young foals that they have great difficulty getting around the stall. These foals are also reluctant to nurse as frequently. For this reason, resin-impregnated plaster (*eg*, Zoroc) is placed over the stockinet, followed by several layers of Light Cast (Merck). The resultant cast is comparatively light yet strong; however, the Light Cast requires exposure to ultraviolet light for curing (Fig 44). Ultraviolet lights are cumbersome and expensive and therefore of no use in the field. However, they are useful in veterinary hospitals. Light Cast is difficult to manipulate but can be applied directly over the damp Zoroc portion of the cast. By the time the Light Cast cures with exposure to UV light, the Zoroc is quite hard. These combination casts do not produce the abrasions associated with casts constructed of fiberglass alone. Placing some acrylic cement (Tech-

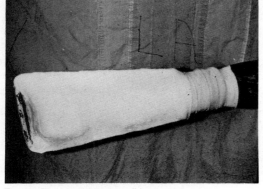

Fig 42. The completed "walking cast."

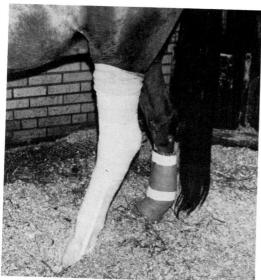

Fig 43. Rear-limb casts are usually quite awkward and should be applied with the limb slightly flexed. About 12 rolls of 6-inch Zoroc and a walking bar are required.

novit:Kyzler) over the sole and toe area prevents excessive wear during normal activity.

Cast Care: Horses wearing a cast should be under direct veterinary supervision at all times. Hospitalization is recommended. Animals kept at home should be inspected daily by a veterinarian unless the owners fully understand the consequences of complications that may occur. Despite such warnings, owners often blame complications of cast application on the veterinarian that applied it originally. The horse should be kept in a dry stall with straw or shavings as bedding. Each day the cast should be inspected closely (not just "eyeballed" through the stall door) for cracks, excessive wear (toe especially) and abnormal or excessive discharges. Cracks can quickly spread, resulting in limb movement and pressure sores. Broken casts should be changed immediately.

The cast should be felt for areas of excessive warmth. There are generally warm spots on the palmar (plantar) aspect of the fetlock and in the carpal area because of blood vessels in those areas; however, excessive heat is abnormal and indicates the need for examination of the limb. A certain amount of experience is required to judge what is in fact abnormal warmth in a cast. Excessive swelling above the cast generally indicates trouble, and the cast should be changed.

The best way to judge how a horse is tolerating the cast is to watch how the animal uses the affected leg. If, on the day after cast application, the horse appears less agile and less confident about bearing weight on the affected leg, there may be a problem. Sometimes a horse may lick or bite the cast. This may be only pruritus but should be regarded as a suspicious sign. One should not rely on changes in the WBC count or a rise in body temperature to predict trouble under a cast. By the time these parameters change, the situation may be irreversible. Horses on drugs like phenylbutazone must be watched even more closely, as the effects of such products can mask problems under the cast.

Pressure Sores: There are 2 common sites at which pressure develops with short casts that extend to the proximal end of the metacarpus/metatarsus. One is the cranial aspect of the cannon bone, just distal to the proximal end of the cast, and the other is the abaxial surface of the sesamoid bones. If the amount of padding is kept to a minimum (no more than outlined above), these areas should be only mildly abraded where the hair has rubbed off. With larger casts that come to the proximal end of the limb, common areas for abrasions are the accessory carpal bone and medial malleolus of

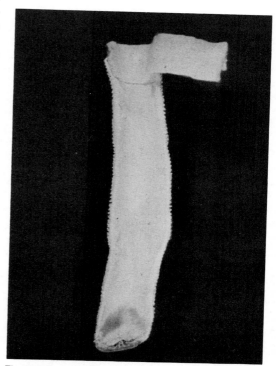

Fig 44. "Combination" casts are light but require ultraviolet light to cure the outer layer of fiberglass.

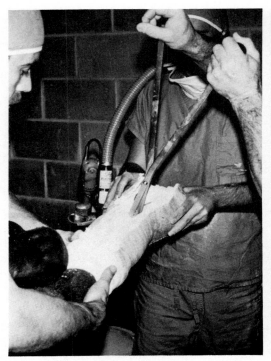

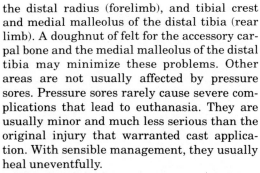

Fig 45. Following removal of the walking bar, the cast is cut in half by cuts on the medial and lateral side. A cast spreader aids removal.

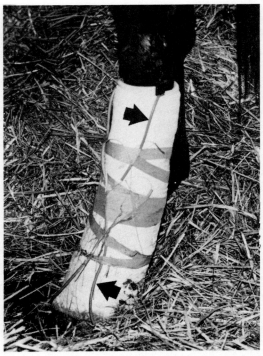

Fig 46. Obstetric wire in polyethylene or rubber tubing (arrows) can be incorporated into the cast to facilitate removal.

the distal radius (forelimb), and tibial crest and medial malleolus of the distal tibia (rear limb). A doughnut of felt for the accessory carpal bone and the medial malleolus of the distal tibia may minimize these problems. Other areas are not usually affected by pressure sores. Pressure sores rarely cause severe complications that lead to euthanasia. They are usually minor and much less serious than the original injury that warranted cast application. With sensible management, they usually heal uneventfully.

When a full-limb cast is to be replaced by a shorter cast (one that ends at the proximal metacarpus/metatarsus), swelling may occur proximal to the end of the smaller cast. Such swelling usually responds to pressure bandages placed on the limb proximal to the smaller cast. Most casts should be changed every 3-4 weeks. In cases of gross contamination or excessive suppuration at the site of trauma, the cast should be changed at intervals of 8-10 days. This interval can be lengthened as the wound heals.

Cast Removal: When the cast has served its function (the wound has healed), it is usually cut off with the horse standing; sedation may

be required in some horses. Fractious animals or those without stockinet under the cast may require general anesthesia for cast removal. However, anesthetized animals must recover from anesthesia without the protection of the cast. This may be detrimental to certain fractures that have not quite healed or lacerations that have not returned to adequate strength. If the cast is cut off in 2 half-shells, the shells can be temporarily placed back on the limb to give support during recovery from anesthesia.

Casts are best removed with an oscillating saw. The walking bar should be removed first with cuts in a sagittal plane. This ensures that a lip of plaster does not remain, which would prevent the 2-inch oscillating saw blade from reaching the full thickness of the remainder of the cast. The cast is then cut in half by cuts on the medial and lateral aspects (Fig 45). Because cast cutters can cut through skin and joints, care must be used during cast removal.

The cast cut should include the foot. It is impossible to cut one side and under the foot, and then crack the cast on the remaining side; the entire perimeter of the cast must be cut. Once the cast has been cut, the stockinet should be cut with bandage scissors prior to cast removal.

Another method sometimes used to facilitate removal of a cast is to insert obstetric wire in polyethylene or rubber tubing and incorporate the tube on the inner surface of the cast (Fig 46). The affected limb generally requires some form of pressure bandage when the cast is removed because limbs placed in a cast usually swell after cast removal. Some fractures require application of a Robert-Jones bandage after cast removal, which provides more immobilization than a pressure wrap.

Commercially Available Leg Braces

An adjustable leg brace is commercially available for limb support in various injuries (Dawson Leg Brace, Petoskey, MI). The metal brace was originally designed to protect an injured limb during recovery from anesthesia but has been used during transport of injured horses as well. The brace consists of vertical rods fastened to horizontal circular members (Fig 47). The brace conforms approximately to the shape of the foreleg but is not as easily adaptable to the rear leg. The brace can be adjusted so the hoof rests on a plate at the bottom of the brace or is suspended above the plate to varying degrees. The main idea behind the brace is that the foot is actually off the ground and axial forces are not transmitted up the leg.

The brace is placed over soft bandages when in use. The limb must be wrapped carefully so the brace can be pulled over the bandages. If too little padding is placed under the brace, the limb lacks stability and moves within the brace. If the brace is clamped too tightly over the bandages, excessive pressure is applied to the skin. The manufacturers are currently designing special pads to avoid this problem.

Optimally the brace must extend to the proximal end of the foreleg and actually rest on the sternum, acting as a crutch. At our clinic we have found some horses too large to achieve this effect.

We have not used the brace on routine orthopedic cases but have found it useful in isolated instances. It is useful in cases of soft tissue infection with concomitant drainage and exudation. The removable brace allows the clinician to rapidly change wound dressings and reapply the pressure wraps and brace. The cost of general anesthesia and a plaster cast are saved if this can be done with the animal standing. The brace is also suitable for support in cases of injury from the carpal joint distad, including soft tissue injuries, fractures and luxations.

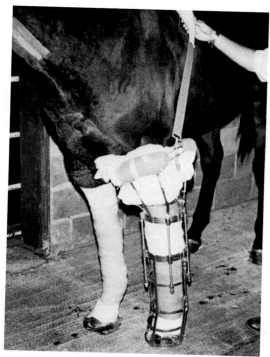

Fig 47. The Dawson leg brace is hinged for quick removal. Its height can be adjusted to suit the size of the horse.

A shoulder strap should be attached to the brace to increase stability of the limb (Fig 47). The strap should be adequately padded to prevent abrasions across the withers. The brace is quite heavy. Most horses can only awkwardly ambulate around their stall. The correct amount of stall bedding should be used for patients wearing the brace. Too much bedding entangles the distal end of the brace and makes it very awkward for the animal. Too little bedding results in decubital sores in horses spending considerable periods recumbent.

The usefulness of this brace is not well defined at this writing. In the author's opinion it does not provide the stability of a well-applied plaster cast.

Compression-Plating in Long-Bone Fractures
by A.S. Turner

A great step forward was made in equine orthopedics when the compression treatment of fractures was applied to horses.[6-10] Several companies manufacture compression-plating equipment, some of which is based on the design of the original Swiss equipment. It is not the point of this section to promote the use of one system over another. In the author's experience, the AO/ASIF (Arbeitsgemeinschaft für Osteosynthesefragen/Association for Study of Internal Fixation) system has the greatest versatility and is most adaptable to equine fracture repair. Compression plating is the only system that has a chance of withstanding the constant forces to which implants are subjected during the healing period.

Compression in Treatment of Fractures

Under normal conditions a fractured bone heals by formation of a periosteal and endosteal callus, which stabilizes the fracture and allows bony union between the fragments. The amount of periosteal and endosteal callus formed depends on the vascular supply, the osteogenic properties of the tissue and, above all, the degree of stability in the area of the fracture. If the fracture is well stabilized, an altered pattern of fracture healing, characterized by haversian remodeling and minimal or no callus formation, occurs. This is so-called "primary bone healing."[11]

The aim of compression plating is to achieve primary bone healing, ideally without callus formation. Great amounts of callus indicate instability at the fracture site. Primary bone healing does not occur commonly in horses, as in humans and small animals, because of the horse's inherently greater body weight. Even in foals, primary healing of long-bone fractures is rare. Callus is usually formed in long-bone fractures repaired by compression plating.

The use of compression plates also minimizes the need for external coaptation (casts, splints). This advantage can be used in foals because the implants can, in most cases, withstand ambulation. In adults, however, internal and external fixation are required because the implants may not be strong enough to withstand ambulation. Minimizing the use of external coaptation allows early movement of adjacent joints, which reduces muscle atrophy, stiff joints and other problems.[11] Foals are particularly prone to complications associated with use of external coaptation. These include abrasions due to the thin skin of foals, weakening of the flexor tendons and associated muscle groups, and pressure injury to the physes of the opposite weight-bearing limb. In my experience, joint stiffness associated with external coaptation is not a major problem in young or old horses.

Compression itself does not stimulate bone healing as was originally thought. Compression merely contributes to stability of the fracture site by providing enough friction to minimize shearing and rotation forces. There is no acceleration of osteogenesis with the use of compression.

The screws available in most compression-plating systems are of the cortical and cancellous types. Cortical bone screws were designed for use in hard bone, as exists in just about every equine long bone. Cancellous screws are used more in the soft bone of foals and occasionally in the metaphyseal area of weanlings and yearlings.

Screws can be applied through the plate into underlying bone or may be used to secure fragments of bone together in the repair of a comminuted fracture. In the latter case the screw is generally inserted using the "lag-screw principle." This achieves maximum compression of the 2 pieces of bone. The hole in the cortex nearer the screw head (gliding hole) is cut so the threads can pass through it without gripping; the threads only grip the other cortex (threaded hole). Compression can also be achieved using a partially threaded cancellous screw, but the threads must not cross the fracture site.[11]

The ASIF dynamic compression plate (DCP) offers several advantages over conventional plates.[12,13] Because the DCP can be used without a removable tension device, it can be placed near the ends of the bones. Another very useful advantage of this plate is the ability to place the screws at angles of other than 90° to the plate. Loss of compression occurred when screws were not placed at exact 90° angles to conventional plates.[12] Another advantage of this plate is that cancellous screws can be used in any hole. This is useful in foals, which have relatively soft bones. Finally, the DCP can be contoured to the bone and the screw heads still fit the holes.

Compression of a long-bone fracture with a plate can be achieved in 2 ways. The plate can be applied as a tension band. In such cases, the plate is applied under tension but the fracture itself is under compression. Such a plate should be placed on the side of the bone under tension if at all possible. If the cortex opposite the plate is intact and the plate is under compression, the tensile forces under the plate are converted to compressive forces. This is the so-called tension-band principle. The plate should be applied according to the methods outlined in the AO manual.[11]

Comminuted fractures are reconstructed using lag screws for interfragmentary compression. The bone plate is then applied between the 2 main fragments of bone, bridging the comminuted area. This ensures that the majority of forces are transmitted from the proximal to distal fragment, thereby reducing unwanted forces on the comminuted area. A plate applied in this manner is called a neutralization plate. Such a plate should be applied under compression; however, excessive compression could disrupt the repair.

Bones should be plated from one metaphysis to the next if possible to avoid stress concentration at the ends of the plates. If double-plating is performed, as is often done in equine fractures, the plates should end in different areas of the metaphysis to avoid stress concentration. Both plates are generally applied under compression to achieve maximum stability.

Intramedullary nailing is recommended for treatment of certain fractures in humans but has limited use in equine fractures.[12] The pin or nail usually cannot be inserted into the bone without penetrating the adjacent joint.[13] The humerus and femur in foals are the only bones amenable to such treatment. Another problem with treatment of fractures using nails is the lack of suitable implants. Large medullary nails are adapted for the relatively long, straight medullary cavity of humans and are either too long or not wide enough for the equine femur and humerus. The other outstanding disadvantage of the use of nails is that they cannot provide the stability and strength to allow for ambulation even in foals.

Transfixation pins, incorporated into plaster casts, occasionally have application in long-bone fractures in horses. However, use of these devices (Hoffman and Wagner apparatus) is extremely limited because of the massive loads encountered in adults during normal ambulation. In foals and ponies with severe comminution and soft tissue trauma, some advantage may be gained by the relatively noninvasive nature of this technic.[14] Problems encountered with transfixation devices are loosening of pins, with subsequent localized osteomyelitis at the pin sites, and occasionally fracture of healing bone through one of the pin sites. Loosening of the pins results in loss of stability at the fracture site, with eventual nonunion. In many cases the localized osteomyelitis at the pin sites resolves but prolonged hospitalization is sometimes required. As with intramedullary nailing, success should be evaluated on how quickly the animal returns to normal ambulation without lameness and on the health of the opposite weight-bearing limb, rather than on fracture healing alone.

Prerequisites of Internal Fixation

The equipment required for internal fixation of equine fractures is very expensive. The operating theater should be of high standard to perform aseptic surgery. The operating table should be at a convenient level to minimize fatigue of the surgeon. The patient should be adequately padded and positioned to minimize problems associated with prolonged recumbency (rhabdomyolysis, etc). Many equine orthopedic procedures require intraoperative radiographs to ensure correct placement of implants. Well-trained assistants and an anesthetist are essential to the success of the procedure.

A full complement of compression-plating equipment is required for optimal repair. The surgeon must be totally familiar with the recommended technics of compression plating, as can be achieved by periodically attending one of the courses presented by the ASIF group in Davos, Switzerland or Columbus, Ohio.

The operation should be carefully planned. If necessary the fracture configuration can be sketched onto cellulose acetate from preoperative radiographs. The fracture can then be mentally repaired before surgery. The approximate dimensions of plates and screws can be ascertained. As well as a mechanical understanding of the fracture repair, the surgeon should become accustomed to thinking in 3 dimensions throughout the surgery. Atraumatic technic should be practiced at all times. To reduce operating time, knowledge of the surgical approach to the fracture site is also an essential requirement. This minimizes the chance of trauma to a vital structure and is the most important contribution to soft tissue handling.[15]

Fractures of Specific Bones
by A.S. Turner

Mandible and Maxilla

Cause: Fractures of the mandible and maxilla are the most common fractures of the head.[16] These fractures are caused by kicks, falls and other trauma. They commonly occur when the teeth are caught under a stationary object, such as a rail, a gate or door latch, and the animal suddenly pulls backward. The design of certain barn door latches may predispose to such accidents.[17] The incidence of these fractures is high in stallions. Occasionally the mandible may be fractured during repulsion of diseased teeth, or a pathologic fracture may occur as a result of alveolar periostitis and local osteomyelitis.

Clinical Signs: The clinical signs of mandibular and maxillary fractures depend on the severity of the fracture. The most obvious sign, common to all except an undisplaced fissure through the horizontal ramus, is malalignment of the incisors. Fracture of only one ramus of the mandible or maxilla may not cause displacement. Crepitation may be evident in some fractures. The bone ends are often visible through the interdental space. Once the initial soreness of the fracture has subsided, affected horses usually develop a keen appetite. The ends of the fractured bones frequently become packed with food material. The tongue sometimes protrudes and saliva dribbles from the mouth. Fractures several days old have the characteristic foul odor of osteomyelitis around the head. Most fractures in this area are open. Radiographs should be taken to ascertain the configuration of the fracture and to check for displacement of fragments not evident on clinical examination. Oblique views are required to delineate the exact configuration of some fractures.

Treatment: Fractured cheek teeth may abscess and require extraction. These cases may eventually come to the attention of the veterinarian long after the original fracture has healed. Difficult mastication, dropping of food and the typical fetid smell of bone necrosis are the presenting signs.

Failure to treat these fractures can result in a number of undesirable sequelae, including malocclusion, abnormal tooth wear, osteomyelitis, sequestration with chronic fistulation, and constant protrusion of the tongue. Conservative treatment may be all that is necessary for fractures with relatively little displacement. Easily digestible, soft food should be fed. Use of analgesics, such as phenylbutazone, may encourage the horse to eat. Antibiotics and tetanus immunization should be administered. Feeding by stomach tube should be reserved for horses not eating or drinking, rapidly losing body weight or becoming dehydrated. Most fractures of the vertical ramus are not severely displaced due to the relatively large amount of protection provided by the pterygoid and masseter muscles. These fractures are also best treated conservatively.

Stabilization is usually required for optimal treatment of compound fractures involving considerable displacement. The condition of dehydrated and debilitated animals should be improved before surgery.[18] This may mean several days of feeding by stomach tube. Preoperative evaluation of the hemogram should be performed in these cases.

General anesthesia is required for repair of nearly all fractures in this region. Fractures of both the mandible and maxilla are best approached with the horse in dorsal recumbency. Lateral recumbency is adequate in some cases. Inhalation anesthesia is currently the safest method and its use is strongly recommended, especially if the procedure will be long and tedious. Tracheotomy can be performed and intubation performed through the tracheotomy to provide additional working room in the mouth.[19] Intravenous anesthesia, with 5% glyceryl guaiacolate and 10% thiamylal sodium, is generally satisfactory for short procedures.[20]

The gums and area of the fracture should be thoroughly scrubbed and irrigated with sterile saline or Ringer's solution. Infected bone ends should be curetted and detached or devitalized pieces of bone should be removed. Debridement is essential in most cases. Gingival lacerations should be sutured if possible, although areas of bone may be completely devoid of soft tissue. This is no cause for alarm since these areas generally heal very rapidly. Use of tetanus antitoxin and antibiotics is indicated.

Fractures of the mandible and maxilla can be repaired in various ways. A complete array of fixation devices should be available during the surgery if possible. The biomechanical principles and various forces involved in mastication must be considered in repair of these fractures. Internal fixation should be used to repair open fractures if it provides the most stability at the fracture site. Transient osteomyelitis usually develops but healing generally occurs even though some movement is present, in contrast to the situation with longbone fractures. Fractures of the mandible and premaxilla are usually easily reduced.

Osteomyelitis may persist as long as implants are present and may be evidenced by a fistulous tract with a malodorous discharge. The infection usually resolves after curettage, sequestrectomy or removal of the implants. Tooth removal may be necessary when the fracture involves the tooth roots.

Wiring the displaced teeth to adjacent teeth may be all that is required for fractures involv-

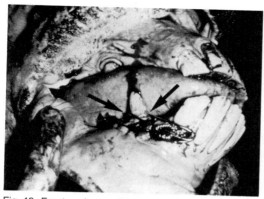

Fig 48. Fractured mandible in a 12-year-old stallion. The fracture occurred in the interdental space, and the bone ends were exposed. The fracture was repaired with 2 Steinmann pins and cerclage wire (arrows) anchored to the canine tooth.

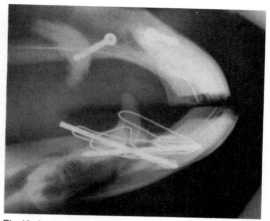

Fig 49. Immediate postoperative radiograph of the fracture in Figure 48. Healing was successful and the implants were eventually removed.

ing the incisor teeth and a relatively small amount of alveolar bone. Very loose or irreversibly damaged deciduous incisors should be removed and permanent teeth realigned to prevent further eruption problems. Holes are made between the teeth at the gingival margin to ensure firm anchorage of wire. In males the canine teeth can be used as an anchor. Most cases requiring simple cerclage wire fixation can be repaired with 18-ga wire. Tightening the wire causes ischemic necrosis of a small amount of gum but is usually of no consequence. In some cases, cerclage wire can be used with Steinmann pins (Figs 48,49).

Fractures of the mandibular symphysis in young animals are generally amenable to fixation with pins and wire. Pins are usually inserted through stab incisions in the gums. A hole slightly smaller than the diameter of the Steinmann pin is drilled and the pin is inserted with a Jacobs chuck.

Excellent results were reported in 9 fractures stabilized with an external thermoplastic brace fixed to the labial side of the incisors.[20] The fractures treated by this method involved a fracture between the central incisors through three-fourths of the body of the mandible, extending rostrelaterad to the junction of the body and horizontal ramus of the mandible, and a fracture between the central and intermediate incisors extending caudolaterad across the body of the mandible in the canine tooth.

Intramedullary pinning alone has been used satisfactorily.[18] The pins are inserted along the ventral surface of each horizontal ramus and directed perpendicularly to the vertical caudal border of each ramus. Intramedullary pinning

of the horizontal ramus of the mandible should be reserved for older animals because of the interference with the tooth roots of younger animals. A Kirschner-Ehmer apparatus has also been used to repair these fractures.[21] Care must be taken to avoid nerve damage with this technic or lip paralysis can result. The outstanding disadvantage of this technic is the awkwardness of the device protruding from the jaw. The apparatus can be deliberately or unintentionally dislodged.

Some mandibular fractures can be treated by compression plating.[22] Stabilization usually results in healing even if osteomyelitis is present at the fracture site. The fracture is approached by an incision directly over the ventrolateral aspect of the horizontal ramus of the mandible. Care should be taken to identify and preserve the parotid duct and facial artery and vein, which pass along the rostral edge of the masseter muscle. The mental nerve should also be avoided as it emerges from the mental foramen.[15] The screws should be placed as low on the horizontal ramus as possible to avoid the roots of the cheek teeth. In an infected fracture, the wound drains until the plate is removed.

Another method of repairing certain mandibular and premaxillary fractures is the U-bar technic.[19,23] This is particularly useful when there is very little bone attached to the incisor teeth for stabilization by conventional methods. The technic requires a U-shaped bar made from 5/16- to 1/4-inch brass rod, which is fashioned before the operation and bent to conform to the dental arcade. The rod is wired to the lower incisors and to the first and second cheek teeth. Gas anesthesia is administered with an endotracheal tube inserted through a tracheotomy. Stab incisions in the cheeks are necessary to drill holes at the gingival margins of the cheek teeth because the commissures of the lips do not extend far enough caudad. The U-bar technic is stable enough to allow the horse to eat normal feed immediately after surgery.

Postoperative care of mandibular fractures usually consists of antibiotics and tetanus prophylaxis. Daily flushing and mechanical removal of food and debris caught in the fixation devices is recommended. Any drainage from the fracture site usually ceases after removal of the implants. Some cases require sequestrectomy and curettage of osteomyelitic areas to encourage resolution of the infection.

Postoperative feeding depends on the individual case. Fractures still fairly unstable after surgery may necessitate placement of an indwelling stomach tube sutured to the nostrils to prevent mastication. A gruel is pumped into the tube with a bilge pump. The tube should be kept plugged, while not in use, to prevent aspiration of air. The gruel can be made from 12.5 kg oats, 1½ bales chaffed oaten hay, ½ bale chaffed alfalfa, 5.5 kg soybeans, 8 kg split peas, 2 kg dehydrated molasses, 2.5 kg powdered milk or casein, 140 g salt, 85 g Ca and 30 g Fe.[18] This mixture should be hammer-milled into a powdery consistency and sieved if necessary. Occasionally $NaHCO_3$ (40-60 g) or oral neomycin powder (2-3 g of active drug) must be added to curb gas production and subsequent colic that sometimes occur from feeding this mixture. A more convenient method currently being used by some veterinarians involves commercial complete pelleted feed (Horse Chow Checkers:Purina) that contains roughage and grain. A crude fiber content of 20-25% is recommended.[24] Dehydrated alfalfa pellets are also suitable but do not have the energy content of the previously mentioned pellets. The pellets are soaked in water overnight and administered as a gruel.

The prognosis for mandibular fractures is good if they are satisfactorily immobilized by the methods described above. Fractures through the temporomandibular joint may result in arthritis and warrant a guarded prognosis.

Skull

Cause: Fractures of the equine skull are relatively common and are usually caused by kicks, running into stationary objects, impact from a moving vehicle and even bludgeoning. Fractures of the cranial vault are often fatal because of associated neurologic problems. Fractures of the facial bones (nasal, frontal, maxilla) are usually amenable to various forms of reconstructive surgery.[17,25-27]

Clinical Signs: Clinical signs of head fractures include deformity of normal facial contours, localized pain and swelling, and unilateral or bilateral epistaxis. Epistaxis is usually caused by laceration of the mucosae of the nasal cavity or sinuses. Instability and crepitus may also be present. Ocular and neurologic signs may accompany these fractures.

Treatment: Failure to diagnose and treat such fractures can lead to sequestration, nonhealing wounds, facial deformity and chronic sinusitis.[26,27] Cosmetic defects are a liability for show horses and impaired respiratory function limits performance.

Because of the edema and hemorrhage at the fracture site, depression and obvious deformity may not be fully appreciated for several days. The deformity becomes progressively worse as the hematoma organizes. The fracture usually heals but the deformity and limitation of respiratory capacity may be permanent.[26]

Radiographs should be taken to eliminate the possibility of more serious fractures, such as fractures of the cranial vault or basosphenoid bone. The fracture is generally visible but several oblique views may be necessary. Some fractures may not be evident until the time of surgery. Head fractures are usually open from an external wound or from laceration of the nasal mucosa. The use of antibiotics is generally recommended but should not replace debridement, hemostasis, generous irrigation and wound closure without tension.[28]

Immediate, primary open reduction produces a better cosmetic result than does repair performed at a later date. Reconstruction should be performed on an elective basis as soon as the patient has been stabilized from the original injury, which is generally a week after the fracture occurred.

Surgery is best performed with the horse under general anesthesia and in lateral recumbency, with the fracture site up. The horse's head should be placed as close to the edge of the table as possible in cases of fractures across the midline of the face. Adequate parenteral fluid replacement should be considered in some cases and horses with considerable blood loss should be crossmatched with suitable donor blood. Manipulation at the time of surgery usually causes considerable epistaxis, which generally subsides by the completion of surgery, unless a major blood vessel is inadvertently lacerated.

The surgical approach for repair of these fractures is through large, curvilinear flap incisions that extend well beyond the margins of the involved bones.[10] Alternatively, generous S-shaped incisions can be used.[27] The extent of the fracture is generally appreciated following reflection of the skin and subcutaneous tissue. The hematoma that usually occupies the fracture site should be removed with moist sponges.

The fracture should be reduced as carefully and patiently as possible. A Langenbeck retractor can usually be inserted into the defect and fragments gently manipulated into normal position.[17] If it is not desirable to disturb the fracture site, large holes can be drilled in healthy bone peripheral to the fracture. An elevator is then inserted in the hole and positioned under the fracture site. Stabilization of the fragments with transosseous 18- to 20-ga wire is necessary in cases with no inherent stability at the fracture site. Wire holes are made with a drill or a small Kirschner wire held in a Jacobs chuck. Care must be taken, when twisting the wire to secure the fragments, not to twist the wire too tightly or it will cut through this relatively soft bone.

Any small, detached fragments of bone devoid of periosteum should be removed because of the likelihood of sequestrum formation. Although defects may exist following repair of these fractures, the result is generally satisfactory if such defects are not very extensive. The large skin flaps are replaced, and the skin and subcutaneous tissues are apposed. Intradermal skin sutures, using fine, synthetic nonabsorbable material, can be used if there is not tension on the suture line. This suture provides a better cosmetic appearance than do other suture patterns. Application of head bandages is recommended during the early postoperative period to minimize chances of subcutaneous emphysema. Bandages should allow normal mastication yet maintain firm even pressure along the surgical site. They are generally left in place until fibrin seals the wound, 3–4 days.

A slight nasal discharge may persist for 1–2 weeks after surgery. This may be the result of a mild sinusitis and sometimes requires antibiotic therapy.

Scapula

Fractures of the scapula are relatively uncommon. They usually occur from collisions with a fixed object or another horse. Varying degrees of lameness result, depending on the configuration and duration of the fracture. Crepitation may be difficult to elicit in acute cases due to extensive soft tissue swelling. Such swelling produces an abnormal contour of the shoulder. Extension of the scapulohumeral joint sometimes elicits a painful response. Varying degrees of supraspinatus and infraspinatus muscle atrophy ("sweeny") occur in chronic cases involving injury to the suprascapular nerve. Some affected animals have sequestration and a chronic, draining wound.[16]

Fracture and displacement of the tuber scapulae usually occur in horses less than a year of age as an epiphyseal separation. This fracture detaches the origins of the biceps brachii and the coracobrachialis muscles. Affected horses have a decreased cranial phase of the stride.[29]

Fractures of the neck of the scapula are usually accompanied with considerable overriding of the bone ends.[16] Fracture of the body of the scapula is rare.

Radiographic diagnosis of a fractured scapula is difficult unless appropriate radiographic equipment is available. Fractures of the tuber scapulae may be visualized, even with portable machines, by silhouetting the point of the shoulder. A posterior-anterior view is necessary to detect fractures of the body of the scapula.[30] Fractures of the scapular neck in foals and small horses can be demonstrated with a portable radiographic machine.

Treatment of a fractured scapula usually depends on the configuration of the fracture. Fractures of the neck are treated conservatively (confinement in a small stall) because the bizarre shape of the bone makes application of internal fixation devices difficult. Also, fractures of the neck of the scapula may cause a variable amount of suprascapular nerve injury. Animals with scapular neck fractures usually remain lame indefinitely.[16]

A fractured and displaced tuber scapulae ideally should be reattached to the neck of the scapula to establish function of the biceps brachii and coracobrachialis muscles. In selected cases this can be attempted using ASIF partially threaded cancellous screws with washers. In larger animals these implants cannot resist the pull of these muscle groups. Resection of the tuber scapulae has been used as a method of treatment of this injury. The severed muscle groups supposedly reattach to the scapula with a fibrous union.[29] More documented cases are needed to evaluate this method of

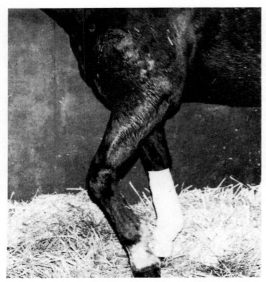

Fig 50. Fractured humerus creates a "dropped elbow" appearance. Soft tissue swelling is also present around the fracture site.

treatment. Details describing the approach to the tuber scapulae are available.[15]

Tuber scapulae fractures should be managed conservatively in breeding animals. Until surgical methods (lag-screw fixation and tuber scapulae resection) are fully evaluated, surgery should be reserved for special cases.

A fracture of the body of the scapula was repaired in a 3-month-old filly using an ASIF semitubular plate.[30] The filly was normal a year later and shows no lameness 4 years after surgery.

Sequestrectomy is usually necessary to eliminate the infection in scapular fractures involving a chronic draining wound.

Humerus

Because of overlying muscle, the humerus is not as prone to fracture as are the bones of the lower limbs. Extremely large forces are necessary to fracture the humerus. Injuries during halter-breaking or collision with another horse or a fixed object may fracture the humerus. The injury may also occur during jumping, in a fall onto the point of the shoulder.

The clinical signs of a fractured humerus are usually quite characteristic and include complete lack of weight-bearing and dragging of the limb in a flexed position. The horse appears to have a "dropped elbow" similar to that seen with a fractured olecranon (Fig 50). Massive swelling in the affected area may muffle crepitation at the fracture site.

In most cases it is impossible to obtain radiographs of the affected area unless high-capacity radiographic equipment is available. In these cases the veterinarian is forced to make a diagnosis based on the history and clinical signs. Because of the grave prognosis for adult horses with humeral fractures, one may elect to euthanize the horse rather than subject the animal to a painful trailer ride to a facility where radiographs can be taken, only to have the horse euthanized.

Fractures of the humerus are usually spiral or oblique, through the diaphysis and rarely compound.[16] Occasionally there is a fracture through the lateral condyle, resembling a Salter-Harris type IV fracture.[31] Humeral fractures are always accompanied by considerable overriding due to muscle spasm. Reduction of these fractures during surgery requires considerable traction. Traction is not achieved merely by applying tension to the distal limb, which may in fact cause displacement of the fracture ends. Fractures of the diaphysis may have varying amounts of radial nerve damage, ranging from contusion to complete severance. The amount of nerve damage may be difficult to determine at the time of injury; prognosis should be withheld until the integrity of the nerve is known. Some cases may take as long as 6 months to regain full neurologic function.

Treatment of humeral fractures is largely dictated by the age of the animal. Because healing time is quite protracted and considerable suffering occurs during convalescence, older animals with humeral fractures should be euthanized. In affected young animals with a future as a breeder, confinement in a small stall for 2-3 months, with good supportive care, is a feasible alternative for such fractures. During this time, the opposite front limb should be supported and the animal should receive good nursing care. Fractures in these young animals eventually heal with considerable callus and some shortening of the bone. The prognosis ultimately depends on the integrity of the radial nerve.

Humeral fractures have been repaired with ASIF cloverleaf nails and with plates.[6,32,33] The bone is difficult to plate because of its extreme shortness and marked curvature of the lateral aspect. In addition, the radial nerve and biceps brachii muscle occupy an awkward position in the lateral aspect of the musculospiral groove. The surgical approach used in humeral fracture repair has been described.[15]

The prognosis of a fractured humerus is largely dependent on the age of the animal. The prognosis is extremely poor in older animals. In foals the prognosis for survival for breeding is quite good if the radial nerve is functional. In many cases the bone may heal but the opposite limb may succumb to angular limb deformities and stretched flexor tendons due to excessive weight-bearing.

Olecranon

Compared with other equine long-bone fractures, fractures of the olecranon are quite common. They are usually caused by trauma from another horse or a fall with the limb outstretched. Fatigue has been implicated in some olecranon fractures.[16] The extent of lameness caused by olecranon fractures depends on the configuration of the fracture. Horses are usually unable to bear weight on the affected limb and may have a "dropped elbow" resembling that seen in radial paralysis (Fig 51). The amount of swelling varies. Crepitation can usually be palpated in the affected area.

The diagnosis of olecranon fracture is by clinical signs and radiographic examination. Anterior-to-posterior and lateral-to-medial views are required. Lateral views, which usually best delineate the fracture, are taken with the leg extended and the x-ray beam directed in a medial-to-lateral direction.

Olecranon fractures assume a variety of configurations, ranging from avulsion of the epiphysis in foals to severe comminution of the ulna, with luxation of the radius craniad (Monteggia fracture). Fractures commonly extend into the semilunar notch. Displacement is sometimes severe in olecranon fractures due to the pull of the triceps brachii muscle.[34,35]

Management of olecranon fractures is conservative or surgical, depending on the configuration of the fracture. For minimally displaced fissure fractures, conservative treatment (absolute stall rest for 6-8 weeks and support of the opposite limb) may suffice. The affected limb should be radiographed periodically to check for displacement of fracture fragments, in which case internal fixation may be indicated. Fractures of the distal ulna, toward the diaphysis of the radius, can also be treated conservatively. Conservative management may be the only reasonable method in extremely comminuted fractures because of large numbers of fragments.

Complications of conservative management of olecranon fractures include contracted flexor tendons of the affected limb, with ankylosis of

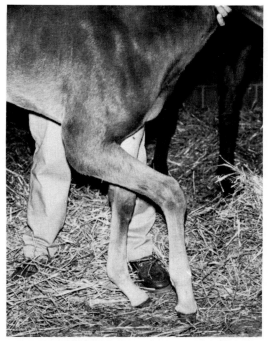

Fig 51. Foal with a fractured olecranon, causing "dropped elbow" appearance.

joints; failure of union due to excessive displacement fragments; permanent pain and stiffness of the elbow joint; and, in young animals, pressure injuries to the physes of the opposite limb due to excessive weight-bearing, with associated angular limb deformities.

The prime indication for surgical intervention in olecranon fractures is to offset the distracting forces of the triceps brachii muscle. Many olecranon fractures create a markedly displaced proximal fragment that can only be repositioned by open reduction and internal fixation. Intra-articular fractures are also an indication for internal fixation to ensure congruency of the articular surface. Most olecranon fractures respond quite dramatically to internal fixation; early return to function is another advantage of surgery.

The most satisfactory technic for repair of the fractured olecranon is application of an ASIF dynamic-compression plate along the caudal aspect of the bone.[36-38] The caudal aspect of the bone is under tension due to the pull of the triceps brachii muscle. The horse is positioned with the affected limb up and the bone is approached, using a muscle-splitting technic, between the ulnaris lateralis and the ulnar head of the deep digital flexor muscle. The ulnaris lateralis is reflected craniad and the ul-

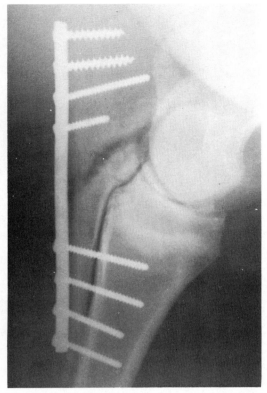

Fig 52. Repair of a fractured olecranon of 3 weeks' duration, using an ASIF dynamic-compression plate, in a yearling Quarter Horse. The horse was completely sound a year later.

nar head of the deep digital flexor caudad, exposing the caudal aspect of the ulna.[15]

The fracture can usually be manually reduced; however, Kirschner wires may be needed to provide temporary fixation of the fragments. The plate is contoured to the shape of the bone. It is sometimes advantageous to shave the caudal aspect of the distal fragment with an osteotome to seat the plate.[39] The plate is applied using the methods recommended by the AO group.[11,12] The bone is quite amenable to application of the tension device because additional exposure is easily obtained along the caudal aspect of the radial diaphysis. Use of the tension device also enables large fracture gaps, typical of this fracture, to be closed by compression (Fig 52). In comminuted fractures at the very proximal aspect of the bone, a portion of the insertion of the triceps muscle must be severed for placement of the plate. The plate is contoured to extend over as much of the olecranon tuber as possible and to ensure maximum compression of the proximal fragment.[36] This minimizes the chances of postoperative detach-

ment of the proximal fragment. No untoward effects have been noticed by detaching this small amount of triceps insertion.

In young animals, cancellous screws should be used in the proximal fragment. If several weeks have elapsed before repair is undertaken in an adult, cancellous screws are also required because the proximal fragment becomes porotic from lack of muscle tension. Cortical screws are usually used distal to the elbow except in the very youngest foals. It is sometimes necessary to bridge the proximal ulnar physis with an implant; this can be done with impunity since very little bone length comes from this growth plate.

Radius

Fractures of the radius are relatively common compared with fractures of other long bones. They result from a variety of injuries, such as kicks, automobile accidents or stepping in holes. Fractures through the shaft of the radius are usually accompanied by extensive edema, soft tissue swelling, and complete lack of weight-bearing. Radial fractures assume many configurations, but oblique fractures are the most common. Compound fractures usually occur on the medial side where the bone lacks soft tissue protection. In young animals the fracture may occur through the proximal or distal radial growth plate, and the metaphysis may luxate craniad.

Radial fractures can be very difficult to immobilize for transport to a facility for further treatment. Fractures of the distal third, including those through the distal radial physis, can be stabilized to some degree in a cast that extends up to and including as much of the elbow as possible.

In some instances, especially fractures involving the proximal two-third of the bone, a cast may exacerbate the instability at the fracture site. In affected foals, a cast incorporated into a Thomas splint sometimes provides enough stability for a trailer ride to a facility where further surgery may be performed.

Diagnosis of a fractured radial shaft is usually obvious upon physical examination. Radiographs are indicated if repair is to be attempted, especially if internal fixation is to be used. Radiographs are also required to confirm the diagnosis if fragments have not separated or a fissure fracture is suspected.

Treatment of radial fractures, like most long-bone fractures, depends upon the age, configuration of the fracture and economics. Adult horses with severely comminuted frac-

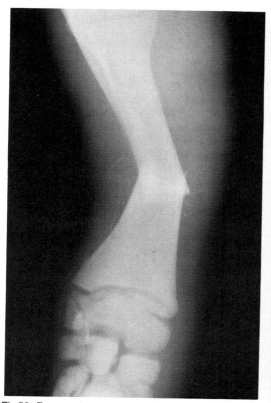

Fig 53. Fractured radius in a 2-week-old Quarter Horse.

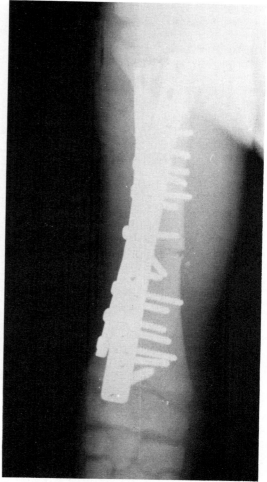

Fig 54. Immediate postoperative radiograph of fracture in Figure 53. Two broad ASIF dynamic-compression plates were used, approaching the bone from the lateral aspect. The foal made a complete recovery.

tures should be euthanized for humane reasons except under exceptional circumstances. Compression plating offers the only realistic chance of successful repair of a fractured radius in an adult. The implants available for internal fixation are not strong enough for most fractures of the radial shaft in adult horses (see Problems Associated with Long-Bone Fractures).

Struggling during recovery from anesthesia presents the possibility of refracture. In fractures of the distal third, a cast up to the axilla can be used to supplement internal fixation. If the fracture is much more proximal than the distal third of the radius, the cast can concentrate the stress on the fracture line and cause refracture at the original fracture site or at the end of the compresson plates. Slings may be of value if the horse's temperament is suitable. If the horse is likely to fight restraint in a sling, the surgeon may elect to allow the animal to recover from the anesthetic, relying solely on the internal fixation for support of the fracture.

If compression plating is used, at least 2 plates and, if possible, 3 plates should be applied, even in foals (Figs 53, 54). Due to the overriding that inevitably occurs with fractures of the shaft of the radius, some form of traction device should be assembled soon after the animal is positioned on the operating table to aid in reduction of the fracture. Steady traction for up to 30-45 minutes may be required to approximate the fracture ends. The plates are applied using a medial or lateral approach and recommended ASIF technics.[11,12,15]

Fractures through the distal radial physis in young animals should be immobilized in a full-limb cast. These fractures sometimes deviate laterad during treatment.[16] However, young animals are capable of considerable remodeling and the result is sometimes quite gratifying. Occasionally a fracture may extend into the radial carpal joint, producing an intra-ar-

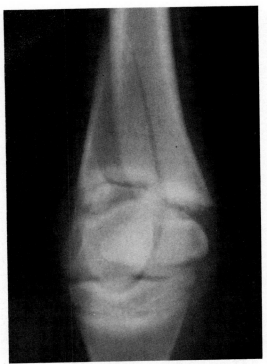

Fig 55. Fracture of the distal metatarsus in a 3-month-old filly. This fracture is a Salter-Harris type-II injury because the fracture line extends across the physis and proximad into the metaphysis.

In foals the prognosis should be withheld until the surgeon has some idea of the amount of stability achieved with the fixation device(s) used to repair the fracture.

Third Metacarpal/Metatarsal Bones

Fractures of the third metacarpal/metatarsal bones are common in horses of all ages. These bones seem quite vulnerable to fracture because of their exposed location.[33] Such fractures are caused by various types of trauma, including kicks, automobile accidents and halter-breaking injuries. The bones are frequently broken in foals when a clumsy mare steps on the foal. Owing to the very limited amount of soft tissue over this bone, these fractures are frequently compound. Similarly, closed third metacarpal/metatarsal fractures are easily converted to compound fractures if the animal struggles or if immobilization is inadequate during transport to a hospital facility.

The diagnosis of metacarpal/metatarsal fractures is generally obvious. Radiographs should be taken to determine the degree of comminution, the presence of an intra-articular fracture and, consequently, if internal or external fixation or both will be necessary in treatment. In some circumstances it may be more prudent to first apply a plaster cast for immobilization during transport to a facility where a more thorough diagnosis and treatment will be performed.

Fractures of the cannon bones assume a variety of configurations, ranging from simple transverse to severely comminuted fractures. Fractures of the second and fourth metacarpal/metatarsal bones usually accompany fractures of the third metacarpal/metatarsal bones. Fractures through the distal metacarpal physis sometimes occur in young animals. These are commonly Salter-Harris type-II fractures (Fig 55).[31] In adults, cannon bone fractures tend to be comminuted; in younger animals the fractures are of more simple configuration.

The treatment of canon bone fractures is dictated by economics and the type of fracture. External coaptation has been used very successfully in many cases. Traction on the limb is usually necessary and is achieved by placing baling wire through the hoof wall (Fig 35). Traction is generally more difficult to apply to the rear limb because of reciprocal apparatus and sometimes causes displacement of fracture fragments. The cast used for external immobilization should encase the entire hoof and should extend to the proximal radius (see Cast Application). In some fractures of the can-

ticular fracture similar to a lateral condylar fracture of the distal metacarpus. Such fractures are best treated with cortical or cancellous bone screws, employing the lag-screw principle. This ensures rigid immobilizaton of the fracture at the articular surface and minimizes the chances of osteoarthritis.

Fractures of the distal third of the radius that do not allow placement of enough screws in the distal fragment because of small size can be immobilized using an ASIF angle-blade plate. Because considerable experience is required to insert the plate, only a surgeon who has worked with the plate should attempt it.

Some surgeons insert transfixation pins into the proximal and distal fragments, and incorporate the pins into an extenal coaptation device. No matter how meticulously these are applied, they lack the stability of compression plates. However, their use could be considered in foals with comminuted fractures too extreme for successful bone plating. Bone grafting should be considered in certain radial fractures (see Bone Grafting).

The prognosis for radial fractures in adults is poor and grave if the fracture is comminuted.

non bones, cast application is indicated to allow the soft tissues to "recover" prior to performing osteosynthesis.[38] Fractures of the cannon bone, particularly in adult horses, are associated with extensive soft tissue injury; immediate internal fixation can lead to devitalization of the skin over the plate. External coaptation is sometimes necessary to augment internal fixation, especially in adults.

Internal fixation is indicated in cases of marked displacement of fragments and in fractures of considerable obliquity. The bone ends in such oblique fractures override and compound within the cast. Any articular component to the fracture is an indication for rigid immobilization to reduce the chances of osteoarthritis from incongruency of the joint surface. In some cases it is less expensive to perform internal fixation because it reduces convalescent time and minimizes the investment in several cast applications otherwise necessary to support the fracture.

Internal fixation of such fractures is best achieved with 1 or 2 ASIF dynamic-compression plates, depending on the size of the horse. In young foals with limited subcutaneous space to cover the implant, a broad plate may be all that can be used (Fig 56).

It is generally possible to use 2 broad dynamic-compression plates in adults. The surgeon must be sure the skin will cover the plates without excessive tension before they are applied or the skin will slough during the convalescent period. These defects can take considerable time to heal by granulation, although osteomyelitis and infection around the implants are more serious sequelae.

Traction on the affected limb should commence as soon as the animal is anesthetized, appropriately positioned and padded. Even in young foals, overriding of the fracture due to muscle and tendon contracture can be difficult to overcome. Slowly applied traction over periods of 30 minutes or more is necessary. The general tendency is for the surgeon to give up after intermittent efforts at traction. Positioning of the horse under anesthesia depends on the configuration of the fracture and the side of the bone to which the plates are applied.

The approach to the metacarpus/metatarsus should be through a large flap-like incision.[15] Large flaps are important to ensure adequate skin coverage of the implants following the osteosynthesis. The plates are applied as outlined by the AO group.[11,12] In young foals it is

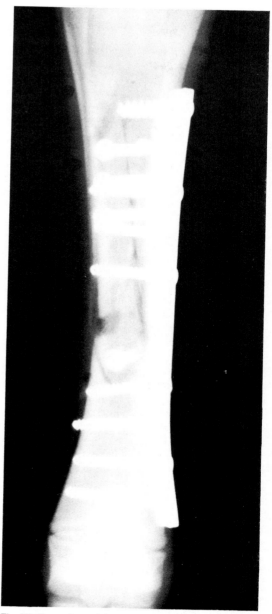

Fig 56. Comminuted fracture of the third metacarpal bone of a 4-week-old Arabian. The fracture was repaired using interfragmentary compression with lag screws, followed by application of a broad ASIF dynamic-compression plate. This plate is functioning as a "neutralization" plate.

sometimes necessary to cross the distal metacarpal/metatarsal physis with the implant to achieve fracture stability. Although an angular limb deformity might result, very little bone growth occurs from the physis after 2½-3 months.[38,39] Loose, detached fragments of devitalized tissue should be removed and thorough

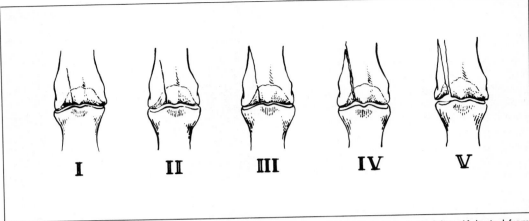

Fig 57. Range of configurations in fractures of the lateral metacarpal and metatarsal condyles. (Adapted from Meagher, DM. Proc 22nd Ann Mtg Am Assoc Eq Pract, 1976)

irrigation performed with internal fixation of compound fractures (see Management of Compound Fractures). Metacarpal/metatarsal fractures with cortical defects or that are extremely comminuted should have cancellous bone grafts. This is essential, especially in adults. Untreated cortical defects persist for many months and represent a weak point in the bone (see Bone Grafting).

Following osteosynthesis, the decision to use external coaptation depends on the case and the stability of the repaired fracture. Some cases require only a Robert-Jones bandage, while others require a full-limb cast. The surgeon may elect to apply a cast for recovery from anesthesia. Some animals, especially adults, require the support of a cast for as long as 2 months. The bones of older horses take 10-12 weeks to heal. The bones of foals heal more quickly and external coaptation should be removed as soon as healing progresses. Prolonged periods in a full-limb cast can lead to atrophy of flexor tendons and associated muscle groups, especially in young foals.

Distal epiphyseal fractures can generally be managed in a cast to the proximal end of the metacarpus/metatarsus for 6-8 weeks. Support bandages are required for 3-4 weeks after cast removal. Internal fixation (lag screws, Rush pins) is occasionally indicated, especially if there is marked displacement of the epiphysis.

Lateral Condyles of the Metacarpus/Metatarsus

Fractures of the lateral condyles of the metacarpus/metatarsus occur in racing Thoroughbreds, Standardbreds and Quarter Horses.[16,40,41] The biomechanics of this fracture have been postulated.[41,42] The configuration of these fractures ranges from a small fissure entering the fetlock joint to complete displacement and separation of the fragment from the cannon bone (Fig 57). Clinical signs vary from acute lameness, with heat, pain and swelling in displaced fractures, to a mild lameness exacerbated by exercise in undisplaced fissure fractures.[40] The fractures predominantly involve the forelimbs, but the rear limbs are occasionally affected, especially in Standardbreds.[6]

At least 4 radiographic views (AP, LM, APLMO, PALMO) of the affected fetlock joint should be obtained for diagnosis. Care should be taken to evaluate the radiographs for concurrent problems. Lesions observed with condylar fractures include axial or apical fractures of the proximal sesamoid bones, osteochondral fractures of the proximal aspect of the first phalanx, periarticular osteophytes indicative of degenerative joint disease, and suspensory desmitis.[6,40] Associated injuries may have a significant bearing on the prognosis with respect to return to racing soundness.

Management of lateral condylar fractures depends on the degree of separation of the fragment and the intended use of the animal. Pressure bandages or a plaster cast, in combination with stall rest, may suffice if the animal is to be retired for breeding and there is minimum displacement of the fracture. Lag-screw fixation with one or more ASIF cortical bone screws is the treatment of choice if there is great displacement of the fragment and the horse is intended for further athletic performance.

The prime aim of rigid internal fixation of such fractures is to: re-establish congruity of the articular surface; minimize the gap that hyaline cartilage must bridge; minimize movement at the junction of the articular cartilage and bone, reducing proliferative change and subsequent joint stiffness; and ensure the original fissure does not enlarge and become displaced.[43] Such fractures should be repaired 24-48 hours after the injury.

The horse is positioned with the affected leg up and the leg is prepared for surgery. An Esmarch bandage and tourniquet are applied. Minimally displaced fractures can be repaired through stab incisions in the skin, whereas displaced fractures are best repaired through an incision over the lateral collateral ligaments of the fetlock joint.[15] The more extensive incision allows visualization of the proximal end of the fracture, which aids alignment at the joint surface. Because these fractures sometimes spiral craniad or caudad, a large incision also gives better visualization of the configuration of the fracture. Blood clots and debris are removed from the fracture site. Any displaced fragment must be manipulated into position; temporary fixation with Kirschner wires is sometimes necessary. All attempts must be made to ensure alignment of the joint surface. The proximal end of the fragment may be used as a guide to determine if the distal end is reduced. If more force is required to reposition the fragment, a 4.5-mm gliding hole is drilled. With the drill bit in place, the fragment is manipulated.

Some surgeons prefer to use the ASIF C-clamp applied to the distal metacarpal/metatarsal tubercles.[6] Its application requires a stab incision on the opposite side of the metacarpus/metatarsus. This clamp ensures that the screw is directed across the greatest diameter of the bone.

Intra-operative radiographs must be taken to ensure alignment of the joint surface. The fragment is then secured to the parent bone using the lag-screw principle (Fig 58).[11] The first screw placed is the one closest the fetlock joint. Once this screw is placed, the ASIF hexagonal-head screwdriver can be left in place and the remaining screws placed free-hand. The 4.5-mm gliding hole must extend beyond the fracture line. In undisplaced fractures, intraoperative radiographs may be required to determine this. With small condylar fractures it may be necessary to place a screw closer to the joint than the tubercles. This necessitates dissection of the collateral ligaments of the fetlock joint

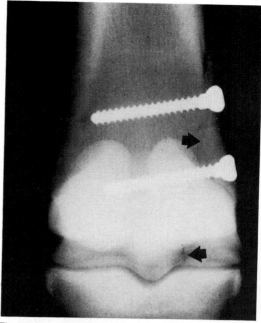

Fig 58. Fractured lateral distal condyle in a Thoroughbred race horse, repaired with 2 ASIF cortical bone screws. The screws were inserted using the lag-screw principle.

and insertion of the screw in the lateral condylar fossa. Countersinking the screw closest to the fetlock joint is usually not required, but countersinking the more proximal screw(s) is necessary because of the dense cortical bone.

The screws are alternately tightened to ensure proper seating of the fragment. Excessive tightening of the screws should be avoided. A washer may be used in the proximal screw if the fragment is thin. A small fragment may break off the proximal end, but this should not affect the prognosis. Radiographs should be taken to ensure proper placement of the screws.

A cast with walking bar is then applied to the limb to prevent possible refracture during recovery from anesthesia. The cast can be removed 1-2 weeks after surgery, depending on the case and on how the horse tolerates the cast. Nonsteroidal anti-inflammatory drugs should be used judiciously during the postoperative period.

Postoperative exercise should be minimal for the first 3 months. Stall rest is recommended during this time. After the first 3 months hand-walking can commence; eventually the horse can be turned out. Training should not recommence for 6-8 months and until follow-up radiographs have been taken.

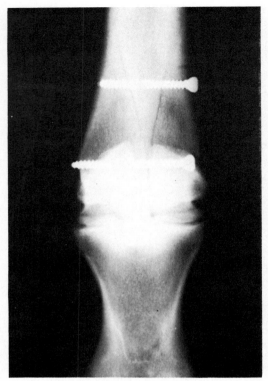

Fig 59. Spiral fracture of the third metatarsal bone in a Standardbred gelding. The fracture was repaired with 2 ASIF cortical bone screws, using the lag-screw principle. The fracture line in the cranial cortex courses mediad and the one in the caudal cortex courses laterad.

The prognosis for future athletic soundness is good following internal fixation of relatively fresh fractures without concurrent injuries and with good alignment of the articular surface.

The implants are generally not removed after healing unless lameness can be directly attributed to their presence. If the screws are to be removed, their location is confirmed with 18-ga disposable hypodermic needles as markers on radiographs. In a series of cases from California, there was no difference in performance between horses that had the screws removed and those that did not. Some horses appear to improve on removal of the implants, while others improve without removal.[40]

Spiral Fractures of Third Metacarpal/Metatarsal Bone

Spiral fractures of the third metatarsal bone are generally more prevalent in Standardbreds. The fracture consists of a fissure in the metatarsophalangeal articulation extending proximad.[41,43] Such fractures cause variable lameness, depending upon the amount of displacement at the articular surface. Forced flexion of the fetlock is usually resented and soft tissue swelling in the distal third of the cannon bone is sometimes evident.

Management of such fractures is similar to that for a lateral condylar fracture. The exact configuration of the fracture, determined by a thorough radiographic study of the entire bone, must be considered during repair. On the radiographs, one fracture line is in the cranial cortex and the other in the caudal cortex. The fracture in the cranial cortex usually courses mediad and that in the caudal cortex courses laterad, resembling some fissure fractures in the first phalanx.

Spiral fractures are best treated by rigid internal fixation with lag screws. One important advantage of using lag screws is that they prevent proximal extension of the fissure.

Rigid immobilization at the level of the articular surface is critical for the same reasons outlined under lateral condylar fractures. An Esmarch bandage and a tourniquet are applied after routine preparation of the limb. The screw closest to the joint is inserted with the aid of an ASIF C-clamp placed at the level of the distal tubercles of the cannon bones. Intraoperative radiographs are taken to ensure correct placement of the C-clamp. The screws are applied using the lag-screw principle. The screw closest to the joint is seated but not tightened. Leaving the screwdriver in the head of the screw, the remaining lag screws are positioned further proximad. These screws usually rotate around the long axis of the bone unless the fracture is perfectly sagittal (Fig 59). The depth of the gliding hole is difficult to estimate unless the fracture is sagittal. A certain amount of guesswork is involved in the placement of the screws up the bone. As many as 7 lag screws have been employed in one case treated by the author.[43]

Postoperative radiographs, including oblique views, are obtained to check for correct screw placement and length. The limb is placed in a cast to the proximal metacarpus/metatarsus to protect against further injury during recovery from anesthesia. The cast should include the hock joint if the fracture extends above the distal third of the metatarsus. Occasionally these fractures extend into the cranial cortex of the cannon bone; violent recovery from anesthesia could result in a more serious fracture if a cast ends in this area. The cast is removed in several days. Pressure bandages are required for

3-4 weeks and the horse is rested in a box stall for several months. Training should commence when the animal is free from lameness and radiographs demonstrate successful healing.

Screw removal is occasionally indicated following repair of such fractures, but should only be performed when there is radiographic evidence of fracture healing. The third metacarpus/metatarsus bones heal slowly; a convalescence of one year should be anticipated before full athletic activity is resumed. Some degree of soreness can be anticipated in cases treated by "lagging" the cranial cortex to the caudal cortex. This occurs because such fixation prevents normal flexion, limited as it may be. Some horses can tolerate the pain caused by fixation of the cranial cortex to the caudal cortex, but others require implant removal to perform successfully. Screw removal is done under general anesthesia; a cast that includes the hock joint should be applied for protection during recovery from anesthesia.

First Phalanx

Fractures of the first phalanx are relatively common in horses.[44-47] Fracture configuration ranges from small fissures into the metacarpophalangeal joint to severe comminution.[46] Comminuted fractures (eg, comminuted second phalangeal fractures) are generally more common in western performance horses (barrel-racing, cutting, etc) because of the stress from sudden turns and slides. Fissure fractures (so-called "split-pattern") are more common in Standardbreds, Thoroughbreds, hunters and jumpers. In these horses the fracture occurs as a result of twisting combined with axial compression.[42] Rarely are first phalangeal fractures compound.

The clinical signs of first phalangeal fractures are variable. Severe lameness and crepitation are evident in severely comminuted fractures. The lameness can be quite subtle in some fractures, especially longitudinal fissures commencing in the fetlock joint. Diagnostic nerve blocks or training in the face of such fissures can result in complete dehiscence of the fracture and a marked decline in the prognosis for future athletic soundness. Such small fissures may even propagate under normal weight-bearing.

The limb should be placed in a large, tightly fitting pressure bandage, with support on the opposite limb, for emergency transport to a facility for definitive treatment. Affected horses usually protect the limb because of extreme

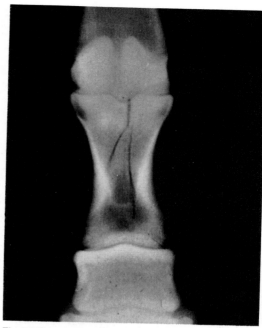

Fig 60. Fractured first phalanx, with duplication of the fracture line due to the different course taken by the fracture in the cranial and caudal cortices. Such a fracture is amenable to internal fixation with lag screws.

pain. Horses to be shipped long distances may require application of a plaster cast prior to transport.

At least 4 radiographic views (AP, LM, APLMO, PALMO) should be taken to confirm the diagnosis. In some fractures there is often duplication of the fracture line due to the different course taken in the cranial and caudal cortices. This may be mistaken for comminution or even sequestration (Fig 60).[46] For fissures close to the articular surface, the x-ray beam should be directed at an angle to minimize interference by the proximal sesamoid bones.

Longitudinal fractures of the first phalanx are candidates for internal fixation because failure to re-establish the congruity of the joint surfaces (metacarpophalangeal and proximal interphalangeal) result in degenerative joint disease. Some clinicians recommend treating small fissures, beginning at the proximal end of the first phalanx and extending no further than 1-2 cm, with a plaster cast.[45] However, the author believes fissures should be treated by internal fixation because microscopic examination reveals continuation of the fissures distad into the remainder of the bone. Periosteal proliferation on the proximal cranial aspect of the first phalanx, resembling "osselets," and demineralization along the fracture line occur in fissures treated conservatively. Such fractures warrant a guarded prognosis.[46]

Comminuted first phalangeal fractures are generally treated by application of a plaster cast encasing the entire foot and extending to the proximal metacarpus/metatarsus. Immobilization for a minimum of 8 weeks is required. Some comminuted fractures require internal fixation to prevent the third metacarpus/metatarsus bone from wedging the fragments apart.

Internal fixation of first phalangeal fractures consists of insertion of one or more ASIF cortical bone screws, using the lag-screw principle.[11] The horse is positioned with the smaller fragment up; the threaded portion of the screw hole is closer to the level of the fetlock joint, resulting in greatest holding power. The positioning of lag screws varies and should be carefully planned to reduce operation time. The screws can be inserted through stab incisions in the skin, although one large incision provides better exposure of the digital vessels and nerves if more than 2 screws are used.[15] Kirschner wires or 2.0-mm drill bits are sometimes useful to estimate the anticipated positions of the lag screws. The technic of lag-screw fixation of a sagittal fracture of the first phalanx is outlined in Figure 61.

Postoperative care after internal fixation consists of application of a cast encasing the entire foot and up to the proximal metacarpus/metatarsus to minimize chances of refracture during recovery from anesthesia. The cast can be removed as early as 10 days postoperatively from minimally displaced fractures, whereas more complicated, potentially unstable fractures require longer periods in a cast. Horses with uncomplicated, minimally displaced fractures benefit from early postoperative mobility of the joints in the affected limb after a short time in the cast. Following removal of the cast, the horse should be confined to a box stall for a length of time, depending on the progression of healing as determined by radiography.

Second Phalanx

Fractures of the second phalanx are relatively common, especially in the western performance horses (barrel-racing, pole-bending, cutting).[47-49] The fracture is relatively uncommon in horses performing other types of work. A rear leg is usually involved but occasionally the second phalanx in a forelimb is fractured. These fractures are usually severely comminuted but rarely compound. Affected horses usually become acutely lame while performing or occasionally become severely lame after strenuous exercise, such as on the way back to the stall. Some affected horses have a history of lameness in the leg prior to the onset of very severe lameness, indicating that some of these fractures may begin as fissures and eventually become comminuted. Horses with heel calks are more prone to such fractures because calks tend to anchor the foot to the ground and prevent slipping.[47-49]

Comminuted second phalangeal fractures are extremely painful on palpation of the area. Complete refusal to bear weight on the affected leg is common. Swelling in the pastern is usually present but may not be immediately obvious. In chronic cases the pastern is enlarged, resembling ringbone, due to callus formation from the original fracture.

Diagnosis of a comminuted second phalangeal fracture is usually confirmed by radiographic examination. Four views should be taken to ascertain the configuration of the fracture and to determine if the fracture extends into the proximal and/or distal interphalangeal joints. Radiographs unfortunately do not give one an appreciation of the enormous soft tissue injury (joint capsule tearing, etc) associated with these fractures.

Fig 61. Diagram of lag-screw fixation of a sagittal fracture of the first phalanx. (A) Location of the fracture (arrows). (B) Insertion of K wires or 2.0-mm drill bits to stabilize the fracture and ascertain correct location of drill holes for screw placement. (C) Insertion of the first lag screw. In some sagittal fractures of the first phalanx, it is necessary to insert the screw closest to the fetlock joint and occasionally the pastern joint first, rather than in the middle of the bone as shown. Here, the 4.5-mm glide hole is drilled to the fracture site. (D) Insertion of the drill sleeve. (E) Drilling the 3.2-mm hole in the opposite cortex. Constant cleaning of the drill bit is necessary to prevent small pieces of bone debris from being forced through the other side of the bone. (F) The hole should be countersunk or the screw head may bend, especially in the area of the first phalanx close to the fetlock joint. (G) The depth gauge is used to determine the correct screw length. Care must be taken not to hook soft tissues on the far cortex or a longer screw than necessary will be chosen. (H) The threads in the 3.2-mm hole in the far cortex are produced with a 4.5 tap. (I) The bone screw is inserted. The screwdriver can be left in place for a reference when drilling the next screw holes. Two more lag screws placed proximal and distal to the one shown would be optimum to stabilize such a fracture.

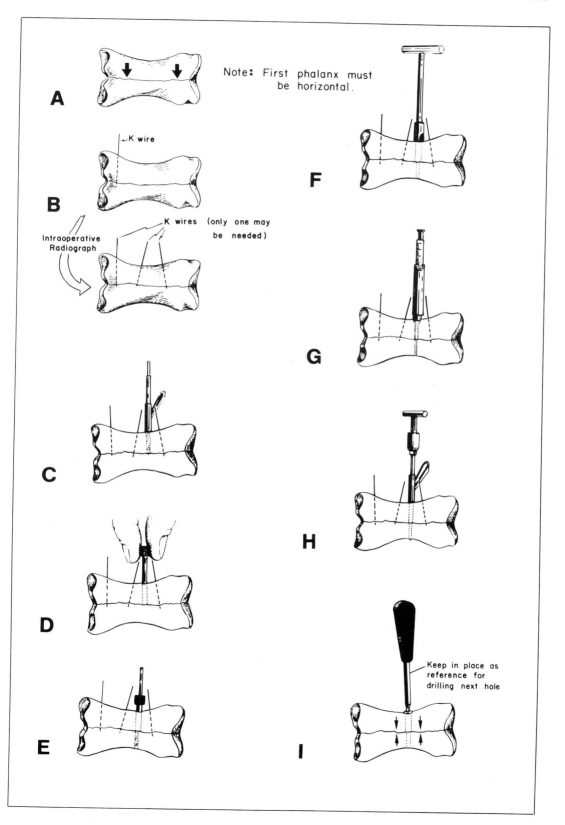

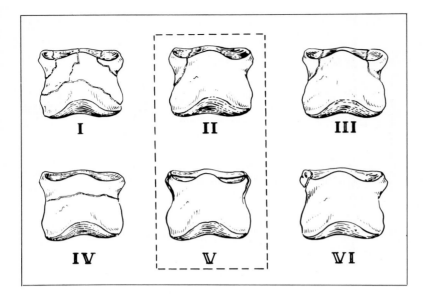

I II III

IV V VI

Fig 62. Common types of second phalangeal fractures. Those enclosed by the dotted line are amenable to internal fixation using lag screws.

The limb should be placed in a large, tightly fitting pressure bandage, with support on the opposite limb, for emergency transport of the animal. These patients are often in considerable pain and application of a walking cast in the standing position is quite difficult due to constant movement of the horse. A cast may be applied to the limb, using general anesthesia, if a long journey is anticipated.

Treatment of comminuted second phalangeal fractures depends on the configuration of the fracture (Fig 62). The prognosis for athletic soundness is quite poor if fractures extend into both proximal and distal interphalangeal joints due to subsequent degenerative joint disease in the distal joint. Animals to be saved for breeding purposes should have the fracture immobilized in a walking cast that encases the entire foot and extends to the proximal metacarpus/metatarsus. The cast is applied and changed with the horse under general anesthesia. The foot should be placed in a natural position. Baling wire, placed through holes drilled in the roof wall, aids in reduction of the fracture and correct positioning of the foot.[16]

The fracture is periodically radiographed to check progression of healing. The limb should remain in a plaster cast for 2-3 months, during which time the cast is changed 3-4 times. Such fractures take considerable time to heal and usually produce a large callus and marked periosteal new bone growth, which may interfere with tendon function. Ankylosis and sometimes arthrodesis of the proximal and distal in-

terphalangeal joints eventually occur during healing of the fracture.

If the fracture does not extend into the distal interphalangeal joint and a rear limb is involved, the prognosis is reasonably good for return to active use. Such fractures of the second phalanx can be treated in other ways. The limb may be placed in a walking cast encasing the entire foot for 8-12 weeks, with management similar to that for a comminuted fracture of the proximal and distal joints. During this time, ankylosis and arthrodesis of the pastern joint occur. This sequence of events takes many months and the period of convalescence can be quite protracted. A number of surgical procedures have been used to encourage ankylosis and arthrodesis of the pastern joint.[47,50]

The limb is prepared for aseptic surgery after application of an Esmarch bandage and a tourniquet. The articular cartilage of the distal first phalanx and proximal second phalanx is stripped using a 3/16-inch drill bit.[47] The drill is inserted between the collateral ligament and common digital extensor tendon between the first and second phalanges, and moved craniad, caudad and mediad as many times as required to destroy the joint. Care must be taken not to traumatize the medial digital artery, vein and nerve with the drill bit.

The pastern joint can be approached from the dorsal aspect of the joint to better expose the joint and to ensure more thorough removal of the articular cartilage.[15] The horse is positioned with the affected limb up, an Esmarch

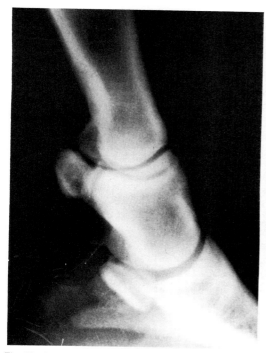

Fig 63. An old, comminuted second phalangeal fracture, with accompanying degenerative joint disease.

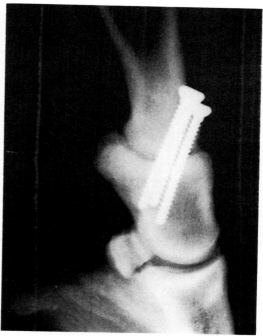

Fig 64. Fracture in Figure 63 after treatment by arthrodesis of the pastern joint, using lag screws and curettage of the joint surfaces.

bandage and tourniquet are applied, and the limb is prepared for aseptic surgery. An I-shaped incision is made over the cranial surface of the first and second phalanges. The proximal part of the incision extends across the middle of the first phalanx and the distal part of the incision is approximately 0.5 cm proximal to the coronary band. The incisions are connected by a sagittal incision on the cranial aspect of the proximal and middle phalanges. The skin is reflected, exposing the common digital extensor tendon and the 2 branches of the interosseous (suspensory) ligaments. A Z-plasty is performed on the common extensor tendon and, if necessary, the branches of the suspensory ligament.[15]

The extensor tendon is carefully dissected away from the joint capsule of the pastern joint and the pastern joint is identified by probing with sterile hypodermic needles. The joint capsule is transversely incised by sharp dissection. The collateral ligaments can be severed to allow exposure of the joint, although this is usually not necessary as there is already enough instability to the joint to permit good visualization. Following arthrotomy a suitable instrument, such as a heavy-duty periosteal elevator,

is used to pry the joint surfaces apart for optimal exposure of hyaline cartilage. A curette or Hall air drill is then used to denude as much cartilage from the bone ends as possible. Flexion of the joint by an assistant allows access to the caudal aspects of the bone. Following cartilage removal, the joint capsule and extensor tendon are reconstructed using #1 or #2 polyglycolic acid or polyglactin 910 sutures in a simple-interrupted pattern. The skin incision is closed and the limb placed in a walking cast that extends to the proximal metacarpus/metatarsus and encases the entire foot.

The period of convalescence can be shortened and greater stability achieved using lag screws.[50] This technic is limited to second phalangeal fractures not severely comminuted and involving only the caudal eminence fractured off. The approach is essentially similar to that already described. Following removal of the articular cartilage, 3-4 lag screws are placed across the pastern joint, engaging as much of the second phalanx as possible. With the avulsion fracture, care must be taken not to direct the screws into the fracture site (Figs 63,64).

In simple fractures in which only one of the caudal eminences has fractured off, a cortical

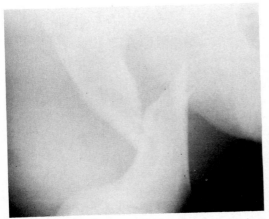

Fig 65. Oblique fracture of the femoral diaphysis in a 2-month-old foal.

bone screw is used to secure the fragment to the parent bone, using the lag-screw principle.[49] Care must be taken not to split the fragment while inserting the lag screw. In some fractures, the fragment is too small to permit screw fixation. In these cases, the surgeon must decide if the fracture is extensive enough to warrant arthrodesis.

In some cases of lag-screw fixation of avulsion fractures, the pastern joint ultimately undergoes ankylosis. This phenomenon occurs because joint capsule tearing and other soft tissue damage at the time of the original injury were not appreciated on the initial radiographic examination.

Longitudinal fractures of the second phalanx, similar to the "split pastern" of the first phalanx, are quite rare. The fracture usually occurs in the frontal plane rather than the sagittal plane. In some cases the fracture does not separate and the horse is presented for a relatively mild lameness similar to that seen with a hairline fracture of the first phalanx. There may be no crepitation or appreciable swelling in such cases. Such fractures are best treated by internal fixation of the fragments with bone screws. This minimizes chances of the fracture lines opening and reduces the likelihood of subsequent degenerative joint disease of the proximal and distal interphalangeal joints.

Because of the proximity of the second phalanx to the coronary band, the approach to the bone for insertion of the lag screws is difficult. A modified approach, similar to the one used for the dorsal approach to the pastern joint (previously described), can be used to insert screws into the dorsal aspect of the bone in fractures on a frontal plane.

Following lag-screw fixation of an avulsion or fissure fracture, the limb should be placed in a walking cast that encases the entire foot and extends to the proximal metacarpus/metatarsus to protect the repair during recovery from anesthesia. The cast may be left in place for a variable time thereafter, depending on the nature of the repair.

Femur

Fractures of the femur are relatively common in horses. Such fractures occur in young animals during halter-breaking or casting procedures. In adults, the fracture is usually comminuted, while in younger animals the fracture is usually simple. Oblique fractures are common in foals, and young animals often fracture the bone through the proximal or distal physes. Fractures of the femoral shaft often involve severe overriding of the fragments, which can present enormous problems at the time of surgery from the standpoint of reduction.

Fractures of the femoral shaft are usually evident on physical examination and are characterized by extreme reluctance to bear weight, crepitation and excessive mobility of the remainder of the limb with respect to the pelvis. The patella is sometimes fixed proximad, especially in fractures of the distal third of the shaft through the distal femoral epiphysis.

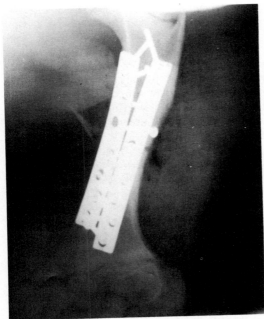

Fig 66. Fracture in Figure 65 immediately after repair with 2 broad ASIF dynamic-compression plates.

Foals with fractures of the proximal femoral epiphysis (slipping of the capital femoral epiphysis) usually bear some weight on the limb and are not as severely lame as with a femoral shaft fracture. Such cases involve swelling in the hip region and crepitation, sometimes referred to the stifle joint.[51]

A rectal examination should be performed, when possible, to detect concurrent fractures of the pelvis. Asymmetry of the pelvis and soft tissue swelling, indicating possible fracture hematoma, should be evaluated.

Although radiographs should be obtained to confirm the diagnosis this is sometimes impossible in adults due to limited capacity of most portable x-ray machines and the massive soft tissue swelling associated with such fractures. In such cases, the course of action must be based on a thorough physical examination. In adults, femoral shaft fractures are impossible to repair by internal fixation due to lack of suitable implants. Only under exceptional circumstances should an adult horse with a femoral shaft fracture be given the opportunity to recover spontaneously. Euthanasia is indicated in most cases. A similar approach should be adopted for yearlings. Some femoral fractures in growing horses may heal during confinement in a small stall.

If repair is anticipated (usually involves animals less than 100 kg), general anesthesia is required to establish the exact configuration of the fracture by radiographic examination. Surgery is undertaken immediately thereafter or the animal is allowed to recover from anesthesia and scheduled for surgery as soon as possible. For humane reasons, adult horses with a fractured femoral shaft should not be anesthetized to confirm the diagnosis and then be permitted to recover from anesthesia. The hip region should be radiographed using a frog-leg position and a 30-60° oblique view through the coxofemoral joint.

Treatment of femoral fractures depends on the age of the horse, the configuration of the fracture, and economics. Compression plating offers some chance of success in young foals if the fracture configuration permits.[32,38,52] Intramedullary pinning is generally unsuccessful because of lack of adequately sized pins to fit the medullary cavity, although stack-pinning and rush-pinning may be possible in some fractures. Pinning is generally difficult in oblique fractures because of overriding that can occur during convalescence. Rotation of fracture

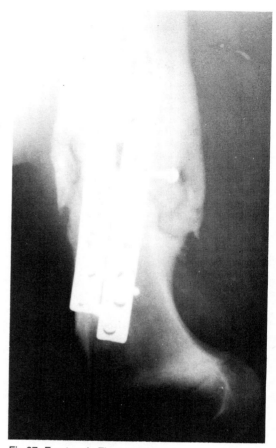

Fig 67. Fracture in Figure 65, showing extensive callus formation. The plates were eventually removed and the foal was completely sound.

fragments and loosening and migration of the implant can occur with the use of pins.

Use of a large intramedullary pin resulted in complete healing of a comminuted oblique fracture of the diaphysis of the femur.[53] If stability cannot be achieved with internal fixation, the animal is best treated by stall confinement.

Compression plating is the treatment of choice in foals if the fracture configuration permits. It is the only method that provides the extreme rigidity necessary and overcomes the severe overriding associated with these fractures. Double-plating is recommended where possible, even in small foals, to allow early return to function and to avoid fracture at the plate ends.

Femoral fractures, even in foals, can be very difficult to reduce. Traction on the distal limb is generally useless and the surgeon must rely on "toggling" and traction of the bone ends at

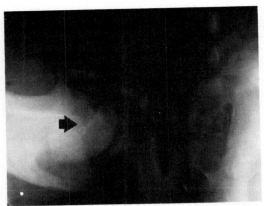

Fig 68. Fracture (arrow) through the capital femoral epiphysis in a 3-month-old foal.

the fracture site. Large forceps, such as Lane or Kern bone-holding forceps, are useful to reduce these fractures. The plates are applied according to standard ASIF technic.[11,12] Oblique fractures can be immobilized initially with one or more lag screws to hold the fracture in reduction while the first compression plate is applied. Once the first plate is in position, the original lag screws are removed and the second plate applied (Figs 65-67).[52] Bone grafting should be used if indicated. One of the few good points about plating the femur is the large soft tissue mass available to bury the implant. Suction drains are sometimes used if accumulation of blood and fluid is anticipated.

The foal should be kept in a small stall with the mare for at least 8 weeks postoperatively. After this time the surgeon may consider follow-up radiographs, obtained under general anesthesia. One must weigh the advantages of follow-up radiographs against the disadvantages of a possible violent recovery from anesthesia and refracture of the bone.

Fractures through the distal femoral physis are difficult to immobilize with internal fixation due to the small size of the distal fragment. Fractures of the Salter type-II configuration may have a large enough metaphyseal fragment to anchor to the parent fragment.

Fractures through the proximal femoral physis are common in foals (Fig 68).[51] These fractures are usually caused by severe trauma, such as rearing over backwards or getting caught under a fence. Once diagnosed, the fracture is repaired by direct pinning or open reduction and trochanteric osteotomy.

Repair of undisplaced fractures of the femoral head, with Knowles pins and radiographic control, has been described.[51] Closed pinning involves an approach between the greater trochanter and third trochanter. Displaced fractures require open reduction to reposition the displaced femoral head in its normal anatomic location. Recovery from surgery is rapid and foals bear weight on the affected limb soon after surgery.

The prognosis for untreated femoral head fractures is extremely poor due to aseptic necrosis of the femoral head, degenerative osteoarthritis and breakdown of the opposite limb. Surgery offers a reasonable alternative to what once was a crippling injury. Femoral head resection, similar to the method used in dogs, enables calves to ambulate until they are slaughtered; however, this is not a feasible alternative for horses and the author cannot recommend it.[16] The prognosis for athletic soundness following surgical repair of a slipped capital femoral epiphysis is guarded.

Tibia

Fractures of the tibia occur with approximately the same frequency as fractures of the radius. The causes of these fractures vary, although kicks are a common cause. Similar to radial fractures, tibial fractures are accompanied by massive edema, soft tissue swelling and complete failure to bear weight on the affected limb. Tibial fractures are usually oblique or spiral and may be comminuted to a varying degree. Tibial fractures are commonly compound due to lack of soft tissue on the medial side of the bone. Sharp fragments due to the oblique nature of the fracture also contribute to the high percentage of open fractures.

Fractures through the proximal and distal growth plates usually occur in foals 1-6 months of age.[54] The proximal growth plate is more commonly fractured than the distal plate. Fractures through the proximal physis usually produce lateral deviation of the limb distal to the stifle joint and are usually type-II Salter-Harris fractures.[31,54] Avulsion of the tibial crest is rare. Care must be taken in diagnosing this radiographically because the physis normally present in this area may mimic an avulsion. The opposite limb should be radiographed for comparison.

Fractures of the tibia, especially of the upper two-thirds can be extremely difficult to immobilize for transport of the animal for further treatment. It is impossible to apply a cast above the stifle joint except in young foals that have not developed the musculature above that joint. Fractures of the distal third of the bone, including those through the distal tibial physis, can be stabilized to some degree in a cast from the ground proximad, including as much of the stifle joint as possible. The cast may be combined with a Thomas splint to safely transport foals. Fractures in the upper half of the bone are virtually impossible to immobilize for transport, especially in adult horses. In fact, a cast may exacerbate the problem by acting like a pendulum.

Diagnosis of a fracture of the tibial shaft is usually by thorough examination of the limb. Radiographs are eventually necessary, if the animal is considered a candidate for internal fixation, to determine the exact configuration of the fracture.

Treatment of a fractured tibia is dictated by the age of the animal, the configuration of the fracture, and economics. Adult horses with a severely comminuted fracture should be euthanized for humane reasons, except under exceptional circumstances.

Young animals with fractures of the distal third of the bone, including fractures through the distal growth plate, can be treated with a full-limb cast extending proximal to the stifle if possible (Fig 69). In these cases the cast should extend as high up the limb as possible. Because fractures of the distal third of the bone in adults are frustrating to treat, many of these animals are eventually euthanized.

Fractures through the proximal growth plate can be treated in a variety of ways. The fracture may heal during confinement in a small stall in cases where there is minimal displacement and the animal is quite young. Fractures in which there is severe displacement can be reduced and stabilized using transversely placed Steinmann pins on each side of the fracture. A Charnley apparatus or turnbuckles placed between the pins on either side can provide mechanical advantage to manipulate and stabilize the fracture.[54] Internal fixation of tibial fractures by compression plating offers a reasonable chance of success, especially in foals.[37,38] The implants available for use in horses are designed for humans and cannot withstand the immense force applied to them by horses over about 100 kg. Repairs of the tibia cannot be suitably supported with external coaptation, except possibly in young foals. Some animals are amenable to support in a sling. Foals that have had the fracture stabilized with compression plates may not need any more external coaptation than pressure bandages.

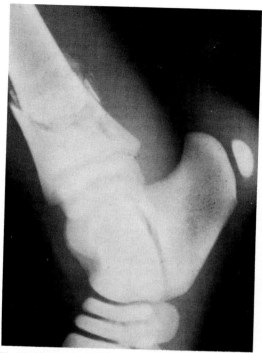

Fig 69. Fractured distal tibia in a 2-week-old American Saddlebred. Because the foal had not developed musculature above the stifle joint, the fracture was immobilized in a cast that included as much of the stifle as possible. The filly was sound a year later.

At least 2 plates and possibly 3 plates should be used to repair tibial fractures, even in foals. The overriding that can occur with fracture through the tibial shaft can present immense problems at surgery. Merely applying traction to the hoof as is done with a fracture of the radius may actually cause distraction at the fracture site due to the reciprocal apparatus of the rear limb. Other factors, such as the oblique configuration of the fracture and the eburnation due to constant movement at the fracture site prior to immobilization, also make these fractures very difficult to reduce. The plates should be applied using recommended ASIF technics and a medial or later approach.[11,12,15] Like the lateral approach to the radius, the lateral approach to the tibia provides a good soft tissue covering for implants and is recommended. Bone grafting should be used where indicated.

The prognosis for a fractured tibia in adults is very poor. In foals the prognosis depends upon the amount of stability achieved by compression plating.

Fibular Tarsal Bone

Fractures of the fibular tarsal bone (tuber calcis) are uncommon in horses and are usually caused by a kick from another horse. The fracture is commonly open and there is usually considerable displacement of fragments due to the pull of the gastrocnemius tendon.[16,55] For this reason, these fractures are difficult to manage with external immobilization alone.

It is quite difficult to appreciably immobilize the stifle joint and thereby eliminate any pull of the gastrocnemius tendon. If the fracture is not severely comminuted and the configuration of the fracture permits, tension-band plating is the best method of treating such fractures.[55] A tension-band plate is a plate placed on the caudal aspect of the bone to neutralize the distracting forces of the gastrocnemius tendon. The equine fibular tarsal bone is under too much tension to withstand repair with wire as in small animals. For this reason, use of a plate is recommended.[55]

It may not be possible to place the plate on exactly the caudal border of the bone because of interference with the function of the superficial flexor tendon. In such cases the caudolateral or even lateral aspect of the bone must be plated.[15]

Although the stifle joint is not completely immobilized, a cast from the proximal tibial region distad to and enclosing the hoof may help prevent undue stress on the repaired bone during recovery from anesthesia.[55] The cast may be used throughout the entire healing period, although some animals may only need a cast during the immediate postoperative period.

Compound fractures of the fibular tarsal bone should be managed accordingly. Sequestrectomy and saucerization may be indicated at various stages of repair. The prognosis is worse if the fracture is open. Bone grafting is indicated if the fracture is comminuted and defects remain following stabilization.

Bone Grafting
by A.S. Turner

Bone grafting, particularly autologous cancellous-bone grafting, is an increasingly popular adjunct to the treatment of certain orthopedic problems. Autologous cancellous-bone grafting has been used for the enhancement of arthrodeses, and repair of delayed unions, nonunions and pseudoarthroses.[56,57] Cancellous bone had a certain innate resistance to infection and is used in humans to treat osteomyelitis.[58] The

technic has potential in the treatment of selected cases of osteomyelitis caused by "navel ill" in foals. Cancellous bone is used to fill the cortical defects and dead space in conjunction with internal fixation of comminuted long-bone fractures. The author uses cancellous bone in any fracture of the third metacarpus/metatarsal bone, in adult horses, that requires a plate for stabilization. These bones heal very slowly and bone grafting considerably enhances healing. Autologous bone has also been used to fill bone cysts. The use of cancellous bone has been advocated in transverse sesamoid fractures as an alternative to lag-screw fixation.[59]

Full-thickness cortical grafts (allografts) are indicated in reconstruction of severely comminuted fractures, particularly of the third metacarpus/metatarsal bones.[60] Unfortunately, comminuted fractures of the third metacarpus/metatarsal bone are usually open.[38] Because dense cortical bone has poor resistance to infection, the application of this technic is limited to closed fractures.

The fate of autogenous cancellous bone following transplantation has been the subject of many studies.[61] It is generally believed that few cells survive the transplantation procedure, although both donor and recipient cells contribute to the new cell population. Most important, the graft stimulates the formation of new bone (osteoinduction). In addition, the graft provides a scaffold for ingrowth of blood vessels and multipotential mesenchymal cells (osteoconduction).[56,61] Capillaries invade the graft fragments after implantation of cancellous bone. Small pieces of cancellous bone are more readily revascularized than are large dense pieces of cortical bone. Host marrow also begins to invade the graft. Cells begin to differentiate into osteoblasts and osteoclasts, and a process of resorption and apposition around the edges of dead trabecular bone begins ("creeping substitution"). Eventually the graft is replaced with new bone and the entrapped cores of necrotic bone are gradually resorbed by osteoclasts. The new cancellous bone becomes lamellar bone and eventually compact bone complete with Haversian systems.

The initial vascularization of homogeneous cancellous bone (allograft) involves a latent period. These grafts do not stimulate as much bone formation as do autogenous grafts. Cancellous allografts require the immediate availability of a suitable donor or some system of storage (bone bank). Autogenous cancellous bone revascularizes more quickly, has earlier and greater production of new bone, and is immunologically more desirable than heterogenous grafts.[61] Full-thickness frozen cortical allografts serve as a trellis for osteoconduction and are ultimately replaced by the host. The graft is invaded by blood vessels, followed by sequential removal of graft bone matrix and gradual replacement with new bone formation. The time taken for revascularization is generally much longer than that required for cancellous transplants. Callus formation and internal repair of the transplant must occur for a successful graft.[61,62]

Harvested cancellous bone is packed into the defect and covered with as much soft tissue or periosteum as possible. Paramount to survival of any bone graft is absolute stability. When used in fracture repair, bone grafting is generally accompanied by some form of internal fixation and/or external coaptation.

The sites most commonly used for harvesting autogenous cancellous bone are the ilium, proximal tibia and rib. The site chosen depends on the actual volume of bone required. The site with the greatest potential yield is the ilium.[56,57]

The harvesting of cancellous bone is generally performed while surgery in another part of the body is being performed, such as internal fixation of a long-bone fracture. The surgery is expedited by the use of 2 surgical teams; prolonged surgery time causes unnecessary exposure of the graft, thereby decreasing graft-cell survival.[57]

The hair over a large area of the tuber coxae should be clipped prior to the induction of anesthesia. Following positioning for the primary surgery, the uppermost tuber coxae is prepared for aseptic surgery in a routine manner. Different technics are used for the initial skin incision. One method is to make a slightly curving incision parallel to the long axis of the tuber coxae with the apex pointing cranioventrad.[56] The incision is about 15 cm long in adults. Another method is to make a straight incision from a caudodorsal position to a cranioventral position across the center of the tuber coxae.[57] The incision is about 25 cm long in adults. The technic preferred by the author is a slightly curved to semielliptical incision about 20 cm long, caudal to the tuber coxae, with the apex directed caudodorsad.[15] The last method minimizes the length of incision directly over the tuber coxae; when the animal is lying in lateral recumbency, most of the incision is not trau-

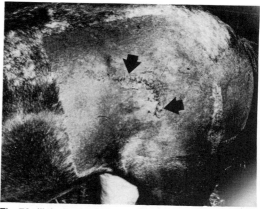

Fig 70. Ilial site for harvesting cancellous bone. The ilium is approached by a slightly curving to semielliptical incision, with the apex directed caudodorsad.

matized. The incision is positioned so that a rectangular piece of bone can be removed from the gluteal face of the ilium (Fig 70).

Following reflection of the incised skin, a straight incision is made in the subcutaneous fascia and superficial gluteal fascia. The incision is continued deep through the gluteus medius muscle, deep gluteal fascia and periosteum on the gluteal face of the ilium. The gluteus medius muscle is subperiosteally elevated, revealing the gluteal face of the ilium. Care must be taken to avoid the iliolumbar vessels, which are close to the ventral border of the wing of the ilium. A window, approximately 4 cm square, is made in the gluteal surface of the ilium or in the end of the ilium itself using a chisel or osteotome. The cancellous bone is then removed in small pieces with a curette. Approximately 50 ml of cancellous bone can be removed from this defect but more can be obtained by scooping out the gluteal and pelvic surfaces. The bone is transferred to a blood-soaked sponge (not into physiologic sterile saline). Once the graft is transferred to the recipient site, further flushing and irrigation should be avoided.[56]

The superficial gluteal fascia and subcutaneous fascia are closed together using a simple-interrupted pattern of 0 or #1 polyglycolic acid or polyglactin 910 sutures. Simple-interrupted sutures of a synthetic nonabsorbable material are used in the skin. In addition, large vertical mattress sutures are placed every 2-3 cm to reduce tension on the incision. Some surgeons advocate the use of stent bandages to help prevent postoperative wound dehiscence. The use of Penrose drains placed subperiosteally has been advocated following the harvesting of cancellous bone.[56] The author does not recommend use of such drains as they may allow infection to ascend into the surgical site. Closed suction drains should be used if removal of excess blood or serum is required.

Other sites of autologous cancellous bone are the proximal tibia and the rib. Harvesting bone from the proximal tibia by the author has on 2 occasions resulted in pathologic fracture through the bone graft site; therefore, this site must be approached with extreme caution. The volume of cancellous bone harvested from the proximal tibia is considerably less than that from the ilium. If only small amounts of bone are required to fill a small bone cyst or the gap between the 2 fragments of a sesamoid fracture, the rib is a suitable site to obtain cancellous bone. However, postoperative pain may be severe if this site is used.

Management of Compound Fractures by A.S. Turner

An open or compound fracture is characterized by communication between the fracture site and the atmosphere. Open fractures are immediately susceptible to infection. The fracture can be compounded by penetration of the skin by a sharp bone fragment or foreign body. Many long-bone fractures are open because the large amounts of energy required to fracture the bone (particularly in adults) invariably cause a break in the surrounding skin. Also, horses have minimal amounts of protective soft tissue covering their lower limbs. Some fractures, as of the tibia, may initially be closed but become open due to penetration of the skin by a bone fragment. Microorganisms enter the wound and settle into the fracture hematoma and devitalized tissue. Such an environment is an ideal medium for bacterial growth. Initially the wound is contaminated but becomes infected if left untreated. The duration of the contamination phase is 6 hours, after which the wound is considered infected.[63] The wound can be surgically converted into a clean wound during this period.

During the initial examination, the veterinarian must be sure there are no other injuries that are more life-threatening than the open fracture. Orthopedic surgeons are renowned for looking at the fracture and not examining the whole animal. The wound should immediately be covered with a sterile dressing to prevent further contamination. If hemorrhage is excessive, further sterile dressings may have to be applied under pressure. Tourniquets should not be used. Analgesics should be used judiciously to relieve pain and prevent excessive movement of the fracture ends and associated tissue damage. Use of hypotensive agents, such as phenothiazine tranquilizers, should be avoided. Suitable antibiotics should be administered. If the horse is relatively tranquil and the equipment is available, a radiograph should be obtained to determine if the fracture is repairable or if the animal should be euthanized.

If the fracture is repairable, the necessary steps should be taken to immobilize the limb. If the fracture is proximal to the distal third of the tibia and radius, any form of temporary immobilization is difficult to apply and may be contraindicated.

A temporary splint, such as a Robert-Jones bandage, should be placed on the limb, the animal anesthetized, the bandage removed and a cast encasing the entire foot applied to immobilize the limb prior to transport of the animal for further treatment. Stabilization of the fracture also contributes greatly to the relief of pain associated with the injury.

If the fracture is to be repaired, the horse should be anesthetized with the temporary cast in place. The cast should then be removed and attempts made to surgically debride the wound. The leg should be clipped and prepared for aseptic surgery in a routine manner. Several assistants are required to stabilize the leg during this procedure to prevent excessive movement at the fracture site and minimize further tissue damage. Every effort should be made to prevent hair and dander from entering the wound. Following preparation of the limb, the surgical team dons gloves, caps and masks, and commences exploration and debridement of the wound. Enlargement of the wound is sometimes necessary to permit thorough inspection. Skin debridement should be conservative but obviously devitalized areas should be trimmed. Through the entire procedure an assistant should irrigate the wound with copious amounts of warm Ringer's solution. An IV set attached to a large syringe and 3-way stopcock provides pressurized irrigation. Antibiotics can be added to the solution. Such antibiotics should be able to kill bacteria on very brief contact and should be compatible with the body tissues and the Ringer's solution.[64]

Excision of devitalized tissue, such as long tags of fascia and crushed muscle, is essential after flushing. Such tissue cannot be removed by phagocutosis and is an ideal medium for bacterial proliferation. Small, detached pieces of bone should be flushed out or removed with forceps.[63] Fragments with periosteum and soft tissue still attached should not be removed. Large fragments should be fitted back into place because they greatly contribute to the stability of the repair. These fragments, if rigidly held in position, act as an autogenous bone graft and are incorporated into the callus by "creeping substitution." Gaps created by removal of fragments do not fill with callus, especially in adults. The tuber coxae should be simultaneously prepared for aseptic surgery in case autogenous cancellous bone is required for bone grafting of such defects.

After thorough debridement, the drapes are removed and the surgical team rescrubs in preparation for fixation of the fracture as a sterile one. The method of fixation of the fracture is the one that provides the most stability. In horses it is limited to compression plating. It was once thought that metal implants act as a foreign body around which bacteria concentrate. However, recent studies have shown that bone heals in the face of infection if absolute rigidity is provided and that stabilization with implants outweighs the foreign-body effect.[65,66]

If plating is performed, the bone should be approached from as far away from the skin defect as possible. The plates are generally easy to apply because much of the soft tissue has been stripped away by the original trauma. It cannot be overemphasized that absolute stability of the fracture site is of utmost importance for successful treatment of an open fracture. Autogenous cancellous bone grafting is almost mandatory in open fractures, especially if cortical defects exist.

Relatively clean skin wounds less than 1 cm long can be sutured. However, in fractures involving considerable tissue loss and trauma to surrounding soft tissues, the wound should be left open and allowed to granulate.[67] Similarly, wounds closed under excessive tension may result in a slough greater than if the wound was left to heal by second intention. Soft tissue closure over plates on the third metacarpus/metatarsal bone can present enormous problems, particularly in open fractures. Delayed primary closure, with skin grafting or other plastic procedures, is performed regularly in open fractures in humans. This level of sophistication has not been reached in equine surgery.

After the fracture is plated, the limb should be supported in a cast, if possible, to provide additional stability. The cast should be changed within 10 days. After this it should be changed according to the amount of discharge from the fracture site. Windows should not be cut in the cast to visualize the wound. Antibiotics should be administered.

Several serious complications may occur after internal fixation of open fractures. Cellulitis is unusual but is usually controlled with antibiotics. Worst of all is contamination that progresses to osteomyelitis at the fracture site. Radiographs should be obtained when the cast is changed to ascertain the presence of osteomyelitis. The implants eventually loosen if the infection is severe. This appears radiographically as lucent areas at the fracture site, under the plate(s) and around the screws. The horse is usually increasingly reluctant to bear weight on the affected limb. At this point the surgeon must decide if the animal should be euthanized or another osteosynthesis performed in an attempt to achieve greater stability. If the latter is chosen, an autologous cancellous bone graft is mandatory.

Formation of a chronic, draining tract is the next most common sequela of internal fixation of an open fracture. If the implants are not loose, they should be left in place; early removal can result in an infected pseudoarthrosis. It is essential that implants be left in place until radiographic and clinical evidence indicates the fracture has healed. Implants that no longer offer stability should be removed and the fracture restabilized. Draining tracts usually disappear when the implants are removed. Irrigation, sequestrectomy and sinus tract debridement may be required as well.

Owners should be warned prior to surgery that a good cosmetic result is the exception, rather than the rule, due to excessive scar tissue formed during healing of open fractures. This is especially important in show animals.

Osteomyelitis and Nonunions
by A.S. Turner

Infection of a fracture site is usually a result of an open fracture or contamination during open reduction of a fracture despite the use of aseptic technic and antibiotics. Infection is more likely to occur if closed fractures are treated with internal fixation; however, in most cases there is no better alternative method of fracture repair.

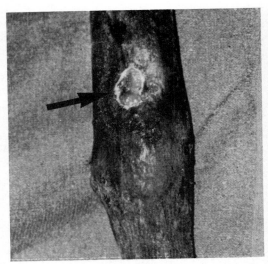

Fig 71. Chronic, draining fistula (arrow) 2 months after repair of a compound fracture of the metatarsus in a 4-week-old Arabian. The bone had healed and the infection was eliminated when the implants were removed.

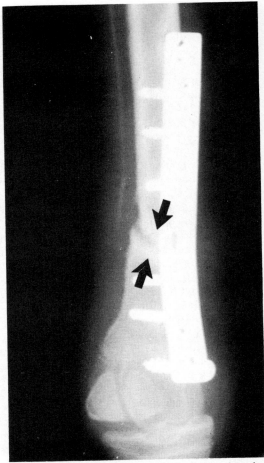

Fig 72. Nonunion associated with internal fixation of a distal metatarsal fracture in a foal. Note the sclerosis in the marrow cavities at the fracture site (arrows). This case was treated by removal of the implant, insertion of a cancellous bone graft and stabilization of the fracture with 2 narrow ASIF dynamic-compression plates.

The clinical signs of bone infection and nonunion of a fracture depend on the duration of infection. In bones stabilized internally, there is an immediate reduction in weight-bearing. If a cast has been applied, the animal becomes less mobile. The limb is hot and painful, and there is usually accompanying fever and leukocytosis. Wound healing at the fracture site is retarded and the skin in the area is thin and generally unhealthy. A draining sinus tract may be apparent (Fig 71).

Radiographs usually reveal osteomyelitis, nonunion or both. Osteomyelitis is characterized by areas of lysis and demineralization, particularly in the area of the fracture. There may also be lysis around the implants; lysis from osteomyelitis must be differentiated from lysis due to plate movement. Variable amounts of periosteal proliferation may be associated with the infection. This may not be evident in adults but is usually present in young animals.

Nonunions are characterized by a complete lack of bone healing at the fracture site or the characteristic "elephant's foot" callus at the ends of the fracture, with sclerosis of the marrow cavity at the fracture site. Nonunions with complete lack of healing at the fracture site are caused by considerable periosteal stripping from large cortical defects associated with comminution. Nonunions with typical elephant's foot callus are rare in horses but are caused by movement at the fracture site (Fig 72).

Osteomyelitis generally does not respond to antibiotic therapy alone and usually requires surgical treatment. A poor response to antibiotic therapy is attributed to avascularity at the fracture site. Nonunions, infected or not, require surgical treatment as well.

Samples for culture should be taken from deep within any sinus tracts. Gram-staining helps determine what type of antibiotic to use while awaiting results of sensitivity tests. The results of sinus tract culture in humans do not always reflect the cause of the osteomyelitis unless the organism is *Staphylococcus aureus*.[68] Antibiotics are useful when there are signs of infection and cellulitis in the affected limb.

The surgical treatment of osteomyelitis and nonunions involves the removal of all necrotic

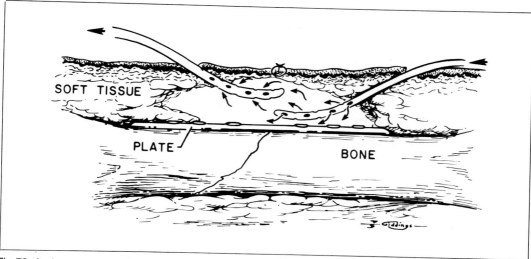

Fig 73. An ingress-egress flushing system. The ingress tubing should be deep in the wound and the egress tubing more superficial.

bone and infected tissue. Loose fragments of bone should be removed unless they contribute to stability of the fracture site. Internal fixation devices still providing rigid internal fixation should be left in place.[11,68-70] Stability must be achieved if the fracture is unstable. Motion at the fracture site promotes the spread and persistence of infection. Because absolute stability cannot be achieved in a plaster cast, some fractures require further internal fixation. However, such action may not be feasible from an economic or humane standpoint. Bone heals under optimum biomechanical circumstances in the face of infection. Application or reapplication of plates is best performed in areas with minimal soft tissue trauma.

Bone grafting should be considered to treat defects created by sequestrectomy. The graft must be placed in a viable bed, such as healthy, bleeding bone or granulation tissue. Ideally the recipient bed should be free of infection, which is mandatory for incorporation of the graft.[71]

Use of negative-pressure drains, such as the Hemovac system (Zimmer), may be indicated in some cases. However these should not be substituted for good hemostasis at surgery. Such drains consist of a multiperforated polyethylene tube placed deep into the cavity. The nonperforated end is brought out through normal tissue as far away from the wound edge as possible and suction applied intermittently with a 3-way stopcock and syringe. These drains usually clot within 12 hours and should be removed when they are nonfunctional or the

amount of fluid retrieved becomes insignificant. An ingress-egress system may be used to maintain continuous suction for longer periods. Such a system involves placement of a perforated ingress drain deep in a surgical wound and a similar egress drain superficially. A solution, such as Ringer's, is infused into the wound through the ingress tube and is evacuated through the egress drain (Fig 73). Bactericidal antibiotics can be used in the ingress solution; however, these systems are effective generally by mechanical cleansing.[71] All blood clots, bone dust and other debris should be flushed from the wound bed prior to insertion of the drains. Tissue fragments, rather than blood clots are probably responsible for drain blockage.

Treatment of postsurgical osteomyelitis and nonunion is usually prolonged.[72] The course is usually expensive for the client and requires good nursing care, husbandry and nutrition. Cases are best handled by well-equipped practices and institutions with a good nursing staff.

Removal of Bone Plates
by A.S. Turner

Occasionally it is necessary to remove the bone plate after fracture repair. Loose or broken implants should be removed if they do not contribute to fracture stability. The most common indication for bone plate removal is persistent soft tissue infection and a draining fistula after repair of a compound fracture.

Such infections usually resolve after removal of the bone plate(s). Localized osteomyelitis may result even though bony union is present. Plate removal is indicated in these cases if the osteomyelitis is to be resolved. Corrosion is rarely a problem with the high-quality stainless steel used for implants. A slight grey discoloration of tissues around the plates often occurs but does not resemble the inflamed appearance around corroding metal. Occasionally lameness disappears when the implant is removed; the cause of this phenomenon in most cases is unknown.

Unless the plates are broken or loose and not contributing to stability, they should be removed only after there is clinical and radiographic evidence of union. Lameness may be the only sign of nonunion. Union is usually evidenced radiographically by disappearance of the fracture gap, although the gap may still be present with no evidence of lameness.

Many equine long-bone fractures are double-plated. Some surgeons first remove one plate and then remove the second months later. During the period between removal of plates, the bone under the plates remodels and strengthens itself. Separate removal of 2 bone plates obviously requires 2 major pieces of surgery. Some cases do not warrant such additional ex-pense and the surgeon may elect to leave the plates *in situ*.

To remove a bone plate, an incision is made directly over the plate. This is usually the easiest in cannon bone fractures. Some cases require an incision over the original incision used to apply the bone plate, in which case wound healing is usually rapid due to the secondary wound healing phenomenon. Interfragmentary screws can also be removed if accessible through the same incision. Removal is usually essential to resolve any localized infection around a screw or plate. Curettage, sequestrectomy and excision of fistulous tracts are necessary in some cases. Placement of drains is advisable following plate removal because large amounts of serum accumulate at the site, especially if soft tissue infection is present around the implants. Pressure-bandaging is generally essential following plate removal, although this is not always possible in areas such as the humerus and femur. Antibiotics are generally not necessary when plates are being removed if good aseptic technic is practiced. Even in cases of considerable soft tissue infection, removal of the implants is the most significant factor contributing to healing of the infection.

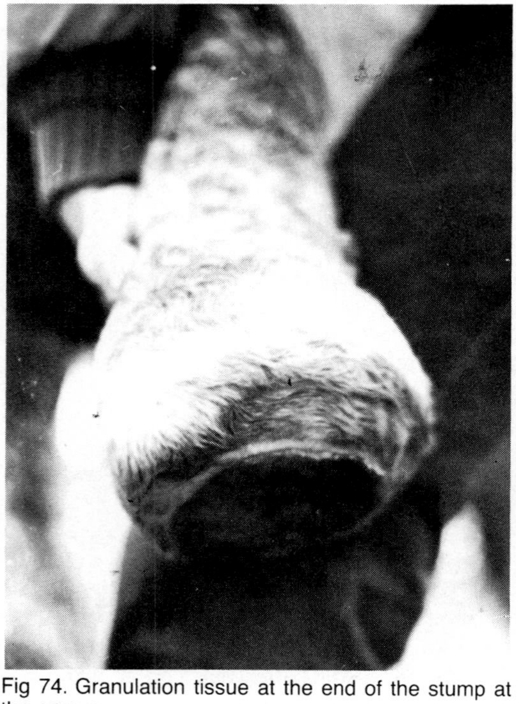

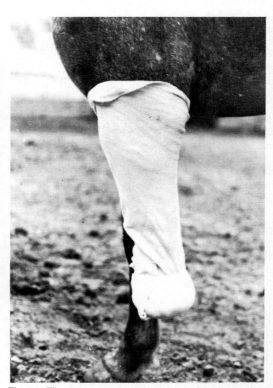

Fig 74. Granulation tissue at the end of the stump at the carpus.

Fig 75. The leg is covered with a stockinet prior to attachment of the prosthesis.

LIMB AMPUTATION AND PROSTHETIC DEVICES
by L.M. Koger

Amputation is occasionally a last resort for complicated fractures or serious degenerative conditions below the carpus or hock. Animals most likely to adapt successfully to partial amputation of a limb are comparatively light, with strong underpinning and enough agility to rise and rest on 3 legs. However, even more important than physical characteristics is the necessity for intelligence and a quiet, gentle, cooperative temperament. Without such a disposition, the best prosthetic attempts will end in frustration and failure. Also, the value of the animal must justify an extended investment of time and money. Therefore, the temperament and character of the owner and handler are likewise critical.

Of 5 successfully treated animals, 4 were mares and the other a gelding. It is doubtful that stallions could be considered good risks for application of a prosthesis; however, an attempt should probably be made under certain conditions.

Amputation Technics
The details of amputation are determined by the nature and location of the fracture and soft tissue injury. Adequate flaps of viable skin are important to obtain a functional stump. The flexor and extensor tendons should be trimmed and sutured over the distal portion of the osseous stump at the joint (carpus or tarsus) to enhance its shape, to improve its capacity to retain the prosthesis, and to protect the weight-bearing osseous stump. Control of hemorrhage, obliteration of dead space, and proper suturing technic are important.

Postamputation Management
The most critical time of the whole procedure is the moment of recovery from anesthesia when the patient expects balance from the affected quarter. Because the horse may panic violently without support on all 4 legs, a temporary prosthesis should be incorporated into a plaster cast constructed to avoid pressure necrosis on the stump.

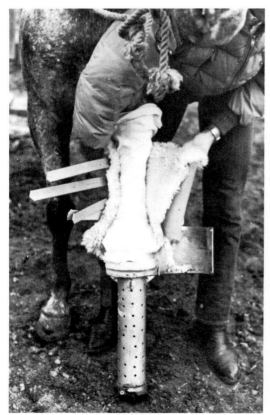

Fig 76. The prosthesis is applied.

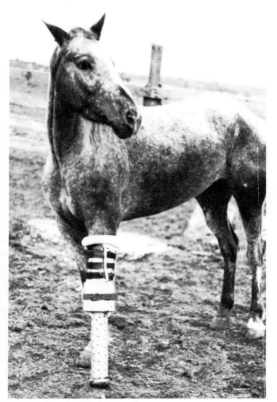

Fig 77. Prosthesis in place on a mare.

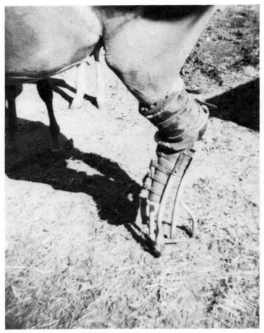

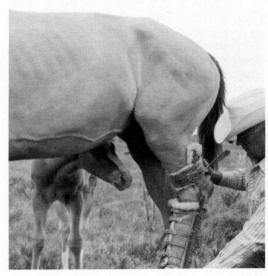

Fig 79. Rear-leg prostheses must provide support above and below the hock. Note the hinge to adapt to movement of the tarsus.

Fig 78. A heel loop on this rear-leg prosthesis provides traction and prevents slipping.

First intention healing has not occurred in our experience, but healing is satisfactory if weight-bearing on the end of the stump is minimized or prevented. The skin of the stump must remain healthy after healing of the surgical wound. Distilled extract of witch hazel, an astringent, is an effective antipruritic and cleansing agent that can be applied as indicated. Powdered calcium hydroxide or slaked lime, an absorbent, desiccating antiseptic material, is a convenient and inexpensive dressing to maintain tough, odor-free skin surfaces. Use of dressing powders with astringent antiseptic properties may also be indicated.

Complications and Hazards

Moist dermatitis and pressure necrosis from the prosthesis are a constant threat and their prevention requires conscientious care. The animal must be kept in quarters in which there is little chance of the prosthesis becoming snagged on an object. Barbed wire, machinery and protruding, sharp points or edges pose greater hazards to amputees than to normal animals.

Fracture of the pelvis caused by falling is a particular hazard; 2 of the 5 amputees previously mentioned were euthanized because of

multiple iliac fractures from falls. One animal had colic and the other panicked after the prosthesis was changed.

Prosthetic Device Design

The device must be as light as possible, self-retaining, nonirritating, and free of pressure on the end of the stump. An open-ended, cone-shaped leather boot, lined with wooled sheepskin to distribute weight-bearing to the maximum area, is attached by encircling buckled straps that conform to the shape of the leg and prevent slippage off the greater diameter of the carpus or tarsus. Aluminum tubing is light and readily available but is expensive to weld and fabricate. The ground surface requires reinforcement, preferably covered with rubberized, nonslip material.

Support for the foreleg is a simple matter of vertical straight-line support (Figs 74-77). Angular conformation is a problem with rear leg prostheses (Fig. 78). The device must adapt to the movement of the tarsus and provide support above and below the joint (Fig 79).

References

1. Anon. Quarter Horse J **1** (1962) 18.
2. Koger, LM *et al*. JAVMA **156** (1970).1600.
3. Armstrong, KL. Appaloosa News (March)(1970) 3.

Other Modes of Therapy
by B.D. Grant

DMSO

Dimethyl sulfoxide (DMSO) has been used to treat skeletal problems in horses since the mid-1960s. The pharmacology of DMSO is described in more detail in Chapter 6 and the drug is only mentioned here to describe its use in the treatment of skeletal conditions. It has been most effective in reducing the acute swelling associated with direct trauma to the lower limbs, especially when applied under an occlusive bandage. The gel form is most convenient and can be reapplied 2-3 times a day, depending on the condition. Its use on breeding animals is contraindicated.

At race tracks or horse shows, DMSO is commonly combined with topical antibiotics and corticosteroids, even though its effectiveness with these products has not been studied. Spontaneous rupture of the superficial digital flexor tendon in 5 of 11 race horses was associated with daily application of a DMSO/dexamethasone combination linament. Many animals suffer local hair loss from chronic use of DMSO and corticosteroids. In addition to affecting the cosmetic appearance, this also predisposes the horse to local skin infections.

It is important to provide proper instructions to the person applying the drug, including the use of rubber or plastic gloves to avoid direct contact with DMSO, especially if the handler is in the child-rearing age group. Also, contact with topical antibiotics, such as nitrofurazone, may sensitize the person to these medications.

Hydrotherapy

Water, either cold or hot, has long been used to treat skeletal conditions. It is probably beneficial to use both cold and warm hydrotherapy, depending on the condition. Many veterinarians, owners and trainers attest to its effectiveness by using it to treat their own ailments.

Water can be applied in many forms, from spraying with a hose for 30-40 minutes daily to elaborate jacuzzi-style containments (Fig 80). Traditionally, cold water or ice has been applied to prevent swelling and, especially in acute injuries, its use on horses with chronic tendon problems has been effective when applied after each workout. Muscle relaxation and increased mobility of arthritic joints are gained from application of warm water.

The following points should be kept in mind when horses are treated with hydrotherapy

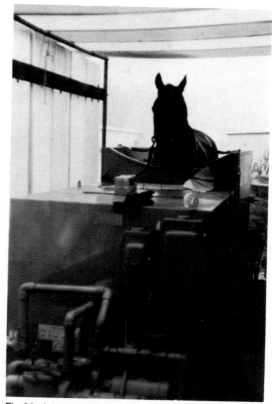

Fig 80. A jacuzzi-type bath for horses. Overuse of this device can lead to an increased incidence of submural abscesses.

over long periods. It is not natural for a horse to spend 1-2 hours a day with its feet in water and there has been an increase in submural abscesses in such cases, perhaps due to maceration of the hoof. The use of iodine-based medications to retain the proper moisture content of the feet in such cases is recommended. Horses with tendon, fetlock or carpal problems benefit most from direct application of cold, either by the use of ice boots, which do not encompass the foot, or the new refrigerated apparatuses (Fig 81). Cooling of injured areas is probably most effective only for 40 minutes at a time since reflex vascularization occurs after this period. It is more prudent to treat animals 2-3 times daily for periods of 30 minutes rather than for 1½ hours at one time.

Hydrotherapy should be used cautiously around open wounds, recently injected joints, or surgical incisions as there are many organisms, such as *Pseudomonas*, that thrive in a wet environment. Open wounds respond to re-

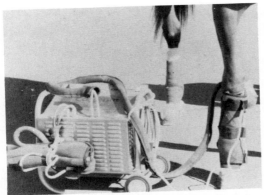

Fig 81. Dry cold therapy is provided by this refrigerating device.

peated hydrotherapy but they tend to swell from increased absorption of water. Horses with open foot wounds should not be stood in water for long periods unless the foot is thoroughly cleaned previously because significant numbers of bacteria can be disseminated throughout the water by the contamination of soil and fecal matter on the foot.

Cryosurgery

In addition to its use for the treatment of neoplasms, especially those of the adnexa, eyes, ears, nose and genitalia, cryosurgery is increasingly used to treat skeletal problems. The ability of cryosurgery to destroy nervous tissue is well known and reports that cryoneurectomy can be performed without an incision have increased its popularity.[73] This technic has a number of problems in that the amount of cryonecrosis needed to disrupt transmission of C-type prereceptors in the distal nerves is usually enough to cause severe necrosis of the skin and subcutaneous tissues, resulting in slow-healing open wounds. Cryosurgery, in combination with a standard posterior digital neurectomy, has been helpful in reducing the incidence of painful neuromas.[74] Excessive use of cryosurgery directly on bone causes osteonecrosis. Its use for treatment of dorsal metacarpal disease is described elsewhere in this chapter.

Ultrasound

The use of ultrasound to treat a variety of skeletal problems in performance horses is widespread. A number of available ultrasound units can deliver ultrasonic waves to the appendages. Reconditioned units often are available through medical/surgical supply houses. When purchasing an ultrasound unit, the size of the applicator head and adequate grounding of the unit are important. The new transistorized models are small, durable and able to withstand the use a busy equine practice or a training stable requires.

Ultrasound therapy is routinely used in postoperative management of splint bone fracture fragment removal and exostoses of the metacarpal bones to reduce the incidence of postoperative dystrophic calcification. It also effectively improves the quality of vascularization, removal of necrotic debris, and appearance of the scar tissue after percutaneous tendon splitting for the treatment of tendinitis in race horses.[75] We routinely begin ultrasound therapy 3 days after tendon-splitting procedures in our clinic. Ultrasound has been satisfactorily used daily on horses in training and afflicted with "splints," villonodular synovitis, spavin, gonitis and trochanteric bursitis. It is also used for muscle conditions and, along with a muscle stimulator, can be used to find so-called "trigger areas" that cause painful spasms of the abaxial muscles.

Ultrasound therapy should not be used over infected areas since this may cause rapid dissemination of the infection. It should not be used over surgical incisions until 14 days after surgery because dehiscence can result. It should not be used over metallic implants since such use often causes excessive heat and loosening of the implant. Finally, it should not be used over the spinal cord because of the possibility of spinal cord damage.

The area should be surgically clipped and shaved, and a liberal application of the disseminating gel applied for transmission of sound waves. Various coupling gels are available; mineral oil is acceptable but somewhat messy. If the unit is properly grounded, treatment can be applied with the leg submerged in water since water is a good conductor of sound waves. Although the patient may object initially to the tingling sensation, sedation with a tranquilizer may be required only for the first 1 or 2 sessions. Care should be taken not to use ultrasound over an area that has been desensitized by neurectomy or local anesthesia. The animal should certainly not have a twitch applied during ultrasound therapy.

To be most effective, ultrasound therapy should be applied for at least 10 days continuously. After this period, alternate-day treatment may be instituted. It is important to note that any reduction in postoperative fibrosis is not usually seen until 10 days after the onset of therapy.

Faradism and Muscle Stimulation

The technic of electrically stimulating painful muscle groups has been used only on a limited basis in this country but much more extensively in England. Faradism involves passage of a small galvanic current through the affected muscle groups to passively stimulate their contraction. This is thought to increase blood flow and allow removal of accumulations of by-products of muscle metabolism.

Radiation Therapy

The use of various forms of radiation to treat skeletal problems has been well documented. Cobalt-60 produces high-quality gamma radiation and is most effective in introducing radiation to a specific area. The use of cobalt-60 is limited by the expense of obtaining the required equipment and the inherent risks of using a radioactive material with a long half-life.

Radon-222 is a gas that emits gamma rays and has a short half-life. It is used as small, gold-encapsulated implants surgically placed in the area to be treated. The use of radon implants requires careful scheduling of implant surgery so the proper dose can be delivered to the patient. The emitted radiation is not of the quality of either cobalt-60 or cesium-37. Use of cesium-37 is similar to that of cobalt-60 in that the emitting source is placed in a boot-like structure and arranged in a predetermined pattern around the treatment sites. Use of radioactive substances requires approval from the appropriate state regulatory agency. They have a significant public health hazard if handled carelessly.

X-Irradiation

The delivery of high-quality x-rays from a rotating anode is possible with the use of sophisticated equipment. "Soft" x-rays can be filtered out with the use of appropriate filters. The major drawback to this is the expense in the purchase of the equipment necessary to safely deliver the proper dose to the patient.

Ionizing radiation causes necrosis of the endothelium of the smaller vessels surrounding an inflamed area. This, in turn, produces necrosis of the usually proliferative area, with a resulting reflex in circulation to remove the debris from initial necrosis. This is a cyclic process that can have 2-3 phases some 30 days apart. Radiation therapy has been used to treat almost all skeletal conditions, with good clinical results but few controlled studies.[76,77] It has been most effective in producing almost complete synovectomy in an area with a distended synovial capsule or sheath.[78] Several cases of tendinitis were successfully treated with intralesional injection of corticosteroids to reduce the amount of inflammatory debris, followed by irradiation 3 weeks later to further reduce fibrosis surrounding the tendon.[79]

Osteoblasts may disappear from treated areas for 3-6 months. For this reason, horses should not be raced or trained after irradiation, to avoid the liability associated with any pathologic fractures that could result.

Radiation therapy should be used with caution in show horses as there is a possibility that it can produce whitening of the hair. It also should not be used in any septic process.

Acupuncture

Acupuncture has recently received a great deal of publicity for its use in various conditions. It is an art that requires a great deal of practice to perfect. However, its efficacy will not be known until clinical trials on known models of equine lameness are performed.[80,81]

Laser Beam

The use of laser light to treat equine lameness is a technic that, like acupuncture, has not been thoroughly evaluated. The availability of laser beam apparatuses is increasing and its use for many conditions is based on the principle of acupuncture. The laser beam is applied to the acupuncture points that control the various structures in the horse's legs. Most units are unable to completely penetrate the dermis of the horse, although they may cause small burns to the skin.

Counterirritation

Although internal and external blisters, thermocautery and sclerosing agents have been used for many years in the treatment of equine lameness, few controlled studies have been performed to assess the efficacy of these methods. Although such modes of treatment can produce beneficial results, careless or imprudent use of such methods can result in further injury to the animal. For this reason, use of these methods should be considered an "art" and should be restricted to those knowledgeable in their application.

References

1. Burke, JF. Postgrad Med **58 (3)** (1975) 65.
2. Yoxall, A. Eq Vet J **9 (4)** (1977) 167.
3. Seropian, R and Reynolds, BM. Am J Surg **121** (1971) 251.
4. Grant, BD. Proc 21st Ann Mtg Am Assoc Eq Pract, 1975. p 95.
5. Hunt, TK *et al.* Ann Surg **170** (1969) 633.
6. Alexander, JT and Rooney, JR. Proc 18th Ann Mtg Am Assoc Eq Pract, 1972. p 219.
7. Clayton-Jones, DG. Vet Rec **97** (1975) 193.
8. Denney, HR. Vet Rec **102** (1978) 273.
9. Gertson, KE *et al.* Vet Med **68** (1973) 782.
10. Winstanley, EW. Vet Rec **95** (1974) 429.
11. Muller, ME *et al.* Manual of Internal Fixation. 2nd ed. Springer-Verlag, Berlin, 1979.
12. Allgower, M *et al*: The Dynamic Compression Plate. Springer-Verlag, Berlin, 1973.
13. Perrin, SM *et al.* Acta Orthoped Scand **125** (1969) 227.
14. Grossman, BS and Nickels, FA. Eq Pract **1(6)** (1979) 13.
15. Milne, DW and Turner, AS: An Atlas of Surgical Approaches to the Bones of the Horse. WB Saunders, Philadelphia, 1979.
16. Fessler and Amstutz, in Oehme and Prier: Large Animal Surgery. Williams & Wilkins, Baltimore, 1974.
17. Wheat, JD. Proc 21st Ann Mtg Am Assoc Eq Pract, 1975. p 223.
18. Wallace, CE. Aust Vet J **47** (1971) 57.
19. Gabel, AA. JAVMA **155** (1969) 1831.
20. Monin, T. J Eq Med Surg **1** (1977) 325.
21. Garner, HE and Thurman, JC. JAVMA **152** (1968) 1402.
22. Panzet, VG and Eisenmenger, E. Wein Tierärztl Monatsschr **60** (1973) 295.
23. Krahwinkel, DJ *et al.* JAVMA **154** (1969) 53.
24. Lewis, LD, Colorado State Univ: Personal communication, 1979.
25. Hertsch, BR *et al.* Dtsch Tier Wschr **83** (1976) 263.
26. Turner, AS. J Vet Surg **8** (1979) 29.
27. Levine, SB. J Eq Med Surg **3** (1979) 186.
28. Smith, in Hardy: Rhoads Textbook of Surgery. 5th *ed.* JB Lippincott, Philadelphia, 1977.
29. Leitch, M. J Eq Med Surg **1** (1977) 234.
30. Goble, DO and Brinker, WO. J Eq Med Surg **1** (1977) 341.
31. Salter, RB: Textbook of Disorders and Injuries of the Musculoskeletal System. Williams & Wilkins, Baltimore, 1970.
32. Valdez, H *et al.* J Vet Orthoped **1** (1979) 10.
33. Vaughan, LC. Eq Vet J **3** (1968) 4.
34. Denny, HR. Eq Vet J **8** (1976) 20.
35. Johnson, JH and Butler, HC. Vet Med **66** (1971) 552.
36. Colahan, PT and Meagher, DM. Vet Surg **8 (4)** (1979) 105.
37. Turner, AS *et al.* JAVMA **168** (1976) 306.
38. Turner, AS. Aust Vet Pract **9** (1979) 43.
39. Fretz, PB. Can Vet J **14** (1973) 50.
40. Meagher, DM. Proc 22nd Ann Mtg Am Assoc Eq Pract, 1976. p 147.
41. Rooney, JR: Mod Vet Pract **55** (1974) 113.
42. Rooney, JR: Biomechanics of Lameness in Horses. Williams & Wilkins, Baltimore, 1969.
43. Turner, AS. JAVMA **171** (1977) 655.
44. Bohm, D and Waibl, H. Tierärztl Wschr **90** (1977) 373.
45. Dubs, B and Nemeth, F. Schweiz Arch Tierheilkd **117** (1975) 299.
46. Fackelman, GE. Vet Med **68** (1973) 662.
47. Adams, OR: Lameness in Horses. 3rd ed. Lea & Febiger, Philadelphia, 1974.
48. Adams, OR. Scope **7** (1962) 2.
49. Turner, AS and Gabel, AA. JAVMA **167** (1975) 306.
50. Schneider, JE *et al.* JAVMA **173** (1978) 1364.
51. Turner, AS *et al.* JAVMA **175** (1979) 1198.
52. Turner, AS. J Eq Med Surg **1** (1977) 180.
53. Stick, JA and Derksen, FJ. JAVMA **176** (1980) 627.
54. White, NA and Wheat, JD. JAVMA **167** (1975) 733.
55. Ferguson, JG and Presnell, KR. Can Vet J **17** (1976) 314.
56. Slocum, B and Chalman, JA. Arch Am Coll Vet Surg (Spring, 1975) 39.
57. Stashak, TS and Adams, OR. JAVMA **167** (1975) 397.
58. DeOliveira, JC. J Bone Joint Surg **53B** (1971) 672.
59. Wheat, JD, Univ Calif: Personal communication, 1979.
60. Jones, RD *et al.* Proc 23rd Ann Mtg Am Assoc Eq Pract, 1977. p 313.
61. Burchardt, H and Enneking, WF. Surg Clin No Am **58** (1978) 403.
62. Albrektsson, T and Albrektsson, B. Acta Orthoped Scand **49** (1978) 1.
63. Jenny, J. JAVMA **147** (1965) 1444.
64. Scherr, DD *et al.* J Bone Joint Surg **54A** (1972) 634.
65. Rittman, WW and Perren, SM: Cortical Bone Healing After Internal Fixation and Infection. Springer-Verlag, New York, 1974.
66. Rittmann, WW *et al.* Clin Orthoped Rel Res **138** (1979) 132.
67. Chapman, MW and Mahoney, M. Clin Orthoped Rel Res **138** (1979) 120.
68. Burri, C *et al.* J Trauma **13** (1973) 799.
69. Clawson, DK and Dunn, AW. J Bone Joint Surg **49A** (1967) 164.
70. Hagen, R. Acta Orthoped Scand **49** (1978) 542.
71. Meyer, S *et al.* J Bone Joint Surg **57A** (1975) 836.
72. Kay, BA *et al.* Can Vet J **17** (1976) 82.
73. Baker, RH. Proc 23rd Ann Mtg Am Assoc Eq Pract, 1977. p 323.
74. Tate, LP and Evans, LH. JAVMA **177** (1980) 423.
75. Marcos, MB and Aswad, A. Eq Vet J **10 (4)** (1978) 267.
76. Grant, BD. Master's thesis, Wash State Univ, 1973.
77. Dixon, RT. Aust Vet J **45** (1969) 389.
78. Paatsama, S *et al.* J Am Vet Rad Soc **10** (1969) 72.
79. Franks, W. Eq Vet J **11 (2)** (1979) 106.
80. Gideon, L. JAVMA **170** (1977) 220.
81. Bowen, J. JAVMA **176** (1980) 500.

THE FOOT
by J.H. Johnson

A thorough knowledge of the anatomy and physiology of the foot is essential to correctly identify the cause of lameness. The foot could be the primary location of lameness or secondarily involved with lameness in another area of the limb. The entire patient should be surveyed as a unit before limiting the examination to a specific limb or foot. The size, shape and angle of the foot can alter the rest of the limb and directly affect the gait. Once the horse has been observed at a walk and trot, and ridden or driven if necessary, the lame leg should be observed closely. A good starting point in any lameness examination is with the foot. Most lameness problems are found in the foot and by starting there with a thorough examination, many embarrassing moments may be avoided.

The Examination

Inspection

The foot should be inspected while bearing weight and compared with the other feet. The inspection should include comparing the size and measuring the angle at which the feet are trimmed. The heel and toe length should be measured. The general conformation of the horse should also be noted, with particular attention to the attachment of the foot to the limb. Does the horse have good conformation or does the foot toe-out or toe-in excessively? Are the shoes applied properly? What is the lo-cation of the clinches? Are they too low or too high? Are the nails the proper size? Are there too many nails? Are they positioned properly?

The bottom of the foot should be slightly concave. If the horse is shod, are the shoes worn properly and is the foot shod level? What is the condition of the frog? Is there any frog pressure when the foot strikes the ground? Are the heels contracted?

Horseshoes, incorrectly applied, may be the most common cause of lameness, both directly and indirectly.[1] Horseshoes not only affect the foot but the entire limb. A shoe is the dominant factor in determining the way in which a limb initially makes impact with the ground. Many horses are shod in an attempt to make the horse artificially better than its abilities.

Close attention should be paid to the nails during inspection of a shod hoof. Only sufficient nails should be used to hold the shoe on properly. The more nails, the more potential problems in that the nails may be too close to the sensitive structures or placed on areas that should not contain a nail. The natural expansion of the hoof is decreased if too many nails are applied. Feet that are shod may expand 1/8-1/2 inch in as little as 30 minutes after the shoes are removed. Hoof expansion is an integral part of the anticoncussive mechanism of the foot and is essential for a sound foot, as well as protecting the rest of the limb.

The manufactured or Keg shoe has 8 closely spaced nail holes, which are probably more than needed. The heel nail holes generally are too far back in manufactured shoes and inter-

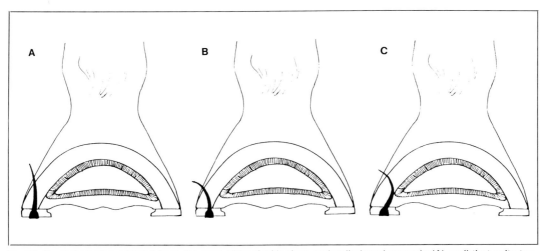

Fig 82. Frontal section, viewed from the rear, of hoof with shoe and nail placed properly (A), nail that exits too low (B), and nail placed too close to sensitive structures and that exits too high on the horny wall (C).

fere with hoof expansion. This problem may be corrected by using a hand-made shoe with 3 properly placed nail holes on each branch, using side or toe clips to help secure the shoe and also help prevent shifting of the foot on the shoe. A manufactured shoe may be improved by filling in the holes and repunching them where needed.

Nails that exit too low and are too shallow in the wall cause splitting and tearing of the hoof walls or loose shoes (Fig 82). This may cause lameness or may lead to problems when the shoe is reapplied and renailed, particularly if the same shoe is used with the same spacing of the nails. To avoid this, the nail holes could be repunched in the shoe, a smaller nail used, or other methods used to help secure the shoes to the wall, such as side or toe clips and, as a last resort, plastic materials. Nails that exit too high on the hoof wall are likely to be driven quite close to sensitive tissue (Fig 82). Those nails may cause an obvious lameness or cause pain each time the hoof strikes the ground.

Small nails should be used on small feet and large nails on large feet. Small, thin nails are less likely to split the hoof wall or penetrate too close to the sensitive structures. Small nails are also easier to control and position properly. Most manufactured shoes require a larger nail to fill the hole than is necessary to hold the shoe on properly. All manufactured shoes, regardless of size, are punched in the same fashion with regard to the depth of fullering and direction and dimension of the holes. The holes are punched perpendicularly to the web of the shoe, as opposed to correctly establishing a proper angle to avoid sensitive tissues. This applies to the last or heel nail more so than to others. This can be corrected by repunching the nail holes and flattening the shoe to change the depth of fullering to accept a smaller nail.

The heel or last nail is most commonly involved in lameness problems, especially the medial heel nail.[1] There are several reasons for this: the wall on the medial quarter-heel region is generally thinner; the wall is also straighter in this area, making it more difficult to drive the nail at the correct angle; manufactured shoes generally have the heel nail hole beyond the bend of the quarter; and it is general practice to bend the medial heel of the shoe toward the midline of the foot to avoid "grabbing" and loosening of the shoe. This problem is alleviated by relocating the heel nail or not using the last nail hole. Nails caudal to the bend of the quarter interfere with proper heel and foot expansion.

Palpation

Digital palpation around the coronary band is used to evaluate swelling, soreness, or an elevation in temperature of the coronary band or hoof. The coronary band area swells before rupture of abscesses. A sunken coronary band in the dorsal area, in conjunction with a digital pulse, may indicate laminitis. Any digital pulse and elevated temperature of the hoof should be compared with those of the other feet. Often more than one foot is involved, as in laminitis, when both front feet may be hot and have a bounding digital pulse.

Percussion

A shoeing or ball-peen hammer can be used to tap around the hoof wall to detect any tender areas caused by inflammation. Light taps are sufficient to elicit pain, using a sound foot as a control. Percussion may not reveal evidence of pain when the horny wall of the hoof is thick and the inflammation mild. All clinches of the nails should be tapped separately in shod horses. After percussing the clinches, the foot should be picked up and the nail heads tapped separately with light blows. Pain is frequently manifested by the horse moving its ears before it jerks the foot.

Paring

The flaky sole should removed with a sharp hoof knife and all black or discolored areas carefully evaluated. The examiner should remember that a foot with the flaky sole removed is more tender than normal. The bottom of the foot should be evaluated as to concavity of the sole, and the nature and consistency of the frog. If the bottom of the foot is flat, the examiner should determine if the foot has been trimmed improperly or if the horse has a flat sole due to some pathologic condition, such as chronic laminitis. Shoes hamper this part of the examination and should be removed unless the lameness is probably not associated with the shoe; the shoes are needed to protect and balance the feet while the horse is being exercised as part of the examination. Any use of the hoof tester on a foot that has not been pared and had the shoe removed is a compromise. It is always wise to have a farrier present for that part of the examination if practical.

Compression

The hands can be used alone or with a hoof tester to compress the hoof. Two sizes of hoof testers should be on hand for a thorough examination: a small pair for applying pressure around the wall and sole, and a larger pair to compress the walls at the heels and to compress the navicular area.

Movement of the sole signifies that enough pressure has been applied. At that point the horse's pain threshold should be established by applying enough pressure to a normal area to make the horse flinch. All feet should then be subjected to less pressure than was needed to establish the pain threshold. The examiner should carefully watch the horse's ears while conducting a hoof tester examination. An ear flicked back could indicate pain before a flinch of the leg. Hoof testers should not be used to hurt the horse but rather to help localize the problem area. Always examine more than one foot with the hoof tester to ensure a complete examination and to prevent the horse from faking a positive response.

Wedges

A wooden wedge about 6 inches wide and with a 30° angle can be used to accentuate a lameness that may not be entirely limited to the foot. The wedge applies more pressure to a limited area of the foot and stretches the opposite collateral ligaments of the joints. The wedge is placed under the lateral wall of the hoof and the opposite foot is held up for 2 minutes to make the horse bear twice as much weight on the affected foot. The rapidity with which the horse removes the foot from the wedge after the raised foot is released is significant. The same procedure is repeated with the wedge under the toe, medial wall and heel. A curved object, such as a short piece of broom handle, can be placed under the frog while the opposite foot is lifted to cause additional pressure over the navicular area

Nerve Blocks

Specific nerve blocks can be used to selectively anesthetize parts of the foot if previous methods of examination are inconclusive. Lidocaine or carbocaine, with or without epinephrine, is generally used for local anesthesia. Procaine generally requires more time to take effect. To prevent postinjection swelling, 1 ml corticosteroid can be added to 10 ml local anesthetic and a bandage applied to the area. Systemic anti-inflammatory agents, such as phenylbutazone or flunixin meglumine, can also be administered to minimize injection site swelling. The site of the palmar digital block

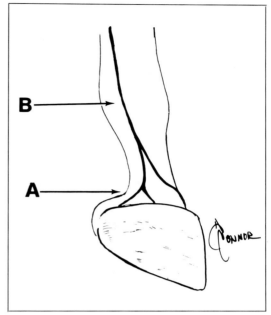

Fig 83. Nerve supply to the foot. The injection site for a palmar digital nerve block is at the level of or distal to the bifurcation of the nerve on the caudal aspect of the foot (A). The injection site for a palmar block is at the level of or proximal to the fetlock (B).

("heel block") is slightly proximal to the lateral cartilage. The nerve is palpated subcutaneously at this point and 2-4 ml local anesthetic are infiltrated around the nerve (Fig 83). This should anesthetize the caudal third of the foot and probably two-thirds of the corium of the sole. Skin desensitization over the heel is considered the measure of an effective nerve block. Only one nerve (medial or lateral) should be blocked at one time. If the palmar digital block is not diagnostic, a ring block can be used just above the coronary band to anesthetize the entire foot.

A palmar nerve block, rather than a ring block, is usually used to anesthetize the entire foot. The palmar nerve is anesthetized proximal to the cul-de-sac of the fetlock joint. The nerve, with the corresponding artery and vein, lies between the suspensory ligament and the deep flexor tendon (Fig 83). The examiner must remember that the caudal aspect of the limb from the sesamoids distal, as well as the coffin joint, is also anesthetized.

Shoes

An equine practitioner is not expected to be a farrier but should at least have a working

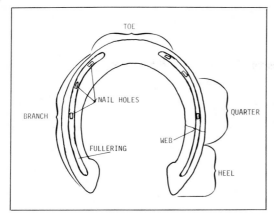

Fig 84. Parts of a horseshoe.

knowledge of how shoes are selected and how they should be applied. The lightest shoe that fulfills the work requirements should be used. The addition of weight to the bottom of the horse's foot can only increase fatigue, decrease agility and exaggerate gaits. The shoe should fit properly and not appreciably decrease the total useful ground surface of the foot. Reduction of the ground surface concentrates the energy of impact to a smaller area and appears to increase dorsiflexion of the fetlock and ventriflexion of the coffin joint, which in turn increases joint rotation and work load.

The width of the web of the shoe is important (Fig 84). A correctly made and applied shoe should contact the hoof wall, white line, and a small portion of the adjacent sole. Most manufactured shoes are too narrow and do not protect the bottom of the foot properly. In a horse in which the sole is not concave, it is not unusual to find the imprint of the shoe in the sole region when the shoe is removed and to detect sensitivity to hoof testers. These horses may be consistently or intermittently lame, especially when worked on a hard surface. The usual "correction" for such cases is the addition of a pad. This may or may not alleviate the problem but encourages an unhealthy situation. A pad can be responsible for reduced foot expansion and commonly causes thrush due to the moist environment between the pad and foot. A shoe with a wider web and a concave sole surface is another and perhaps better way to help a horse with flat feet. Such a shoe can be made by hand from bar stock or by reshaping a manufactured shoe in a forge, flattening the web and grinding or hammering the sole part of the shoe so that it does not touch the sole. A steel training plate can also be shaped by hammering the inner

thin edge of the shoe toward the ground surface of the shoe.

Accessories can be added to shoes, such as calks, toe grabs, bars and borium. All of these are a potential hazard if used incorrectly or placed on the shoe improperly. High or long heel calks could create 5 abnormal situations: reduction of total ground surface; concentration of the energy of impact to a rather small area when horses are working on hard surfaces; alteration of the foot axis by elevating the caudal aspect of the foot, causing overrotation of the coffin and fetlock joints; inside heel calks on rear feet often cause interference in flat-racing horses; and calks may cause fractures of the first or second phalanx or the third metacarpal/metatarsal bone in horses that make sudden turns because the foot remains stationary while the limb rotates.[1]

Heel calks should only be used when needed and should be low or short. Other types of shoes, such as full-rim or full-fullered shoes, may serve the same purpose.

Toe grabs or other additions at the toe also may alter the gait and change the angles of the joints. The toe of the shoe should always be examined for abnormal wear. Toe grabs decrease surface contact and, if not positioned properly, alter normal foot breakover. Toe grabs are worn abnormally in cases of abnormal foot breakover.

If a grab is to be used, the foot should be balanced and the grab centered at the breakover point of the hoof. A toe grab should only be big enough to serve as intended. If the grab is too high, it can be rasped down or the shoe changed to a full-rimmed or full-fullered shoe.

Lesions of the Wall of the Foot

Wall Cracks

Most cracks in the horny wall are fissures parallel to the laminae. The crack may originate at the distal surface of the wall and extend varying distances up to the coronary band or may originate at the coronary band and extend varying distances down to the distal surface. Cracks that originate at the coronary band are a result of hoof growth disruption due to injury to the coronary band. A permanent hoof defect may result if the coronary band is severely injured. When the bearing surface is the origin of the crack, the cause is usually drying of the wall or improper foot trimming.[3,4] A properly functioning foot has a certain amount of elasticity in the wall and sole, and moisture is the key to flexibility. The normal hoof wall contains about 25% water, the sole about 33%, and the frog about 50%.[5]

Cracks on the quarter and heel are usually the most severe and may involve the sensitive laminae. Affected horses usually are lame, and hemorrhage from the crack is common after exercise.

Toe Cracks

Cause: In the absence of other pathologic conditions, such as chronic laminitis, toe cracks usually originate at the distal surface because the foot is too dry. Toe cracks that originate at the coronary band result from an injury that interrupts wall growth.

Diagnosis: The horny wall is disrupted at the toe and the horse becomes lame if the crack involves the sensitive laminae. A hoof tester and nerve blocks help confirm the diagnosis if the horse is lame.

Treatment: If the crack does not extend into the coronary band, a transverse groove rasped through the horny wall proximal to the crack and application of a shoe prevent the crack from extending proximad up the wall. In some cases, toe clips can be applied on each side of the crack to prevent expansion of the wall at the site of the crack (Fig 85). If the crack extends down into the sensitive laminae, it should be pared out in a dovetail fashion, laced with stainless-steel wire or strong suture and filled with plastic (see Quarter Cracks). If the crack originates at the coronary band, a transverse groove down to the white line below the crack prevents it from extending to the distal surface. When the coronary band is intact, new wall grows distad at ¾-1 inch/month.

Quarter Cracks

A crack in the quarter of the hoof wall is referred to as a quarter crack.

Cause: Excessive growth of the hoof wall and improper care of the hoof can result in the wall's splitting at the distal surface. Trauma to the coronary band, such as when a base-narrow horse strikes the coronary band with the opposite foot, can cause temporary disruption of growth or tearing away of the hoof wall and result in a quarter crack.

Diagnosis: Affected horses may or may not be lame. Hemorrhage from the crack after exercise indicates that the crack extends into the sensitive laminae. Purulent material may exude from chronic cracks when pressure is applied to the wall. Because of the inflammation,

the hoof wall and adjacent coronary band are usually warmer than the rest of the foot. Injection of local anesthetic into the soft tissue immediately above the crack aids in diagnosis if the animal is lame.

Treatment: Cracks that result from improper foot care and that do not extend into the sensitive laminae can be controlled by proper trimming and creation of a transverse groove through the horny wall proximal to the crack as in treatment of toe cracks. Shoeing is beneficial. The wall caudal to the crack should be trimmed shorter than the rest of the foot so it does not bear weight until the crack has healed by hoof growth.

Cracks originating at the coronary band that do not extend into the sensitive laminae or to the distal weight-bearing surface may be treated by removing a triangular section of the horny wall, with the base of the triangle at the coronary band. This section of wall can be removed with an electric tool equipped with a burr.

If a crack causes lameness, hemorrhage or suppuration and if it extends from the coronary

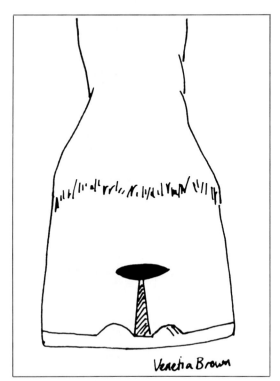

Fig 85. Treatment of a toe crack originating at the distal weight-bearing suface. A transverse groove has been pared down to the depth of the white line proximal to the crack, and a shoe with 2 toe clips has been applied to limit expansion of the crack.

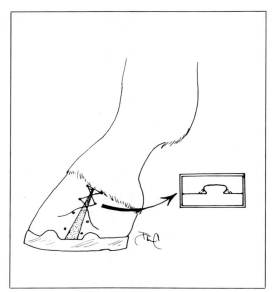

Fig 86. A quarter crack has been pared out in a dovetail fashion (inset) and laced in preparation for application of plastic.

band to the distal surface, the crack should be pared to the sensitive laminae with a burr, and the edges dovetailed and filled with plastic.[3,6] In preparing the crack, small holes are drilled on each side of the pared-out crack, starting in the normal wall and extending to the depths of the dovetailed area (Fig 86). These holes should be placed approximately ½ inch apart, and 20-ga stainless-steel wire used to close the crack. The wire laces help hold the crack together and serve as a matrix to contain the plastic. The hoof should be dry and free of hemorrhage and exudates before the plastic is applied. Slight hemorrhage can be stopped with silver nitrate applicators. It is best to bandage the foot until the infection is controlled in cases of suppuration. Soaking the foot in a supersaturated solution of magnesium sulfate usually is helpful. Swabbing the area with full-strength formalin just before applying the plastic material helps prevent infection. The entire defect is then filled with plastic and rasped down, after the plastic hardens, to resemble a relatively normal foot.

Prognosis: The prognosis depends on the cause of the crack. It usually is favorable if there is no disruption of the coronary band.

Heel Cracks and Avulsions of the Wall at the Heel

The term "heel crack" refers to disruption of the horny wall at the heel of the foot.

Cause: A heel crack may result from the same causes as quarter cracks, but trauma is the most common cause. The horse may step on or kick a sharp object and tear away a portion of the heel.

Diagnosis: The diagnosis usually is obvious as a small amount or up to the entire quarter of the horny wall is partially torn away from its laminar attachment.

Treatment: Repairing this type of crack is seldom practical. The horny wall is generally separated from the sensitive laminae at the bearing surface. The horny wall caudal to the crack is removed following injection of a local anesthetic over the palmar digital nerve. The horny wall separates from its laminar attachment quite easily. A pair of nippers is used to grasp the wall and peel the wall proximad in the direction of the coronary band. The foot is then covered with antibacterial ointment and a pressure bandage to control hemorrhage for 3-5 days. After the bandage is removed, a drying agent, such as 10% formalin, can be applied to the lesion. A bar shoe helps protect the heel until new growth covers the area.

Transverse Cracks

Cause: Transverse cracks in the horny wall result from injury to the coronary band or from infection that migrates up the white line from the distal surface and causes the horny wall to separate from the coronary band.

Diagnosis: The lesion is obvious and usually secondary to another condition.

Treatment: The primary underlying condition deserves first consideration because in time the transverse crack grows out and is trimmed out. If suppuration is present in the crack, the opening should be widened, purulent material removed, and a drying agent applied. The underside of the foot should be examined for an object in the white line area.

Puncture Wounds of the White Line

This condition is generally referred to as "gravel." Infection introduced by penetration at the white line follows the line of least resistance proximad up the white line, resulting in drainage above the coronary band.[7] A small piece of gravel may be found when paring out the wound, hence the term gravel. It was once thought that a stone entered the bottom of the foot, then migrated and erupted above the coronary band. The presence of the stone is now thought to be incidental.

Cause: A puncture wound or crack at the white line may allow infection to enter. The white line may be widened at the toe due to rotation of the third phalanx following chronic laminitis; this predisposes to gravel.

Diagnosis: Before the wound opens above the coronary band, the lesion consists of a puncture or break in the white line. This usually is represented by a very black area that, when explored, leads to an accumulation of pus. The horse usually is severely lame as the pressure of the exudate increases but becomes sound when the lesion opens proximal to the coronary band. The foot is hot and the adjacent soft tissues may be swollen.

Treatment: Drainage of the abscess is essential. In severe cases, both the wound proximal to the coronary band and the causative wound can be enlarged to allow good drainage. If only a puncture wound in the white line is present, application of a poultice or supersaturated solution of magnesiuim sulfate helps reduce the swelling and promotes drainage of the exudate. The foot should be bandaged until the drainage has stopped and the wound is dry. A shoe with a full pad should then be applied to prevent material from being packed into the ventral hole. Unless laminitis is a complication, the prognosis is favorable. Systemic antibiotics should be administered if warranted. Tetanus toxoid should be administered as outlined in Chapter 2.

Keratoma

A keratoma is a tumor that usually grows from the inner aspect of the horny wall and causes lameness as it encroaches on the sensitive laminae. There may or may not be a change in the shape of the foot.

Cause: The exact cause is unknown. Keratomas have not been associated with injury or irritation, and in some cases regrow after being surgically removed.[8]

Diagnosis: The tumor may be present for some time before lameness is evident. Any bulging of the horn begins at the coronary band. Deviation of the white line toward the center of the foot could lead one to suspect this condition. Fistulous tracts may also be present.

Treatment: Treatment involves surgically removing the entire affected area. Parallel cuts are made in the horny wall on both sides of the tumor from the coronary band to the distal surface. A large pincer is used to grasp the distal border and the entire section of horny wall is removed by reflecting it proximad to the coronary band. Initially the foot is bandaged, and is shod when the horse goes sound. Plastic can be used to fill the defect and protect the sensitive laminae until new hoof growth covers it.

Lesions of the Sole

Bruised Sole

Cause: The sole can be bruised by stones or an improperly fitted shoe.

Diagnosis: In the acute stage, the foot is inflamed and lameness is apparent. Pressure applied over the involved area elicits pain. An area of hemorrhage is evident on paring the sole and may later develop into a seroma. The cause of this lameness must be differentiated from fracture of the third phalanx and a subsolar abscess. Radiographs are helpful in establishing a diagnosis.

Treatment: Initial therapy consists of application of cold packs or antiphlogistic packs and administration of anti-inflammatory drugs, such as phenylbutazone. The horse should be worked on a smooth surface free of small stones, or a full pad should be applied between the shoe and foot until the lameness subsides.

Bruised Heels or Corns

The heel at the angle between the wall and bar is frequently traumatized and the resultant lesions are referred to as "corns." They occur most frequently on the medial angle of the front feet and rarely on the rear feet.

Cause: Improper shoeing is the most common cause of bruised heels, particularly when the shoes are left on too long. The hoof wall forces the heels of the shoe into the wall and causes excessive pressure on the sole at the angle of the wall and bar. This condition is most common in horses worked on hard surfaces.

Diagnosis: The horny wall grows over the shoe and an area of hyperemia is evident when the flaky sole is removed. The hyperemic area is extremely sensitive to application of hoof testers, and a palmar digital nerve block relieves the pain.

Treatment: The shoes should be removed and the feet trimmed if improper shoeing or overgrown feet are the cause. Shoes should not be reapplied until inflammation in the bruised area subsides. The undermined sole should be removed and the foot bandaged if an abscess develops in the bruised area. Applying a properly fitted shoe with a full pad and packing the sole of the foot with pine tar and oakum or a commercial hoof packing helps shorten the convalescence of moderately affected horses.

A radiograph helps determine if the third phalanx is involved and helps predict the length of the recovery period required. If there is no osseous involvement and the feet are properly trimmed and shod, the condition can be corrected before permanent changes are observed in the third phalanx.

Puncture Wounds of the Sole

Cause: Puncture wounds or breaks in the sole occur when a horse steps on a sharp object.

Diagnosis: Lameness is the most consistent sign of a puncture wound of the sole. It develops acutely but may not occur immediately after the puncture has occurred. The horse becomes obviously lame when enough exudate accumulates to cause pressure. As the exudate accumulates, the horny sole is undermined from the corium and exudate drains at the heel.

Puncture wounds or breaks in the sole always result in a black dot or line at the site of injury. The penetrating object is often found embedded in the sole. If the object is not in the foot, the flaky sole should be removed and all discolored areas thoroughly explored. A hoof tester is helpful in locating the affected area.

Treatment: The original puncture site in the sole must be pared out in a conical shape at least 2 cm in diameter. The entire undermined area of the sole should be removed. If the subsolar abscess is small and the related structures of the foot are not involved, lameness disappears when the abscess is drained. The frog is commonly involved and the undermined area of this structure should be removed. The removed horny sole and frog regenerate without leaving defects in the foot. If the entire sole is undermined, it can be removed in stages over 2-3 days. A local nerve block is indicated if the horse shows pain during the procedure.

Medical treatment of subsolar abscesses varies widely. Administration of tetanus antitoxin or a toxoid booster is indicated. The usefulness of systemic antibiotics is questionable. A support bandage may be used if the leg is swollen. Soaking the foot in a supersaturated solution of magnesium sulfate or applying a poultice (retained in a boot) is beneficial until the acute inflammation subsides. If removing a large portion of the sole causes considerable hemorrhage, an antibacterial ointment should be applied under a bandage while the wound is suppurative. Astringents are of value after suppuration is controlled and may be the only treatment in acute puncture wounds with little accumulation of exudate. Equal parts of phenol,

formalin and strong tincture of iodine usually dry the lesion in 3-4 days when applied under a bandage. If suppuration still occurs during this period, removing more of the sole or probing the wound to its depths is indicated.

The development of complications depends on the area of sole involved and the depth of the penetration. Involvement of the third phalanx could result in a small area of necrosis or a pathologic fracture. Tenosynovitis or septic arthritis may develop if the coffin joint, navicular bursa or tendon sheath is penetrated. Daily flushing of the involved joint or bursa with an antibiotic and administration of systemic antibiotics may be more effective than opening the navicular bursa or tendon sheath. The deep flexor tendon sheath can be flushed by inserting a needle on each side of it. A local nerve block is helpful before trying this. The tendon sheath should be flushed every other day for a total of 3 times before the tendon sheath is opened. The approach for the surgery is to remove a generous portion of the apex of the frog down to the sensitive laminae. The laminae are incised down to the tendon sheath and a section of the tendon sheath is removed. The wound is treated as an open wound with daily flushing and bandage changes. If the third phalanx is involved, necrotic bone should be removed by curettage down to bleeding bone.

Throughout the period of treatment, the foot should be covered and the horse kept in a clean stall. A shoe with a piece of sheet metal that slips under the toe and fastens with screws to the heel can be used instead of a bandage while the foot is treated. This is of particular value if the horse does not wear a bandage well or if the coronary band is irritated by the bandage.

A shoe with a full pad can be applied when the wound is dry and there is no evidence of exudation around the edges of the pared sole. The sole should be packed with an antibacterial ointment before the pad and shoe are applied. Warm pine tar should be poured under the pad twice weekly until the shoe is reset in 4-6 weeks. The decision to reapply the pad when the shoe is reset depends on the amount of sole growth at that time.[7-10]

Prognosis: A guarded prognosis is warranted if the navicular bursa, tendon sheath or coffin joint is involved. When the penetration is only through the sole and slightly into the corium, the response to proper treatment usually is good even though a portion of the sole and frog must be removed. Prompt treatment of a penetration always produces a more rapid response.

Other Lesions of the Foot

Thrush

This condition primarily involves the central and lateral sulci of the frog. It is characterized by a fetid, grey to black discharge that usually is associated with disintegration of the horn.

Cause: Poor sanitation and improper trimming of the feet predispose the foot to thrush; *Spherophorus necrophorus* is most commonly involved. This organism multiplies and invades healthy tissue when the feet are not cleaned regularly.

Diagnosis: The odor and dark discharge in the sulci of the frog are typical. The sulci may be deeper than normal when they are cleaned; in advanced cases the sensitive tissues of the foot may be exposed. Affected horses resist hoof cleaning because of pain in the area. In severe cases, the horse may be lame due to involvement of the sensitive tissues. Swelling of the legs ("stocking up") may be seen. Generally the rear legs are most frequently involved.

Treatment: This condition is best prevented by keeping stalls clean and providing proper care of the feet, such as cleaning them daily and trimming them monthly. A horse with thrush should be stabled on a dry surface and the affected frogs should be trimmed to achieve drainage. Astringents, such as formalin or copper sulfate (Kopertox), applied to the infected area are sufficient treatment in early cases. When the condition is advanced, soaking the bandaged foot in a supersaturated solution of magnesium sulfate may be necessary until the infection is controlled. Tetanus immunization should be kept current.

Prognosis: A favorable prognosis can be made if the feet are properly treated before extensive involvement of sensitive tissue occurs.

Canker

This condition is a chronic, hypertrophic, moist pododermatitis with a characteristic fetid odor. It usually begins at the frog and slowly extends to the sole and wall. The condition is most common in draft breeds and usually involves the rear feet.[8]

Cause: Canker occurs when horses are kept on bedding soaked with urine, feces or mud, and when foot care is neglected. Spirochetes and other bacteria have been isolated from diseased tissue, but a specific causative agent has not been identified.

Diagnosis: Thrush is the only condition that must be differentiated from canker. Canker, unlike thrush, may involve the entire foot and may result in separation of the horn of the foot from the sensitive laminae. Degree of lameness is related to the extent of involvement.

Treatment: Treatment of canker involves removal of diseased tissue and bandaging the foot in an antiseptic pack. Use of systemic antibiotics is indicated in severe cases, *eg*, 3 million IU penicillin daily.[11] Application of chlortetracycline powder directly on lesions results in a 96.5% recovery rate and few relapses.[12] The foot should be bandaged until the lesion has healed or until the animal is placed on a clean, dry surface.

Prognosis: The prognosis is guarded due to the intensive care and prolonged therapy required.

Pedal Osteitis

Osteitis, an inflammation of bone, is manifested by decalcification and subsequent increase in periosteal new bone.

Cause: Inflammation of the feet due to repeated concussion on a hard or uneven surface results in chronic pedal osteitis. Pedal osteitis may be the sequel to a severe sole bruise, corns, laminitis or puncture wound.

Diagnosis: The degree of lameness depends on the severity of the condition. The front feet are primarily involved because they support more weight than the rear. The condition may be unilateral if it is secondary to a severe bruise or a puncture wound. Hoof testers applied over the toe cause the horse to pull the foot away. The condition could be confused with laminitis. Radiography may be helpful in establishing a diagnosis. However, radiographs of the solar border and measurement of the vascular channels in the third phalanx should not be used as the sole basis of diagnosis unless radiographs are compared with those of normal horses. The extent of roughening of the solar border of the third phalanx may vary, depending upon the radiographic projection. The lateral solar border usually appears more rough than the medial border. Oblique projections are required to adequately evaluate the lateral and medial borders of the third phalanx.[13]

Treatment: Primary lesions, *eg*, puncture wounds, should be treated. If use on a hard or uneven surface is the cause, the feet should be medicated topically with something that toughens the sole, such as equal parts phenol, formalin and iodine. Protection of the sole with a full pad applied between the shoe and foot also helps.[9] The horse should also be rested. A long convalescence is common in advanced cases in which the third phalanx sustains a

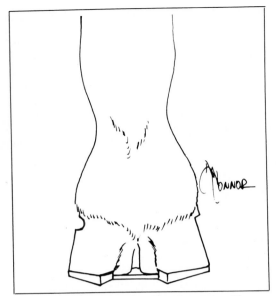

Fig 87. Three methods of expanding a foot with contracted heels. On the right the wall has been rasped thin distal to the coronary band and tapered to the distal weight-bearing surface. On the left the hoof is grooved to allow for expansion. The shoe has been tapered at the web to allow for expansion.

pathologic fracture from demineralization of the bone.

Prognosis: The prognosis of pedal osteitis depends on the stage of development and the cause. A dramatic response to therapy is unlikely when the condition becomes chronic.

Fractures of the Third Phalanx

Fractures of the third phalanx most commonly affect the front feet.

Cause: Trauma, such as stepping on a rock on a race track is the usual cause. In a rear foot it could be caused by kicking an uneven, solid object.

Diagnosis: Most fractures of the third phalanx cause acute lameness. The bounding digital pulse and increased foot temperature associated with this condition may resemble those seen in subsolar abscesses or laminitis. Nerve blocks should not be used when a third phalanx fracture is suspected because exercise may cause fragment displacement and delayed healing. Radiography is the definitive method of diagnosis. However, some fractures are not readily visible initially on standard views. Additional oblique views should be taken before a third phalanx fracture can be ruled out. Some fractures follow vascular channels, confusing the diagnosis even more. Others occur as wing,

articular or other fractures anywhere around the perimeter of the bone.

After the initial inflammation has subsided, diagnosis of a third phalanx fracture may be a diagnostic challenge. Lameness from fractures of the bone in a rear limb may appear to originate more proximal in the limb due to the stance of the horse; however, a thorough physical examination should pinpoint the problem in the foot.

Some fractures of the third phalanx apparently do not heal, as viewed radiographically, even though the horse is not lame. Chronic fractures may not cause lameness while the horse is shod but may do so after the shoe is removed.

Treatment: Therapy is aimed at immobilizing the fracture using a bar shoe with side clips or a rim on a shoe that fits around the entire horny wall. This prevents expansion of the foot and reduces movement of the phalanx. Use of a lag screw may be considered if the fracture is sagittal and involves the coffin joint in a horse over 4 years of age. This technic consists of trimming the foot and applying a bar shoe with side clips preoperatively. The shod foot is wrapped in an antiseptic solution for 12 hours preoperatively. After a series of radiographs with radiopaque markers applied to the hoof, the appropriate area of the hoof is trephined and removed to gain entry to the third phalanx. A Kirschner wire is directed through the third phalanx and a lag technic used to place a screw across the fracture site. The removed piece of hoof wall can be placed over the defect and held in place with plastic, or the hole can be left open and the entire foot wrapped for several weeks until new growth covers the area. Contrary to published reports, this technic of lag fixation of fractures of the third phalanx has been used successfully in yearlings. The fracture heals in about 3 months, at which time the screw is removed.

If the fracture involves a wing of the third phalanx, a neurectomy of the ipsilateral palmar digital nerve may relieve the lameness if the fracture fails to heal with the use of a bar shoe with heel clips. Fractures on the perimeter of the third phalanx generally only cause lameness for 2-3 weeks, at which time the horse may be sound if shod with a pad. If fractures occur at the tip of the third phalanx, the opposite foot should be radiographed to see if it is similarly affected. If so, the fractures may be due to avascular necrosis caused by thrombosis of small vessels in the corium.

Third phalanx fractures may also occur in cases of laminitis or deep puncture wounds. These fractures are probably due to thrombosis of the smaller vessels in the corium, causing demineralization of the third phalanx.

Contracted Heels

Although the name of this condition indicates the heels are narrower than normal, the entire foot may be involved. The front feet are more commonly affected.

Cause: Contracted heels usually result from a lack of proper frog pressure, due to improper foot care or to a pathologic condition of one or both front feet severe enough to cause the horse to avoid bearing weight properly on the heels. Contracted heels are seen frequently in Tennessee Walking horses and American Saddlebred horses if their feet are allowed to grow long for show purposes. Proper frog pressure is hard to maintain with excessively long feet. Contraction of the heels might accompany a case of thrush involving the entire frog.

Diagnosis: Contracted heels usually occur secondary to another condition. The primary lesion or cause should be identified before a diagnosis of contracted heels is made. A unilaterally affected foot is typically smaller than the opposite one, particularly in the heel. The frog is recessed and atrophied. A difference in size may not be apparent when both feet are involved.

Treatment: The primary lesion responsible for the contracted heels should be treated in conjunction with therapy for the heel. The object of therapy is to re-establish normal frog pressure. Corrective trimming after shoe removal is helpful in some cases. The horny wall over the quarters should be rasped thin to allow expansion and a hoof dressing applied to keep the foot soft. The quarters should be rasped very thin (½ inch) distal to the coronary band and tapered so the distal surface is of normal thickness.

Slipper shoes should be applied when corrective shoeing is necessary. These are shoes in which the web in contact with the wall at the quarter is tapered. When the foot bears weight, the walls slip laterad from the midline (Fig 87). A heel spring of spring steel can be applied to keep constant pressure on the bar of the foot (Fig 88).[2,9,14] This spring is applied under a full pad and shoe to keep it in position. It may cause lameness for a few days after the shoe is applied but phenylbutazone helps alleviate the lameness. Another way to expand the quarter

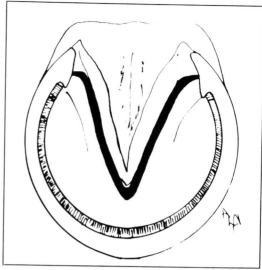

Fig 88. A heel spring helps expand the heels. This spring should always be used with a full pad and shoe.

is to groove it with a series of vertical lines, with the first line at the cranial tip of the lateral cartilage. The wall is then trimmed short in the quarter and a pressure "T" bar shoe is applied. This shoe has a bar that causes considerable pressure on the frog (Fig 89).

Prognosis: The prognosis depends primarily on correction of the condition that caused improper frog pressure.

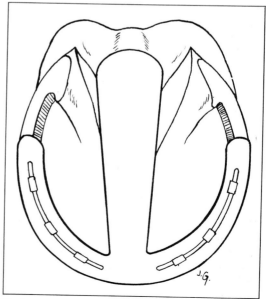

Fig 89. A T-bar shoe.

Sheared Heels

Improper balancing of the foot is a major source of lameness. The foot is balanced when its position in relation to the limb is such that the weight is equally distributed over the foot.

Cause: Improper trimming and shoeing are the most common causes of sheared heels. For example, it is difficult for a right-handed farrier to avoid lowering the lateral heel of the left front foot more than the medial side due to the difficult position required to nip or rasp the medial side of the heel. The reverse is true on the opposite foot or with a left-handed farrier.[15]

Diagnosis: Viewing the feet from directly behind the horse is a good way to assess the heels. The coronary band should be viewed with the horse bearing full weight on the feet to see if the heels have the proper flair. Observe the horse at a walk, trot and with a rider if needed. A local nerve block may be helpful in confirming the diagnosis.

Treatment: Therapy is aimed at restoring proper heel alignment and foot balance.[15] A shorter toe and an elevated heel may help correct the problem, but the simplest method is to remove the shoes.[16]

Burst Heels

This is a condition in which one or both sides of the heels, at the junction of the heel and frog, crack and become quite sore. The rear feet are more commonly affected.

Cause: Affected horses typically have large frogs that are compressed against a dry, contracted hoof. Over-reaching is another cause.

Diagnosis: Visual inspection of the affected hoof is sufficient.

Treatment: Restoration of normal hoof moisture to allow proper hoof expansion and trimming the sides of the frog are of some benefit. Application of topical medication to relieve inflammation and to keep the lesion dry is also beneficial.

Navicular Bursitis

Inflammation of the navicular bursa is seen most frequently in young horses (2-3 years old) that are beginning training.

Clinical Signs: It may appear as an acute or intermittent lameness of one or both front feet. Affected horses usually favor one foot over the other, are reluctant to move and have a short, choppy gait. Discontinuing training, even for a short time, usually results in improvement. Acutely affected horses may spend a great deal of time lying down or pawing and pulling a pile of bedding up under the heels of the front feet and bracing their rear against the stall wall. The horse may be presented for apparent shoulder or rear-leg lameness.

Diagnosis: Navicular bursitis is difficult to diagnose since it must be differentiated from other conditions of the caudal third of the foot. Differential diagnoses include improper trimming and shoeing, bruised heels, subsolar abscess, severe thrush, and fractures of the third phalanx or navicular bone.

The shoeing must be evaluated carefully as to when the shoes were reset, additions or changes in the shoes, and altered joint angles. A hoof tester is useful in assessing painful areas of the foot.

Palmar digital nerve blocks are very helpful in establishing the location of the primary lameness. Negative radiographic findings, in conjunction with an improvement in gait following a palmar digital nerve block, may suggest a diagnosis of navicular bursitis after other conditions are ruled out.

Treatment: Since the cause of navicular bursitis is probably a combination of direct trauma and improper trimming and shoeing, therapy is aimed at preventing the initiating cause. Rest is important during the acute phase and exercise should be limited. Corrective shoeing to establish the proper angle may help if the horse has minimal heel; if the feet are long, the toe may be trimmed and the feet left bare.

Administration of nonsteroidal anti-inflammatory drugs, such as phenylbutazone, meclofenamic acid, naproxen or flunixin meglumine, provides some relief. These drugs may be used separately or in combination to effect. The dosage recommended by the manufacturer should be used initially, but can be increased to up to twice the recommended dosage if there is no apparent effect.

Local (juxtabursal) injections of orgotein should be considered in conjunction with systemic medication or in lieu of systemic medication if the horse cannot be treated daily or refuses to eat oral medication. Local injections, when effective, may relieve the condition sufficiently to resume training. If one injection does not help, a second may be tried within 5-7 days. Other methods should be tried if there is no improvement within 2 days of the second injection. Local injection of orgotein helps to some degree in 70-75% of cases with no radiographic changes.

Another method of treating navicular bursitis is direct (intrabursal) injection of the bursa with orgotein or a corticosteroid (see Navicular Disease). Extreme care should be taken when entering the bursa to prevent sepsis and to avoid damaging the articular cartilage. These factors make the juxtabursal technic preferable.

Cryogesia of the palmar digital nerves may be considered as an adjunct to therapy to allow time for proper foot care. This noninvasive cryotherapeutic technic consists of applying a small probe to the skin to block the nerve after the area has been aseptically prepared. The nerve may be palpated easily over the lateral border of the sesamoid and can be held over the base of the sesamoid with a finger while the blunt cryoprobe is applied. The probe is pressed against the skin over the nerve until the nerve "sticks" or freezes to the deeper structures and cannot be moved or rolled with the finger. The duration of application varies with the cryosurgical unit used, ambient temperature and humidity. A period as short as 20 seconds or as long as 2 minutes may be required to produce the desired ice ball. When the ice ball thaws, a second application is necessary to produce the desired effects. Skin necrosis may result if the cryoprobe is held in contact too long. Although the blood supply to the foot is decreased during ice ball formation because the nerve is so close to the artery and vein, the short duration of decreased blood supply does not result in complications. Aftercare consists of application of an antibacterial ointment and support bandage. A small blister may form within 12-24 hours and rupture, leaving a raw lesion that forms a scab and heals in 7-10 days. White hair grows in the area where the probe was applied. This technic offers the advantages of being noninvasive and not causing neuroma formation. The disadvantages are the growth of white hair, inconsistent efficacy and short duration (2-4 months) of efficacy. Some horses do not respond at all and others respond only for a few days, with less than 50% showing some improvement in gait for up to 4 months. In the case of navicular bursitis, this may be sufficient time for the horse to recover from the initial inflammation and also allow enough time for the feet to grow and be trimmed properly.

Neurectomy of the palmar digital nerves should be considered only as the last resort since navicular bursitis is seen primarily in young horses.

Navicular Disease

Navicular disease or podotrochleosis describes a number of pathologic conditions af-

fecting the distal sesamoid or navicular bone. This shuttle-shaped bone is situated on the caudal aspect between the distal interphalangeal joint and deep flexor tendon. The navicular bone has 2 surfaces that articulate with the second and third phalanges on one side and the deep flexor tendon on the other. The distal interphalangeal joint and the navicular bursa, situated between the navicular bone and deep flexor tendon, do not communicate.[18]

Cause: The factors that contribute to navicular disease are not clearly defined, although several have been incriminated. Pathologic changes occur on the side that contacts the tendon and not on the side that articulates with the distal interphalangeal joint.[19,20] This condition does not fit the description of an osteoarthritic disease. Although conformation and injury could be the most important etiologic factors, nutritional and hormonal influences should not be excluded.

Certain conformation, such as an upright pastern and shoulder, increases concussion on the navicular bone. The weight transmitted to the navicular bone by the first and second phalanx forces the navicular bone against the deep flexor tendon. Articular cartilage and deep flexor tendon damage results when vibration of the navicular bone against the deep flexor tendon causes excessive friction.[21] A horse with a small foot in proportion to body size is predisposed to this condition since the small foot must absorb proportionately more concussive forces.

Recent work suggests that navicular disease is caused by ischemia of the navicular bone due to progressive arterila occlusion. At least 2 primary arteries, with some involvement of the collateral blood supply, must be occluded before lameness occurs.[22]

Diagnosis: Most affected horses are 4-9 years old. Males are more often affected than females, geldings more often than stallions, and Quarter Horses more often than other breeds.[23] Navicular disease usually involves both front feet, but the lameness in one foot is more severe. The more severely affected foot is contracted in chronic cases.

In the initial stages of navicular disease, the horse does not stride out properly, wears the toes excessively, and is inclined to stumble. This is followed by slight lameness which, with exercise, may disappear; gradually over a period it does not. When resting, the horse may point one toe or stand with both feet extended further outward than normal. Barefooted horses wear their toes short and square, bruise their toes and grow their heels long. Shod horses wear the toes of the shoes excessively.

When lameness becomes continuous, the horse takes short strides and the rider may report that the animal is sore in the shoulders. Secondary bicipital bursitis may develop, and the horse exhibits pain when digital pressure is applied to the bicipital bursa. Lameness is accentuated when the horse is jogged on a hard surface in tight circles. Hoof testers applied over the navicular bursa usually elicit pain.

A palmar digital nerve block, excluding the caudal branch just proximal to the alteral cartilage, helps diagnose this condition. This block minimizes the possibility of anesthetizing too much of the foot. If the nerve is blocked close to the cranial branch, the anesthetic solution may spread and block the entire foot. One must avoid improperly diagnosing navicular disease when lameness is relieved by a palmar digital nerve block.

Radiographs of the navicular area aid in diagnosis and prognosis. Careful attention should be given to positioning the navicular bone for radiography.[24] If the radiographs of the navicular area are interpreted as normal, other problems that could affect the heel must be considered in the diagnosis, such as bruised heels or corns. Navicular bursitis also has negative radiographic findings.

A distinction should be made radiographically as to the bony changes before giving a prognosis and speculating on successful therapy. Normal vascular channels on the distal border of the navicular bone are cone-shaped, whereas pathologic changes create a "lollipop" appearance of vascular channels.[25] Spurs on the lateral borders of the navicular bone denote tearing of the collateral ligaments. Bone cysts appear as large osteolytic areas generally close to the distal border of the bone. There is no correlation between the radiographic changes and the type of work for which the horse has been used.[23] Often the foot with the more severe lameness is not the foot with the most obvious radiographic changes. Therefore, both front feet should be radiographed when navicular disease is suspected.

Treatment: True navicular disease is incurable, but palliative measures may alleviate pain and prolong the horse's usefulness. Rest and correct shoeing may be beneficial in cases of navicular bursitis with no radiographic changes of the navicular bone. Corrective shoeing consists of keeping the toe short and

the heels elevated. The toe can be square and rolled or rockered to help the foot break over faster. The heels of the shoe are elevated with heel calks or the branches of the shoe are rolled back to increase their height. If a bar shoe is used to protect the frog, the web of the shoe should be slippered so the foot can expand when it contacts the shoe. Contracted heels can occur with a bar shoe unless the shoe is made and reset properly. Some lameness attributed to navicular disease may be relieved when a heel spring is applied under a full pad. This spring puts constant lateral pressure on the bars of the feet and allows the foot to expand. Its application should be considered if there is any sign of contracted heels and can be used in conjunction with a bar shoe.

Horses with navicular disease should be exercised. Any horse with a chronic lameness needs a certain amount of exercise daily, such as long walks or ad libitum exercise in a large paddock, for proper hoof growth and maintenance of muscle tone.

Anti-inflammatory medication, such as phenylbutazone, meclofenamic acid, flunixin meglumine or naproxen, can be used alone or in combination. The response of individual horses varies, so trial and error is the only way to find the best drug or combination. Horses not ridden consistently should only be treated before exercise and should not receive medication continuously. For horses in training, drug administration should be correlated with days of strenuous exercise. For example, a race horse that is to "breeze" should receive medication in the feed the evening before the day of the work, if needed, and then not receive it for the next 3-4 days. Corticosteroids can be used in navicular disease but are not recommended over nonsteroidal drugs because of the side effects of long-term therapy. Short-term therapy with moderate doses usually has no side effects.

Local and/or systemic injections of orgotein provide relief in some cases of navicular disease.[26] Horses with the poorest response to this therapy are those with cysts or "lollipops" on the distal border of the navicular bone. The technic for local injection of orgotein is to block the foot with a palmar nerve block and surgically scrub the heel. A 20-ga, 1-inch needle is inserted on the midline just dorsal to the heel in the direction of the toe, with the horse supporting weight on the limb. Picking up the opposite limb during this procedure may be helpful. The injection can be given using a nose twitch as the only restraint, but this may compromise needle placement. The hub of the needle and the syringe should be held tightly to prevent spillage while 1 ml orgotein is injected at the full depth of the needle. The needle should be repositioned if injection is difficult. If injection is extremely easy, the orgotein is probably being injected into the deep flexor tendon sheath.

Horses with "lollipop" lesions on the distal border have a poor prognosis and a neurectomy may be required to return them to usefulness. Palmar digital neurectomy involves surgically preparing the limb 24 hours before surgery and wrapping the limb with a sterile wrap after application of povidone iodine or comparable bacteriocidal solution. The limb is prepared a second time immediately before surgery. Neurectomy can be performed using local anesthesia of the palmar nerve several inches proximal to the incision site or a general anesthetic can be administered before positioning the horse in lateral or dorsal recumbency.

The site for incision is the lateral border of the deep flexor tendon distal to the level of the middle of the first phalanx. The nerve should be located by palpation before making the incision. A short incision, up to an inch long, is made parallel to the deep flexor tendon and a hemostat is used for blunt dissection. Care should be taken not to damage the digital artery and vein, which are in close proximity to the nerve. The nerve should not be confused with the ligament of the ergot. Once the nerve is located it can be positively identified by rolling it with the thumb nail over the hemostat; it should roll like a cable or rope with its many fibers. If in doubt, a small-gauge needle (22-25 ga) can be inserted to see if the structure contains blood. If doubt still remains, suture material can be placed around the structure and retracted until the artery, vein and nerve are identified. The nerve is severed and a hemostat is used to pull the nerve distad before transecting it proximad. At least an inch of nerve should be removed. The cut nerve should retract up the limb subcutaneously away from the incision site; this helps prevent a painful neuroma. Painful neuromas are the most frequent complications following neurectomy.

The technic that probably results in the least number of painful neuromas is the neurolemma sheathing technic. With the horse under general anesthesia, the nerve is transected and the severed proximal end grasped with a hemostat. A small scalpel blade is used to carefully incise the epineurial (perineurial) sheath

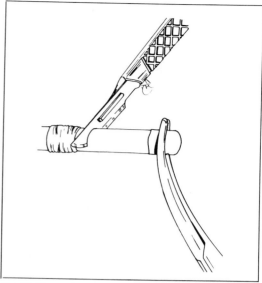

Fig 90. The exposed neurofibrils are transected distal to the reflected neurolemma sheath.

around the entire nerve. The sheath is carefully teased proximad up the nerve for ½-1 inch and the exposed nerve fascicles are transected just distal to the reflected sheath (Fig 90). The loose end of the sheath is ligated over the nerve stump using 3-0 to 5-0 silk, and the subcutaneous tissue and skin are closed in 2 layers. A recent report describes use of a double freeze-thaw cycle on the exposed nerve fascicles after the epineurial/perineurial sheath is reflected.[28] The sheath is then pulled over the end of the fascicles and secured with a single suture. The incidence of painful neuroma was 15% when this technic was used on horses with painful neuroma and only 4% in horses with no previous neurectomy. The legs are wrapped until the sutures are removed in 7-10 days. Additional wrapping may be necessary if the legs swell due to inactivity. Exercise is restricted to hand-walking for 10-15 minutes twice daily for 3 weeks after suture removal, at which time the horse can be returned to light training or turned out. Postoperative rest for 4 weeks appears to lessen the degree of painful neuroma formation.[27]

An alternative to neurectomy in treatment of horses with "lollipop" lesions is a regimen of anticoagulation therapy.[25] Dicumarol (warfarin sodium) is administered PO daily at 0.018 mg/kg body weight. It is important to establish the individual dosage since overdosage can be fatal. In doing so, a base-line, one-stage prothrombin time (normal range 10-16 seconds) must be established. The dicumarol is then administered daily and prothrombin time is monitored twice weekly with the objective of a 2- to 4-second increase; the prothrombin time should not double. If the prothrombin time is not prolonged after 10 days, dosage should be increased by not more than 20%. Once the dosage is established, which may take up to 6 weeks, a prothrombin time should be conducted every 2 months as long as the horse is on medication. The dosage may vary with feeding and management practices. This therapy may prolong the life of affected horses considerably and is completely effective in 80% of the cases treated. Phenylbutazone must not be administered in conjunction with anticoagulant therapy because of the risk of fatal hemorrhage or hemorrhage into a joint.

Navicular Bone Fracture

Cause: Transverse fractures of the navicular bone are thought to be traumatic in origin, as from stepping on a small stone while traveling at a fast pace. Rear-leg navicular fractures could occur from kicking a solid object. The cause of small fractures of the distal border is uncertain. They could be associated with circulatory problems, as mentioned under Navicular Disease, since these are usually observed in horses in the navicular disease age group.

Diagnosis: An acute transverse navicular fracture could be confused with a subsolar abscess, fracture of the third phalanx, or congenital "nonfusion" of the navicular bone. The pain is relieved with a palmar digital nerve block. Definitive diagnosis is by radiography.

Treatment: Transverse navicular fractures offer a poor prognosis because synovial and joint fluid at the fracture site delay healing. Acute fractures may be treated the same as third phalanx fractures by using a bar shoe and side clips. If there is no improvement after 4-6 months of confinement and use of this shoe, a palmar digital neurectomy may be the treatment of choice. Old fractures may not appear healed radiographically, but the horse no longer favors the limb.

Small distal border fractures are probably best treated by a palmar digital neurectomy since all affected horses have radiographic evidence of navicular disease.

Other Navicular Diseases

Congenital absence of part or all of the navicular bone has been observed. Affected horses may or may not be lame; however, the prognosis for normal function is poor. Separate centers of ossification of "nonfusion" of the navicular bone must be distinguished from navicular fractures.

Laminitis

Laminitis is defined as an inflammation of the pedal laminae. All 4 feet can be affected but the front are involved more frequently. The acute stage is manifested by extreme pain, a bounding digital pulse, and warm or hot feet. The chronic stage is manifested by intermittent or persistent lameness and a diverging growth pattern around the hoof wall. The sole of the foot is usually dropped due to rotation of the third phalanx.

Cause: Recent research has made progress in identifying some of the changes that occur in this multifaceted disease process.[29] Overeating grain appears to be the most common cause of laminitis. Retained placenta can cause refractory laminitis. Drug-induced laminitis has been observed when conditioned horses in training are treated with corticosteroiods systemically or locally and stressed after such therapy. Laminitis has also been related to excessive water consumption immediately after exercise ("water founder") and related to exercise ("road founder"). Excessive trimming of all 4 feet has also caused laminitis.

Horses and particularly ponies may develop laminitis ("pasture founder") in the spring when grass is lush. Although affected horses and ponies have probably grazed the same pasture for several years, there is a drastic change in feed content when the new grass comes out in the spring. These horses are usually fat and may have a thick, fat (cresty) neck. Such horses may be hypothyroid and usually suffer from chronic laminitis after the acute episode. The laminitis flares up each spring as the pasture changes unless the time on pasture is restricted. After 1-2 weeks of adjustment, the horses can be left on the pasture. This same cycle of recurrence can repeat itself if the season is dry and considerable rain allows new grass growth.

In the case of carbohydrate overload, lactic acid-producing bacteria proliferate in the cecum. These bacteria (*Lactobacillus, Streptococcus* and *Bacillus*) subsequently release an abundance of lactic acid, causing the intracecal pH to decline from 7 to 4 within 24 hours. The lactic acid may be absorbed into the extracellular fluid to produce lactic acidosis. The rapid decline in intracecal pH kills the *Enterobacteria*, causing liberation of endotoxins in the cecum.

High levels of lactic acid and endotoxin probably result in severe mucosal damage to the intestine. The endotoxin absorption could then be related to the severity of mucosal damage. Therefore, laminitis could be due to the combined effects of increases in plasma lactate and endotoxin levels. Changes in the cecal lactate and endotoxin levels can be observed as soon as 3 hours after carbohydrate overload. The lameness associated with carbohydrate overload is thought to occur 16-24 hours postingestion.[30] Aortic blood flow, heart rate and mean arterial pressure were significantly higher in experimentally induced laminitis and mean plasma volume was significantly decreased.[31] There is an increase in blood flow to the digit but the blood is shunted by arteriovenous shunts and does not reach the laminae.[32,33] This conclusion is supported by the finding of ischemic necrosis in histopathologic studies of the laminar architecture.[34] Serum testosterone levels were elevated in geldings and mares with clinical signs of laminitis. The elevation in serum androgen levels in mares and geldings suggests adrenal involvement.[35]

Diagnosis of Acute Laminitis: The front, rear or all 4 feet may be affected in acute laminitis. Lameness develops rapidly. If only the front feet are involved, the horse places the rear limbs under the body to take weight off the front feet. The abdominal and back muscles are tensed to help support the weight on the hind limbs. If only the rear feet are involved, the horse generally shifts its weight continually from one rear foot to the other. If all 4 feet are involved, the horse stands with all 4 feet under

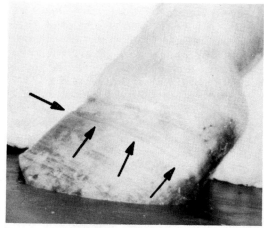

Fig 91. A hoof with divergent growth lines as a result of chronic laminitis. Heel growth has exceeded toe growth.

its body, occasionally shifting weight, and is very reluctant to move. Severely affected horses may be recumbent and only stand when forced.

The feet are very hot and the digital arteries pulsate quite strongly. Some affected horses have signs of endotoxic shock and diarrhea. If the coronary band is sunken, the case is probably beyond the acute phase.

Diagnosis of Chronic Laminitis: The condition may become chronic after the acute phase has passed. Severe lameness may or may not be evident and acute recurrence is not uncommon. Fat horses and ponies turned out to pasture may become acutely lame due to the sudden change in pasture as the lush grass returns in the spring, as previously mentioned.

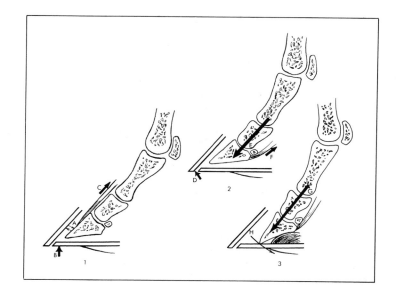

Fig 92. (1) The normal hoof is supported by the interlocking force (A), reciprocal force (B) and lifting force (C). (2) Os pedis rotation involves the tearing force (D), driving force (E) and pulling force (F). (3) The animal's weight (G) tends to force the laminae (H) away from the horny wall, while the deep flexor tendon and digital cushion act as a fulcrum.

The hemogram and total serum cholesterol and SGOT levels should be monitored in intractable cases of chronic laminitis. Evidence of fatty infiltration of the liver, hypercholesteremia and increased SGOT activity should prompt therapy besides care of the feet.[36,37]

A dropped sole, bilateral lameness and a diverging growth line in the hoof wall at the heel indicate chronic laminitis (Fig 91). A diverging line indicates more heel growth when compared with toe growth because the blood supply to the toe is decreased in the initial phase, interfering with biosynthesis of hoof keratin. Rotation of the tip of the third phalanx, as a result of the deep flexor tendon's pull against the inflamed laminae, can be demonstrated radiographically (Fig 92). A separation between the wall and sole may be found at the toe in the region of the white line. The bottom of the foot is not concave as normal and may be flat. The white line at the toe is wider than at the heel due to separation of the laminae as the third phalanx rotates.

Although a diagnosis of laminitis is usually not difficult to make, a palmar nerve block is useful in some cases. It alleviates lameness provided the feet are not grossly overgrown. As in all lameness examinations, a palmar digital nerve block should be done first to rule out other conditions; this block may result in some improvement in gait.

Treatment of Acute Laminitis: The first consideration in treatment is to control the basic cause, such as enterotoxemia and endotoxic shock associated with grain overload. Fluid volume replacement can be critical and should be assessed immediately. The use of corticosteroids may be indicated in the initial shock therapy only as a one-time treatment since prolonged use may worsen the condition. One dose of furosemide may be beneficial, but daily administration could produce chronic laminitis and alter electrolyte balance. Mineral oil should be given for its laxative effect and to prevent further absorption of endotoxins.

A palmar nerve block re-establishes blood supply to the toe so keratin synthesis is not disturbed.[38] The sole should be filled with plaster of Paris to help prevent third phalanx rotation. A limited amount of exercise may be beneficial in early cases, such as 10 minutes every hour until the horse walks sound or 24-36 hours have passed. In the latter case, the laminitis is probably more chronic in nature than was initially thought. The laminae are permanently damaged and the blood supply cannot be entirely restored after the local nerve block if laminitis has existed for more than 12-18 hours. In some cases it may be necessary to repeat the local block 2-3 times daily for no more than 2 days. If nerve blocks are impractical, a mixture of DMSO and local anesthetic painted from the carpus to the hoof has produced almost the same effect. Anti-inflammatory drugs should be given in larger than normal doses, such as 4-6 g phenylbutazone BID for adult horses. The use of corticosteroids is contraindicated because they delay or inhibit keratin synthesis.[38]

Adrenocorticotropic hormone (ACTH) is reportedly effective in the treatment of acute laminitis because of its indirect effect on blood osmolarity.[17] It has also been used as an adjunct to other therapy for chronic laminitis.[36]

Although antihistamines have been reported to be effective in treating some horses with acute laminitis, the results of recent studies do not support the use of antihistamines in treating laminitis.[39-41]

Since there is a lack of perfusion to the pedal laminae, standing acutely affected horses in cold water may be beneficial to decrease the O_2 requirements of the ischemic laminae.

Administration of heparin at 30-40 million U/kg body weight every 4 hours until the partial thromboplastin level is increased 4 times normal level may help prevent thrombosis in the capillaries.[42] This may benefit acutely affected horses before laminar ischemia has caused irreversible changes.

Arterial blood pressure is elevated in acute laminitis and may be lowered with small doses of a phenothiazine tranquilizer and removal of all salt from the ration.[43] Venous blood has been withdrawn in various volumes and injected into cervical and limb muscles. The injected blood is thought to stimulate adrenal gland secretion of glucocorticoids, which may improve the horse's gait.

Treatment of Chronic Laminitis: Standing the horse in a cool stream has been a traditional treatment for chronic laminitis. There is no clear contraindication for such treatment if the sole is intact, since it may help relieve pain.

Corrective trimming should be the main approach to making the horse sound enough for work. The heels should be lowered but not to the point of standing solely on the frog, since this compresses the existing blood supply in that area and may cause additional problems. The toe should be rasped down over the cranial aspect if the wall is deviated or concave ("dished"). Radiography is essential to assess the rotation and condition of the third phalanx. Corrective shoeing may be used to improve the angle of rotation of the third phalanx. Repair of the wall defect can be accomplished with acrylic but this practice is not as popular now as previously.[6,37] A reverse-wedge pad and a wide bar shoe are used most frequently (Fig 93). The bar of the shoe should begin at the apex of the frog and extend to the heel. The sole should be trimmed first so there is some concavity left and the bar does not compress the wall-sole-frog. If the sole is tender, it should be painted with equal parts phenol, formalin and iodine ("sole paint"). A compressing bar could cause necrosis and rupture of the sole, with the corium penetrating through the opening, due to compromise of the impaired blood flow.

Additional therapy depends on the individual horse and the damage produced to other body systems during the acute attack. A hemogram and a blood chemistry profile may provide guidance for additional therapy. Hypertensive horses should be put on a salt-free diet and the ration should be supplemented with 1 oz KC twice daily in the water. Grain intake should be restricted or eliminated and a good-quality (preferably alfalfa) hay should be offered free choice. Supplementation of methionine (10 g daily) is useful in treating laminitis since it and cystine are essential for keratinization of the hoof.[44]

Horses that repeatedly have acute recurrences of laminitis while on lush grass in the spring should be fed dry feed during this period. Thyroid extract may be beneficial if these horses are overly fat.[45-47]

If the corium of the sole or the third phalanx penetrates through the sole, the chance of recovery beyond hobbling around is very slim (Fig 94). Inferior check desmotomy or deep flexor tenotomy has been attempted with varying degrees of success. Application of sole paint over a very tender sole that appears ready to open may toughen it and, with a thickly padded bandage, may prevent the corium from perforating the sole. Once the corium is exposed, the feet must be protected with a strong, clean bandage. A supersaturated solution of magnesium sulfate should be applied if there is any evidence of purulence. If the exposed corium is relatively dry, it should be painted with sole paint and kept wrapped. A shoe and pad can be applied if the horse responds in a week or so.

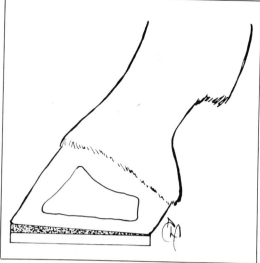

Fig 93. Proper trimming and shoeing with a reverse wedge pad in chronic laminitis.

Antibiotics should be administered to all affected horses over a period of several weeks due to the high incidence of abscesses. If the horse does not have decubiti from being recumbent, administration of isoniazid at 4-6 mg/lb body weight for 2 weeks, then at 2-3 mg/lb for 30-60 days, may also help. Nonsteroidal anti-inflammatory medication should be administered in sufficient amounts to control severe pain and to aid in getting the horse on its feet. The legs should be massaged at least once daily and

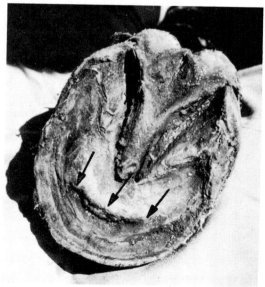

Fig 94. Os pedis rotated through the sole.

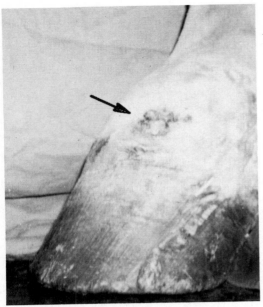

Fig 95. Draining tract proximal to the coronary band as a result of necrosis of the lateral cartilage.

wrapped if they swell. Exercise should be limited to short walks or turning out in a small paddock. Daily vigorous foot care is needed; if this is not available, it may be best to euthanize the horse. Continued weight loss during the course of laminitis indicates a malabsorption problem. A glucose-tolerance test is indicated to diagnose such a development. These horses eat continuously, pass voluminous amounts of feces and constantly lose weight. The eventual outcome is death.

Prognosis: Some horses with acute laminitis respond to therapy without developing secondary complications, such as os pedis rotation; however, others develop complications that may cause recurrent problems. Although horses with chronic laminitis are prone to acute attacks, they can usually be kept reasonably sound by trimming their feet, shoeing them properly and providing a proper ration.

The prognosis is poor when the tip of the third phalanx rotates and penetrates through the sole. Some affected animals recover, but their lameness is usually quite evident. Therapy is futile in some cases and euthanasia may be the only approach.

Ossification of the Lateral Cartilages

Cause: The cause of ossification of the lateral cartilages ("sidebones") is not always clear, but conformation, concussion and direct trauma have been incriminated.[8,9] Ossification of the lateral cartilages occurs primarily in the front feet.

Diagnosis: Sidebones usually is diagnosed by palpation or radiography. Lameness is not common, but inability of the foot and lateral cartilages to expand normally can predispose to corns or other lesions, such as contracted heels. Although large ossified cartilages may cause lameness by impinging on the second phalanx, several oblique radiographs should be obtained before sidebones is incriminated as the origin of a lameness.

Treatment: No treatment is required if neither pain nor lameness is associated with an ossified lateral cartilage. An ossified cartilage can be removed surgically, but in most cases this is done for cosmetic reasons. A fractured ossified cartilage, not to be confused with 2 separate ossification centers on radiographs, requires surgical intervention or confinement of the horse to a stall.[48]

When an affected foot is contracted, the walls at the heel should be rasped thin or grooved to allow expansion (see Contracted Heels). If the foot is shod, the web of the shoe should be slipped to allow expansion and the last heel nail omitted.

Prognosis: The prognosis is favorable unless the exostosis impinges on the second phalanx. An affected foot appears deformed unless the calcified cartilage is removed.

Necrosis of the Lateral Cartilage

"Quittor" is the term used to describe purulent inflammation and necrosis of a lateral cartilage.

Cause: The most common cause of lateral cartilage necrosis is a puncture wound or laceration proximal to the coronary band in the region of the lateral cartilages. Necrosis results because the cartilage has a limited blood supply and the wounds are usually contaminated. Either deep puncture wounds of the sole or an interfering gait may also result in necrosis of a lateral cartilage.

Diagnosis: This condition should be suspected with any painful swelling over a lateral cartilage and when lameness improves after rupture of such swelling, followed by drainage of a purulent exudate (Fig 95). The degree of lameness increases every month or so as the pressure of the purulent exudate increases and decreases when the lesion drains.

Treatment: The treatment of choice is surgical removal of the necrotic cartilage and surrounding affected tissue.

Pyramidal Disease

This condition refers to periostitis of the extensor or pyramidal process of the third phalanx. The term "buttress foot" is also used to describe the lesion.

Cause: The periostitis that develops around the pyramidal process results from tearing of fibers of the common digital extensor tendon at its insertion on the pyramidal process of the third phalanx.

Diagnosis: Heat, swelling and sensitivity are apparent in the early stages at the coronary band on the dorsal midline of the foot. The horse may be lame when worked and point the foot when at rest. As the condition progresses, a bulge becomes evident at the coronary band; in time the foot contracts. The appearance of the foot is suggestive of a buttress.

This condition could be confused with fracture of the pyramidal process of the third phalanx because the associated lamenesses are similar. Nerve blocks help localize the lesion, and radiographs can differentiate between periostitis and fracture of the pyramidal process.

Treatment: In the early stages, rasping the hoof wall distal to the coronary band at the toe may relieve pressure and be of temporary benefit. Radiation therapy should be considered to curtail excessive periostitis. Blistering the area has been advocated, but its value is doubtful. Although anti-inflammatory drugs may relieve clinical signs temporarily, the lameness is eventually only relieved by a cranial neurectomy or bilateral low-volar neurectomy, which could result in such complications as loss of the hoof wall.[10] Surgical removal of the fragment should be considered if there is a chip fracture at the pyramidal process.

Prognosis: The prognosis is unfavorable.

Fracture of the Extensor Process of the Third Phalanx

This fracture occurs primarily in the front feet. It is frequently seen in both front feet; therefore, radiographs should be taken of both feet before deciding on therapy.

Cause: The etiology, other than trauma, is not clearly defined. If lesions are seen in both front feet, for example, conformation must be considered as part of the problem. Separate ossifying centers may also weaken the extensor process and allow separation.

Diagnosis: In the acute stages with only one foot involved, lateral radiographs readily reveal such fractures. The hoof wall may change shape in the chronic stage. Excessive perios-

teal new bone growth is present radiographically, lameness is apparent and pain may be evidenced on palpation of the coronary band.

Treatment: Therapy is usually of little value if both front or rear feet are involved, as evidenced by radiographic evaluation. If only one foot is involved, the fracture is acute and the fragment large, one should consider attaching the fragment to the parent bone using a lag screw.[9] Fragment removal may be the best treatment if the fracture is chronic or the fragment too small to use a lag screw. Surgical removal of the fragment is usually of limited value if periosteal new bone growth is excessive on the third and the second phalanx.

Fragment removal involves rasping the hoof wall down to the white line from the coronary band distad down the hoof for about an inch. The hoof should be thoroughly scrubbed and bandaged in an antiseptic bandage for 12 hours preoperatively. This surgery is best conducted under general anesthesia with the horse in lateral recumbency. An incision is made on the midline starting about an inch proximal to the coronary band extending through the coronary band and distad into the hoof itself. The extensor tendon is divided longitudinally between the fibers to expose the fragment, which is removed by blunt dissection with a periosteal elevator. The extensor tendon fibers are pulled back together with 0 or 00 absorbable sutures. The subcutaneous tissue is closed in a separate layer and the skin is closed with nonabsorbable sutures in an interrupted pattern. A snug bandage should be applied to cover the entire foot. If a screw is used to secure a large fragment, a cast is applied before recovery from anesthesia. The cast should be changed in 2-3 weeks and reapplied for an additional 2-3 weeks, at which point radiography may help dictate continued use or removal of the cast.

Horses that are not surgical candidates may benefit from corrective shoeing, such as a short rolled toe.

Prognosis: The prognosis should be guarded to poor in all cases. Periodic radiographs are of benefit in prognostication.

Osteoarthritis of the Distal Interphalangeal Joint

The term "ringbone" refers to any bony enlargement below the fetlock, whether or not a joint is involved (Fig 96). "True ringbone" refers to osteoarthritis of the proximal or distal interphalangeal joint, and "false ringbone" to periarticular periostitis of the involved pha-

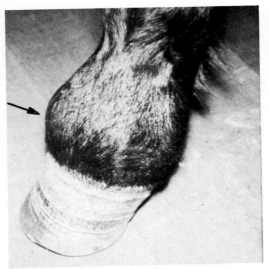

Fig 96. Enlargement proximal to the coronary band (ringbone).

lanx. "True or articular low ringbone" affects the coffin joint, and "true or articular high ringbone" involves the pastern.

Cause: Trauma is the usual cause of osteoarthritis. When the joints are injured severely enough to cause articular lesions, there usually is some tearing of the collateral ligament and fibrous joint capsule. This results in a periosteal reaction that is later evident grossly.

Conformation can predispose a horse to excessive trauma on one area of a joint and lead to articular involvement and collateral ligament stretching or tearing. In base-narrow horses, for example, more weight is borne on the lateral articular cartilage; the opposite is true with a base-wide conformation. When a base-narrow or base-wide conformation exists in conjunction with toeing-in or toeing-out, the consequent rotating effect on the joint stretches or tears the collateral ligaments.[9,21] The cause of osteoarthritis from osteoporosis and breakdown of subchondral bone is undetermined. Rarefaction of subchondral bone may result from impaired blood supply to the area. This lesion may be observed early, suggesting osteochondritis dissecans.

Diagnosis: Osteoarthritis may affect all 4 limbs, but the front are more commonly involved. A history of acute lameness and swelling of the affected joint is typical of osteoarthritis of the interphalangeal joint. In some cases the lameness may develop gradually.

Extreme flexion of the limb accentuates lameness. Nerve blocks or ring blocks are very helpful in diagnosing and localizing the lesion. Radiographs also help identify and locate the lesion unless periostitis has not developed. Periarticular osteophytes develop in advanced cases, making it difficult or impossible to determine whether the primary lesion was articular or periarticular.

Treatment: Treatment involves attempts to temporarily relieve pain or ankylosis of the involved joint. The coffin joint can be ankylosed but this procedure results in permanent lameness. Pain may be relieved temporarily by injecting the joint with a corticosteroid or by administering phenylbutazone. Either treatment has limited value and may lead to further destruction of the joint.

Prognosis: A poor prognosis is indicated. Some movement is necessary in the coffin joint for the horse to walk sound.

Periostitis of the Distal Interphalangeal Joint

This condition has been referred to as "false or periarticular low ringbone."

Cause: Tearing or stretching of the collateral ligaments can result in perarticular periostitis. Toe-in or toe-out conformation predisposes to this condition by excessive strain on the collateral ligaments.[9]

Diagnosis: Sudden tearing or stretching of the collateral ligaments causes severe lameness. The lesion may be located by heat, pain and swelling around the coronary band. A ring block just proximal to the coronary band usually relieves the pain. There is no radiographic evidence of an acute lesion for about 3 weeks, after which time periostitis becomes apparent.

If lameness develops gradually, it is likely that conformation and the type of work performed are involved. The diagnosis is based on the results of nerve blocks or a ring block proximal to the coronary band and radiographic evidence of active periostitis of the distal portion of the second phalanx and proximal portion of the third phalanx.

Treatment: Phenylbutazone given systemically and a poultice applied to the limb help relieve acute inflammation. Local infiltration of corticosteroids is beneficial if the lesion is not contaminated as a result of a puncture wound. The horse should be confined to a small area and radiographed in 3-4 weeks to help determine the need for further therapy.

Therapy is aimed at arresting the periosteal inflammation when the lesion is chronic and there is active periostitis. Radiation therapy is especially useful in treating this condition because the hoof interferes with other forms of therapy.

Prognosis: The prognosis is guarded to poor.

References

1. Moyer, W and Anderson, JP. JAVMA **166** (1975) 42.
2. Szabuniewicz, M and Szabuniewicz, JM. VM/SAC **70** (1975) 205.
3. Keown, G. Proc 8th Ann Mtg Am Assoc Eq Pract, 1962. p 143.
4. Layton, EW. VM/SAC **60** (1965) 248.
5. Butzow, RF. Illinois Vet **4** (1961) 98.
6. Jenny, J *et al.* JAVMA **147** (1965) 1340.
7. Johnson, JH. VM/SAC **65** (1970) 147.
8. O'Connor, JJ: Dollar's Veterinary Surgery. 4th ed. Baillière, Tindall and Cox, London, 1960.
9. Adams, OR: Lameness in Horses. 2nd ed. Lea & Febiger, Philadelphia, 1966.
10. Frank, ER: Veterinary Surgery. 7th ed. Burgess Publishing, Minneapolis, 1964.
11. Mason, JH. J So Afr Vet Assoc **23** (1962) 223.
12. Banic, J and Skusek, F. Berl Münch Tierarzt Wschr **73** (1960) 186.
13. Rendano, VT and Grant, B. Am Vet Rad Soc **19** (1978) 125.
14. Lungwitz, A and Adams, JW: A Textbook of Horseshoeing. 11th ed. JB Lippincott, Philadelphia, 1913.
15. Moyer, W and Anderson, JP. JAVMA **166** (1975) 53.
16. Rooney, JR. Mod Vet Pract **58** (1977) 708.
17. Lambert, RW Jr. VM/SAC **62** (1967) 903.
18. Calishar, T and St. Clair, LE. JAVMA **154** (1969) 410.
19. Schebitz, H. Proc 13th Ann Mtg Am Assoc Eq Pract, 1967. p 263.
20. Wilkinson, GT. Br Vet J **109** (1963) 55.
21. Rooney, JR: Biomechanics of Lameness in Horses. Williams & Wilkins, Baltimore, 1969.
22. Colles, CM: Personal communication, 1979.
23. Ackerman, N *et al.* JAVMA **170** (1977) 183.
24. Jones, SL. Rad Tech **41** (1969) 31.
25. Colles, CM and Hickman, J. Eq Vet J **9** (1977) 150.
26. Coffman, JR *et al.* JAVMA **174** (1979) 261.
27. Evans, LH. Proc 16th Ann Mtg Am Assoc Eq Pract, 1970. p. 103.
28. Tate, LP and Evans, LH. JAVMA **177** (1980) 423.
29. Garner, HE *et al.* Eq Vet J **10** (1978) 249.
30. Garner, HE *et al.* J Anim Sci **45** (1977) 1037.
31. Garner, HE *et al.* Am J Vet Res **38** (1977) 725.
32. Hood, DM *et al.* J Eq Med Surg **2** (1978) 439.
33. Robinson, NE *et al.* Am J Vet Res **36** (1975) 1249.
34. Garner, HE *et al.* Am J Vet Res **36** (1975) 441.
35. Amoss, MS *et al.* J Eq Med Surg **3** (1979) 171.
36. Coffman, JR. Proc 12th Ann Mtg Am Assoc Eq Pract, 1966. p 275.
37. Coffman, JR *et al.* JAVMA **155** (1969) 45.
38. Coffman, JR *et al.* JAVMA **156** (1970) 76.
39. Chavance, J. Vet Med **41** (1946) 199.
40. Robinson, NE: Personal communication, 1980.
41. Robinson, NE *et al.* Proc Soc Exp Biol Med 149 (1975) 805.
42. Hood, DM *et al.* Paper presented at AVMA mtg, 1980.
43. Garner, HE. Vet Clin No Am **2** (1980) 25.
44. Urmas, P. Finak Vet **74** (1968) 11.
45. Britton, JW. Calif Vet **15** (1959) 17.
46. Frank, ER: Personal communication, 1970.
47. Irvin, CHG. Proc 12th Ann Mtg Am Assoc Eq Pract, 1966. p 197.
48. Lundvall, RL. Proc 11th Ann Mtg Am Assoc Eq Pract, 1965. p 319.

THE PASTERN JOINT
by B.D. Grant

The proximal interphalangeal (pastern) joint can be the source of a number of problems, ranging from painful fractures and infections to nonpainful enlargements that have only cosmetic implications.

Osteochondrosis

Subchondral cyst-like lesions are seen occasionally on routine radiographs of the pastern joint. Their clinical significance should always be questioned (see Carpal Osteochondrosis).

Fractures

These fractures vary in size and location. They are usually the result of excessive torque applied to the bone through such trauma as getting a foot wedged between 2 immovable objects. Pastern fractures usually cause lameness, the severity of which is related to the type and size of the fracture. Early surgical removal of even quite large fragments has been more satisfactory than screw fixation or cast application. Comminuted fractures of the first and second phalanx and involving the pastern joint are discussed in the sections on fractures of those bones.[1]

Osteoarthritis

Degenerative osteoarthritis of the pastern joint was more common when use of draft horses was routine but is still a significant condition in rodeo horses. There often is a history of having the foot caught between 2 immovable objects. Affected horses often have a considerable amount of dystrophic calcification at the attachments of the collateral ligaments.

Physical examination typically reveals an enlarged pastern, with reduced mobility and a painful response to flexion. The lameness is usually improved with the use of a low volar nerve block. Intra-articular anesthesia in advanced cases is not usually effective. Radiography is the definitive diagnostic method and

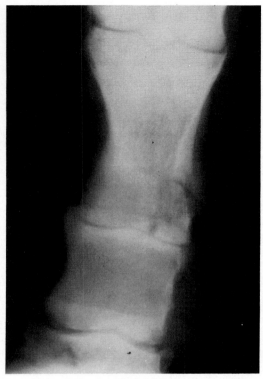

Fig 97. Suppurative arthritis of the pastern joint, osteomyelitis of the first phalanx, and a pathologic fracture of the medial condyle.

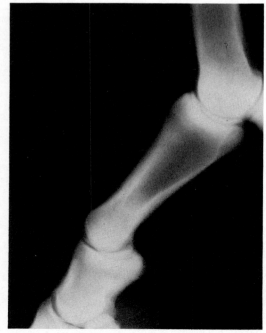

Fig 98. Subluxation of the pastern joint ("Thoroughbred ringbone").

reveals a narrowed joint space, osteophytes and dystrophic calcification.

Therapy depends upon the intended use of the horse and the severity of the lameness. Some affected animals respond to application of shoes that allow early breakover (rolled toes, swedged heels), administration of phenylbutazone, and avoidance of exercise involving excessive turns (figures 8's, "roll backs"). In the more severe cases, surgical arthrodesis and lag-screw fixation are required (Fig 97).[2]

Luxation and Subluxation

Luxation of the pastern joint is rare and usually associated with multiple fractures of the second phalanx. Subluxation of the pastern joint is more common and often referred to as "Thoroughbred ringbone" because of the frequency with which it occurs in race horses with a previous injury to the stabilizing tissues of the fetlock joint (Fig 98). Contraction of the straight distal sesamoidean ligament also may be a contributing factor. Subluxation of the pastern joint also occurs after suspensory desmotomy as treatment for subluxation of the fetlock joint associated with digital flexor tendon contraction.

Treatment of pastern joint subluxation has not been described. It is possible to section the origin of the distal sesamoidean ligament, using the same approach as for annular ligament resection. This treatment did not relieve the subluxation in one chronically affected horse treated by the author. Because subluxation of the pastern joint is secondary to other conditions, use of thermocautery and counterirritants may produce more pathologic changes.

References

1. Colahan, PT et al. JAVMA **178** (1981) 1182.
2. Schneider, JE et al. JAVMA **173** (1978) 1364.

THE FETLOCK JOINT
by B.D. Grant

Pathologic changes in the metacarpophalangeal (fetlock or ankle) joint may cause severe lameness and joint distension or subtle lameness with only slight joint distension. The more subtle conditions are characterized by stumbling, "not grabbing the race track," interference, "running down behind," "bearing in," and "bearing out." Although an accurate history and thorough physical examination are essential in diagnosis of metacarpophalangeal problems, the diagnosis is usually confirmed by

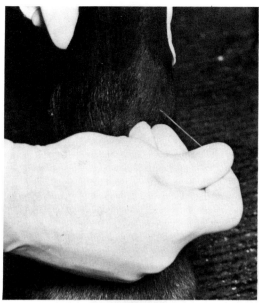

Fig 99. Site for arthrocentesis of the fetlock joint from the cranial aspect.

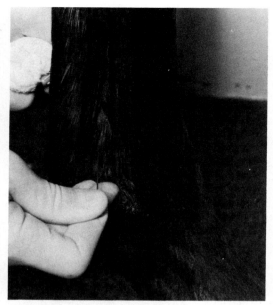

Fig 100. Site for arthrocentesis of the caudal cul de sac of the fetlock joint.

radiography. Xeroradiography, contrast arthrography, cinematography or electrogoniometry may be required in some cases.

The fetlock can be determined as the source of pain by intra-articular injection of local anesthetics (Fig 99). The cranial aspect of the joint is the preferred injection site to minimize chances of iatrogenic hemarthrosis that can occur from injection of the caudal cul de sac (Fig 100). Moderate physical restraint (twitch) should be applied and the area aseptically prepared before introduction of a 20-ga or smaller needle. Clipping or shaving the area is usually not necessary. The character of the synovial fluid should be observed as it flows from the needle. Digital pressure on the caudal cul de sac aids collection of the fluid; aspiration with a syringe is usually unproductive.

Osslets

Osslets is a general term for enlargement of the cranial aspect of the fetlock (Fig 101). Before the use of radiography became common, all enlargements of the fetlock were diagnosed as osslets (Fig 102). The common treatment was counterirritation in the form of thermocautery (firing), blistering or both. In this text the term osslets refers to enlargements of the cranial aspect of the joint, with no intra-articular abnormalities.

Chronically affected joints become firm and have limited movement due to dystrophic cal-

cification. This process usually occurs subsequent to hemorrhage from trauma.

Treatment: Although chronically affected animals can perform successfully, conservative therapy is indicated in acute cases. Conserva-

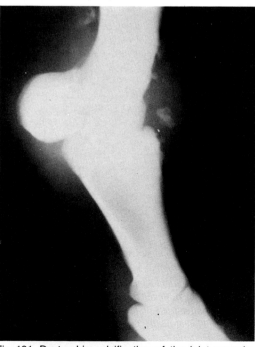

Fig 101. Dystrophic calcification of the joint capsule (osslets).

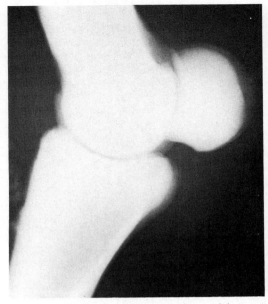

Fig 102. Soft tissue enlargement on the cranial aspect of the fetlock and dystrophic calcification of the insertion of the lateral digital extensor tendons. The clinical diagnosis would be osselets.

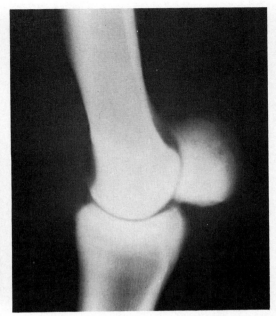

Fig 103. Typical scalloped appearance of the third metacarpal bone due to pressure osteolysis from a villonodular mass.

tive management of osselets involves ruling out other conditions that may cause fetlock enlargement and avoiding activities that predispose to the condition. Young racing horses should rest 2-3 months to allow the torn fibrous portion of the joint capsule to heal. A better cosmetic appearance of the fetlock can be obtained with the use of support wraps and greatly restricted exercise. Moderate doses of phenylbutazone may be used over long periods to inhibit the enzymatic destruction of the joint cartilage that can occur with traumatic arthritis. The prognosis for recovery is usually guarded; however, properly managed young race horses have been able to return to the highest level of competition.

Villonodular Synovitis

This condition is characterized by a firm enlargement to the cranial aspect of the fetlock joint, synovial distension, reduced joint motion, and a painful response to flexion. Affected racing animals have a history of fetlock trauma, bearing in or out, and inability to obtain traction. The characteristic villonodular masses are enlargements of the proximal fibrous tabs of the joint capsule and are often associated with osteochondral fractures of the proximal first phalanx. The condition is often not recognized because radiographic examination of the

joint does not reveal any fractures. The characteristic radiographic abnormality is the scalloped appearance of the third metacarpal bone (Fig 103). The masses are often evident on deep digital palpation. The diagnosis can be confirmed by using a contrast agent to demonstrate a radiolucent soft tissue mass (Fig 104).

Treatment: Conservative management of villonodular synovitis consists of intralesional injection of corticosteroids, long-term use of phenylbutazone, and ultrasound therapy. Using adequate restraint, a 20- to 22-ga needle is used to inject 2-3 ml corticosteroids into several areas of the mass. Concurrent use of ultrasound also helps reduce the size of the lesions. The use of radiation therapy alone has also reduced the size of such masses. While a conservative approach may permit continued training, it usually does not resolve the problem.

Surgical treatment usually consists of removal of the mass.[1] The approach most often used is that for repair of proximal first phalanx fractures (Fig 105). An extended incision is made to fully explore the dorsal compartment of the fetlock joint. The masses are grasped with Allis tissue forceps and excised with curved dissecting scissors. The underlying degenerated bone is curetted down to a smooth, bleeding surface. The proximal aspect of the first phalanx should be inspected for rough-

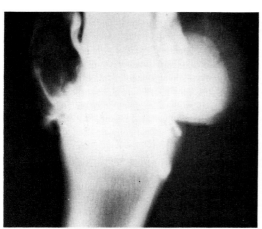

Fig 104. Contrast arthrogram of the fetlock in Figure 103. The teardrop-shaped villonodular mass is outlined with contrast medium.

ened projections, which may have caused the original irritation to the proximal fibrous tab. The closure is the same as that described for proximal first phalanx fractures.

Aftercare consists of application of support bandaging for 6-8 weeks and stall rest. Hand-walking may begin on the second postoperative week. The use of ultrasound therapy beginning 12 days postoperatively reduces the size of the fetlock and results in a more acceptable cosmetic appearance. As in the treatment of other conditions, one should avoid early use of ultrasound since it can cause dehiscence of wounds and can be responsible for an acute lameness if a subacute septic condition exists. Radiation therapy has been beneficial. Training can be resumed 3 months postoperatively; about 80% of operated animals make a full recovery.

Fractures of the First Phalanx

Fractures of the cranial aspect of the proximal first phalanx are a common source of synovial distension of the fetlock joint. They are most commonly seen in racing animals, especially Thoroughbreds racing on hard western tracks. Horses racing on the softer eastern tracks are not as commonly affected.

During the first 24 hours after injury, the horse is obviously lame and experiences pain upon flexion of the distended fetlock joint. Arthrocentesis of the fetlock joint 2-3 hours after the injury reveals hemorrhagic synovial fluid. It is generally not necessary to use intra-articular anesthesia to confirm the source of lameness. The diagnosis is most often confirmed by radiographic examination. Considerable care should be taken to correctly label

the oblique markers so that the proper surgical site can be selected.

Treatment: Treatment of fractures from the cranial aspect of the proximal first phalanx remains controversial since many horses with radiographic abnormalities are successfully treated.[2] Some clinicians advocate fragment removal while others advocate 3 months of rest but no surgery. After some experience in dealing with this type of injury, clinicians may gain certain insights into which types of fractures respond to conservative therapy and which are candidates for surgery.

Many affected animals are treated with intra-articular injections of corticosteroids and return to racing.[3] However, the veterinarian should inform the owner of the possibility of further injury to articular surface of the joint and the possibility of septic arthritis. Veterinarians may become involved in litigation if a treated animal falls during a race and injures riders and other animals. The use of combinations of counterirritants and rest may be indicated to stabilize the fracture without surgery.

If surgical treatment is elected, it is especially important to carefully review the label-

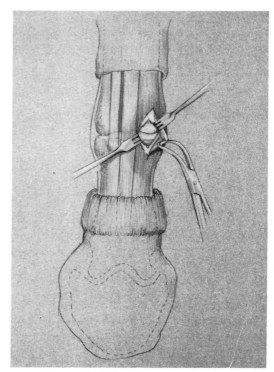

Fig 105. Surgical approach for removal of osteochondral fracture fragments from the medial aspect of the proximal first phalanx and villonodular masses from the distal metacarpus.

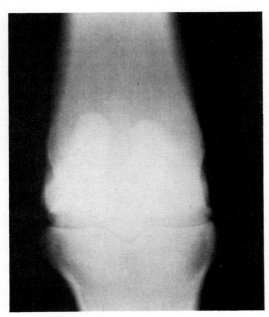

Fig 106. Narrowed fetlock joint space.

ing of the radiographs to determine if a fracture is medial or lateral to the common digital extensor tendon and exclude the possibility of fractures on both sides of the common digital extensor tendon.[4] Once the surgeons are confident of the location of the fracture, the animal is placed in lateral recumbency on the side that affords the best visualization of the fracture. The surgery is best performed using an Esmarch bandage and tourniquet.

After sterile preparation, the incision site is surrounded with sterile towels and a drape, and an impervious surgical barrier is applied. If the fracture is medial to the common digital extensor tendon, a curvilinear incision (with the apex toward the medial aspect) is made over the joint (Fig 105). The skin flap is reflected with a towel clamp or skin hook. The joint capsule is incised with a sterile blade in a vertical plane approximately 4-5 mm from and parallel to the common digital extensor tendon. The fibrous portion of the joint capsule is usually thin but may be thickened in chronic cases.

Proximal displacement of the fracture fragment often obscures visualization of the articular surfaces. After the fragment is removed by sharp dissection, the articular surfaces are easily examined. The articular cartilage should be white and glistening. Any "wear lines" or yellow discoloration in the opposing cartilage decreases the chance of a return to normal

function. The fracture site should be carefully curetted down to smooth, bleeding subchondral bone. The proximal recess of the joint should be examined for the presence of a villonodular mass, which is removed if present. The tourniquet is released after the joint capsule is closed and any bleeders ligated. After skin closure, the joint is dressed and bandaged as previously described.

Postoperative management consists of administration of phenylbutazone for 10 days and antibiotics for 5 days, passive flexion twice daily for 10 days, and stall rest. Bandage changes should be delayed until the seventh postoperative day to prevent contamination of the incision. After the initial bandage change, a hyperosmotic ointment applied in the form of a sweat and changed every second day greatly improves the cosmetic appearance of the wound.

Fractures of the caudal aspect of the proximal first phalanx are discussed under Fractures of the Basilar Sesamoid Bones.

Degenerative Joint Disease

Degenerative osteoarthritis or degenerative joint disease (DJD) of the fetlock joint is most commonly seen in performance animals, especially those with long racing careers and those subjected to repeated intra-articular injections of corticosteroids.[7] Because chronic joint trauma is an important factor in the pathogenesis of this condition, the intra-articular use of corticosteroids worsens the situation by decreasing the protein synthesis and causing a loss of strength of the collagen fibers in the weight-bearing surfaces of diarthrodial joints.[5] Affected horses are usually presented with an obvious lameness, often at a walk. Although the lameness may initially respond to the use of anti-inflammatory agents, the condition gradually becomes refractory to medical treatment. Joint motion and effusion are limited, and passive flexion causes a painful response.

Radiographic examination reveals a narrowed joint space, especially on the medial or caudal aspect (Fig 106). This narrowing of the joint space is sometimes difficult to detect and one should carefully inspect all radiographs, especially the AP projection. The articulation between the metacarpal and sesamoid bones can also be involved, especially with basilar sesamoid or condylar fractures (Fig 107). All lateral films should be carefully inspected for loss of convexity of the condyle as this usually indicates a degenerative, unresponsive condition of the fetlock joint. Xeroradiography has been useful in demonstrating these changes.

Villonodular synovitis and dystrophic calcification of the joint capsule can also occur with degenerative osteoarthritis. Adjuncts to diagnosis include cytologic examination of the synovial fluid, contrast arthrography, cinematography and electrogoniometry.

Treatment: Medical treatment of DJD involves intra-articular injection of hyaluronic acid to increase the normal metabolism in the joint and the continuous use of phenylbutazone to inhibit enzymatic destruction of articular surfaces.[6-8]

If the patient is to be used for breeding and is not responding to medical management, surgical arthrodesis may be indicated. Various methods of fusion of the fetlock joint have been recommended, including injection of irritants, placement of lag screws and bone plugs, removal of the articular cartilage, and combinations of all of these. One of the most successful methods of arthrodesis is described elsewhere in this chapter. If the cartilage damage is confined to the third metacarpal bone or first phalanx, a prosthesis can be surgically implanted to reduce the pain. However, this procedure has not been fully evaluated in clinical trials.

Bursitis

Some horses have a bursa, associated with the common digital extensor tendon on the cranial aspect of the fetlock joint, that may become inflamed and distended, usually due to trauma to the fetlock area. The condition is usually not responsible for any lameness but is often mistaken for joint disease or osslets, and should be differentiated so that an accurate prognosis can be given. In any case of bursitis, the association of the horse with cattle and the possibility of concurrent *Brucella* infection should be determined. It is also possible that the bursitis may have been the result of surgical intervention of the craniomedial aspect of the fetlock joint. Contrast agents should be used if survey radiographs fail to disclose any osseous abnormality. If a communication of the bursa with the joint is suspected, injection of contrast media into the volar pouch of the fetlock joint is indicated. Drainage and injection with corticosteroids can be performed in uncomplicated cases if a cosmetically appealing appearance is necessary. Radiation therapy or surgical removal can be attempted in unresponsive cases.

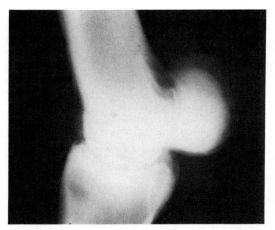

Fig 107. Two osteochondral fractures of the proximal first phalanx, and narrowing and loss of convexity of the caudal aspect of the condyle.

Epiphysitis

Enlarged fetlock joints are seen in most fast-growing young horses and are considered a normal occurrence. However, some cases are associated with pathologic changes of the distal metacarpal epiphyseal region (Fig 108). Such horses are affected with a varying degree of lameness, which may consist of only stiffness

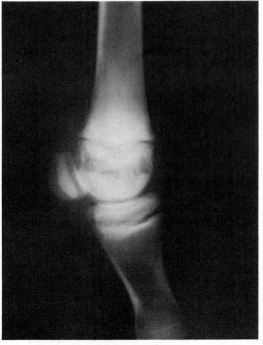

Fig 108. Marked osteolysis and destruction associated with suppurative epiphysitis.

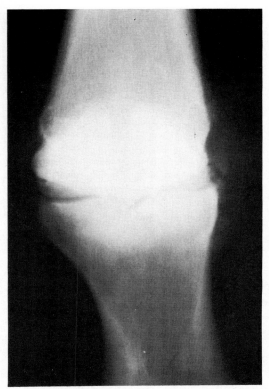

Fig 109. Dystrophic calcification of the collateral ligaments, collapse of the medial articular surface, and widening of the lateral surface in a mare with a varus deformity.

noglobulins. Acute lameness usually occurs with extension of the septic condition into the fetlock joint. Therefore, aspiration of the fetlock joint should always be performed under sterile conditions. The aspirate should be cultured and cytologically examined (see Septic Arthritis). The prognosis for recovery for animals with septic epiphysitis is unfavorable. Involvement of more than one joint worsens an already poor prognosis.

Luxation of the Fetlock Joint

Complete luxation of the fetlock joint most commonly occurs in severe lacerations or racing injuries in which the supporting structures have been severely damaged. Most medial or lateral subluxations are associated with trauma to the medial or lateral collateral ligaments (Fig 109). Contraction of the suspensory ligament and/or flexor tendons produces a cranial or caudal subluxation (see Diseases of the Tendons).

The degree of lameness depends on the severity of the luxation and the cause. Animals with contracted tendons have very upright forelegs, with subluxation of the fetlock joints and reluctance to exercise freely if the condition is due to a dietary problem, or total reluctance to bear weight if the condition is septic in nature. A CBC and radiographs are certainly indicated in all cases. When treating an infection of any synovial or osseous structure in a young foal, immunoglobulin levels should be evaluated since failure of passive transfer of colostral antibodies is common.

Treatment: Reduction of caloric intake, by avoiding the feeding of grain or weaning the foal from a heavily lactating mare, is indicated if the cause is dietary. Short periods of moderate exercise are beneficial. The use of small doses of phenylbutazone and support bandages is also indicated in cases of bilateral involvement. If there is no response after 3-4 weeks, radiographs should be obtained for re-evaluation. Long-term use of phenylbutazone in foals may cause gastric ulcers;[10] any change in the stool should be viewed suspiciously.

Animals with septic epiphysitis usually have a fever, an increased WBC count and fibrinogen level and, in many cases, a lack of immu-

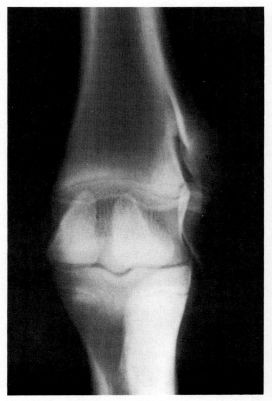

Fig 110. A supernumerary digit.

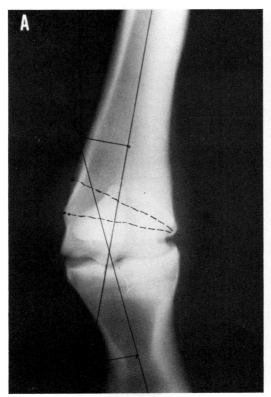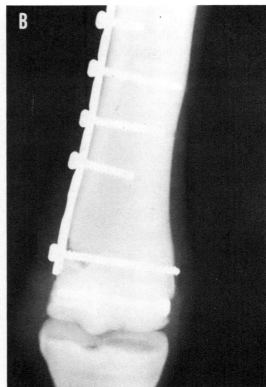

Fig 111. Presurgical appearance of a varus deformity, with calculations for the size of the wedge to be removed (A), and the postoperative appearance (B).

at every step or intermittently causing an audible "click." Flexion of the fetlock joint and digital pressure on the sesamoids are usually painful but animals usually bear weight on the affected limbs. There is no medial or lateral loss of stability of the joint.

In cases of medial or lateral instability, there is a marked varus or valgus deformity of the forelimb and an increased range of motion of the digit relative to the fetlock joint. The amount of fibrous tissue is often increased on the affected side. Affected animals have pain on flexion but can walk to some degree.

Diagnosis of fetlock luxations should be confirmed by a complete radiographic examination so the presence of concurrent fractures, collapse of joint space, and degenerative disease can be evaluated. It is advantageous to obtain radiographs in a stressed position to demonstrate the loss of integrity of the collateral ligaments.

Treatment: Cranial or caudal subluxations can be treated by the methods described for flexor tendon contracture. The prognosis varies with the condition and duration, but the pres-ence of degenerative joint disease and sesamoiditis worsens the prognosis. Treatment can consist of application of corrective shoes that provide increased medial or lateral stability to the joint. In human medicine, surgical reconstruction of the torn ligaments and application of a cast are the treatments of choice. Casts should not be left on for long periods since they tend to weaken the soft tissue support to the joint. After the cast has been removed, additional support with corrective shoes or splints should be applied. A long period of stall rest and application of support bandages are also indicated since the repair time of ligaments is especially prolonged.

Osteochondrosis

Subchondral bone cysts and osteochondritis dissecans of the metacarpophalangeal joint are most often recognized only after radiographs are obtained (see Carpal Osteochondrosis). Therefore, their clinical significance should be properly evaluated before treatment is begun.

Neoplasia

Reports of fetlock neoplasms are rare.[11] One such case was an Arabian mare with an enlarged rear fetlock that was painful to flexion. Radiographs demonstrated a number of radiolucent areas. Biopsy and necropsy results determined the masses to be a chondrosarcoma.

Congenital Anomalies

Supernumerary digits (polydactylism) occasionally occur in horses (Fig 110). Most cases only result in an altered cosmetic appearance; however, in one case the supernumerary digit caused an angular deformity of the fetlock.

Surgical removal of the extra digit has been described and is usually rewarding.[12] Care should be taken to identify all the structures in the neurovascular bundle. The closure of any connecting synovial structure is recommended.

Angular Deformities

Varus or valgus deformities of the fetlock joint necessitate thorough radiographic examination to determine the cause. These deformities and their treatment are discussed elsewhere in this chapter. In older animals, rupture of a collateral ligament or collapse of the medial or lateral articular cartilage may be a cause. In selected cases a wedge osteotomy may be performed (Fig 111).

Hypertrophic Pulmonary Osteoarthropathy

Bilateral osseous enlargements of the distal extremities have been associated with intrathoracic lesions. In 2 reported cases the enlargements developed secondary to a thoracic abscess and granular-cell myoblastoma.[13,14] Less obvious forms of this syndrome are manifested as limb edema that develops during recovery from viral or bacterial pneumonia.

References

1. Nickels, FA et al. JAVMA 168 (1976) 1043.
2. Milne, FJ. Can Vet J 13 (1972) 33.
3. McKay, AG and Milne, FJ. JAVMA 168 (1976) 1039.
4. Adams, OR. JAVMA 148 (1966) 360.
5. Noyes, FR et al. Clin Orthoped Rel Res 123 (1977) 197.
6. Asheim, A and Lindblad, G. Acta Vet Scand 17 (1976) 379.
7. Swanstrom, OG. Proc 24th Ann Mtg Am Assoc Eq Pract, 1978. p 345.
8. Torbeck, RL and Prieur, DJ. Am J Vet Res 40 (1979) 1531.
9. Grant, BD et al. J Eq Med Surg 1 (1977) 206.
10. Snow, DH. Vet Rec 105 (1979) 26.
11. Riddle, WE and Wheat, JD. JAVMA 158 (1971) 1674.
12. Behrens, E. JAVMA 174 (1979) 266.
13. Goodbary, RF and Hage, TJ. JAVMA 137 (1960) 602.
14. Alexander, JE et al. JAVMA 146 (1965) 703.

Arthrodesis of the Fetlock Joint
by L.R. Bramlage

The indications for surgical fusion of the fetlock joint include mechanical disability due to loss of soft tissue or bony support of the joint, and functional disability, in which the joint remains anatomically intact but weight-bearing on the arthritic joint elicits severe pain. Most indications involve chronic injuries, in which conservative therapy has failed to reduce pain to a tolerable level, or acute conditions, in which anatomic disruption risks further injury. Examples of such situations include nonresponsive degenerative arthritis, chronic caudal subluxation due to rupture of the suspensory apparatus, degenerative joint disease due to metastatic osteomyelitis, and vascular damage due to acute suspensory apparatus rupture. The objectives of surgical fusion are to obliterate the joint surfaces and stabilize the members of the joint so union can occur.

Technic

The patient is positioned in lateral recumbency with the injured leg down to allow a medial approach. A tourniquet may be used if the surgery is elective or if there is no vascular damage. The surgery should be performed without a tourniquet if vascular damage is a possibility.

A curvilinear skin incision is made from the proximal end of the third metacarpal bone to the coronary band. The deep incision follows the skin incision through the fetlock joint capsule, just cranial to the medial collateral ligament. As the extensor branch of the suspensory ligament is encountered, the deep incision should be curved craniad parallel to the ligament. The tendon is split longitudinally when the midline of the extensor tendon is reached. The periosteum and fetlock joint capsule are separated from the bone by subperiosteal and subcapsular dissection.

Contouring and positioning of the implant is done before the normal architecture is disrupted. The cranial surface of the first phalanx is dorsiflexed about 10° and the plate is contoured to fit this surface. The natural tapering of the first phalanx from proximal to distal results in an overall angle of about 30° to the long axis of the leg when the phalanx is stabilized in this position. The plate is centered on the long axis of the leg and 4 screws are inserted into the first phalanx. If a tension-band wire is to be used in fixation, 2 holes are drilled in the bone to accept the wire. Both holes are drilled

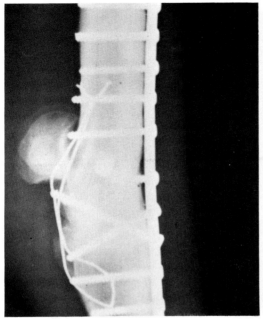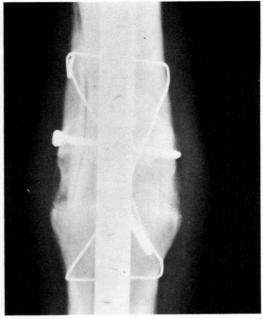

Fig 112. Radiographs obtained 13 weeks after arthrodesis of the fetlock joint, using tension-band wire for caudal support.

from medial to lateral in the frontal plane. The plate is removed and an oscillating bone saw is used to remove a segment of the condyle as thin as possible but thick enough to allow lag screw replacement without danger of comminution. The cranial surface of the osteotomized fragment is elevated and reflected caudad, which disarticulates the joint and exposes the articular surfaces. Removal of all articular cartilage is then possible using hand curettes or power instruments.

After the articular cartilage is denuded, a 2-mm drill bit is used to perforate the distal metacarpal and proximal phalangeal subchondral bone at 1-cm intervals. This establishes a communication between the osteoblast-rich metaphyseal area and the joint surface.

If tension-band wire is used, it should be inserted before the iatrogenic luxation is reduced. Care should be taken to thread the wire flat against the caudal aspect of the phalanx. The wire should be crossed immediately caudad to the joint surface.

The joint is then reduced and a lag screw is inserted into the predrilled condyle to restore the normal anatomy. The tension-band wire is tightened at this time (Fig 112). If the sesamoids are used to create the tension band, lag screws are inserted through the metacarpus into the sesamoids (Fig 113). The leg should be

in slight ventriflexion when the tension band or sesamoid screws are placed.

Once the tension band is in place caudal to the joint, compression can be applied to the joint surface by attaching the plate to the cranial surface of the bone in tension, using the tension device. The remaining screws are then inserted and tightened. The screws on either side of the joint are inserted as lag screws across the joint surface. The skin and soft tissue are replaced and sutured over the plate, and a drain is placed alongside the plate.

In adult horses a cast is applied to the foot, ending just distal to the carpus for support during recovery from anesthesia. Juvenile animals require only support wraps during recovery. The drain is removed in 2-3 days and the cast is changed or removed in 10-14 days, at which time the sutures are removed. Difficult aftercare is avoided because minimal external coaptation is necessary when using this technic. The stability achieved provides immediate pain reduction and an immediately functional limb for protection of the sound limb.

Arthrodesis of the fetlock functionally lengthens the affected limb and the horse must adjust to the lack of fetlock flexion. Therefore, arthrodesis should be undertaken early to protect the sound limb rather than waiting until damage has already occurred.

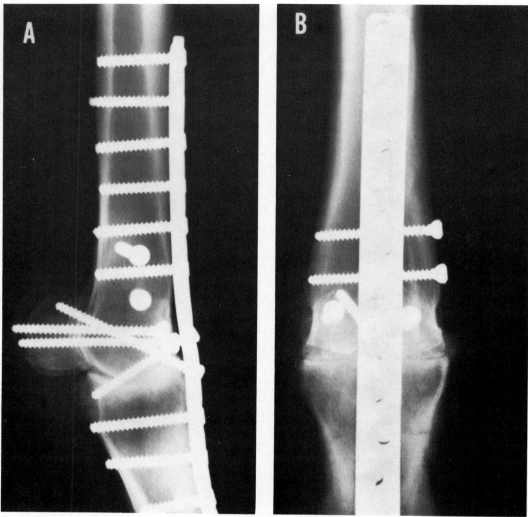

Fig 113. Radiographs obtained 15 weeks after arthrodesis of the fetlock joint, using lag-screw fixation of the sesamoid bones for caudal support.

THE SESAMOID BONES
by B.D. Grant

Disease of the proximal sesamoid bones is a common cause of lameness and poor performance. Pathologic changes usually cause a distended metacarpophalangeal joint and pain upon flexion and digital palpation over the attachments of the suspensory ligament, which are usually enlarged. Specific nerve blocks cannot be used to isolate sesamoid injuries but lameness decreases with intra-articular anesthesia of the metacarpophalangeal joint, and with high volar and ulnar nerve blocks. A posterior digital nerve block may also reduce lameness caused by sesamoid bone fracture.

Therefore, if no disease can be found in the foot and lameness is reduced by a posterior digital nerve block, a lesion of the sesamoid bones should be suspected.

Radiography is the most definitive diagnostic method. In examining radiographs of the proximal sesamoids, one should bear in mind that variations in the vascular channels in the sesamoids are related to the horse's degree of performance. An excellent review of the radiographic appearance of the proximal sesamoids has been published.[1] The opposite forelimb should be radiographed to compare the vascular channels in the normal sesamoid bones before implicating sesamoid disease as a definitive cause of lameness. Further diagnos-

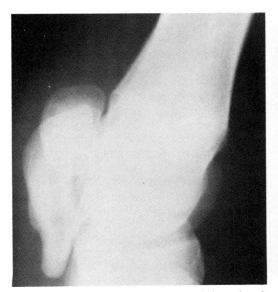

Fig 114. An unusual, elongated sesamoid bone in a 3-month-old foal.

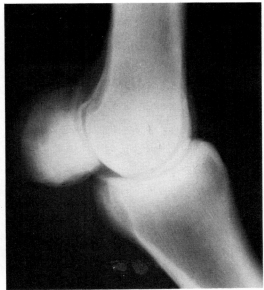

Fig 115. Circular, cyst-like area in the proximal sesamoid bone.

tic tests include electrogoniometry, xeroradiography and cinematography.

Congenital Lesions

Very few congenital abnormalities are associated with sesamoid bones. An elongated sesamoid was observed in a 3-month-old mustang with no obvious pain in the fetlock (Fig 114). Osteochondritis dissecans can occur in the proximal sesamoids and is characterized by cyst-like lesions on radiographs (Fig 115). The presence of such cysts is not necessarily an ominous sign.

Osteomyelitis

Although the sesamoids are usually protected from most penetrating wounds, a pitchfork or nail can penetrate the flexor canal to produce a localized area of infection in the sesamoids. The diagnosis is based upon a history of penetration and localized osteolysis on radiographs (Fig 116). Treatment consists of radical curettage using an approach through the flexor canal as described in the section on Diseases of the Tendons.

Fractures

Fractures of the sesamoid bones are relatively common injuries in performance horses and are classified as apical, abaxial, body and basilar. Affected animals usually have a history of lameness after an athletic event. Apical and abaxial sesamoid fractures commonly cause lameness an hour or so after a race, a distended

joint capsule, and pain upon flexion and palpation. Arthrocentesis of the fetlock joint reveals hemorrhagic synovial fluid and radiographs disclose the fracture. Body and basilar fractures often cause horses to "break down" on the race track or to be "eased" and removed from the track by ambulance.

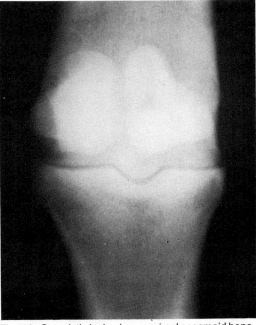

Fig 116. Osteolytic lesion in a proximal sesamoid bone.

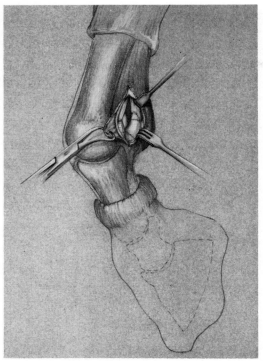

Fig 117. Surgical approach for removal of osteochondral fracture fragments from the sesamoid bones and the caudal aspect of the proximal first phalanx.

Apical Fractures: Apical sesamoid fractures not associated with osteoarthritis in the fetlock joint usually have a guarded to favorable prognosis if the fragment is removed within 2 weeks of injury. A prognosis should not be issued until the amount of articular cartilage damage is evaluated at surgery. If the articular cartilage has retained its normal marble-white, glassy appearance, with no wear lines, the prognosis for recovery is good. Many affected animals have been able to return to racing at the same level of competition.

The standard preoperative orthopedic procedures, as previously described, are performed. Using general anesthesia, the patient is placed in lateral recumbency with the affected sesamoid up. A curvilinear skin incision is made caudal to the third metacarpal bone, distal to the splint bone, and cranial to the suspensory ligament and proximal sesamoid to the distal border of the sesamoid (Fig 117). The joint is entered by incising the proximal volar pouch to the fetlock joint with a sterile blade. Traditionally, apical sesamoid fracture fragments have been removed by palpation through this pouch with blunt, almost blind dissection. However,

continuation of the incision through the collateral sesamoidean ligament affords better inspection of the fracture site and precludes the use of fingers in the joint. More visualization is achieved by flexion of the fetlock and caudal retraction of the proximal sesamoid.

After the sesamoid fracture fragment is removed by sharp dissection, the fracture site is curetted smooth to reduce postoperative ossification. The fracture site is smoothed with a bone rasp if necessary. Use of bone wax helps reduce bone hemorrhage and subsequent dystrophic calcification. Closure consists of preplacement of horizontal mattress sutures of nonabsorbable material in the collateral sesamoidean ligament and the fibrous portion of the volar pouch. Injection of 1 million IU potassium penicillin in 7-10 ml saline helps determine the integrity of the joint capsule closure. If the injected fluid readily escapes, the site should be noted and additional sutures used. The subcutaneous tissues are best closed using nonabsorbable material in a simple-continuous pattern. Use of an everting pattern is recommended for skin closure. As in all orthopedic cases, postoperative radiographs should be made.

Heavy cotton bandages are applied to prevent damage during recovery from anesthesia. If there is no febrile response or edema in the leg, the bandages can be left on for 6-7 days before the first change. The bandages should be changed rapidly to prevent swelling and contamination of the surgical site. Passive flexion of the fetlock starting the day of surgery produces a more mobile joint. Suture removal is usually in 12-14 days. The use of ultrasound after postoperative day 14 to prevent excessive soft tissue proliferation and dystrophic calcification is recommended.

If the fracture is fresh, the articular cartilage normal, and the postoperative period without complication, the animal can return to training within 3 months.

Abaxial Fractures: Abaxial fractures are characterized by the same clinical signs and history as apical sesamoid fractures except that digital palpation of the affected area produces a much more painful response. Although affected animals can race successfully after only 3-4 months rest if the articular surface is not involved, surgical removal of the fragment is recommended if the articular surface is involved. A good prognosis can be given if care is used in dissecting the fragment from the attachments of the suspensory ligament. Intraoperative radiographs are best taken to

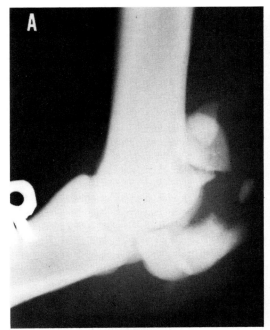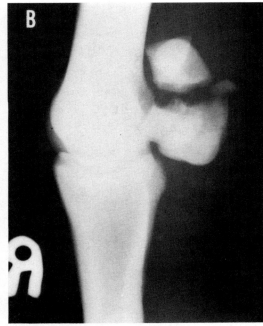

Fig 118. Comminuted sesamoid fractures before (A) and after (B) application of a Hitchcock splint.

demonstrate complete removal of all fragments. Postoperative management is the same as for apical sesamoid fractures.

Basilar Sesamoid and Caudal Proximal P1 Fractures: Small basilar and caudoproximal fractures of P1 cause the same signs as apical sesamoid fractures, including joint distension after physical exertion, and pain upon flexion and deep palpation. The AP radiographs of suspected basilar fractures should not be underexposed since many times what is thought to be a large basilar fracture is actually a T-shaped fracture of the basilar portion. This drastically changes the method of treatment in that placing a screw into what one thought was a large fracture would not be successful.

The best treatment of basilar sesamoid or proximal P1 fractures is immediate surgical removal. If the animal is only to be used for pleasure riding or breeding, surgical intervention is probably not indicated. These fractures do not heal well in horses that have even had a long period of rest and are often refractured with moderate galloping. The use of internal counterirritation (*eg*, Osteum:Schering) has been advocated but results have not been documented. The surgical approach for the removal of basilar sesamoid and caudal P1 fractures is the same as described for apical sesamoid fractures (Fig 117). The fragments

are embedded in the deep cruciate ligament in such cases.

Body Fractures: Fractures of the body can involve one or both sesamoids (Fig 118). The amount of fragment displacement usually corresponds to the amount of tearing of the intersesamoidean ligament and tension exerted by the suspensory and distal sesamoidean ligaments. Affected horses become extremely lame immediately after an athletic event, and have a swollen, painful fetlock. Arthrocentesis produces bloody synovial fluid.

Surgical intervention is required if the fracture is in the middle or distal third of the sesamoid and the athletic ability of the animal is to be preserved. If the animal is not to be used for racing and there is little fragment displacement, 3-4 months of stall rest are beneficial. Application of a plaster cast to prevent further displacement may be indicated. However, consideration should be given to severing the suspensory ligament that attaches to the affected sesamoid.

Screw fixation of body fractures is quite difficult and should only be attempted by experienced surgeons. The same approach as that for basilar sesamoid fractures is used, with the addition of a continuation of the skin incision caudad over the base of the sesamoid.[2] The neurovascular bundle is retracted caudad and an

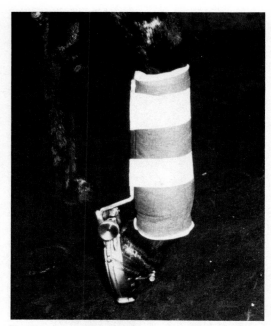

Fig 119. Application of a Hitchcock splint prevents further damage to the lower limb after comminuted fracture of the proximal sesamoids.

incision is made in the distal sesamoidean ligament to allow introduction of the index finger to palpate the basal border of the sesamoid. The small depression in the basal border is the site for introduction of the drill guard. The fragments are apposed with the use of bone clamps. Care should be taken not to drill completely through the apical portion into the suspensory ligament since this often results in dystrophic calcification of the suspensory ligament. The 4.5-mm drill should not be used in the proximal fragment as there is usually just enough room for a significant number of threads of the screw under the best of circumstances. As the screw is tightened one should observe the articular margins of the fracture for adequate reduction. Closure is the same as for apical sesamoid fractures. A plaster cast and walking bar are applied from the bottom of the foot to just ventral to the carpus to reduce the amount of traumatic separation that could occur during a stormy recovery from anesthesia.

Fractures of the bodies of both sesamoids occur commonly in "broken-down" horses on the race track and are a common cause for destruction due to severe trauma to the support apparatus of the lower limb and the possibility of damage to the vascular supply of the foot. Such horses must be treated vigorously from the on-

set of the injury.[3] These injuries become much more severe during the ride in the horse ambulance to the stable area if proper fixation is not previously applied (Fig 119).

If an affected animal is to enter a breeding program or is a successful racing gelding with much sentimental value, the limb should be placed in a plaster cast or splint until metacarpophalangeal arthrodesis can be attempted (Fig 118). It is advisable to postpone surgical intervention for 4-5 days to allow the patient to adapt to the cast and recover from the initial stress of the injury. Small fragments of the proximal sesamoid, especially those apparently devoid of blood supply, are best removed. A pain-free arthrodesis should be accomplished in 8 weeks to avoid compensatory rotation of the third phalanx in the opposite limb.

Complications of Sesamoid Fractures: Several complications may occur with screw fixation or removal of sesamoid fracture fragments. Postoperative sepsis has been noted, especially in animals that have received preoperative intra-articular corticosteroid injections. If there is any question as to this possibility, one should try to overcome the inhibitory factors of the corticosteroids with the use of oral vitamin A preparations.[4]

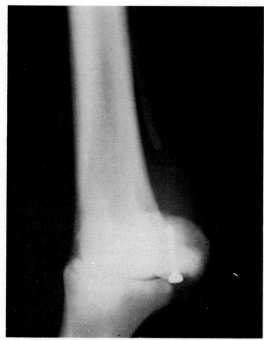

Fig 120. Marked enlargement of the small metacarpal bone after surgical stabilization of a sesamoid bone with a compression screw.

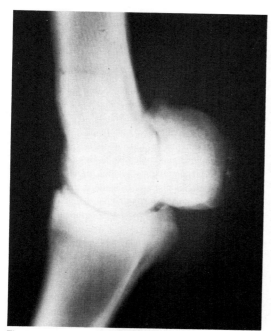

Fig 121. Large apical osteophytes on the proximal sesamoids.

suspensory desmitis is enlargement of the distal end of the small metacarpal bone on the affected side (Fig 120). If the metacarpal bone is enlarging and its extremity has been displaced into the suspensory ligament, early surgical removal of the distal splint bone provides a much better chance for recovery.

Osteophyte formation on the apical aspect of the sesamoid bone is common with chronic instability of the metacarpophalangeal joint, especially with condylar fractures of the third metacarpal/metatarsal bone. They can often be large enough to cause pressure lysis of the caudal aspect of the third metacarpal/metatarsal bone. Osteophytes are an indication of degenerative joint disease and must be assessed before recommending specific therapy. Surgical removal is indicated if the condylar fracture with which they are associated is healed and the osteophytes do not respond to conservative medical management (Fig 121). The osteophytes are removed with a sharp osteotome using the same approach as for apical sesamoid fracture repair. The osteotomy site should be smoothed with a bone rasp or air drill and have bone wax applied.

References

1. O'Brien, TR *et al*. J Am Vet Rad Soc **7** (1971) 75.
2. Fackelman, GE. J Eq Med Surg **2** (1978) 32.
3. Wheat, JD and Pascoe, JR. JAVMA **176** (1980) 205.
4. Grant, BD. Proc 21st Ann Mtg Am Assoc Eq Pract, 1975. p. 95.
5. Asheim, A and Lindblad, G. Acta Vet Scand **17** (1976) 379.
6. Swanstrom, OG. Proc 24th Ann Mtg Am Assoc Eq Pract, 1978. p 345.

Postoperative degenerative joint disease is a common complication when sesamoid fracture fragments have been removed after the first 10-12 days after injury. Degenerative joint disease can be controlled by the early and consistent use of support bandages and therapeutic doses of phenylbutazone. Radiation therapy has been used to prevent excessive amounts of dystrophic calcification but no control studies have been reported. The use of ultrasound is indicated if the proliferation is not due to a subacute septic process or joint instability. Hyaluronic acid injection may be a useful adjunct.[5,6]

The screw may back out of the drill hole in cases of over-drilling. In such cases the screw should be replaced with a larger screw. In some cases the proximal portion is comminuted by screw placement; removal of the fragments and screw can result in recovery.

Suspensory desmitis can result from the inflammation that occurred at the original time of injury and subsequent to forceful dissection of fracture fragments. This is often exacerbated by the inadvertent removal of a portion of the cartilage that is mistaken for bony fragments by inexperienced operators. This fibrous cartilage is located between the apex of the sesamoids and its very firm consistency mimics that of a fracture fragment. Another cause of

DISEASES OF THE TENDONS
by S.J. Selway

Tendons consist of dense connective tissue and connect muscle to some other tissue, primarily bone. Tendons can localize, spread or change the direction of tension from muscle contraction. They consist of fibroblasts and bundles of fibers lying approximately parallel to their long axis, and are composed mainly of collagen and associated ground substance.[1,2] The tendon bundles are composed of smaller bundles arranged in 3-dimensional networks or helices, with interweaving of these bundles and cross-branching between loops.[3] These smaller bundles are composed of primary fibers of tropocollagen, which in turn is composed of

3 protein chains of great but unknown lengths.[1,4] The type of collagen normally present is type 1, whereas scar tissue (the end result of secondary healing) is composed of primarily type-3 collagen.[5]

The epitendon, a thin layer of connective tissue, covers the tendon and continues into its interior as the endotendon, intervening between tendon bundles and carrying small blood vessels, lymphatics and nerves. Where the tendon is not within a sheath, external to the epitendon is a layer of loose connective tissue, rich in elastic fibers, called the peritendon. A sheath is present where there is increased friction, such as at bony prominences and joints. The sheath is composed of a fibrous layer and a synovial layer similar to a joint capsule. The mesotendon attaches to the tendon within and outside the tendon sheath. Blood supply, innervation and lymphatics enter the tendon primarily through the mesotendon. Bursae are occasionally found where increased protection and decreased friction are necessary and a tendon sheath is not present.

The loose connective tissue structures of the muscle are continuous with the corresponding tissues of the tendon. Fibrocartilage is often found at tendon insertions and over bony prominences at points of considerable friction. Retinacula (bands of dense connective tissue) extend externally over a tendon similar to a staple on a wire fence wherever there is a change in direction of tension as a result of muscle action. These structures keep the tendon in place and decrease vibration somewhat.[7]

Tendons are essentially nonextendible but have an absolute elastic phase when forces are applied below the critical stress point.[1,3,8] Their action is primarily passive in nature. The absolute tensile strength of tendon is probably in the range of 5-10 kg/mm^2.[3,9,10]

Tendon exhibits stress decay and, when loaded over the critical stress point without sufficient time for recovery, may exhibit a marked decay of percent strain in relation to load.[3] This may be related to the occurrence and recurrence of tendinitis.

Tendons do not heal from within but must depend on the tendon sheath, peritendon or adjacent connective tissue for capillary and fibroblastic ingrowth and ultimate repair. The result of this healing is the formation of adhesions between the tendon and adjacent structures.[11-13] Thus, a secondary type of wound repair occurs. If an impervious material is placed around a tendon for much more than 1.5 cm, blood and new fibroblasts cannot reach the area, resulting in avascular necrosis of the tendon.[14] Similarly, if a tendon is severed within a tendon sheath, healing will not occur if the ends are kept apart and not allowed to contact the tendon sheath itself.[14,15]

Trauma to the surface of a tendon causes considerable adhesion formation.[1,16] Adhesions are more severe where a peritendon rather than a sheath is the blood supply and fibroblasts are readily available.[6,15] The highly elastic peritendon loses its elastic fiber content and marked fibroblastic proliferation follows. It is desirable that resultant adhesions be long and gliding rather than short and restrictive.[1,14,16] The idea of "breaking down" adhesions is probably undesirable due to the damage caused and the increased magnitude of reaction, resulting in more adhesions. Rather, lengthening or stretching of adhesions is more desirable.[1,17]

Various materials and methods have been used in attempts to prevent restrictive adhesions, as well as various drugs, surgical procedures and postoperative regimens.[1,2,18-22] The results of these preventive measures for the most part have been inconsistent and sometimes damaging.[7,22,24-26]

Tendon repair tissue differs structurally and biochemically from the tissue it replaces.[1,5,27] Some investigators believe the results of tendon repair are inferior to the condition of the tendon before trauma.[1,28] There is no proof of this assumption.

It has been proposed that once an injured tendon has healed, the tissue differentiates to its previous structure and function.[1] In some areas, particularly in areas of a large amount of tendon excursion and/or friction (eg, flexor tendons), as well as with prolonged immobility of the area, lack of tissue differentiation results in chronic tendinitis.[15,17,29]

Tendon injuries may result in sharp, complete or partial transection. Blunt or partial transection can occur with or without the skin being broken. Rupture, rather than laceration, can occur due to abnormally high, sudden stress forces. Damage to the tissue surrounding the tendon can lead to eventual primary damage due to adhesions causing disruption of normal tendon architecture.[29] Tendons can also be injured by kicks from other horses, improper bandaging, and overreaching during locomotion.

Flexor Tendinitis

Tendinitis and related tendon disorders usually dictate a guarded to unfavorable prognosis for return to sustained soundness or racing and jumping.[29] Flexor tendinitis ("bowed tendons") occurs most commonly in race horses, especially Thoroughbreds.

Anatomy: The superficial flexor tendons of the front limbs are most commonly affected.[21,30] Tendinitis most commonly occurs at the level of the middle of the third metacarpal bone.[12,28]

The flexor tendons lie within tendon sheaths in the carpal region and from the metacarpophalangeal joint distad. However, no sheath is present in a majority of the metacarpal region. The structures composing the carpal canal proximad and the annular ligament of the fetlock distad are the associated retinacula. There is no tendon sheath nor retinacula between these previously mentioned proximal and distal areas (Fig 122). As described earlier, where a tendon is not within a tendon sheath, external to the epitendon is a layer of loose connective tissue, the peritendon. This peritendon is rich in elastic fibers and is an essential element in the free, gliding tendon.[29]

Tendinitis between the proximal and distal flexor sheaths is called a "bow." Tendinitis involving the proximal tendon sheath is a "high bow," and tendinitis within the distal flexor sheath is a "low bow." Tendinitis within a tendon sheath is generally accompanied by distension of that sheath. Tendinitis involving the proximal flexor sheath is occasionally associated with damage to the deep flexor tendon and/or inferior check ligament. Tendinitis within the distal flexor sheath usually involves one or both branches of the superficial flexor tendon where it divides to allow the deep flexor tendon to continue to its insertion on the third phalanx.

Cause: The common causes of tendinitis include direct trauma (blunt or sharp), improper bandaging, and actual tearing of the tendon. The last cause is most serious as far as successful treatment is concerned. However, it is important to note that unless tendinitis is promptly and properly treated, the result of all 3 causes is chronic recurrent tendinitis.

The clinician must also recognize predisposing factors to be corrected if possible if treatment of tendinitis is to be successful. Improper shoeing, with the weight-bearing surface of the foot too far forward (long toe and collapsed heels), or extremely high heels, resulting in a broken foot axis, predisposes to tendinitis. Lameness in the opposite limb produces greater weight-bearing on the tendons of the sound limb, which may lead to tendinitis. An abnormally long pastern places more stress on the

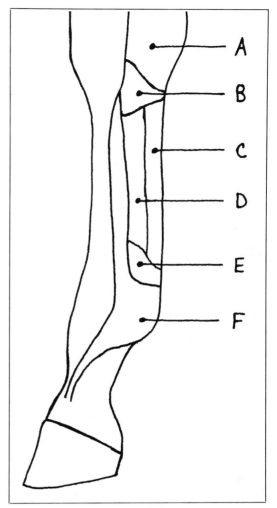

Fig 122. Retinacula and tendon sheaths associated with flexor tendons. A. Volar annular ligament of the carpus and deep fascia of the metacarpus. B. Proximal flexor tendon sheath. C. Superficial flexor tendon. D. Deep flexor tendon. E. Distal flexor tendon sheath. F. Annular ligament of the fetlock.

flexor tendons. An abnormally long metacarpal area results in a larger area with no retinacula or tendon sheath and increased vibration. Fatigue from too much strenuous exercise results in failure of the muscle/tendon unit (possibly stress-decay). Exercise on uneven terrain causes sudden, abnormally high stress forces. Finally, a calf-kneed, tied-in at the knee conformation predisposes to tendinitis.

Due to the lack of retinacula in the metacarpal area, from a strictly mechanical aspect there is a predisposition to damage occurring in this area when the tendons are stressed by overextension during running. Along with the

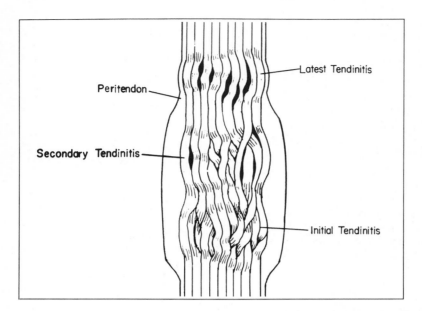

Fig 123. Pathologic changes in the tendon sheath.

obvious direct stress force predisposition are the factors of vibration of the fatigued muscle/tendon unit and the so-called fetlock "bounce" observed in the laboratory.[33]

In normal horses the peritendon of the superficial flexor is very elastic.[29] In horses afflicted with tendinitis of long enough duration so fibrous adhesions have formed between the tendon and the peritendon, the peritendon is tightly adhered to the tendon and the freedom of movement between the tendon and peritendon is lost.[29] The uninhibited movement of the tendon is lost and there is additional force stress placed on the tendon laterally rather than longitudinally.

The breaking strength of the superficial flexor tendon is significantly great when the tendon is loaded longitudinally.[34] However, when the load force is exerted laterad, much less force is needed to disrupt tendon architecture. When one recalls the structural description of the tendon fiber bundles and considers the longitudinal force placed on the tendon when a horse runs, primary tendon damage can occur as a result of horizontal tendon-peritendon adhesion strain.

Circumferential adhesions may cause healing scar tissue in the tendon parenchyma to orient, not in a longitudinal direction as in normal tendon, but along lines of stress.[17] The adhesion phenomenon is even more interesting considering the location in the tendon in which damage is most often observed. The most commonly damaged area in tendon is just proximal or distal to the previous lesion at the level where the tendon/peritendon union is more normal or more loosely attached (Fig 123).[29]

The literature abundantly describes acute areas of inflammation, degeneration, hemorrhage and repair in chronically involved tendons.[31,35] A hypothesis has been set forth that acute Achilles tendon damage in human athletes and onset of acute clinical signs are the results of restrictive adhesions from previous, often subclinical or at least unnoticed tendon damage.[35] This also agrees with findings in tendons of apparently normal horses.[28,29] Failure of the peritendon to return to a normal, loose connective tissue arrangement, but rather remaining a compact, well-organized nonelastic, restrictive structure, may be due to microtrauma, with intermittent stimulus for reaction of the peritendon tissue.[21,28,29] Thus, an initial tendon injury may never assume its original function and structure because of continuous tearing of adhesions and normal tendon tissue.[1,37]

Numerous studies of normal and abnormal equine flexor tendons have been undertaken to substantiate the theory of poor blood supply as the cause of recurrent tendinitis.[12,28,35] However, results of such research have indicated serious doubt to the validity of this theory. This is not to say blood supply is not important, but assumptions of avascular degeneration and necrosis have not been proven.

In summary, the initial cause of tendinitis may be more closely related to physical phenomena (stress/strain, frequency, creep, subcellular metabolism and structure of the limb itself) than to avascular necrosis or poor blood supply.[29] Fetlock "bounce" occurs during weight loading, which is a third-order acceleration.[33] Muscle is the active component of the muscle/tendon unit; when fatigued, considerable vibration develops since the muscle is no longer able to exert its dampening effect.[34] The character of the gait itself is altered by fatigue.[38] Also, one must not ignore the principle of stress/decay which, when in combination with the aforementioned factors, can cause primary tendon fiber damage.[3] It has been further proposed that the resulting restrictive adhesions and alteration in tendon and peritendon architecture are much more significant than inadequate blood supply in recurrence of tendinitis.[29] In other words, overhealing occurs, with resultant loss of structure and function.

Clinical Signs: Acute tendinitis is characterized by varying degrees of heat, pain and swelling. Not infrequently the history reveals one or a combination of these signs to a slight (approaching subclinical) degree prior to the presenting incident.[31] Heat is a common finding, although it might be very slight initially. Pain is one of the earliest and most useful signs to aid early diagnosis and to monitor the results of treatment and physical therapy. Pain must be evaluated when the limb is not bearing weight. Use of digital pressure, applied to the individual flexor tendons over their entire length, is recommended. Comparing the reaction obtained from palpation of the opposite limb is also advisable. The initial lameness in acute, nonrecurrent cases subsides very rapidly, causing many trainers to resume training too early.

Treatment: Various methods have been used to treat tendinitis. Prolonged rest, application of external and internal irritants, tendon-splitting, peritendonectomy, tendon transplants, fascia implantation, carbon fiber implants, irradiation, ultrasound and transection of the palmar (plantar) annular ligament have been used with varying degrees of success.[1,11,12,20,21,25,32,39-51]

At this writing, the recommended treatment of tendinitis uses noninvasive methods commencing immediately upon diagnosis of the condition to decrease the amount of restrictive adhesions formed.[29,32,52] A retrospective study indicated that just over 5% of affected horses treated conservatively raced 2 or more times without recurrent tendinitis; use of invasive procedures, primarily percutaneous tendon-splitting, only increased this percentage to approximately 10%.[53] A recent study indicated

that 70% of horses affected for the first time and over 35% of horses with recurrent tendinitis responded to the following conservative therapy.[52] Horses without recurrent tendinitis after conservative therapy resumed racing within 1-2 months; those with recurrent tendinitis required 4-6 months for recovery.

When minimal or no swelling is present, immediate conservative treatment and controlled physical therapy are usually successful. When more swelling is present as a result of more extensive peritendon and/or tendon damage caused by edema and hemorrhage, the prognosis for uncomplicated recovery is significantly decreased due to the ensuing fibrous reaction.

Use of systemic and topical corticosteroids may not be desirable if surgery is a possibility in the near future. Prednisolone acetate, DMSO, 9-fluoroprednisolone acetate, hydrodiuril, phenylbutazone and other similar drugs have proven useful. Application of ice packs or cold water is also beneficial. The affected area should be kept firmly bandaged between hydrotherapy sessions to minimize swelling.

Significant fibrous adhesions develop 10-14 days after tendon injury. During this time attempts should be made to minimize the reaction to the injury and the possibility of further injury. Stall rest is recommended. After a rest period of 10-14 days, exercise is initiated, starting with walking, then gradually increasing the duration and speed of exercise as quickly as possible without reinjuring the tendon.

As discussed previously, the signs of heat, pain and swelling must be evaluated both before and after exercise. Particular attention must be paid to pain, as pain is the most reliable indicator. If palpation reveals pain, exercise must be slowed or stopped for a few days and resumed when pain has subsided. Close observation and proper amounts of exercise should result in no recurrence of swelling. This requires close observation but is very rewarding. If the horse is not exercised enough, restrictive adhesions occur rather than adhesions that allow for the normal gliding movement of the tendon.

Initially, swimming is the ideal controlled exercise, followed by gradually increasing periods of track exercise and decreasing periods of swimming. Since the degree of damage to the tendon and peritendon varies from case to case, a rigid time table of physical therapy increase is not possible. As a rule of thumb, the nearer the horse comes to the level of exercise to which

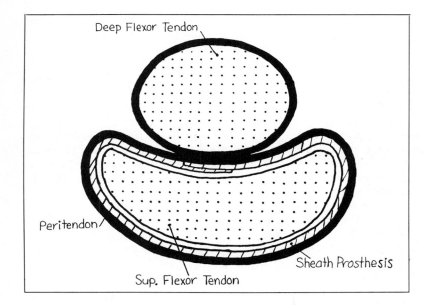

Fig 124. Cross-section of tendon, showing placement of a Teflon prosthesis.

it will be maximally subjected, the less the likelihood of recurrence.

When such conservative therapy is employed in recurrent tendinitis, one must expect setbacks in that adhesions and/or tendon tissue itself will be torn. The object is to decrease the inflammation from this tearing as soon as possible and to follow with controlled exercise to prevent reformation of restrictive adhesions. This conservative, noninvasive treatment regimen requires not only close observation and patience, but also cooperation of the horse and owner involved. The conservative approach outlined above appears to be the most successful treatment for bowed tendons.

Two more areas of investigation may prove fruitful in the treatment of tendinitis. The first is the biochemical control of fibroblastic prolif-

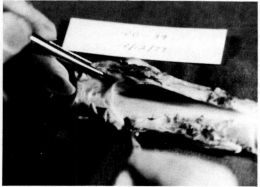

Fig 125. A few long, gliding adhesions allow normal excursion of the tendon.

eration and collagen metabolism.[54-56] The second area of investigation is placement of an inert material between the highly reactive peritendon and the tendon, thereby regulating the quantity and quality of fibrous ingrowth and preventing massive restrictive adhesions (Fig 124).[29,32,44,57] This delicate balance of allowing enough capillaries and fibroblasts through the material to facilitate repair, but not so much ingrowth as to cause restriction of normal tendon glide, has been achieved using one inert material (Fig 125).[32] Of 34 horses subjected to surgery for placement of a Teflon implant, only one horse experienced recurrence of tendinitis.[29,32] This horse was being pushed much too rapidly in the postoperative exercise program. Three horses were not returned to training due to mismanagement of the cases during the first 4 weeks after surgery. However, the studies of Teflon implants in treatment of tendinitis involve too few cases with insufficient followup to draw conclusions as to success rate.

Deep Digital Flexor Tendinitis

Tendinitis of the deep flexor tendon alone is not common. Involvement of this tendon is observed more in draft horses and to some extent in Standardbred race horses.[30] The areas most commonly involved are at the level of the inferior check ligamentous attachment and at the pastern. Often there is also involvement of the other flexor tendon and ligaments (superficial digital flexor tendon, inferior check ligament, suspensory ligament).

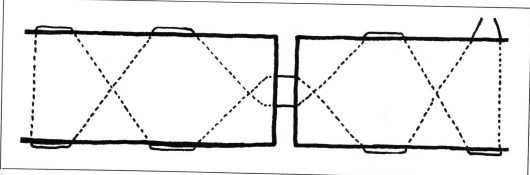

Fig 126. Bunnell suture pattern in tendon.

Cause: This injury may occur when the horse stumbles, thereby overextending the fetlock with the carpus flexed. Tearing of the inferior check ligament and/or the origin of the suspensory ligament, with associated fibrosis, may cause secondary tendinitis due to adhesions eventually involving the deep flexor tendon. Chronic, recurrent superficial flexor tendinitis may result in deep flexor tendinitis by increased stress placed on the deep flexor tendon when the superficial flexor tendon is torn severely or by adhesions involving the deep flexor tendon secondarily. However, examination of horses with severe chronic tendinitis usually reveals very little adhesion between these 2 flexor tendons.[29,32]

Clinical Signs: Signs include a low-grade, chronic progressive tendinitis rather than the immediate signs observed in superficial flexor tendinitis. This is particularly true of involvement at the inferior check ligament attachment.

Treatment: In acute cases, conservative treatment may be successful, as recommended for superficial flexor tendinitis, such as anti-inflammatory, systemic and topical treatment, with 10-14 days' rest, then gradual return to training. Chronic cases usually involve considerable fibrosis and have often been treated by methods that further increase restrictive fibrosis and result in recurrence.

Prognosis: The prognosis of deep digital flexor tendinitis is similar to that of superficial flexor tendinitis. Chronic cases have a tendency to recur.

Flexor Tendon Transection

Results of complete transection of the flexor tendons depend upon which structures are severed. If the superficial digital flexor tendon is severed, the fetlock is slightly to moderately dropped and the foot remains flat on the ground.

When the suspensory ligament is severed, the fetlock is moderately to severely dropped and the foot remains flat on the ground. If the deep digital tendon is severed, there is no significant drop in the fetlock and the toe comes up off the ground when the horse walks.

Treatment: Treatment consists of thorough debridement of the area, liberal flushing with sterile saline with or without antibiotics, and adequate stabilization of the limb. Tendons severed within a tendon sheath receive priority for suturing providing the treatment principles are fulfilled. However, it is often difficult to determine if a tendon has been severed. It is wise to treat such cases initially as outlined above, then wait until you are more certain infection is not present before reuniting the ends with sutures or synthetic materials, such as carbon fibers or Teflon.[33,48] Use of this same procedure is advisable when a tendon not enclosed by a sheath is severed. Use of tenolysis, with Teflon sheath implantation after the tendon has healed, may also be considered.[29,32] A physical therapy program is also essential.

The caudal aspect of the pastern is a common area of injury due to wire cuts and kicking or falling through objects, such as partitions, windows and floors. Extensive debridement and anti-infective measures must be employed before defects in the tendon sheath are sutured. If this cannot be done satisfactorily, the sheath should not be sutured. If suturing a severed tendon is attempted, use of a Bunnell suture pattern of nonabsorbable, nonreactive, flexible suture material is recommended (Fig 126).[30] Adequate stabilization is extremely important for proper healing and any hope of return to athletic activity. Casts may be employed with or without walking bars; however, casts do not allow easy access to the damaged area for adequate treatment and close observation. Also,

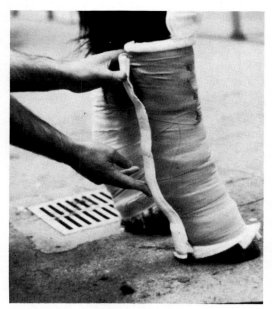

Fig 127. Orthoplast splint applied to the caudal aspect of the limb.

with significant instability of the lower limb, pressure sores are more likely to develop under a rigid cast. If severe soft tissue damage and vascular compromise are present, cast complications are likely. Strong consideration should be given to use of a Robert Jones bandage, with splints or a walking bar, for support during transport of the animal to a facility for definitive treatment. This decreases the chances of further damage and contamination.

After thorough debridement and cleansing of the wound, consideration should be given to the use of specially designed shoes with or without attachable devices.[30,58] A good support bandage with or without splints is also necessary. A thick cotton support bandage is applied after the sterile dressing is applied. Significant additional support can be obtained by making 2 splints (3-4 thicknesses each) of Orthoplast (Johnson & Johnson). The width of these splints should be 3-4 inches, the length being dictated by the length of the area bandaged. One splint should extend from the ground or weight-bearing surface of the foot up the cranial aspect of the limb, and the other up the caudal aspect of the limb. The Orthoplast is heated in hot water or in an oven to make it pliable. When pliable, the splints are placed on the limb external to the bandage and affixed to the bandage with elastic bandages or elastic tape (Fig 127). Care should be given to keep the splints truly cra-

nial and caudal during application. This technic adds considerable stability to the limb and allows easy access to the damaged area. It is also inexpensive in that the splints can be reused. Such splints are not adequate for treatment of complete transections and must be combined with a special shoe or wood angle-block (Fig 128).

Care must be exercised in selecting a shoe if the front limb is involved. A shoe that extends beyond the back of the hoof very far is likely to be torn off by a hind foot. Also, use of an excessively heavy shoe apparatus can lead to disastrous damage if the horse does not tolerate it, particularly when recovering from general anesthesia (Fig 129). A combination of a shoe and caudal board or sling splint can be employed (Figs 130, 131).[30,58] When these types of stability appliances are used, it must be certain that excessive local pressure does not occur on the cranial aspect of the limb. Care should also be exercised to prevent damage to the caudal aspect of the limb at the proximal end of the splint.

Prognosis: The prognosis for these transecting wounds depends upon the location, structures damaged, presence of infection, damage to blood vessels, nerves and lymphatics, and damage to adjacent soft tissue including the skin. The prognosis is generally guarded for return to sustained athletic soundness.

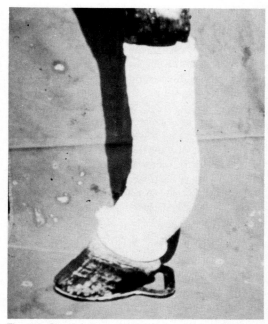

Fig 128. Special shoe applied to correct instability.

Extensor Tendon Transection

Extensor tendon transections usually involve less soft tissue damage than do flexor tendon transections. If the wound involves the area of a tendon sheath or joint capsule, these structures must be evaluated for damage. Extensive flushing, debridement and antibiotic therapy are very important in such cases. Unless one of these structures is opened and infected, the prognosis for return to athletic activity is favorable.

The principles of thorough debridement, flushing and stabilization, as used for flexor tendon transections, also apply to extensor tendon transections. Thorough debridement often necessitates removal of the common or long digital extensors (occasionally the lateral digital extensor, anterior tibialis and peroneus tertius) for several centimeters if the tendon is damaged or contaminated and the distal end is separated from the limb. Healing is slowed and fibrosis increased if this damaged, contaminated tissue is not removed. Occasionally there is some initial instability (partial flexion or cranial subluxation) of the fetlock joint. This decreases as healing of the soft tissue occurs. The affected limb initially knuckles over but the animal rapidly begins to accommodate for this by flipping the distal limb craniad so it lands flat. Care should be taken when turning the patient around, when first moving the horse off, and when walking the horse over uneven ground. A good support bandage extend-

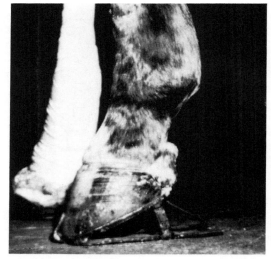

Fig 129. This special shoe is much too heavy and extends too far caudad, especially when applied to a front foot.

ing to the proximal aspect of the hoof is sufficient during transport of the horse for definitive treatment.

Not infrequently a portion of the third metacarpal/metatarsal bone is exposed. Care should be taken after debridement and flushing to keep the exposed bone moist. The skin flap can be debrided and used as a cover for the bone even if some of the flap eventually dies. Sequestration is likely if the exposed bone is not kept moist and healing is delayed (Fig 132).

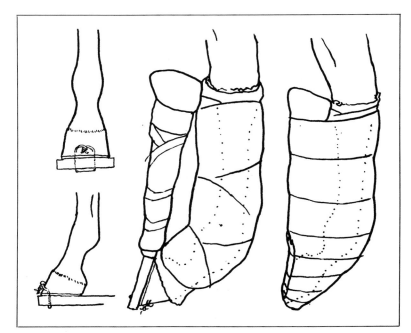

Fig 130. Combination shoe and caudal board.

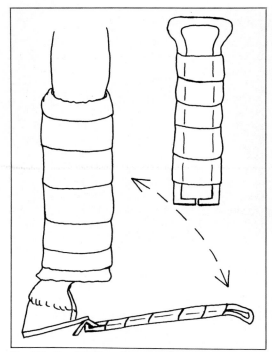

Fig 131. Combination shoe and sling splint.

Skin grafting is often necessary or at least advisable (see Chapter 16). The split-thickness pinch or mesh technics are relatively simple and save time for the clinician and money for the owner. The result is superior and the chronic, inelastic scar deformity and breakdown with subsequent excessive granulation is avoided.

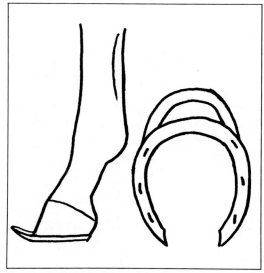

Fig 133. Shoe with extended toe for horses with a severed extensor tendon.

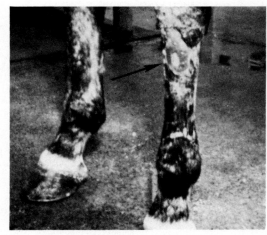

Fig 132. Sequestrum of exposed bone.

This is especially true over the cranial aspect of the tarsus and proximal metatarsus.

Adequate immobilization of transected extensor tendons is important but not as difficult as with flexor tendon transections. A toe extension on the shoe is generally adequate to prevent knuckling over (Fig. 133). The extension should be turned up at the end because a flat extension may predispose to knuckling rather than prevent it.[30] Another means of preventing knuckling is to attach a piece of twine or strapping from the toe extension up to the caudal aspect of the proximal metacarpal/metatarsal area, providing this area is adequately bandaged. In addition to the shoe, serious consideration should be given to a bandage/Orthoplast splint to further guard against knuckling over. Application of an Orthoplast splint or cast to extensive wounds of the cranial aspect of the hock is essential to achieve satisfactory results, particularly cosmetically. Casting necessitates general anesthesia and the disadvantages mentioned concerning flexor tendon transections apply. In addition, a significant number of horses do not tolerate a full-leg cast on a hind limb and destroy the cast or themselves no matter how it is constructed or reinforced. Orthoplast splinting all the way up the cranial aspect and up to the level of the hock on the caudal aspect works quite satisfactorily. Care should be taken not to apply the elastic adhesive bandage too tightly over the tuber calcis but just cover the cotton (Fig 134).

Tendon Rupture

Ruptured tendons occur as a result of infection, sudden, very forceful stress, trauma by blunt objects (particularly where the tendon

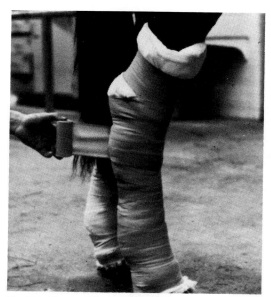

Fig 134. Elastic adhesive bandage applied loosely over the tuber calcis.

lies directly over bone), the effects on tendon of rough degenerative bone or bone fragments, and injection of certain corticosteroids into tendon tissue.[10,37,54,59]

Treatment depends on the location, cause and the amount of damage present, as does the prognosis. The prognosis for ruptured tendons is guarded at best. Carbon fiber implantation, tenolysis and implantation of a Teflon sheath could be beneficial.[29,32,48] Also, use of the last procedure alone after natural healing of the rupture may improve the prognosis in some cases. The following are some examples of tendon ruptures occasionally seen in horses.

Rupture of the Deep Flexor Tendon: This rupture usually occurs at or near the insertion. Infection, usually from a puncture wound of the sole or frog and extending to the tendon itself, can cause rupture. This condition is also indirectly caused by posterior digital neurectomy in horses with severe navicular bone disease. Feeling no pain in the area, the horse exercises and "saws" the tendon during locomotion.

The toe is raised off the ground as the horse walks and bears weight on the affected limb. The digital flexor sheath may be distended due to infection or inflammation. If infection is present, evidence of such is present and the horse is extremely lame, possibly necessitating local nerve blocking to ascertain if the tendon is ruptured, providing the horse has not had a neurectomy.

Prognosis for a ruptured deep flexor tendon is poor and euthanasia is recommended.

Rupture of the Tendon of the Extensor Carpi Radialis:[60,61] This type of rupture usually occurs at the proximal level of the carpus or just above the carpus. Tenosynovitis is often concurrent. This condition can occur when young horses, confined to a stall, become nervous and strike a firm object, such as a stall screen or a bucket. It also has been observed in horses with chronic degenerative joint disease of the carpus, particularly of the radiocarpal joint. Large spurs and chip fractures of the distal radius can erode the tendon sheath and cause direct trauma to the tendon itself. Of course, any direct trauma to this area can damage and rupture the tendon and sheath.

Clinical signs include acute heat, swelling, pain and marked distension of the tendon sheath (Fig 135). Palpation may reveal a rupture. Examination should be made during manual flexion and extension of the carpus. Lameness is usually present initially. The gait deficit is that of a somewhat stiff and less efficient extension of the limb. In chronic cases the distal limb may be flipped craniad during locomotion, somewhat similar to movement in

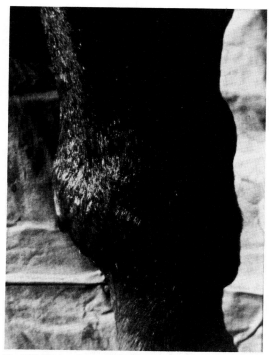

Fig 135. Distension of the sheaths of the extensor carpi radialis.

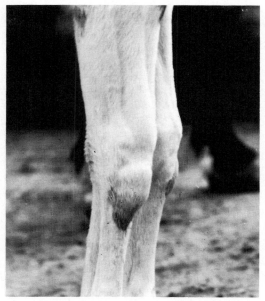

Fig 136. Rupture of the common digital extensor tendon in a foal.

common digital extensor tendon rupture; however, no knuckling of the distal limb occurs. Radiographs should be taken to ascertain any underlying bone disease and contrast studies can be employed to confirm communication between carpal joints and the tendon sheath.[60] Calcification may occur in the damaged area.

If extensive chronic degenerative joint disease is involved, treatment is usually impractical. Joint surgery may be considered if joint damage is not severe. Tenolysis (severing restrictive adhesions to free the tendon) and a partial tenosynovectomies may be beneficial in some cases. Tenosynovectomies may be cosmetically beneficial if chronic multicystic tenosynovitis is present. Partial rupture may necessitate debridement at the time of tenolysis. Complete ruptures have been sutured but results have not been encouraging. The use of carbon fiber and/or a Teflon sheath may be considered. The limb should be placed in a cast for 4 weeks if the tendon is ruptured.

The prognosis must be guarded because a significant chronic gait deficit, due to restrictive fibrosis in the area and chronic bone and joint involvement, is usually present after treatment. Cosmetic surgery for distension of the sheath may not yield satisfactory results.

Rupture of the Common Digital Extensor Tendon in Young Foals:[30,61] This condition may be due to excessive running with the mare

when the foal is only a few days old or from sudden stress forces as the foal is getting up and moving around unsteadily in the stall.

There is swelling over the cranial aspect of the carpus and just proximal to the carpus (Fig 136). The tendon completely or partially ruptures at the musculotendinous junction and retracts distad into the tendon sheath. Usually the severed end of the tendon can be palpated. The foal may be able to stand and walk quite stiffly but cannot extend the distal limb. The foal may knuckle over onto the dorsal (cranial) aspect of the distal limb. In such cases the condition could be mistaken for contracted tendons unless the foal is adequately examined.

Suturing the tendon ends after debridement and placing the limb in a cast for 30 days has been successful. Surgical debridement with cast application and cast application alone have been used successfully.

The prognosis is guarded for return to athletic activity.

Rupture of the Peroneus Tertius:[30,61] The peroneus tertius is entirely tendinous in the horse and, as part of the reciprocal apparatus, is responsible for simultaneous hock and stifle flexion. If the tendon is ruptured at its origin, the long digital flexor tendon may also be affected since it has a common origin, resulting

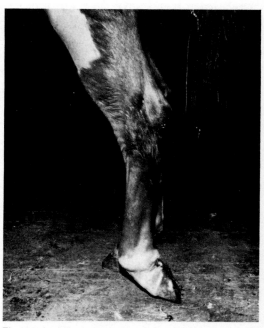

Fig 137. Inability to extend the lower limb due to rupture of the peroneus tertius and long digital flexor tendon at their origins.

in inability to extend the lower limb (Fig 137). The most common site of rupture is between the stifle and hock, usually just above the hock. Ruptures at the insertion are usually partial.

Rupture can result from a kick, hyperextension of the hock, kicking through a partition and getting the leg caught, or missing a jump. There may also be a conformational predisposition to partial tearing at the insertion. A very straight hock or one that is "tied-in" may predispose to a jerking motion of hyperextension as the horse drives off the limb.

Signs vary with the severity of damage. The hock is overextended with normal flexion of the stifle and the gastrocnemius tendon area is flaccid, especially when the hock is extended. In severe cases the hock may jerk up slightly and caudad as the limb is brought craniad without flexion of the hock. Partial tearing at the insertion may produce exostosis (Fig 138). If an overextension instability persists, degenerative arthrosis of the cranial aspect of the proximal intertarsal, distal intertarsal and tarsal joints may occur.

Use of stall rest for a mimimum of 2 months has been recommended as treatment.[30] The more severe the damage, the longer the stall rest period, particularly in complete ruptures and ruptures at the origin. Initially it may be beneficial to prevent the horse from lying down. If some overextension of the hock persists and/or is predisposed by conformation, use of a 1-2° wedge pad, with the thickest part at the toe, may decrease the jerky motion of hyperextension. The pads can be applied temporarily to check for improvement.

Most of these ruptures heal with time; however, ruptures at the origin may not progress satisfactorily. Reinjury, possibly due to restrictive adhesions, has been noted when the initial damage was at the level of the proximal aspect of the tarsus. Some instability may persist and may be predisposed by conformation. Degenerative joint disease of the distal 3 joints of the tarsus may become clinically significant.

Rupture of the Achilles Tendon: Rupture of the gastrocnemius tendon alone or in combination with the superficial flexor tendon and the soleus may occur.[30] Partial ruptures are more common than complete ruptures, although both are uncommon.

Hyperflexion of the hock, from falling with the leg under the body, may cause this condition. This injury has occurred when horses have tried to get up too soon after general anesthesia.[61] This area can also be damaged from

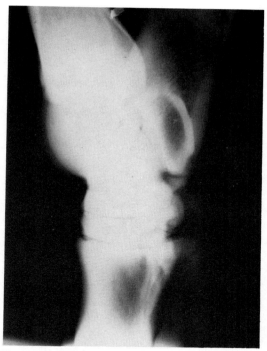

Fig 138. Exostosis due to tearing of the insertion of the peroneus tertius.

improper cast application and bandaging over the tendon.

The horse cannot bear weight on the limb in complete rupture and the hock overflexes markedly. In partial ruptures the horse may be able to bear weight and hyperflexion of the hock may be difficult to detect. Palpation aids evaluation of the extent of the injury. Pressure necrosis may be present if a cast or bandage is to blame. Crepitus in the area may indicate a tuber calcis fracture, and radiographs are then indicated.

Stall rest for a minimum of 2 months is recommended if a partial tear is present. Treatment generally is unsuccessful, as far as return to athletic activity is concerned, in cases of complete rupture.[62]

The prognosis is guarded, depending on the degree of tearing and the presence of bone and muscle disease.

Luxation of the Rear Superficial Flexor Tendon:[30,61] Luxation of the superficial flexor tendon at the level of the tuber calcis usually occurs on the lateral aspect. The luxation is usually due to rupture of the medial insertion of the superficial flexor tendon onto the tuber calcis. Retinacula associated with the tendon may also be damaged.

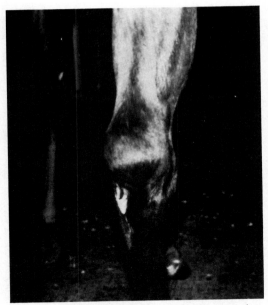

Fig 139. Luxation of the rear superficial flexor tendon.

Application of a sudden force to the area, particularly when the hock is flexed, can cause this injury. Wheeling on the rear legs or kicks are common causes.

The tendon is displaced and usually moves back and forth, returning to its normal position during locomotion (Fig 139). Heat, swelling and lameness are present initially. Overflexion of the tarsus may or may not be present.

Application of a cast or splint and 1-3 months of stall rest have been employed successfully.[30] Surgical correction involves suturing the ruptured tendon attachment and inserting a Steinmann pin into the tuber calcis just lateral (or medial) to the main part of the tendon. The pin is left protruding from the tuber calcis enough to keep the tendon in place. The tendon must not be returned to its original position for the horse to be sound. However, chronic movement of the tendon (luxation) can produce chronic lameness.[61] Reinjury of the involved structures and/or adhesions in the area can cause recurrent lameness.

The prognosis for return to sustained athletic soundness is guarded.

Rupture of the Tendons of the Shoulder: The infraspinatus and supraspinatus tendons are most commonly involved. External trauma, such as a kick or running into a stationary object, is the cause. Lateral instability of the affected shoulder is characteristic. Radiographs may be warranted if crepitus and/or bone involvement are suspected. Treatment consists

of stall rest for 2-4 months, with hand-walking after 3-4 weeks. The prognosis is somewhat guarded, depending on the amount of damage and instability present.

Rupture of the Prepubic Tendon: This condition is observed in pregnant mares approaching or just after parturition (Fig 140). No specific treatment is indicated other than stall rest. It may be necesary to assist delivery of the foal with or without cesarean section.

Multiple Congenital Exostosis and Superradial Exostosis

These exostoses may affect tendons and their sheaths. The most common site for this damage is the flexor sheath and associated tendons proximal to the carpus. Extensive distension of the carpal flexor sheath is usually present. Radiographs are indicated. Surgical removal of the offending exostosis has resulted in successful return to athletic activity. Careful examination for other exostoses should be performed. Histologic examination of the exostosis, as well as evidence of other sites of exostosis, differentiate the 2 conditions. Severe damage and complications from previous corticosteroid injections may adversely affect the prognosis. Primary tendon ossification, possibly congenital, has been reported.[63]

Tenosynovitis

Distension and inflammation of a tendon sheath is called tenosynovitis.

Cause: The cause may be chronic or acute external trauma or a shearing force on the tendon sheath, particularly where the sheath attaches to the tendon.

Clinical Signs: Heat, swelling and possibly pain on palpation, particularly at tendon sheath margins, are present in acute cases. Lameness may or may not be present. In chronic cases only distension is usually present. Extensive distension may cause lameness through interference with normal motion.

Treatment: Systemic and local anti-inflammatory treatment is indicated in acute cases. Bandaging of the affected site (if possible) is recommended. The animal should be examined for predisposing causes, such as poor conformation, improper shoeing, improper training, overloading of the limb due to disease in the opposite limb, and disease adjacent to or within the involved sheath.[64] The predisposing cause should be eliminated if possible.

Aseptic drainage of the distension, with or without injection of a corticosteroid, may be employed. This treatment is less successful in chronic cases, in which the tendon sheath is stretched and associated bone and soft tissue disease is present.[64] Cosmetic partial tenosynovectomies have been attempted. The patient must be cooperative and adequate immobilization of the area is essential. Postoperative problems may yield poor results.

Suspensory Desmitis

The suspensory ligament differs from tendon histologically in that the ligament contains considerably more elastic fibers and also contains muscle fibers. The main function of the suspensory ligament is to support the fetlock. Desmitis may occur at the origin, body or branches of the suspensory ligament going to each sesamoid bone, particularly just proximal to the bifurcation. Suspensory ligament disease is observed most frequently in Standardbred race horses, in which it occurs in the rear or front limbs. In Thoroughbred race horses, the front limbs are more frequently involved and the rear limbs rarely involved.

Cause: A "toed-in" conformation may predispose development of the desmitis by overstressing the lateral aspect of the suspensory ligament, particularly at its origin and sesamoid insertion; "toeing-out" results in increased stress on the medial aspect. A very long pastern predisposes to desmitis, particularly just proximal to the bifurcation, as does improper shoeing that places the weight-bearing surface too far craniad. Medial or lateral foot imbalance can cause desmitis, particularly at the origin and the insertion at the sesamoid, and may compound the increased stress placed on the ligament by faulty conformation. Of course, exercise on uneven terrain, causing uneven landing of the limb, may be a factor. The "rolling" type of gait observed in the pacer could cause increased stress on the ligament.

Two bony structures directly associated with the suspensory ligament are the sesamoid bones and splint bones. Disease of any of these structures generally results in involvement of the other 2 if not treated adequately. Thickening of the suspensory ligament can cause the splint bone to pull away from the third metacarpal/metatarsal bone and thicken significantly. Desmitis at the insertion of the suspensory ligament causes abnormal stress on the sesamoid bones, with sesamoiditis as a possible result. Conversely, sesamoiditis may also lead to suspensory desmitis. This becomes a vicious cycle in that more involvement in one structure causes more involvement in the other. A fractured splint bone often instigates

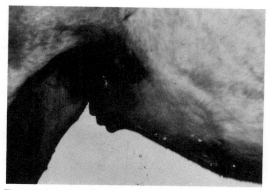

Fig 140. Rupture of the prepubic tendon.

the cycle. A splint bone pulled away from the third metacarpal/metatarsal bone not only thickens and exerts pressure on the ligament but is also more likely to become fractured; the resulting large callus from nonunion causes more desmitis. Avulsion fractures of the proximal sesamoid bones are observed with desmitis and can cause suspensory desmitis.

Clinical Signs: Initially the desmitis may be subclinical in that no significant heat or swelling is present. As in tendinitis, one of the first signs is pain on digital palpation of the limb when it is not bearing weight. Pressure should be applied down the medial and lateral aspects of the ligament from origin to insertions at the sesamoid bones. The suspensory ligament should also be examined by placing a finger on each side (caudal and cranial) and tracing it from origin to insertion with the limb bearing weight. This tracing should be done on the medial and lateral aspects of the limb. The thickness should remain constant all the way to the sesamoid bones. Slight thickenings can be detected in this manner. A gait deficit similar to lameness from a knee or shoulder problem is frequently caused by damage to the origin of the ligament.

Inflammation at the origin may involve the inferior check ligament and the interosseus ligament of the splint bone, particularly in chronic inflammations. Chronic suspensory desmitis results in considerable restrictive adhesions in the area, and recurrence is not uncommon. Damage to the body of the suspensory ligament is more easily detected since swelling and heat in the area are greater.

Inflammation at the insertion on the sesamoid bone is most easily detected by palpation with the leg bearing weight as described above. The splint bones and seasmoid bones should also be palpated due to their relationship to pathologic changes in the area. Radiographs are usually indicated. Signs, such as lameness, dropping of the fetlock, and calcification of the ligament, vary with the amount and longevity of damage.

Treatment: Treatment of only the suspensory desmitis yields poor results if a splint bone or a sesamoid bone is also involved. If a splint bone is fractured or displaced, the distal portion should be removed to the point at which it is firmly attached to the third metacarpal/metatarsal bone. Removal of the fragments is usually recommended in apex fractures of the proximal sesamoids. Treatment of the desmitis is more successful once the associated bone disease has been treated.

Anti-inflammatory topical and systemic treatment is recommended in acute suspensory desmitis. This treatment should begin immediately since the longer the swelling in the suspensory ligament is present, the more likely is the "triad cycle" of involvement. Stall rest for 3-4 weeks to several months is recommended, depending on the amount of pathologic change present. In severe cases of desmitis, 6-9 months are often needed before training can be resumed. In fact, the amount of suspensory ligament damage present should decide the time of return to training after splint bone and sesamoid surgery.

Treatment of damage at the origin of the suspensory ligament can be frustrating due to recurrence. Radiation therapy, along with 3-6 months of stall rest has been quite successful although sometimes impractical. Rest alone, local injection of corticosteroids, topical anti-inflammatory drugs, topical counterirritants, and local injection of counterirritants have been used with mixed results. A combination of rest, local injection of corticosteroids, and topical anti-inflammatory therapy has yielded quite satisfactory results.[65] In a series of over 400 cases, less than 2% recurrence was noted in a 4-month followup period.

Injection of 200-400 mg methylprednisolone acetate (Depo-Medrol:Upjohn) between the proximal splint bone and the involved origin of the suspensory ligament is accomplished using a 22-ga, 1½-inch needle, with the leg not bearing weight. Injection of 50-100 mg methylprednisolone in the area of the inferior check ligament at the same time can be employed if this area shows involvement. Asepsis is strictly observed and a sterile bandage applied. The horses should receive stall rest for 3-4 weeks, during which time a topical sweat of DMSO containing prednisolone acetate at 2 mg/ml DMSO is applied. The sweat is applied for one week, skipped for a week, and then applied for another week.

Use of topical and locally injected counterirritants may increase the amount of restrictive adhesions formed, although this form of treatment has been quite popular.

In chronic desmitis, percutaneous splitting of the thickened suspensory ligament is successful, as far as return to racing is concerned, 75% of the time (primarily in Standardbred race horses).[21,42,66] The higher success rate, as compared to those for treatment of tendinitis, may be due to considerably less excursion of the suspensory ligament in this condition; therefore, the resultant adhesions are not as significant. Also, scar tissue contraction decreases the size of the suspensory ligament.

This procedure can be performed under local anesthesia with the horse standing. Strict asepsis must be observed. The special bistoury is directed at a right angle to the limb through the skin and through the involved ligament, with the cutting edges running longitudinally with the ligament fibers. The bistoury handle is then rotated proximad and distad until the cutting edge is felt under the skin. This produces a semicircular splitting of the ligament in the direction of its fibers. The knife is then removed and inserted at a distance proximal to the initial incision so that the next semicircular split overlaps the first half-circle by the length of the radius of the half-circle (Fig 141). The splitting is performed every 0.75-1 cm of the thickness of the ligament. This procedure is repeated on the other side of the suspensory ligament if that branch and/or the body of the ligament is involved. A sterile bandage and pressure wrap are applied after hemorrhage has subsided. A 6- to 10-month rest period is recommended before return to racing.

Prognosis: The prognosis varies greatly with the amount of damage, location and involvement of the triad of structures. Standardbred race horses apparently can race significantly more successfully with suspensory ligament damage than can Thoroughbreds. The prognosis is guarded in Thoroughbreds with extensive desmitis since recurrence is likely.

Sesamoidean Desmitis

Desmitis of the 3 paired sesamoidean ligaments may occur with or without fracture of the corresponding base of the proximal sesamoid bone. Radiographs are indicated.

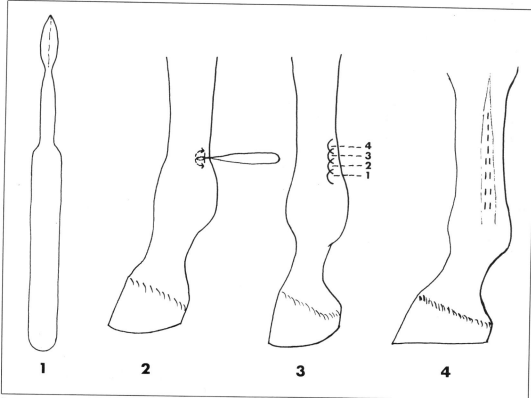

Fig 141. Percutaneous splitting of the suspensory ligament. 1. Bistoury. 2. Insertion and movement of the bistoury in the suspensory ligament. 3. Positions of the bistoury, showing overlap of splitting movement. 4. Pattern of insertions of the bistoury.

Cause: The cause is a sudden, twisting torque force at the time weight is placed on the limb.

Signs: In acute cases, heat, pain, and swelling are present, while in chronic cases, fibrotic enlargement may be the only sign.

Treatment: Cases not involving sesamoid fractures are treated with 2-10 months' rest, with local and systemic anti-inflammatory therapy and a supportive bandage initially. The distal fragment may be removed if fractures of the distal portion of the sesamoid bone are present.

Prognosis: Recurrence of the desmitis is not uncommon, and return to sustained soundness as far as racing is concerned is generally unfavorable after removal of a distal sesamoid bone fragment.

Miscellaneous Conditions

Other conditions in which a tendon is involved directly in surgery include cunean tenectomy or tenotomy for degenerative arthrosis of the distal 3 joints of the tarsus ("bone spavin"), tenectomy of the lateral digital extensor tendon for the condition "stringhalt," and medial patellar desmotomy for upward fixation of the patella.[61] These 3 conditions are discussed elsewhere in this chapter.

Severe ruptures of the distal components of the stay apparatus (superficial digital flexor, deep digital flexor, suspensory ligament and sesamoidean ligaments in particular) are occasionally observed in Thoroughbred race horses. There are often a variety of sesamoid bone fractures present, as well as occasional fractures of the cranioproximal aspect of the first phalanx.

The prognosis for return to racing is poor and for salvage as a breeding animal is guarded. The key factor as to whether the horse can be saved is an adequate blood supply to the lower limb, which must be evaluated very closely before surgery to stabilize the distal limb.

If an attempt is to be made to save the horse, a Robert Jones bandage, with Orthoplast splints, and a special shoe or shoe/brace combination should be employed.[30,58] A cast should not be used because of the extensive soft tissue damage present; periodic evaluation is impossible with the cast on, an adequate cast cannot be put on the standing horse, and infection is usually present because of skin lacerations.

Careful consideration of the behavior of the patient and the orthopedic capabilities of the surgeon and instrumentation is essential before surgery is contemplated. A conservative approach using special shoes and braces may be more rewarding in some cases.

References

1. Peacock, EE and van Winkle, W: Surgery and Biology of Wound Repair. WB Saunders, Philadelphia, 1970.
2. Webbon, PM. Eq Vet J 10 (1978) 253.
3. Elliot, D. Biol Rev 40 (1965) 392.
4. Dale, WC et al. Experientia 28 (1972) 1293.
5. Gunson, DE. Eq Vet J 11 (1979) 97.
6. Chaplin, DM. J Bone Jt Surg 55B (1973) 369.
7. Mayer, L. Ann Roy Coll Surg II (1952) 69.
8. Evans, JH and Bartenel, JC. Eq Vet J 7 (1975) 1.
9. Blanton, PL and Biggs, NI. J Biomech 3 (1970) 181.
10. Cronkite, AE. Anat Rec 64 (1936) 173.
11. Fackelman, GE. Proc 18th Ann Mtg Am Assoc Eq Pract, 1972. p 237.
12. Fackelman, GE. Eq Vet J 5 (1973) i.
13. Klein, L et al. J Bone Jt Surg 54A (1972) 1745.
14. Potenza, AD. J Bone Jt Surg 45A (1963) 1217.
15. Potenza, AD. J Am Med Assoc 187 (1964) 99.
16. Verdan, CE. J Bone Jt Surg 54A (1972) 472.
17. Forrester, CP. Proc 1st Int Symp Wound Healing, 1975. p 59.
18. Bader, KF and Curtis, JW. Plastic Reconstr Surg 47 (1971) 576.
19. Davis, L and Aries, LJ. Surg 2 (1937) 877.
20. Morcos, MB and Aswad, A. Eq Vet J 10 (1978) 128.
21. Nilsson, G and Bjorck, L. JAVMA 155 (1969) 920.
22. Peacock, EE et al. Am J Surg 122 (1971) 686.
23. Brooks, DM. Proc Roy Soc Med 63 (1970).
24. Grant, BD et al. Eq Vet J 11 (1978) 509.
25. Knudsen, O. Eq Vet J 8 (1976) 101.
26. Webbon, PM. Eq Vet J 11 (1979) 264.
27. Silver, IA. Eq Vet J 11 (1979) 93.
28. Stromberg, B and Tufuesson, G. Clin Orthoped 62 (1969) 113.
29. Selway, SJ. Proc 20th Ann Mtg Am Assoc Eq Pract, 1975. p 53.
30. Keown, in Catcott: Equine Medicine and Surgery. 2nd ed. American Veterainary Publications, Santa Barbara, 1972.
31. Stromberg, B. Acta Rad Suppl 305 (1971) 1.
32. Selway, SJ, Pembroke Pines, FL: Unpublished data, 1981.
33. Rooney, JR. J Eq Med Surg 3 (1979) 376.
34. Rooney, JR. J Eq Med Surg 3 (1979) 50.
35. Norberg, AI et al. Proc 13th Ann Mtg Am Assoc Eq Pract, 1967. p 243.
36. Snook, GA. Med Sci Sports 4 (1972) 155.
37. Peacock, EE. N Engl J Med 275 (1967) 680.
38. Leach, DH et al. J Eq Med Surg 3 (1979) 436.
39. Selway, SJ, Pembroke Pines, FL: Unpublished data, 1980.
40. Balasubramaniam, P et al. J Bone Jt Surg 54A (1972) 729.
41. Ketchum, L. Plastic Reconstr Surg 47 (1971) 471.
42. Nilsson, G. Eq Vet J 1 (1969) 111.
43. Proctor, in Catcott: Equine Medicine and Surgery. 1st ed. American Veterainary Publications, Santa Barbara, 1963.
44. Snyder, CC. Proc 1st Surg Forum Am Coll Vet Surg, 1973.
45. Stromberg, B and Tufuesson, G. Eq Vet J 9 (1977) 231.
46. Stromberg, B et al. JAVMA 164 (1974) 57.
47. McKibben, LS. Backstretch (July 31, 1971) 26.
48. Littlewood, HF. Vet Rec 105 (1979) 223.
49. Hunter, JM and Salisbury, RE. J Bone Jt Surg 53A (1971) 829.
50. Franks, PW. Eq Vet J 11 (1979) 106.
51. Adams, OR. VM/SAC 69 (1974) 327.
52. Selway, SJ, Pembroke Pines, FL: Unpublished data, 1981.
53. Beech, J, Univ Penn: Unpublished data, 1980.
54. Dupis, PR and Uhthoff, HK. Union Med Can 101 (1972) 1763.
55. Jackson, DS. Eq Vet J 11 (1979) 102.
56. Lane, JM et al. J Surg Res 13 (1972) 135.
57. Homsy, CA. J Biomed Mat Res 2 (1968) 209.
58. Wheat, JD and Pascoe, JR. JAVMA 176 (1980) 205.
59. Wrenn, RN et al. J Bone Jt Surg 36A (1954) 588.
60. Llewellyn, JR. Eq Vet J 11 (1979) 90.
61. Mason, TA. Eq Vet J 9 (1977) 186.
62. Webbon, PM. Eq Vet J 9 (1977) 61.
63. Meagher, DM et al. JAVMA 174 (1979) 282.
64. Edwards, GB. Eq Vet J 10 (1978) 97.
65. Selway, SJ, Pembroke Pines, FL: Unpublished data, 1981.
66. Jones, RD and Fessler, JR. Can Vet J 18 (1977) 29.

Tendon Disorders of Young Horses
by C.W. McIlwraith

Flexor Tendon Flaccidity or Weakness in Foals

This condition of newborn foals is generally mild and affects the rear legs or all 4 legs. Primary systemic illness and lack of exercise have been implicated as causes of the musculotendinous weakness.[1] Affected foals walk on the caudal part of the hoof, do not bear weight on the toe, and essentially rock back on the bulbs of the heel (Fig 142).

Treatment involves corrective trimming and forced exercise. The heels are trimmed to eliminate the "rocker" effect and to provide a flat weight-bearing surface (Fig 143).[2] The toes should not be trimmed. If the heels are not trimmed, the foal rocks further back on its heels and subluxation of the distal interphalangeal joint may result. The use of protective bandages or casts exacerbates tendon flaccidity. The use of some form of heel extension has been described but is seldom indicated.[3]

Digital Hyperextension in Foals

This extreme form of the flaccid flexor tendon syndrome is apparent at or shortly after birth and is characterized by extreme dorsiflexion of the phalangeal joints.[4] Severely affected animals bear weight on the ventral surface of the sesamoids. The etiology is unknown. It is reportedly often seen in foals from poorly nourished mares but has also been observed in foals from well-fed mares.[4] It is less common than congenital flexor contracture.

Conservative methods of treatment, such as the use of elongated shoe branches and support bandaging, are not generally successful. A surgical procedure for shortening the superficial and deep flexor tendons has been described.[4] From the clinical nature of the condition and the response to surgical shortening of the flexor tendons, it has been implied that the cause of this condition is a flexor musculotendinous defect. However, electromyographic examinations have not demonstrated any pathologic changes in the musculature of the flexor group.[4]

Contracted Tendons or Flexion Deformities

The term "contracted tendons" may be a misnomer since the defect is not necessarily in the tendon itself. At least in acquired cases, the effective functional length of the musculotendinous unit is less than necessary to maintain normal limb alignment and a flexion deformity results. However, "contracted tendons" has become common usage and the author considers its use justified provided the user is aware of all the possible pathogenetic mechanisms.

Tendon contractures are considered congenital (apparent at or close to the time of birth) or acquired (developing during the growth period). Various etiologic factors have been incriminated in each group.

Congenital Flexor Tendon Contracture: Cases of congenital contracture have been classically attributed to uterine malpositioning. While this is possible, it is likely that such cases are the result of other more complex influences, including genetic factors and insults during the embryonic stage of pregnancy.

Genetic defects involving various degrees of skeletal abnormality have been described. One report described 8 foals with severe fetlock

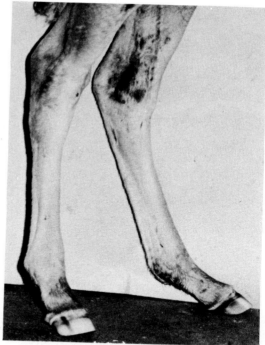

Fig 142. Flaccid flexor tendons in the rear limbs of a foal. The problem was treated with corrective trimming. (Courtesy of Dr JF Fessler)

flexion, most likely resulting from a recent dominant gene mutation in the sire.[5] A reported contracted foal syndrome involved torticollis, scoliosis, hypoplasia of the vertebral articular facets and distal extremities of the third metacarpal and metatarsal bones, and flexion contracture of the fetlock, carpal and tarsal joints.[6] The etiologic basis of the syn-

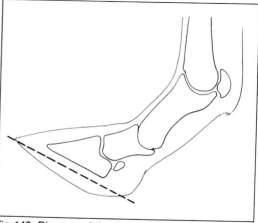

Fig 143. Diagram of the line of hoof trimming for the treatment of flaccid flexor tendons.

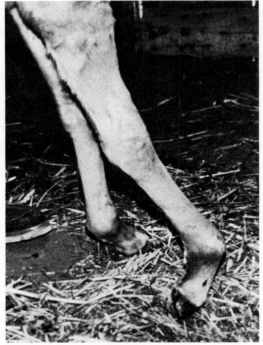

Fig 144. Congenital flexion deformity of the fetlock in the right forelimb of a foal.

genital flexion deformities of the carpus also occur (Fig 145). Individual tendon involvement is difficult to define in these cases. The ulnaris lateralis and flexor carpi ulnaris units have been incriminated but contraction of the carpal fascia is frequently an important component.

Some foals with congenital flexion deformities improve spontaneously. Treatment should be initiated as soon as possible. The basic principle of treatment is forced extension of the limb using splints or casts to induce the inverse myotatic reflex, with relaxation of the flexor muscles.[8] Gutter splints of yucca board or cut sections of PVC tubing may be used (Fig 146). A commercial corrective appliance (Badame Corrective Appliance) has been used in young foals.[9] Generally, if the splint enables the foal to walk on the sole of the foot so that tension forces are constantly applied to the flexor units, flexor relaxation may be quickly induced. However, all splinting devices require careful use of padding and constant changing of the splints to prevent skin necrosis. When the limb cannot be extended with splints, this treatment is generally unsatisfactory.

Casts may also be used to provide extension. In severe contractions that cannot be extended completely, casting may weaken the muscles

drome is unknown. It was hypothesized that the flexion deformities originated with joint instability, which in turn was due to bone malformations. In a report of 2 cases of tendon contracture in Clydesdale foals, one of the foals had severe extension deformities rather than flexion deformities.[7]

Arthrogryposis in other species produces a flexion deformity that can be difficult to differentiate from contracted tendons. This disease has been associated with specific etiologic agents.[1] One author reported 3 cases of congenital contracture in foals from mares on a farm with an influenza outbreak; the mares were in the embryonic stage of pregnancy at the time of the outbreak.[1] Although only circumstantial, such evidence underscores the need for continuing investigation into the role of toxic and infectious agents in congenital deformities.

Congenital flexion deformities may affect one or more limbs. The most common manifestation is fetlock flexion deformity. Some foals can stand but knuckle over at the fetlock (Fig 144). Severely affected foals cannot stand or they walk on the dorsal surface of the fetlock. Generally both the superficial and deep flexor tendons are involved in these cases. Involvement of the deep digital flexor alone and con-

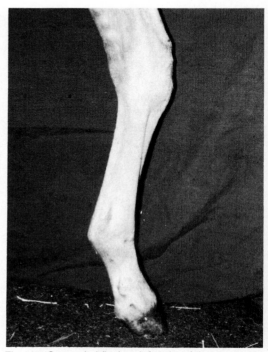

Fig 145. Congenital flexion deformity of the carpus.

enough to allow sufficient extension at cast changing. However, the prognosis is generally poor in all such cases. Cast application commonly results in problems. A plaster cast is very heavy for a foal. Fiberglass is light but full-length fiberglass casts commonly cause pressure sores. The use of 2 layers of Zoroc plaster to give internal molding, followed by application of fiberglass, is a good compromise. In this respect, a new light casting material applied wet without any special apparatus (Cutter Cast) would be preferable for most practitioners compared to the material requiring special equipment for hardening.

The final alternative in treatment of congenital contractures is surgery. Flexor tenotomy and inferior check desmotomy have been used successfully (methods described under Acquired Flexor Tendon Contracture). However, the prognosis becomes less favorable as the surgical treatment becomes more drastic.

Acquired Flexor Tendon Contracture: Acquired contracted tendons are unilateral or bilateral and usually occur as flexion deformities of the fetlock or coffin joint.

The pathogenesis of acquired contracted tendons is frequently related to pain. Any pain in the limb initiates the flexion withdrawal reflex, which may lead to flexor muscle contraction. Pain can arise from epiphysitis, osteochondritis dissecans, arthritis, soft tissue wounds or hoof infections with or without pedal bone involvement. Epiphysitis is common in animals with contracted tendons. Contracted tendons have been associated with osteochondritis dissecans in the shoulder and stifle.

Poor nutritional management constitutes the most common cause of contracted tendons in young growing foals; overfeeding and imbalanced rations have been implicated.[10,11] Epiphysitis, osteochondritis dissecans and contracted tendons are increasingly recognized in association with the intake of excess energy during growth. Excess energy intake has also been implicated in the pathogenesis of cervical vertebral stenotic myelopathy.[12] Pathologic changes were observed within the growth plate as well as the bone and articular cartilage.

The 2 potential pathways by which faulty nutrition may be involved in the pathogenesis of contracted tendons are illustrated in Figure 147. Faulty nutrition may contribute to contracted tendons by a direct pathway as well as being involved in the pathogenesis of epiphysitis and osteochondritis dissecans, which may in turn, cause contracted tendons.[13,14] The au-

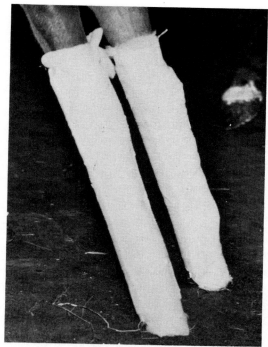

Fig 146. Treatment of bilateral congenital flexion deformities with gutter splints of yucca board bandaged to the legs. Sections of PVC tubing also serve as suitable gutter splints.

thor of a discussion on overfeeding and lack of exercise as related to tendon contracture believes that the term "contracted tendons" is a misnomer and that rapid bone growth without exercise results in a failure of tendons and ligaments to develop at the same rate as bone lengthening.[11] The foal develops flexion de-

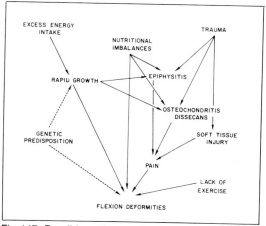

Fig 147. Possible pathogenetic pathways in acquired flexion deformities (contracted tendons).

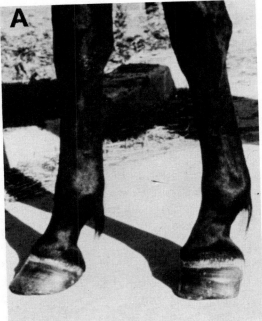 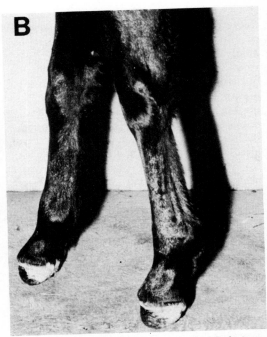

Fig 148. A. The typical "club-foot" appearance of stage-1 contracture of the deep digital flexor tendon. B. A stage-1 deep digital flexor tendon contracture that has not responded to hoof trimming. Both cases responded to inferior check desmotomy.

formities because flexor tension exceeds extensor tension.

Regardless of which pathway is involved, the major nutritional error involved in the pathway of contracted tendons is excess energy. This situation may arise soon after birth when the mare has large amounts of milk or an excessive energy intake, or it can develop when the foal is allowed access to unlimited amounts of high-energy creep ration. The third insult is the well-known situation of owners pushing their animals after weaning with commercial concentrates and grain to achieve a big yearling. So-called "high-protein" rations have been blamed by some clinicians for causing contracted tendons. However, rations such as Purina's "Big-Un" and Carnation's "Super Foal" are well-balanced rations with a 16-17% protein content (requirement 16%) and balanced Ca:P proportions. Foals on these rations may be simply overfed, with the consequent provision of excess energy.

Any possible specific effect of excess protein in addition to excess energy warrants investigation. In studies in other species, excess dietary protein has a calciuretic effect and could induce a Ca-deficient state. A study in humans revealed an eight-fold increase in urinary Ca excretion when dietary protein intake was increased to 10 times the daily requirement.[15] High levels of dietary protein may contribute to flexor contracture in horses by inducing an increased secretion of growth hormone.[16] In young horses, the feeding of the high-protein rations, such as Calf Manna (25% protein) and, more particularly, soybean meal (44% protein), may require careful monitoring.

Another nutritional error implicated in the pathogenesis of contracted tendons is Ca:P imbalance. A Ca or P excess exists if the Ca:P ratio is outside 3:1 to 0.8:1. Commercial concentrates are well-balanced for these minerals. However, grain is relatively low in Ca and hay is relatively low in P.

Although less common, contracted tendons also occur in poorly fed individuals. Possible nutritional factors involved in these cases include protein and P deficiency.

There are 2 somewhat distinct clinical entities. The first is so-called contracture of the deep digital flexor, which causes a raised heel and a "club foot" (Figs 148, 149).[1,10] For purposes of prognosis and therapy evaluation, deep digital flexor contracture has been subdivided into stage 1 and stage 2.[18] Stage-1 contracture is used when the dorsal surface of the hoof has not passed beyond vertical (Fig 148). When the dorsal surface of the hoof passes beyond vertical, the situation is classified as stage 2 (Fig 149).

The primary abnormality in deep digital flexor contracture appears to be a relative shortening of the deep digital flexor musculotendinous unit. However, once the problem has progressed to that of a stage-2 contracture, pathologic changes soon develop in the joint capsular and cartilaginous tissues of the coffin joint. An irreversible state develops if these cases are not treated promptly (Fig 150).

The other clinical entity, classically referred to as contracture of the superficial digital flexor, is characterized by knuckling at the fetlock, with the hoof itself in normal alignment (Fig 151). There may be deep digital flexor involvement in these cases as well; the deep digital flexor is contracted but fetlock knuckling allows the heel to remain on the ground. It would probably be more appropriate to describe the condition as combined superficial digital flexor-deep digital flexor contracture. In long-standing cases, the suspensory ligament becomes involved secondarily and degenerative changes occur in the fetlock joint.

The "club foot" type of deep digital flexor contracture has been described as typically found in foals and weanlings and the fetlock knuck-

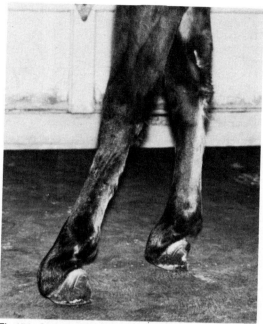

Fig 150. Severe, chronic stage-2 deep digital flexor tendon contracture with irreversible changes.

ling type as typically found in animals 1-2 years old.[11] Such a distribution was thought to be related to the suspensory ligament losing muscle fiber content, and therefore elasticity, during the first year of life. In foals, the extensor tendon and extensor branches of the suspensory ligament stretch as the distal interphalangeal joint flexes under the influence of deep digital flexor contracture. After one year of age, the extensor branches of the suspensory ligament cannot stretch and the extensor tendon can only stretch proximal to its junction with the extensor branches of the suspensory ligament. In such cases, knuckling of the fetlock occurs.[11] Some of these assumptions are controversial and the sequence of events requires investigation. In another study, fetlock knuckling occurred in older animals; however, deep digital flexor contracture was observed in animals over 12 months of age.[17]

In all cases of tendon contracture, the legs should be palpated carefully in the standing and flexed positions to determine which structures are involved.

Conservative methods of treatment, such as dietary changes, exercise and hoof trimming are appropriate if affected animals are presented early enough. A profound reduction in feed intake for rapidly growing horses has been recommended.[11] Ideally, animals should be

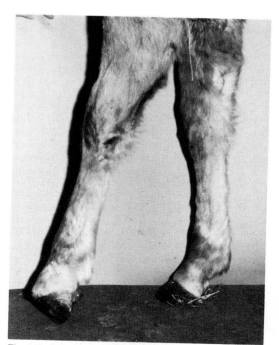

Fig 149. Stage-2 contracture of the deep digital flexor tendon. The dorsal surface of the hoof has passed beyond vertical. This case was successfully treated with deep flexor tenotomy.

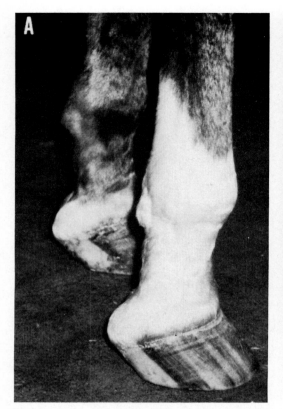
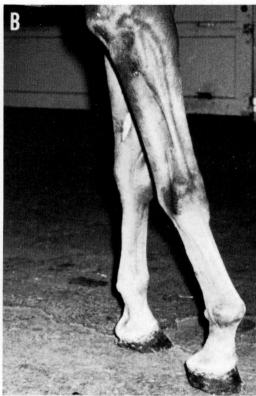

Fig 151. A. Combined superficial and deep digital flexor contracture. This horse was successfully treated with a combination of superficial flexor tenotomy and inferior check desmotomy. B. Severe combined superficial digital flexor tendon and deep digital flexor tendon contracture that failed to respond to surgical treatment. Joint capsule contracture was confirmed at necropsy.

turned out to pasture and fed only grass and water. If this is not feasible, feeding concentrates should at least be avoided. Affected animals may be fed alfalfa hay to provide adequate protein intake while energy intake is lowered. Grass hay provides the maximum decrease in energy intake. A high-P mineral supplement should also be available since a grass hay diet is deficient in P.[13] The animal should be exercised and phenylbutazone used judiciously if pain is a cause of the problem.

Animals with deep digital flexor contracture should have the heels trimmed short so that tension is placed on the flexor tendons to induce the inverse myotatic reflex.[8] For the superficial digital flexor or superficial digital flexor-deep digital flexor type, it has been generally recommended to raise the heel by corrective shoeing. It was thought that raising the heel creates a relative relaxation of tension in the deep flexor tendon, which in turn leads to selective overloading of the remaining support

structures and dropping of the fetlock.[16] However, some recent research indicates that although mean tendon strain in the deep digital flexor tendon changes with hoof angle, there is no significant difference in strain in either the superficial digital flexor tendon or suspensory ligament with changing hoof angle.[18] According to these findings, the real value of hoof angle change in a fetlock flexion deformity is questionable.

Surgical intervention is indicated in cases unresponsive to conservative methods of therapy. Immediate surgical intervention is also indicated on initial presentation of some cases when rapid correction of the flexion deformity is necessary to prevent the development of permanent degenerative joint changes.

Stage-1 deep digital flexor contractures should be treated by inferior check ligament desmotomy. This technic has furnished excellent results and is described below.[17] Normal limb alignment is often attained immediately following surgery. In other cases, flexor relaxation progresses for 7-10 days postoperatively as the digital flexor muscles relax in response to increased tensile forces imposed on them after section of the check ligament. Some cases in which the dorsal surface of the hoof is beyond vertical (mild stage 2) may respond to inferior check desmotomy if a toe extension is applied postoperatively to increase the tensile force on the deep flexor tendon.

Compared with tenotomy of the deep digital flexor tendon, inferior check ligament desmotomy causes less postoperative pain, has a superior postoperative appearance, and the long-term functional capability of the operated limb is much improved. Horses have raced following check ligament desmotomy as youngsters.

Deep flexor tenotomy is indicated for severe, long-standing cases of deep digital flexor contracture, including most stage-2 deep digital flexor contractures. This surgery corrects the flexion deformity in some animals, but in others fibrosis and contraction of the joint capsule and associated ligaments does not permit proper realignment. In addition, the cosmetic appearance following tenotomy is frequently unsatisfactory and the functional ability of the limb is often limited because of the surgical induction of a severe "bowed tendon."

In these situations some people consider a tendon-lengthening procedure more appropriate since spontaneous regeneration is not required to the same extent between the cut ends.[19] The actual functional advantages are uncertain. In the author's opinion, the cosmetic appearance is improved little by tendon-lengthening compared to tenotomy. Tenotomy is simple and, in an animal with a poor prognosis (as animals requiring tenotomy generally are), the use of simple tenotomy has advantages. Methods of tenotomy and tendon-lengthening are described below.

The results of surgical treatment of fetlock flexion deformities or superficial digital flexor-deep digital flexor contracture are more frequently unsatisfactory than for deep digital flexor contracture. A number of surgical treatments are available. If the superficial flexor tendon is the most taut, superficial flexor tenotomy may be performed. The technic is simple and not as drastic in terms of cosmetic appearance and postoperative functional ability as deep flexor tenotomy.

Superior check desmotomy has provided some good results for the treatment of acquired flexion deformities of the fetlock.[16,20] However, the

surgery is more difficult than inferior check desmotomy, and recontracture and carpal canal problems may develop postoperatively. In cases of failure of a superior check desmotomy or a superficial flexor tenotomy, some cases may be successfully managed by also performing an inferior check desmotomy. In other cases of fetlock flexion deformities, the deep digital flexor tendon seems to be the most affected; such cases may respond to inferior check desmotomy as the sole surgical procedure. These instances provide further testimony to the role of the deep digital flexor tendon in superficial flexor contracture.

Suspensory desmotomy may be considered in some cases but is a drastic final measure. Subluxation of the proximal interphalangeal joint is an anticipated sequela. However, it has been claimed that fibrosis of the pastern joint capsule occurs and appears to adequately stabilize the articulation.[16]

Surgical Treatment of Acquired Flexor Tendon Contracture: Inferior check desmotomy is performed with the patient under general anesthesia and in lateral recumbency. A lateral approach is used to avoid the common digital (medial palmar) artery medially. However, a medial approach is feasible and may be used so that any blemish that develops is on the medial side of the limb.

A 5-cm skin incision is made over the cranial border of the deep digital flexor tendon from the proximal quarter of the metacarpus half way down the metacarpus. The subcutaneous fascia and paratenon are incised and reflected to identify the deep digital flexor tendon and inferior check ligament (Fig 152). A cleavage plane between the proximal part of the deep digital flexor tendon and the inferior check ligament is used to dissect the check ligament clear in preparation for desmotomy (Figs 153, 154). This surgical manipulation sometimes results in disruption of the synovial sheath of the carpal canal, the distal extremity of which extends most of the way down inside the cleavage plane. This seems to be of little consequence.

Following separation of the check ligament from the deep digital flexor tendon, the ligament is severed with a scalpel and the foot is manually extended (Fig 155). The ends of the check ligament become separated after all parts of the check ligament have been completely severed (Fig 156). The paratenon and subcutaneous fascia are closed with synthetic absorbable sutures and the skin is closed with nonabsorbable sutures. The limb is bandaged

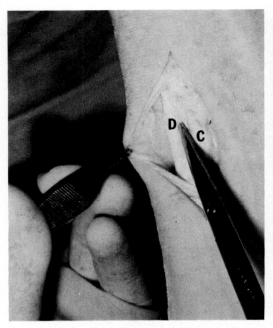

Fig 152. Inferior check desmotomy. The incised para-
tendon and superficial flexor tendon have been reflected and the points of the scissors are placed
between the deep digital flexor tendon (D) and the inferior check ligament (C).

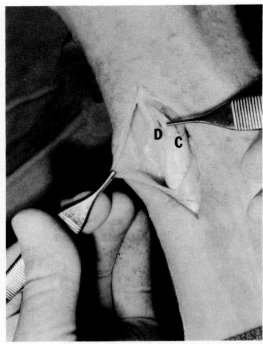

Fig 153. The cleavage plane between the deep digital
flexor tendon (D) and the inferior check ligament (C)
is identified.

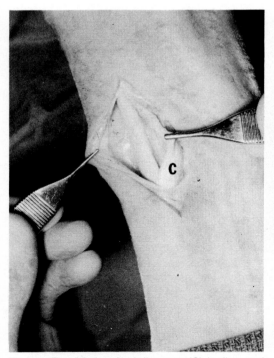

Fig 154. The inferior check ligament (C) is dissected
free from the deep digital flexor tendon.

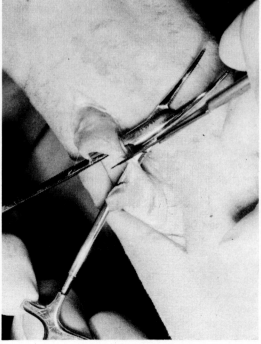

Fig 155. Forceps are inserted under the check ligament
to isolate it prior to severance with a scalpel.

from the proximal metacarpus to the coronary band and the hoof trimmed to normal conformation. Phenylbutazone (1-2 g) is administered IV to reduce postoperative pain and facilitate lowering of the heel. Antibiotics are not administered routinely. Toe extensions may also be used in severely affected animals.

Superior check desmotomy is performed with the horse under general anesthesia and in lateral recumbency. A 10-cm skin incision is made medially between the common digital vein and the caudal aspect of the distal radius. A branch of the vein that penetrates the antebrachial fascia in the central area of the superior check ligament is a useful landmark. This branch is incised between ligatures and the antebrachial fascia is incised to expose the check ligament. The synovial sheath of the carpal canal borders the distal aspect of the check ligament. The check ligament is carefully severed in a proximal direction (the small arteries of the rete carpi volare beneath the check ligament must be avoided in the proximal portion). The antebrachial fascia and subcutaneous tissue are closed with absorbable synthetic sutures in an interrupted pattern and the skin is closed with nonabsorbable sutures. The limb is bandaged and phenylbutazone is administered postoperatively.

Superficial flexor tenotomy may be performed under local analgesia in selected patients or in lateral recumbency under general anesthesia. The mid-metacarpal area is surgically prepared and a small skin incision, sufficient to admit a tenotomy knife, is made. The tenotomy knife blade is introduced and manipulated between the superficial and deep flexor tendons. When the position is considered satisfactory, the blade is turned 90 degrees and the tendon is severed. Alternatively, a 2-cm skin incision may be made so that the tendon can be visualized before insertion of the tenotomy knife. Following tenotomy, only the skin is sutured.

Deep digital flexor tenotomy may also be performed in the mid-metacarpal region. The author prefers exposure of the tendon. A tenotomy knife is used and care is taken to avoid the palmar arteries, veins and nerves.

An alternative technic for deep digital flexor tenotomy uses an approach through the digital tendon sheath at a level immediately proximal to the bulbs of the heel.[21] The tendon sheath is opened and trimmed back to facilitate healing of the severed tendon. The result is considered

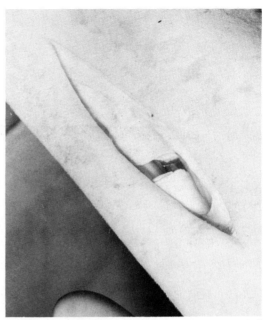

Fig 156. The ends of the check ligament are separated after complete severance.

cosmetically and functionally superior to results of other technics.[21]

Tendons can be lengthened by Z-plasty or Z-tenotomy.[19] The tendon is exposed in the mid-metacarpal region and a longitudinal incision of approximately the same length as that of the lengthened tendon is made in the center of the tendon. Transverse incisions are then made at each end of the central incision but on opposite sides (Fig 157). The tendon is lengthened and the long ends sutured together with interrupted sutures of 00 monofilament nylon. The paratenon is not sutured. The skin is closed with synthetic nonabsorbable sutures.

Summarizing the treatment of acquired flexor contractures, many cases respond to conservative therapeutic measures. However, some contractures rapidly worsen and timely surgical intervention is indicated in cases that are not responding or are getting progressively worse. Inferior check desmotomy provides good results in most cases of deep digital flexor contracture in which the dorsal surface of the hoof is at an angle of 90 degrees or less to the ground. More severe cases may respond to deep digital flexor tenotomy but the prognosis for later performance is less favorable. Fetlock flexion deformities associated with superficial digital flexor-deep digital flexor contracture do

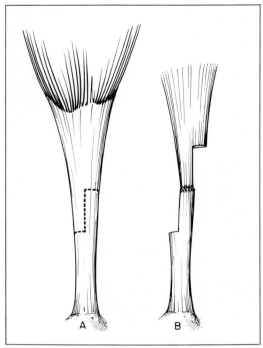

Fig 157. Z-tenotomy technic for tendon-lengthening. A. Dotted line marks incision in tendon. B. Long ends are sutured with simple-interrupted sutures.

not respond to surgical treatment as consistently as do deep digital flexor contractures. Superficial tenotomy or superior check desmotomy and/or inferior check desmotomy are the treatments of choice in such cases.

Rupture of the Common Digital Extensor Tendon

This condition is usually bilateral and is generally present at birth or develops within the first few days after birth.[22] Affected foals may have carpal flexion deformities with normally extended fetlocks and may knuckle over at the fetlocks when they move. The characteristic feature of this condition is the presence of a swelling over the craniolateral aspect of the carpus (Fig 158). Depending on the amount of synovial fluid present in the synovial sheath of the common digital extensor tendon, one may or may not be able to palpate the enlarged ends of the ruptured tendon. If the ruptured common digital extensor tendon is not recognized, the problem may be diagnosed as solely attributable to contraction of the flexor tendons.

Rupture of the common digital extensor tendon may be accompanied by contraction of the flexor tendons. In a series of 10 cases, severe contraction of the flexor tendons of the front

legs was present in 4 foals at birth, mild contraction was present in 3, while no contraction was present in the other 3 foals.[22] It is therefore difficult to decide in some cases if the extensor tendon ruptures secondary to flexor contracture or if flexor contracture occurs because the extensor tendons rupture.

Affected foals may have concomitant multiple birth defects, including prognathism, underdeveloped pectoral muscles and hypoplasia of the carpal bones.[22] The implication here is that the extensor tendon rupture may be one of a complex of congenital defects.

In general, foals without severe contraction of the flexor tendons recover spontaneously with stall rest. The use of protective bandaging is indicated to prevent abrasive damage to the dorsum of the fetlock. The separated tendon ends may still be palpable in some foals that have recovered clinically. Suturing of the tendon ends has been reported but is not considered to be indicated.[19] The use of splints or casts may be appropriate if contracted flexor tendons exist. As mentioned before, careful management and supervision of cast application is necessary in foals to avoid complications. The author prefers the use of splinting with PVC tubing. The prognosis is guarded when the contraction of the flexor tendons accompanies extensor tendon rupture.

Angular Limb Deformities in Foals
by C.W. McIlwraith

An angular limb deformity is a condition in which the conformation of an extremity is abnormal. The deviation is generally in a medial-lateral plane as opposed to the cranial-caudal deviations associated with tendon contractures and ruptures as previously described.

Angular deformities arise in foals of all breeds.[23-26] A high incidence has been reported in Quarter Horses.[26] Colts were more affected in one report but in another report the sex distribution was in proportion with that of the general patient population.[25,26] The condition may be unilateral or bilateral and may be congenital or acquired when the foal is a few weeks to several months old.

Etiology and Pathogenesis

Physeal Growth Imbalances: Most angular deformities, particularly acquired ones, are due to imbalances of metaphyseal and epiphyseal growth. The problem is considered to stem from asymmetric pressure on the metaphyseal

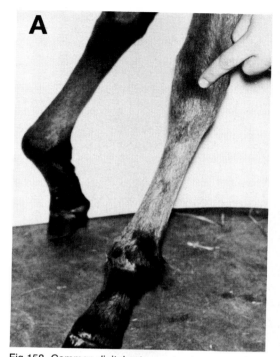
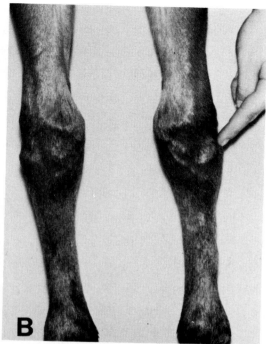

Fig 158. Common digital extensor tendon rupture in a foal. A. Note the fetlock knuckling on the right leg and the worn skin over the dorsal aspect of the left fetlock. The finger is placed in the indentation caused by the lack of continuity of the common digital extensor tendon. B. The bulging distal end of the tendon can be seen on both limbs.

growth plate or physis.[27,28] This axis deviation is present at birth or develops in the early postnatal growth period.

Excessive pressure on an area of the metaphyseal growth plate impairs the blood supply, resulting in delayed production of chondrocytes on the epiphyseal side of the plate and consequent retardation of new bone production on the metaphyseal side of the plate.[29,30]

The postulated causes of asymmetric pressure on the growth plate include malpositioning in utero, an earlier deformity associated with defective ossification, joint laxity, poor conformation, and lameness in the opposite leg.[27] Affected animals are often fast-growing, heavily-muscled, overweight or excessively active. Quarter Horses are evolving into a breed of horses with heavy bodies on comparatively small limbs. This relatively excessive weight can cause a progressive tilt to the epiphysis[31] Young, growing foals with unlimited access to a high-energy creep ration often become overweight, which may cause increased trauma to the metaphyseal growth plate. An increased growth rate from over-feeding could also cause problems in bone formation at the growth plate itself. The role of Ca:P imbalances is uncertain.

The growth plates of the distal radius and distal metacarpus are commonly involved in angular limb deformities. The growth plate of the distal tibia is occasionally affected but much less so than those of the radius and metacarpus.[26] The distal metatarsal physis may be similarly affected.

The situation described above is the common cause of an angular deformity in a foal. However, other problems are manifested as an angular deformity and their differential diagnosis is important in forming a treatment protocol and prognosis.

Defective Ossification: Incomplete or defective ossification of the carpal bones has been recognized as a cause of angular deformity in the carpus.[32] The terms hypoplasia and necrosis of the carpal bones have also been used but these have not been histologically confirmed. Because ossification of the carpal bones occurs late in fetal development, any delay in ossification or a premature birth results in abnormal forces on the incompletely ossified cartilage, with subsequent deformities.

Angular deformities due to defective carpal bone ossification are typically encountered in the newborn. Problems have been recognized

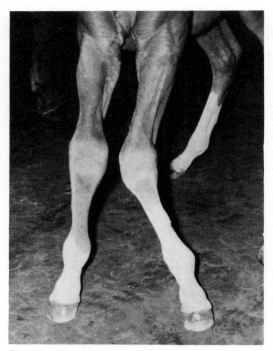

Fig 159. Bilateral carpal valgus in a foal.

in the radial, intermediate, ulnar, third and fourth carpal bones; 2 or more bones are commonly involved. The author has observed carpal bone defects and radial epiphyseal defects in the same limbs; in such cases it is difficult to ascertain which was the primary lesion. Carpal bone defects have also been observed in foals with concomitant tarsal bone collapse.[33]

Collateral Ligament Laxity: Laxity of the collateral ligaments of a joint may cause an angular deformity, typically in a newborn foal. This may also contribute to a physeal problem by causing asymmetric pressures.

Trauma: Traumatic luxation and fractures of the carpal bones also cause angular deformities. A true Salter type-V injury may occur and cause an angular deformity. In such cases there is an absolute cessation of growth in the affected area of the growth plate. This injury is rare in foals.

Whatever the cause of the initial angular deviation, the problem may be exacerbated as growth is further retarded on the compressed side of the growth plate.[27]

Clinical Signs

Valgus and varus deformity are the terms commonly used to describe an angulation deformity. Valgus is a deformity in which the an-

gulation of the distal part is away from the midline of the body, and varus is one in which the angulation of the distal part is toward the midline. For example, carpal valgus or "knock knees" refers to a lateral deviation of the metacarpus, with medial deviation of the distal radius (Fig 159). Carpal varus is a medial deviation of the metacarpus, with lateral deviation of the distal radius (Fig 160). Fetlock varus is a medial deviation of the phalanges and lateral deviation of the distal end of the third metacarpal bone (Fig 161). Tarsal valgus is a lateral deviation of the metatarsus, with medial deviation of the distal tibia (Fig 162).

Carpal valgus and fetlock varus are most common. In a recent study of 55 joints examined for angular deformity, the incidence of carpal valgus was 49%, of carpal varus was 7%, of fetlock valgus was 0%, and of fetlock varus was 44%.[26]

Angular deformity due to flaccidity or damage to periarticular supporting tissues may be clinically differentiated from deformity from other causes by a return to a normal axis on manipulation of the limb.[32]

When more than one physis in a limb is involved, a complex deformity results. Multiple limb involvement also may occur (Fig 163).

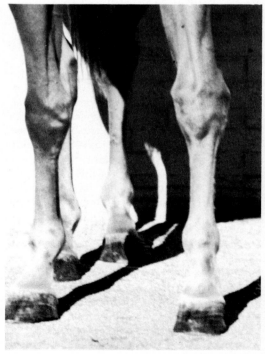

Fig 160. Carpal varus in the left forelimb. (Courtesy of Dr AS Turner)

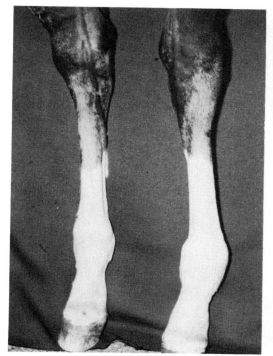

Fig 161. Fetlock varus in the left hindlimb.

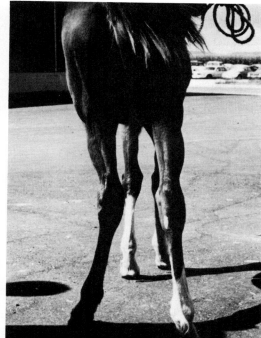

Fig 162. Tarsal valgus in the left hindlimb.

Affected animals are not usually lame but the history may reveal that lameness of another limb had been noticed previous to the development of the angular deformity.[26] Angular deformities directly attributable to excess weight-bearing are more typically varus.

Radiographic Findings

A good radiographic study is important to characterize the angular deformity and to differentiate it from other problems such as ossification abnormalities or fractures of the carpal bones. A craniocaudal radiograph, centering the carpus on a 14 x 17-inch cassette, should be taken for all carpal deviations. For additional information, the outlines of the radiograph may be traced on a clear cellulose acetate sheet and lines drawn parallel to the radius and third metacarpal bone.[26] The angle of intersection is measured with a protractor and provides a measure of the angular deformity. When the intersection of the 2 lines is within the epiphysis, the angular deformity is generally considered due to abnormal growth of either the distal radial metaphysis or distal radial epiphysis and therefore amenable to surgical treatment (Fig 164). However, an angle of intersection within the radial carpal joint or distal to it indicates cuboidal bone ab-

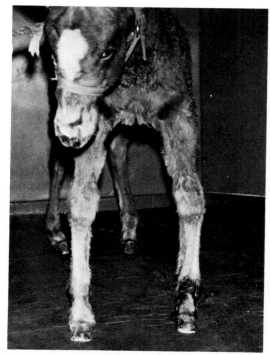

Fig 163. Bilateral carpal varus in the front limbs and bilateral fetlock varus in the hindlimbs of a foal.

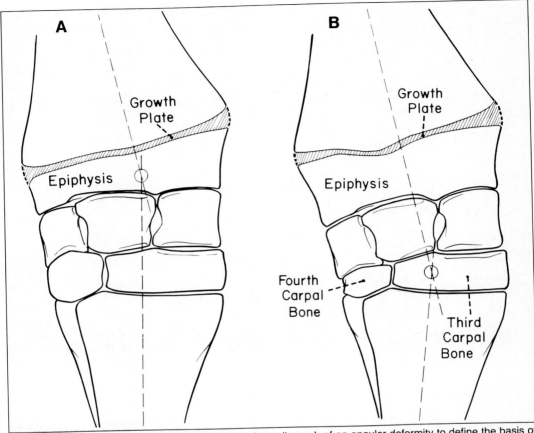

Fig 164. Plotting the intersection of lines drawn on the radiograph of an angular deformity to define the basis of the problem. A. The lines meet within the epiphysis in a metaphyseal growth plate problem. B. In a case of defective ossification of the fourth carpal bone, the lines intersect within the carpus itself.

normalities or ligamentous laxity; these abnormalities may or may not be obvious on the films. In some situations, growth plate and carpal bone defects, as well as ligamentous laxity, may be present in the same joint; defining the point of intersection helps assess the status of these joints. The fetlock is radiographed similarly and the angular deformity is measured.

In addition to epiphyseal wedging and metaphyseal asymmetry, various radiographic changes may be observed in cases of epiphyseal and metaphyseal growth imbalance. In carpal valgus, these changes include widening of the physis on the medial side, metaphyseal lipping on the lateral or compressed side, metaphyseal sclerosis, and metaphyseal and diaphyseal cortical thickening on the lateral side (Fig 165). Carpal varus involves changes on the opposite sides. In young foals, secondary radiographic changes are usually not present. Additional radiographic lesions, considered secondary to the

abnormal forces, are sometimes observed and include chip fractures of the carpal bones, bone necrosis on the compressed side, and wedging of the carpal bones (Figs 166-168). In fetlock varus, the epiphysis of the third metacarpal or metatarsal bone is wedged on the medial side, the physis may be widened on the lateral side and the metaphysis may be flared, lipped or sclerotic on the medial side (Fig 169).

Radiographic findings in a cuboidal bone problem include absence or decrease in ossification and an abnormal shape of affected carpal bones (Fig 170).

Treatment

Correction of angular deformities associated with growth plate defects in foals is desirable to improve conformation as well as to prevent degenerative changes that may arise secondary to abnormal stress on the deviated limb. Many foals born with minor angulations recover spontaneously within a few weeks. Other young foals may respond to conservative treatment, including stall confinement, corrective hoof trimming and nutritional mangement.[3,26,34] Stall rest helps foals by decreasing trauma to the growth plate. Corrective hoof trimming corrects hoof balance and assists limb alignment. For example, a foal with carpal valgus wears the inside of the hoof and needs trimming of the outside hoof wall. Nutritional management should include restricted feeding of concentrate, and alfalfa and a high-P mineral supplement fed free-choice.

Although the use of splints, casts and hinged braces has been recommended, the author does not favor their use in the treatment of angular limb deformities associated with growth plate abnormalities.[32] Although application of a cast decreases stress on the growth plate, it also inhibits recorrection of normal alignment. Management of a limb deviation using splints is difficult and the results are sometimes disastrous. However, the use of casts is appropriate in the treatment of angular deformities associated with cuboidal bone abnormalities or collateral ligament laxity (described later).

Temporary transphyseal bridging is indicated in young foals that do not respond to conservative treatment, that have severe deviations, or in foals 2 months or older. One author feels that any time after 2 weeks is an excellent time to initiate surgical correction.[25]

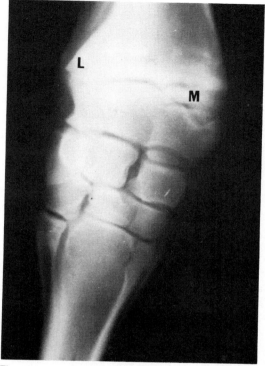

Fig 165. Carpal valgus attributed to a distal radial growth plate problem. Changes include wedging of the epiphysis, widening of the metaphyseal physis on the medial side (M), metaphyseal lipping on the lateral side (L), metaphyseal sclerosis, and increased density of cortical bone on the medial side.

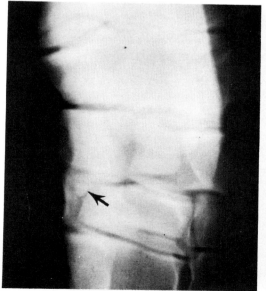

Fig 166. Chip fracture (arrow) of the third carpal bone in carpal valgus. Note the wedging of the radial epiphysis.

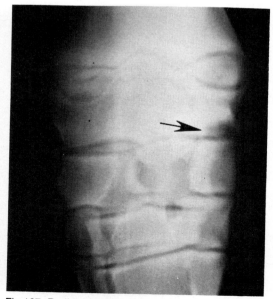

Fig 167. Radiolucent defect (arrow) attributed to pressure necrosis on the compression side of the distal radius in a case of carpal valgus.

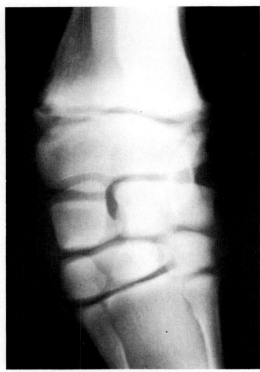

Fig 168. Wedging of the third carpal bone in a 1-month-old foal with carpal valgus attributed primarily to a growth plate problem.

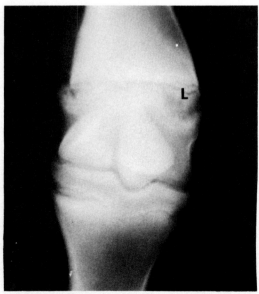

Fig 169. Fetlock varus in a 3-month-old foal. There is wedging of the distal epiphysis of the metacarpus, widening of the physis on the lateral side (L), metaphyseal sclerosis, and reactive bony change on the medial (compressed) side.

Primary angular deformities at the distal radius or tibia can produce a secondary rotational deformity of the fetlock, probably because of torque.[25] Since the growth plate of the distal metacarpus or metarsus closes much earlier than that of the distal radius or tibia, it is argued that early correction of the primary defect is indicated.[24,25]

The principle of temporary transphyseal bridging is to retard longitudinal bone growth on the side being bridged. Internal growth pressure builds up against the restraining device and production of new chondrocytes in the germinal side of the growth plate is inhibited in the same fashion that asymmetric pressure on an area of the plate is considered to produce the initial defect.[35] The use of staples, or tension-band wire and screws has become accepted technic in the correction of angular deformities in foals.

Either of the technics described below can effectively straighten the limb if there is sufficient growth potential remaining in the bridged physis. This is an important aspect of evaluating the potential use of surgery in a particular patient. Although the distal radial growth plate does not close until 24 months of age, growth only continues until 18 months and 71% of the growth takes place within 12 months.[36,37] Surgical correction should therefore begin before this stage. Treatment at 2-3 months is recommended to prevent rotational deformity and osteoarthritis due to asymmetric biomechanical loading.

The distal growth plate of the metacarpus begins to close at 5 months and is completely closed by 7-7½ months.[36] However, there is little growth after 3 months and most cases in foals older than 3 months may be beyond correction.[27] Slightly deviated fetlocks can be treated if the animal is not older than 2 months, while severe deformity at this age is probably already beyond correction. Other authors have set the upper limit before which surgery should be performed as 6 months.[38]

Transphyseal Stapling: Using a carpus valgus as an example, the medial aspect of the carpal area is prepared for aseptic surgery and draped. A curvilinear incision is made over the medial aspect of the physis, with the apex directed caudad. A skin flap with the incision caudal to the bony prominence reduces pressure on the incision line. The flap is reflected, the physis is located by probing with a sterile 18-ga needle and the position of the needle in

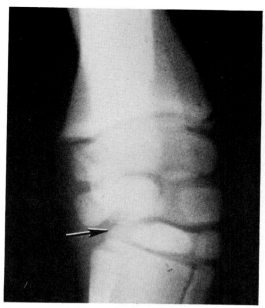

Fig 170. Carpal varus in the right forelimb of a newborn foal from absence of a normal fourth carpal bone (arrow). (Courtesy of Dr AS Turner)

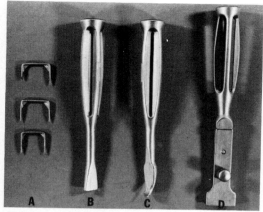

Fig 171. Instruments used in transphyseal stapling: (A) Vitallium staples (various sizes); (B) staple set; (C) staple extractor; and (D) staple-holder.

the physis is confirmed with a craniocaudal radiograph.

The use of heavy-shouldered vitallium staples is preferred. The use of angulated vitallium staples has been recently recommended because of their superior "fit."[28] The legs of the staple are placed equidistant proximal and distal to the physis. The number and size of the staples used depends on the size of the animal. At least 2 staples should be used in the distal radial physis on the craniomedial and caudomedial aspects. Special instruments facilitate placement of the staples (Fig 171). The staple-holder enables more accurate staple placement and provides a firm grasp to drive the staple against the bone. Removal of soft tissue between the legs of the staple facilitates setting the staple to the bone. Radiographs are taken after the staple is seated to ensure correct positioning and to check that the legs of the staple have not bent or deviated during seating (Fig 172). Subcutaneous tissue is closed with synthetic absorbable sutures and the skin is closed with synthetic nonabsorbable sutures. The limb is carefully bandaged in the postoperative period and skin sutures are removed 10-12 days postoperatively.

Stapling of the distal tibia requires accurate staple placement because of the size and shape of the distal tibial epiphysis. The distal leg of the staple must be shortened or it penetrates the tibiotarsal articulation. Angled staples need not be altered.

The owner is instructed to observe the animal weekly and return when the limb is

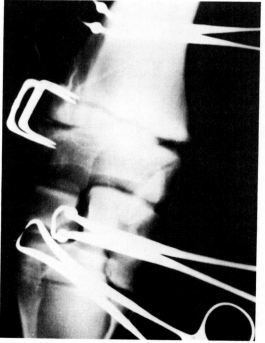

Fig 172. Radiograph obtained during placement of 2 staples across distal radial growth plate. Note needle placed in physis to act as a guide.

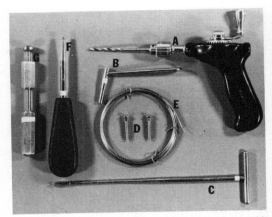

Fig 173. Equipment used in transphyseal bridging with screws and wires: (A) drill with 3.6-mm drill bit; (B) drill guide; (C) 6.5-mm cancellous tap; (D) 6.5-mm cancellous screws; (E) cerclage wire; (F) screwdriver; (G) wire-tightener.

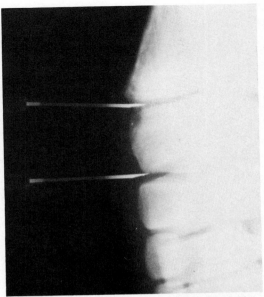

Fig 174. Radiographic confirmation of needle positioning in physis and radiocarpal joint prior to insertion of screw in epiphysis.

straight. The owner should be instructed to walk the foal during examination at home. The hooves should also be trimmed as necessary. Exercise should be restricted to reduce trauma to the growth plate from overactivity.

The staples are removed under general anesthesia when the limb is straight. Staple removal can be quite difficult because of fibrous deposition over the staple. Bone may also envelop the staples and may even lead to a Salter type-VI injury. The staples are located and elevated with a staple-remover or screwdriver. The wound is closed in a routine manner.

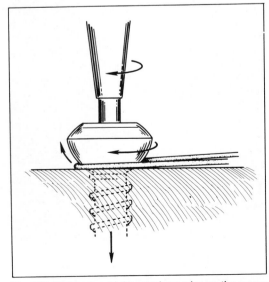

Fig 175. Tightening of the cerclage wire as the screw head is rotated.

Transphyseal Bridging with Screws and Wire: This technic was initially used to treat carpal valgus.[39] More recently the technic was used for treatment of carpal valgus, carpal varus and fetlock varus.[26] Use of the technic to treat tarsal valgus has been described.[40] The equipment used in the procedure is illustrated in Figure 173.

The same skin incision and approach to the physis is made as described for stapling. The physis and adjacent joint are located using sterile 18-ga needles and a craniocaudal radiograph is made to ascertain their position (Fig 174). Holes for the 6.5-mm ASIF full-threaded cancellous bone screws are drilled above and below the physis with a 3.6-mm drill bit using a 4.5-mm tap sleeve as a drill guide. The distal hole is centered in the epiphysis and drilled to a depth of 38-40 mm using the needles to direct position. The drilling of this hole is critical in terms of positioning. The drill hole is tapped with a 6.5-mm cancellous tap and the cancellous screw is inserted but not tightened. Placement of the proximal screw is less critical. The hole is drilled approximately 2 cm from the physis and passes through one cortex to a depth of about 40 mm. A radiograph may be made at this stage to check screw placement. Stainless-steel cerclage wire (18- to 20-ga) is then placed in a figure-8 pattern around the 2 screw heads and tightened with a cerclage wire tightener.

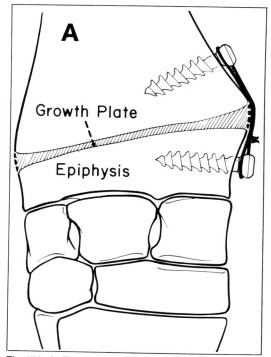
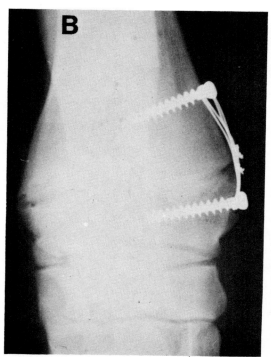

Fig 176. A. Transphyseal bridging using screws and wire. B. Craniocaudal radiograph following transphyseal bridging.

The author routinely uses 2 wires. The twist should be made so that it lies in the middle of the figure-8 rather than adjacent to the screw heads. The screws are then tightened another turn so that the wire slides up the screw head, resulting in increased tension (Fig 175). The result is illustrated by Figure 176.

Application of the screw and wire technic in cases of tarsal valgus requires special care in distal screw placement. Because of the limited amount of epiphysis available and the risk of penetrating the tibiotarsal joint, a 4.5-mm cortical screw is used and radiographic monitoring of screw positioning is mandatory (Fig 177).

Following correction of the deviation, the screws and wire can be easily removed on an outpatient basis. In certain patients, removal can be performed under local analgesia with the animal standing. The screw heads are usually palpable but the distal screw may be slightly covered by fibrous tissue. The screws are removed through stab incisions. The cerclage wire is then removed by retraction through the proximal incision (Fig 178).

Results of Surgical Treatment

It has been suggested that the screw and wire technic produces immediate compression at the physis, which in turn could lead to more rapid straightening.[40] However, biomechanical data are lacking and a comparative study did not indicate a faster correction rate with screws and wire.[27] The same study, using regression plots of foal age vs degrees of correction per day, demonstrated that younger foals are more responsive to temporary transphyseal bridging than are older foals. In addition, large deviations have insufficient time for correction before closure of the growth plate in older foals. This aspect is an important consideration in selection of surgical candidates. A retrospective study indicated the average correction time in relation to age at which surgery was performed.[25] Foals up to 3 months of age required 4 weeks for correction, foals 3-6 months old required 8½ weeks, foals 6-9 months old required 12 weeks, and foals over 9 months old required over 12 weeks for correction. These figures are averages and the response of individual animals depends on the amount of angulation present.

Although the overall success rate between the use of staples or screw and wire has been evaluated and shown not to differ, the occurrence of surgical complications varied.[27] The major complication of stapling is a soft tissue blemish in terms of excessive fibrous tissue de-

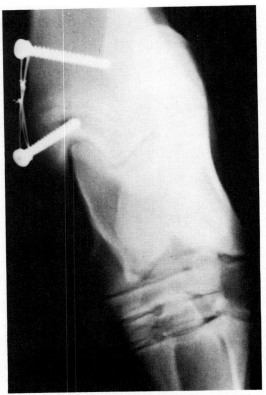

Fig 177. Tarsal valgus following transphyseal bridging with screws and wire. In this case, thicker cerclage wire should have been used.

position following surgery. This is only a cosmetic problem but may be significant, particularly in halter horses. Theoretically, the problem can be eliminated with good technic and lack of staple motion, but this situation rarely exists.[3] The degree of soft tissue blemish is less with the screw and wire technic.[27]

Mechanical insufficiencies may develop with both technics. Spreading and extrusion of the staples occasionally occur. Mechanical insufficiency in staples can be handled by increasing the number of staples used but this also increases the bulk of the implants. Wire breakage may also occur in the screw and wire technic. The author now uses 2 pieces of wire routinely. Care should also be taken that the wire is twisted evenly; breakage typically occurs in the area of wire twisting. Although use of the screw and wire technic with tarsal valgus is convenient for placing an anchor in the distal tibial epiphysis and the results are generally good, wire breakage has occurred even

when using 2 strands of 18-ga wire. Increasing the size of the implant is not ideal since the implant lies immediately below the skin and soft tissue problems may develop. An alternative to staples or screw and wire is that of using a small bone plate.[41]

Another potential complication of both technics, particularly with staple insertion and removal, is the development of periosteal new bone that forms a bridge between the metaphysis and the epiphysis. This causes continued growth restraint and leads to overcorrection of the deformity. This situation has been described as a Salter type-VI injury.[42] Such fusion may be irreversible. Care must be taken when placing the implant, and especially when attempting to remove it, that trauma to the periosteum is minimized.

Removal of the screw and wire apparatus is easier than removal of staples and is a major advantage. Use of the technic in tarsal valgus is an illustration of its versatility in that the distal screw can be angled to avoid the joint space.

Despite early and effective correction of valgus deformities in the carpus, rotational deformities remain a problem in a few cases. The author has also observed exacerbation or development of rotation after correction of the angular deformity. This suggests that the forces producing rotation are not solely due to the original angular deformity. There is still a place for an improved treatment method for these rotational problems.

Recently another technic has been proposed for the correction of carpal valgus in young foals. The procedure involves screw fixation of the lateral styloid process to the epiphysis.[28] The rationale is based on a theory that before

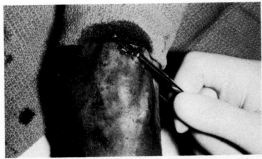

Fig 178. Removal of screws and wire after correction of angular deformity. Following removal of screws through stab incisions, the cerclage wire is removed through the proximal incision.

fusion, the styloid process (distal ulnar epiphysis) is unstable and there is a lack of support to the ulnar carpal bone. This in turn could contribute to carpal valgus and some rotation in the joint.[28] Although correction occurred in all treated foals, the animals were all young and spontaneous correction could have occurred regardless of treatment. A more thorough evaluation is necessary to assess the validity of the suggested pathogenetic mechanism and the treatment.

As previously suggested, most cases of fetlock varus in foals older than 3 months are beyond correction by transphyseal bridging because of early closure of the growth plate. The author treated one case of severe varus deformity with a closed distal metatarsal physis by performing a wedge osteotomy and reuniting the epiphysis to the metaphysis by bone plating. The results of this case encourage further use of this technic when the situation is no longer amenable to transphyseal bridging.

Treatment of Angular Deformities Not Caused by Epiphyseal/Metaphyseal Growth Problems

Angular deformities due to incomplete or retarded ossification of the carpal bones are treated by manually reducing the deviation if possible and retaining the limb in its corrected position with plaster or fiberglass casts until ossification occurs.[32] The use of tube casts over the carpus suspended by "cast braces" has been described.[32] Leaving the limb free distal to the fetlock has advantages over complete limb immobilization (lack of muscle atrophy and flexor tendon weakness). Cast application and the results should be carefully monitored; casts should be replaced in 10-14 days. Casts may also be used for treatment of angular limb deformities associated with collateral ligament laxity. If encountered early enough, an angular deformity due to a fractured carpal bone may also be amenable to reduction and cast application.

References

1. Fessler, JF. Archives (Vet Surg) **6** (1977) 19.
2. Myers, VS and Lundvall, RL. JAVMA **148** (1966) 1523.
3. Adams, OR. Lameness in Horses. 3rd ed. Lea & Febiger, Philadelphia, 1974.
4. Fackelman, GE and Clodius, L. VM/SAC **67** (1972) 1116.
5. Hutt, FB. Cornell Vet **58** (1968) 104.
6. Rooney, JR. Cornell Vet **56** (1966) 173.
7. Boyd, JS. Eq Vet J **8** (1976) 161.
8. Breazile, in Swenson: Duke's Physiology of Domestic Animals. 8th ed. Cornell University Press, Ithaca, 1970.
9. Badame, GF. Proc 9th Ann Mtg Am Assoc Eq Pract, 1963.
10. Johnson, JH. Mod Vet Pract **54** (1973) 67.
11. Owen, JM. Eq Vet J **7** (1975) 40.
12. Mayhew, IG *et al*. Cornell Vet **68** Suppl **6** (1978) 71.
13. Lewis, LL. Proc 25th Ann Mtg Am Assoc Eq Pract, 1979.
14. Moore, JD and McIlwraith, CW. Vet Rec **100** (1977) 133.
15. Morgen, S *et al*. Am J Clin Nutr **26** (1974) 584.
16. Fackelman, GE. Comp Cont Ed **1** (1979) 51.
17. McIlwraith, CW and Fessler, JF. JAVMA **172** (1978) 293.
18. Lochner, FK. Master's thesis, Ohio Stater Univ, 1977.
19. Johnson and Lowe, in Oehme and Prier: Textbook of Large Animal Surgery. Williams & Wilkins, Baltimore, 1974.
20. Fackelman, GE, Univ Penn: Personal communication, 1979.
21. Fackelman, GE and Auer, J, Univ Penn: Personal communication, 1980.
22. Myers, VS and Gordon, GW. Proc 21st Ann Mtg Am Assoc Eq Pract, 1975. p 67.
23. Heinze, CD. Proc 9th Ann Mtg Am Assoc Eq Pract, 1965. p 203.
24. Heinze, CD. Proc 11th Ann Mtg Am Assoc Eq Pract, 1965. p 273.
25. Heinze, CD. Proc 15th Ann Mtg Am Assoc Eq Pract, 1969. p 59.
26. Fretz, PB *et al*. JAVMA **172** (1978) 281.
27. Turner, AS and Fretz, PB. Proc 23rd Ann Mtg Am Assoc Eq Pract, 1977. p 175.
28. Heinze, CD. Proc 23rd Ann Mtg Am Assoc Eq Pract, 1977. p 287.
29. Trueta, J and Trias, A. J Bone Joint Surg **43B** (1961) 800.
30. Rooney, JR. Cornell Vet **53** (1963 567.
31. Tschantz, P *et al*. Clin Orthoped **123** (1977) 271.
32. Fackelman, GE *et al*. Proc 21st Ann Mtg Am Assoc Eq Pract, 1975. p 161.
33. Turner, AS, Col State Univ: Personal communication, 1979.
34. Guffy, MM and Coffman, JR. Proc 15th Ann Mtg Am Assoc Eq Pract, 1969. p 47.
35. Sieffert, RS. J Bone Joint Surg **48-A** (1966) 546.
36. Myers, VS and Emerson, MA. J Am Vet Rad Soc **1** (1966) 39.
37. Heinze, CD and Lewis, RE. Proc 14th Ann Mtg Am Assoc Eq Pract, 1968. p 213.
38. Vaughan, LC. Vet Rec **98** (1976) 165.
39. Fackelman, GE and Frolich, D. Proc 19th Ann Mtg Am Assoc Eq Pract, 1972. p 325.
40. Campbell, JR. Eq Vet J **9** (1977) 116.
41. Foerner, JJ, Naperville, IL: Personal communication, 1979.
42. Salter and Harris, in Rang: The Growth Plate and Its Disorders. Williams & Wilkins, Baltimore, 1969.

DORSAL METACARPAL DISEASE
by G.L. Norwood and P.F. Haynes

The term "bucked shins" has traditionally been used to describe painful periostitis of the dorsal cortex of the third metacarpal bone associated with exercise, particularly training or racing. Early thoughts on the pathogenesis of this disorder related to periosteal tearing, subperiosteal hematoma formation and microfractures.[1] A much greater appreciation of this disease has developed in recent years. The current consensus on the pathophysiology of exercise-induced disease of the dorsal cortex of the third metacarpal bone is that this spectrum of diseases is caused by excessive compression on a bone that has not adequately remodeled to withstand such stress. The greatest incidence of this disease is in 2-year-old Thoroughbreds, and reportedly occurs in 70% of that age group.[2] The incidence is lower in Quarter Horses and is only occasional in Standardbreds. Bilateral forelimb involvement is the rule in the 2-year-old, although this syndrome tends to occur only in the left forelimb of older Thoroughbreds. Rarely, the hindlimbs may be involved.

Pathogenesis: Young and untrained horses have a metacarpus that tends to be relatively symmetric mediad and laterad, with a thicker

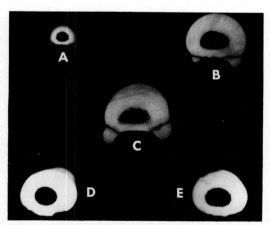

Fig 179. Radiograph of mid-shaft cross-sections of the left metacarpus of a 300-day-old fetus (A), a yearling (B), a 4-year-old actively racing (C), a 2-year-old with Grade-II dorsal metacarpal disease (D), and a 3-year-old with Grade-III dorsal metacarpal disease (E). These cross-sections demonstrate the normal thickening of the dorsal and dorsomedial cortices of the metacarpus (A-C). Diffuse subperiosteal new bone growth is present in the dorsomedial aspect of section D, characteristic of Grade-II dorsal metacarpal disease. A fracture line is visible in the dorsolateral aspect of section E, affected with Grade-III dorsal metacarpal disease.

dorsal cortex (Fig 179). This observation is understandable as the dorsal cortex experiences greater compression than the caudal cortex and thus requires greater strength. [3,4] Horses exposed to heavy exercise (stress), such as training or competition, experience remodeling characterized by increased thickness of the dorsomedial cortex (Fig 179). Bone remodeling is a response to increased stress (maximum load transmission). In a cylindric structure, this stress is greatest at the outer surface or periphery.[5] The medial surface of the forelimb is under greatest stress and therefore undergoes the greatest degree of remodeling.[3]

Development of a painful dorsal cortex in young horses is a function of bone failure since the stress is greater than the remodeled bone can withstand. Damage occurs faster than it can be repaired. Horses that are calf-kneed or back-in-the-knee are predisposed to dorsal metacarpal disease. It is reasonable to postulate that this failure in young horses results in microfracture(s).[1,6-10] The term fatigue (stress) fracture may be applicable as it defines a progressive failure of material under cyclic or fluctuating loads resulting from repeated stress rather than a specific traumatic episode.[11,13] This disease most often occurs bilaterally, although the left leg is often more severely involved. Excessive stress on that limb is related to left turns during exercise. Quarter Horses are not predisposed to severe limb involvement. Seldom are such fractures demonstrable radiographically in the acute disease in 2-year-olds. A greater subperiosteal callus ("shin splint") results if the insult is severe, if training was intentionally continued or if the disease was not diagnosed (Figs 180, 181).

Thoroughbreds, as old as 2 years or older, occasionally incur dorsal metacarpal disease of a more dramatic nature. This disorder is a frank and radiographically demonstrable fracture, typically of the left leg, that occurs in the dorsolateral cortex at the junction of the middle and distal thirds of the third metacarpal bone. This fracture has been referred to as a fatigue, stress, saucer, tongue, shear or fissure fracture.[3,7,14] It is apparently an acute manifestation of a chronic insult in the metacarpus that has caused dorsomedial remodeling. Such horses often have a history of recurrent dorsal metacarpal disease. The dorsolateral cortex, inherently of less substance than the dorsomedial cortex due to remodeling as explained above, may be weaker and experience greater relative stress, leading to failure.[3] Excessive compres-

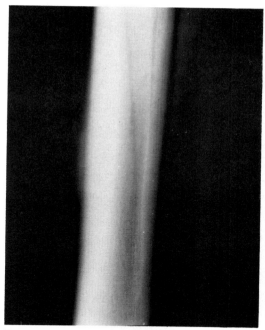

Fig 180. An APLMO radiograph of a left metacarpus with typical Grade-II dorsal metacarpal disease reveals broad-based subperiosteal new bone growth.

The disease is relatively acute in onset and may become obvious after intense exercise. At this time the animal is seldom obviously lame but may have a mild bilateral gait deficit. Palpation of the dorsal cortex reveals focal pain. Radiographs taken during this acute phase are usually negative, although fractures are occasionally observed.

The subacute or chronic form (Grade II) of dorsal metacarpal disease develops if the acute form does not respond to conventional therapy or is unrecognized. This form occurs more often in horses 26-42 months of age. The remodeling process previously discussed has usually taken place at this time, resulting in thickening of the dorsomedial cortex of the third metacarpal bone. Varying degrees of painful periostitis are palpable over the dorsal and/or dorsomedial aspect of the bone. Pain is more pronounced after heavy exercise or racing; the horse may not be obviously lame. As in Grade I and Grade III, the left leg is more severely affected. Most of the focal pain and gait deficit, if present, resolve within days or a few weeks, only to recur if heavy exercise is resumed. Occasionally, with continued heavy exercise, the condition

sion of the lateral aspect of the distal limb occurs during a counterclockwise exercise pattern. This increased lateral compression on the left forelimb, coupled with the suspected decrease in elasticity of the maturing and remodeled third metacarpal bone, may also contribute to the location of this fracture.

Fracture of the dorsolateral cortex is most suggestive of failure in compression due to shear forces and results in fractures at an angle of 35-45° from the long axis of the bone.[10,15] It is imperative that this disease be differentiated from the traditionally accepted "bucked shin" based upon age group and location of pathologic changes.

Clinical Signs: It is most convenient to categorize dorsal metacarpal disease into 3 grades: Grade I involves an acutely painful dorsal metacarpus without radiographic lesions; Grade II involves a subacute and mildly painful dorsal metacarpus, with radio-graphic evidence of subperiosteal callus; Grade III is a dorsal cortical fracture.

Grade I dorsal metacarpal disease is usually seen in race horses 18-36 months of age. The acute form has been observed in older horses (3-5 years) that did not train strenuously or race as 2-year-olds. However, most cases in horses over 2 years are of Grades II and III.

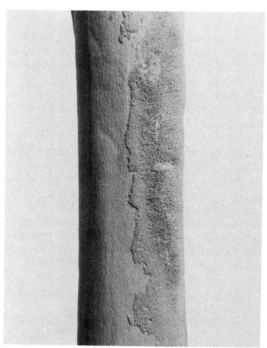

Fig 181. Macerated specimen of the right metacarpus, demonstrating typical craniomedial subperiosteal new bone growth associated wtih Grade-II distal metacarpal disease. This patient's left metacarpus is seen in cross-section in Figure 179D.

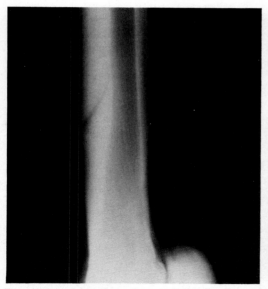

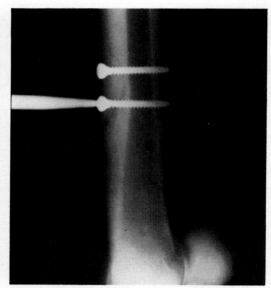

Fig 182. Lateral radiograph of left metacarpus with Grade-III dorsal metacarpal disease. The fracture enters the dorsal cortex in typical fashion and progresses proximad.

Fig 183. Postoperative lateral radiograph of the left metacarpus of the patient in Figure 182 demonstrating intercortical fixation of Grade-III dorsal metacarpal disease. This is nearly a true "saucer" fracture.

progresses to Grade-III disease (dorsal cortical fracture).

Diagnosis: Radiographic findings include thickening of the dorsal or medial cortex, with demineralization of the subperiosteal surface, a single focus or multiple foci of subperiosteal new bone growth, and an endosteal response in advanced cases (Fig 180).

Horses with a distinct dorsal cortical fracture(s) (Grade-III dorsal metacarpal disease) usually have a fairly typical history. Most fractures occur in horses over 2 years of age, and often these patients have had chronic and persistent Grade-II disease. Pre-existing fractures may have gone undiagnosed. While there may be some variation in the presenting complaint, veterinary assistance is usually solicited when acute, severe lameness occurs after intense exercise or competition. Less often, there is concern about a persistent, moderately painful focal elevation on the dorsal cortex of the third metacarpal bone. As previously mentioned, the left leg is predisposed to this type of fracture in Thoroughbreds.

A raised and painful area can be identified if the fracture causes noticeable lameness. Radiographic examination is essential to characterize the nature and extent of the fracture. A series of at least 4 radiographic views should be taken: anterior to posterior (AP), lateral to

medial, anterior to posterior lateral to medial oblique (APLMO), and anterior to posterior medial to lateral oblique (APMLO). Because of the usual location of the fracture, lateral and APMLO views best characterize the fracture. Slight variation in the above views may be required after assessment of the initial series. Repeated radiographic examinations at 7- to 10-day intervals may be necessary when a fracture is suspected but is not obvious. Demineralization along the fracture line after 14-21 days usually allows definitive diagnosis.

The fracture most frequently seen is a relatively straight or slightly concave (dorsad) fracture line that enters the dorsal cortex and proceeds proximad at an angle of about 35-45° (Fig 182). Seldom is the medullary cavity entered, but rather the fracture may extend proximad in a more vertical direction and occasionally proceed toward or exit through the dorsal cortex (saucer fracture) (Fig 183). Multiple fracture lines may radiate from the distal point of entry, although this is not common. Subperiosteal callus is frequently present and is a function of the duration and extent of the insult. Endosteal proliferation may help confirm the location of the fracture and should be appreciated.

Treatment: Regardless of the extent of dorsal metacarpal disease, a period of inactivity is required to allow resolution of inflammation. Daily walking is acceptable and activity can be increased when the metacarpus is no longer painful to firm palpation of the involved area. A reasonable adjunct to management during this period is local hypothermia. The duration of this convalescent period may range from 21-30 days (Grade I) to as long as 60-90 days in more extensive cases.

The return to exercise might be termed a controlled exercise program. The intent of controlled exercise is to allow the third metacarpal bone an opportunity to remodel prior to resumption of heavy exercise. The animal can be exercised without a rider (ponying) or slowly galloped, depending on the severity of disease. Exercise intensity is increased as long as the metacarpus remains nonpainful; close patient assessment is therefore imperative. During this period it may be beneficial to have the horse shod without toe grabs. In mild cases, a full exercise program may be resumed in 15-30 days.

Grade-II disease can be the most difficult and frustrating to manage because of extensive damage to the bone (multiple microfractures). Some patients may experience pain on palpation the remainder of their racing careers, while others may take a year or longer to become sound.

Most acute dorsal cortical fractures, particularly in young athletes, resolve with conservative management as outlined above. The duration and extent of the fracture dictate the convalescent period preceding extended work. This period is usually 4-6 months, although it may be prolonged in refractory cases.[14] Older horses with dorsal cortical fractures, particularly those with a history of recurrent dorsal metacarpal disease, may be considered candidates for surgical intervention with compression-screw fixation.

Fracture healing can only be evaluated by serial radiographic examinations. It is most important that serial identical views be compared since, unless the fracture line is penetrated by the primary beam, the radiographic study may give the false impression of fracture resolution or healing. The small (second and fourth) metacarpal bones should be closely scrutinized for their radiographic positioning relative to the third to establish that comparable views are being evaluated. Serial studies should be conducted at 30- 45-day intervals until the lesion is totally healed. Fracture lines are usually more evident 30 days after occur-

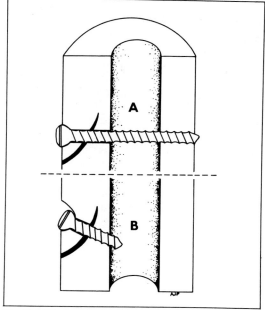

Fig 184. Diagram of intercortical (transcortical) (A) and intracortical (unicortical) (B) fixation technics for repair of Grade-III dorsal metacarpal disease. The fracture line depicted is most common.

rence because of the initial demineralization during the normal healing process.

Two surgical technics have been suggested to treat refractory cases of dorsal cortical fracture of the third metacarpal bone.[14,16] Fracture compression is accomplished by placing a screw across the fracture line within the dorsal cortex (intracortical or unicortical fixation) or by compressing the fracture line by fixation in the palmar cortex (intercortical or transcortical fixation) (Fig 184). While both procedures have been used successfully, compression within the cranial cortex is suggested as more physiologic in that it allows independent movement of the dorsal and palmar cortices during weight-bearing.[16] Refracture may occur more often with the intercortical technic than with the other, although documented studies are unavailable.

Fracture fixation is accomplished under general anesthesia, and intraoperative radiography is necessary. The approach, dependent on fracture location, is usually by a vertical incision between the common and lateral digital extensor tendons over the area of prominent swelling.

Placement of markers (needles) and intraoperative radiographic examination are required to identify the exact location of the fracture. The lag-screw principle is used and the ASIF system is suggested for optimal mechanical advantage. The intercortical technic allows compression of the fracture against the dorsal cortex by anchoring the screw in the palmar cortex (Fig 183). The intracortical technic involves precise measurements to ensure that the fracture line is compressed against the parent cortex. While the screw should be placed at right angles to the long axis of the third metacarpal bone with the intercortical technic, the screw should be as close to perpendicular to the fracture as possible in the intracortical technic to provide maximum holding power. The metacarpus may be protected during recovery by a low-leg cast, which can be removed in 48-72 hours. Healing of the surgical site is usually uneventful.

Postoperative management includes limited exercise until the surgical site is nonpainful. Controlled exercise follows thereafter, with the extent of work based upon radiographic determination of fracture resolution.

The results of internal fixation of this fracture have been variable. Both technics have been used successfully, although intercortical fixation may predispose to demineralization about the head of the screw, with attendant pain, after 6-12 months of racing. However, removal of the screw, followed by rest, may result in refracture when training or racing is resumed. Intracortical fixation may decrease the incidence of demineralization by reducing relative motion of the screw. At this point, without the benefit of documented studies, it is important to appreciate that internal fixation is not without potential complications. The prognosis in these cases is guarded.

Other methods of therapy include thermocautery (pin-firing), chemical vesication (blistering), injection of osteogenic substances (sodium oleate), and cryotherapy (point-freezing). These treatments have resulted in varying degrees of success. Regardless of which approach is selected, an adequate period of metacarpal remodeling is necessary to reduce the incidence of recurrence.

Prevention: Young horses on a sound and deliberate training schedule experience a lower incidence of dorsal metacarpal disease than do others.[17] Furthermore, an adequate interval between periods of heavy exercise allows the horse to adjust to the increased stress by dynamic remodeling and resolution of insults to the third metacarpal bone. Young horses should be examined carefully after every workout.

The horse's work schedule should be reduced if pain or inflammation is detected. Continued exercise at a lower intensity allows remodeling to continue. While complete inactivity allows microfractures to heal, remodeling is slowed to the point that recurrence may be a problem. Therefore, continued low-intensity exercise is indicated once inflammation has resolved.

Race tracks should strive to create racing surfaces with adequate cushioning to allow rotation of foot on impact. Hard surfaces may prevent the hoof from cutting in and the resulting sliding effect develops a longer compression phase on the third metacarpal bone.[18] "Cuppy" tracks also apparently enhance the incidence of dorsal metacarpal disease.[10] Horses that only compete on grass seldom experience dorsal metacarpal disease, which supports the "sliding" theory.

Any variation in hoof care that delays breakover predisposes to distal metacarpal disease. The toe grab and long-toe, low-heeled hoof shape ("race-track foot") both delay breakover. This results in reduced ability to absorb shock and increases stress on the metacarpus.

References

1. Johnson, in Catcott: Equine Medicine and Surgery. 2nd ed. American Veterinary Publications, Santa Barbara, 1972.
2. Norwood, GL. Proc 24th Ann Mtg Am Assoc Eq Pract, 1978. p 319.
3. Rooney, JR. Mod Vet Pract **59** (1978) 633.
4. Turner, AS *et al.* Am J Vet Res **36** (1975) 1573.
5. Albright, JA, Louisiana State Univ: Unpublished data, 1978.
6. Devas, MB. J Bone Jt Surg **49B** (1967) 310.
7. Fackelman, GE: Surgical Diseases of the Equine Musculoskeletal System. Paper presented at Louisiana VMA meeting, 1978.
8. Lingard, DR. VM/SAC **64** (1969) 895.
9. Milne, FJ. Proc World Vet Cong, 1971. p 1124.
10. Rooney, JR: Biomechanics of Lameness in Horses. Williams & Wilkins, Baltimore, 1969.
11. Carter, DR and Hayes, WC. J Biomech **9** (1976) 227.
12. Carter, JR and Hayes, WC. Clin Orthoped Rel Res **127** (1977) 265.
13. Walter, NE and Wolf, MD. Am J Sports Med **5** (1977) 165.
14. Fackelman, GE: Treatment of Saucer Fractures of Equine Metacarpus by Internal Fixation. Paper presented at Annual Forum, American College of Veterinary Surgeons, Chicago, 1976.
15. Chamay, A. J Biomech **3** (1970) 263.
16. Fackelman, GE, New London, PA: Personal communication, 1978.
17. Maderious, WE. Proc 18th Ann Mtg Am Assoc Eq Pract, 1972. p 451.
18. Rooney, JR. Mod Vet Pract **55** (1974) 217.

THE SMALL METACARPAL AND METATARSAL BONES
by D.O. Goble

Metacarpal II and IV or metatarsal II and IV are commonly referred to as splint bones in the horse. These small bones represent remnants of the other 2 digits horses had prior to the evolutionary change from a 3-digit animal to a soliped. Although only vestiges, the bones are an important part of the supporting and stabilizing structures of the horse's pectoral and pelvic limbs.

General Considerations

The small metacarpal or metatarsal bones are positioned on the caudomedial and caudolateral surface of metacarpal III or metatarsal III. The suspensory ligament lies in the groove formed by these small bones. Metacarpal II articulates proximad with the second and third carpal bones (type-B articulation), while metacarpal IV articulates with the fourth carpal bone.[1] Each of these bones also articulates with metacarpal III. Metatarsal II and IV articulate proximad with the tarsus and metatarsal III. Metatarsal II is a more slender bone than metatarsal IV and articulates with the fused first and second tarsal bones. Metatarsal IV articulates with the fourth tarsal bone.

The small metacarpal and metatarsal bones have been overlooked as to their function in support of the carpus or tarsus. This is especially true when considering the front limb. The small metacarpal bones support not only the carpus but also reinforce metacarpal III in much the same way that floor joists function in the construction of a house. The caudal cortex of metacarpal III is markedly thinner in its proximal portion where the splint bones add support (Fig 185). This fact is of special importance when ostectomy is performed to remove 75% or more of the distal small metacarpal bone.

There are numerous factors associated with or predisposing to diseases of the small metacarpal or metatarsal bones. Conformation, nutrition, body weight, exercise, improper shoeing and trauma have all been incriminated as contributing factors. Disease of the small metacarpal or metatarsal bones is more frequent in young horses and occurs most commonly when 2- or 3-year-old horses are put into training.

Conformation of a type that increases stress on the medial side of the front limb increases the frequency of disease of metacarpal II. Bench knees are a conformational fault that predisposes to the formation of splints (periostitis of the splint bones).[2] Conformation that predisposes to interference, such as base-narrow toe-out, can traumatically induce splint formation. Improper shoeing may unbalance the feet and produce interference. This is not an unusual problem when the farrier is attempting to correct some other pre-existent conformational fault.

Malnutrition, such as an imbalance in Ca and P intake, and overfeeding are often associated with splint bone problems. Fast-growing, young, overweight Quarter Horses often develop splints because of increased weight-bearing at an early age.

Trauma associated with direct injury from kicks or interference during a race accounts for many fractures in the small metacarpal or metatarsal bones. Generally these fractures are of metacarpal IV or metatarsal IV.

Pathologic Conditions of the Splint Bones

Due to variations in terminology of disease involving the small metacarpal or metatarsal bones, certain terms must be defined.

True Splint: The splint bones rely in part upon the interosseous ligament between the splint bone and metacarpal or metatarsal III for stabilization. In addition, the annular and collateral ligaments of the joint also add support and maintain normal alignment. The interosseous ligament is present in the proximal half of the splint bone. Tearing or straining of the interosseous ligament and the resulting periostitis between these 2 bones is termed a true splint. As normal healing occurs, an enlargement forms at the site of injury. This swelling is initially composed of fibrous connective tissue and later a portion of it calcifies to become

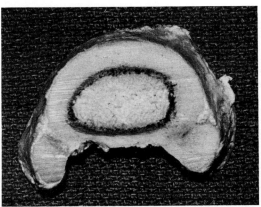

Fig 185. Cross-section of metacarpals II, III and IV 4 cm distal to the carpus. Note the thin caudal cortex of metacarpal III.

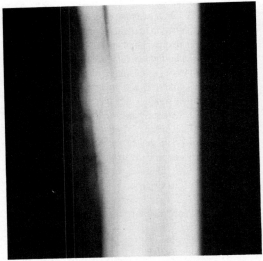

Fig 186. The most common location of splints, 6-8 cm distal to the carpus.

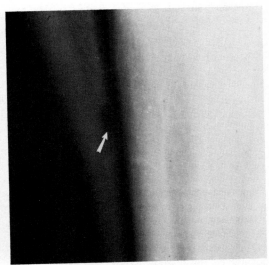

Fig 187. Osteolysis (arrow) associated with a blind splint.

bone. Histologically, the interosseous ligament changes from predominantly collagen fibers prior to injury to chondroid tissue after injury.[1] True splints most commonly occur as a firm enlargement 6-8 cm distal to the carpus between metacarpal II and III (Fig 186).

Blind Splint: Blind splint is a rather ambiguous term applied to an inflammation of the interosseous ligament that is not readily detectable externally by observation or palpation. Radiographically these appear as areas of decalcification between the splint bone and metacarpal or metatarsal III (Fig 187). Often the enlargement is between the splint bone and suspensory ligament.

Periostitis of the Splint Bone: Trauma to the splint bone often irritates the periosteum and produces proliferative periostitis (Fig 188). Injuries associated with kicks or interference are the most frequent cause. This same type of injury may also involve the large metacarpal or metatarsal bone in conjunction with the splint bone. These injuries are usually superficial and unlikely to cause severe lameness; however, they result in a blemish. Cosmetic removal is occasionally requested but the result is often

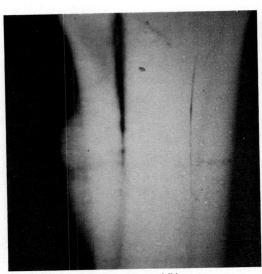

Fig 188. Periostitis of metacarpal IV.

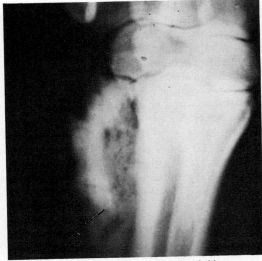

Fig 189. Knee splint, with associated arthritis.

less than satisfactory. Recurrence is common when interference is the initiating cause.

Knee Splint: The splint bones articulate proximad with the carpus/tarsus and metacarpal/metatarsal III. When the most proximal portion of the splint bone is injured, arthritis may develop (Fig 189). This is the most serious problem of the splint bones and the prognosis for full functional soundness of affected horses is unfavorable.

Fractured Splint: Fractures of the splint bones most frequently occur in the distal third of the bone (Fig 190). Such fractures produce mild lameness, swelling and heat for only a few days. If the horse is rested and treated with leg wraps or sweats, the leg may appear normal in a week. As soon as the horse is returned to work, however, the problem recurs. Horses with chronic suspensory desmitis may be prone to fractures of this type. Fractures of the splint bones occur more frequently in the front legs.

Fractures of the proximal half of the splint bones are usually incurred by trauma, such as with interference in gait, a kick from another horse or some form of direct trauma. Fractures of this type produce greater pain, swelling and lameness than those associated with the distal third of the splint bone. Radiographs must be taken to determine the presence of such fractures. These fractures often lead to osteomyelitis due to the fact that the causative trauma frequently lacerates the skin and contaminates the injury (Fig 191).

Diagnosis of Splint Bone Lesions

Any lameness in a horse presents a certain challenge in determining the exact location of the associated lesions. The presence of a splint does not necessarily mean it is the source of lameness. Nor does the physical size of the splint indicate the severity of the problem. Many large splints produce no lameness, while some very small ones produce severe lameness. Therefore, a thorough physical examination of each affected horse is of utmost importance.

As in the diagnosis of most lamenesses, the horse must be observed while in motion. A horse with splints is not usually lame at a walk and stands without favoring the affected leg. The lameness is best seen by trotting the horse on a hard surface. Splint bone lesions cause a supporting-leg lameness, *ie*, when the front limbs are involved the horse drops its head as the sound limb bears weight at a trot. Lameness of the rear limb may be more difficult to detect and detection of an area of soreness on

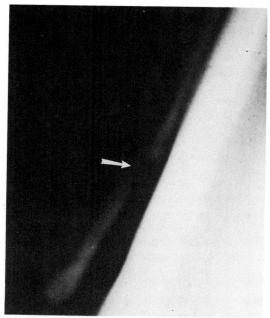

Fig 190. Fracture (arrow) of the distal portion of a splint bone.

the rear limb may be the first sign observed. Close observation as the horse is trotted straight away may show that the hip of the sound limb drops slightly lower when it bears weight than does the hip on the affected side.

Physical examination of the splint bone must be done with the leg flexed. This allows palpation of the entire length of the bone, including the medial and lateral borders. It is of

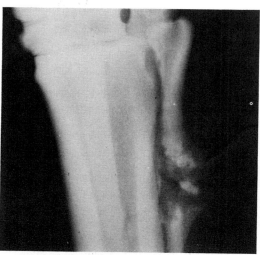

Fig 191. Fracture of the proximal portion of a splint bone. Osteomyelitis and a sequestrum are evident.

extreme importance when palpating the small metacarpal or metatarsal bones to closely examine the suspensory ligament at the same time. When a splint is present, the degree of involvement with the suspensory ligament often determines if chronic lameness will evolve. Palpation over the area of the splint should elicit pain if this is the cause of lameness. Assessing the degree of pain in response to the severity of clinical lameness must also be attempted. Pain associated with a splint may be a secondary problem and not the primary cause of lameness. If palpation of the splint reveals mild pain but the horse is markedly lame, one should look elsewhere for additional and possibly more severe lesions.

Most splints can be diagnosed by the presence of heat, pain and swelling in the affected area. Occasionally it is necessary to locally anesthetize a splint to determine if it is the true cause of lameness. Once a tentative diagnosis is made, radiographs are necessary to determine if a fracture is present. Generally, a fractured small metacarpal/metatarsal bone causes greater pain and swelling than a simple or uncomplicated splint.

Radiographs of the splint bones should be taken in the lateral-medial, anterior-posterior and oblique views. The anterior-posterior view allows more complete evaluation of the medial portion of the splint bone and possible impingement upon the suspensory ligament. However, this view is unsatisfactory to determine the presence of fractures, interosseous ligament damage or possible joint involvement. Therefore, the oblique and lateral-medial views are an absolute necessity to fully evaluate the splint bone and surrounding structures.

Treatment

Methods of treating splint bone problems are widely diversified but basically include the use of anti-inflammatory agents, counterirritation, and surgical excision and/or stabilization.

Anti-Inflammatory Treatment: Anti-inflammatory substances include cold water, ice packs, antiphlogistics, corticosteroids, phenylbutazone and other items too numerous to mention. These agents are most effective in the acute or peracute stage of inflammation.

In the treatment of acute splints, the use of cold water and support wraps is an excellent method to reduce the heat, pain and swelling. The use of whirlpool boots and ice twice daily for 45 minutes for the first 5-7 days is beneficial. The splint should also be massaged for 10

minutes after each treatment and then placed in a support bandage. After 10-14 days (or when splint is cooled out), a mild liniment may be applied and the support bandages changed daily. Close observation must be maintained to avoid irritation from either the bandages or the liniment. Affected horses should have stall rest for 30-45 days, with 15-20 minutes of hand-walking twice a day.

If the splint is a result of interference, splint or shin guards may help prevent further injury during training. Corticosteroids injected directly into the area of inflammation have been employed.[2] This method is generally not satisfactory because the problem commonly recurs unless the horse is given an extended period of rest. Systemic use of phenylbutazone improves the lameness but a period of at least 45 days' rest is still mandatory to allow healing.

Counterirritation: This is probably the most frequently used method of treatment. Some form of counterirritation has been used for centuries to treat splints. Counterirritants include pyropuncture (firing), sclerosing agents, blisters (internal and external), acids, radiation and other caustics. Their function is to convert a chronic or low-level inflammatory process to an active, acute inflammatory response.

Firing is probably still the most common method of counterirritation treatment of a true splint. This method is often unacceptable on show horses due to scarring and is more frequently used on race horses. Firing, however, is not effective in treating blind splints involving the suspensory ligament because the area involved is not accessible to the firing iron. Injectable iodine counterirritants or sclerosing agents may be of benefit when applied on the medial side of the splint bone.[3] In general, treated horses should have at least 30 or more days' rest after a counterirritant is applied, depending on the extent of the original damage. No form of counterirritation should be administered for at least 45 days following local treatment with corticosteroids.

Surgery: Surgical intervention is a common treatment of disease of the small metacarpal and metatarsal bones. The risks associated with surgery must be clearly explained to the client, as well as the prognosis if surgery is not done. Although descriptions of removal of fractured splint bones in the standing horse have been published, this procedure has little merit in the realm of modern equine surgery.[4] The chance of infection is increased and it is difficult to treat the soft tissue properly when attempting surgery under such conditions.

It has been suggested that any time more than 50% of the distal segment of the splint is removed, the proximal portion should be immobilized.[5] Screw-fixation can be a difficult task because many splint bones lack sufficient substance in which to place a screw, except in the proximal third of the bone. It is probably more reasonable to consider internal fixation only if the distal 75% of the bone is removed. This allows placing a screw in a larger mass of bone, with less chance of fragmentation on compression. It should also be stressed that screw-fixation is contraindicated in cases of osteomyelitis and sepsis due to external trauma. The opportunity for osteomyelitis of metacarpal or metatarsal III is greatly enhanced by placing a screw through the cortex.

Twelve hours prior to surgery, the leg should be clipped with a #40 surgical clipper from below the fetlock to the carpus. The leg is then scrubbed with surgical soap. The entire area must be rinsed free of all soap because some horses react to the soap as to a blister. An alcohol bandage should then be placed over the leg and a support wrap applied.

At the time of surgery the wrap is removed and a surgical scrub completed. The incision is made directly over the splint bone from approximately 3 cm proximal to the fracture site to 3 cm distal to the tip of the splint bone. The incision is continued in the same plane through the periosteum on the proximal segment. The periosteum may be difficult to identify and elevate if a proliferative periosteal reaction or large callus is present. Use of a periosteal elevator facilitates this portion of the surgery.

The soft tissue should be carefully dissected free of the splint bone with a sharp scalpel, while avoiding further injury to the suspensory ligament if it is adhered to the fracture site. After the soft tissue is dissected free, the site is chosen at which the bone is to be resected. A sharp osteotome and mallet are used to transect the bone so that the proximal segment is beveled at an approximate 40° angle to its long axis (Fig 192). Care is taken that metacarpal/metatarsal III is not traumatized when making this cut. The distal segment of the splint bone is then elevated from any bony attachment and removed.

Soft tissue damage to the suspensory ligament and deep flexor tendon is evaluated at this time. Since most splint bone fractures are in the distal third of the bone, adhesions of one

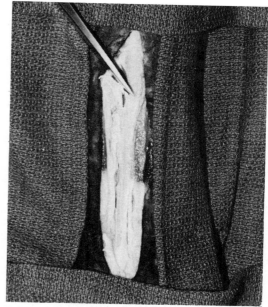

Fig 192. Resection of the distal portion of a splint bone using an osteotome.

strand of the suspensory to the caudal border of metacarpal/metatarsal III are common. Any adhesions between the suspensory ligament and surrounding structures should be freed. When the suspensory ligament is very fibrotic, longitudinal splitting may be beneficial.

The periosteum is closed with 00 absorbable suture material if it is identifiable and intact. An effort should be made to obliterate all deadspace to reduce postsurgical calcification. If this is not possible, a drain is placed for 3-5 days after surgery. The drain can usually be removed with the first bandage change. A continous subcuticular suture pattern with 00 absorbable suture material also aids in closing deadspace. The skin is then closed with an interrupted vertical-mattress pattern of 0 nonabsorbable monofilament suture. The surgical site is dressed with an antibiotic ointment, sterile combine roll and a support wrap. The wrap can be left in place for 5 days if it remains dry and clean. Additional sheet-cotton and elastic wraps may be applied to protect the leg during recovery.

Special precautions must be taken if 75% or more of the distal splint bone is removed. Removal of part of the supporting structure could increase the chance of fracture during recovery. This is especially true in the front legs of large horses. A temporary cast can be applied from the foot to the elbow on the front leg. Preconditioning the horse 24 hours prior to surgery with a full-leg Robert-Jones bandage accustoms the horse to having the leg immobilized. The temporary cast can be removed 24-36 hours postoperatively.

Aftercare includes the use of phenylbutazone and hand-walking 10-15 minutes twice daily from the first postoperative day to reduce formation of adhesions and impaired suspensory ligament function. The sutures are removed in 14 days and work can be resumed in 45 days if there are no complications.

References

1. Rooney, JR et al. Cornell Vet 56 (1966) 259.
2. Adams, OR: Lameness in Horses. 3rd ed. Lea & Febiger, Philadelphia, 1974.
3. Johnson, in Catcott: Equine Medicine and Surgery. 2nd ed. American Veterinary Publications, Santa Barbara, 1972.
4. Lundvall, in Catcott: Equine Medicine and Surgery. 1st ed. American Veterinary Publications, Santa Barbara, 1963.
5. Heinze, in Catcott: Equine Medicine and Surgery. 2nd ed. American Veterinary Publications, Santa Barbara, 1972.
6. Jones, RD and Fessler,, JF. Can Vet J 18(2) (1977) 28.

THE CARPUS
by B.D. Grant

The carpus or knee is a complex arrangement of 2 rows of at least 7 cuboidal bones that form 3 synovial joints. The radiocarpal and middle carpal joints do not communicate and are regarded as ginglymi (hinge joints). The carpometacarpal joint is an arthrodial (sliding) joint with little movement. It communicates with the middle carpal joint.[1]

Diagnosis of Carpal Lameness

Diagnosis of carpal lameness is based upon the history and the results of physical examination and supplementary diagnostic technics. The history should include information on the onset of lameness and any previous use of intra-articular corticosteroids. Physical examination is performed as described in Chapter 1.

Synovial distension is the hallmark of carpal joint disease. Synovial distension of the radiocarpal joint produces a soft, fluctuant swelling on the cranial, caudal and proximal aspects of the carpus. Such a distension can be distinguished from distension of the carpal sheath by

its inability to be palpated distal to the carpus. Synovial distension of the middle carpal joint is evident craniad, as well as caudolaterad distal to the accessory carpal bone.

Carpal lameness can be confirmed with intra-articular injections of 6 ml of a local anesthetic, such as mepivacaine, into each joint after the withdrawal of synovial fluid. Local anesthetic should not be injected into joints from which homogeneously dark red fluid is withdrawn because of the probability of fractures in such cases. The injection site is aseptically prepared and joint fluid is aspirated with a 20-ga needle (Fig 193). A new vial of local anesthetic should always be used to prevent injection of contaminants. At least 20 minutes should elapse before evaluation of lameness to allow for adequate absorption of local anesthetic. Support bandages should be applied after injection to minimize swelling.

The presence of suspected carpal lesions can be confirmed with the use of AP, lateral, APLMO and PALMO radiographs.[2] A flexed lateral view aids detection of osteochondral fractures of the carpal joints. Tangential projections are useful when no lesions are evident on standard views (Fig 194).

Sedation with xylazine or acepromazine may be necessary to ensure motion-free images. Intra-articular anesthesia and a dorsal ulnar nerve block may be necessary to obtain radiographs of the flexed carpus in cases of large carpal fractures.

Electrogoniometry, cinematography and arthroscopy are also useful in assessing carpal lesions.

Carpal Fractures

Lateral Distal Radius

The lateral surface of the distal radius is a common fracture site because of its projecting conformation (Fig 195). Recent fractures cause synovial distension, pain on palpation and flexion, and head-bobbing at a jog. Old fractures may be asymptomatic despite radiographic evidence of a fracture.

The proximal intermediate carpal bone should also be radiographically examined with tangential views since that area is often concurrently fractured with lateral distal radial fractures. Fragments of the proximal intermediate carpal bone should be removed if the joint has not undergone degenerative changes. If

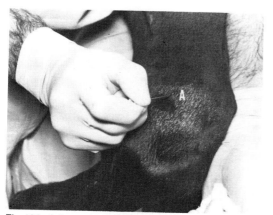
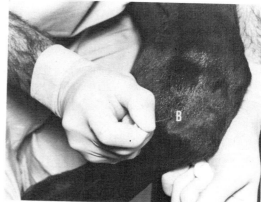

Fig 193. Arthrocentesis sites between the extensor carpi radialis and the common digital extensor tendons for the radial carpal joint (A) and the middle carpal joint (B).

only the distal radial fracture is present, 3 months of stall rest followed by 3 months of paddock rest may result in recovery.

In cases requiring surgical intervention, a curvilinear skin incision is made between the common digital and extensor carpi radialis tendons, with the joint slightly flexed (Fig 196). Carpal flexion is reduced after the joint is entered and the fracture site is evaluated. Palpation with a blunt instrument usually reveals the loosely attached fragment(s). After the fragments are removed, the fracture site is smoothed by curettage. Fractures of the intermediate carpal bones are treated similarly. The joint is flushed and closed as previously described. The area is bandaged with Telfa pads, Elastikon and a stovepipe bandage, with extra cotton over the carpus (Fig 30).

Aftercare consists of administration of antibiotics for 5 days, moderate doses of phenylbu-

tazone, and passive flexion of the carpus for the first 10 days. Hand-walking is begun on day 10 and continued as long as necessary. Sutures are removed at 12-14 days.

Medial Distal Radius

Fractures of the medial surface of the distal radius tend to be larger and not as common as

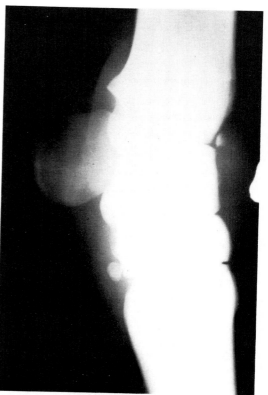

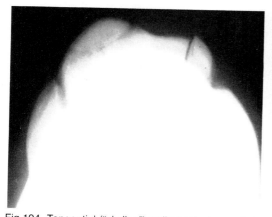

Fig 194. Tangential ("skyline") radiograph demonstrating 2 osteochondral fractures of the third carpal bone.

Fig 195. Large osteochondral fracture on the lateral aspect of the distal radius.

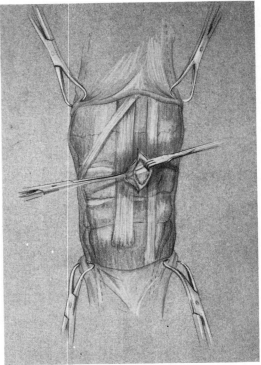

Fig 196. Surgical approach for removal of osteochondral fracture fragments from the lateral aspect of the distal radius and proximal intermediate carpal bone.

those on the lateral surface. Most fragments are firmly attached, with little displacement, and a conservative approach is usually indicated (Fig 197).

Surgical treatment of fractures of the medial distal radius is similar to that for those on the lateral surface. The skin incision is medial to the extensor carpi radialis tendon. The tendon sheath of the abductor policus longus may be entered but is not a serious problem. Fragment removal, closure and aftercare are similar to that for fractures of the lateral radius.

Radial Carpal Bone

The distal aspect is usually involved in fractures of the radial carpal bone. Recent fractures are characterized by obvious lameness, synovial distension, and pain on palpation and flexion. Chronic fractures are not as painful but result in poor performance and degenerative osteoarthritis due to fragment displacement (Fig 198).

Recent fractures of the distal radial carpal bone are best treated by surgical removal of fragments. A guarded to favorable prognosis can be issued if the articular cartilage is white and undamaged. The prognosis is poor for recovery from a chronic fracture in which chondromalacia is evident at surgery.

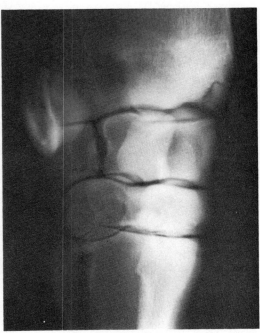

Fig 197. Large osteochondral fracture on the medial aspect of the distal radius.

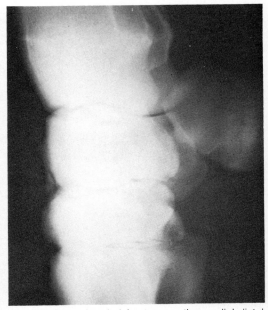

Fig 198. Osteochondral fracture on the medial distal aspect of the radial carpal joint and traumatic dystrophic calcification at the attachment of the dorsal carpal ligament.

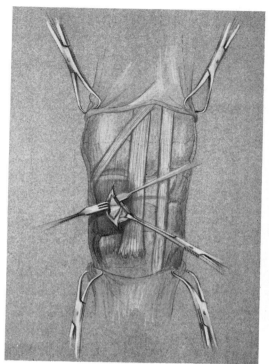

Fig 199. Surgical approach for removal of osteochondral fracture fragments from the distal medial aspect of the radial carpal bone and proximal third carpal bone.

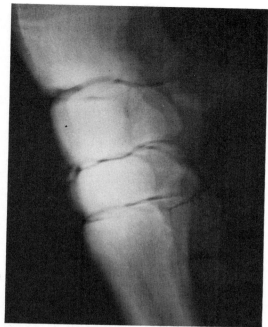

Fig 200. "Saucer" osteochondral fracture of the third carpal bone.

Surgical treatment entails a curvilinear skin incision toward the medial surface of the middle carpal joint, which is marked by a depression (Fig 199). The fragments are removed as previously described and the fracture site smoothed with a Hall drill. The joint capsule and skin are closed after the joint is closely inspected for debris and flushed. •

Third Carpal Bone

Fractures of the third carpal bone are described as saucer, slab or comminuted (Figs 200-202). Recent fractures cause joint distension with hemorrhagic fluid, varying degrees of lameness, and pain on palpation and flexion. Comminuted fractures are characterized by a varus deformity and obvious crepitus. The diagnosis is confirmed by radiographic examination, including tangential views.

Undisplaced, noncomminuted slab fractures that cause minimal lameness can heal after 6 months of stall rest. Analgesics are not administered in an effort to prevent excessive use of the limb. Radiographs should be obtained 2 and 4 weeks after the injury to detect possible displacement and early osteophyte production.

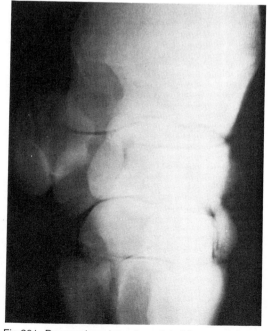

Fig 201. Dorsopalmar lateral-medial oblique projection reveals a displaced, unstable "slab" fracture fragment of the third carpal bone a month after a racing injury. Osteolysis of the fragment, dystrophic calcification and a concurrent fracture of the distal radial carpal bone are evident.

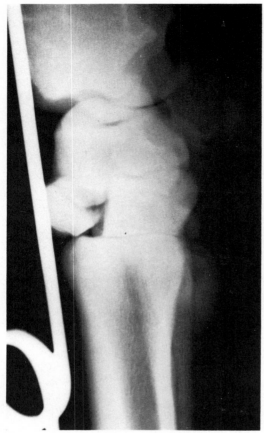

Fig 202. Comminuted fractures of the second and third carpal bones resulted in collapse of the middle carpal joint space and a varus deformity.

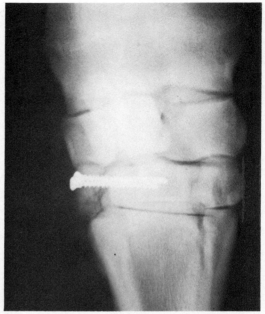

Fig 203. Postoperative radiograph of a comminuted fracture of the fourth carpal bone, treated with a lag-screw technic.

Saucer and displaced fractures of the third carpal bone require immediate surgical intervention. The patient is placed in lateral recumbency with the affected leg down or in dorsal recumbency, with the affected limb extended. A skin incision is made similar to that for distal radial carpal surgery (Fig 199). After the fracture is identified, the limb is fully flexed to minimize fragment displacement. A small stab incision is made in the extensor carpi radialis tendon 5-6 mm distal to the articular border to facilitate drill and screw entry.

If a fragment is large enough for lag-screw compression, the screw hole is drilled through the fragment into the third carpal bone. The hole should be drilled as parallel as possible to the articular surface and radiographs obtained to check hole placement. After a properly sized screw is placed, radiographs are obtained to check screw position. Excessive compression should be avoided.

Fragments too small for lag-screw fixation can be removed. After fragment removal, rough edges are smoothed, bone wax is applied to bleeding subchondral bone, and the joint is flushed, closed and bandaged as previously described. Aftercare is similar to that for other fractures but ultrasound therapy should be avoided if metal implants were used. Screws are not removed unless determined to be a source of chronic pain.

Fourth Carpal Bone

Fractures of the proximal aspect of the fourth carpal bone shold be assessed with oblique radiographs to determine if they also involve the lateral aspect of the third carpal bone or the medial aspect of the fourth carpal bone (Fig 203). The distal end of the intermediate carpal bone is often concurrently fractured. The history and clinical signs of affected animals are similar to those for fractures of the third carpal bone. Fractures of the fourth carpal bone should not be confused with osteophytes associated with radial carpal fractures and joint instability.

Early surgical treatment is indicated in horses with athletic potential. A skin incision is made over the middle carpal joint between the extensor carpi radialis and common digital extensor tendons. Slab or comminuted fractures are treated by fixation or fragment removal as previously described.

Second Carpal Bone

Fractures of the second carpal bone are uncommon and typically comminuted (Fig 202). Affected animals have a varus deformity, a grade-IV lameness, a diffusely enlarged carpus, and pain on palpation and flexion. Animals to be salvaged for breeding should be treated as described for other comminuted carpal bone fractures.

Multiple Comminuted Carpal Fractures

Multiple, comminuted carpal fractures occur most commonly in racing and jumping horses during athletic events. Affected animals are obviously lame and have severe pain on flexion and palpation. Arthrocentesis produces homogeneously bloody synovial fluid. A varus or valgus deformity may be present, depending on which bones are fractured.

Treatment should only be undertaken on animals with breeding potential or great sentimental value since few affected horses fully regain athletic abilities. The affected limb should be immediately stabilized and radiographs obtained to determine the nature of the fractures and the number of fragments. Lag-screw fixation is usually very difficult in these cases owing to the large number of small fragments. Arthrodesis is usually indicated in severe, multiple comminuted fractures, followed by 3-6 months immobilization in a cast to ensure ankylosis. Phenylbutazone should be used to prevent compensatory rotation of the contralateral third phalanx. Use of an acrylic radial carpal prosthesis has been described.[3]

Other Carpal Diseases

Osteochondrosis

Osteochondrosis or cyst-like lesions are often noted on examination of carpal radiographs (Fig 204). Their clinical significance should always be questioned. If intra-articular anesthesia results in improvement in the lameness and no other lesions can be demonstrated, such cyst-like lesions can be assumed as the cause of lameness. Conservative management consists of longer, slower training periods and judicious use of phenylbutazone.

Degenerative Joint Disease

This condition can affect any or all of the carpal joints and usually occurs secondary to trau-

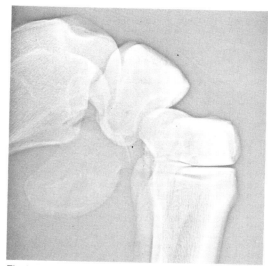

Fig 204. Xeroradiograph of the carpus of a 2-year-old Thoroughbred with a subtle lameness associated with the carpus. Note the well-defined cyst-like lesion. (Courtesy of Dr JH Cannon)

matic osteochondral fractures. Intra-articular use of corticosteroids in the presence of such fractures hastens the onset of degenerative joint disease.[4] It occasionally occurs as a primary entity.

Diagnosis is based upon response to intra-articular anesthesia, changes in synovial fluid character, and radiographic appearance of a narrowed joint space (Fig 205). Intra-articular injection of hyaluronic acid is indicated if the animal is to be retained as a performance

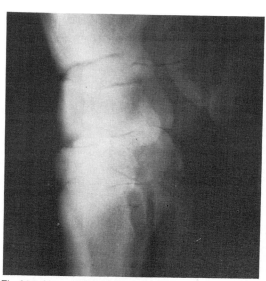

Fig 205. Narrowed middle carpal joint space.

horse.[5,6] Use of a middle carpal prosthesis benefited an arthritic aged mare.[7]

References

1. Sisson, S and Grossman, JD: Anatomy of the Domestic Animals. 4th ed. WB Saunders, Philadelphia, 1953.
2. Thrall, DE *et al*. JAVMA **158** (1971) 1366.
3. Winstanley, EW and Gleeson, LN. JAVMA **165** (1979) 87.
4. Meagher, DM. Proc 16th Ann Mtg Am Assoc Eq Pract, 1970. p 405.
5. Asheim, A and Lindblad, G. Acta Vet Scand **17** (1976) 379.
6. Swanstrom, OG. Proc 24th Ann Mtg Am Assoc Eq Pract, 1978. p 345.
7. Grossman, BS *et al*. Vet Surg **9** (1980) 93.

THE ACCESSORY CARPAL BONE
by K.J. Easley, Jr.

The accessory carpal bone is the most prominent structure on the caudal aspect of the equine carpus. This bone does not directly bear weight as do the other 6 carpal bones. If functions as a sesamoid bone, interposed in the course of the tendons of the flexor carpi ulnaris and ulnaris lateralis muscles. Its position enables these 2 muscles to act at a mechanical advantage in flexing the carpus. In a horse with normal joint conformation, the dorsal border of the accessory carpal bone is perpendicular to the long axis of the limb. Four alterations are associated with hyperextension of the carpus: ventral angulation of the accessory carpal bone in relation to the long axis of the radius; periosteal new bone growth on the lateral and caudal surface of the distal portion of the radius; cranial displacement of the proximal end of the radius; and alterations of the joint capsule on the dorsal surface of the radiocarpal joint.[1] Repeated carpal hyperextension at impact may predispose to arthrosis and fractures of the dorsal surfaces of the carpal bones.

The flexor carpi ulnaris inserts on the proximal aspect of the accessory carpal bone by a short, strong tendon and blends with the flexor retinaculum. The ulnaris lateralis inserts on the lateral and proximal palmar border of the bone. The accessory carpal bone is the lateral point of attachment of the carpal fascia that completes the flexor retinaculum and carpal canal, in which lie the digital flexor tendons, carpal synovial sheath, medial palmar or second common palmar digital artery and nerve.

A smooth groove crossing its proximal part contains the long tendon of the ulnaris lateralis. This small, round tendon in a synovial sheath passes distad and slightly dorsad to insert on the fourth metacarpal bone (Fig 206).

The accessory carpal bone is firmly attached to adjacent bones by 4 ligaments (accessorioulnar, accessoriocarpoulnar, accessorioquartal and accessoriometacarpal) that firmly anchor the dorsal aspect of the bone to the carpus but not the area palmar to the lateral groove (Fig 207). The accessory carpal bone is richly supplied with blood through its tendinous and ligamentous attachments that completely surround the body of the bone. Most of the structures are supplied by the caudal interosseous, collateral ulnar and median arteries, as well as branches of the brachial artery.

The nerve supply to the accessory carpal bone and communicating structures is derived from the ulnar nerve. This nerve divides into 2 terminal branches just proximal to the carpus. The dorsal branch emerges between the tendons of insertion of the flexor carpi ulnaris and ulnaris lateralis, and ramifies on the fascia and skin of the dorsolateral aspect of the carpus. The palmar branch unites with the median nerve to course distad.

Accessory Carpal Bone Fractures

Incidence and Type: Fractures of the carpal bones are common. Accessory carpal bone fractures are relatively uncommon, occurring in 1-10% of carpal fractures reported.[2,3] The characteristic fracture of the accessory carpal bone is in the vertical plane. Usually the fracture is more or less through the center of the bone so that a considerable portion remains attached to the dorsal or articular segment. Occasionally the fracture line is such that two-thirds of the accessory carpal bone are separated at the cranial margin of the lateral groove. This fracture is quite often comminuted, with bone fragments found at either the proximal or distal border, adjacent to the fracture line, or on both sides of the fracture. The other plane of fracture occurs transversely. A transverse fracture is rare and has a grave prognosis if the proximal portion is displaced by the tension of the flexor muscles attached to its proximal border.

Cause: Its prominent position renders the accessory carpal bone most liable to fracture from trauma of all the carpal bones. Types of trauma include kicks from other horses, loose stirrups and polo mallets, or getting a leg caught over a fence. A case reported in a draft horse during

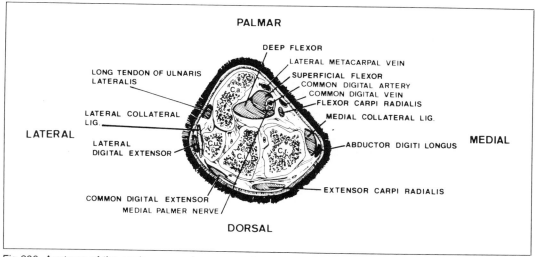

Fig 206. Anatomy of the equine carpus in cross-section.

work was thought to result from excess muscle contracture. The incidence of accessory carpal bone fractures tends to be higher in race horses, especially steeplechasers.

Several theories have been advanced as to the etiology of this type of fracture.[4-7] This fracture may occur from a combination of mechanical factors. The 4 ligaments firmly support and stabilize the segment of bone dorsal to the groove of the long tendon of the ulnaris lateralis. The accessory carpal bone is narrowest, and therefore probably weakest, in the area of this groove. The pull of the ulnaris lateralis and flexor carpi ulnaris and the push of the flexor tendons from within the carpal canal are concentrated in the area palmar to the lateral groove. When the leg is fully loaded in a partially flexed position, the concentrated forces stress the palmar segment beyond its tensile strength, thus causing the fracture.

Clinical Signs: The variation of clinical signs is striking. Some horses become 3-legged lame while others are only slightly sore and continue to perform. The position of the accessory carpal bone favors diagnosis by palpation, but crepitation on movement may not be present. If the animal is examined immediately after the accident, there is a greater chance to manipulate the bone; however, this soon becomes impossible due to extensive swelling. The carpal sheath may be distended and bulging between the digital extensors and ulnaris lateralis. There is sensitivity to sharp flexion or extension of the limb disproportionate to or exclusive of a supporting-leg lameness.

It is not uncommon for accessory carpal bone fracture to accompany other injuries. Quite often one of the ligaments of the accessory carpal bone is also ruptured. The intercarpal ligament is often ruptured in jumpers and steeplechase horses suffering this type of injury. Thickening of the tendons in the carpal

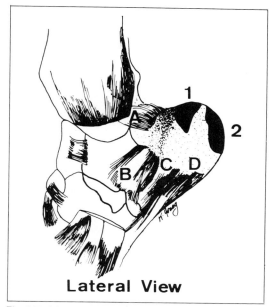

Lateral View

Fig 207. Ligamentous and tendinous attachments of the accessory carpal bone. 1. Attachment of the main tendon of the ulnaris lateralis. 2. Attachment of the flexor carpi ulnaris tendon. A. Accessorioulnar ligament. B. Accessoriocarpoulnar ligament. C. Accessorioquartal ligament. D. Accessoriometacarpal ligament.

canal and fibrosis of the caudal carpal annular ligament at the level of the fracture are common early adjuncts to accessory carpal bone fracture. Villous synovitis, with adhesions between the lateral digital extensor tendon and its sheath, has been reported.[8]

Diagnosis: Diagnosis is usually confirmed by radiography. Radiographs are not useful in identifying the stage of healing of the fracture. If the fracture has healed with a fibrous union, the fracture line is still easily discernible. Ulnar nerve block, while not dependable, may aid in the diagnosis of this type of fracture.[9]

Treatment: Treatment of accessory carpal bone fractures has progressed from conservative therapy or humane destruction to surgical repair by removal of the fracture fragments, bone grafts, or reduction and stabilization of the fracture by internal fixation.[5,6,10-14] Most surgeons prefer conservative treatment of accessory carpal bone fractures. The prognosis varies with conservative treatment. Some surgeons feel the fracture heals with a painless, fibrous union and that the animal can become sound after 12-18 months of rest. Others feel that while the bone heals by a fibrous union following rest, a bony callus never forms and the animal is likely to reinjure the bone with exercise. Still others contend that the prognosis is poor, with little chance of recovery following conservative therapy.

Bandages and splints should not be used to stabilize this type of fracture because increased tension on the muscles attaching to the proximal border of the bone may add to displacement of the fracture fragments.[15] Complete rest

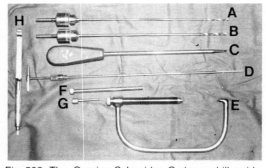

Fig 208. The Carnine-Schneider C-clamp drill guide and elongated instruments. A—Elongated 3.2-mm drill with 5-mm calibrations on shaft. B—Elongated 4.5-mm drill with 5-mm calibrations on shaft. C—Elongated hexagonal screwdriver. D—Elongated 4.5-mm cortical bone tap. E—C-clamp drill guide. F—4.5-mm drill guide sleeve. G—3.2-mm drill guide sleeve. H—ASIF screw hole-measuring device.

is required. The animal should be kept comfortable and bearing weight on the leg, thus keeping the leg fully extended and the fracture fragments in proper alignment.

Some authors feel the most effective treatment of the typical vertical, centrally placed fracture is removal of the separate palmar portion of the bone.[5,6] Interruption of the insertion of the flexor carpi ulnaris or removal of the palmar quarter of the accessory carpal bone produced signs of carpal hyperextension and arthrosis.[1] Therefore, it is not advisable to remove the palmar portion of the bone in repair of this type of fracture. Several old fractures have been successfully treated after the fracture site was packed with a corticocancellous bone graft.[12] Special care must be taken not to narrow the carpal canal with this bone graft.

Lameness associated with accessory carpal bone fractures that have healed following conservative therapy may be due to excessive pressure on structures within the carpal canal ("carpal canal syndrome").[4] A longitudinal strip of the volar carpal annular ligament can be removed to relieve this pressure. This procedure is performed with the animal in lateral recumbency and the affected leg down. After the leg is surgically prepared and draped, a 15-cm skin incision is made on the medial aspect of the leg from 3 cm proximal to 5 cm distal to the accessory carpal bone, parallel and caudal to the common digital vein. A longitudinal elliptical strip of the volar carpal ligament about 1 cm wide is removed from between the common digital vein and the lateral metacarpal vein. The length of the strip should be no longer than the zone of thickening. The subcutis and skin are closed in layers and the leg placed in a properly padded bandage.

The typical vertical fracture of the accessory carpal bone with little or no comminution heals best if repaired by internal fixation.[16] The basic principles of internal fixation rely on specific landmarks and precise placement of the implants. This is especially important in an area, such as the carpus, in which damage to structures medial or lateral to the fixation could lead to permanent disability. The following procedure allows for precise screw placement if meticulous attention is paid to details.

It is essential that fracture fragments be aligned with the limb in a hyperextended position and maintained there by an assistant. A tourniquet should not be used proximal to the carpus since it creates tension in the flexor muscles, which would tend to displace the caudal fragment proximad. The lateral aspect of the groove of the common digital extensor tendon at the distal radius lies in the same median plane as the dorsal articulations of the accessory carpal bone. The lateral aspect of this groove is the landmark for placement of the dorsal point of the equine C-clamp (Fig 208).[17] This landmark allows for accurate screw placement related to the articular area on the dorsal surface of the bone. The caudal fragment should be retracted as far laterad as possible while placing the screws to provide maximum space in the carpal canal when the fracture is stabilized. There is little chance of excessive retraction due to the strong attachment of the flexor retinaculum to the accessory carpal bone. Retraction may be aided by placement of a temporary K-wire in the caudal fragment to facilitate manipulation. The dorsal point of the C-clamp is left in the same position at the most distal aspect of the radius for placement of both screws. This allows the screws to be placed at an angle and not parallel, thus creating better mechanical stability of the fragments.

Technic: Following proper procedures for the preparation of the orthopedic patient, the animal is anesthetized and placed in lateral recumbency with the affected leg up. The leg is prepared and draped, leaving the entire carpus exposed. A 15- to 20-cm elongated, C-shaped skin incision is made on the lateral aspect of the carpus, starting just proximal and dorsal to the emergence of the dorsal branch of the ulnar nerve, gently curving dorsad and distal to the lateral digital extensor sheath at the proximal row of carpal bones. The incision then courses in a palmar direction to just distal to the carpus over the second metacarpal bone. The skin, subcutaneous fascia and dorsal branch of the ulnar nerve are reflected in a palmar direction to expose the lateral and palmar aspect of the accessory carpal bone. All skin and subcutaneous vessels are clamped or ligated.

The proximal and distal aspects of the accessory carpal bone should be identified at this time. A 2-cm longitudinal skin incision is made over the dorsal aspect of the radial carpal joint just lateral to the sheath of the extensor digitorum communis. The affected limb is supported in a hyperextended position by an assistant. A large C-clamp is applied across the accessory carpal bone and radial carpal joint (Fig 209). The cranial point of the clamp is inserted into the dorsal skin incision and held by the assistant just lateral to the sheath of the extensor digitorum communis at the level of

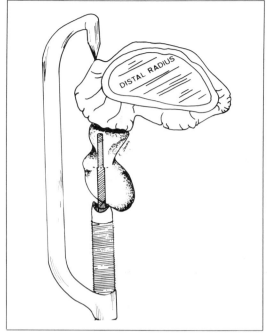

Fig 209. Proper placement of the C-clamp in the median plane. A 4.5-mm guide hole is drilled to the fracture line and a 3.2-mm hole is drilled to the dorsal cortex of the bone.

the radial carpal joint. This position is checked periodically by the surgeon, verifying that the point is in line with the prominent groove for the tendon on the distal aspect of the radius. The caudal point of the C-clamp is placed 5 mm distal to the most proximal aspect of the accessory carpal bone on its caudolateral border. The caudal set of the C-clamp is adjusted and rested on the lateral aspect of the fascial covering of the bone 5-10 mm dorsolateral to its most palmar aspect. The assistant secures the C-clamp in this position while applying traction on the caudomedial aspect of the bone.

The fascia is incised down to the bone under the caudal set of the C-clamp. A 4.5-mm drill with 5-mm calibrations on the shaft is inserted into the barrel of the C-clamp and a hole is drilled to the approximate predetermined depth of the fracture line (about 10 mm). A 3.2-mm calibrated drill is used to drill a hole to the approximate depth of the dorsal cortex of the accessory carpal bone (about 45-50 mm). The screw hole is tapped with an elongated 4.5-mm bone tap and the drillings are flushed from the area with sterile saline solution. A 4.5-mm cortical bone screw of the approximate length to reach the far cortex of the bone but not to pen-

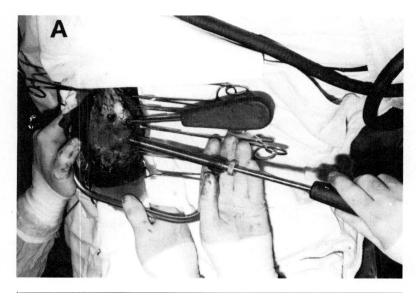

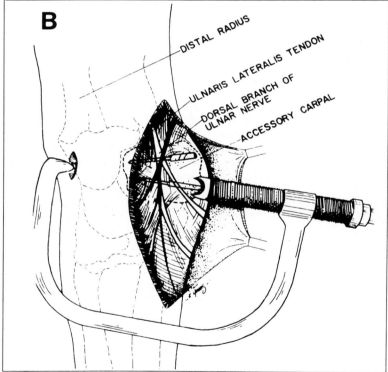

Fig 210. A. The C-clamp is in place and the distal screw is seated into the accessory carpal bone. The short screwdriver turns the proximal screw. B. Illustration of the C-clamp in place and the holes drilled in the accessory carpal bone.

etrate it when tightened (usually 36-46 mm) is placed in the hole and tightened firmly. The C-clamp is loosened and the caudal set swung distad. The assistant, while keeping the leg in full extension, steadies the C-clamp. The C-clamp is placed with the caudal set 5-10 mm proximal to the most distal aspect of the accessory carpal bone. (Because the bone is slightly thicker distad, the screw may be placed slightly more medial on the bone).

The holes are drilled, tapped and screws placed as described for the proximal fixation (Fig 210). When the screws are tightened, the heads disappear beneath the fascial covering of the bone. The procedure for screw placement is performed under radiographic control. The area is flushed with sterile saline to remove all bone debris. The skin flap is brought back over the incision and the subcutaneous fascia closed in a simple-continuous pattern using 00 synthetic absorbable suture material. The skin is closed in an interrupted pattern using 00 non-absorbable suture material. A sterile dressing of elastic gauze and elastic tape is placed over the carpus, with padding around the accessory carpal bone. The limb is then placed in a stacked compression bandage from the coronet to mid-radius.

Aftercare consists of stall confinement for 90-120 days, followed by 60-90 days of paddock rest. If the animal is not completely sound when returned to training, carpal canal syndrome should be suspected and dealt with surgically.

References

1. Manning, JP and St. Clair, LE. Proc 18th Ann Mtg Am Assoc Eq Pract, 1972. p 173.

2. Thrall, ED *et al*. JAVMA **158** (1970) 1366.

3. Wyburn, RS and Goulden BE. N Zeal Vet J **22** (1974) 133.

4. Mackay-Smith, MP *et al*. JAVMA **160** (1972) 993.

5. Roberts, JE. Proc 3rd Br Eq Vet Assoc Congress, 1964. p 18.

6. Roberts, JE. Vet Rec **76** (1964) 137.

7. Rooney, JR: Biomechanics of Lameness in Horses. RE Drieger, Huntington, NY, 1970.

8. Mason, TA. Eq Vet J **9** (1977) 186.

9. Wheat, JE. Univ Calif: Personal communication, 1978.

10. Share-Jones, JT: Surgical Anatomy of the Horse. WR Jenkins, New York, 1907.

11. Kirby, RO: Veterinary Medicine and Surgery in Diseases and Injuries of the Horse. Wood, New York, 1883.

12. Sornichsen, HV, Copenhagen, Denmark: Personal communication, 1978.

13. Schneider, JE, Kansas State Univ: Personal communication, 1979.

14. Von Salis, B, Usslingen, Switzerland: Personal communication, 1979.

15. Baker, RH, Chino, Calif: Personal communication, 1978.

16. Easley, KJ and Schneider, JE. JAVMA **178** (1981) 219.

17. Carnine, B. Master's thesis, Kansas State Univ, 1977.

THE UPPER FOREARM
by M. Leitch

The Shoulder Joint

Articular Fractures of the Scapula

Glenoid Fossa: Vertical fractures of the scapula, originating in the glenoid fossa, comprise the majority of scapular fractures. These may develop as single or multiple fissures that dissect proximad into the neck and body of the

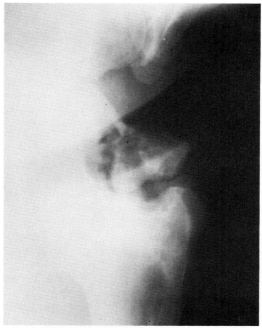

Fig 211. Chronic fracture of the tuber scapulae (supraglenoid tubercle), with associated degenerative joint disease.

scapula. Diagnosed most frequently in Throughbred race horses, they occur with or without direct trauma to the shoulder area. They have also been seen in young horses that collide with each other or obstacles while at pasture.

Depending upon the configuration of the fracture and the amount of comminution, degree of lameness and reluctance to use the limb may vary from moderate to total. The range of motion of the cranial phase of the stride is limited. Accompanying soft tissue swelling may also vary and crepitance is usually appreciable with comminuted fractures. Manipulation of the joint produces pain.

The prognosis is grave for future soundness in all cases; however, although there are no reports of such, the undisplaced singular fissure may heal adequately with stall rest to permit pasture soundness. There are no reports of attempts to stabilize these fractures and euthanasia is generally recommended.

Tuber Scapulae (Supraglenoid Tubercle): The cranial and distal aspect of the scapula, cranial to or including the cranial rim of the glenoid fossa, is not an unusual site of scapular fracture in young horses (Fig 211). The fracture often follows the course of the physis of the tuber scapulae/coracoid process, which does not fuse with the parent portion of the scapula until the horse is 10-12 months of age. The fracture usually results in cranial and rotational displacement of the fracture fragment and effectively detaches the origins of the biceps brachii tendon and coracobrachialis muscle from the scapula. Nonetheless, horses so injured retain the ability to extend the shoulder joint and, although they are lame at the walk and have an associated reduced cranial phase of the stride, they are not reluctant to bear weight on the limb while standing. Associated swelling is usually minimal, and the fracture may go undiagnosed initially because of the mild signs and rapid clinical improvement. Radiographic evaluation of the joint confirms the diagnosis.

If left untreated, these horses usually become pasture sound and may even be suitable for light work since the resulting fibrous union provides an attachment for the biceps tendon not anatomically far removed from the normal site.[1] However, the degenerative joint disease and mechanical obstruction to full extension of the limb that develop usually prohibit these individuals from becoming sound performance horses.

There are no reports of successful surgical repair; however, excision of the fracture fragment produces no articular instability.[1] Surgery should be limited to those individuals with recent fractures.[2]

Luxation

Luxation of the shoulder joint is rare and is usually associated with slipping and falling. The humeral head dislocates laterad and muscular contraction causes it to shift proximad to a level parallel with the glenoid fossa. Affected horses are reluctant to bear full weight on the limb but may use it as a prop.

On palpation of the region, the distal aspect of the scapular spine becomes indistinguishable and the head of the humerus is more prominent than usual. The degree of soft tissue swelling is variable.

While the prognosis for correction and subsequent soundness must be poor, successful closed reduction of the luxation has been possible in several cases diagnosed early. With the horse in dorsal recumbency and under general anesthesia, tension is exerted on the distal limb in line with the long axis of the limb until the humerus is reduced adequately to permit it to relocate. The weight of the horse provides adequate countertraction and the limb can be attached to a pulley to provide the force necessary for extension of the limb.

Recovery from anesthesia should be assisted with a sling, but it has not been necessary to maintain the individuals in a sling postoperatively. Stall rest is recommended for a minimum of 4 weeks, followed by a gradual return to activity. If luxation recurs, further efforts to reduce it have not been successful and euthanasia is recommended.

Osteochondrosis Dissecans

Osteochondrosis dissecans involving the humeral head was originally reported in 1965 and has since been described in several additional reports.[3-7] The condition usually occurs as a unilateral or bilateral lameness in horses under one year of age. The etiology remains controversial; however, the primary defect appears to be the disturbance of endochondral ossification, with thickening of the articular cartilage. Contributing influences may include genetic and nutritional factors.

The lameness has swinging and supporting phase components. Chronicity, prior to diagnosis, results in associated atrophy of the shoulder girdle and hoof. At rest, unilaterally affected individuals do not bear full weight on the limb and stand with the carpus in partial flexion. Passive manipulation of the leg is painful and accentuates lameness. Intra-articular anesthesia is diagnostic.

The radiographic appearance of the lesion is variable, ranging from apparent flattening of the humeral head to osteolytic lesions in the caudal third of the articular surface, often accompanied by a margin of underlying bony sclerosis. Periarticular osteophytes may be present in more severely advanced cases. Radiographic evaluation of both shoulder joints is recommended, even in those individuals with unilateral clinical manifestations, since the condition is usually bilateral.

The prognosis for working soundness is guarded to poor. There is only one report of successful surgical excision of the osteochondral defect and associated osteophytes.[5] The approach to the shoulder joint recommended by those authors is through a 35-cm skin incision extending from a point 15 cm proximal to the joint distad along the spine of the scapula and shaft of the humerus. The brachiocephalicus muscle is then reflected craniad and the dissection continued deeply to separate the deltoideus and infraspinatus muscles. The tendinous insertion of the infraspinatus muscle is then isolated, transected and reflected dorsad, leaving an adequate stump distad to permit reattachment. A 5-cm curved incision is made in the joint capsule.

Manipulation of the humerus permits examination of the majority of the caudal half of the humeral head. Excision of the osteochondral fragment, curettage of the underlying subchondral bone, beveling of the cartilaginous margins of the defect, and excision of the periarticular osteophytes with rongeurs may then be accomplished. Liberal lavage of the joint is followed by closure of the joint capsule with preplaced, simple-interrupted sutures of 0 monofilament nylon. The infraspinatus bursa over the lateral tuberosity of the humerus is removed by sharp dissection and the tendon of infraspinatus is reapposed using a Bunnell suture of #1 braided steel in conjunction with horizontal mattress sutures. The tendon is also sutured to the peritendinous fascia. The muscles and fascia of the shoulder are anatomically reapposed and sutured with simple-interrupted sutures of 0 chromic gut and the skin is closed with similar sutures of 0 nylon.

Recovery from anesthesia is assisted by use of a sling. Sling support is maintained for 3 weeks postoperatively. Stall rest is recommended for an additional 5 months, followed by pasture exercise. Twelve months after surgery, the colt described was training successfully, with no signs of lameness.

Necropsy reveals widely variable lesions of the humeral head, ranging from clinical asymptomatic dimpling of the articular cartilage to osteochondral defects of most of the joint surface. In chronic cases, dissolution of the fragment may occur, with subsequent eburnation of the underlying subchondral bone and opposing damage to the glenoid fossa.

Degenerative Joint Disease

Primary degenerative joint disease affecting the shoulder joint has not been reported and is an extremely rare necropsy finding despite the inordinately high frequency of "shoulder lameness" diagnoses. The single report of favorable response to intra-articular injection of corticosteroids in horses exhibiting signs compatible with a diagnosis of dysfunction of the suprascapular nerve ("sweeny") may reflect development of degenerative joint disease of the shoulder joint secondary to neurogenic muscular dysfunction.[8] Each horse in the cases reported had the classic signs of supraspinatus and infraspinatus muscle atrophy, accompanied by lateral subluxation of the shoulder joint, secondary to trauma to the region. Intra-

articular injection of corticosteroids (30 mg triamcinolone acetonide; 100 mg methylprednisolone acetate and 30 mg triamcinolone acetonide; 10 mg flumethasone; or 300-400 mg prednisolone acetate) resulted in the regression of lameness and muscle atrophy, and successful return to competition. This is the only available report of successful treatment of this condition, which is otherwise afforded a uniformly poor prognosis.

Neoplasia

Neoplasia of the shoulder joint is rare. A single report of disseminated malignant melanosarcoma described involvement of the head of the humerus, bicipital bursa, elbow joint, and nearly all abdominal viscera.[9] Chronic foreleg lameness, with associated shoulder girdle atrophy, was the primary presenting sign. The horse succumbed to the disease shortly after presentation.

Bicipital Bursitis

The bicipital or intertuberal bursa is a large synovial structure that underlies the tendon of biceps brachii as it passes over the intertuberal or bicipital groove. It extends around the edges of the tendon to partially envelop the superficial face of the tendon.[10] Its function is to facilitate movement of the biceps tendon during flexion and extension of the shoulder joint.

Inflammation of the bursa may develop from direct trauma to the area and the abnormal gait that accompanies navicular disease.[11] The associated lameness is variable, ranging from reluctance to bear full weight on the limb, with toe-dragging, to a mild decrease in the range of protraction. Tenderness on palpation of the region of the bursa is likewise variable; however, lameness is usually accentuated by flexion of the shoulder and extension of the elbow produced by pulling the leg caudad.

Intrabursal anesthesia is diagnostic. Radiographic evaluation is of little value; however, calcification of the bursa has been observed in chronic bursitis.

In acute primary bursitis, rest and intrabursal injection of corticosteroids can be effective. Systemic use of anti-inflammatory drugs, such as phenylbutazone, is also beneficial. The local use of counterirritants has not produced satisfactory results. Chronic bursitis is usually unresponsive to even repeated systemic and local treatment. Bursitis secondary to foot lameness, particularly navicular disease, seems to subside with successful treatment of the primary cause of lameness. Radiation therapy of the condition, previously popular in humans, may benefit chronically affected horses whose value warrants such expenditure.

There is a single report of neoplastic invasion of the bicipital bursa by metastatic malignant melanoma, which resulted in inflammatory changes in the bursa.[9]

Ossification of the Tendon of Biceps Brachii

A developmental anomaly resulting in heterotopic bone formation in the tendon of biceps brachii in a 4-year-old Quarter Horse resulted in bilateral foreleg lameness consisting of reluctance to extend the limbs and dragging the front feet.[12] Associated shoulder girdle atrophy was present, as was abnormal wearing of the toes. Intra-articular anesthesia of the shoulder joint reduced the degree of lameness and radiographs confirmed the presence of bilateral ossification of the bicipital tendons, with associated degenerative joint disease.

Necropsy revealed heterotopic bone formation in both bicipital tendons, with destruction or agenesis of the intermediate ridge of each bicipital groove. Marked atrophy of the biceps brachii muscles and associated degenerative joint disease of both shoulder joints were also present.

The Elbow Joint

Degenerative Joint Disease

Degenerative joint disease of the elbow is rare, although it has been observed accompanying an osseous cyst-like lesion of the proximal radius. The lesion communicated with the articular surface and with an osteochondrotic lesion of the humeral condyle. Frequently it is secondary to articular fractures or joint sepsis.

The accompanying lameness consists of a supporting and swinging component, with a decrease in the range of the cranial phase of the stride. Flexion of the elbow joint is painful and accentuates the lameness. Intra-articular anesthesia is diagnostic. Radiographic evaluation reveals periarticular osteophyte production and loss of joint space in chronic cases.

Prognosis for working soundness is poor. Rest may be the only effective therapy.

Septic Arthritis

Septic arthritis is not an infrequent sequela to traumatic wounds in the region of the elbow joint because the joint capsule is quite superficial as it inserts on both the cranial and caudal borders of the lateral collateral ligament.[10]

Vigorous treatment is indicated since the resultant lameness and disability may necessitate destruction of the animal.

While the details of an appropriate regimen for the treatment of septic arthritis are available in the literature, the basic principles include aspiration and lavage of the affected joint, culture and sensitivity of the aspirate to determine appropriate antibiotic therapy, intra-articular infusion of a broad-spectrum bactericidal antibiotic, and institution of systemic antibiotic therapy for at least 10 days.[13] Repeated aspiration and lavage of the joint may be necessary to control infection and inflammation before cartilage damage of an intolerable magnitude occurs.

The elbow joint is accessible via the joint capsule that inserts on the lateral collateral ligament. With the horse under general anesthesia, a needle or catheter (14-ga) is introduced into the joint cranial or caudal to the collateral ligament. The joint is lavaged with buffered polyionic electrolyte solutions and antibiotics are introduced. Access can also be achieved through a communicating wound if one is present.

The prognosis must be guarded. Failure to institute rapid, aggressive therapy can be fatal because of the debility that usually accompanies the progressive degenerative joint disease of septic arthritis. Two horses successfully returned to competition after such vigorous therapy.[14]

Luxation

Although rare in horses, luxation of the elbow joint occurs in several configurations: cranial displacement of the radius, with associated separation or fracture of the shaft of the ulna; caudal displacement of the radius and ulna as a unit; or medial displacement of the ulna and head of the radius, with fracture of the proximal radius. One has been successfully treated;[15] however, because disruption of the collateral ligaments is complete and stability is difficult, if not impossible, to restore, euthanasia is usually recommended.

References

1. Leitch, M. J Eq Med Surg 1 (1977) 234.
2. Leitch, M, Cochranville, PA: Unpublished data, 1979.
3. Schebitz, H. Proc 11th Ann Mtg Am Assoc Eq Pract, 1965. p 359.
4. Meagher, DM et al. Proc 19th Ann Mtg Am Assoc Eq Pract, 1973. p 247.
5. Schmidt, GR et al. VM/SAC 70 (1975) 542.

6. Rejno, S and Stromberg, B: Osteochondrosis in the Horse. Pathology, Sweden, 1976.

7. Mason, TA and MacLean, AA. Eq Vet J **9** (1977) 189.

8. Miller, RM and Dresher, LK. VM/SAC **72** (1977) 1077.

9. Grant, B and Lincoln, S. VM/SAC **67** (1972) 995.

10. Sisson, in Getty: Sisson and Grossman's The Anatomy of the Domestic Animals. 5th ed. WB Saunders, Philadelphia, 1975.

11. Adams, OR: Lameness in Horses. 3rd ed. Lea & Febiger, Philadelphia, 1974.

12. Meagher, DM *et al.* JAVMA **174** (1979) 282.

13. Leitch, M. JAVMA **175** (1979) 701.

14. Edwards, GB and Vaughan, LC. Vet Rec **103** (1978) 227.

DISEASES OF THE REAR LEGS
by R.D. Norrie

Fractures of the Pelvis

Pelvic fractures can occur at any age and usually result from falls. They have also occurred while a horse was galloping on a track.

Clinical Signs: Pelvic fractures cause acute lameness, the degree of which is determined by the location and severity of the fracture. In most cases there is marked lameness. Horses recumbent after fracturing the pelvis are often reluctant to rise. The horse may bear partial weight on the leg at rest if the fracture is not through the coxofemoral joint. Most affected horses are reluctant to advance the leg and have a very short stride. Crepitus and local swelling may be evident. Muscle atrophy may develop in the hip and croup area on the affected side as early as 2-3 weeks after the injury, causing an asymmetric conformation.

Diagnosis: Rectal examination often reveals bone displacement or crepitation. The hand is placed in the rectum and the horse is rocked from side to side or walked a few steps to reveal crepitation. In addition, hematoma formation results in a palpable enlargement at the fracture site.

Fracture of the wing of the ilium is probably the most common pelvic fracture and usually the most severe. This type of fracture is often comminuted, with marked displacement of fragments and a large pelvic hematoma. Fractures of the ilium may also include fractures through the acetabulum. Occasionally laceration of the iliac vessels by fracture fragments results in internal exsanguination.

Fractures of the ischium usually result in less severe lameness than fractures of the ilium or acetabulum. Local swelling is typically less obvious and rectal examination findings less dramatic.

Radiography of the pelvis requires general anesthesia, expensive equipment and trained personnel. Recovery from anesthesia may result in marked displacement of a relatively undisplaced fracture, which in turn can cause extensive internal hemorrhage. However, if the clinician is inclined to substantiate his diagnosis for prognostic evaluation, radiography is a necessary adjunct.

Treatment: Some fractures, such as comminuted fractures of the ilium and acetabulum, are severe enough to require euthanasia for humane reasons. Rest and supportive care, including analgesics, are all that can be offered for most affected horses. Use of a body sling, if tolerated by the horse, is often beneficial since it allows the horse to rest without having to lie down. Recovery takes several months.

Prognosis: Pelvic fractures heal with a bony union if there is no extensive fragment displacement; however, few affected horses return to complete working soundness. Fractures of the ischium offer the best prognosis for returning to soundness. Fractures through the acetabulum commonly result in coxofemoral arthropathy and a very poor prognosis for soundness. Development of a large hematoma or callus formation around displaced fracture fragments can sufficiently reduce the size of the pelvic canal in mares to jeopardize use of the animal as a broodmare.

Fracture of the Tuber Coxae

This condition, also referred to as a "knocked-down hip," is often caused by the horse rushing through a narrow door or gate opening and hitting one side.

Clinical Signs: When a portion of bone fractures off, the tuber coxae is usually displaced ventrad by tension of the internal abdominal oblique muscle. There may be lacerations and usually soft tissue swelling locally. Affected horses often bear weight, but are very reluctant to advance the leg (shortened cranial stride). When viewed from behind, the tuber coxae area is asymmetric.

Diagnosis: Palpation occasionally reveals crepitus. Rectal examination is rarely helpful diagnostically.

Treatment and Prognosis: Analgesics are often required for the first 2 weeks to keep the horse comfortable. Relative confinement for 3-4 months usually provides time for sufficient healing, and many horses return to working soundness. Surgical removal of necrotic sequestra has been necessary in some cases, but this should not alter a fair prognosis for return to soundness.

Coxofemoral Luxation

Coxofemoral luxations can occur at any age but are more common in foals. The usual cause is a fall.

Clinical Signs: Because the head of the femur typically luxates dorsad and slightly craniad, the leg appears shorter, with the foot and stifle turned laterad and the point of the hock turned mediad. Affected horses occasionally bear some weight on the leg but are generally very lame.

Diagnosis: The trochanter of the femur is usually more easily palpable than normal and in a different position from the unaffected side. Asymmetry may be evident.

A slipped capital femoral epiphysis in a foal causes many of the signs of coxofemoral luxation and radiography is often necessary to distinguish them.

Treatment and Prognosis: Surgical repair is difficult if not impossible. Even with extreme muscle relaxation under anesthesia, replacement of the femoral head into the acetabulum is difficult. Furthermore, luxation is often associated with fracture of the dorsal rim of the acetabulum, so reluxation is likely. Femoral head removal does not result in soundness. Definitive diagnosis is important if surgical repair of a slipped capital femoral epiphysis in a foal is to be considered.[1]

Sacroiliac Subluxation

This condition occurs infrequently and causes a rather obscure rear-leg lameness, characterized by a short stride in one or both rear legs. Digital palpation may reveal soreness in the loin and croup areas.

Diagnosis: When the flat of the hand is placed over the sacroiliac articulation and the horse is walked, movement is felt as the sides of the ilium move independently. This movement can often be seen as the horse walks.

Treatment and Prognosis: Treatment yields fair results and involves injection of counterirritants or sclerosing agents deep into this area. Healing reduces movement and often takes months.

Trochanteric Bursitis

Cause: The trochanteric bursa lies beneath the tendon of the middle gluteal muscle as it passes over the greater trochanter of the femur. Middle gluteal tendinitis is also occasionally involved. Trochanteric bursitis ("whorlbone lameness") occurs in horses racing on small tracks where turns are close together, horses racing on deep tracks, and horses that work off their hind limbs, *eg*, western reining horses. Horses shod or trimmed with very little heel behind seem quite prone to gluteal muscle soreness and associated trochanteric bursitis. Trochanteric bursitis can also occur secondary to lameness lower in the rear leg, most notably, hock soreness.

Diagnosis: Thumb or palm pressure applied directly over the trochanter of the femur produces a painful response. In a pure case of trochanteric bursitis, the horse carries the limb mediad and lands on the medial aspect of the foot. Characteristically, the horse "dog trots," moving the rear end away from the involved leg. The gait is altered accordingly if there is an associated myositis or bone spavin. In chronic cases there may be atrophy of the gluteal muscles.

Treatment and Prognosis: When trochanteric bursitis is associated with myositis or lower-leg lameness, those conditions must be treated before significant response can be expected. Injection of corticosteroids into the bursa or bursal area often gives relief in acute cases (Fig 212). In chronic cases, injection of counterirritants into the area effects a more rapid response. Topical counterirritants are not adequate treatment.

The prognosis for cases treated early is favorable. Those that develop muscle atrophy do not have a good prognosis for long-term soundness.

Coxitis

Arthropathy of the coxofemoral joint is not common and usually results from an old fracture through the acetabulum or rupture of the round ligament.

Clinical Signs: The condition is usually insidious in onset and generally seen in older horses. Because of its chronic nature, there is usually muscle atrophy over the affected hip. Characteristically the foot and stifle are turned laterad and the horse often stands with the leg slightly under and moved craniad. Affected horses move with a much shortened stride, moving the leg in the turned-out fashion just described. The rear end is carried away from the affected side, so the horse travels in a somewhat diagonal manner.

Diagnosis: Rectal examination is of little value other than to rule out pelvic fracture. Aspiration of more than 10 ml fluid upon arthrocentesis of the coxofemoral joint, using a 6- to 8-inch needle, is considered abnormal. Injection of local anesthetic into the joint often reduces lameness.

Radiographs of the coxofemoral joint may be diagnostic in severely affected animals and may be indicated for prognostic evaluation.

Treatment: Aspiration of the joint and intraarticular injection of corticosteroids often temporarily relieve much of the discomfort but rarely produce soundness. There is a poor prognosis for soundness.

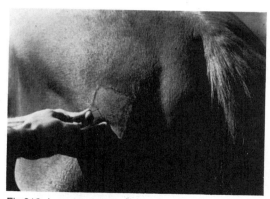

Fig 212. Location for injection of the trochanteric bursa.

Patellar Fixation

In this condition the medial patellar ligament becomes fixed proximal to the medial trochlea of the femur. The condition should not be referred to as "patellar luxation."

Cause: It is most common in horses with a straight-legged conformation behind (very little angle between the tibia and femur) or in horses with poor muscling through the stifle area. Patellar fixation also occurs as a result of stretching of the patellar ligament from injury to the leg. The same condition is also seen in horses abruptly taken out of training and confined to a stall. The apparent rapid loss of tone in the stifle muscles and ligaments allows for increased range of movement of the patella, with resultant fixation. A return to exercise immediately improves the situation.

The condition is often bilateral. Once patellar fixation occurs, the frequency and ease of fixation seem to increase.

Clinical Signs: The severity of this condition varies widely. In the most severe form the patella becomes fixed and the horse cannot flex the leg. Any attempt to move results in dragging the toe on the ground. In some cases the horse cannot relieve this situation and manual, forceful dislodgment of the patella is necessary before the horse can move normally. In a less severe form, the patella becomes fixed but spontaneously comes free only to "lock" again in a few steps. This occurs most frequently when the horse turns toward the affected leg. This form of patellar fixation has been confused with stringhalt because, as the horse begins to advance the leg, the patella pops free and the leg jerks craniad in rapid flexion.

The least obvious form of patellar fixation is momentary fixation of the patella, causing a slight hesitation in the gait. It also seems a horse begins anticipating the catching of the patella and thus avoids full extension of the limb, with consequent shortening of the stride. The horse also moves with a low foot arc, resulting in dragging of the toe.

Although this is a mechanical problem, severe or prolonged fixation can result in gonitis or arthropathy of the femoropatellar joint.

Diagnosis: The signs are characteristic and only in the subtle form does the diagnosis present difficulty. In the mild or subtle form, the diagnosis can be aided by manually forcing the patella (with the palm of the hand) proximad and laterad. This may cause the patella to become fixed; as the horse moves forward the patella pops free.

Treatment and Prognosis: Treatment varies with the severity of the fixation. Horses with a locked stifle and unable to flex the leg require a medial patellar desmotomy, which involves transection of the medial patellar ligament at its tibial attachment. The procedure is not difficult and, in tractable individuals, can be done in the standing position with a local anesthetic. Unless the condition is absolutely unilateral, the desmotomy should be performed bilaterally.

In the standing patient, the hair is clipped and the site aseptically prepared. Local anesthetic is injected SC over the tibial attachment of the middle patellar ligament, then mediad and deep to the medial patellar ligament. It is important to have the limb bearing weight during the entire procedure. A stab incision is made over the middle patellar ligament. Through this incision a slightly curved, blunt-ended bistoury is passed behind the medial patellar ligament. Thumb pressure is placed on the ligament and the bistoury is rotated la-

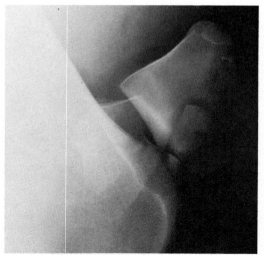

Fig 213. Relatively undisplaced fracture of the patella.

terad, cutting the ligament; often the stifle pops craniad when the ligament is cut. Several simple-interrupted sutures are placed in the skin incision.

The gait is slightly altered in some horses as a result of the desmotomy; therefore, 3-6 weeks should be allowed for accommodation to the functional loss of this ligament. Scar tissue forms between the cut ends of the ligament but seldom causes recurrence of the problem. The prognosis following surgery is good.

Horses with infrequent patellar fixation can also be treated by patellar desmotomy. However, an alternative, and perhaps more desirable, form of treatment involves the injection of a counterirritant into the middle and medial patellar ligaments. This causes some tightening of the ligaments and reduces the range of motion of the patella.

The injection procedure can be performed on most standing horses using mild sedation and a nose twitch. Commonly used counterirritants are iodine (eg, Hypodermin:Haver-Lockhart, McKay's Liniment:Spohn). Small amounts should be injected in about 6 sites along the length of the medial patellar ligament for a total of 6-15 ml, depending on the concentration of the product. About half this amount should also be injected directly into the middle patellar ligament.

Most horses are slightly stiff for the first few days and local swelling may be evident in some. The horses should be provided daily mild exercise so as not to lose all muscle tone. In most cases the response to treatment is good, although retreatment may be necessary in

some horses. A serious relapse may necessitate patellar desmotomy.

In unconditioned horses with mild patellar fixation, vast improvement occurs as the horse is conditioned (develops muscle tone) and often no treatment is necessary. Increased trotting, especially uphill or in deep sand, is beneficial.

In the same respect, immature horses often outgrow the condition as their muscles develop. However, if these animals are locking their stifles frequently, a desmotomy may be indicated to avoid injury to the joint.

Patellar Luxation

Lateral luxation of the patella is congenital. Affected foals are unable to extend the leg. Bilaterally affected foals move around in a semi-crouched position. Luxation occurs as a result of a shallow intertrochlear groove and hypoplasia of the lateral trochlea of the femur. There is no successful surgical treatment.[2]

Fracture of the Patella

Patellar fractures are caused by direct trauma to the area, usually a kick from another horse. Marked lameness, local swelling and increased synovial effusion are usually evident. There may be considerable displacement of fracture fragments (Fig 213).

Surgical implants may be used to repair this type of fracture in some cases.[3] If displacement of fragments is not too great and articular damage not too severe, the horse can achieve pasture soundness in several months. The prognosis for working soundness is very poor.

Osteochondritis Dissecans

Osteochondritis dissecans (OCD) lesions occur on both the trochlea and condyle of the femur, but the lesions are dissimilar. In the femoropatellar joint the lesion is almost exclusively on the lateral trochlea and takes the typical OCD form as an avascular portion of bone "dissected" free from the underlying bone. Although the exact etiology is not completely understood, it is believed to be a developmental abnormality often manifested after injury. The condition occurs primarily in yearlings and is rarely seen after 2 years of age.

Clinical Signs: The femoropatellar joint has pronounced synovial effusion. Lameness is present in varying degrees and is usually more severe in the initial stages.

Diagnosis: There is nothing specific about the lameness but OCD should be suspected in any lame yearling with acute distension of the femoropatellar joint. Radiographs are needed for definitive diagnosis; both stifles should be radiographed since the condition may occur bilaterally. A free fragment of bone, with a defect in the lateral trochlear ridge, is evident on radiographs. Occasionally the bone fragment(s) is at the bottom of the joint. In some cases a bone fragment is not visible but only an osseous defect in the trochlear ridge that is surrounded by dense subchondral bone (Fig 214).

Treatment and Prognosis: Over several weeks the fluid distension and lameness often subside. Soundness may return in several months, although few horses completely recover. Radiographically there is often evidence of healing, characterized by filling of the osseous defect.

Surgical removal of bone fragments has been performed. Although the benefit of this surgery for long-term working soundness remains to be fully evaluated, it does seem to be beneficial. Generally speaking, the prognosis for soundness is guarded but many do make substantial improvement.

In the femorotibial joint the OCD lesion is on the articular surface of the femoral condyle and almost exclusively the medial condyle. This is also a condition of yearlings and 2-year-olds, and is considered a developmental abnormality. Although the condition has been diagnosed in full siblings, heritability has yet to be proven.

There is no fluid distension of the joint and nothing abnormal about the appearance of the leg. The lameness is typically variable: one day the horse is very lame and the next is only mildly lame. Lameness is often best seen when circling with the affected leg on the outside of the circle.

Definitive diagnosis must be made radiographically. Radiographs reveal a well-circumscribed, circular lesion on the articular

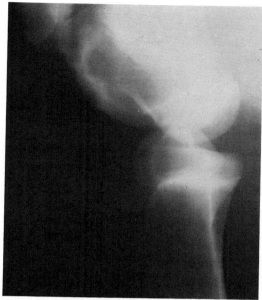

Fig 214. Osteochondritis dissecans of the stifle, characterized by osteolytic lesions of the lateral trochlea of the femur, with sclerosis of underlying subchondral bone.

surface of the condyle; there is no associated free fragment of bone. Both stifles should be radiographed since the condition can occur bilaterally (Fig 215).

There is no specific treatment. In some cases, improvement occurs over a few months, seen radiographically as a decrease in the size of the osseous lesion. The prognosis for return to working soundness is poor.

Gonitis

Gonitis, inflammation of the stifle, is often used as collective term for stifle lameness in which a specific etiologic diagnosis has not

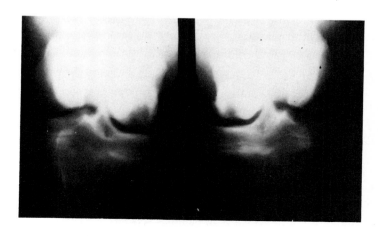

Fig 215. Bilateral osteochondritis dissecans of the stifle, characterized by osteolytic lesions of the medial condyle of the femur.

been made. The degree of lameness varies with the severity of the injury.

Diagnosis is made by careful observation, palpation and elimination of other causes of lameness. In many cases there may be no obvious joint effusion (palpable between the patellar ligaments); however, careful palpation and comparison with the opposite stifle may reveal thickening of the joint capsule or increased synovial effusion. Radiographs are often only diagnostic in cases of fracture or chronic osteoarthritis but are a valuable diagnostic aid. Intra-articular injection of local anesthetic is occasionally rewarding but a lack of response to the anesthetic should not distract from a diagnosis of stifle lameness.

Conditions that may cause gonitis include the following:

Chronic Patellar Fixation: Chronic patellar fixation produces mild lameness by inflammation in the femoropatellar joint; increased synovial effusion is not characteristic. The response to intra-articular injections of corticosteroids is usually good and in many cases should be included as part of the treatment for upward fixation of the patella. The most severe form of this condition, chondromalacia of the patella, responds poorly to treatment.

Cruciate Ligament Injury: The diagnosis is difficult to make unless there is complete rupture of the ligament(s). Ligament rupture may be associated with fracture of the crest of the tibia and can be visualized radiographically. If there is complete rupture, manipulation may reveal abnormal craniocaudal movement of the stifle joint. Even with prolonged rest the prognosis for soundness is poor.

Collateral Ligament Sprain: This is usually associated with trauma. Careful palpation and manipulation often elicit a painful response. Minor sprains may heal satisfactorily with rest. Healing of severe sprains may occur with rest but chronic instability of the joint often results in osteoarthritis and a poor prognosis for soundness.

Meniscal Injury: Meniscal injuries undoubtedly occur but are difficult to diagnose. These injuries quite likely lead to chronic osteoarthritis in the femorotibial joint.

Some cases of stifle lameness may be a combination of the previously mentioned conditions, especially with acute injuries. In cases in which radiographs reveal fracture fragments, caution should be used in advocating surgical removal of the fragments until the presence of additional stifle injuries has been ruled out.

Additional soft tissue injuries could jeopardize a favorable postsurgical prognosis; the more severe the lameness, the more likely are additional stifle injuries.

Cunean Bursitis

The cunean bursa is situated on the medial aspect of the hock between the intertarsal bones and the tendon of insertion of the tibialis anterior muscle (cunean tendon). Cunean bursitis is one of the most common forms of hock lameness and is often a precursor to spavin lameness. This condition occurs in nearly every type of horse. It may be more common in horses with abnormal rear-limb conformation but also occurs frequently in individuals with normal conformation. It is also quite common in young horses.

Clinical Signs: In many cases lameness can be quite subtle and may be manifested as the horse "not using its hocks." Those actually lame have signs similar to spavin lameness, although often not as pronounced. The cranial phase of the stride is shortened, with a toe-stabbing gait. The leg is usually carried mediad when advanced and lands more on the lateral aspect of the foot; therefore, the toe and lateral branch of the shoe show increased wear. The spavin test often elicits a positive response. The condition often occurs bilaterally and in such cases the horse has a short, choppy gait behind, often resulting in muscle soreness through the lower loin and croup area, as well as soreness in the trochanteric area. Soreness in these areas may complicate the appearance of the lameness. Unilaterally affected horses often prefer to rest the leg when standing. There may be a painful response to thumb pressure applied over the cunean bursa (rolling cunean tendon under the thumb).

Diagnosis: Radiographs are rarely of benefit since this is a soft tissue lesion, but occasionally there are early spavin lesions in the distal intertarsal joint. The diagnosis can be confirmed if the lameness improves after injection of local anesthetic into the cunean bursa. The cunean tendon is located by palpation, and a 22-ga needle is inserted on the lower edge of the tendon. When bone is encountered, the needle is backed out slightly and the anesthetic is injected. The anesthetic should flow easily when in the bursa, which distends above and below the tendon if 4-5 ml anesthetic are used. In acute cases there may be a small amount of fluid in the bursa, but this is unusual.[4]

Treatment: Treatment is by injection of long-acting corticosteroids into the bursa. In some cases a single injection is all that is required; in others the lameness recurs as the drug dissipates. Repeated injections may be necessary. The necessity of repeated injections or an increasingly poor response to bursal injections often indicates early joint involvement (tarsitis or spavin) (Fig 216).

Response to corticosteroid injection appears less effective if it immediately follows injection of local anesthetic into the bursa. It is better to wait a few days after local anesthetic injection to inject corticosteroids, or to treat without using a diagnostic anesthetic injection.

Cunean tenectomy is an alternative treatment for recurrent cunean bursitis. Surgery should not be performed until all effects of corticosteroid injection have worn off, since the presence of corticosteroids encourages wound dehiscence. Horses can usually return to training 3-4 weeks after cunean tenectomy. The response to tenectomy is usually good and the prognosis favorable.

Prolonged periods of rest are seldom beneficial or necessary unless the horse has become very sore through the back and hip areas. Use of nonsteroidal anti-inflammatory drugs during this rest period often hastens recovery.[5]

Cunean Tenectomy Technic: The cunean tendon is palpable as it obliquely crosses the medial aspect of the hock. After the hair is clipped and the site aseptically prepared, 4 ml local anesthetic are injected into the cunean bursa. The subcutaneous tissue is infiltrated with local anesthetic and a 3-cm vertical skin incision made over the tendon. Subcutaneous tissue is dissected to identify the upper and lower edges of the tendon. Forceps are passed under the tendon from the top edge and the tendon is transected at the distal end. The free end of the tendon is then rolled craniad and the tendon is transected more proximad. At least 2 cm of tendon should be removed. The skin is closed routinely with simple-interrupted sutures. Bandaging helps reduce postoperative swelling. Most horses always have a small bump of fibrous tissue at the tenectomy site.

Bone Spavin

This is a degenerative arthropathy of the distal intertarsal joint and occasionally also of the proximal intertarsal or tarsometatarsal joint. The lameness is usually insidious in onset and clinical signs are as described for cunean bursitis, except the toe-stabbing gait may be more

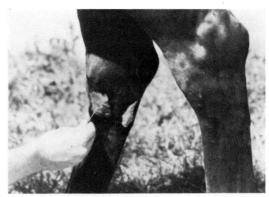

Fig 216. Location for injection of the cunean bursa.

prevalent. Initially the horse warms out of the lameness but the lameness is usually persistent as the condition progresses and may be exacerbated by use.

Diagnosis: Visual examination of the hock is usually not diagnostic. The bony enlargement of the medial hock typically described for spavin is seen in only very long-standing cases and usually represents the end stage of the disease.

The injection of 2-3 ml local anesthetic into the intertarsal joints is often of benefit diagnostically. Reduced lameness after anesthetic injection indicates that corticosteroid injection of these joints may be an effective treatment.

Radiographically the condition begins as irregularity and widening of the craniomedial aspect of the joint and progresses to complete collapse of the joint space. The lesions typically begin mediad and may progress across the entire joint space. Occasionally there are also bone production mediad and bone spurs on the articular edges. The severity of radiographic changes does not necessarily reflect the degree of lameness.[4]

There are several alternatives for treatment. Based upon response from local anesthetic injection, corticosteroid injection of the cunean bursa and intertarsal joints is often indicated and should be repeated if necessary.

Depending upon the degree of the intra-articular changes, some horses respond better than expected to cunean tenectomy. Corrective shoeing is often used in conjunction with other treatment procedures. The shoeing involves a short toe and slightly elevated heel to aid breakover. A lateral trailer on the shoe is occasionally used to assist breaking over the inside toe.

Surgical arthrodesis of the intertarsal joints has been performed to hasten fusion of these

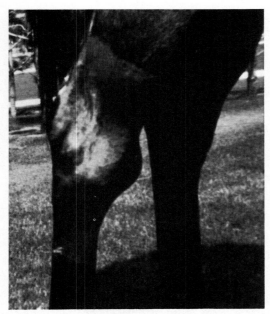

Fig 217. Fluid distension of the tibiotarsal joint capsule, commonly referred to as bog spavin.

joints.[6] The period required for osseous fusion of the joints is usually several months. Although arthrodesis may improve the degree of lameness, the prognosis for performance soundness is not favorable since some hock action is often lost.

Prolonged periods of rest help very lame horses but many such animals do not return to soundness. Horses that do not respond to other treatments often also do not recover with rest. Rest theoretically allows progression of the disease to the point of complete joint fusion, but this does not happen often. If at all possible, the horse should be worked through the active part of the joint disease with some of the treatment procedures described earlier.

Systemic use of nonsteroidal anti-inflammatory drugs is often beneficial for mildly affected horses and may be used in conjunction with other treatment procedures.

The prognosis for bone spavin varies with the individual but is guarded to fair.[5]

Fracture of the Distal Tibia

The fracture described here is a fragment from the distal dorsal (cranial) articular surface of the tibia, which rides between the trochleas of the tibial tarsal bone. Some clinicians feel this is not a true fracture but rather an example of osteochondritis dissecans in the hock joint. It is a condition commonly seen in horses under 2 years of age and can occur bilaterally.

The horse is usually examined because it has a very "boggy" hock rather than because of lameness, although many are slightly lame. Radiographs are needed to make the diagnosis. Usually a single bone fragment, not much displaced, is involved. The bone fragment(s) may be located at the bottom of the joint.

In older horses this lesion is occasionally an incidental finding in radiographs of the tibiotarsal joint taken for some other problem; there is no "bogginess" of the hocks in these older horses. For this reason there has been some question as to the significance of this lesion and whether surgical removal is justified. Synovial distension decreases after surgical treatment.[7]

Bog Spavin

This term refers to fluid distension of the tibiotarsal joint and is a poor term since it more describes a sign rather than a specific condition. Distension of the joint can be caused by different conditions, such as infection, articular fracture and joint injury, and for unexplained reasons in some young horses. In the last instance, affected horses are usually 2 years of age or less, often have a straight-legged conformation behind, and are fast-growing or heavy-bodied. The "boggy" hock occurs spontaneously and is usually bilateral in such horses (Fig 217).

Lameness may or may not be present and is determined by the nature of the underlying cause. Radiographs and aspiration of joint fluid for analysis are indicated to better define the condition.

"Boggy" hocks in young horses can be difficult to treat but are more of a cosmetic than a functional problem. Many improve as they mature. Affected horses should be given uncontrolled exercise and provided a maintenance ration only. Topical treatment has variable results but is generally unsuccessful. Aspiration of all fluid from the joint, followed by intra-articular corticosteroid injection and bandaging, is seldom rewarding and should not be performed without first obtaining radiographs.

Capped Hock

This is an acquired sacculation of bursal fluid in the bursae associated with the point of the hock. It often results from kicking stall walls or kicking in a trailer. The condition is strictly cosmetic and not a dysfunction. A mild case is characterized by a localized edematous swelling that usually subsides in a few days. In chronic cases there may be no fluid accumulation but just thickened, mushy tissue. Lateral luxation of the superficial flexor tendon from the tuber calcis should be ruled out in unilateral cases.

Any pockets of fluid must be removed to resolve the condition. Needle aspiration of the fluid, injection of a corticosteroid, and snug bandaging for 3 days often are satisfactory. If the condition is chronic, with a large fluid accumulation, or if the sacculation has been drained several times previously, the best treatment is to provide drainage through an incision in a dependent part of the sacculation. Swabbing the lining of the sacculation with strong iodine when the fluid is drained often prevents recurrence. Control of kicking is obviously necessary to prevent recurrence.

Curb

Curb is desmitis of the plantar ligament and appears as a firm swelling on the plantar aspect of the hock. In some horses the head of the lateral splint bone is very prominent and can give the appearance of the hock being "curby." Palpation of the area reveals this is not a true curb. Curb can occur traumatically, as from kicking a pipe fence. It is also caused by extraordinary stress on the ligament, as in abnormal conformation, such as sickle hocks. Mild lameness may be present initially.

Treatment is directed at reducing swelling and preventing recurrence. Systemic anti-inflammatory drugs and topical treatment should be used for the first several days to reduce swelling. Counterirritation (blistering or firing) 10-14 days after injury may be beneficial. In many cases the cosmetic appearance is never normal but the prognosis for returning to soundness in a few months is good.

Stringhalt

This condition is manifested as an involuntary hyperflexion of the rear leg as the limb is advanced. Hyperflexion can be quite mild or so severe that the fetlock nearly hits the abdominal wall. The true etiology in most cases has never been adequately explained. Lathyrism was the etiologic diagnosis in one case. The lateral digital extensor muscle or tendon is believed to be involved since tenectomy of the same cures many horses.

The horse may only show signs intermittently. The abnormal gait is most frequently seen when the horse is turning or backing, and appears entirely mechanical since there is no

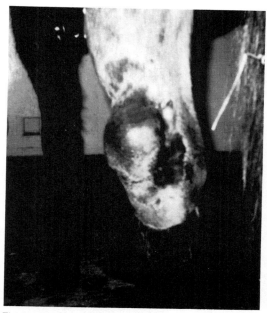

Fig 218. A large thoroughpin or fluid distension of the deep flexor tendon sheath at the point of the hock.

evidence of pain on movement. Horses with only mild involvement can often be ridden without problems.

The only treatment is lateral digital extensor tenectomy. Tenectomy is much preferred to tenotomy. Most horses show immediate improvement or complete recovery. The horse can be used again when healing of the incision is complete in 2-3 weeks. A few horses seem to take much longer to improve and some show no improvement at all.

Lateral Digital Extensor Tenectomy Technic: Tenectomy is performed where the tendon crosses the lateral aspect of the hock. In the standing horse, the site is aseptically prepared and local anesthetic is injected SC over the lateral digital extensor tendon. A second anesthetic injection is made proximal to the hock at the musculotendinous junction of the lateral digital extensor. A 3-cm incision is made through the skin and SC tissue at each site of anesthetic injection and the tendon is identified. In the distal incision forceps are passed under the entire tendon and the tendon is transected. Similarly, forceps are passed under the tendon through the proximal incision. The forceps are then grasped on either side of the tendon and pulled sharply dorsad to free the tendon from any attachments across the hock. The tendon is exteriorized and transected proximad at the dorsal end of the incision. Nonabsorbable skin

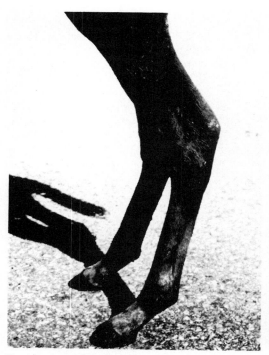

Fig 219. Increased angulation of the hock joints associated with collapse of the third tarsal bone.

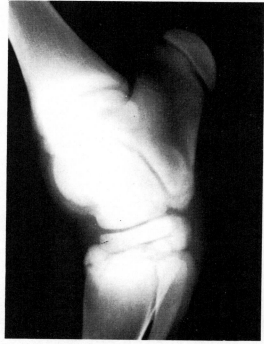

Fig 220. Collapse and fragmentation of the third tarsal bone.

sutures are used to close the incisions. Bandaging is not necessary.

Thoroughpin

Thoroughpin is a fluid distension of the deep flexor tendon sheath, evident just cranial to the point of the hock (Fig 218). The condition can appear quite suddenly and is more of a cosmetic problem than a functional one; there is rarely associated lameness. Radiographs may be indicated to rule out an underlying osseous lesion of the sustentaculum tail.

In chronic cases, surgical exploration has revealed clotted fibrinous material in the deep flexor tendon sheath. Removal of this material and liberal saline lavage of the sheath improved the condition. However, chronically affected horses often have a thickened synovial lining that is difficult to completely resolve. Drainage of the tendon sheath fluid, followed by injection of corticosteroid into the sheath, may provide temporary improvement, but the condition often recurs. Repeated injection of corticosteroids into the tendon sheath is not advisable since this can damage the tendon itself. Topical medication and bandaging are seldom effective treatment.

Tarsal Bone Necrosis and Collapse
by C.W. McIlwraith

Tarsal bone collapse causes a flexion deformity of the hock joint from collapse of the distal tarsal bones rather than from any problem in the tendons. It occurs in young foals and was initially described as aseptic necrosis of the third tarsal bone from infarction, followed by secondary collapse of the affected bone.[8] According to 2 other reports, the condition was observed in foals with hypothyroidism, and the central and third tarsal bones were affected.[9,10] The localized bone lesions were thought to be related to the hypothyroidism. The condition has also been observed in association with defective ossification and collapse of the carpal bones, suggesting that both conditions share some common developmental pathogenesis.

Clinical signs include swelling, pain and angulation of the hock (Fig 219). All signs are not necessarily present in affected foals. The earliest radiographic sign is decreased density of the third tarsal bone. The third tarsal bone becomes progressively compressed craniad on a lateral view. In more severe cases, fragmentation of the cranial aspect of the third tarsal bone occurs (Fig 220). Other secondary degenerative changes may also develop.

There is no treatment. Euthanasia is generally indicated in severe cases. Some affected foals have been turned out and become functionally sound; however, the prognosis should remain guarded in all cases.[8]

References

1. Turner, AS et al. JAVMA 175 (1979) 1198.
2. Rooney, JR et al. Cornell Vet 61 (1971) 849.
3. De Bowes, RM et al. Eq Pract 2 (5) (1980) 49.
4. Gabel, AA. JAVMA 175 (1979) 1079.
5. Gabel, AA. JAVMA 175 (1979) 1086.
6. Adams, OR. JAVMA 157 (1970) 1480.
7. Birkeland, R and Haakenstad, LH. JAVMA 152 (1968) 1526.
8. Morgan, JP. JAVMA 151 (1967) 1334.
9. Rooney, in Catcott: Equine Medicine and Surgery. 2nd ed. American Veterinary Publications, Santa Barbara, 1972.
10. Shaver, JR et al. J Eq Med Surg 3 (1979) 269.

DISEASES OF THE SPINE
by P.C. Wagner

Examination of the Spine

Clinical signs of equine spinal disease include lameness, neurologic abnormalities and altered performance or appearance. Neurologic signs may aid in localization of the lesion in the spine; however, many bone lesions result in only vague signs of discomfort or altered performance. Abnormalities of the equine vertebral column may be caused by trauma, infection, congenital defects, stenosis of the vertebral canal and aging. A thorough examination of the spine often reveals the location and helps establish the nature of the lesion.

History

History-taking should include questions regarding changes in attitude or behavior, traumatic incidents associated with the complaint, and pain or ataxia exhibited when the animal moves, lowers its head to eat, micturates or defecates.[1] Loss of performance or change in performance preference, and resentment of tightening of the girth or mounting by rider should be noted. Abnormal body movements, resentment to having legs lifted, shaking of the head or tail, or intermittent lameness may be complaints by owners of horses with back pain. Signs of ataxia, spasticity, paresis and loss of proprioception may be noticed with bony defects that impinge upon the spinal cord. Efforts should be made to determine the chronicity and progressiveness of the signs.

Physical Examination

The equine spine consists of 51-57 vertebrae. The vertebrae of each area of the spine have unique osseous structures but all have a body, processes and an arch. The horse has 7 cervical, 18 thoracic, 6 lumbar, 5 sacral and 15-21 coccygeal vertebrae.[2] Variations in the number of thoracic and lumbar vertebrae have been noted.[3]

Inspection of the horse's back as the animal stands squarely should reveal any asymmetry, lumps, swellings, scars, sores, or obvious muscle spasms. Palpation of the dorsal portion of the spine is possible from the thoracic vertebrae to the sacrum. Pressure applied over the candal thoracic region normally causes spinal dorsiflexion at the mid-back, while pressure over the sacral region causes ventriflexion. Pain is evidenced by grunting or moving away from the pressure. Areas of pain response or muscle spasm, as well as abnormal curvature, should be noted. A rectal examination should be performed; however, only gross lesions of the caudal spine are palpable rectally.

The horse should be moved at a walk, trot and canter in a straight path as well as in a circle. Gait disturbances, such as loss of hock action, toe-dragging, jerky movements, poor tracking with the rear legs and abnormal muscle spasms, may indicate chronic back pain. If a horse with a spinal column lesion is backed, pain may cause toe-dragging. Exercise should be continued to determine if the signs worsen or improve. When possible, the horse should be mounted to demonstrate any resentment to weight. Exercise that the owner feels causes signs of back pain should be performed.

Other Diagnostic Methods

Local Nerve Blocks: Blocking pain with local anesthesia has been used to confirm pain caused by overlapping spinous processes seen radiographically.[4] Injection of lidocaine has also been used to confirm the diagnosis of sacroiliac subluxation.

Radiographic Examination: Diagnostic radiographs of the cervical spine are possible under anesthesia, using a grid when the thickness of the neck is greater than 11 cm. Radiographic examination of the thoracic, lumbar and sacral spine has been described using a 200 kV/100

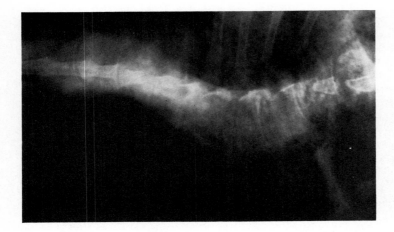

Fig 221. Scoliosis of the thoracic and lumbar spine in a foal.

mA-tube, an 8:1 cross-hatch grid, ultrahigh-speed screens and x-ray film of high speed.[4]

Congenital Lesions of the Spine

Congenital lesions are, by definition, present at birth and may be either hereditary or due to some event during gestation.

Scoliosis

The most common congenital condition of the spine is lateral deviation (Fig 221). The degree of deviation varies and foals with minor cases can adapt. Some minor deviations present at birth straighten with age.[4] Horses with severe scoliosis often have other deformities in the appendicular skeleton, such as contracted tendons.

The cause of scoliosis is not known and there is no treatment. Some time should be allowed for mild cases to correct spontaneously.

Lordosis

Lordosis, or ventral curvature of the spine, causes a dipped or sway-backed appearance (Fig 222). The condition does not appear to cause pain unless so severe that dorsal spines override. The ventral deviation of the back begins at about T_5-T_7.

The caudal articular facets of the first affected thoracic vertebrae, as well as the cranial and caudal facets of successive thoracic vertebrae, are hypoplastic. Hypoplasticity of the articulation allows overextension at the joint. The curvature is ventral due to the greater strength of the longissimus dorsi muscles compared to the abdominal muscles.[5] In at least one case the dam of an affected foal had produced other foals with lordosis.

There is no treatment for lordosis. The condition may not interfere with performance and some affected horses have raced quite successfully; however, some authors feel the curvature may predispose these animals to back trouble under heavy work.

Kyphosis

Congenital kyphosis, or roaching-up of the back, has not been described as an isolated entity; however, kyphoscoliosis (Fig 223) has been seen in a foal.[6] The deviation began in mid-thorax and included lateral deviation, rotation of the spine and kyphosis. Acquired kyphosis may occur secondary to chronic pain in one or more limbs, especially in the rear legs.

There is no treatment for the congenital form of this condition. Acquired kyphosis can subside if the cause of the pain is removed.

Occipitoatlantoaxial Malformations

Several malformations involving the skull and first 2 vertebrae have been described.[7-9]

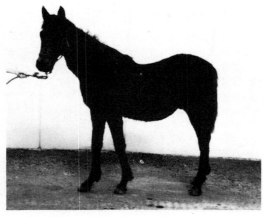

Fig 222. Lordosis in a young horse.

The most commonly reported syndrome is familial in the Arabian breed. The defects include occipitalization of the atlas, with atlantalization of the axis. The atlas is hypoplastic and fused to the occipital bones. The axis is also hypoplastic, with the dens blunted and the transverse processes widened to resemble the wings of the atlas. Asymmetric deformities of the skull and atlas are less common.

Affected foals may have tetraparesis at birth or progressive ataxia from a young age. A clicking sound from flexion of the unstable atlantoaxial joint is due to the dens moving ventral to the caudal edge of the atlas and back into position on extension. Luxation between the atlas and axis is common because normal movement at the atlantooccipital joint is impossible. Radiographically the atlas is incorporated into the occipital bones and the axis resembles an atlas.

There is no treatment. Because of the familial tendency of this trait, inbreeding should be avoided.

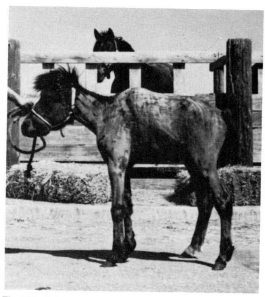

Fig 223. A foal with congenital kyphoscoliosis.

Spina Bifida

Spina bifida is a defect in or loss of the dorsal vertebral arches (Fig 224). The spinal cord may be normal (bifida occulta), the spinal membranes may protrude (meningocele), or the spinal cord itself may protrude (myelomeningocele). The spinal cord may be normal or cavitated (syringomyelia or hydromyelia). Large bony defects are usually associated with abnormalities of the cord and CNS disorders.[10,11]

Affected foals may have an abnormal gait and posture, especially hopping on rear legs and standing base-wide behind. Presenting signs, other than gait abnormalities, may include soft fluctuant masses over the vertebral arch cleft.[12] Radiographs reveal loss of bony arches and myelograms show extrusion of subarachnoid space.

Attempts at surgical correction in horses have not been reported; however, closure in human patients is frequently performed.

Hemivertebrae

This is a congenital defect of the spine in which one side of a vertebra more or less completely fails to develop (Fig 225). One affected foal had a sharply deviated neck at the level of the hemivertebra (C_5), an atonic esophagus and subsequent aspiration pneumonia.[13] Radiographs showed angulation of the spine at the affected area.

There is no treatment for this condition.

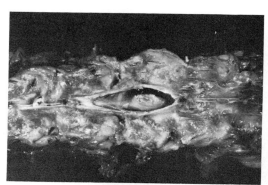

Fig 224. Spina bifida in a foal showing undeveloped lamina of the spinal column. (Courtesy of Veterinary Orthopedics)

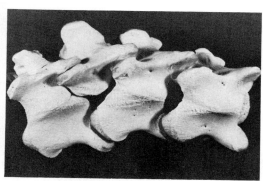

Fig 225. A hemivertebra at C_5.

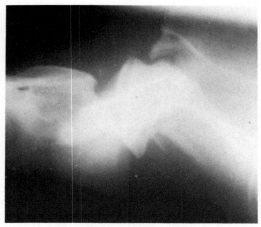

Fig 226. Fracture of the cranial epiphysis of C_2. (Courtesy of Dr L. Enos)

Traumatic Lesions of the Spine

Fractures

Vertebral fractures occur when the horse falls or collides with objects with considerable force. Foals are more susceptible to vertebral fractures than are adult horses, and the cervical vertebrae are more vulnerable to trauma than the rest of the column.[14,15]

Cervical Fractures: The most common cervical fractures occur at the dens and vertebral epiphyses. Ataxia, tetraparesis or tetraplegia may occur, depending on the degree of impingement of fracture fragments upon nervous tissue. Abnormal angulation of the neck and swelling of soft tissue often indicate the site of involvement, although crepitation is often not palpable.[3,16]

The dens is considered embryologically to be the body of C_1 and is attached to C_2 by one of the cranial epiphyses of C_2. When fractured, the dens is usually displaced dorsad and compresses the spinal cord (Fig 226). If death does

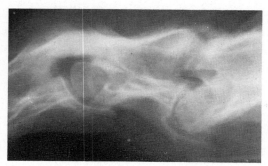

Fig 227. Epiphyseal fracture in the cervical vertebrae.

not occur immediately, incoordination of all 4 limbs, stumbling and falling usually become progressively worse over a short period. The diagnosis is confirmed by cervical radiographs.

The caudal epiphyses of the bodies of C_2-C_6 do not close until the horse is 4-5 years old. Therefore, trauma to the neck may result in fracture of the ventral portion of the epiphysis. The strong fibrocartilage disc carries the fracture fragment caudad (Fig 227). If the trauma is severe, the caudal dorsal facets fracture, the spinal canal angulates dramatically, and severe cord compression results. If the facets do not fracture, cord trauma may be limited to spinal shock.

Treatment of cervical fractures depends upon the amount of nervous tissue damage. An assessment period of 1-7 days may be necessary to determine if the cord trauma is reversible. In cases where dorsal facets have not been fractured and angulation is slight, some return to function may be expected even if the horse is tetraplegic at the incident.

Treatment with diuretics and anti-inflammatory agents to help reduce CNS edema should be initiated immediately. Glycerol given PO at 2 g/kg diluted in water reduces edema in as little as one hour. Treatment should be repeated at least 3 times a day. A 20% solution of mannitol at 3 g/kg has been used; however, this must be repeated 4-5 times a day. In addition to diuretics and anti-inflammatory agents, analgesics such as phenylbutazone at 6 mg/kg, and good nursing care are essential. Massive IV doses of glucocorticoids are effective in 2-12 hours, depending upon the form given.

If the fractures are unstable, manual reduction may be possible under anesthesia (Figs 228, 229). Surgical stabilization has been achieved with Steinmann pins.[17] In cases where spinal cord damage is not severe, stall rest and feeding and watering the horse from an elevated position may suffice. Stabilization has been attempted by fashioning of a neck brace that partially immobilizes the neck from C_2 to C_7. Torticollis and some degree of ataxia may be permanent sequelae to cervical fractures.

Thoracolumbar Fractures: Fracture of the dorsal spinous processes of the thoracic vertebrae occur most often when the horse falls over backwards.[4] The processes usually fracture between T_4 and T_{10}, with T_6 being the most frequently affected at the high point of the withers.[18] Such fractures occur most often in young animals in which the tips fracture and displace laterad in the soft tissue.

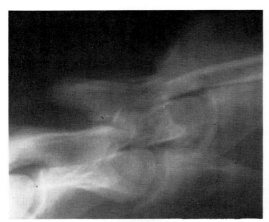

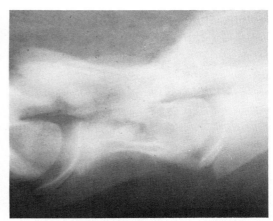

Fig 228. Fracture of the body of C_3. (Courtesy of Dr L. Pickering)

Fig 229. Fracture in Figure 228 after reduction with tension.

Clinical signs include heat, pain and swelling in the affected area, with no signs of neurologic involvement. If neurologic signs are seen, an interbody thoracic fracture should be suspected.[19] Diagnosis may be confirmed by lateral radiographs of the thoracic dorsal spinous processes (Fig 230). The epiphyses of the spines are still readily apparent in mature horses and must not be mistaken for fractures.

Treatment is usually limited to stall rest because most spinous fractures resolve uneventfully. A persistent swelling over the fractures may require use of a special saddle for riding.

Removal of the fracture fragments may be necessary if infection and osteomyelitis develop at the fracture sites. The horse is placed under general anesthesia in lateral recumbency and the dorsal midline is clipped and prepared for sterile surgery. The skin incision is made on dorsal midline and continued through the subcutaneous tissue and the funicular portion of the ligamentum nuchae that inserts on the summits of the spinous processes. The ligamentum nuchae is divided longitudinally to remove the fragments and should not be severed transversely so as to avoid interruption of the attachment to the lumbosacral part of the supraspinous ligament. Loss of this attachment could result in inability to completely extend the neck and elevate the head.

All pieces of necrotic bone are removed. Incisions lateral and ventral to the midline incision are made to allow adequate ventral drainage. Penrose drains are placed in the ventral incisions for several days to ensure good drainage. The wound may be left open to heal by second intention. Care should be taken not

to extend incisions behind the blade of the scapula because drainage may cause cellulitis and infection between the scapula and body wall. Healing of this wound may be prolonged. Daily cleaning and treatment with antibiotic ointment should be continued until the wound granulates completely.

Fractures of the transverse and dorsal spinous processes of the lumbar vertebrae usually heal uneventfully.[20]

Fractures of the body of the thoracic and lumbar vertebrae most commonly occur at T_1-T_3, T_{11}-T_{13} and L_1-L_3.[18] The most frequently reported cause is somersaulting over a high jump. Such injuries occur more commonly in females. A displaced fracture may sever the cord or the cord may be functionally transected by hemorrhage and edema. Very rapid onset of paraplegia of the rear legs, with inability to rise without assistance but with withdrawal reflexes in the rear legs and good anal tone, suggests fracture displacement. Onset of neu-

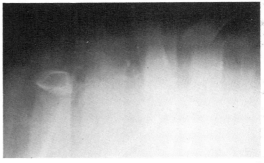

Fig 230. Fracture of the dorsal spinous processes of T_6-T_{11}.

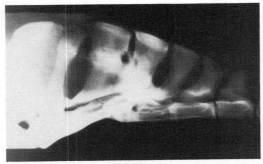

Fig 231. Fracture with displacement of the sacrum. Callus formation caused pressure on the cauda equina. (Courtesy of J Eq Med Surg)

rologic signs after a short delay or paraplegia after the horse lies down also suggests fracture followed by displacement. Pain due to periosteal tearing, and ataxia without paraplegia may indicate an undisplaced fracture. Clinical signs usually indicate the diagnosis. Radiographs of the spine in affected young horses may confirm this. Rectal examination may disclose a ventral enlargement in the iliopsoas area caused by trauma to those muscles.

If paraplegia occurs immediately, the prognosis is usually unfavorable; however, 24 hours of treatment with anti-inflammatory agents, diuretics and analgesics are appropriate to determine what, if any, improvement might occur. Pain can be controlled but decubitus formation, urine and fecal retention, and pulmonary edema must be considered in caring for paraplegic horses over long periods. If no improvement has occurred after several days of care, the prognosis is very unfavorable. If the horse is only ataxic or paretic, movement of the spine should be minimized by placing the horse

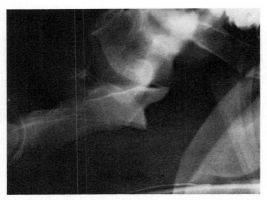

Fig 232. Atlantoaxial luxation. Tearing of the dorsal ligament allows the dens to slip ventral to the atlas.

in a sling or cross-tying to prevent the horse from lying down and displacing the fracture. Healing time is 2-3 months.[4,21]

Sacral Fractures: These fractures usually occur when the animal goes down behind suddenly, as in backing out of vans or going over backwards in a starting gate.[21,22] Clinical signs vary, depending on the level of the fracture and the amount of impingement on the cord or cauda equina (Fig 231). Relaxation of the anal and bladder sphincters, loss of the motor control of the tail, loss of sensation in the perianal region and atrophy of the gluteal muscles may occur. Gait disturbances may occur in more cranial fractures. The defect can be palpated rectally in some cases of severe displacement. Electromyography of the involved muscles may help to locate the level of the lesion.

Sacral fractures may be confused with neuritis of the cauda equina and sorghum poisoning.

Treatment with systemic anti-inflammatory agents may result in some improvement. Fecal material must be manually evacuated several times daily if the anus is flaccid. The legs should be protected from urine scalding if bladder sphincter control is lost. If neurologic signs persist for more than several weeks, the prognosis for recovery becomes less favorable.

Luxations

Atlantoaxial Luxation: Atlantoaxial luxation occurs when the dens moves cranioventral to the body of the atlas.[23] This occurs rarely because in most cases the dens or atlas fractures first, resulting in atlantoaxial subluxation. The dens articulates within the atlas and its ligament is very strong. Atlantoaxial luxation has been reported in a foal and was thought to be the result of 2 traumatic incidents; the first weakened the ligament without dens fracture and the second allowed luxation. Atlantoaxial luxation causes immediate prostration and possible respiratory failure. Diagnosis may be confirmed by radiographs (Fig 232). Treatment has not been reported.

Atlantoaxial Subluxation: Atlantoaxial subluxation occurs in fracture of the cranial epiphysis of the axis. The dens remains in normal position or is elevated from the floor of the atlas and the axis moves ventrad, causing cord compression.[17,24] Clinical signs include pain, crepitation, ataxia, and recumbency. Surgical stabilization with Steinmann pins was successful in one case.[17] In a second case, extensive hemilaminectomy of C_1 and durotomy provided good results.[24]

Sacroiliac Subluxation: The diarthrodial joint between the sacrum and the wings of the ilium is roughened and crossed by many fibrous bands as well as the ventral sacroiliac ligament.[25] The sacroiliac ligament is very strong and provides stability and immobility to the joint. The dorsal sacroiliac ligament between the tuber sacrale and the dorsal spines on the sacral vertebrae also helps stabilize this area by immobilizing the joint. Damage of these ligaments may cause subluxation and pain until healing occurs by fibrosis. Subluxation occurs when the animal falls, slips or twists in unusual movements. The fibers of the cranial portion of the sacroiliac ligament stretch and the ilium moves craniodorsad. Therefore, the tuber sacrale is higher on the affected side if the condition is unilateral. If the condition is bilateral the tuber sacrale is visible on both sides (Fig 233).

Signs of subluxation include prominence of the tuber sacrale, chronic pain, stiffness and shortening of the stride in the rear legs, unilateral or bilateral rear leg lameness, and rolling motions of the hip.[26,27] Pain may be elicited if movement is induced by pressure on the tuber coxae or the sacroiliac joint. Affected horses may be reluctant to jump.

Rectal examination is usually not rewarding but should be attempted. Crepitation may be present; however, muscle spasms may stabilize the articulation making movement difficult to feel. Rectal examination should be performed with the horse in motion so that the examiner may feel movement and crepitation. The tubera sacrale may move relative to each other if one side is affected and the other is not. Prominence of the tuber sacrale in an asymptomatic horse may indicate an old sacroiliac subluxation. Scar tissue that has filled the area is not as strong as the ligament it replaces and damage may recur.

Stall rest for at least one month is recommended to allow healing of the sacroiliac ligament. If joint damage is severe, fusion takes up to 6 months. Injection of sclerosing agents into the damaged ligament may speed scar formation and soundness. This area is difficult to reach with a needle and attention to asepsis and anatomic accuracy in deposition is important.

Overriding and Crowding of the Dorsal Spinous Processes: Impingement of the dorsal spines of the thoracic vertebrae usually occurs

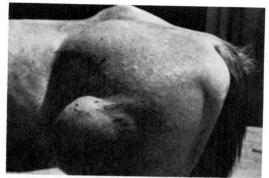

Fig 233. The characteristic "hunter's bumps" of a bilateral sacroiliac subluxation.

in the area under the saddle, at T_{12}-T_{17}. The cause of the pain is not well understood but apparently occurs when jumping or extreme exertion causes periosteal damage as the processes override. A secondary pseudoarthrosis or bursitis may result.

Affected horses usually have a history of chronic back pain. The condition is most common in heavy Thoroughbreds used for jumping or dressage.[1,4] Although the onset of severe signs may be associated with a fall, careful history-taking may elicit reports of an insidious onset. The owners may recall decreased performance, change in attitude toward exercise and a reluctance to lie down that preceded the onset of overt signs. Back pain is not always evident on palpation; however, loss of back flexibility is seen. Alternate pressure on the caudal thoracic and cranial coccygeal vertebrae causes dorsoflexion and ventroflexion in a normal horse, but little movement in a horse with overriding spines. In long-standing cases the muscles of the back may have some atrophy. Clinical findings may be substantiated with radiographs of T_{12}-T_{17} (Fig 234). Sensitive points between spines, with evidence of periosteal response or

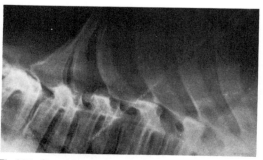

Fig 234. Overriding dorsal spines in the thoracic region.

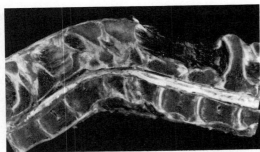

Fig 235. Vertebral osteomyelitis is usually extradural. Neurologic signs are referable to vertebral collapse.

pseudoarthrosis formation, substantiate a clinical diagnosis of overriding. Overriding occurs in some horses without clinical signs.

Injection of lidocaine into the affected area further confirms the diagnosis.[1,4] Using an 18-ga needle, 5-10 ml 2% lidocaine are injected between affected spines. The horse is tested for increased performance after 5-10 minutes.

Injection of corticosteroids into the affected area has been suggested as a palliative measure. Surgical removal of the summit of the affected spinous processes results in clinical improvement if the condition has responded to local nerve blocks.

The horse is placed in lateral recumbency under general anesthesia and the area over the affected spines is clipped, shaved and prepared for aseptic surgery. A longitudinal paramedian incision is made and the supraspinous ligament is identified and dissected away from the spinous process. The supraspinous ligament should not be transected. Enough of the process is removed to relieve pressure on the adjacent spine. If 3 spines are involved, removal of only one may be required. A bone saw, rongeurs or wire may be used to remove the process.

Stall rest is necessary for 2 months after surgery. Improvement may not be evident at the end of that time but should be seen after several months of riding.

Spinal Ankylosis: The significance of spinal ankylosis, especially in the lumbar area, has been questioned.[28,29] The condition was observed in 50% of race horses necropsied in one study; however, it has never been seen in the spine of wild equidae. The pathogenesis is thought to be fusion secondary to inflammation and excessive movement caused by the weight of a rider. It has been reported in horses as young as 3 years of age.

There is no correlation between clinical signs and pathologic findings. Some horses may suffer from low-grade, chronic back pain for most of their working lives until ankylosis is complete. Pain should subside once fusion occurs.

Diagnosis of low-grade pain in the lumbar area may sometimes be made by rectal examination. Upward pressure on the sublumbar muscles in the area of L_3-L_6 may elicit pain. Spinal dorsiflexion and ventriflexion elicited by pressure over the caudal thoracic and sacral spines, respectively, may cause the horse to "grunt."

Use of anti-inflammatory agents and analgesics may allow affected horses to perform. Movement in the area may actually hasten fusion of the lumbar spine. Return to soundness may be anticipated once fusion is complete.

Infectious Lesions of the Spine

Vertebral Osteomyelitis

Vertebral osteomyelitis is relatively rare in horses. This type of lesion is most common in young animals. Some affected animals have a history of an affected limb joint.

Intervertebral and costovertebral joint infection, with collapse of adjacent bone, leads to cord compression and neurologic deficits (Fig 235). The dura is rarely invaded; pressure from epidural abscesses or vertebral collapse causes the neurologic signs. Organisms cultured include *Corynebacterium*, *Actinobacillus*, *Brucella* and *Mycobacterium tuberculosis* var *bovis*.[30-34] In one case, failure of passive transfer of colostral antibodies preceded the appearance of vertebral osteomyelitis.[34]

Gait abnormality and stiffness of the neck or back may be common features of vertebral osteomyelitis. Pyrexia, dullness and inappetence are inconsistent findings. A mild to moderate leukocytosis, with a left shift, and increased total plasma protein levels are typical laboratory findings. The cell count, protein level and examination for bacteria in the CSF are normal if the infection is extradural. If the dura is invaded, meningitis and encephalitis occur and signs are progressive. Confirmation of a suspected case of osteomyelitis is by radiographic examination of the area. Most reported cases have been in the cervical vertebrae. The reason for this is unknown but accessibility of this area to trauma from blows, kicks and injections must be considered.

If aspiration of the abscess is possible, identification of the organism may be achieved and treatment with the appropriate antibiotic initiated. Surgical drainage of interbody cervical abscesses has been suggested but not described. The approach and establishment of ventral drainage of osteomyelitis in the bodies of C_2-C_6 would be possible using the surgical approach for ventral cervical spine fusion.[35,36]

Stenotic Lesions of the Spine

Cervical Vertebral Malformation

Cervical vertebral malformations or variations from normal occur in up to 10% of the Thoroughbred population.[37] Malformations usually go unnoticed until they result in spinal cord compression and associated symmetric ataxia, paresis, spasticity and dysmetria, commonly referred to as "wobbles" (Fig 236).

The signs of focal cervical cord compression usually are noted in young, rapidly growing animals. Thoroughbreds are most commonly affected and the age of onset of signs is 6-18 months. Affected animals are usually well-fed or over-fed. Affected males outnumber females 3:1. In many cases the owner recalls a traumatic incident associated with the onset of signs, which may be acute or insidious. The rear legs are often affected more severely than the forelegs. Cerebral spinal fluid from cisterna magna and lumbosacral aspirations is normal.[21,36-43]

Radiographs of the neck in extension and flexion may reveal the compressive lesion. In some cases the area of cord compression is readily apparent on survey radiographs (Fig 237). If the stenotic area is questionable, the area of focal cord compression can be localized by myelography.

Myelography is performed under general anesthesia. Prior to anesthesia, the horse is given 20 mg dexamethasone and 4 g phenylbutazone to reduce meningeal inflammation. Under general anesthesia, the atlantooccipital area is clipped and surgically prepared. An 18-ga, 3-inch spinal needle with a stylet is inserted through the skin, ligamentum nuchae and interarcuate ligament into the subarachnoid space of the cisterna magna with the bevel directed caudad. The head is then elevated 6-8 inches using an incline and 20-30 ml CSF are removed with a syringe. Cytologic analysis of the CSF is performed to rule out meningitis. Over 2-4 minutes, 3-6 g of the contrast medium, metrizamide (Amipaque: Winthrop), are injected. The needle is removed and the head is lowered for radiographs with the neck flexed

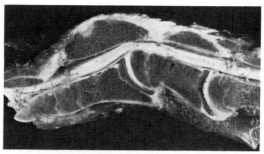

Fig 236. Spinal cord compression at C_2-C_3.

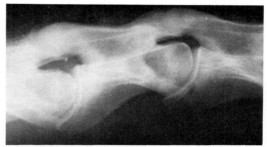

Fig 237. Dynamic lesion at C_3-C_4, with narrowing of the canal upon flexion of the neck.

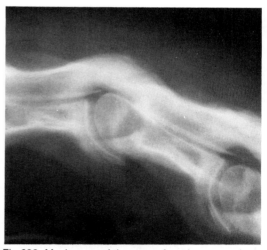

Fig 238. Myelogram of the area of cord compression.

and extended. The head is elevated for recovery. Elevation of the head during injection and recovery discourages reflux of the contrast medium into the lateral ventricles of the brain.

Subluxation, vertebral instability and spondylolisthesis are seen most commonly at C_3-C_4 and clinical signs occur at 6-18 months of age. The cranial end of C_4 moves dorsad during flexion to narrow the cervical cord canal. A positive myelogram reveals a 50% or greater

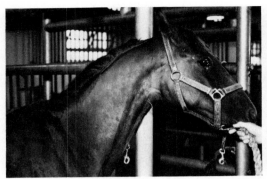

Fig 239. Angulation of the neck from a lesion at C_2-C_3.

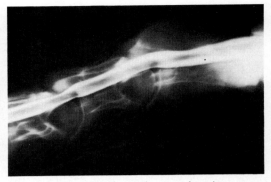

Fig 240. Myelogram of a static area of cord compression. Dorsal decompression, rather than ventral stabilization, may be helpful in such cases.

narrowing of both the ventral and dorsal dye columns on flexion (Fig 238).[21] The compression is alleviated when the neck is extended.

Subluxation at C_2-C_3 has been seen. The horse has a characteristic angulation to the neck (Fig 239) and under anesthesia the subluxation cannot be reduced. This malformation appears to be congenital.

If the cord compression occurs only when the neck is flexed, surgical stabilization of this ar-

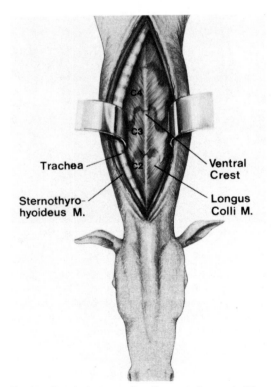

Fig 241. Surgical approach to the ventral aspect of the cervical spine.

ticulation in the extended position prevents further damage and results in clinical improvement in 90% of operated horses.[35]

Intravertebral stenosis with focal cord compression may occur as a static lesion when the cranial or caudal orifice of the vertebral canal is narrowed. The orifice is considered narrow when the measurement is less than 16 mm.[21] Because of the variability of the absolute size of the canal diameter due to age and breed, myelography is helpful to determine the presence of cord compression (Fig 240). When the canal is narrowed by intravertebral stenosis, very minor misalignment may cause cord compression. Myelograms with the neck extended and flexed allow evaluation of the degree of static versus dynamic lesion. If cord compression is apparent in the extended and flexed positions, subtotal dorsal laminectomy should be considered.

Medical treatment of cervical cord compression is aimed at decreasing inflammation and preventing further pressure on the cord. Dexamethasone and phenylbutazone have been used to alleviate clinical signs but recurrence of ataxia often occurs when therapy is discontinued. Recent trials in human spinal trauma therapy have prompted veterinarians to try DMSO IV at 100 ml/1000 lb once daily to decrease edema; however, this treatment should be considered experimental.

Surgical treatment for dynamic cervical instability in horses, using the Cloward technic of cranial cervical fusion, has been reported.[35,36,44] The ventral surface of the neck is clipped and prepared for surgery and the horse is placed in dorsal recumbency with the neck in extension over a brace to open the vertebral canal as widely as possible. Needles are placed in the

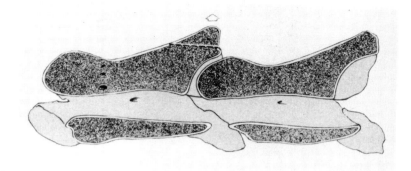

Fig 242. The ventral crest is removed.

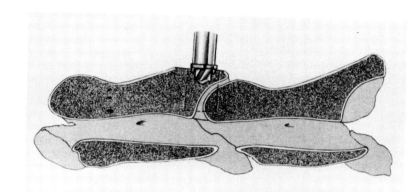

Fig 243. The guide hole is drilled with a 16-mm twist drill.

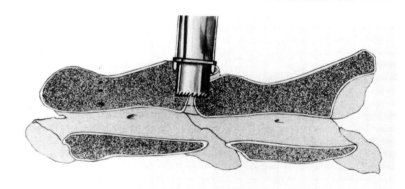

Fig 244. A core saw is used to enlarge the hole.

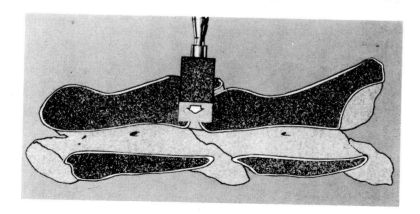

Fig 245. A bone dowel from a cadaver ilium is used to stabilize the vertebrae.

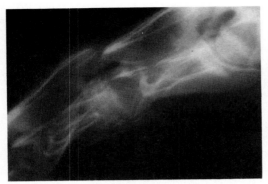

Fig 246. The operative site on the horse described in Figure 240, 3 months after surgery. The disc space has been obliterated.

skin and a lateral radiograph made to locate the articulation to be fused. After surgical preparation and draping, a 30-cm skin incision is made on the ventral midline beginning 20 cm caudal to the wing of the atlas. The incision is continued between the sternothyrohyoideus muscles, which are then retracted. The deep cervical fascia between the trachea and the carotid sheath is divided longitudinally using blunt dissection. The trachea is retracted to the left and the right carotid sheath is retracted to the right to allow palpation of the ventral crest through the longus colli muscles (Fig 241).

The longus colli muscles are retracted following separation from the bone using a periosteal elevator. The ventral crest is exposed

and removed with rongeurs to prepare a level bed for the drill guide (Fig 242). The 16-mm drill guide is placed over the area of the disc space and, using a 16-mm Cloward twist drill on a Hudson cranial drill brace, a guide hole is drilled (Fig 243). Measurements made from the radiographs give an estimate of the depth of the hole to be drilled. Drilling is stopped when the depth of the hole is ¾ to ⅞ the depth of the vertebral body. Disc material, recognized by its white fibrous appearance, is removed.

Using a 25-mm core saw, the hole over the disc is enlarged and all debris removed (Fig 244). The bone dowels for fusion are obtained from equine cadaver ilia and are preserved in antibiotic solutions at −70 C until used. After the hole is complete, a bone dowel is anchored on the dowel driver and driven into the hole with a mallet (Fig 245). The dowel is countersunk with a tamper.

After routine closure of the muscles, subcutaneous tissue and skin, the horse is allowed to recover from anesthesia and a postopertive radiograph is taken. A protective bandage is applied to the neck and left in place for 5-7 days. Antibiotics are given; no analgesics are required. The horse is fed and watered from elevated containers to discourage flexion of neck.

Follow-up radiographs are taken 6-8 weeks postoperatively to evaluate fusion (Fig 246). Improvement in clinical signs occurs as early as 3 months postoperatively and may continue for a year.

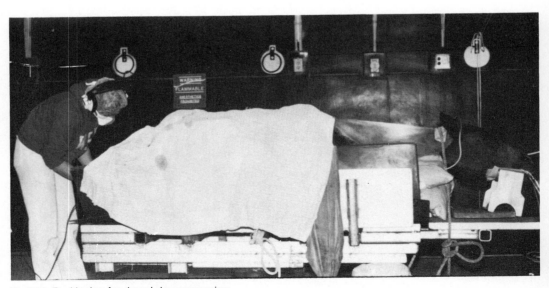

Fig 247. Positioning for dorsal decompression.

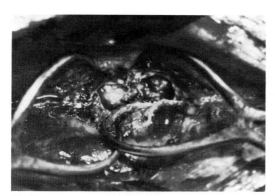

Fig 248. Area of cord decompressed.

A dorsal decompressive laminectomy may be performed to alleviate compression in horses with intravertebral stenosis or a compressive lesion in extension and flexion. After removal of the mane and hair from the dorsal neck, the horse is placed in sternal or lateral recumbency (Fig 247). Needles are placed in the skin of the neck and radiographs made to determine the area to be decompressed. After surgical preparation and draping, a 30-cm incision on the dorsal midline of the neck is made. The incision is continued through the subcutaneous tissue and fat until the funicular portion of the ligamentum nuchae is reached. This is divided longitudinally and the deep lamellar portion separates easily to expose the muscles overlying the dorsal lamina of the spinal column. The multifidus muscle is then elevated from the dorsal lamina of the vertebral arch. When the area is free of soft tissue, a Hall drill is used to describe the area to be removed. A plate of bone as long as the compressed area and most of the width of the laminar arch should be removed to effectively decompress the cord (Fig 248). If the compression does not involve the entire vertebra, the lamina not compressing the cord should be left for stability. Extreme care must be taken to avoid perforation of the dura under the thin dorsal lamina and trauma to the cord. After the plate of bone has been removed, a portion of body fat is placed over the cord and the ligamentum nuchae, subcutaneous tissue and skin are closed over the laminectomy site. Broad-spectrum antibiotics are given for 5-7 days and the horse is fed from elevated containers.

Dorsal decompression must be considered a highly experimental surgery in horses. Of 9 cases attempted at Washington State University, only 3 showed clinical improvement. Two horses suffered postoperative fractures of a dorsal facet, leading to more severe cord compression and 4 horses had an increased neurologic deficit after surgery. Three horses developed postsurgical myositis, which was so severe in 2 horses that humane destruction was advised. One case of wound dehiscence was treated as an open wound and healed after a period of 6 weeks.

Postsurgical exercise after either cervical stabilization or decompression should be limited to hand-walking for 6 weeks. Gradual increase in exercise and training is advisable after that period.

The neurologic signs and diagnosis of cervical vertebral malformation are also discussed in Chaper 21.

References

1. Jeffcott, LB. Eq Vet J **7** (1975) 69.
2. Sisson, S and Grossman, ID: The Anatomy of the Domestic Animals. 4th ed. WB Saunders, Philadelphia, 1953.
3. Morgan, JP et al. Calif Vet **26** (3) (1972) 15.
4. Jeffcott, LB. J Eq Med Surg **2** (1978) 9.
5. Rooney, JR and Prickett, ME. Cornell Vet **57** (1967) 417.
6. Lerner, DJ and Riley, G. JAVMA **172** (1978) 274.
7. Whitwell, KE. Eq Vet J **10** (1978) 125.
8. Mayhew, IG et al. Eq Vet J **10** (1978) 103.
9. Leipold, HW et al. VM/SAC **69** (1974) 1312.
10. Cho, DY and Leipold, HW. Eq Vet J **9** (1977) 195.
11. Bailey, CS. JAAHA **11** (1975) 426.
12. Leathers, C et al. J Vet Orthoped **1** (1979) 55.
13. Klaassen, JD and Wagner, PC: Hemivertebra in a Foal. Eq Pract. *In press*, 1981.
14. de Lahunta, A. Proc 19th Ann Mtg Am Assoc Eq Pract, 1973. p 25.
15. McGrath, JT. Proc 8th Ann Mtg Am Assoc Eq Pract, 1962. p 157.
16. Morgan, JP. JAVMA **147** (1965) 521.
17. Owen, R and Smith-Matie, LL. JAVMA **173** (1978) 854.
18. Jeffcott, LB and Whitewell, KE. Proc 22nd Ann Mtg Am Assoc Eq Pract, 1976. p 91.
19. Moyer, WA and Rooney, JR. JAVMA **159** (1971) 1022.
20. Stecher, BM. Am J Vet Res **23** (1962) 939.
21. de Lahunta, A: Veterinary Neuroanatomy and Clinical Neurology. WB Saunders, Philadelphia, 1977.
22. Wagner, PC et al. J Eq Med Surg **1** (1977) 282.
23. Guffy, MM et al. JAVMA **155** (1969) 754.
24. Slone, DE et al. JAVMA **174** (1979) 1234.
25. Rooney, JR et al. Eq Vet J **1** (1969) 287.
26. Adams, OR. Proc 15th Ann Mtg Am Assoc Eq Pract, 1969. p 198.
27. Adams, OR: Lameness in Horses. 3rd ed. Lea & Febiger, Philadelphia, 1974.

28. Stecher, RM and Goss, LJ. JAVMA **138** (1961) 248.

29. Smythe, RH. Mod Vet Pract **43** (**9**) (1962) 50.

30. Evans, LH *et al*. JAVMA **53** (1968) 1085.

31. Kelly, WR *et al*. J Am Vet Rad Soc **13** (1972) 59.

32. Collins, JD *et al*. Vet Rec **88** (1971) 321.

33. Chladek, DW and Ruth, GR. JAVMA **168** (1976) 64.

34. Kittleson, SL *et al*, Pullman, WA: Unpublished data, 1980.

35. Wagner, PC *et al*. Vet Surg **8** (**3**) (1979) 7.

36. Wagner, PC *et al*. Vet Surg **8** (**3**) (1979) 84.

37. Rooney, JR: Biomechanics of Lameness in Horses. Williams & Wilkins, Baltimore, 1969.

38. Dimock, WW and Errington, BJ. JAVMA **95** (1939) 261.

39. Steel, ID *et al*. Aust Vet J **35** (1959) 442.

40. Eraser, H and Palmer, AC. Vet Rec **80** (1976) 338.

41. Rooney, JR. Cornell Vet **53** (1963) 411.

42. Prickett, ME. Proc 14th Ann Mtg Am Assoc Eq Pract, 1968. p 147.

43. Beech, J. Proc 22nd Ann Mtg Am Assoc Eq Pract, 1976. p 79.

44. Cloward, RB. J Neurosurg **5** (1958) 602.

21

The Nervous System

by I.G. Mayhew and R.J. MacKay

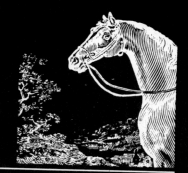

NEUROLOGIC EVALUATION

The most fundamental component of equine neurology is the neurologic examination. To identify neurologic deficits and determine the anatomic sites(s) and extent of lesion(s) are the goals of such an examination. The diagnosis of the cause of the disease and appropriate treatment of the horse are the rewards of mastering the neurologic examination. To achieve these goals, the equine clinician must have a basic knowledge of nervous system structure and function. This is perhaps more important than with any other organ system because in neurology, it is the *site* of the lesion(s) more than the *cause* of the disease that determines the clinical signs.

A logical, practical, repeatable neurologic examination allows the clinician to begin the examination at the nose and conclude at the tail, considering the anatomic site of the lesion(s) as the examination proceeds.

It must be understood that consideration of the chief complaint, signalment, history and physical examination must precede the neurologic examination. In addition, routine and special diagnostic aids may be used and several specific principles of therapy followed to successfully manage a horse with a nervous system disease.

Chief Complaint

The events related to the onset of signs, the progress of all neurologic signs and any therapy given are part of this aspect of the evaluation. Acute onset of signs must be distinguished from the initial observation of signs. Signs resulting from trauma and vascular disorders (*eg*, infarcts, equine herpesvirus-1 myelitis) are acute in onset and usually stabilize or improve within 24 hours. The first sign reported by an owner of a horse with spinal cord disease

is often that the animal fell, stood up, and was ataxic and weak. In fact, it is often more likely that spinal cord disease caused the fall.

Many metabolic diseases (*eg*, hepatoencephalopathy), lesions resulting in brain or spinal cord edema (especially trauma and space-occupying lesions), and a few toxic diseases (*eg*, lead encephalopathy—neuropathy) result in signs that fluctuate markedly. Convulsions must be characterized as to evidence of asymmetry and localized signs; the examiner may not have the benefit of observing a convulsion. A chief complaint that includes signs of progressive, multifocal lesions is characteristic of several infectious diseases (*eg*, protozoal myeloencephalitis, rabies).

Response to previous therapy is helpful. Many diseases respond to corticosteroid therapy, although the long-term effect on most infectious diseases is probably harmful.

Signalment

The age, breed, sex, use and color of the neurologic patient can be very significant factors. Congenital malformations of nervous tissue usually result in signs at birth that are nonprogressive. However, congenital malformations of the calvarium and vertebral column may result in signs of nervous system involvement at several months of age. Cervical vertebral malformation with stenosis of the vertebral canal occurs most frequently at 6-30 months of age. Neuritis of the cauda equina, hepatoencephalopathy resulting from acute hepatic necrosis, and protozoal myeloencephalitis all usually affect mature horses. Narcolepsy-cataplexy ("fainting foal" syndrome) has only been seen in Shetland ponies, Suffolk horses and their crosses. Particular cerebellar degenerations are described in the Arabian, Gotland pony and Oldenburg breeds. Also, Arabian horses may have a specific congenital occipi-toatlantoaxial malformation. Cervical verte-bral malformation is seen more frquently in males than in females, particularly in Thor-oughbreds that are large for their age. Proto-zoal myeloencephalitis is most common in young adult horses at breeding and racing/training establishments, and is most common in Thoroughbreds and Standardbreds. Grey horses have a predisposition to melanoma for-mation and these tumors occasionally invade the central nervous system (CNS).

History

This includes an assessment of the environ-ment, management, nutrition, parasite control and vaccination status as well as past trau-matic, medical and surgical events.

Prevailing winds may significantly deter-mine which horses are exposed to lead fallout from industrial wastes. Exposure to toxins and poisonous vegetation, such as corn that is moldy with *Fusarium* spp, cattle feed contain-ing monensin, yellow star thistle, and tremor-genic ryegrass and Dallis grass pastures, is important to document. Perinatal manage-ment may be important in the pathogenesis of such diseases as neonatal maladjustment syn-drome, and meningitis associated with failure of passive transfer of immunity. Rapid growth associated with *ad libitum* feeding of a high-energy ration may be one of the predisposing factors in cervical vertebral malformation. To-gaviral encephalitis (eastern, western and Venezuelan) vaccines protect for up to 6 months, although equine herpesvirus-1 (EHV-1, rhin-opneumonitis) vaccines may not protect against the neurologic form of the disease.

A history of recent trauma can obviously be significant. Also, trauma weeks or months pre-viously may be associated with post-traumatic cerebral scarring causing seizures, or repara-tive exostoses from vertebral injury compress-ing the spinal cord. Enzootic strangles infection or EHV-1 syndromes (abortion, upper respira-tory inflection, fever) are important anamnes-tic facts when evaluating a horse with a *Streptococcus equi* cerebral abscess or EHV-1 myelitis, respectively. Often historical evi-dence of medical problems, such as aural dis-charges in a horse with otitis media-interna or diarrhea in a foal with *Salmonella* vertebral osteomyelitis, is helpful. Horses with tetanus, epidural empyema and even botulism of wound origin may have histories of traumatic epi-sodes or surgical wounds.

Physical Examination

Many toxic, metabolic, neoplastic, traumatic and infectious diseases affecting the nervous system have signs related to other systems that should be detected during physical exam-ination. Irregular respiratory patterns may be associated with brainstem lesions and meta-bolic encephalopathy. Inhalation pneumonia may occur in horses with dysphagia resulting from guttural pouch mycosis, lead-induced neuropathy or forage poisoning (presumptive botulism).

Signs of musculoskeletal disease can mimic those of neurologic disease. These signs are usually those of disuse or weakness. A detailed musculoskeletal examination can be time-con-suming and may be included in the neurologic examination. A thorough lameness evaluation is often required in horses with vague gait def-icits. A rectal examination should be per-formed to identify sublumbar muscle tenderness, masses involving lymph nodes or sacrocaudal vertebrae, pelvic fractures and urinary bladder distension. A distended blad-der may be observed in horses recumbent for any reason.

Neurologic Examination

The neurologic examination is completed by evaluating each of the following components in the order listed, irrespective of whether the horse is recumbent or ambulatory:

1. head
   a. behavior
   b. mental status
   c. head posture and coordination
   d. cranial nerves
2. gait and posture
3. neck and forelimbs
4. trunk and hindlimbs
5. tail and anus

Evidence of a brain lesion is sought by as-sessing the behavior, mental status, head pos-ture, coordination and cranial nerve function of the patient. The presence of such "head signs" indicates a lesion in the brain, cranial nerves and/or muscles of the head. Evaluation of the gait follows. Lesions in the brainstem and cerebellum can result in gait deficits (weakness, ataxia, spasticity and hypermetria). However, in the absence of head signs, any gait deficit is most likely due to a lesion in the spinal cord, peripheral nerves or muscles.

Close evaluation of the neck, forelimbs, trunk, hindlimbs, tail and anus follows to de-

VETERINARY MEDICAL TEACHING HOSPITAL
UNIVERSITY OF FLORIDA

NEUROLOGIC EXAMINATION OF LARGE ANIMALS

OUTPAITENT:	STALL NO.:
DATE:	TIME:
CLINICIAN:	CHARGES:
STUDENT:	ACCOUNT:
HISTORY:	

PHYSICAL EXAMINATION:

NEUROLOGIC EXAMINATION

HEAD: Behavior:
Mental Status:
Head Posture:
Head Coordination:
Craniel Nerves:

EYES	LEFT	RIGHT
Ophthalmic Examination:		
Vision; II:		
Menace; II-VII, Cerebellum:		
Pupils, PLR; II-III:		
Horners; Symp:		
Strabismus; III, IV, VI, VIII:		
FACE		
Sensation; Vs, cerebrum:		
Muscle mass, jaw tone; Vm:		
Ear, eye, nose, lip reflex; V-VII:		
Expression; VII:		
Sweating, Symp:		
VESTIBULAR—EAR		
Eye drop:		
Nystagmus; resting:		
positional:		
vestibular:		
Hearing:		
Special vestibular:		
TONGUE		
Tone, mass, fasciculations; XII, cerebrum:		
PHARYNX, LARYNX		
Voice; IX, X:		
Swallow; IX, X:		
Endoscopy:		
Slap test:		

GAIT:	LEFT		RIGHT	
	FORE	HIND	FORE	HIND
Paresis:				
Ataxia:				
Spasticity:				
Dysmetria:				
Total deficit:				
Other:				

NECK & FORELIMBS	LEFT	RIGHT	TRUNK & HINDLIMBS:	LEFT	RIGHT	TAIL & ANUS:	LEFT	RIGHT
Hoofwear:			Hoofwear:			Strength:		
Posture:			Posture:			Muscle Mass:		
Strength:			Strength:			Tone:		
Muscle Mass:			Muscle Mass:			Reflexes:		
Tone:			Tone:			Sensation:		
Reflexes:			Reflexes:			Rectal:		
Sensation:			Sensation:					
Sweating:			Sweating:					

ASSESSMENT

SITE OF LESION(S): General (circle): cerebrum, brainstem, peripheral cranial nerves, cerebellum, spinal cord, peripheral nerves, muscles, skeleton

Specific:

CAUSE OF LESION(S):

PLAN

DX:
RX:
EX:

SIGNATURE:	DATE:

Fig 1. Sample form for neurologic examination of horses.

tect localizing signs of lesions in the C_1-T_2, T_3-S_2 and S_3-Cy spinal cord segments or their associated peripheral nerves or muscles, respectively. A lesion at C_1-T_2 usually results in tetraparesis and a lesion at T_3-S_2 usually results in paraparesis. A lesion at S_3-Cy does not cause a gait deficit but results in neurologic deficits in the tail, anus, bladder and rectum. Peripheral nerve and muscle diseases result in signs only in the limb or area affected.

Results of the neurologic examination must be recorded, not risked to memory. A sample neurologic examination form is shown in Figure 1. Repeated examinations are often necessary to detect progression or spread of the lesion, signs of another lesion and response to therapy. Such changes alter the working etiologic diagnosis, therapy and prognosis.

Each component of the neurologic examination is detailed below.

Head

Behavior: Information obtained from the owner about the horse's behavior is very important. Age, breed, sex and use can influence behavior. Occasionally horses recumbent as a result of brain, spinal cord, muscle or orthopedic disease become quite violent and aggressive in their struggles to get up. Seizure activity is often altered or ceases with a change in environment; therefore, close observation may be required to see such changes. Auditory and tactile stimuli may induce seizures and in mares periodic seizures may occur more frequently during estrus. Seizure activity that is asymmetric or initially involves one part of the body suggests a focal, acquired lesion.

The frequency and duration of seizures is important in determining the progress of the disease and response to therapy. Aggression, wandering, circling, head-pressing, changes in voice and continual yawning are easily recognized behavioral changes indicative of cerebral disease. Remarkable alterations in behavior frequently occur with the togaviral (eastern, western and Venezuelan) and rabies encephalitides, and with hepatoencephalopathy. Foals with neonatal meningitis or neonatal maladjustment syndrome can have subtle behavioral changes, such as wandering away from the dam and inappropriate, ineffective nursing behavior, and may vocalize abnormally or have seizures. Such foals are referred to as "wanderers," "dummies," "barkers" and "convulsives," respectively. Horses with an asymmetric cerebral lesion (*eg,* cholesterol granuloma, moldy

corn leukoencephalomalacia, cerebral abscess) tend to circle toward the side of the lesion.

Mental Status: The mental status is the level of consciousness and awareness. This level of responsiveness to the external and internal environments is controlled by the cerebral cortex and the ascending reticular activating system (ARAS) in the brainstem. Because these areas are affected by sensory stimuli, the response of a depressed horse to visual, auditory, tactile, painful, olfactory and gustatory stimuli helps determine its mental status.

A comatose horse is completely unresponsive to noxious stimuli and may have a large lesion in the cerebrum or brainstem, particularly the midbrain. Semicoma is a state of partial responsiveness to noxious stimuli and some voluntary movements usually occur with stimulation. Horses with less profound levels of altered mental status are described as obtunded, somnolent, lethargic or depressed. The terms stuporous and delirious imply additional inappropriate movement or vocalization. Horses that are recumbent due to vestibular, spinal cord, peripheral nerve or muscle disease may be depressed from exhaustion, dehydration, decubiti and myopathy.

Temporary coma often results from head trauma and vascular accidents such as intracarotid injection and *Strongylus vulgaris* embolic showers to the brain. This does not mean that irreversible damage to the ARAS or cerebrum has occurred. Other neurologic signs (*eg,* cranial nerve deficits are just as important in determining a prognosis. Involvement of the ARAS or cerebrum by diseases, such as eastern equine encephalitis (EEE), western equine enciphalitis (WEE), neonatal bacterial meningitis or hemorrhage, characteristically results in some loss of consciousness.

Head Posture and Coordination: Normal horses maintain their heads in certain natural postures and maneuver them smoothly and accurately to perform tasks such as drinking and prehension of food. Diseases of the vestibular system often affect the mechanisms that help maintain normal head posture and result in a head tilt. Such a vestibular head tilt is characterized by one ear closer to the ground and rotation of the poll about the muzzle. The head is usually tilted toward the side of the lesion. Blindfolding a horse with vestibular disease almost always exaggerates any head tilt. A horse with a cerebral lesion usually has its head turned and circles toward the side of the lesion (Fig 2). Scoliosis and torticollis due to

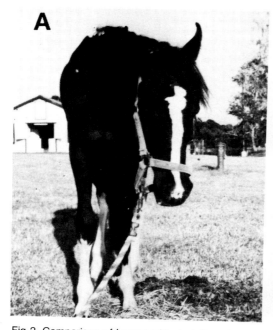 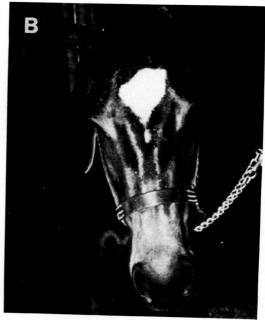

Fig 2. Comparison of horses with deviation of the head and neck (A) and a head tilt (B). The horse in (A) has a diffuse, symmetric central disease and holds its head and neck to the right. The animal also wanders in circles to the right. The horse in (B) has otitis media-interna, which results in a slight head tilt to the right with the poll held to the right of midline. This is characteristic of vestibular disease. The horse in (B) also has right facial paralysis.

musculoskeletal disorders must be considered in horses with abnormal head posture.

Bilateral vestibular disease can result in wide swaying movements of the head and neck. The cerebellum modulates movement of the head and limbs. Fine control of head movement is often lost with cerebellar disease, resulting in awkward, jerky movements. Even in a horse at rest, the lack of control is apparent as bobbing of the head. Such a head bob can be exaggerated by attracting the horse's attention with food, water or some visual or auditory stimulus. The resultant fine jerky movements of the head are known as an intention tremor. Cerebellar degeneration in Arabian foals classically results in these cerebellar signs as well as a cerebellar gait deficit.

Cranial Nerves: In keeping with the format of neurologic examination, the cranial nerves are examined by starting with the most rostral and proceeding caudad. The cranial nerves and their nuclei are spread along the entire brainstem and their function is frequently affected by lesions involving the brain. Therefore, this part of the examination is vital in localizing brain lesions. Lesions of the medulla oblongata frequently produce tetraparesis with ataxia

identical to that caused by cervical spinal cord lesions. Subtle cranial nerve deficits may be the only indication that the lesion is in the brainstem rather than the spinal cord.

I. *Olfactory Nerve.* Loss of the ability to smell (anosmia) is rare. The ability to smell food or the examiner's hand is regarded as normal functioning of these nerves and the olfactory lobes. Ammonia and cigarette smoke irritate the nasal mucosa and may be used to assess the sensory branches of cranial nerve V. Further evaluation of smell entails the use of pure aromas, such as citrol.

II. *Optic Nerve.* The menace, blink or eye-preservation response is used to evaluate the visual pathway. A menacing gesture with the hand to each eye in turn results in the horse closing the eyelids and frequently jerking the head away. In the horse, there is essentially a total crossover of fibers in the optic nerves at the optic chiasm. Therefore, vision in one eye is perceived in the contralateral visual (occipital) cortex. The incoming (afferent) pathway for the menace response is from the ipsilateral eyeball and optic nerve to the contralateral optic tract, lateral geniculate nucleus (thalamus), optic radiation and occipital cortex. The outgoing (efferent) pathway is from the contra-lateral occipital cortex to the ispsilateral facial nucleus, which effects the blink.

It is important not to touch the face or create air currents that a blind horse might feel when performing this test. Performing the test out-side where a continual breeze obviates extra air currents can be an advantage. Depressed, stoic, or excited horses may respond poorly to this test. By tapping the side of the face lightly, the examiner can attract such a patient's at-tention to perform the test adequately. Neo-nates have vision but may become refractory to repeated menace response testing.

If a menace response deficit is suspected, an obstacle course should be used to detect true visual deficits. This is done by blindfolding each eye in turn to detect unilateral deficits. Unilateral blindness can be difficult to detect and often necessitates silently approaching the horse's stall and making visual gestures from one side, then the other.

Very depressed horses and those with vesti-bular disease may stagger or bump into objects without being blind. An ophthalmoscopic ex-amination of each optic fundus is part of the examination of the optic system. Congenital optic nerve hypoplasia and optic nerve atrophy associated with head trauma and blood loss can be detected easily with an ophthalmoscope. These lesions and others of the eye and optic nerve, such as recurrent uveitis, optic nerve neoplasia and periorbital masses, can result in ipsilateral blindness. In contrast, lesions of the optic tract, lateral geniculate nucleus and oc-cipital cortex result in contralateral blindness.

Space-occupying cerebral lesions, such as *Streptococcus equi* abscesses and hematomas, can produce unilateral blindness due to direct involvement of the optic pathways. More fre-quently the blindness is contralateral to the le-sion or bilateral and is the result of forebrain swelling and compression of the occipital vi-sual cortex caudad against and ventral to the rigid tentorium cerebelli, which separates the cerebrum from the cerebellum.

The visual pathways may be affected by focal lesions such as protozoal myeloencephalitis, cerebral infarction from *Strongylus vulgaris* embolic showers and *Hypoderma* larval migra-tion. The visual deficit associated with such central blindness is contralateral to the lesion and pupillary light reflexes are intact. This is in contrast to the ipsilateral blindness and ab-normal pupillary light reflexes seen with le-sions involving the eyeball and optic nerve.

Horses with diffuse cerebellar lesions, such as Arabian foals with cerebellar degeneration, do not blink when menaced. This menace re-sponse deficit does not indicate blindness be-cause these animals can see, blink when their eyelids are touched and have no other signs of forebrain disease. The efferent pathway of the menace response from the visual cortex to the facial nucleus and nerve may pass through the cerebellar cortex; therefore, cerebellar lesions can interfere with the response.

III. *Oculomotor Nerve.* Parasympathetic fi-bers in the oculomotor nerve innervate the pupillary constrictor muscles and maintain constrictor tone according to the amount of light entering the eyeball. Opposing this is the dilator tone to the pupil, which is maintained according to sympathetic input (*eg,* fear and excitement) to the brainstem. A sympathetic tract passes down the brainstem and cervical spinal cord to synapse on the preganglionic neurons in the first few thoracic segments. Pre-ganglionic sympathetic fibers exit the spinal cord there, pass up the neck in the vagosym-pathetic trunk and synapse in the cranial cer-vical ganglion on postganglionic neurons, which innervate the pupillary dilator muscles. These opposing functions are considered together.

After ensuring that no lesions such as cata-racts or iris adhesions might affect light enter-ing the eyeball or movement of the iris, the pupils are examined for size and symmetry. Al-lowances must be made for the amount of am-bient light and the emotional status of the patient. The pupillary light reflex is then tested for each eye, preferably in a dimly lit place. This test consists of directing a bright light into each eyeball and observing immedi-ate reflex constriction of the pupil in the same eye (direct reflex) and in the opposite eye (con-sensual reflex). The pathway for these reflexes is from the retina and optic nerve into both sides of the midbrain without passing through the lateral geniculate nuclei or visual cortices, and to both oculomotor nuclei and nerves ef-fecting constriction of both pupils. Lesions that affect the central visual pathways, therefore, do not affect the pupillary light reflexes. Also, midbrain lesions may interfere with this reflex to cause pupil dilation without blindness. A horse with normal vision and a dilated pupil (mydriasis) but no response to light directed into either eye most likely has a lesion in the midbrain or oculomotor nerve on the same side as the mydriasis. In such cases, light directed through the dilated pupil causes consensual constriction of the opposite pupil with intact oculomotor connections.

Cranial trauma frequently results in midbrain damage and monitoring pupillary function is a vital part of the evaluation of such cases. Also, the oculomotor nerves exit from the ventral midbrain and are predisposed to compression along their intracranial course by any process that produces brain swelling, such as cranial trauma and cerebral abscesses. Asymmetric swelling of the forebrain often results in anisocoria (asymmetric pupils), usually with the dilated pupil on the same side as the swollen cerebrum because of pressure applied to the ipsilateral oculomotor nerve. Progressive, bilateral pupillary dilation (eg, following head trauma) usually indicates severe midbrain and oculomotor damage, and warrants a bad prognosis.

Lesions of the eyeball or optic nerve that result in peripheral blindness also effect pupillary changes. The pupil on the affected side is slightly dilated when compared with the contralateral pupil, and neither pupil constricts when light is directed through it. Both pupils constrict when light is directed into the eye on the unaffected side. However, a retrobulbar lesion that involves not only the optic nerve but also the oculomotor nerve causes ipsilateral blindness and mydriasis, and no constriction of either pupil in response to light directed into the eye on the affected side. Also, constriction of the pupil only on the unaffected side occurs when light is directed through it.

Anisocoria also results from lesions of the sympathetic supply to the pupils. This is referred to as Horner's syndrome and is characterized by ipsilateral pupillary constriction (miosis), a drooping upper eyelid (ptosis), and a slightly sunken eyeball (enophthalmos) with protrusion of the nictitating membrane (Fig 3). These changes are caused by loss of sympathetic tone to the pupillary dilator muscles, the elevator muscles of the upper eyelid and the periorbital smooth muscles, respectively. Horner's syndrome in horses also includes dilated facial blood vessels, and elevated facial and cervical temperature with localized sweating. This is discussed in more detail below.

IV. *Trochlear Nerve,* VI. *Abducens Nerve.* These 2 nerves, together with the oculomotor nerve, innervate the extraocular muscles that retain the eye in its normal position and move it within the bony orbit. Their function is tested by observing for normal eye position and movement.

Movement of the eye is stimulated via the vestibular system by moving the head slowly from side to side and observing the normal rhythmic horizontal movement of each eyeball, known as normal vestibular nystagmus. Each full arc of head movement produces 4-5 horizontal eye movements. The slow phase of eye movement occurs in the direction opposite to the direction of head movement and the fast phase occurs in the same direction as head movement. In addition, when a horse's head is extended on the neck, the eyeballs rotate ventrad within their bony orbit and essentially maintain a horizontal orientation. As the head is lowered, the eyeballs return to a central position within the bony orbit. A normal, vertical vestibular nystagmus is stimulated by increasing the range and rate of head elevation.

Abnormalities in these eye responses are frequently seen with vestibular disease. In particular, there is often a ventral or sometimes dorsal deviation of the eyeball on the side of the vestibular lesion. Such a vestibular strabismus is usually exaggerated by elevation of the head. In contrast to true strabismus resulting from paralysis of cranial nerves III, IV or VI, vestibular strabismus is characterized by eye movement in the direction opposite the deviation. Paralysis of particular extraocular muscles results in deviation of the eyeball (strabismus) opposite to the direction of muscle pull. Such forms of strabismus are present with the head in any position and the eyeball cannot be moved out of the deviated position, even during the above maneuvers. The nature of the strabismus and the syndrome that occurs with paralysis of cranial nerves III, IV and VI are not known for the horse. By extrapolation from observations of other species, paralysis of the oculomotor nerve may result in lateral and ventral strabismus, and ptosis of the upper eyelid, in addition to the mydriasis and decreased pupillary light reflex described above. Paralysis of the trochlear nerve may result in dorsal rotation of the medial pupillary angle (dorsomedial strabismus) and paralysis of the abducens nerve may produce medial strabismus. Loss of function in all of these nerves probably results in inability to retract the globe into the bony orbit and no reflex closure of the nictitating membrane when the cornea is touched with the eyelids held open (corneal reflex).

Some horses with severe asymmetric cerebral and probably thalamic lesions walk in circles toward the side of the lesion and, with any stimulus, turn sharply in the same direction. In addition to the head turning and body leaning, the eyeballs may also be drawn in the same direction. Such asymmetric behavior and movement is described as the "adversive" syndrome. Again, the eyeballs are not fixed in the deviated position.

V. *Trigeminal Nerve*. This largest cranial nerve contains sensory nerve fibers of the head in its mandibular, maxillary and ophthalmic branches, and motor nerve fibers to the muscles of mastication in its mandibular branch.

The sensory function of this nerve is tested by eliciting facial reflexes and by assessing sensory perception of the face. Facial reflexes are tested by lightly touching the ear, eyelid, external nare and labial commissure on each side of the face, and observing flicking of the ear, closure of the eyelids, flaring of the nostril and withdrawal of the labial commissure. Sensory impulses for these reflexes are carried in branches of the trigeminal nerve. In the pons and medulla, impulses pass from the sensory trigeminal nucleus to the facial nucleus, and then to the muscles of the ear, eyelids, nostril and lips within the facial nerve on each side. Consequently, these reflexes are deficient with lesions involving cranial nerve V or VII or the pontomedullary nuclei of those nerves. The corneal reflex has been referred to above.

Facial sensation is tested by observing a cerebral response, such as retraction of the head, to pricking the ear, eyelids, nostril and lips on each side. Sensation in the nasal septum should be tested, particularly in extremely depressed or stoic patients, as this is the most sensitive area on the face. Horses with facial nerve (VII) paralysis have deficient facial reflexes and cannot move the ear, eyelid, nare and lips on the affected side, but have normal facial sensation.

Damage to sensory branches of cranial nerve V results in variable loss of facial sensation and facial reflexes, and packing of feed in the cheeks; however, facial movement and expression remain unaffected. Lesions of the sensory nucleus of nerve V can result in the same syndrome. This nucleus is very large and is not often totally destroyed by most diseases. However, space-occupying lesions in the lateral pons and medulla oblongata, cranial trauma, rabies and protozoal myeloencephalitis can do so. In addition, total facial (and body) hypalgesia may occur in severe diffuse encephalopathy, such as hepatoencephalopathy and togaviral encephalomyelitides, presumably through involvement of the sensory cortices.

More selective facial hypalgesia or analgesia, including the very sensitive nasal septal mucosa, occurs with extensive focal lesions of the cerebrum, probably of the parietal sensory cortex. This has resulted from cerebral embolic infarction due to intracarotid injections or *S vulgaris* thromboarteritis, cerebral trauma and laceration, and very large cholesterol granulomas of the lateral ventricles. Such sensory deficit occurs on the contralateral side of the face and, because there is no lesion in the medulla oblongata, the facial reflexes remain intact. Some horses that are head-shy, throw their head, tilt their head or continually rub the side of the face may have facial hyperesthesia, referred to as trigeminal neuralgia. However, this has not been documented. Some cases are associated with guttural pouch lesions.

Motor function of the mandibular nerves is evaluated by observing chewing movements, assessing the strength of mouth closure, and determining the mass of the muscles of mastication. Bilateral dysfunction of the motor branches of cranial nerve V results in a dropped mandible, with the tongue dropped cephalad between the teeth, and drooling of saliva and feed from the mouth. Ultimately the masseter, temporal and distal belly of the digastricus muscles atrophy. Unilateral lesions of the pontine motor nucleus of cranial nerve V, as in protozoal myeloencephalitis, or of the motor fibers in one mandibular nerve, as in cranial neoplasms, result in slightly weak mouth closure that is difficult to detect until muscle atrophy develops. In some horses with unilateral lesions of the motor branches of cranial nerve V, the mandible is deviated somewhat toward the unaffected side.

VII. *Facial Nerve*. This cranial nerve distributes motor fibers from the facial nucleus in the medulla oblongata to the muscles of facial expression via its auricular, palpebral and buccal branches. Its function is tested, along with that of the sensory branches of the trigeminal nerve, in the facial reflexes described above. Facial nerve function is also tested by observing the ability to move the ears, close the eyelids, flare the nostrils during inspiration, and move the lips and muzzle during food prehension. Unilateral facial nerve paralysis causes asymmetric facial expression and movement, and is evident as ipsilateral ptosis, drooped ear, lack of flaring of the naris, drooped lips, and contralateral retraction of the muzzle (Fig 3).

In addition, facial muscle hypotonia results in poor closure of the eyelids when the cornea

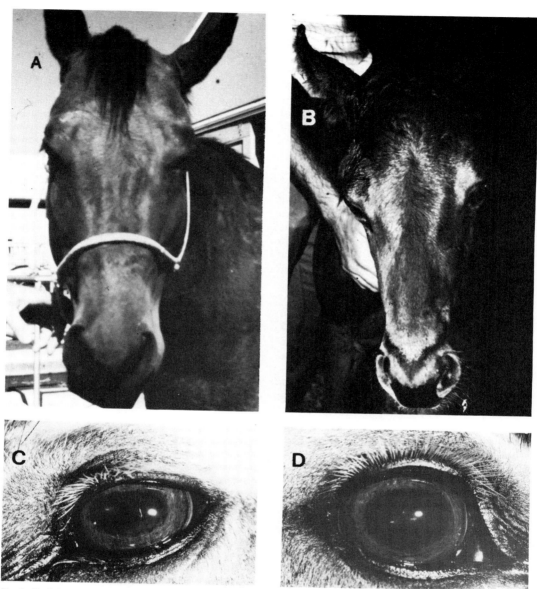

Fig 3. Facial paralysis and Horner's syndrome. The horse in (A) has right facial paralysis involving all branches of the nerve. The right ear, eyelid and lips droop. All of these structures are flaccid and the muzzle is pulled to the left (unaffected side). The foal in (B) has Horner's syndrome on the right side. Ptosis is evident on the right. Sweating is also visible (and hyperthermia palpable) on the right side of the face and cranial aspect of the neck, and is most prominent at the base of the right ear. In (C) and (D), the right (affected) and left (unaffected) eyes of another horse with Horner's syndrome on the right side are illustrated. Ptosis and slight miosis are evident on the affected (C) side.

is gently touched, loss of normal wrinkling around the nares and muzzle, and drooling of saliva from the labial commissure. Food, particularly hay, often remains in the labial commissure and sometimes in the buccal pouches. This difficulty in prehension must be differentiated from other causes of dysphagia. Lesions of the facial nucleus usually result in some de-

gree of ear, eye, nose and lip paresis or paralysis. Lesions of the proximal facial nerve to the level of the facial canal in the temporal bone result in the same signs. In the latter cases there are no other signs of brainstem involvement, such as semicoma or hemiparesis.

Because the facial nerve separates into its major branches prior to rounding the caudal border of the mandible, peripheral lesions most frequently involve one of the branches. Damage to the buccal branches results in ipsilateral drooping of the lip and contralateral retraction of the muscle.

Some normal horses have an asymmetric muzzle and external nares, which can be confused with partial facial paralysis. Specific aspects of disease producing facial paralysis are discussed under Neurologic Problems.

VIII. *Vestibulocochlear Nerve.* The vestibular branch of the cranial nerve VIII supplies the major input to the vestibular system. Originating in the inner ear, the vestibular nerve passes through the petrosal bone, penetrates the medulla oblongata and terminates in the vestibular nuclei. Some fibers terminate in small areas of the cerebellum. Input to the vestibular system also comes from the cerebellum and other brainstem centers.

The vestibular system controls balance by orienting the head, body, limbs and eyes in space. Signs of vestibular disease are seen with lesions of any part of the vestibular apparatus. In the acute phase of vestibular disease, there is very often a rhythmic nystagmus in conjunction with the head tilt and strabismus as described above. This spontaneous nystagmus may occur when the head is in a normal position (resting nystagmus) or when the head is placed in an unusual position, such as grossly tilted or elevated (positional nystagmus). The direction of nystagmus is defined by the direction of the fast phase of movement. With lesions of the central components of the vestibular system, nystagmus may be horizontal, vertical or rotary. Nystagmus may be directed toward or away from the side of the lesion and often is altered in rate and direction by changes in head position.

Spontaneous nystagmus from peripheral vestibular lesions involving the vestibular nerve or inner ear is almost always horizontal, with the fast phase directed away from the side of damage. A wide-base stance and staggery gait are frequently seen with vestibular disease because of a loss of balance. These signs may be quite remarkable and the disorientation may account for the frantic struggling of some horses during the acute phase of the disease. Central and peripheral vestibular disease frequently causes increased extensor tone in the contralateral limbs. This often results in a tendency to lean, fall and roll toward the side of the lesion. Only with central vestibular disease are there other signs of brainstem involvement such as profound weakness and ataxia of the ipsilateral limbs.

The cochlear division of cranial nerve VIII is involved with hearing. Hearing deficits are exceedingly difficult to detect in these horses.

Specific diseases involving the vestibulocochlear nerve are discussed under Vestibular Syndrome.

IX. *Glossopharyngeal Nerve,* X. *Vagus Nerve,* XI. *Accessory Nerve.* These 3 nerves contain sensory and motor fibers that innervate the pharynx, larynx, esophagus and much of the remaining viscera. They are closely associated as they leave the swallowing centers in the caudal medulla, exit the calvarium and pass by the caudal aspect of the guttural pouch. A major function of these nerves is to control swallowing and phonation, which are assessed by observing normal swallowing, palpating the larynx externally for normal muscle mass, listening for a normal voice and observing normal structure and function of the larynx and pharynx through a fiberoptic endoscope. Swallowing can be observed when the horse is offered food and water, and can be elicited by touching the pharynx with a nasogastric tube and observing swallowing movements with passage of the tube into the esophagus.

The predominant signs resulting from lesions of any part of these nerves or their medullary nuclei are dysphagia and laryngeal paralysis. Unilateral lesions result in partial dysphagia, with ipsilateral laryngeal hemiplegia and food in the nostrils. Laryngeal hemiplegia is seen particularly with selective involvement of the recurrent laryngeal nerve, which emerges from the vagus nerve in the thorax, ascends the neck and innervates the intrinsic muscles of the larynx except the cricothyroid. The resulting syndrome usually includes a roaring sound on forced inspiration. Bilateral involvement of the swallowing centers of cranial nerves IX and X results in dysphagia, with food and water passed out the nostrils. Endoscopy reveals food (and usually exudate) in the pharynx and larynx. Swallowing or coughing cannot be elicited when the pharynx and larynx are touched, and the soft palate is frequently displaced above the epiglottis. Secondary inhalation pneumonia is a common sequel.

Dysphagia may result from selective involvement of one or more of these nerves in the region of the guttural pouch or from involvement of the pharyngeal muscles. Ineffective swallowing, with food held in the mouth and pharynx and sometimes appearing at the nostrils, results from diffuse or large focal lesions of the forebrain that also cause depression. In such horses there may be no lesions of the swallowing centers and the swallowing reflexes are intact, but the voluntary effort required for effective swallowing is weak. This deficit is referred to as supranuclear palsy and is seen in diseases such as hepatoencephalopathy, cerebral infarction from *S vulgaris* thromboembolism, and large space-occupying cerebral lesions.

The form of dysphagia described here must be differentiated from difficulties in grasping, masticating and swallowing food caused by other diseases, such as pharyngeal and laryngeal obstructions, and by lesions affecting the trigeminal, facial or hypoglossal nerves.

XII. *Hypoglossal Nerve.* The last cranial nerve provides motor pathways to the lingual muscles and originates from its motor nucleus in the caudal medulla oblongata. Bilateral dysfunction results in profound lingual weakness and atrophy. The tongue remains out when it is pulled from the mouth and the horse cannot pass feed to the back of the mouth for swallowing, which results in feed dropping from the mouth (quidding). Unilateral lesions involving the medullary nucleus or the hypoglossal nerve result in mild lingual weakness and hemiatrophy but very little difficulty with prehension and swallowing.

Supranuclear palsy involving the tongue also results in mild dysphagia and feed dropping from the mouth. This is more common than the supranuclear palsy affecting cranial nerves IX, X and XI, as described above, but is seen with similar severe cerebral lesions involving descending voluntary motor pathways to the hypoglossal nucleus and nerve. In these horses the tongue is left protruding when placed out of the mouth, although it can be pulled back into the mouth when stimulated. There is no atrophy of lingual muscles.

Gait and Posture

There are 4 primary components of a neurologic gait deficit: paresis (weakness), ataxia (incoordination), spasticity (stiffness or hypometria) and hypermetria (overreaching). These signs are present in various combinations for different neurologic diseases.

This phase of the examination is an overall evaluation of limb motor function and limb somesthetic or proprioceptive input to the CNS. If the patient cannot stand, the examiner proceeds to the next phase of the examination. Lesions affecting descending motor pathways interrupt voluntary effort and consequently cause paresis caudal to the lesion. Because these descending motor pathways normally have a suppressive effect on spinal reflexes, damage to them can also result in overactive reflexes, seen as a spastic (stiff) gait.

Ascending proprioceptive fibers in peripheral nerves or white matter of the spinal cord and medulla relay information on limb position in space. Damage to these fibers results in degrees of ataxia or incoordination in the muscles and limbs caudal (distal, in the case of peripheral nerves) to the lesion. Such lesions also interfere with other proprioceptive information destined for the cerebellum. This results in poor cerebellar control of voluntary effort and is seen as overreaching and limb hyperflexion, known as hypermetria. Musculoskeletal disease can be confused with neurologic disease because the former also may result in weakness and spasticity. However, musculoskeletal disease rarely results in ataxia and hypermetria and never results in all 4 types of deficit simultaneously.

Gait deficits occur with lesions of the brainstem from the midbrain caudad, and examination of the head usually indicates if such a lesion is present. If there is a gait deficit in all 4 legs but no evidence of brainstem involvement, such as cranial nerve deficits, the lesion (or one of the lesions) may be in the spinal cord from C_1-T_2 or diffusely throughout the spinal cord, peripheral nerves or muscles. Also, if such a lesion exists between C_1-T_2 and involves only the white matter on one side, a gait deficit occurs in the ipsilateral fore- and hindlimbs.

Grading of the degree of gait deficit in each leg assists in identifying the site and particularly the extent of the lesion in many cases of spinal cord disease. A grade of 1+ defines a gait deficit barely evident in a limb. Grade 2+ defines a deficit easily seen at normal gaits and exaggerated readily with maneuvers such as turning tightly on a slope. Grade 3+ defines a deficit severe enough to make the horse stumble and possibly fall when maneuvered. A limb deficit is graded 4+ when the horse stumbles or falls while walking in a straight line.

With most lesions of white matter in the brainstem and between C_1-T_2, the gain deficit is about one grade worse in the hindlegs than in the forelegs. Lesions also involving ventral horn cells in the grey matter supplying the forelegs (C_6-T_2) cause marked foreleg weakness and a more severe grade of foreleg gait deficit when compared with the hindlegs. A similar profound weakness, but involving restricted muscle groups, occurs with peripheral nerve disease. Selective sensory deficits may be present in such cases. A focal, compressive cervical spinal cord lesion caused by trauma or cervical vertebral malformation may be mild enough to result in only a 1+ deficit in the pelvic limbs and no visible signs of neurologic dysfunction in the thoracic limbs. However, if such a lesion is more severe and results in a 2+ deficit in the pelvic limbs, a mild (1+) neurologic deficit is visible in the thoracic limbs. On the other hand, diffuse spinal cord diseases such as WEE, EHV-1 myelitis and, in particular, equine degenerative myeloencephalopathy may result in neurologic signs as severe in the thoracic limbs as in the pelvic limbs. Also, a horse with a 4+ gait deficit in the pelvic limbs and a 1+ deficit in the thoracic limbs must have more than one lesion. In such animals, a severe lesion is probably present between T_3 and S_2, and another mild lesion cranial to T_3.

Paraplegic and tetraplegic horses should be encouraged to stand and walk unless there is a suspicion of a vertebral fracture. A horse paraplegic from spinal cord disease that can "dog-sit" for several minutes at a time usually has a lesion between T_2-S_2.

To detect these neurologic deficits, a horse should be observed while standing still and moving under various conditions. Horses with proprioceptive deficits often stand with their feet wide apart or crossed for prolonged periods. Limb weakness is often seen as muscle tremors and a tendency to buckle over on the affected limb. Tetraparetic horses usually drag the toes of each foot while walking in a straight line. Ataxia is usually seen as swaying of the pelvis and sometimes the trunk, and also as swinging of the feet in or out while they are advanced. This results in faulty foot placement in an abducted or adducted position.

Stumbling from scuffing the ground with a foot may be the result of weakness and/or ataxia. Hypermetria and spasticity may be evident at this stage. A difference in stride length is most easily detected by walking next to or behind the horse, matching stride for stride. A shorter than normal stride is usually seen in a spastic leg and a longer than normal stride in a weak leg. Weakness in a pelvic limb is often confirmed by walking beside the horse and pulling laterad on the tail. Normal horses can resist a considerable amount of lateral pulling but weak horses are easily pulled to the side

and put off stride. Trotting a horse in a straight line sometimes exaggerates ataxia, and sharply turning an ataxic horse while trotting often results in a wide circumduction of the outside pelvic limb and even interference.

Many horses with marked gait deficiencies due to spinal cord, brainstem or cerebellar disease have a tendency to pace at a walk and while attempting to trot. Weak horses often drag the toes on the ground at a trot; however, some normal horses have this characteristic gait at a trot and are referred to as "daisy cutters." Therefore, caution must be used in interpreting this finding. The horse should be walked in tight circles. Any tendency to circumduct or cross the limbs is often accentuated and implies a proprioceptive deficit.

The horse's head should be elevated while walking in straight lines and in circles on a slope. These 2 maneuvers are extremely helpful because they frequently exacerbate a subtle gait disorder. In particular, hindlimb ataxia and slight forelimb spasticity or hypermetria are exaggerated. Typically, horses with a very mild cervical spinal cord lesion and normal forelimb gait on flat ground show signs of a forelimb deficit when maneuvered on a slope with the head elevated. These signs often include lack of carpal flexion while the horse descends the slope akin to a marching tin soldier. Such horses also show some delay in forefoot placement while turning and stab the toes into the ground when ascending the slope. While being turned as tightly as possible, a horse may leave a forelimb or hindlimb in one place and pivot on it. This is interpreted as marked ataxia or as weakness in that limb. Tendencies for a horse to circumduct, cross and step on its own limbs are also exaggerated by this maneuver.

Horses with marked limb spasticity often leave that limb fixed to the ground when attempting to back up. This results in awkward posturing and possibly a fall, and also may be seen when one or more limbs are profoundly weak. Spastic, hypermetric hindlimb flexion (stringhalt-like action) is usually exaggerated by backing the horse.

The horse should be walked over small obstacles or a curb to evaluate foot placement. Horses with marked ataxia often "clip" such obstacles, but most horses with subtle spinal cord disease signs perform rather well in such a test.

It is sometimes necessary to observe a horse while jumping to detect subtle gait deficits.

This is particularly so when the owner's complaints refer to such activity.

Most horses with spinal cord disease do not show any marked gait deterioration when blindfolded. This is in contrast to horses with vestibular and some cerebellar diseases, which usually have a greater degree of spasticity and ataxia (staggering) when blindfolded.

Finally, it can be helpful to look for gait deficits while a horse is running free in a paddock. The spastic, hypermetric gait frequently seen with cerebellar disease can become profound when the affected horse attempts to run. Horses weak and ataxic due to diseases at various sites often sink down in the pelvis when stopping suddenly from a canter and the limbs are often flung wildly about just prior to stopping.

Neck and Forelimbs

Having completed the evaluation for head signs and gait abnormalities, the clinician should know if there is (are) a brain, cranial nerve, spinal cord, peripheral spinal nerve or muscle lesion(s). This phase of the examination focuses attention on the neck and thoracic limbs to localize the lesion(s) to a particular spinal cord segment between C_1 and T_2, neck or forelimb peripheral nerve, or neck and forelimb muscle. The same examination procedure is used with minor variations for ambulatory and recumbent patients.

The neck and forelimbs are inspected closely for signs of malformation, deviation, muscle atrophy, and the degree of strength and voluntary effort. A horse standing with its head continuously held close to the ground may have a painful or restrictive cervical lesion. More frequently this is a sign of diffuse cervical muscle weakness seen in lower motor neuron diseases such as forage poisoning. A tetraplegic horse that can lift its head and neck off the ground most likely has a lesion at C_7-T_2. In contrast, a tetraplegic horse with a severe focal lesion at C_1 or C_2 usually cannot lift its head and cranial part of the neck off the ground. If such a lesion is at C_4 or C_5, the horse can usually lift its head and cranial neck off the ground with sufficient stimulation but the caudal part of the neck remains on the ground. At this stage, any sign of excessive sweating (hyperhidrosis) should be evident, which usually indicates involvement of the sympathetic supply to the affected skin areas. Horses with Horner's syndrome (see Neurologic Problems) usually show sweating on the lateral aspect of the cranial part of the neck. Peripheral cervical nerve

lesions usually result in well-demarcated strips of sweating on the neck at the level of the lesion(s) and concomitant localized hypalgesia, hyporeflexia and muscle atrophy in the area of hyperhidrosis. Horner's syndrome, in conjunction with sweating over the entire neck and body, indicates a total interruption of the descending sympathetic pathway within the brainstem or spinal cord cranial to T_3.

The neck and forelimbs should be palpated to assess muscle mass and bone symmetry. The articular and, more frequently, the transverse processes of the cervical vertebrae are palpable and are often prominent at C_4-C_6 in a thin horse. Greatly enlarged, asymmetric articular processes can be palpated and asymmetric atrophy of the lateral cervical musculature, especially the caudal part of the branchiocephalicus muscle, has been palpated in conjunction with several types of lesions of the caudal cervical spinal cord grey matter. When palpating cervical muscle mass, the neck and head must be held straight and moved from side to side since asymmetric posture can markedly alter the muscle tone and apparent muscle bulk. This is of greatest importance when palpating muscles of the forelimbs in a standing horse; slight changes in posture make considerable differences in palpable muscle volume.

Cervical muscle tone can be difficult to evaluate objectively. In a recumbent horse, forelimb muscle tone is assessed by passively flexing and extending all joints while noting the amount of resistance to movement. A limb totally flaccid to such manipulation, with palpably atonic (flabby) muscles, may be caused by a lower motor neuron lesion (spinal cord ventral grey matter, peripheral nerves or muscles) in that limb. Such lesions cause profound weakness, greatly reduced voluntary effort and depressed reflexes. Also, muscle atrophy develops in the affected limb within 1-2 weeks.

Limb and neck manipulation assists in detecting musculoskeletal defects. Many horses without cervical spinal cord or cervical nerve lesions are reluctant to have their necks flexed laterally. Therefore, caution is required in interpreting such a finding, and repeated observations and manipulations are required to determine if there is reluctance or inability to flex the neck for reasons other than true neck pain. The latter has been detected unequivocally with spinal meningitis, cervical vertebral osteomyelitis, greatly enlarged articular processes associated with degenerative joint disease, neurofibromas of cervical nerves and cervical soft tissue foreign bodies. The fore-limbs cannot always be manipulated if the patient is standing, but this must be done if there is a marked gait deficit in only one forelimb. Squeezing and pressing down on the withers causes a horse with marked weakness in one or both forelimbs to buckle in the affected limb(s).

Postural reactions cannot be performed on adult horses but should be considered at this stage of the examination of foals. Wheelbar-rowing is performed by lifting the hindlegs off the ground and making the foal walk forward on only the forelegs. Hopping reactions are evaluated by lifting each forelimb in turn, as well as both hindlimbs, off the ground and making the foal hop sideways. These sensitive tests exaggerate subtle neurologic deficits due to asymmetric brain and spinal cord lesions that may not be detected during gait evaluation. These reactions require intact ascending proprioceptive pathways from the forelimbs to the cerebellum and brainstem, and descending motor pathways from the brainstem to the forelimbs. Also, the motor neurons, peripheral nerves and muscles must be functioning. A lesion any place along these pathways may result in delayed onset of movement and slow limb placement. Foals with spastic or hyper-metric gaits from cervical spinal cord or cere-bellar disease, respectively, may perform these reactions with exaggerated lifting of the feet after delayed initiation of movement.

Neck and forelimb spinal reflexes and sen-sation are next assessed. It is a common mis-take to stimulate the neck or forelimbs with hemostats or a needle and interpret the result-ing neck or forelimb movement as evidence of intact sensation. In fact, such responses occur in tetraplegic horses with the spinal cord sev-ered at C_1. Assessment of stimulus perception requires observation of a cerebral/behavioral response such as head and body movement away from the stimulus, phonation or attack directed toward the stimulus or examiner. In recumbent patients a pronounced raising of the upper eyelids or an attempt to elevate the head is evidence of perception of a noxious stimulus to the neck and forelimbs. Localized sensory deficits on the neck or forelimbs of an ambula-tory patient usually indicate a peripheral nerve lesion. Horses tetraplegic from a severe spinal cord lesion have cervical and thoracic limb hy-palgesia or analgesia caudal to the lesion.

There are several consistent responses when the skin on the lateral aspect of the neck is tapped with a blunt instrument such as hemo-stats. The subcutaneous musculature of the neck contracts, causing localized flicking of the skin. In addition, other lateral cervical mus-cles, such as the brachiocephalicus, contract if the stimulus is strong enough. Brachiocephal-icus muscle contraction is most prominent when the skin over the muscle is tapped in the caudal part of the neck, which results in the shoulder jerking forward and sometimes in slight head retraction toward the side of the stimulus. In conjunction with these local re-sponses there is twitching of the lips (grima-cing) and flicking of the ear on the same side as the stimulus. The lip twitch may be more prominent if the caudal part of the neck is stimulated, whereas the ear flick may be prom-inent when the cranial part of the neck is stim-ulated. The exact pathways for these responses are not known, although suppressed and ab-sent responses have been detected with various lesions in the cervical spinal cord. Localized deficits tend to occur caudal to the level of the lesions. Markedly exaggerated responses have been seen in a horse with protozoal myeloen-cephalitis lesions in the medulla oblongata and in a foal with cranial neck, C_1 and C_2 nerve root, and vagosympathetic trunk injury on the side of hyperresponsiveness. Interpretation of this finding is difficult.

An interesting response has been observed consistently in normal horses and undoubtedly requires certain pathways in the cervical spinal cord to be intact.[1] By slapping a normal horse firmly just behind the scapula on the dorsolat-eral aspect of the withers, the contralateral ar-ytenoid cartilage momentarily adducts as seen through a fiberoptic endoscope. This is known as the "slap test." Initial adduction is followed by abduction of the arytenoid cartilages and vocal folds. If the stimulus is excessive, both arytenoid cartilages and even the entire larynx and pharynx may move. Some horses with cervical vertebral malformation or protozoal myeloencephalitis involving the medulla ob-longata and cervical spinal cord have poor or absent slap test responses. Several horses with asymmetric cervical spinal cord lesions and those with laryngeal hemiplegia have asym-metric responses.

Thoracic limb spinal reflexes are assumed to be present in horses that can walk with the forelimbs. An important spinal reflex in the forelimbs that should be tested in all foals and in recumbent horses is the withdrawal reflex. This is performed by pinching the skin of the pastern with a pair of hemostats and observing for flexion of the fetlock, knee, elbow and shoulder, and subsequent limb withdrawal. This reflex tests the afferent sensory fibers in the median and ulnar nerves, grey matter at C_6-T_2 and efferent motor fibers in the axillary, musculocutaneous, median and ulnar nerves. Lesions along this pathway result in a depressed or absent withdrawal reflex. This and all other spinal reflexes involving the limbs must not be assessed while the horse is lying on the limb. Also, these reflexes are depressed in horses recumbent for any reason.

Pastern stimulation may result in extension of the contralateral limb in addition to very active withdrawal of the ipsilateral limb. Such a crossed extensor reflex, if prominent and repeatable, is good evidence of a lesion in the descending motor pathways cranial to C_7 because these motor pathways have a calming influence on many spinal reflexes; loss of this inhibiting effect results in hyperactive reflexes. In this case the normally inhibited tendency to extend the contralateral limb is expressed.

Peripheral nerve lesions in the thoracic limbs result in well-defined syndromes as discussed below under Neurologic Problems. The more distal the site of damage to these and any other peripheral nerves, the more precise the deficits of weakness, muscle atrophy, reflex and sensory loss, and localized sweating.

Trunk and Hindlimbs

Lesions of the white matter in the brainstem, cerebellum and spinal cord between C_1-T_2 cause gait deficits in the hindlimbs and forelimbs. By this stage of the examination, lesions within those areas have been localized. If the only deficit detected by this stage is a hindlimb gait deficit, there is most likely a spinal cord lesion between T_3-S_3 or in the hindlimb peripheral nerves or muscles. This phase of the examination is an attempt to more precisely localize such a lesion. As suggested above, a small lesion of the white matter of the brainstem or spinal cord from C_1-T_2 may result in subtle hindlimb ataxia and weakness, but no forelimb neurologic signs. In such a case, close examination of the trunk and hindlimbs does not reveal evidence of a lesion between T_3-S_3; the examiner is then able to state only that there is a lesion in the spinal cord cranial to S_3, or in the hindlimb peripheral nerves or muscles.

The trunk and hindlimbs are observed from each side and the back for evidence of musculoskeletal malformations, vertebral column deviations and muscle atrophy. Mild to moderate lordosis and kyphosis are often present with no neurologic deficits, but relatively severe asymmetric lesions of the thoracolumbar spinal cord result in scoliosis with the concave side directed away from the side of major involvement. Gluteal muscle atrophy is a frequent finding in protozoal myeloencephalitis and is the result of lesions of the ventral grey column at L_6. Gluteal atrophy may be seen with any lesion involving L_6 or the cranial gluteal nerve, and is of course also seen with several musculoskeletal diseases of the pelvis.

The degree of effective voluntary effort in the pelvic limbs should be assessed in recumbent horses. If such a horse can attain a dog-sitting posture for several minutes at a time, there is most likely a lesion between T_2-S_2. Wherever possible, paraplegic horses should be assisted to stand and walk to assess voluntary effort. However, reasonable voluntary effort should not be equated with the ability to support weight. For example, after several days a foal with a severely lacerated spinal cord at T_{14} may support weight on its pelvic limbs, which are spastic and have hyperactive reflexes, without being able to step normally. Quite often when there is very mild ataxia and weakness in the forelimbs and a profound neurologic gait deficit in the hindlimbs, the forelimb signs are excused as being the effect of the hindlimb signs. In most cases this is not so and there is a lesion cranial to T_3. Any areas of localized sweating are important to note at this stage as they frequently indicate a lesion of the peripheral nerve and its sympathetic fibers supplying the skin.

The muscles, vertebrae and limb bones should be palpated to detect musculoskeletal malformation and muscle atrophy. The horse should be made to support weight on each hindlimb while the limb muscles are palpated because muscle volume changes markedly with changes in posture and weight-bearing. Muscle tone is assessed in recumbent patients, and passive flexion and extension of the relaxed limbs indicate whether the limbs are flaccid or spastic. Total flaccidity of a limb in a paraplegic horse strongly suggests a lower motor neuron lesion in the limb, whereas limb stiffness, even when the paraplegic horse appears relaxed, suggests an upper motor neuron lesion of white matter cranial to L_4.

If the patient is ambulatory, a loin pressure maneuver should be performed by quickly pinching and pressing down with the fingers on the loin and dorsal hip region. Weak horses usually sink down in the hindquarters, whereas strong horses extend and fix the vertebral column and hindlimbs to resist the pressure. Pulling the tail to each side as the horse walks allows detection of a weak pelvic limb. Such horses are easily pulled toward the affected side and are put off stride. As for the forelimbs, postural reactions should be considered when examining foals. The hopping reaction is performed by elevating the forelimbs and one hindlimb off the ground and observing the hopping movements of the other hindlimb when the foal is moved to the side. Subtle degrees of ataxia and weakness become evident during this test. In addition, hemiwalking is useful to detect subtle degrees of asymmetric deficits in the limbs on one side of the body compared with those on the other side. Both limbs on one side of the body are supported and the foal is made to hop sideways. Paresis and ataxia are apparent as slow initiation of lateral stepping and a tendency to stumble.

Sensory perception in the flanks, back, pelvis and hindlimbs is assessed in recumbent as well as ambulatory patients. A line of hypalgesia on one or both sides of the flanks and back is a very helpful localizing sign. There may be a strip of hypalgesia or analgesia if the dorsal grey matter, dorsal nerve roots or spinal nerves are damaged. Hypalgesia of the body may occur caudal to the level of a major lesion of a large part of the spinal cord. The latter situation warrants a very poor prognosis because the multisynaptic fibers transmitting pain impulses appear to be most resistant to damage; therefore, there must be a severe spinal cord lesion to result in this sign.

Partial hypalgesia of the pelvic limbs (except the medial stifle area) occurs with sciatic nerve lesions. Specific areas of hypalgesia resulting from peroneal and tibial nerve lesions are difficult to detect. Proximal lesions of the femoral nerve result in hypalgesia of the medial stifle and tibial area, which is innervated by the saphenous nerve. It is occasionally necessary to use as an electric prod to assess sensation in a horse recumbent for some time.

Prominent skin flicking over the thorax and flank occurs in normal horses in response to prodding these areas with a blunt object and is known as the panniculus response. The pathway for this response is assumed to be via segmental sensory nerves into the thoracolumbar spinal cord, ascending in white matter tracts to the caudal cervical segment and to the subcuticular muscles of the thorax and flank (panniculus muscle) via the lateral thoracic nerve.

Severe lesions of the thoracolumbar spinal cord result in despression of this reflex over the thorax and flank caudal to the level of the lesion due to interruption of the sensory fibers ascending the spinal cord. Various asymmetric lesions of the caudal cervical spinal cord result in asymmetric suppression of the panniculus response. The suppression is most obvious on the side of the body in which the spinal cord lesion is more severe.

Hindlimb spinal reflexes should be evaluated in all foals and recumbent horses. The patellar reflex is readily elicited by supporting the partly flexed limb and tapping the middle patellar ligament with a firm instrument such as a short piece of iron pipe 3 cm in diameter or a large pair of needle holders. The reflex initiated is momentary extension of the stifle and back from contraction of the quadriceps muscle. Sensory and motor pathways for this reflex are contained in the femoral nerve and pass through the nerve roots and ventral grey matter column at $L_{4.5}$. This sensitive reflex is frequently exaggerated and may cause clonus (bobbing of the limb as it continues to extend after the initial reflex) with lesions of the white matter cranial to L_4.

The hindlimb withdrawal reflex is performed by pinching the skin of the pastern with a pair of hemostats and observing flexion of all hindlimb joints. This reflex involves sensory and motor pathways in the sciatic nerve and passes through the L_6-S_1 segments. Full hip joint flexion in this reflex requires intact lumbar spinal cord segments, segmental lumbar nerves and sublumbar muscles. As for the forelimbs, a brisk response with extension of the contralateral limb may occur with lesions of the descending motor pathways to the L_6-S_1 segments due to loss of the calming influence of upper motor neurons.

It is very difficult to interpret limb reflexes if the horse is lying on the limb. Also, recumbency in adult horses very quickly leads to suppressed limb reflexes as a result of decubitus formation, ischemia and exhaustion. Recumbent horses should be turned frequently and reflexes evaluated in the upper limbs.

Specific neurologic deficits from lesions of peripheral nerves to the hindlimbs are discussed under Neurologic Problems.

Tail and Anus

This phase of the neurologic examination is likely to be just as rewarding as any other phase, yet it is surprising how often it is omitted. An ambulatory horse with a cranial nerve or forelimb gait deficit with muscle atrophy, or hyporeflexia analgesia of the perineum must have more than one lesion. Such a finding is consistent with an infectious or inflammatory mechanism as opposed to degenerative, neoplastic or metabolic disease.

The caudal body region can be inspected for symmetry of bony prominences and muscle mass. Some horses with no evidence of neurologic disease hold their tail to one side when moving. Although some horses are natural "tail-wringers," this somewhat disturbing trait may be acquired. Some horses with severe spinal cord disease and profound gait deficits elevate their tail and hold it to one side. This is apparently an acquired abnormal tail carriage. Some urogenital and painful musculoskeletal diseases may result in tail-wringing or tail elevation, and a few cases of mild, nonsuppurative myeloencephalitis have been associated with it. The cause frequently remains unknown. Many non-neurologic diseases cause a horse to rub its perineum, but this is also seen with neuritis of the cauda equina.

Tail muscle tone is remarkably variable among normal horses and may be affected by age, breed, sex and use. Mild degrees of hypertonia or hypotonia probably go undetected. Tail muscle atony is caused by trauma and neuritis of the cauda equina that damage the sacrococcygeal motor nerves. This is often accompanied by analgesia, areflexia and finally muscle atrophy if the lesion is severe.

Anal and tail reflexes are tested by gently prodding the perineum and observing reflex contraction of the anal sphincter and clamping down of the tail. The anal reflex requires intact pudendal nerves and S_1-S_3 segments, and the tail reflex requires intact sacral and coccygeal segments and nerves. A severe spinal cord lesion may cause total analgesia of the tail and anus but reflexes are intact and possibly hyperactive if the lesion is cranial to S_1. Therefore, as with all spinal reflex testing, sensory perception of the stimulus must be assesed separately from reflex action. For example, a foal with massive spinal cord lesion at C_1 due to trauma is tetraplegic, with no voluntary effort in the limbs. After several hours to days, spinal reflexes in the forelimbs, hindlimbs, tail and anus are present and hyperactive. Moderate stimulation of the hindquarters with hemostats often results in flicking of the tail and paddling movements of the limbs. This is the result of a spread of reflex activity within the spinal cord and should not be equated with voluntary effort. In such a case, if total limb and body analgesia is present 48 hours after the injury, the prognosis is totally hopeless despite reflex spinal movements.

Rectal palpation should be performed during this phase of the examination to evaluate rectal and urinary bladder content and tone. These structures are innervated by the sacral segments and nerves, particularly S_1-S_3. Lesions of the ventral grey column at S_1-S_3 or of the sacral or pelvic nerves result in rectal flaccidity and bladder atony, with subsequent accumulation of feces and urine. Horses with such a lesion may pass feces with considerable straining and urine may passively flow from the overdistended bladder; however, obstipation, incontinence and retention cystitis usually result. Diffuse spinal cord lesions may result in urinary incontinence possibly due to the inability to posture and void urine. Sudangrass toxic myelopathy and EHV-1 myelitis frequently result in this sign. Recumbent horses usually develop a distended urinary bladder which, if not periodically emptied, results in necrotic cystitis and possible bladder rupture.

The equine spinal cord terminates at the middle of the sacrum. Caudal to that point there are only sacral and coccygeal nerve roots that pass caudad to exit at their corresponding intervertebral foramina. Therefore, a cranial sacral lesion results in denervation of the tail, perineum, anus, rectum and bladder.

Lesion Location

It cannot be overemphasized that it is the *location* of the lesion(s) that is first elucidated by the neurologic examination. After the lesion is localized, the possible causes can be considered, and a diagnostic and therapeutic plan instituted. The following is a summary of neurologic signs seen with lesions in specific locations.

Cerebrum

Behavioral abnormalities, depression, coma, central blindness with intact pupillary light reflexes, and seizures characterize cerebral lesions. Horses with unilateral lesions often circle and hold their head toward the side of the lesion, and there may be contralateral blindness and contralateral facial hypalgesia. Seizures may be localized (contralateral face or body), generalized, or localized with secondary generalization. Dysphagia associated with poor voluntary jaw, facial muscle, tongue and pharyngeal movement is common. In the peracute phase, a mild gait deficit may be evident in the contralateral limbs. This may be more evident in foals as poor performance in postural reaction testing. Gait and postural reaction changes are always mild and temporary.

Brainstem

The most prominent signs of brainstem lesions are marked depression, cranial nerve deficits and gait abnormalities that vary with location of the lesion.

Rostral Brainstem (Thalamus): Lesions in this area cause variable depression and behavioral abnormalities, and a tendency to circle toward the side of the lesion with any stimulation; this is the adversive phenomenon. Generalized seizures may be seen. Central, contralateral blindness with intact pupillary light reflexes are also seen with unilateral thalamic lesions. Severe bilateral lesions of the optic tracts produce blindness and dilated, unresponsive pupils. Localized lesions of the optic nerve (II) produce ipsilateral blindness and a dilated pupil unresponsive to light directly shone in it but consensually responsive. There may be hypalgesia of the body, particularly of the head. Any gait deficits are usually subtle and temporary, as with cerebral lesions.

Mid-Brainstem (Midbrain): Severe depression or coma with pupillary changes are most common with lesions of the midbrain. Lesions of an oculomotor nerve or nucleus produce an ipsilateral dilated pupil that is unresponsive to light shone into either eye; however, the ipsilateral eye has vision. The eyeballs may be deviated and there is usually tetraplegia or spastic tetraparesis that may be asymmetric.

Caudal Brainstorm (Pons and Medulla): Lesions in this region result in variable degrees of depression, cranial nerve deficits, head tilt, ataxia and asymmetric spastic tetraparesis. Cranial nerve deficits cause facial hypalgesia and hyporeflexia (V sensory), masseter muscle atrophy (V motor), facial paralysis and hyporeflexia (VII), head tilt, nystagmus and eye deviations (VIII), and dysphagia (V, VII and particularly IX, X and XII). Damage to peripheral cranial nerves results in various combinations of these signs but there is no depression or gait deficit, except for a staggering gait with vestibular nerve (VIII) damage.

Cerebellum

Diffuse cerebellar disease results in depressed menace responses without blindness, head tremor and hypermetric or spastic ataxia of all 4 limbs, with preservation of strength. With asymmetric cerebellar lesions, these signs are more pronounced ipsilateral to the more severe part of the lesion. The neck and trunk may sway at rest. Vestibular signs occur occasionally and may be more evident contralateral to a unilateral cerebellar lesion.

Spinal Cord

Diseases affecting the spinal cord white matter result in various degrees of ataxia, weakness, spasticity and hypermetria in the ipsilateral limb(s) caudal to the most cranial aspect of the lesion. Paraplegia or tetraplegia results from massive lesions. Mild to moderate lesions between C_1-C_6 result in a gait deficit usually more evident in the hindlimbs than in the forelimbs. In addition, spinal reflexes in the limbs caudal to such a lesion may be hyperactive. Severe cervical and thoracic cord white matter lesions may result in poor cervical and panniculus responses, respectively. There may be hypalgesia of the neck or trunk caudal to the level of severe lesions. Additional lower motor neuron signs, such as profound weakness, hypotonia, hyporeflexia, muscle atrophy, and localized sensory deficits and sweating, are strong indications of spinal cord grey matter (or peripheral nerve) involvement. Such signs in the forelimbs indicate a lesion between C_7-T_2 and such signs in the rearlimbs indicate a lesion between L_4-S_2. Urinary incontinence may occur with spinal cord lesions cranial to S_4. This sign is prominent with lesions of the grey matter at S_1-S_3, and is typically accompanied by rectal and anal flaccidity. Lesions of the grey matter or nerve roots from S_1 caudad result in a flaccid, areflexic tail.

Peripheral Nerves and Muscles

Muscle diseases and those that damage peripheral nerve motor fibers produce hypotonia, areflexia, profound weakness and muscle atrophy in the affected limb or muscle, all of which characterize lower motor neuron disease. With involvement of sympathetic and sensory fibers, peripheral nerve lesions result in localized sweating and occasionally sensory deficits. Both signs may be well demarcated when a peripheral nerve is involved but are usually poorly defined with spinal nerve root lesions.

Diffuse lower motor neuron diseases, such as polyneuropathy and polymyopathy, may result in head, limb, body and tail signs.

Cause of the Lesion

After deciding on the presence, location and extent of the neurologic lesions(s), the most likely etiologic mechanism should be considered and a list of differential diagnoses constructed. From this point, the clinician can develop a diagnostic and therapeutic plan, and give the client a realistic prognosis. Etiologic mechanisms have certain distinguishing characteristics as follows:

Malformation

Congenital malformations of nervous tissue result in neurologic signs by the time the animal walks. Not all congenital malformations are hereditary, but may be due to *in utero* toxic, nutritional, physical and infectious processes. Developmental malformations are acquired for the most part. Nervous tissue may be compressed by a malformed calvarium or vertebral column. Under these conditions the signs may not be detectible at birth but have a later onset, and may be progressive or intermittent with repeated compression of nervous tissue. Radiographs are very useful to demonstrate skull and vertebral malformations.

Infection and Inflammation

These mechanisms include diseases caused by viruses, bacteria, fungi, helminths and arthropods, as well as inflammatory and granulomatous diseases of immunologic and unknown etiology. These diseases may be acute or chronic and are usually progressive, although spontaneous healing may occur. Outbreaks can occur and often affect certain age groups. Asymmetric and multifocal lesions are characteristic of these mechanisms. Clinicopathologic evidence of systemic involvement and abnormal results of CSF analysis are helpful in diagnosis. Serologic and microbiologic examination may assist in definitive diagnosis.

Trauma

The initial signs of nervous system trauma are acute in onset, usually stabilize within 24 hours and improve thereafter. Secondary effects of CNS edema, hematoma or reparative callus formation may alter the course of events following nervous system trauma. Lesions are usually well localized but multifocal trauma may easily mimic an acute infectious process. Radiographic evaluation and improvement with time and therapy are useful diagnostic and prognostic aids in trauma cases. Repeated nervous system trauma may result from malformation of the calvarium or vertebral column.

Toxic, Nutritional, Metabolic

These mechanisms frequently result in symmetric signs that are acute or subacute in onset and that vary in location and intensity with time. Systemic involvement is the rule rather than the exception and herd outbreaks can occur.

Removal of offending poisons and specific therapy often result in spectacular improvement.

Vascular

Vascular accidents in the nervous system may result from thrombi, emboli, aneurysms, and inflammatory and immune-mediated vasculitides. There is usually an acute onset of signs that stabilize within 48 hours and frequently regress. The end result of vascular accidents is leakage of plasma or blood from vessels. The clinical course and changes in CSF composition associated with nervous system vascular disease may mimic those of trauma.

Degeneration

This mechanism includes many diseases of unknown etiology. As specific causes become known, such diseases can be redefined as congenital, traumatic, toxic, metabolic, nutritional, endocrine, immunologic or vascular processes. Some degenerative diseases involve a hereditary deficiency of a specific metabolic enzyme, resulting in defective metabolism and often in characteristic morphologic features. These processes tend to progress and result in symmetric, diffuse lesions.

Neoplasia

Neoplasms that produce neurologic signs are rare in horses. Those that involve the CNS are almost always secondary and include lymphosarcoma, melanosarcoma and hemangiosarcoma. Clinical signs resulting from such tumors are generally chronic but may have a surprisingly rapid onset. Primary nerve sheath tumors, such as neurofibromas, occur in the peripheral nervous system and result in specific deficits that often include localized pain.

Adenomatous changes in the pars intermedia of the pituitary are common in old horses but rarely result in signs recognizable during neurologic examination.

Diagnostic Aids

Organ biopsy and function testing, and hematologic, microbiologic, radiographic and serologic examination assist in diagnosis and management of neurologic diseases. Cerebrospinal fluid analysis, neuroradiographic examination, electrodiagnostic testing, and peripheral nerve and muscle biopsy are diagnostic aids in neurologic case management.

Cerebrospinal Fluid Analysis

The procedures for obtaining a CSF sample from the atlanto-occipital and lumbosacral sites in horses have been described.[2,3] Samples

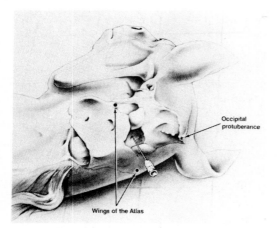

Fig 4. For CSF collection from the atlanto-occipital site, the horse is placed in lateral recumbency and the head is positioned 90° to the median axis of the neck. The needle is inserted at the intersection of a line drawn between the cranial edges of the wings of the atlas (black circles) and the midline, indicated by the occipital protuberance (black cross). (Courtesy of the Cornell Veterinarian)

of CSF can be obtained from the lumbosacral site in standing horses, and from the atlanto-occipital and lumbosacral sites in recumbent horses under general anesthesia.

A CSF sample can be obtained from the atlanto-occipital site by needle insertion at the middle of a line drawn between the cranial borders of the wings of the atlas (Fig 4). The subarachnoid space is entered with a 3½-inch, 18- or 20-ga spinal needle at a depth of 1-2½ inches and is felt as a sudden loss of resistance to needle passage. Ten ml of CSF can be removed safely. The area for needle insertion at the lumbosacral site is the palpable depression on the dorsal midline just caudal to the spine of L_6, just cranial to the sacral spines and between the paired tubera sacrale (Figs 5, 6). This site is about level with the highest points of the rump. A 6- to 8-inch 18-ga spinal needle is required because the subarachnoid space is at a considerable depth. A change in resistance may be felt when this space is entered and usually there is some response by the horse, such as a flick of the tail to indicate correct placement of the needle.

The WBC and RBC are counted using a hemacytometer and diluting fluid, and a differential WBC count is performed if there are more than 5 WBC/μl CSF. A cytocentrifuge or microfiltration technic may be used to prepare a slide of the cells for differential morphologic classification. These methods are not always

available and, because WBC in CSF degenerate rapidly, a simple sedimentation chamber can be used (Fig 7). One ml of CSF is placed in the chamber and left to stand for 25 minutes. The supernatant is then aspirated off, the glass cylinder is snapped off the slide, the remaining CSF is removed with bibulous paper gently applied to the center of the paraffin ring, and the wax is removed with a scalpel blade. The sample of sedimented cells is then fixed and stained with a blood smear stain, dried and covered with a mounting medium and cover glass. The CSF protein content should be determined using a technic standardized between 0-200 mg/dl. Normal values for equine CSF analysis are shown in Table 1.

Increased opening CSF pressure values are not often detected in the horse. The CSF pressure can be high due to a space-occupying mass within the calvarium or as a result of CSF flow obstruction within the vertebral canal. Excessive flexion of the neck during measurement may produce falsely elevated readings.

Normal CSF is clear and colorless. Protein contents above 150 mg/dl and WBC counts

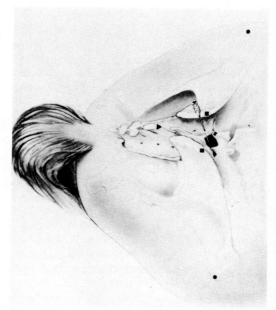

Fig 5. The approximate site of CSF collection from the lumbosacral site is the midpoint of a line joining the caudal borders of the tubera coxarum (black circles). The exact site is a palpable depression bordered craniad by the caudal edge of the sixth lumbar vertebra (black cross), laterad by the tubera sacrale (black squares), and caudad by the cranial edge of the first or second sacral vertebra (black triangle). (Courtesy of the Cornell Veterinarian)

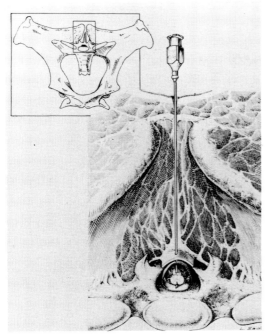

Fig 6. Lumbosacral CSF collection from the horse. Cranial view of the pelvis, sacrum and area of dissection (insert). In the transverse dissection through the lumbosacral articulations, the spinal needle passes through the skin, thoracolumbar fascia adjacent to the interspinous ligaments, interarcuate ligament, dorsal dura mater and arachnoid, dorsal arachnoid space and conus medullaris. The needle point is in the ventral subarachnoid space. (Courtesy of the Cornell Veterinarian)

some degenerative, toxic, nutritional and metabolic diseases. Bacterial meningitis results in neutrophilic pleocytosis, whereas most viral CNS diseases produce a lymphocytic to macrocytic response. Neutrophils appear in the CSF in the early stages of EEE virus infection. Mononuclear cells, particularly macrophages containing phagocytic vacuoles, occur in CSF processes that result in tissue damage. Eosinophils are present in the CSF of horses with helminths in the CNS and occasionally in horses with protozoal myeloencephalitis.

The clinical range for protein content in normal equine CSF is 20-85 mg/dl. Occasionally a horse without CNS lesions has a CSF protein content outside this wide range (Table 1). It is, therefore, of some help to compare protein contents of CSF obtained from the atlanto-occipital and lumbosacral sites. A difference of more than 20-25 mg/dl is good evidence of a CNS lesion. The source of protein (lesion) is likely closer to the site from which the sample with the higher protein content was obtained. Leakage of blood or plasma into CSF raises the protein content and occurs in traumatic, vascular, inflammatory and some degenerative diseases. Also, globulin production within the CNS can raise the protein content. This is usually seen only in chronic infectious and possibly in some immune-mediated diseases.

Refractive index, measured with a handheld refractometer (American Optical), is a simple measurement roughly related to protein content. A CSF sample that registers a protein content of 300 mg/dl or more on a urine dipstick test and has a refractive index of 1.3350 or more almost certainly has an elevated protein content.

Neuroradiographic Examination

The use of plain radiography is vital to document fractures, luxations, malformations and

above 50/μl result in opacity. A few thousand RBC per μl result in a pink discoloration. Xanthochromia (yellow discoloration) results from the presence of blood pigments or hemoglobin breakdown products and usually indicates trauma or leakage of plasma or RBC from damaged vessels, such as in vasculitis with EHV-1 myeloencephalitis. A slightly pink discoloration that disappears after centrifugation was probably due to CSF contamination with RBC at the time of collection. Pre-existing subarachnoid hemorrhage rapidly results in xanthochromia from RBC breakdown.

The most important factor in determining the significance of excess RBC in a CSF sample is assessment of the collection procedure. If the first few drops of CSF collected are pink but subsequently collected CSF is clear, the RBC were likely present because of trauma during collection.

Excessive numbers of WBC are present in CSF in traumatic, infectious, neoplastic and

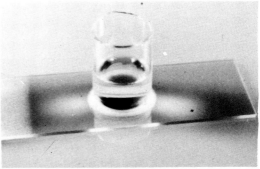

Fig 7. CSF cytology sedimentation chamber.

Table 1. Normal CSF Values

opening pressure (atlanto-occipital site, recumbent)	100-500 mm H_2O
clarity	clear
color	colorless
RBC	0/μl
WBC	0-6/μl
protein (atlanto-occipital or lumbosacral site), 95% confidence limits absolute range	20-85 mg/dl 5-115 mg/dl
protein, atlanto-occipital-lumbosacral difference refractive index	± 25 mg/dl 1.3347-1.3350

occasionally infections and neoplasms of the skull and vertebral column. Objective measurements of the vertebral canal diameter are useful to determine the probability of spinal cord compression in horses with the wobbler syndrome. [4,5]

New radiographic contrast media have made positive-contrast myelography a clinically feasible procedure for investigating spinal cord disease in horses. [5,6] Nevertheless, performance of this procedure is not without possible complications. Some expertise is required to perform a myelogram and experience is required in interpreting the radiographs. Consequently, it is suggested that myelography be done in a horse only when the results of the study could alter the course of action taken in the management of the case. This does not detract from the importance and value of this procedure. It is also suggested that, except for some vertebral fracture repairs, vertebral column and spinal cord surgery should not proceed without myelographic confirmation of the site, extent and nature of the lesion(s). Similar comments are offered for vertebral phlebography, which has some value in identifying the cranial extent of cervical spinal cord compression. [4]

The procedure of myelography is discussed in Chapter 20.

Electrodiagnostic Testing

Needle electromyography (EMG) is a useful diagnostic test in horses to help localize a nervous system lesion (see Chapter 19). [4] The procedure involves placing needle electrodes in the cranial, paravertebral and limb muscles to detect the presence of muscle fibers displaying abnormal electrical activity due to disruption of their nerve supply. With some myopathies and damage to motor neurons in the ventral grey column or in peripheral nerves that innervate muscle fibers, affected muscle fibers undergo a change in their electrical characteristics. After about a week, these denervated muscle fibers develop spontaneous electrical discharges that include excessive insertional activity, positive sharp waves, fibrillation potentials and bizarre high-frequency discharges. Collectively these phenomena are termed denervation potentials and are detected with a needle EMG. Consequently, with certain grey matter lesions and peripheral nerve diseases, an EMG can provide evidence of the presence, location and extent of a lesion and is helpful in the management of such cases. The methodology for needle EMG is the same in all species and interested readers are referred to other sources for details. [7,8]

Electroencephalography (EEG) is used in horses to record the electrical activity of the brain as a superficial montage of summated electrical potentials from the cerebrum. [9] Once the normal patterns are clearly understood, any abnormal EEG readings can be identified. There are particular changes in EEG tracings characteristic of hydrocephalus, encephalitis and space-occupying lesions, such as hematomas, abscesses and neoplasms. The reader is referred to other sources for more information on EEG. [7,8]

Several methods of electrodiagnostic testing have been adapted from human neurology for use in small animals. [10,11] Peripheral nerve conduction velocities have been determined for the horse. [12] These technics, when refined, will assist in defining the extent and nature of certain neurologic disorders for a particular species; however, it will be many years before they are used widely in equine neurology.

Peripheral Nerve and Muscle Biopsy

The reader is referred to other sources for discussions of these procedures. [13,14]

Necropsy

Necropsy of horses affected by neurologic disease often results in localization of suspected lesions and/or discovery of unsuspected lesions of the nervous system. Unlike postmortem examination of other body systems, the CNS within the skull and spinal column presents great difficulties in field necropsy. For this reason, it is probably best to remove the head and take it to your office for examination. The only reasonable way to recover the cervical spinal cord and to examine the vertebrae for wobbler and other lesions is to disarticulate the neck. It is virtually impossible to remove the thoracolumbar spinal cord entirely in the field; however, the renderer may be willing to assist you.

The removal of the brain and spinal cord from the skull and cervical spinal column, respectively, is illustrated in Figure 8.

A good hacksaw or band saw is required for removal of the brain and spinal cord. If a band saw is not available to obtain spinal cord samples for histologic examination, a hatchet and hammer are needed. From the ventral side, the hatchet is set at about a 45-degree angle at the junction of the vertebral body and arch, and the hatchet is struck sharply with the hammer. The process is repeated on the opposite side. The vertebral body is removed after the intervertebral discs are cut with a knife. The spinal cord is then exposed and is cut at each end with a sharp knife and removed with the intact dura. If a band saw is available, a dorsal laminectomy is carefully performed to expose the spinal cord in the dura, and both are removed.

NEUROLOGIC DISEASE

Malformations

Hydrocephalus

Although hydrocephalus has a wide variety of causes, it is apparently very rare in horses. Hydrocephalus is most conveniently described as an increased CSF volume within the ventricular system or subarachnoid space of the head. This condition may be either congenital or acquired, and normotensive or hypertensive. Normotensive hydrocephalus is usually incidental to hypoplasia or loss of brain parenchyma after destructive prenatal or postnatal infection or injury. The CSF volume passively expands to fill the space normally occupied by brain tissue. Therefore, normotensive, compensatory hydrocephalus is the result of, not the cause of, CNS disease. Normotensive hydrocephalus may be expected following massive cerebral destruction in horses surviving diseases such as viral encephalitis or leukoencephalomalacia due to moldy corn poisoning.

In contrast, hypertensive hydrocephalus may cause progressive overt CNS disease by damaging tissue adjacent to expanding ventricles. Hypertensive hydrocephalus is generally a consequence of obstruction of the CSF conduit (especially the mesencephalic aqueduct and lateral apertures) between the sites of production in the third and lateral ventricles, and the sites of absorption by the arachnoid villi in the subarachnoid space. Blockage may be due to hypoplasia or aplasia of a conducting part, or acquired due to inflammation and swelling of, or injury to, the ependymal lining of the aqueduct, lateral apertures or arachnoid villi. Inflammation can be acute, as in neonatal bacterial meningitis, or chronic and proliferative, as in the granulomatous ependymitis of equine infectious anemia. Also, any space-occupying mass, such as a cerebral abscess or large choroid plexus cholesterol granuloma, may result in progressive, hypertensive hydrocephalus. Regardless of the etiology, the end result is usually increased CSF pressure and dilation of the third and lateral ventricles. However, by the time the animal is evaluated, the pressure is usually normal.

Clinical Signs: Hypertensive, obstructive hydrocephalus may cause enlarged calvaria with open sutures in young animals. It should be remembered, however, that many normal neonatal foals, especially those of the Arabian breed, have slightly domed foreheads.

The CNS signs observed are referable to pressure-induced attenuation of cerebral white matter. Most conspicuous are mental disorders such as diminished learning ability, lack of affinity for the dam, and reduced or absent desire or ability to suckle. If the signs are progressive the foal may suffer menace response deficits, loss of vision and profound depression. Animals that survive for extended periods are regarded as "dummies," difficult to train and often unthrifty.[15]

Diagnosis: Plain lateral radiographs may show a characteristic homegeneous, "ground glass" appearance of the cranial cavity.[16]

Direct lateral ventricular paracentesis may be performed at a point 1-2 cm lateral to the intersection of lines drawn from each ear to the lateral canthus of the opposite eye. After surgical preparation, a needle with stylet is intro-

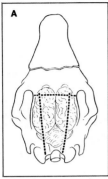

A. Dorsal view of skull showing location of brain. Remove major muscle masses from area of incisions (dotted lines).

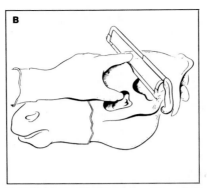

B. Hold head with thumb in eye socket and index finger on saw blade. Cut transversely through frontal bone caudal to supraorbital process.

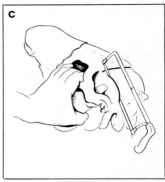

C. Place head on right side. Second cut is sagittal, just medial to left occipital condyle.

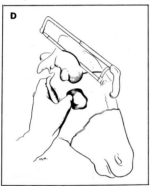

D. Place head on left side for right sagittal cut. Place nose toward you, thumb in eye socket and fingers around mandible.

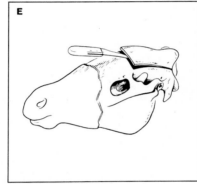

E. Pry up and remove skull cap.

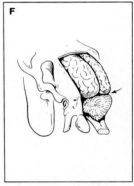

F. Be sure tentorium cerebelli (arrow) and other limiting dura are removed.

Fig 8a. Necropsy technic for removal of the brain. [Adapted from Mod Vet Pract 60 (1979) 109]

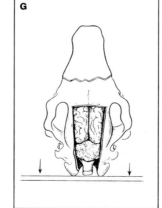

G. With head in upright position, tap it lightly on table to loosen brain.

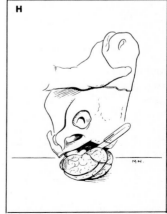

H. Cut olfactory tracts and cranial nerves as brain is removed. Tilt head so that brain *rests* on table. Section, label and place in formalin.

Fig 8b. Necropsy technic for removal of the spinal cord.

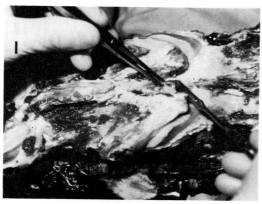

I. Trim soft tissues from cervical vertebral column. Proceed to step L if no bone or joint lesions are suspected. Expose each dorsal intervertebral space, remove epidural fat and grasp dura mater so spinal cord is severed cleanly.

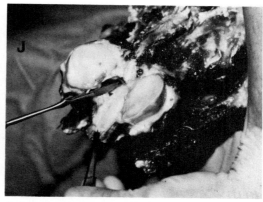

J. Cut spinal nerve roots with thin scalpel inserted from each end of vertebra. Grasp dura mater to expedite severance of spinal nerve roots and pull spinal cord segment free. Split dorsal dura mater longitudinally. Label each section separately and place in formalin.

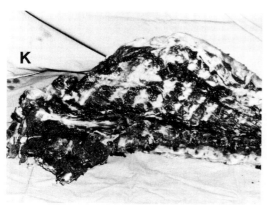

K. Trim soft tissue from thoracic, lumbar and sacral sections of vertebral column and trim down bone with saw. If no band saw is available, place 6- to 12-inch sections in formalin. Pathologist completes removal after fixation.

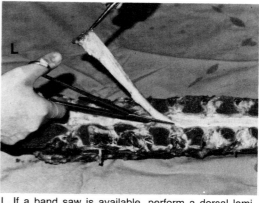

L. If a band saw is available, perform a dorsal laminectomy and remove spinal cord in dura by cutting spinal nerve roots. Split dorsal dura mater longitudinally, label spinal cord and place in formalin.

duced through a hole in the skull made by a guarded Steinmann pin. Easily aspirated fluid indicates probable enlargement of the lateral ventricle. Air can be introduced into the ventricle after removal of a small amount (10-20 ml) of CSF to help outline the ventricular system radiographically.

Treatment: Progressive hydrocephalus might be rationally treated with glucocorticoids, which have been shown experimentally to reduce CSF production in dogs. Excess pressure may first be relieved carefully via ventricular paracentesis. This is followed by the IM administration of dexamethasone (or equivalent) at

0.05 mg/kg body weight twice daily, then once daily after a week. Dexamethasone administration is discontinued after 3 weeks if a satisfactory response is obtained.[15]

Infectious Diseases

Togaviral (Arboviral) Encephalomyelitides

According to recently revised nomenclature, the insect-borne viruses previously known as arboviruses have been grouped in the family Togaviridae, comprising the genera *Alphavirus* and *Flavovirus*.[17-19] The alphaviruses include the agents of western equine encephalomyelitis (WEE), eastern equine encephalomyelitis (EEE), Venezuelan equine encephalomyelitis (VEE) and Semiliki Forest encephalitis, which were previously called Group-A arboviruses.[20]

Several flaviviruses (formerly Group-B arboviruses) affect horses and characteristically cause serologic evidence of infection without associated clinical disease (eg, St. Louis encephalitis, Murray Valley encephalitis).[17,20] The agents of Japanese B encephalitis and louping ill may cause typical signs of viral encephalomyelitis in a small percentage of infected horses.[21-23] The life cycle of flaviviruses requires the use of insect vectors, usually mosquitoes (Japanese B encephalitis, St. Louis encephalitis) or ticks (louping ill, Russian spring-summer encephalitis).

Equine Encephalomyelitis

The loss of hundreds of thousands of horses to the major alphaviral encephalomyelitides (WEE, EEE and VEE) during the last century has had considerable economic and social impact within the American continent.[24] In recent years the importance of these diseases has declined as reliance on horses for transport and agriculture has diminished. As recently as 1971, however, the threatened spread of VEE into the US was of sufficient importance to warrant the declaration of a national state of emergency and the mobilization of the considerble resources of the Department of Defense.[25] These viruses are not only equine pathogens but cause potentially lethal disease in humans.

In general the alphaviruses are maintained in nature by incompletely defined sylvatic cycles involving mosquito vectors and bird or rodent reservoirs. Periodically these viruses "spill" out of their focal reservoirs and infect a wide range of vertebrate hosts, of which the horse is the most severely affected, resulting in epizootics of occasionally devastating proportions.

An extremely productive research effort followed major outbreaks of all 3 diseases during the 1930's, and resulted in the isolation and identification of the agents and the development and widespread use of effective, albeit crude, formalized vaccines.[18]

History and Distribution: Epizootics of WEE have occurred primarily in the western and midwestern US, with the first well-documented outbreaks occurring in Kansas and adjacent states in 1912.[19] An unrelenting series of outbreaks began in California's San Joaquin Valley in 1931 and culminated in the summer

of 1938 with the death of over 180,000 horses.[17,26] Isolation of the virus and development of a successful vaccine quickly followed, as did a rudimentary understanding of the natural history of the disease.

Notable epizootics of WEE have occurred more or less regularly since World War II, but total morbidity has steadily dropped with the decline in horse numbers and the widespread use of effective vaccines. The disease has been recognized in horses in every state west of the Appalachians and in isolated cases in the eastern US, and has caused regular epizootics in western Canada, and Central and South America.[19,27]

The distribution of EEE is more restricted within the US than is WEE, although some overlap (in Florida, Louisiana and Texas) does occur. Since the first putative descriptions from Massachusetts in 1831 and from Long Island in 1845, there have been epizootics in all states on the eastern seaboard and Gulf Coast, and virus isolations in Michigan, Wisconsin and Alberta.[17,19] Serious outbreaks have also occurred in the Caribbean, Dominican Republic, Haiti, Panama, and Central and South America, and there is questionable serologic evidence of the disease in horses in the Philippines.[17,19] The virus was isolated in 1933.[19]

The VEE virus was first isolated during an epizootic in 1938 in Venezuela.[24,25,28] Extremely severe and widespread outbreaks traditionally swept through Venezuela, Colombia, Ecuador and Peru at about 10-year intervals; however, in 1969 an epizootic erupted on the Pacific coastal plain near the Guatamala-El Salvador border and spread to reach Costa Rica in 1970 and the southwest corner of Texas in 1971.[24,25,29] Approximately 1500 horses died of VEE in Texas before further spread of the disease in the US was halted by the immunization of horses with an attenuated vaccine, resulting in an "immune belt" across the southern US.[24,25,29]

No further cases of epizootic VEE have been reported in the US since the 1971 outbreak, although a focus of enzootic Type-II VEE virus exists in the Everglades region of Florida without associated equine disease (see epizootiology section).

Epizootiology: The viruses of WEE and EEE form a relatively homogeneous group with only minor antigenic variations detectible serologically among isolates from North and South America. Some cross-reactivity is encountered between WEE and EEE viruses when using hemagglutination inhibition (HI) and complement-fixation (CF) tests.[18] The prevalence of equine disease due to these agents depends on the size and status of the reservoir, vector, amplifying and "target" (equine) hosts. For successful transfer of virus from reservoir to equine host with subsequent expression of disease, a number of physically conducive conditions must be present.[19]

In nature, WEE and EEE viruses are maintained between epizootics in reservoir hosts that probably include certain birds, rodents and reptiles.[27] Whether these viruses persist as chronic relapsing infections, by occult reservoir host-mosquito cycling, or by some other mechanism is not clear, although persistent infections in a variety of birds and reptiles occur.[19] The viruses periodically spread from rather focal reservoirs out into the general bird population where they are propagated and amplified by rapid bird-mosquito-bird transmission. The mosquito vector for WEE is usually *Culex tarsalis*, and several species of mosquitoes including *Culiseta melanura* are known to transmit EEE among birds.[19] Many avian species become infected, and develop high-order viremia and high serum titers, but do not usually become ill. However, some exotic species, including Chinese pheasants and chukar partridges, may suffer high morbidity and mortality, particularly when infected by EEE virus.[17,19]

Cases of encephalomyelitis usually begin to occur in susceptible horses 2-3 weeks after spread into the bird population.[19] *Culex tarsalis*, an omnivorous feeder, is also responsible for transferring WEE virus from bird to horse. Different vectors are required for EEE transfer, including *Aedes sollicitans* and *Aedes vexans*.[19] The viremia of infected horses is of such low order that further infection of feeding mosquitoes cannot occur.[18] For this reason, horses are often described as "dead end" hosts.[27,30]

Epizootics of EEE and WEE are rather variable with respect to area and time of onset but tend to occur in mid- to late summer when weather conditions (especially warmth and humidity) favor breeding, longevity and mobility of mosquito vector populations.[19] Standing surface water for mosquito larval development, bush cover for wild hosts and the immune status of the various hosts also affect the timing and magnitude of equine epizootics. Many of these physical factors are significantly affected by the cultivation, clearing and irrigation of land, and by drainage of swamps.[19] The equine epizootic usually declines with the onset of cool or dry weather unsuitable for mosquito and/or bird activity and with the depletion of suscep-

tible equine hosts (by death or the development of immunity among survivors).[19]

Many other vertebrate species become infected and seroconvert during an equine epizootic but rarely with serious disease or viremia sufficient to infect feeding mosquitoes.

It is impossible to discuss VEE as a single entity because of the wide variety of subtypes and variants. In general, the VEE complex of viruses can be separated into enzootic and epizootic groups according to their natural history and virulence in horses.[29,30]

The enzootic group, although important in the overall view of VEE, are not known pathogens of horses. They persist in focal, isolated wild rodent-mosquito cycles in South and Central America and Florida.[25] The mosquito vectors of enzootic VEE almost exclusively belong to the *Culex (Melanconion)* subgenus.[28,31] Horses living in close proximity to a focus of enzootic VEE activity usually become infected and seroconvert but do not have signs of disease. In fact, horses with serum titers to enzootic VEE virus may be protected from the virulent epizootic virus.[25]

The natural history of epizootic VEE viruses may resemble WEE and EEE insofar as interepizootic maintenance may depend on silent vertebrate-mosquito cycling, *eg*, possible *Culex*-rodent cycles. Persistent, chronic relapsing, or immune-tolerant infections are likewise possible mechanisms of viral persistence. The fundamental difference between VEE and the North American encephalomyelitides in the evolution of an epizootic is the role of the horse not only as a victim but as a powerful amplifying host.[24,25] Because of the very high viremia developed by infected horses, all that is needed to sustain an epizootic once it has begun is a variety of mosquitoes and a population of susceptible horses.[22,26] There is little evidence yet that birds are important in the dissemination of epizootic VEE, and most species are resistant to experimental infection.[25,28,29]

Noncontiguous dispersal is a consistent feature of VEE outbreaks and may be due to the movement of apparently healthy infected horses away from the disease center. Transmission by birds or other vertebrates has also been postulated but most animals do not develop illness or sufficiently high viremias to further distribute the virus to mosquito vectors. Notable exceptions are laboratory rodents that are extremely susceptible to experimental VEE infection.[25]

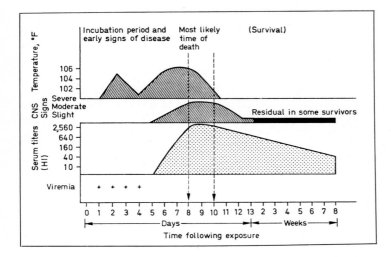

Fig 9. Clinical, virologic and serologic responses of horses to EEE viruses. HI = hemagglutinin inhibition. (From Proc 3rd Int Conf Eq Inf Dis, 1972. Courtesy of S. Karger AG, Basel)

Pathogenesis, Clinical Course and Immunity: The sequential clinical and serologic events following infection with EEE, WEE or VEE virus are similar, and differ only in detail and lethality. Infected horses respond in any or all of the following ways.[18,19,25,28,30]

Inapparent infection with a very low-grade viremia and fever may occur about 2 days after inoculation. Mild lymphopenia and neutropenia are usually present. This sequel may be quite common according to serologic surveys and probably represents the initial viremia following viral proliferation in regional lymph nodes.[18]

Generalized febrile illness (up to 41 C) with anorexia, depression, tachycardia, diarrhea (in the case of VEE), and profound lymphopenia and neutropenia may be observed. This stage is associated with the relatively high-grade secondary viremia that follows viral proliferation in various body organs. Although some horses may die during the generalized form, veterinary attention is not usually sought during inapparent or generalized febrile illness.[18,28]

Encephalomyelitis is the classic form of the disease. The onset is associated with the febrile crisis described above. The first signs usually occur about 5 days after infection and most deaths occur 2-3 days later.[18,28] Biphasic febrile episodes preceding the onset of CNS signs are commonly recorded after experimental WEE and EEE infections but are less clearly defined during VEE (Fig 9).[18,28] Early CNS signs are quite variable and referable to diffuse or multifocal cerebral cortical disease; evidence of brainstem and spinal cord involvement becomes more obvious as the illness progresses.

Often the first thing noticed is a change in behavior. Docile animals may become irritable and even bite their handler; other horses may seem somnolent or fail to respond to their owner's call. Food and water are usually refused. Further signs of dementia often follow, including head-pressing, leaning against a wall or fence, or compulsive walking, often in a circle (especially around the inside of a stall or small paddock). Blindness and lack of a menace response may be noted at this stage. Unilateral or bilateral cranial nerve deficits, including nystagmus, facial paralysis and lingual and pharyngeal paresis often occur as the disease progresses, and ataxia and paresis of the trunk and limbs result in a progressively more unsteady gait.[26,29]

The rapidity of deterioration and eventual outcome vary among individual horses and among the 3 diseases. Mortality rates range from 75-90% for EEE, 19-50% for WEE and 40-90% for VEE.[19,24,30] Death, if it occurs, is usually preceded by a period of recumbency during which the horse may be semicomatose and convulsing.[28] Surviving horses gradually recover over a period of weeks but may have residual signs of CNS damage such as dullness and diminished learning capacity. Such horses are often referred to as "dummies."

Neutralizing, HI and CF antibodies are usually present at the onset of encephalitic disease and may be present in high levels at death.

Diagnosis: The togaviral encephalomyelitides must be distinguished from other diseases characterized by diffuse cerebral signs with or without brainstem signs. The most important are hepatoencephalopathy, rabies, protozoal myeloencephalitis, verminous encephalitis and leukoencephalomalacia.

A presumptive diagnosis is usually made clinically, especially in areas where these diseases are prevalent during the mosquito season. Characteristic clinicopathologic changes, including increased cell numbers (neutrophils acutely, then mainly lymphocytes) and protein in the CSF, lymphopenia and neutropenia, may contribute to antemortem diagnosis.[25,28]

Both HI and CF antibody tests have been developed, and a 4-fold rise in titer between acute and convalescent sera is considered positive, although a very high acute titer in an unvaccinated animal is probably sufficient to establish a diagnosis. Results of acute and single serologic tests must be interpreted very cautiously if there is a history of vaccination against the encephalomyelitides.

Fresh or frozen brain is probably the best tissue for virus isolation.[32] The test inoculum is injected intracerebrally into mice, guinea pigs or wet chicks and produces CNS disease and death in 2-7 days if positive.[15,19,29] Alternatively the inoculum is placed directly into cell cultures to test for characteristic cytopathic effects. Neutralization tests with appropriate antisera are then used to identify the virus.[19]

Very strong supportive evidence for the diagnosis is obtained if characteristic histologic changes are present in the brain. Gross necropsy lesions are usually minimal and nonspecific (see below).

Treatment: Treatment is largely supportive. Affected horses should be placed in a shaded and well-bedded area. Free-choice water and feed should be provided. During the severe stage of the disease, IV fluids may be neccessary to maintain hydration. An indwelling stomach tube may facilitate feeding of dysphagic horses. Recumbent animals should be encouraged to assume a sternal position and any decubiti should be treated vigorously. Some veterinarians prefer the use of a sling to assist the animal to remain standing; however, affected horses should not be allowed to hang in the sling.[30]

Convulsions can be controlled by sedative doses of chloral hydrate, glyceryl guaiacolate or barbiturates. Specific hyperimmune antisera are of no value in treatment because affected animals usually have high antibody titers at the onset of clinical signs.[18] Vaccination of horses in the early stage of VEE with TC-83 vaccine protects against severe diseases in some cases.[24]

Necropsy Findings: Gross findings are nonspecific and are mainly congestion of most organs and slate-grey discoloration of the brain and spinal cord, especially obvious on section of formalin-fixed tissue.

Histologically there is evidence of diffuse meningoencephalomyelitis. There is a predominant involvement of grey matter with diffuse neuronal degeneration, gliosis, perivascular and neuroparenchymal infiltrates, and meningitis. Neutrophils are prominent in acute EEE and VEE lesions, whereas lymphocytes predominate in older lesions. Lymphocytes are usually the primary inflammatory cell in WEE lesions.

Disease in Humans: The WEE, EEE and VEE viruses can produce an influenza-like syndrome in humans, with symptoms of sore throat, myalgia, fever and headache; CNS signs may follow, ranging from mild disorientation to fulminant encephalitis and death.[25] Children and aged people are more susceptible. Mortality rates of up to 75% for EEE, 20% for WEE and less than 10% for VEE have been reported for people who develop encephalitis.[19,25]

It is important to remember that the horse is not a source of WEE and EEE for human infection, whereas VEE virus is readily transmitted to humans directly or via a mosquito vector.[24]

Control: The EEE and WEE viruses will probably never be eradicated from the US because reservoirs exist in many areas and do not depend on horse infection for their maintenance. For these reasons, continual vigilance and conscientious immunization programs will always be necessary to minimize and contain epizootics in horses. Despite some early work with attenuated viruses, inactivated chick embryo or tissue culture origin vaccines are now used almost exclusively.[18] Monovalent, bivalent (containing EEE and WEE) or trivalent vaccines (containing EEE, WEE and VEE) are available, and choice of the appropriate product for a particular area depends upon the prevalence or likely occurrence of the 3 diseases. Horses should be vaccinated at least a month before the anticipated risk period or prior to the onset of vector mosquito activity.[18] This time varies with latitude, rainfall and to some extent with altitude, ranging from January or February in Florida and Mexico to May or June in parts of Canada and the northern US.[18] Clinical evidence suggests a maximum of 6 months' protection following vaccination against EEE or WEE, so revaccination during the summer is necessary in warm areas with long mosquito seasons.

General control measures aimed at reducing mosquito vector populations significantly diminish but do not eliminate the risk of equine infection. These measures include good agricultural and engineering management of cultivated land, drainage and/or insecticide treatment of mosquito-breeding areas, and application of insect repellent to horses, especially at night.[19]

Routine surveillance of the virus pool with sentinel chickens often provides early warning of an impending outbreak and allows time for vaccination of susceptible horses.

The principles of control outlined above generally apply to epizootics of VEE. In marked contrast to EEE and WEE, a VEE outbreak requires quarantine of horses.[24,25] No horse should be considered free of the disease until 3 weeks after vaccination; even this assumes that vaccination is synonymous with immunization. Until recently, only the attenuated TC-83 vaccine was used to protect horses in the US, mainly because a large store of this vaccine had been made available by the government during the 1971 Texas outbreak.[24,25] The attenuated vaccine has the advantage of providing protection within 3 days of vaccination, compared with 7 days for formalin-inactivated vaccines. However, there has been concern that attenuated virus could infect mosquitoes feeding on vaccinated horses and even revert to virulence if passed sufficiently often.[24,33] Also, the presence of antibodies to heterologous alphaviruses (EEE and WEE) suppressed antibody response to VEE vaccination. As a result, the TC-83 vaccine has now been largely supplanted by a formalinized product incorporated into a trivalent vaccine with EEE and WEE antigens.[34,35]

Septic Meningitis

Leptomeningitis (inflammation of the arachnoid and pia mater) occurs as a component of many diffuse, infectious CNS diseases such as viral and verminous encephalitides. Clinically recognizable meningitis, however, is generally caused by bacteria that spread hematogeneously, by direct extension of suppurative process in or around the head, or as a result of penetrating wounds of the skull.

The profound neurologic deficits often associated with septic meningitis are a reflection of the diffuse involvement of the superficial parenchyma and nerve roots of the brain and spinal cord. The secondary development of hypertensive obstructive hydrocephalus may further complicate the clinical picture.

Focal pachymeningitis (inflammation of the dura mater) may accompany epidural abscessation.

Approximately 30-50% of all equine deaths during the first 8 weeks postpartum are due to infectious conditions.[32,36,37] Of these, only a relatively small proportion are due to meningitis, although the condition is probably underdiagnosed.[17] Meningitides usually occur in foals as a result of hematogenous dissemination of organisms from a primary site of sepsis, such as the placenta, umbilical stump or GI tract.

Predisposing causes for meningitis in foals include maternal uterine infections, early placental separation, unhygienic conditions (eg, in the foaling barn), failure of passive transfer of maternal immunoglobulins, and adverse environmental conditions (including extremes of temperature and humidity). The bacteria involved are those most commonly causing neonatal septicemica. Beta-hemolytic streptococci, *Antinobacillus equuli*, *Escherichia coli* and, more rarely, *Klebsiella pneumoniae* and coagulase-positive staphylococci are likely causes of meningitis during the first month of life.[36,38] Meningitis caused by *Salmonella* spp, especially *S typhimurium*, occurs more frequently in older foals.[39]

The prodromal bacteremic phase of meningitis is characterized by fever, lethargy and lack of affinity for the mare. Early meningeal involvement may be suggested by behavioral changes such as aimless walking, depression and abnormal vocalization (wanderer, dummy and barker). Progression of signs is often rapid, leading to blindness, loss of suckling reflex, diffuse cranial nerve deficits, ataxia and paresis of the trunk and limbs. Pain is manifested by trismus and reluctance to move the head or neck. The initial cutaneous hyperesthesia, muscular rigidity and tremors may be followed by diffusely diminished sensation and reduced spinal reflexes. If the foal is untreated, recumbency, coma and seizures can quickly occur. Coincident signs of septicemia include hypopyon, polyarthritis, dyspnea and abnormal lung sounds.

Bacterial meningitis in foals is a medical emergency and requires rapid and meticulous management, so early diagnosis and indentification of the causative organism are essential. The diagnosis is confirmed by finding bacteria, increased numbers of inflammatory cells (especially neutrophils), and high protein and low glucose levels in the CSF. A gram stain, culture and antibiotic sensitivity test should also be performed on CSF. If CSF cannot be collected or gram stain and culture results are negative, related sites of sepsis, such as umbilical abscess, urinary sediment, septic joint fluid, feces or blood, should be checked for bacteria. Antimicrobial treatment is preferably based on gram stain and culture results. Otherwise, large doses of broad-spectrum antibiotics or antibiotic combinations are indicated. Typical regimens include various combinations of the following drugs given IV divided in 4-6 daily treatments: potassium k penicillin G at 100,000-200,000 IU/kg body weight/day; sodium ampicillin at 100-200 mg/kg body weight/day; and chloramphenicol succinate at 100-200 mg/kg body weight/day. Dosages of renally excreted antibiotics (especially aminoglycosides) should be reduced in azotemic foals.

Treatment should continue for at least 5 days. Intrathecal medication is often advocated but is seldom advantageous and can be dangerous. Supportive treatment is important and is aimed at avoiding or correcting dehydration (by oral or IV fluids) and treating severe hyperthermia (with alcohol baths, fans, etc). Metabolic derangements, such as azotemia, hyponatremia (<120 mEq NA/L), hyposmolality (<260 mOsm/L) and hypoglycemia (<50mg/dl), are often present and can exacerbate nervous signs. Such disorders should be identified and corrected. Seizures may be controlled by manual restraint; otherwise a test dose of 5-10 mg diazepam should be given IV and repeated as necessary. Intractable seizures may necessitate sedative to anesthetic doses of chloral hydrate or Na pentobarbital. Although usually contraindicated, the slow IV use of 20% mannitol (0.25g/kg) and/or corticosteroids (dexamethasone at 0.2 mg/kg) must be considered in recumbent, convulsing comatose foals with meningitis. Rapidly progressive signs are often caused by severe brain edema of obstructive hydrocephalus, which can be fatal unless aggressively treated.

Cryptococcal meningitis is caused by the encapsulated yeast-like fungus *Cryptococcus neoformans,* a saprophyte found commonly in soil, especially in avian habitats.[40] Several extraneural infections have been recorded in horses, including myxomatous lesions of the lips, nasal mucosa and lungs.[41,42] It is likely that meningeal localization occurs after hematogenous or direct spread from a benign or clinical focus in the respiratory tract. Signs of cryptococcal meningitis may be acute or insidious in onset but usually progress rather slowly.[41,43-45] The clinical picture is typical of a diffuse meningitis with dementia, blindness, dysphagia, initial hyperesthesia and rigidity, with progression to ataxia, weakness, recumbency, convulsions, coma and death. An unusual case involved localized grey matter/peripheral nerve signs, including gluteal muscle atrophy, pelvic limb gait deficits, atony and areflexia of the tail and anus, and perineal hypalgesia. This was due to involvement of the cauda equina and lumbosacral nerve roots and dura.

Antemortem diagnosis can be made by finding the encapsulated organism in an India ink preparation or routine laboratory stain of CSF sediment, or by positive culture on most routine laboratory media. Histologically the characteristic budding, yeast-like organisms are readily found in the meninges and around vessels in the brain parenchyma surrounded by a predominantly lymphocytic and giant cell reaction. Clinical evidence of a primary cryptococcal infection should be sought, including culture and India ink preparations of any nasal or tracheal exudates.

The disease is effectively treated in humans by the systemic or intrathecal use of antifungals, such as amphotericin B and flucytosine (Ancoben:Roche), either alone or in combination.[46] Because of the high cost and potential nephrotoxicity of systemically administered amphotericin B in horses, intrathecal treatment seems to have the most promise.

Diffuse, fatal meningitides have been associated with *Streptococcus equi* and *Actinomyces* spp infections.[47,48] Purulent meningitis due to *S equi* has occasionally been noted at necropsy in horses without clinical evidence of CNS disease.[47]

Cerebral Abscess

Cerebral abscesses occur sporadically in horses, most commonly during epizootics of *Streptococcus equi* (strangles) or *Actinobacillus mallei* (glanders) infection. Such abscesses may be clinically silent, associated with overt meningitis or cause signs of a space-occupying cerebral lesion. The cerebral hemispheres have a considerable capacity to accommodate large masses without clinically impaired function, but signs of cerebral disease become apparent with sufficient compression and attenuation of cerebral tissue.

The onset of neurologic signs may be acute or insidious, and the clinical course is often characterized by marked fluctuations in severity. Most obvious are behavioral changes such as depression, head-pressing, aimless wandering or sudden unprovoked excitement. Affected horses may circle or stand with the head and neck toward the side of the abscessed cerebral hemisphere. With progression there can be episodes of unconsciousness, recumbency and seizures. Consistent early signs are contralateral impaired vision, deficient menace response and decreased facial sensation (best appreciated by comparing the response to stimulation of each side of the nasal septum). Sufficient abscess enlargement and/or severe associated cerebral edema may cause signs of brainstem compression, such as asymmetric pupillary constriction, ataxia and weakness.

The condition must be distinguished from other causes of asymmetric cerebral disease such as protozoal myeloencephalitis, trauma, aberrant parasite migration, parasitic thromboembolism and cholesterol granuloma. Diagnosis is largely based on a consideration of history (eg, prior strangles infection) and clinical signs. Elevations of fibrinogen and plasma globulin levels, and peripheral WBC count should be expected. Changes in CSF depend on the degree of meningeal or ependymal involvement. In most cases there is xanthochromia and moderate elevation of protein levels, reflecting cerebral compression and damage. There are elevated numbers of inflammatory cells (particularly neutrophils) in the CSF if there is associated meningitis or ependymitis.

Therapy is based on the prolonged use of large doses of appropriate antimicrobials. For a cerebral abscess caused by *Strep equi*, a suggested treatment regimen is potassium or sodium penicillin at 100,000-400,000 IU/kg body weight divided in 4 daily doses for 1-2 weeks, followed by IM procaine penicillin at 22,000 IU/ kg body weight every 12 hours for at least 4 more weeks. With careful surgical technic, the contents of a cerebral abscess might be aspirated via a small trephine hole if the abscess is adequately localized. Recovered horses may have residual deficits such as impaired vision and decreased facial sensation contralaterally.

Verminous Encephalitis

Verminous encephalitis is caused by the rather random intracranial wanderings of one or more parasites and is therefore an extremely variable clinical entity. Depending upon the number, size and location of the parasites and the duration of their migration through the brain, a spectrum of signs is possible ranging from a nonprogressive localizing neurologic deficit to rapidly fatal, diffuse encephalitis. Parasite migration through the spinal cord occurs less commonly and is discussed below (see Spinal Cord Diseases). Verminous encephalitis usually occurs sporadically and is most commonly associated with *Strongylus vulgaris, Hypoderma* spp, *Micronema deletrix* and *Setaria* spp infections.

Encephalitis due to *Strongylus vulgaris* is probably a consequence of aberrant intimal or subintimal migration of fourth stage larvae to the proximal aorta or left ventricular endocardium. From verminous thrombi at these sites, larvae can be carried to any part of the brain by the circulation to continue migration and development.[49,50] Disintegration of a verminous thrombus occasionally results in massive embolic showering, which causes infarction and edema, particularly of the ipsilateral forebrain.

Clinical signs are abrupt in onset and progression depends upon the further disposition of the nematode(s) that may die or migrate out of the CNS, leaving only residual neurologic impairment.[51] More often, however, the signs progress as further migration within the brain occurs. A series of 6 fatal cases was described involving clinical courses from 3 hours to 22 days and a variety of neurologic signs that included depression, limb paresis, ataxia, various cranial nerve defects, convulsions and recumbency.[49] Larval migration through the brainstem or cerebellum is likely to cause more severe and progressive signs than is migration through the forebrain.[50] However, massive embolic showering of the brain may cause peracute recumbency followed by signs of diffuse cerebral disease, such as blindness, circling, head-pressing and dysphagia.

A definitive diagnosis of *S vulgaris* encephalitis is usually only made at necropsy but should be suspected in any case of acute-onset CNS disease with signs referable to a single lesion in the brain or a diffuse cerebral lesion and no history of trauma. Changes in CSF are not specific or consistent in cases of *S vulgaris* migration in the brain, but some hemorrhage into the CSF and increased numbers of inflammatory cells, including eosinophils, are expected. Marked CSF xanthochromia and protein level elevation accompany the cerebral infarction syndrome. No data on therapy are available but treatment of suspect horses with thiabendazole at 440 mg/kg body weight or fenbendazole at 30 mg/kg body weight daily for 2 days and anti-inflammatory drugs such as dexamethasone at 0.1-0.25 mg/kg body weight every 6 hours during the acute phase of the disease is probably justified.

Intracranial myiasis by *Hypoderma* spp in horses was first described in England in 1842 and has since been reported in Europe and the US.[52,53] The horse is not a normal host for *Hypoderma* (the cattle grub or warble) since successful pupation seldom occurs following tissue migration. Aberrant migration of first instar larvae through the foramen magnum (or other cranial foramina) can result in neurologic signs referable to a brainstem or cerebellar lesion. One such affected horse had severe depression, a dilated left pupil, lingual paresis, left-sided facial paralysis, and ataxia and paresis of the left limbs.[52] These signs were caused by extensive migration of a 12.5-mm x 2-mm *H lineatum* larva through the left side of the brainstem from the region of the oculomotor nucleus.

Clinical signs of *Hypoderma* migration are usually characterized by sudden onset, a short course and death within a week. The diagnostic difficulties described for *S vulgaris* encephalitis apply equally here, but the disease should be considered in areas where cutaneous myiasis by *Hypoderma* is common. There is some evidence that certain pour-on insecticides for cattle (eg, Ruelene:Dow with 13.4% crufomate) effectively prevent grub infestation of horses.[54]

There have been at least 6 reports of *Micronema deletrix* infection of horses in the US and Egypt since the first description in 1965.[54-58] In each instance there was invasion of cranial tissues; the parasites were found in the brain of 4 horses, in the nasal soft tissues and maxilla of one horse, and in the gingiva of another. Two horses with brain involvement also had renal lesions. Regardless of the tissue involved, the characteristic response to invasion by this parasite was granulomatous inflammation. *M deletrix* is a tiny (250-350μ) rhabditid nematode closely related to several saprophytic species. The life cycle is not well known but *M deletrix* is generally thought to be a facultative parasite. Massive invasion of most or all of the brain by hundreds of *M deletrix* adults results in acute signs of diffuse encephalitis, including severe dementia, blindness and incoordination progressing to recumbency, coma and death after a short course. Although CSF sampling was not performed in the reported cases, it is reasonable to expect a marked pleocytosis with some eosinophils and even larvae or larval fragments in the CSF. All stages of the *M deletrix* life cycle, including gravid females, larvae and ova, may be found in the brain, especially in the Virchow-Robin spaces surrounded by a predominantly mononuclear and giant cell reaction. This disease is important because of its antemortem similarity to the viral encephalitides; however, the histologic findings at necropsy are diagnostic.

Central nervous system diseases caused by *Setaria* spp are known by a variety of names (eg, kumri and enzootic cerebrospinal nematodiasis) throughout the Orient, India and Sri Lanka, and cause significant losses to the horse industry in these countries.[59] Aberrant migration of one or more immature *Setaria* nematodes through the brain or spinal cord causes signs indistinguishable from those described above for *S vulgaris* migration. This disease is seasonal in occurrence, corresponding with fly vector activity. In Japan mosquitoes have been shown to carry *Setaria digitata* microfilariae from the natural hosts, cattle, to abnormal hosts including horses, sheep and goats. A case of kumri was recently reported in the US.[60]

Diethylcarbamazine at 20-40 mg/kg body weight for 1-3 days has been successfully used as a prophylactic or therapeutic microfilaricide during periods of vector activity.[24]

Necropsy Findings: S. vulgaris arteritis, endocarditis and resultant thromboembolic showering of the brain may cause multifocal arterial infarction that may be ischemic or hemorrhagic, and may result in diffuse brain edema and swelling. *S vulgaris*, *Hypoderma* spp and *Setaria* spp usually create destructive, tortuous, hemorrhagic soft tracts through brain parenchyma. The cellular reaction varies from hemorrhage, with neutrophils in the peracute lesion, to cavitating necrotic areas, with macrophages, eosinophils, lymphocytes and reactive glial cells in the more advanced stages. The more diffuse lesions seen with *M deletrix* infection are characterized by perivascular cuffing with macrophages, plasma cells and eosinophils.

Rabies

Rabies has long been the most feared of all diseases. Although traditionally associated with mad dogs, vampire bats and hydrophobic humans, rabies can affect any warm-blooded animal and has been reported in horses in most parts of the world.

Cause: The disease is caused by a large neurotropic rhabdovirus.[61] A distinct but related rhabdovirus known as Nigerian horse virus has been isolated from the brain of a horse that showed signs resembling rabies.[62] In developed countries, the rabies virus pool is largely maintained by transmission among certain wildlife species.[63] Susceptible domestic animals are occasionally infected by contact with sylvan hosts and then have the potential for further transmission of the disease to humans and other animals.

The patterns of rabies infection and disease are constantly changed by immunization programs and wildlife population shifts brought about by disease and human-related pressures.[63] In Europe, Russia and Canada, the fox is the most important wildlife reservoir and the most likely vector of equine rabies.[63,64] Rabid foxes are also found in Alaska and the eastern US. In the midwestern states, Texas and northern California, skunks are by far the most common vector.[63,64] The marked aggression and fearlessness shown by rabid skunks make this species especially dangerous.[65] An isolated pocket of raccoon rabies exists in the southeastern US (mainly Florida and Georgia) but the prevalence of rabies among domestic animals in this area remains low.[64]

In North America the economic importance of equine rabies is negligible, with only 18 cases reported in the US and 32 cases in Canada in 1977.[64] However the disease is still a devastating killer of horses (and cattle) in large areas of Central and South America extending from northern Argentina to northern Mexico and into the Caribbean.[66] In Mexico, tens of thousands of horses died annually of rabies in the early 1960's and at least 1800 horses perished in a small area of Brazil between 1913-1918.[66,67] The vector of these rabies epizootics was usually the blood-sucking vampire bat, although fruit and insect bats can also transmit the disease.[66,67] Bats also carry rabies in the US and are becoming more important in the northeastern US and northern California.[64] Some measure of rabies control has been achieved in South America over the last decade by the increased vaccination of livestock.[63,65] Recently the vampire bat population has been decimated in some areas by the use of intraruminal anticoagulants (*eg,* diphenadione) in exposed cattle.[63,66] Continued application of this control method should decrease the prevalence of rabies in horses and other animals in Central and South America.

Several countries, including Australia and New Zealand, have never recorded a case of rabies and Great Britain, Scandinavia and Hawaii are currently free of the disease.

Pathogenesis: Rabies is usually transmitted by salivary contamination of a bite wound, although infection by inhaled, oral or transplacental routes has been demonstrated in some species.[68] The virus multiplies at the site of infection and, after a variable period of eclipse, moves centrally (centripetally) in the axons of peripheral nerves to reach the dorsal horn of the grey matter of the brainstem or spinal cord.[65] Hematogenous dissemination of virus does not usually occur. Spread throughout the rest of the CNS and sympathetic chain is quite rapid, and is due in part to multiplication and active spread of the virus in neurons and probably also passive transport in CSF.[68] The salivary glands are usually infected before the onset of clinical signs by "centrifugal" spread of virus from the CNS via cranial nerves.[68]

The incubation period for rabies in horses has seldom been documented but probably varies from 2 weeks to several months. Rabies virus is already widespread in the CNS by the time the first nervous signs are seen, although the most severe morphologic lesions are usually found in the brainstem or spinal cord at the point of virus entry.[68] Signs observed in horses probably depend on the age, size and immune status of the affected animal, the dose of virus, and the site and source of infection.

Clinical Signs: The signs of rabies, at least terminally, are those of diffuse or multifocal CNS disease. However, even from the small amount of literature describing equine rabies, it is clear that the presenting signs and clinical course are extremely variable. The initial signs have included depression, mania, forelimb lameness or weakness, ataxia, hindlimb paralysis and colic.[67,69-76] Fever (up to 40.6 C), anorexia, icterus and injected mucosae were variably present. Whatever the presentation, the disease was rapidly progressive and resulted in death 3-5 days after the onset of signs. One recovery has been recorded in a presumptive case of experimentally produced rabies in a donkey.[73]

During the course of the disease, rabid horses may have predominantly encephalitic signs or signs of spinal cord disease. This distinction is by no means absolute. Horses in the latter group often have an ascending flaccid paralysis, beginning with knuckling and crossing of the hindlimbs and swaying of the hips. There is usually flaccid paralysis of the tail and anus, retention of urine and feces, and loss of spinal reflexes and sensation as the signs advance. The front limbs are soon involved and affected horses progressively lose the ability to stand and finally to remain sternal. There may be no disturbance of behavior or appetite until the final stages, during which signs of encephalitis (eg, mania, dysphagia) frequently appear.[25,72] The disease transmitted by vampire bats is almost invariably this paralytic form of rabies.[67]

Horses with the encephalitic form of rabies usually manifest some early behavioral changes such as profound depression or unprovoked excitement. Maniacal horses are particularly dangerous because they may ignore restraint, charge at bystanders and bite themselves and their surroundings.[74] Other signs of brain disease are often present such as dysphagia, facial paresis, nystagmus and altered vocalization. Tetraparesis and ataxia appear early and progress quickly to recumbency. Horses with either form become comatose or convulse and thrash violently before dying.

Cerebrospinal fluid from rabid horses is frequently normal but may show moderate elevations in protein content and mononuclear cell numbers.[69,76]

Diagnosis: The clinical diagnosis of rabies may be difficult but should be considered in any horse showing rapidly progressive CNS signs, especially in areas where rabies is enzootic. Signs of severe grey matter disease, such as flaccid limbs, tail paralysis, analgesia and loss of spinal reflexes, strongly suggest rabies. Consequently, this disease must be differentiated from other conditions with signs of grey matter damage, such as cauda equina neuritis, EHV-1 myeloencephalitis, protozoal myeloencephalitis, and sorghum-sudangrass poisoning. The encephalitic form of rabies may resemble togaviral encephalomyelitides, hepatoencephalopathy, brain trauma, protozoal myeloencephalitis or moldy corn poisoning. If rabies is suspected, the brain should be halved sagittally, and half placed in 10% formaldehyde for histologic examination and the other half frozen and submitted for a fluorescent antibody (FA) and/or mouse inoculation test.

Histologically there is diffuse nonsuppurative polioencephalomyelitis, which is often surprisingly mild in horses. The hippocampus, brainstem, cerebellum and spinal cord grey matter are frequently affected, and there is often a ganglionitis, particularly of the trigeminal ganglia. Lesions consist of neuronal degeneration, gliosis and lymphocytic perivascular cuffing. Large eosinophilic cytoplasmic inclusions (Negri bodies) occur in ganglion cells and neurons, and are of diagnostic significance.

The FA test is the most widely used test in diagnostic laboratories and identifies at least 98% of rabies-infected brains.[77] Fluorescein-conjugated rabies antiserum is used to identify rabies antigen in brain tissue. The hippocampus and cerebellum are most commonly chosen for examination. Fluorescent antibody straining of corneal scrapings may be a useful antemortem test for rabies.[78]

The mouse inoculation test is the most accurate diagnostic test for rabies.[79] Test homogenates of brain or salivary gland are injected intracerebrally into weanling mice. Mice developing nervous signs after the fifth postinoculation day are slaughtered and the brains examined for evidence of rabies by histologic or FA technics. Alternatively, mice are killed after day 5 before clinical signs develop.

Prevention and Treatment: The efficacy of rabies vaccines in horses is unknown. Horses in high-risk areas should be vaccinated annually with ERA-strain tissue culture origin vaccine. Serum neutralizing antibody titers can be measured to assess the humoral response to vaccination.

If a horse is bitten by a suspect rabid animal, the wound should be thoroughly washed with soapy water and swabbed with iodine or alcohol. If available, rabies antiserum (usually equine origin) can be infiltrated around the wound. Even in humans, the value of postexposure vaccination is questioned;[62] however, horses bitten by rabid animals might rationally be given up to 5 doses of vaccine daily for 14 successive days, followed by booster vaccinations 10, 20 and 90 days later. This is based on current World Health Organization recommendations for postexposure treatment of humans. Once a horse shows nervous signs, there is no effective treatment. Strict precautions must be taken to prevent exposure of people handling affected horses.

Fungal Encephalitis

Cerebral and cerebellar infarction due to disseminated, fulminating phycomycosis occurred in a horse that may have been immunosuppressed by prolonged corticosteroid therapy.[80]

Fungal encephalitis occasionally follows guttural pouch infection by *Aspergillus*.

Toxic Diseases

Leukoencephalomalacia (Moldy Corn Poisoning)

The syndrome of equine leukoencephalomalacia (LEM) was probably first described in the US in 1850 and has since been associated with many sporadic cases and several major epizootics of fatal disease.[81] The best known epizootic occurred in Illinois, Iowa, and other midwestern states in the winter of 1934-35 and resulted in the death of more than 5000 horses, mules and donkeys.[82-84] Circumstantial clinical evidence and experimental studies during the 1934 outbreak suggested that moldy corn or cornstalk ingestion was the cause of equine LEM and more recent work has incriminated *Fusarium monoliforme* as the specific toxigenic fungus.[85] Toxicosis due to *monoliforme* is manifested as either LEM or as a fulminant, fatal hepatopathy, depending upon the dosage and duration of intake.[86]

The course of reported epizootics has paralleled the supply of moldy corn and is most severe during the 6 months after harvest of a damaged corn crop.[83,84] Outbreaks in Egypt have occurred after annual flooding of the Nile.

Clinical signs are first seen 2-24 weeks (average 3 weeks) after the initial ingestion of moldy corn.[86] In general, the initial signs are referable to a cerebral lesion(s) and include depression, unresponsiveness, head-pressing, circling, aimless wandering, blindness and occasionally unprovoked excitement and frenzy. The signs are frequently asymmetric. Further progression may be associated with pharyngeal paralysis, incoordination and finally recumbency, paddling, coma and death. The clinical course is usually less than a week but may be much longer in horses that recover.

Horses with uncomplicated LEM are not usually febrile, a fact that helps distinguish this disease from the clinically similar viral encephalomyelitides.

The lesions seen at necropsy are usually diagnostic and consist of focal areas of liquefactive, hemorrhagic necrosis in the white matter of one or both cerebral hemispheres (up to several cm in diameter).[87] Malacic areas within the grey or white matter of the brainstem and spinal cord are less frequently encountered but may be expected in cases marked by profound weakness and ataxia of the trunk and limbs.[83]

Treatment of affected horses is only supportive. Contaminated feed should be removed from exposed horses and an effort made to eliminate toxin already in the alimentary tract by the use of laxatives and activated charcoal.

Locoweed Poisoning (Locoism)

Locoism is a chronic, progressive neurologic disorder of horses, cattle and sheep grazing the rangelands of western North America.[88-90] It is caused by prolonged ingestion of certain species of *Astragalus* and *Oxytropis* legumes (locoweed). The toxic principle has been partially identified as an alkaloidal locoine.[90] Outbreaks of locoweed poisoning occur when normal forage is scarce, in conditions of overgrazing or drought. There is a tendency for horses eating locoweed to develop a craving for them, even to the exclusion of other feeds.[89] Clinical signs begin abruptly and indicate diffuse CNS disorder. There is marked dementia and periods of depression alternating with frenzied excitement when affected horses are disturbed. Variable visual impairment, head-nodding, and dysphagia with lingual and labial paresis are also observed. Gait deficits may be severe and characterized by high-stepping, toe-scuffing, stumbling and swaying. These signs are exacerbated by excitement and mildly affected horses may seem normal until disturbed or handled. Weight loss occurs quickly and often progresses to emaciation and death.

There is said to be no recovery from locoweed poisoning, even following removal of the offending plants.[89] Slightly affected animals remain unsafe for riding and show nervous signs when excited. Excellent results have recently been reported in treating several horses with a combination of mood elevators (tranylcypromine and protryptaline) and repeated reserpinization.[90] Clinical recovery was rapid and treated horses remained essentially normal for 2 years following treatment. More research is required to confirm the value of this therapy.

Gross necropsy findings are unremarkable, but histologically there is widespread neurovisceral cytoplasmic vacuolation.[91] These changes affect most organs and virtually all neurons of the CNS. In protracted cases, there is neuroaxonal dystrophy.[92] Locoism is probably a plant-induced lysosomal storage disease similar to *Swainsona* spp poisoning.[93]

Darling Pea (*Swainsona* spp) Poisoning

Outbreaks of *Swainsona* spp poisoning in horses have been reported following early spring or fall rains in eastern and western Australia.[92,94] There are no obvious differences between *Swainsona* spp poisoning in Australia and locoweed poisoning of horses in North America. Prolonged ingestion of darling pea causes a chronic disease characterized by neurologic disturbances, weight loss and addiction to the plant. Histologically there is widespread cellular vacuolation.[94]

Recent research in sheep indicates that the vacuolation (and toxicosis) represents aberrant lysosomal storage of various glycoproteins secondary to inhibition of α-mannosidase by a plant compound. Darling pea poisoning is therefore comparable to hereditary mannosidosis of humans and cattle.

Vascular Disease

Intracarotid Injection

The close proximity of the common carotid artery to the jugular vein makes accidental intracarotid (IC) injection a very real hazard. The injected material may travel in the carotid distribution to the ipsilateral forebrain to cause acute cerebral disturbance.[95,96] A violent reaction typically occurs within 30 seconds of IC injection, with signs ranging from sudden unprovoked activity in the standing position (eg, head-shaking, kicking, running) to recumbency and loss of consciousness for a variable period. Most affected horses recover in minutes to hours, although prolonged coma, convulsions and death occasionally occur. Very consistent but frequently overlooked findings are decreased facial sensation, blindness and deficient menace response, all contralateral. These findings, which may be transitory or permanent, reflect ipsilateral cerebral damage. Marked cardiovascular changes, such as bradycardia, arrhythmias and blood pressure fluctuations, may accompany CNS signs.

Most drugs commonly used IV can cause this reaction if injected IC. Those incriminated include phenothiazine tranquilizers (acetylpromazine, promazine, etc.), barbiturates, chloral hydrate, xylazine, phenylbutazone, calcium gluconate, oxalic and malonic acids, and sodium iodide.[96,97]

The morphologic changes caused by accidental IC injection are typical of acute cerebral ischemia and include marked edema, vascular endothelial damage and hemorrhage, and neuronal degeneration.

Treatment is largely symptomatic. Appropriate padding and sedation are indicated in thrashing delirious horses. If signs of severe cerebral edema and brainstem compression occur, medical decompression of the CNS should

be attempted. The use of mannitol may be contraindicated because of the concomitant cerebral hemorrhage, but dexamethasone at 0.1-0.25 mg/kg body weight may be useful. Atropine at 0.04 mg/kg may reverse the severe bradycardia and arrhythmia accompanying accidental IC injection of xylazine.

Noninfectious Space-Occupying Lesions

The signs caused by space-occupying lesions within the CNS depend upon the type, size, number, rate of growth and position of the lesions within the CNS. Such masses may cause neurologic dysfunction by compression, invasion and/or replacement of neural tissue. Obstruction of CSF outflow from the ventricular system can cause ventricular enlargement and signs of hydrocephalus.

The cerebral cortices and diencephalon (thalamus, hypothalamus) can often accommodate small masses without clinical effects. In contrast, space-occupying lesions of the caudal brainstem and spinal cord usually cause neurologic impairment. Clinical signs may begin insidiously or acutely (even with slowly growing masses). A focal lesion is usually suggested by specific neurologic signs, although certain masses involving the brain may cause generalized seizures. The rate of progression of signs varies greatly but clinical fluctuations are often noted, reflecting variable CNS edema and inflammation.

Space-occupying lesions involving peripheral nerves usually result in well-defined motor, sensory, proprioceptive and sympathetic signs that may include hyperpathia or localized pain.

Neoplasia

Primary Neoplasms: Primary neoplasms of the nervous system are very uncommon in horses.[98] General conclusions regarding the relative incidence and behavior of such tumors cannot easily be drawn. Nervous system neoplasms have been classified according to their origin as tumors of nerve cells, neuroepithelium, glia, peripheral nerves and nerve sheaths, mesodermal structures and endocrine organs.[99]

A single sympathetic ganglioneuroma (also containing cells of the glial type) is apparently the only neoplasm of nerve cell origin reported in horses.[100] Tumors of neuroepithelial origin have included ependymoma, choroid plexus papilloma and malignant medulloepithelioma.[101-107] Among glial cell neoplasms described in horses are optic disc astrocytoma, retinoblastoma and nicroglioma.[108-110] Neoplasms of peripheral nerves and nerve sheaths may be more common than CNS neoplasms. In a survey of 11 North American university veterinary hospitals, all 28 recorded nervous tissue tumors found in horses involved peripheral nerves. Most reported peripheral nerve neoplasms have been neurofibromas or neurofibrosarcomas.[111-115] Neurofibromas are often found cutaneously. The most common sites are the pectoral region, abdomen, neck and face.[116]

The most commonly reported mesodermal neoplasm is the meningioma.[99,117-119] Neoplastic reticulosis, a lipoma in the mesencephalic aqueduct, an angioma in the cervical spinal cord, and a melanoblastoma of the cerebellar meninges have also been described.[101,120-122]

Adenoma of the parts intermedia of the pituitary gland is common; however, any clinical signs observed are usually referable to endocrine dysfunction.[117] Benign neoplasms of the pineal gland (pinealomas) have occasionally been reported.[117,123,124]

Secondary Neoplasms: Secondary neoplasms may penetrate through the cranial vault or vertebrae, grow through osseous foramina, or reach the nervous system by metastasis. Resulting clinical signs are due to pressure-induced destruction, direct invasion and/or compromise of blood supply to nervous tissue. Extraneural tumors may also infiltrate or encroach upon peripheral nerves.

Lymphosarcoma is the most common secondary neoplasm affecting the nervous system of horses. This tumor has been found in the epidural space (usually lumbar) as a cause of compression myelopathy, in the brain and olfactory tracts, and infiltrated into various peripheral nerves.[125-129]

Melanomas occasionally invade the CNS of white or grey horses. Usually these tumors are found in the epidural space after contiguous spread from melanomatous sublumbar lymph nodes.[130-133] These are also reports of melanomas of the spinal meninges and brain that have occurred after metastasis of cutaneous melanomas.[116,117,134]

Among sarcomas, hemangiosarcomas are generally considered to metastasize most frequently to the brain.[101] Two such cases in horses have been reported.[135]

Adenocarcinomas may invade the brain by direct spread from a primary site in the nose or paranasal sinuses, or by metastasis from a distant site such as the adrenal gland.[136-138] Benign tumors of bone, such as the osteoma, or of bone marrow, such as the plasma-cell myeloma, involving the skull or vertebrae can cause compression of the brain or spinal cord.[139,140]

Malformation Tumors

Malformation tumors include epidermoids, dermoids, teratomas and teratoids. These growths originate from heterotopic tissues that usually lie close to embryonic lines of closure.[101]

Epidermoid cysts (epidermoid cholesteatomas) are slowly enlarging, encapsulated structures that arise during embryonic life from ectopic epithelial tissue. These tumors are usually situated near the midline in the angle between the cerebrum and cerebellum. Epidermoid cysts are usually incidental necropsy findings but occasionally grow large enough to cause CNS signs.[141-143] There are also a number of reports of intracranial tooth heterotopias, which are not true teratomas.[144] A true teratoma has been described, although the identification was somewhat questionable.[145]

Cholesterol Granuloma of the Choroid Plexus (Cholesteatoma)

Cholesterol granulomas are often found in the choroid plexuses of old horses, most commonly within the lateral ventricles of the brain. They may represent a chronic granulomatous reaction to cholesterol crystals associated with chronic vascular leakage. Mature cholesterol granulomas are generally circumscribed, yellowish brown, firm and granular, with a glistening "pearly" appearance on the cut surface.[146,147] Most of these masses remain clinically silent but some grow large enough to compress brain tissue directly or block CSF drainage and cause obstructive hydrocephalus. Cholesterol granulomas often occur bilaterally but one is usually larger.

Clinical signs are typically insidious in onset. Signs may be intermittent but are usually progressive, asymmetric and referable to impaired cerebral cortical function. Early reports often described affected horses as "stupid" or "confused."[148] One well-documented case was in a 7-year-old Arabian mare that experienced several brief attacks of ataxia, weakness, recumbency and unconsciousness in the previous 2 years.[149] Before a particularly severe episode, the mare circled to the right and had a reduced menace response and facial hypalgesia on the left side. These signs could be explained clinically by a right-sided cerebral lesion and at necropsy a large (4 cm in diameter) cholesterol granuloma was found within the right lateral ventricle, causing severe cortical atrophy. There was a smaller granuloma in the left lateral ventricle. A CSF sample was markedly xanthochromic and had a very elevated protein level (322 mg/dl). These CSF changes were not specific but a diagnosis of cholesterol granuloma should be considered when a mature horse shows signs of slow onset or intermittent CNS (especially cerebral) disease without evidence of related trauma or infectious disease.

Medical therapy is unlikely to be curative but temporary relief of signs might be expected with corticosteroid treatment.

Cholesterol granulomas of the chorid plexus must be distinguished from the much rarer and histologically unrelated epidermoid cholesteatomas (see Malformation Tumors).[148,150]

Miscellaneous Lesions

Congenital venous malformation in a Welsh Cob foal caused spinal cord malacia and ataxia.[151]

Idiopathic Diseases

Neonatal Maladjustment Syndrome

There is now a substantial body of literature describing a clinically recognizable, noninfectious cerebral syndrome of newborn foals characterized clinically by gross behavioral disturbances and morphologically by ischemic cerebral necrosis, and cerebral edema and hemorrhage.[32,152-157] Attempts to classify the disease according to clinical signs have led to the popular use of such descriptive but nonspecific terms as "barkers," "wanderers," "dummies" and "convulsives."

The cause of this syndrome, now known as neonatal maladjustment syndrome (NMS), is not yet clear but the resulting brain lesions are most likely associated with a perinatal cerebral circulatory derangement.[155] Recent investigators speculate that increased intracranial vascular pressure during delivery could induce NMS.[158] Paradoxically, most cases of NMS occur in foals after a rapid, uncomplicated delivery.[155] However, certain obstetric procedures such as clamping of the umbilical cord have been suggested as causes. Despite initial comparisons between some cases of NMS of foals and the respiratory distress syndrome of children, the cardiopulmonary and metabolic abnormalities sometimes seen in NMS are now considered to be various manifestations of the common underlying pathogenesis of NMS.[159,160]

The neonatal maladjustment syndrome usually occurs in otherwise normal foals during the first 24 hours postpartum. Signs are abrupt in onset and referable to diffuse cortical impairment. Sudden stiff, jerky movements of the head and body are seen first, progressing to extensor spasms of the neck, limbs and tail. There is complete loss of the suckling reflex. If able to stand the foal may wander aimlessly, oblivious to its surroundings and apparently blind. Hyperexcitability, grinding of the teeth, exaggerated "gulping" of air, and abnormal vocalization ("barking") have been noted during this stage. The rate of progression of signs varies but affected foals often become recumbent and semicomatose, with paddling and clonic convulsions. Close observation may reveal constricted or dilated asymmetric pupils. Some animals are tachypneic, with or without pulmonary atelectasis, and often have metabolic or respiratory acidosis with a venous pH of 7.0 or less. The hemogram should be relatively normal for foals of this age.

With reasonable care, at least 50% of foals with NMS recover after a course of from several hours to several weeks. Neurologic functions return in the reverse of the order in which they were lost, ie, consciousness, standing position, vision and awareness, recognition of dam, and finally suckling ability. Recovery is complete if the foal survives, although occasional relapses have been reported.

Management and treatment should be conservative and aimed at providing water and nutrition, maintaining body temperature and controlling convulsions. Ideally, the foal is fed its dam's milk, with an emphasis on providing colostrum during the first 12 hours of life.[156] Warm milk or milk replacer is fed hourly in volumes of 8-10% of body weight daily. This is facilitated by placement of an indwelling nasoesophageal catheter with the distal end cranial to the gastric cardia. The foal should be placed on a warm surface (eg, straw bedding) and, if necessary, woolen or electric blankets or heat lamps can be used. Acidosis, if present, should be corrected by calculated doses if IV or oral bicarbonate solutions. If laboratory data are not available, foals with NMS that are in respiratory distress should probably receive humidified 100% O_2 at 10 L/minute by nasal tube and 5% $NaHCO_3$ at 5 ml/kg body weight given IV. Unnecessary stimuli, such as bright lights and loud noises, should be avoided. Most convulsions can be controlled manually without excessive restraint; however, if convulsions are severe or cause hyperthermia or distress, chemical control with 5-10 mg diazepam IV can be repeated as necessary. For long-term control, phenytoin has been used successfully IV, IM or PO at 5-10 mg/kg, followed by maintenance dosages of 1-5 mg/kg every 2-4 hours; the dosage interval is reduced after 12 hours to 6- or 12-hour intervals.[32]

Seizures

Seizures are the result of sudden, abnormal discharging of neurons in part or all of the cerebral cortex. These bursts of cerebrocortical activity cause paroxysmal movements and profound behavioral alterations. On the basis of their clinical appearance and progression, seizures are classified as generalized, partial or partial with secondary generalization.

Generalized seizures reflect diffuse cerebral disturbance. The onset of a generalized seizure may be signaled by a short period of restlessness and disorientation, with chewing, teethgrinding or other bizarre behavior. This is followed by generalized muscular rigidity (often beginning in the neck), recumbency and unconsciousness. There are usually clonic, paddling movements and signs of autonomic activity such as salivation, urination, and defecation. Diffuse cortical disturbances due to inflammation, metabolic disorders and toxicities may produce generalized seizures.

Signs of a partial seizure depend on the portion of the cerebral cortex discharging. The origin of the abnormal electrical activity is known as the seizure focus. When the seizure focus is in the motor cortex, there may be tremors or involuntary jerking on the other side of the head or body. Seizure foci in other parts of the brain may result in behavioral abnormalities such as exaggerated gulping of air, apparent blindness, confusion, viciousness, unprovoked excitement or unconsciousness. Between seizures, other localizing neurologic deficits may be apparent. Focal lesions in the diencephalon (thalamus, hypothalamus) or cerebral hemispheres, from trauma, inflammation, ischemia or compression, may initiate partial seizures.

Partial seizures may progress to generalized seizures if the electrical discharge spreads through the entire cerebral cortex. Localizing signs are usually apparent before the onset of such generalized seizures. For example, with a seizure focus in the motor cortex an animal may turn its head to the side or flick its leg before falling on its side unconscious in a generalized seizure.

Recurrent seizures without evidence of an active underlying disease, known as epilepsy, may result from residual cerebral damage after trauma, encephalitis, aberrant parasite migration or ischemia. Partial seizures or partial seizures that secondarily generalize are the usual manifestations of acquired epilepsy. This condition is rare in the horse. If a clinical or pathologic cause for recurrent seizures cannot be found, the syndrome is described as idiopathic epilepsy. Good evidence for such a syndrome has not yet been found in horses. However, it has been observed in several weanling foals, particularly Arabians, that recurrent seizures may suddenly begin. These usually respond to medication and it appears that the foals "grow out" of the seizures and do not require permanent medication.

Seizures are most often the result of some underlying disease process in horses. The following conditions may be associated with seizure activity.

Inflammation/Infection: togaviral encephalitis (EEE, WEE, VEE), rabies, meningitis, verminous encephalitis, protozoal myeloencephalitis

Compression: cholesterol granuloma, cerebral abscess, hydrocephalus, neoplasm

Vascular Disorders/Ischemia: parasitic thromboembolism, intracarotid injection, neonatal maladjustment syndrome, hypoxia

Trauma

Toxicity: moldy corn poisoning

Metabolic Disorders: hepatoencephalopathy, hyposmolality, hyperosmolality, hypocalcemia, hypoglycemia

If a horse is in a continual seizure state (status epilepticus), the seizures should be controlled with drugs, such as glyceryl guaiacolate, chloral hydrate or sodium pentobarbital, before proceeding with further evaluation. Diazepam in IV doses of 5-100 mg is expensive but often effective in short-term treatment of seizures. Complications of seizure activity, such as self-inflicted trauma, hyperthermia, acidosis and ventilatory difficulties, can then be managed. Prevention of further seizure episodes depends on the identification and successful treatment of underlying disease.

Because idiopathic and acquired epilepsy are rare in horses, there is little information available on the chronic use of oral anticonvulsants. Phenobarbital may be given IV or PO to effect at up to 2 mg/kg body weight.

Traumatic Disease

Cranial Trauma

Because of their nervous temperament, horses are quite prone to head injuries. Most often these injuries result from kicks from other horses, running into posts, or rearing and falling over backwards to strike the poll. Any resulting neurologic signs depend on the sites and severity of brain concussion, contusion, laceration or hemorrhage.[161]

Three broad but clinically recognizable neurologic syndromes have been observed following cranial trauma in the horse: the cerebral, midbrain and medullary-inner ear syndromes.[161] These syndromes are by no means precisely defined or invariable but their recognition is helpful as part of a rational and organized approach to cranial trauma.

Cerebral Syndrome: Signs referable to cerebral damage occur most frequently after trauma to the frontal or parietal areas of the head. This is often the fate of an overly inquisitive foal kicked by an older horse. Compound fractures of the frontal or parietal bones cause cerebral laceration and hemorrhage.

After an initial period of coma the horse regains consciousness in minutes to hours. Subsequent neurologic signs tend to fluctuate with the degree of cerebral edema. Affected horses are usually depressed and may wander in circles, usually toward the side of the damaged cerebral hemisphere. Characteristically there is blindness and sometimes decreased facial sensation contralaterally, which is best appreciated by stimulating the contralateral nasal septum or ear. Pupillary light responses should be brisk, although there may be some asymmetry and fluctuation of the pupils and a tendency toward miosis. Apart from depressed menace responses and possible lingual paresis, all other cranial nerve responses should be intact. Obvious signs of ataxia are generally absent. The appearance of gait deficits suggests progression to other parts of the brain. Genuine seizure activity or random, uncontrolled motor activity (thrashing, paddling) is most often seen in delirious or semicomatose recumbent horses and is difficult to accurately correlate with the site of the brain lesion. True seizures in horses probably indicate a forebrain lesion. If the cerebral hemispheres swell sufficiently, they can herniate caudad against the midbrain to cause signs such as dilated, unresponsive pupils (see below). The development of the midbrain syndrome is an unfavorable prognostic sign. In most cases, however, recognition of the cerebral syndrome warrants an optimistic prognosis. Injury to the cerebral hemispheres is less critical than brainstem damage and response to treatment for brain swelling is usually good.

Midbrain Syndrome: Closed head injuries (*ie,* no skull fractures) often result in midbrain hemorrhage, and severe cerebral edema can cause compression of this area (see above). Profound neurologic signs and a poor prognosis accompany damage to the midbrain. After an initial period of coma, there is marked depression due to involvement of the rostral part of the ascending reticular activating system. Extensive midbrain injury causes recumbency, and "decerebrate" posturing with generalized extensor rigidity. If the horse is ambulatory, gait deficits of ataxia and weakness are present. Affected horses may have vision but pupillary light responses are sluggish or absent, in contrast to those with the cerebral syndrome. Depending upon the extent of damage and the area of the midbrain involved, the pupils may be "pinpoint-sized" and fluctuant (tectum) to dilated and fixed (oculomotor nuclei and/or nerves). With unilateral lesions, the ipsilateral pupil is affected initially and later involvement of the opposite pupil suggests an enlarging lesion. Progression from miosis to bilaterally dilated, unresponsive pupils is a very unfavorable sign. Injury to the nuclei or connections of cranial nerves supplying extrinsic eye muscles can cause the deviations (strabismus) and vestibular nystagmus. Spontaneous nystagmus is not usually seen with midbrain lesions.

Bizarre respiratory patterns, cardiac arrhythmias and bradycardia may occur with severe lesions of the midbrain pons or medulla.

Medullary/Inner Ear Syndrome: Trauma to the back of the head may cause hemorrhage around the medulla and/or into the inner ear. This is often seriously complicated by fractures of the occipital and petrosal bones, or by separation of the occipital and petrosal bones, or by separation of the basioccipital and basisphenoid bones ventral to the pons and medulla (Fig 10). The resulting neurologic signs are often asymmetric and quite variable depending upon which cranial nerves are affected and the extent of medullary parenchymal damage. Hemorrhage into the middle and inner ear cavities causes vestibular and facial nerve signs such

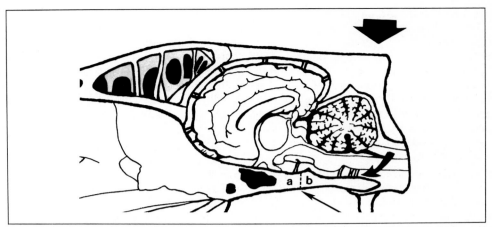

Fig 10. Median section of the equine skull and brain. Trauma to the occipital protuberance (wide arrow) can result in transfer of forces to the temporal bone, with subsequent fractures of its petrosal portion and the basioccipital bone. Separation of the basioccipital (a) and basisphenoid (b) bones often occurs at the suture (long arrow). The facial and vestibulocochlear nerves (curved arrow) are in close proximity to the basioccipital and petrosal bones. Consequently, facial paralysis and/or vestibular signs can result from trauma to the poll and subsequent fracture of these bones or hemorrhage in or around the medulla oblongata.

as head tilt, circling and leaning toward the affected side, ipsilateral facial paralysis, and spontaneous horizontal or rotary nystagmus with the fast phase away from the side of the lesion. Vestibular nystagmus may be abnormal or absent. Bleeding may extend into the external ears and guttural pouches.

Hemorrhage in or around the medulla causes additional signs such as depression, ataxia, weakness, recumbency, and other vestibular and cranial nerve signs. Horses with acute vestibular signs occasionally thrash and struggle violently in an effort to stand. Not uncommonly, horses with this kind of injury (eg, a blow to the poll) develop a head nod or coarse head tremor especially obvious during eating or drinking. This is probably due to direct cerebellar injury.

Neurologic Evaluation: A systematic approach to examination of patients with cranial trauma is essential; otherwise, important signs can be missed.[162] Sedative doses of drugs such as chloral hydrate or sodium pentobarbital (in the foal) may facilitate examination of a thrashing, delirious horse.

If possible, a thorough history should be obtained including a description of the accident, subsequent progression of signs and any treatment given. A general physical examination should be performed to evaluate other abnormalities (eg, fractures, hemorrhage, cardiac arrythmias). The state of consciousness should be assessed. Standard nomenclature arbitrarily grades increasing loss of consciousness as depression, obtundation, stupor, delirium, semicoma and coma. These states are defined by the horse's responsiveness to various visual, auditory and noxious (painful) stimuli. Comatose horses do not respond to any stimulus.

The head and neck should be closely examined, noting position, symmetry and evidence of trauma or fractures. Cranial orifices should be checked for evidence of bleeding, particularly the external ear canals (eg, with a finger), nostrils and, if possible, guttural pouches (with a rhinolaryngoscope). When evaluating vision and menace responses, remember that horses with cerebellar injury or facial nerve paralysis can see but may not have menace responses. Conversely, horses with ocular damage may be blind but have intact central visual pathways.

The eyes should be observed for position, nystagmus, and pupillary size, symmetry and responsiveness. These signs should be interpreted cautiously if there are indications of uveitis, such as corneal damage and edema or iridal adhesions. The other cranial nerves should be evaluated, especially V-VII reflexes (ear, eyelid, nose and lip), and tongue (XII) and jaw (motor V) tone and movement. When checking facial sensation, remember that cortical perception is being evaluated as well as pontomedullary reflex (V-VII) function. Emphasis is placed on the symmetry of responses.

If the horse is ambulatory, look for gait abnormalities (weakness, spasticity, incoordination, dysmetria). Voluntary effort, spinal reflexes and muscle tone can be evaluated in recumbent animals.

Aids to diagnosis include a hemogram, serum biochemical tests, skull radiographs and CSF sampling. A CSF sample should not be obtained from the atlanto-occipital site if there is evidence of brain swelling (see above).

Management: Unless there is clear radiographic evidence of a condition requiring surgical intervention (*eg,* depressed skull fracture), early management is supportive and medical. The main objective of medical treatment is to reduce or minimize brain swelling and, to a minor extent, intracranial hemorrhage. Life-threatening conditions, such as blocked airway, severe bleeding or fractured ribs with a ruptured lung, should be immediately treated. Seizures may be controlled with 5 mg (foal) to 100 mg (horse) diazepam, repeated as necessary. Intractable seizures may require sedative to anesthetic doses of chloral hydrate, glyceryl guaiacolate and thiamylal sodium, or sodium pentobarbital. Xylazine must be used cautiously because it results in transient hypertension that may exacerbate CNS hemorrhage.

All horses with CNS signs following cranial trauma should probably receive dexamethasone (or equivalent) at 0.1-0.25 mg/kg body weight. This should decrease brain edema and CSF production within several hours. The dose can be repeated every 4-6 hours for 1-4 days. Horses presented in a coma or semicoma should receive a slow IV infusion of 20% mannitol at 0.25 g/kg body weight. Improvement should be seen within 30 minutes. Mannitol administration can be repeated every 4-6 hours for up to 24 hours if clinical improvement follows its use. Intracranial bleeding, especially subdural, is exacerbated by the use of mannitol. Subdural hematomas are very difficult to diagnose but fortunately are rare in horses.

The IV use of 40% dimethyl sulfoxide (DMSO) has shown great promise in relieving cerebral edema in experimental models using dogs and monkeys.[163] A dose of 1-4 g/kg can be given slowly IV with dexamethasone and/or mannitol. Mild cholinergic-like effects (muscle tremors, sweating) have been occasionally noted during IV infusion of DMSO in horses.

Remember that renal-acting diuretics (*eg,* furosemide) remove fluid from the intravascular space, whereas osmotic diuretics (*eg,* mannitol) remove fluid primarily from the extravascular compartment. The possible usefulness of furosemide in reducing CSF production and decreasing systemic blood pressure in horses with brain injury is unknown.

Hypoxia and hypercapnia should be avoided. A reduction in arterial pO_2 exacerbates brain swelling and an elevated pCO_2 can increase intracranial blood pressure and hemorrhage.[163] The airway must remain patent. Recumbent horses should be rolled to the opposite side often to minimize pulmonary arteriovenous shunting and ventilation-perfusion abnormalities. Humidified 100% O_2 may be given via a nasal tube or mask. If possible, the head should be kept at heart-base level or above to avoid hypostatic intracranial congestion.

The use of antimicrobials after skull fractures in humans is controversial.[164] However, horses with fractures associated with significant skin damage should receive a standard course of broad-spectrum antibiotics.

Other supportive treatment includes maintenance of hydration and correction of electrolyte abnormalities. Overhydration must be avoided as it can exacerbate brain edema. Fever (*eg,* as a result of convulsions) increases brain edema and should be treated with alcohol baths, fans or antipyretics (phenylbutazone, dipyrone). Decubiti and traumatic skin and eye lesions should be treated. Lubricant ointments should be used on the corneas of horses with facial paralysis.

Monitoring is very important and constant re-evaluation is necessary to assess response to treatment. If there is improvement within 6-8 hours, treatment should be repeated. If there is deterioration or no improvement, more aggressive medical or surgical treatment should be considered. An exploratory craniotomy is often the only way to identify and deal with serious (*eg,* parenchymal or subdural) bleeding. Decompressive procedures can be performed. Small animal texts describe procedures that can be modified for equine patients.[163] If a comatose patient does not improve or continues to deteriorate for 36 hours after injury or surgery, euthanasia is usually indicated.

Sleep Disorders

Narcolepsy-Cataplexy

Narcolepsy-cataplexy or the "fainting foal" syndrome is a rare congenital sleep disorder of foals that has been reported in the Shetland pony and Suffolk breeds,[165,166] Narcolepsy and cataplexy refer to the acute onset of transient periods of sleep and loss of muscle tone, respectively. These attacks are provoked by excitement or stimuli such as smelling or eating food, rubbing, grooming or forced movement. Following stimulation, the response of affected foals ranges from drowsiness to collapse (cataplexy) and sleep (narcolepsy) with recovery in minutes to hours. Between attacks, such foals are clinically normal.

This condition is probably a disorder of the ascending reticular activating system and associated "sleep centers" in the brainstem. It is generally incurable but the signs may be controlled with the use of drugs such as dextroamphetamine (Dexedrine:SKF), phenelzine (Nardil:Warner-Chilcott), methylphenidate (Ritalin:CIBA) and imipramine (Tofranil: GEIGY).

Cranial Nerve Disorders

Facial Nerve Paralysis

The muscles of facial expression are innervated by fibers of the facial nerve (VII) in distinction to the muscles of mastication, which are supplied by the trigeminal nerve (V). Facial nerve fibers originate from a motor nucleus in the floor of the medulla oblongata and course dorsad, rostrad, then caudolaterad to exit the medulla in close association with the vestibulocochlear nerve (VIII). Within the medulla, cranial nerve VII is related to the reticular system, vestibular nuclei, descending motor tracts and ascending proprioceptive tracts. After entering the internal acoustic meatus with cranial nerve VIII, the facial nerve traverses the petrous temporal bone within the facial canal. During its passage through the facial canal, the nerve courses in the caudal wall of the middle ear and contributes secretomotor branches to the lacrimal glands via the geniculate nucleus. The facial nerve emerges from the skull through the stylomastoid foramen, then crosses the dorsal aspect of the guttural pouch where branches originate deep to the parotid salivary gland to supply the caudal ear muscles (caudal auricular nerve), eyelid muscles and cranial aspect of the ear (auriculopalpebral nerve). The remainder of the nerve crosses the vertical ramus of the mandible about 5 cm ventral to the temporomandibular joint and divides into dorsal and ventral buccal nerves, which supply the cheeks, nose and lips.[167]

Paresis or paralysis of the muscles of facial expression is common in horses. The facial nerve may be damaged centrally or peripherally, on one or both sides. Depending upon the site of damage, some or all of the facial muscles can be affected. Complete unilateral facial paralysis is evident as deviation of the nose toward the normal side, reduced flaring of the ipsilateral nostril during inspiration, and ipsilateral drooping of the lip, eyelid and ear. Reflexes involving cranial nerve VII, such as the lip, eyelid, corneal, menace and ear reflexes, are reduced. Inability to close the eyelid causes exposure keratitis, which may be particularly severe when there is also reduced tear formation due to damage of the secretomotor fibers of the facial nerve at or proximal to the geniculate ganglion.[168,169] Tear production can be evaluated by the Schirmer tear test.[170] Slight bilateral facial paresis may be difficult to detect because of the symmetry of signs. Complete bilateral facial paralysis may cause some difficulties in prehension of food. Defective nasal flaring increases upper airway resistance, resulting in an abnormal inspiratory noise and reduced exercise tolerance.

Determination of the site of a facial nerve lesion is very important in terms of prognosis and therapy, and is based upon consideration of concurrent clinical signs.

Lesions of the facial nerve or nucleus within the medulla usually cause all the components of facial paralysis (ie, of the lip, nose, eyelid, ear); however, various facial muscles may be unequally affected. For example, the ipsilateral ear and eyelid may droop without obvious deviation of the nose. Generally there are other signs of medullary disease, including depression, limb paresis, ataxia and other cranial nerve deficits (especially vestibular). Bilateral facial paresis is often a feature of diffuse brain diseases such as the metabolic encephalopathies, and infectious encephalitides and meningitides. Facial paralysis may accompany more localized damage to the brainstem as in protozoal myeloencephalitis, aberrant parasite migration and caudal head trauma.

Lesions of the facial nerve proximal to the vertical ramus of the mandible cause total facial nerve paralysis. Damage within the facial canal often causes concurrent vestibular signs, such as a head tilt, nystagmus and circling.[168] Tear production may be reduced by damage at or proximal to the geniculate nucleus.[168,169]

Proximal facial nerve paralysis is usually caused by extension of fracture of the petrous temporal bone and/or hemorrhage into the middle/inner ear, otitis media/interna, arthritis of the temporohyoid joint, guttural pouch mycosis, parotid lymph node abscessation, inflammation or neoplasia of the parotid salivary gland, or fracture of the vertical ramus of the mandible.[168,169]

The facial nerve may be affected in polyneuritis equi (neuritis of the cauda equina) or chronic lead poisoning. Temporary idiopathic facial paralysis occurs without clincial evidence of any of the above and may represent a viral neuritis.

Distal facial nerve damage is usually due to direct injury from a blow or lateral recumbency. Often the nerve or its branches are damaged as they cross the mandible or zygomatic arch. Facial paresis following recumbency during general anesthesia is common and usually involves only the nose and lips. Occasionally there is also drooping of the ear and/or eyelid, probably as a result of local damage to the nerve branches supplying these muscles, or to damage of the muscles themselves.

The prognosis for return of facial nerve function depends on the site and severity of the causative process. There is a fair chance of recovery with facial nerve deficits caused by trauma to the caudal aspect of the head. Other central facial nerve lesions usually warrant a poor prognosis. Facial nerve deficit is often permanent with middle ear disease, whereas the associated vestibular signs often improve. In the absence of severe skin laceration, the prognosis for peripheral facial paralysis is good and recovery takes from several days to several months. If there is skin damage and section of the nerve, the ends should be identified and either surgically repaired immediately or tagged (eg, with stainless steel sutures) for future identification. Idiopathic facial paralysis generally resolves after 2-4 weeks.

Vestibular Disorders

Each side of the vestibular system consists of a receptor, cranial nerve and central nuclei.[167] The labyrinthine vestibular receptor occupies the inner ear with the auditory receptor (cochlea) and is contained within the petrous temporal bone. The vestibular nerve passes from the receptor to the medulla through the internal acoustic meatus with the cochlear (auditory) division of cranial nerve VIII. In each side of the medulla are 4 vestibular nuclei with major connections to the cranial nerves control-

ling eye movements (III, IV, VI), and to spinal nerves affecting muscle tone of the neck, trunk and limbs. Connections are also made with small parts of the cerebellum.[167]

The function of the vestibular system is to maintain appropriate orientation of the trunk, limbs and eyes with respect to the position and movements of the head. Therefore, vestibular disease results in disturbed equilibrium and ataxia, usually without paresis. Vestibular disorders tend to be unilateral or asymmetric and are caused by either peripheral or central lesions. Peripheral disease causes a head tilt toward the affected side, abnormal vestibular nystagmus, spontaneous horizontal or rotatory nystagmus with the fast phase away from the affected side and, with elevation of the head, exaggerated eye drop ipsilaterally. There is usually a staggering, dysmetric gait with a tendency to lean or circle toward the affected side as a result of increased extension of the contralateral limbs.

Horses with any acute peripheral or central vestibular disease sometimes fall or even roll to the side of the lesion and may panic and thrash wildly in an effort to stand. Central lesions generally cause pronounced gait deficits, and nystagmus may be variably horizontal, vertical or rotatory. The fast phase of the nystagmus can be away from or toward the side of the lesion and may alter direction with changes in head position. Bilateral vestibular disease causes dysmetria, severe ataxia and complete absence of normal vestibular nystagmus. The horse may have wide swinging movements of the head. As with any vestibular disorder, signs are markedly exacerbated by blindfolding. Deafness is also apparent when there is bilateral involvement of the cochlear division of cranial nerve VIII.

Central Vestibular Disease

In addition to vestibular signs, central vestibular disease frequently involves adjacent brainstem structures to cause depression (reticular system), paresis (motor tracts), and other cranial nerve deficits (eg, cranial nerve VIII). With severe depression and recumbency, abnormal eye positions and movements may be the only indicators of vestibular disease.

Conditions causing central vestibular signs include diffuse brain disease caused by head trauma, infectious meningoencephalitides and metabolic encephalopathies, and focal brainstem diseases, such as protozoal myeloencephalitis and aberrant parasite migration.

Certain fungal toxins, some of which are known as tremorgens, have a predilection for the central vestibulocerebellar system and are probably responsible for the signs seen in ryegrass staggers and phalaris staggers.[171]

Peripheral Vestibular Disease

Signs of peripheral vestibular disease are usually unilateral and acute in onset. Central accommodation often occurs over a period of weeks and affected animals may even return to racing. Signs of vestibular disease may still be elicited by blindfolding, however.

Otitis Media-Interna: This condition is uncommon in the horse but can occur by hematogenous spread of bacteria or by direct extension of pharyngeal, guttural pouch, bone or external ear infections.[168] In addition to vestibular signs, there may be fever and a hemogram indicative of bacterial infection (leukocytosis, neutrophilia and elevated plasma fibrinogen levels). Concurrent ipsilateral facial paralysis is common due to extension of the suppurative process from the middle and inner ear to the adjacent facial canal containing cranial nerve VII. Although apparently rare in horses, it is possible for infection to spread through the internal acoustic meatus to involve the lateral medulla. Rupture of the tympanic membrane usually causes discharge from the external ear. Rhinolaryngoscopy may disclose pharyngitis or guttural pouch disease and radiographs can detect sclerosis of the affected tympanic bulla in chronically affected horses. Any ear, guttural pouch or pharyngeal exudates must be cultured. Beta-hemolytic streptococci and penicillin-resistant staphylococci have been cultured from middle ear infections, but other organisms may be cultured, including *Aspergillus* spp, with extension of guttural pouch mycosis.[168]

Treatment of associated diseases is essential (*eg,* guttural pouch, pharynx), and intensive, prolonged antimicrobial therapy is necessary for a cure. If streptococcal infection is suspected or if signs improve with penicillin therapy, high levels of penicillin should be maintained for 2-6 weeks. Other appropriate drugs are ampicillin, sulfas, trimethoprim-sulfa combinations, and oxacillin or cephalothin for penicillin-resistant staphylococci. There may be an indication for short-term (12-48 hr) corticosteroid use at the initiation of therapy for acute otitis interna. Surgical drainage of empyema of a tympanic bulla should be considered in cases resistant to medical therapy.

Middle-Inner Ear Hemorrhage: Vestibular signs due to hemorrhage into the middle-inner ear with or without fracture of the petrous temporal bone often follow trauma to the head, especially to the poll.[168] There may also be bleeding into the guttural pouch and external ear. The prognosis for recovery is good if there are no associated fractures of the floor of the calvarium or of the frontal bones, or other complications such as hemorrhage into the medulla or midbrain. Therapy is outlined in the Head Trauma section.

Vestibulocochlear Neuritis: Vestibulocochlear neuritis in association with polyneuritis equi may result in signs of peripheral vestibular disease.[172]

Idiopathic Vestibular Syndrome: Horses are occasionally presented with acute signs consistent with unilateral peripheral vestibular disease. There are no other neurologic signs and no history or evidence of trauma. These animals can be treated as occult head trauma cases. Irrespective of therapy, the signs resolve in 1-3 weeks. This may be the result of a transient disease of the vestibular nerve, possibly a viral neuritis or labyrinthitis.

Dysphagia

Dysphagia is often defined as "difficult swallowing" but in this section is used in its broadest sense to mean difficulty in eating or drinking, and includes disorders of prehension, mastication and swallowing.[173] Only primary neurologic dysphagia is discussed; dysphagia from other causes is covered in other chapters.

Central control of eating is mostly by specific medullary centers and their afferent and efferent pathways in the trigeminal (V, muscles of mastication, and facial sensation), facial (VII, muscles of the lips and cheeks), glossopharyngeal and vagus (IX and X, pharynx and larynx), and hypoglossal (XII, tongue) nerves. The voluntary effort in eating and drinking is initiated in the cerebral motor cortex and the basal nuclei. Therefore, disorders of the forebrain, medulla and cranial nerves V, VII, IX, X and XII can cause dysphagia.

Forebrain Disease

Forebrain diseases do not cause actual paralysis of the muscles involved in eating but can impair voluntary control of these muscles, resulting in incoordinated, dystonic and/or weak movements of the face, tongue, mouth and pharynx.

Diffuse cerebral disease can cause dysphagia in addition to other gross behavioral and attitudinal abnormalities (eg, depression, head-pressing, circling, blindness). There is characteristically some weakness and protrusion of the tongue, drooping of the lower lip and drooling of saliva. Foals lose the suckling reflex. Included in this group are the togaviral (arboviral) encephalitides, rabies, hepatoencephalopathy, diffuse meningitis, neonatal maladjustment syndrome, head trauma with brain swelling, leukoencephalomalacia and hydrocephalus.

Dysphagia caused by lesions of the basal nuclei occurs commonly in the western US as a result of yellow star thistle or Russian knapweed poisoning (see below under nigropallidal encephalomalacia), but can also be caused by the focal lesions of protozoal myeloencephalitis or migrating nematode larvae. Prehension and mastication are impaired but affected animals can usually swallow. Other brain signs may be mild or absent.

Medullary Disease

The signs of dysphagia seen with medullary lesions depend on the specific cranial nerve nuclei affected. Manifestations of various cranial nerve deficits affecting eating are discussed below. There are usually other, often asymmetric signs of medullary disease such as depression (reticular system), gait deficits (motor and proprioceptive tracts) and other cranial nerve signs (eg, vestibular, facial). Specific causes include protozoal myeloencephalitis, migrating parasites and trauma to the back of the head with medullary hemorrhage. Diffuse brain diseases with medullary components, such as the togaviral encephalitides, rabies, meningitis, locoweed poisoning and hepatoencephalopathy, are also included here.

Peripheral Cranial Nerve Disease (V, VII, IX, X, XII)

Trigeminal Nerve: Bilateral involvement of the motor branches of cranial nerve V causes paralysis and eventually atrophy of the masseter muscles (also of the temporalis, pterygoid and distal bellies of the digastricus muscles). The resulting weak jaw tone causes difficulty in mastication and allows the tongue to hang from the mouth. Unilateral trigeminal paralysis does not cause significant dysphagia but may result in slight deviation of the jaw away from the affected side. Damage to the sensory branches of cranial nerve V from the face and mouth does not produce severe dysphagia but may cause food accumulation in the cheeks.

Facial Nerve: Paralysis of the lips due to facial nerve damage causes minor problems in prehension of food, especially pasture or grain. Saliva may dribble from the labial commissure and food often adheres to the gingivae and lips.

Glossopharyngeal and Vagus Nerves: Bilateral paralysis of the pharyngeal and palatine muscles, innervated by cranial nerves IX and X, makes swallowing impossible. Attempts at eating are followed by choking, dorsal displacement of the soft palate and the appearance of food and saliva at the nostrils. Unilateral paralysis causes less severe signs. Aspiration of food may lead to necrotic bronchopneumonia and is particularly likely if there is concurrent paralysis of the larynx due to damage of the laryngeal fibers of cranial nerve X. Collapse of the atonic pharyngeal walls, displacement of the soft palate, and poor abduction of the vocal folds causes abnormal respiratory noises, especially during exercise.

Hypoglossal Nerve: Damage to cranial nerve XII causes lingual paralysis and eventual atrophy (unilateral or bilateral), with "quidding," drooling and poor tongue retraction. There may also be persistent lingual fasciculations even when the tongue is totally relaxed.

Combinations: Various combinations of cranial nerve deficits may have synergistic effects in producing dysphagia (eg, V with XII, and VII with XII).

Cranial nerve damage and dysphagia may follow guttural pouch mycosis (IX, X), ruptured rectus capitis ventralis muscle (IX, X), fractured hyoid bone (V or XII depending on site of fracture), excessive traction on the tongue (XII), and retropharyngeal lymph node abscessation (IX, X, XII). All interfere with chewing and swallowing.[174,176] These horses usually have other signs of the primary disease in addition to dysphagia.

Polyneuritis equi can cause dysphagia by affecting any or all of cranial nerves V, VII, IX, X or XII. Dysphagia is a common sequel to chronic lead poisoning.

Botulism and diseases resembling botulism (postanesthesia myasthenia and the shaker foal syndrome) are associated with generalized paresis of striated muscles, including those of prehension, mastication and swallowing. The toxins produced by *Clostridium botulinum* block neuromuscular transmission by interfering with the action of acetylcholine.

The neurotoxin produced by *Clostridium tetani* facilitates firing of motor neurons throughout the CNS. This toxin has a slight predilection for the medullary nuclei, which control eating. Thus, besides generalized muscle tetany, there is hypertonicity of the muscles that control eating, particularly the masseter muscles, resulting in trismus (lockjaw).

Guttural Pouch Mycosis

Most of the diverse clinical signs of guttural pouch mycosis are caused by fungal damage to any of a number of vital structures lying adjacent to the caudodorsal aspect of the medial compartment of the guttural pouch. Pseudomembranous mycotic lesions characteristically arise ventral to the tympanic bulla and medial to the great cornu of the hyoid bone.[177] Contained within a fold of the guttural pouch at this site are the internal carotid artery, glossopharyngeal (IX) and vagus (X) nerves, and cranial cervical sympathetic trunk and ganglion. The spinal accessory (XI) and hypoglossal (XII) nerves are also in this area. Mycotic lesions rarely originate in the lateral compartment of the guttural pouch or spread across the roof from the medial compartment to the area of the internal maxillary artery (a major branch of the external carotid artery), facial nerve (VII) and mandibular nerve (a branch of cranial nerve V).[178,179]

Clinical Signs: Of 59 cases of guttural pouch mycosis surveyed in the literature, 11 (19%) were in horses with dysphagia as the primary complaint, vs 30 (51%) with epistaxis.[176-180] Another 17 horses (29%) later developed obvious dysphagia, with regurgitation of food and water from the nostrils. Three horses with dysphagia also developed necrotic bronchopneumonia as the result of food aspiration. Some signs reported in horses without obvious dysphagia, such as dorsal displacement of the soft palate during exercise, coughing during feeding and bronchopneumonia, may also have reflected damage to cranial nerves IX and X with partial pharyngeal and/or laryngeal paresis. Twelve horses had endoscopic evidence of laryngeal hemiplegia and all but one involved the left side, although there was an approximately equal incidence of left- and right-sided guttural pouch lesions.[181] This finding is interesting in view of the predisposition to left-sided laryngeal hemiplegia in the general horse population. No mention was made of lingual paresis or atrophy in the cases surveyed.

Surprisingly there were only 2 convincing descriptions of Horner's syndrome in association with guttural pouch mycosis.[168,182] One of these followed accidental inclusion of sympathetic fibers in ligatures around the internal carotid artery during a successful surgery for epistaxis.[182] In another report, 3 horses had ptosis ipsilaterally and one had miosis, but the description did not include other important criteria of Horner's syndrome (*eg*, ipsilateral facial sweating and hyperemia) and could have been consistent with subtle ipsilateral facial nerve damage.[181]

In 2 horses, facial paralysis followed secondary abscessation of the parotid lymph nodes adjacent to the affected guttural pouches, but there was only one report of facial paralysis that could be directly attributed to mycotic invasion of the dorsolateral aspect of the ipsilateral guttural pouch.[179,181] There was also hemorrhage from the internal maxillary artery at this unusual site. Facial paralysis was occasionally associated with other complications of guttural pouch mycosis (see below). To date there have apparently been no reports of masseter paresis or atrophy as a result of mandibular nerve damage in horses with guttural pouch disease.

Various unusual complications of guttural pouch mycosis have been reported. Bony structures adjacent to typical mycotic lesions may become diseased and cause additional cranial nerve involvement. Examples include proliferative osteitis of the great cornu of the hyoid bone with or without fracture, avulsion of the insertion of the rectus capitis ventralis muscle (IX, X damage), mycotic lesions of the tympanic bullae that may extend into the middle ear (damage to VII and VIII in or around the middle/inner ear), and osteoarthritis of the temporohyoid joint.[168,174,179,181] It is not clear whether fungal lesions cause or are secondary to bony damage. Intracranial invasion occurred in 2 instances, once by direct extension of a guttural pouch lesion through the basal cranial bones and by embolic dissemination via the internal carotid artery in the other horse.[183,184] The latter horse had profound encephalitic signs in addition to peripheral facial paralysis and laryngeal hemiplegia.

Prognosis: If the affected horse does not succumb to blood loss or inhalation pneumonia, there is some capacity to accommodate to unilateral pharyngeal paresis, although residual signs of regurgitation and coughing during feeding are likely to remain.[181] Other neurologic signs, such as those of sympathetic or facial nerve damage, are unlikely to improve.

Guttural Pouch Empyema

Guttural pouch empyema *per se* does not usually cause neurologic deficits, although transient dysphagia that responds to treatment is not uncommon. If empyema is associated with adjacent lymph node abscessation, various cranial nerve signs are possible, including cranial nerve IX, X or XII deficits with retropharyngeal lymph node abscessation and cranial nerve VII damage as a result of parotid lymph node abscessation.[181]

Further details of guttural pouch disease are contained in Chapter 15.

Nigropallidal Encephalomalacia (Yellow Star Thistle Poisoning)

Prolonged ingestion of yellow star thistle (*Centaurea solstitialis*) or Russian knapweed (*C repens*) produces a neurologic syndrome in horses known as nigropallidal encephalomalacia (NPE). Yellow star thistle poisoning was first described in 1954 in northern California and has since been reported in southern California, southern Oregon, Argentina and Australia.[185] In 1969, NPE due to Russian knapweed ingestion was confirmed in western Colorado and more recent cases have been reported from eastern Utah and eastern Washington.[186] Most cases of NPE occur during the later summer and fall in horses grazing dry, weedy pastures where *Centaurea* spp provide most of the available forage.[186]

Clinical signs are peracute in onset and reflect bilateral dystonia of the muscles of prehension and mastication. Affected structures include the masseter, digastricus and facial muscles, and the tongue. Animals with NPE hold the mouth partly open with the lips retracted and the tongue partially protruded, resulting in a peculiar "wooden" expression. There are frequently tremors of involved muscles and purposeless chewing movements. The tongue may be moved in and out of the mouth or may be curled in the form of an open tube.[187] Despite a normal appetite, most affected horses are unable to move food back to the pharynx to be swallowed and wads of food may be packed around the tongue and gums. Weight loss and debility quickly follow. Many horses can drink water by totally immersing their muzzles and some mildly affected animals maintain condition by adopting unusual eating methods.[188] Behavioral abnormalities, such as circling, depression, yawning or frenzied activity, are common during the first few days after onset of NPE but can be seen at any time. Most affected horses are readily aroused from a state of drowsiness. Cranial nerves are intact and the gait is usually normal, although at rest the legs may be inappropriately placed.[185]

There is no effective treatment for NPE and most horses are euthanized or die within weeks from dehydration, starvation or intercurrent disease. Mildly affected horses can sometimes accommodate adequately and should be provided with pelleted complete feeds or grain that can be scooped into the mouth and swallowed more easily than hay or pasture.

The necropsy findings to which the disease owes its name are quite characteristic and consist of sharply circumscribed areas of coagulative or liquefactive necrosis in the substantia nigra and/or globus pallidus that are almost always bilaterally symmetric.

Chronic Lead Poisoning

Peripheral neuropathy is a common effect of lead poisoning.[189] Clinically this is apparent as pharyngeal and laryngeal paralysis with dysphagia, abnormal respiratory noises ("roaring") and inhalation pneumonia.

Horses appear quite susceptible to poisoning by prolonged low-level ingestion of lead. Clinical data suggest a daily intake as low as 1.7 mg/kg body weight for several months causes typical signs of lead intoxication.[190] Acute lead poisoning is rare in horses apparently because of their selective feeding habits.[190] Generally, affected horses live within the fallout or "smoke" zone of lead mining or processing industries and are poisoned by eating pasture contaminated by aerial fallout of lead.

The earliest clinical sign of lead poisoning may be an abnormal inspiratory noise during exercise or coughing during feeding, with persistent "chokes" and regurgitation of food through the nostrils. Pneumonia often occurs due to food inhalation.[190-194] These signs are all referable to dysfunction of cranial nerves IX and X. Bilateral facial (VII) paresis and limb weakness occasionally occur.[191]

Anorexia, weight loss and poor haircoat soon follow, and other rather variable clinical signs have been reported, including transient colic, lameness, protein-losing nephropathy with ventral edema, and a blue "lead line" along the gingival margins of the teeth.[191] Anemia is a common finding and is occasionally accompanied by the appearance of immature RBC and basophilic stippling of RBC.

Diagnosis is usually based on the clinical signs and history, but lead assays of blood and urine may be diagnostic.[193,194] Because 90% of lead in blood is bound to RBC in an inactive form, blood lead levels of anemic or hemoconcentrated animals should be interpreted cautiously.[195] Blood levels do not always reflect the

Table 2. Lead Levels in Various Equine Tissues[193,194,197]

	Controls (Pb ppm wet matter) $\overline{X} \pm SD$	Intoxication (Pb ppm wet matter) range
blood	0.1007 ± 0.085	0.1 - 0.47
bone	7.33 ± 3.01	340 - 375
liver	0.83 ± 0.35	20 - 33
kidney	0.23 ± 0.08	55 - 86

total body content of lead in chronic poisoning because the distribution in and mobilization from tissues are affected by the status of other substances, including Ca, P, vitamin D and Zn.[191,194,196] Urine lead levels are rather variable but the concentration of lead may dramatically increase in the urine of affected animals after chelation treatment with Ca versenate (EDTA). The diagnostic value of this finding is uncertain.[39,193] Other assays of the biochemical activity of lead, such as serum aminolevulenic acid dehydrase, urine delta-aminolevulenic acid and urine porphyrins, have not been adequately evaluated in horses.[195]

Tissue levels of lead are consistently elevated in horses with chronic lead poisoning. The best tissues for analysis are bone, liver and kidney (Table 2).[193,194,197]

Chelation of the lead in soft tissues by the use of Ca versenate appears to be the most effective treatment. Intermittent dosage may be more effective than constant administration. A daily dosage of 2% Ca versenate at 50-100 mg/kg body weight in a slow IV drip has been used successfully. This was repeated daily for 3 days, then repeated for 3 days again after an interval of 4 days. The concurrent use of acidifying agents may promote resorption of lead from bone.[191]

Cerebellar Diseases

The cerebellum receives proprioceptive information from all parts of the body and projections from the brainstem motor centers. By continuous assimilation of this and other information, the cerebellum regulates the quality of motor activity via its efferent pathways. Therefore, cerebellar disorders are generally expressed as errors in the rate, range and force of movement.[198] These errors are most obvious as delayed and exaggerated (hypermetric) movements, increased extensor tonus (spasticity), and intention tremors. Despite profound dysmetria, normal strength is preserved. Sensorium and vision are normal, although the menace response may be absent due to interruption of the pathway from the occipital cortex to the facial nucleus as it passes through the cerebellum.

Congenital and/or hereditary cerebellar disorders can be classified according to cause as genetic or idiopathic malformations, destruction due to viral disease (in utero or early neonatal) or degeneration (abiotraphy).[198] The only well-defined syndromes reported in horses thus far are the familial cerebellar abiotrophies of the Arabian horse and Gotland pony breeds.[199-205]

Cerebellar Abiotrophy of Arabian Horses

This condition of Arabian or part-Arabian horses has been recognized since 1966 and is caused by degeneration of the cerebellar cortex during late fetal or early neonatal life.[202] Signs of cerebellar disease may be present at birth but usually develop during the first 6 months. Progression of signs is variable but often slow or inapparent after an initial rapid deterioration. Affected foals develop a spastic, ataxic gait and pronounced hypermetria ("goose-stepping"), especially of the front limbs. At rest they may stand base-wide with rhythmic swaying of the trunk and neck from side to side or backward and forward. These signs are exaggerated during walking or excitement. Blindfolding has no effect on posture or gait. Hopping responses are delayed and hypermetric. Spinal reflexes are normal or increased. If the head is elevated, the foal may buckle in the rear limbs or fall over backwards. There is usually a fine head tremor exaggerated by voluntary movements such as reaching to suckle the mare or to sniff at feed offered by the examiner. Careful observation may reveal an intention tremor of the eyes and tongue. As expected in a diffuse cerebellar disorder (see above), the menace response is usually absent bilaterally, although vision is unaffected. In contrast to those diseases caused by lesions of the spinal cord or brainstem, there is no paresis.

Cerebellar abiotrophy appears to be an inherited disorder with a reported incidence of up to 8% in foals of certain families.[199] There is no treatment and most affected horses are destroyed before maturity. Gross necropsy findings are usually unremarkable and histologic abnormalities are confined to the cerebellar cortex. There is diffuse reduction in numbers, degeneration and disorientation of Purkinje cells, often accompanied by thinning and depletion of the granular and molecular layers.

Cerebellar Abiotrophy of Gotland Ponies

The clinical signs and underlying pathologic changes of this inherited condition appear similar if not identical to the Arabian horse syndrome. Signs of spastic ataxia without weakness appear during the first 6 months of life. Surprisingly, no mention is made of a head tremor or menace response deficit in published reports.[204] The disease is probably inherited as an autosomal recessive gene.

Other Cerebellar Disorders

Cerebellar hypoplasia has been reported in New Zealand in a Thoroughbred foal unable to stand after birth.[205] Another isolated case of cerebellar hypoplasia in a Thoroughbred foal was reported in the US, but details were not provided.[200] An acute, rapidly progressive cerebellar syndrome of 1- to 2-month-old Oldenberg foals was first described in Germany in 1949.[206] The morphologic basis for this disease is not clear but one investigator described grey-red areas in the cerebellum evident histologically as foci of demyelination.

Signs of cerebellar dysfunction are also seen with diseases such as protozoal myeloencephalitis, verminous encephalitis and brain trauma. In these acquired disorders the signs are often asymmetric.

Infectious Disease

Tetanus

Tetanus is a highly fatal infectious disease caused by the toxin of *Clostridium tetani*. The disease causes muscular rigidity, hyperesthesia and convulsions in horses of all ages. Despite the ready availability of cheap and effective prophylaxis, tetanus continues to cause sporadic equine mortality throughout the world.

The vegetative form of *Cl tetani* is a slender, motile gram-positive bacillus requiring anaerobic conditions for growth and replication. The organism exists largely in spore form and is commonly found in the intestinal tract and feces of animals, and in soils rich in organic material. Spores are resistant to most environmental extremes, chemical disinfectants and antimicrobials, but can be destroyed by heating to 115 C (239 F) for 20 minutes.[207]

The most common route of infection is by wound contamination with *Cl tetani* spores.[207] Disease results when favorble conditions exist for germination and proliferation of the organism, and toxin is subsequently elaborated. Lowered O_2 tension is the most important of these requirements and is most often found in the depths of puncture wounds or in wounds associated with considerable necrosis, impaired blood supply, foreign bodies or concomitant pyogenic bacterial infection.[208] Neglected puncture wounds are especially dangerous but any break in the skin or mucous membranes is a potential portal of entry for *Cl tetani*. Castration wounds, metritis following dystocia and/or retained placenta, and the use of contaminated hypodermic needles have all been associated with the development of tetanus.[209] An infected umbilicus is the usual site of *Cl tetani* proliferation and toxin formation in neonates.[210,211] The potential danger of tetanus infection in the normal or inflamed GI tract is not known. Spores are viable in tissues for many months and may germinate long after a wound has healed if appropriate conditions are met (*eg*, after reinjury).[207] This accounts in part for the wide variability among individuals in the time between wound contamination and onset of signs of tetanus. The incubation period is usually 1-3 weeks but may range from several days to several months.[207,208]

Cl tetani is a noninvasive organism and signs of tetanus are due to the potent exotoxin (tetanospasmin), which is produced locally and acts principally on the CNS. Tetanospasmin is a water-soluble protein that appears to reach the CNS hematogenously and by passage along peripheral nerves.[212,213] The toxin localizes in the ventral horn of the grey matter of the spinal cord and brainstem where it binds irreversibly to gangliosides within synaptic membranes.[214] The main action of tetanospasmin is to block the release of the inhibitory neurotransmitter. Therefore, reflexes normally inhibited by descending inhibitory motor tracts or by inhibitory interneurons (polysynaptic reflexes) are greatly facilitated, resulting in tetanic contractions of muscles after normal sensory stimulation.[215]

Tetanus toxin has been shown experimentally to have a number of peripheral effects including sympathetic nervous system stimulation, neuromuscular blockade during the later stages of tetanus, and alterations of catecholamine and adrenocorticoid metabolism.[208,215,216] The relevance of these findings to tetanus in horses is not known.

Clinical Signs: The severity and rate of progression of clinical signs depend on the dose of toxin and the size, age and immune status of the affected animal. The signs of tetanus reflect spasticity of striated muscles. The earliest clinical signs depend on the specific muscle groups first affected. In many cases, a slightly stiff gait is the initial sign; some horses are reluctant to feed off the ground due to spasm of cervical muscles. Overreaction to normal external stimuli is another early sign. Spasm of the muscles of mastication (trismus) may cause difficulty in eating, and facial muscle spasm results in an anxious expression with retracted lips, flared nostrils, prolapsed nictitating membranes and erect ears. External stimuli, particularly a hand clap or tap on the forehead, or attempts at eating may provoke further spasms of facial and masticatory muscles. Other striated muscles are progressively affected, causing a very stiff, stilted gait with rigid extension of the neck, limbs and tail ("sawhorse" stance). Spasms of paraspinal musculature often result in ventral or lateral arching of the neck, back or tail. Colic is occasionally the presenting sign or complicates the course of tetanus and may reflect sympathetic overactivity. Spastic paralysis of pharyngeal muscles sometimes results in regurgitation or aspiration of food.

Inability to posture appropriately causes retention of urine and feces. Once an affected mature horse falls, it is generally unable to regain its feet. Attempts at standing cause further tonic-clonic muscle spasms and distress. In lateral recumbency, increased extensor tonus results in rigid extension of extremities and dorsiflexion of the neck (opisthotonus) and back (lordosis). Foals may often be assisted to stand in this remarkably abnormal posture. Even slight stimulation can cause prolonged generalized muscle spasms. Insensible water losses and energy expenditure are greatly increased by this activity, resulting in rapid cachexia, dehydration and metabolic acidosis.

Death usually occurs after 5-7 days and is often caused by asphyxia due to spastic paralysis of respiratory mucles, laryngospasm or aspiration pneumonia. Complications of recumbency and intense muscle spasms, such as decubitus formation, rhabdomyolysis with myoglobinemia, and fractures, can also be lethal. If death does not occur, signs usually stabilize after about a week. Recovery is gradual and takes about 6 weeks in most cases.[207,211,217] If recovery occurs, it is complete and without residual signs. Recovered animals are *not* protected from further episodes of tetanus.

Treatment: The current approach to treatment of tetanus is based on the premises that the toxin-ganglioside bond is chemically irreversible and that recovery is due to the gradual replacement of altered gangliosides by normal metabolic processes.[213] For these reasons, treatment is generally symptomatic and supportive, with particular emphasis placed on good nursing care.

The main objectives of therapy are destruction of *Cl tetani* organisms, neutralization of unbound toxin, control of muscle spasms, and general support.[217]

Destruction of *Cl tetani* organisms and neutralization of the toxin traditionally involves the IV, IM or SC administration of large amounts of homologous tetanus antitoxin, plus penicillin or tetracycline therapy and wound debridement to destroy the remaining organisms. The suggested dosages for antitoxin have been rather arbitrary, ranging up to 220 IU/kg body weight every 12 hours.[207] Repeated massive doses are very expensive and probably unnecessary since circulating toxin levels are usually very low. An IV or IM dose of 5,000-10,000 IU is probably adequate. In addition, tetanus toxoid is administered at a separate site because protective humoral immunity is not induced by the natural disease. High doses of penicillin, up to 200,000 IU/kg body weight of potassium penicillin G divided in 4 daily doses, are used for the first 2-4 days to destroy vegetative *Cl tetani* organisms in poorly perfused necrotic tissue. If a wound or infection is found, it should be minutely debrided and irrigated with hydrogen peroxide or another disinfectant solution.

Intrathecal (subarachnoid) administration of tetanus antitoxin has been used for many years in humans and animals with tetanus with variable success.[209,212,217-220] The rationale for its use has not been clearly defined but some clinical trials indicate that progression of the disease may be arrested and survival rates improved by this therapy.[219,220] It is worth emphasizing that signs of tetanus may be stabilized but probably not reversed, so intrathecal treatment of affected horses should be most useful if performed early in the disease (ie, before recumbency).[216] Current recommendations are for the administration of 30,000-50,000 IU homologous tetanus antitoxin at the cisternal or lumbosacral site after slow removal of 30-50 ml CSF.[220] The addition of 20-100 mg prednisone succinate is optional and has not yet been evaluated in horses.

Muscular rigidity and reflex spasms are controlled by placing affected horses in a quiet, dark environment to minimize external stimulation.[217,221] Ideal chemical control would provide relief of anxiety, muscle relaxation and control of convulsions. However, few commonly used drugs meet these needs.

Strong sedatives, such as chloral hydrate, magnesium sulfate, and sodium pentobarbital, are useful to diminish anxiety and response to stimulation but cause problems with eating and ambulation when used in doses sufficient to produce muscle relaxation.[221] Ataractics, such as promazine (0.5-1.0 mg/kg body weight every 4-6 hr), chlorpromazine (0.4-0.8 mg/kg body weight every 4-6 hr), and acepromazine (0.05-0.1 mg/kg body weight every 4-6 hr) are probably most commonly used in treating equine tetanus and provide useful muscle relaxation and sedation while maintaining the standing position.[217,221] Oil preparations of d-tubocurarine given IM have been used quite successfully in standing animals at 0.25-0.5 mg/kg body weight daily but the dangers of overdose and respiratory or limb paralysis are great.[209,221,222]

Potentially more practical are the centrally acting muscle relaxants, such as methocarbamol and glyceryl guaiacolate, which inhibit polysynaptic reflex activity in the brainstem and spinal cord. Glyceryl guaiacolate has a relatively short duration of action (25-30 minutes) and is difficult to use in standing animals.[223] However, careful titration of its effect by slow IV drip may produce adequate relaxation without recumbency. Methocarabamol (10-20 mg/kg body weight every 8 hr) is convenient and relieves muscular pain and rigidity in mild cases, and can be safely used in combination with a variety of sedatives. Diazepam has not been properly evaluated in horses with tetanus but it is the drug of choice in human patients.[219,224] It effectively relieves muscular spasms and anxiety in horses with tetanus but is expensive to use in mature animals (50-200 mg IV every 4-6 hr). Diazepam can be used alone or in combination with sedatives (the dose of diazepam must be reduced accordingly). The use of xylazine (0.5-1.0 mg/kg body weight) may facilitate brief procedures such as nasogastric intubation or IV catheter placement.

Horses presented in lateral recumbency (especially neonates) have very little chance of recovery and early euthanasia should be considered. Complete paralysis with curariform drugs and total respiratory and nutritional support may be considered for valuable neonates at hospitals with the facilities. Paralysis for 1-3 weeks may be necessary.

Good general nursing care is the most important aspect of tetanus treatment. Dysphagic horses can be fed through an indwelling nasoesophageal tube or conceivably via a surgically created esophageal fistula. Animals that can eat should be fed and watered from containers placed well above the ground.[211] Placement of an indwelling IV catheter minimizes the stress of repeated blood sampling and injections. Serum electrolyte levels and the hemogram should be monitored regularly and any abnormalities corrected. Infections, such as aspiration pneumonia and cystitis, must be vigorously treated. Manual rectal evacuation and bladder catheterization may be necessary. Slinging is indicated for animals in danger of falling.[211,217]

Prophylaxis: Active immunization against tetanus is reliably achieved with potent commercial aluminum hydroxide-adjuvanted toxoids. The usual recommendations are for a second vaccination 3-4 weeks after the first. followed by annual revaccination, with boosters after lacerations or other tetanus-prone wounds. Although annual revaccination is probably advisable, recent work indicates that protective antibody titers persist for at least 4 years after the first booster.[225]

Equine-origin tetanus antitoxin (TAT) is widely used to protect unvaccinated horses after injury. The usual prophylactic dose is 1500 IU given SC or IM. There have been occasional reports of acute, fatal hepatic necrosis (Theiler's disease) in horses 2-3 months after administration of TAT.[226] In areas where this disease occurs, owners should be advised of the attendant risk when TAT is administered. Nevertheless, wounded, unvaccinated horses everywhere should receive TAT and tetanus toxoid (at separate sites) initially, followed by a toxoid booster 3-4 weeks later, and annually thereafter. Hopefully the institution of conscientious and widespread tetanus vaccination programs will reduce the need for TAT use.

Tetanus toxoid and TAT can be given simultaneously, in separate syringes at separate sites, to achieve a combination of immediate protection and active immunization. (Remember, tetanus spores can germinate months after a wound has healed.) Passively acquired, circulating TAT may interfere with the immune response to tetanus toxoid vaccination.[227] For this reason, foals that have received colostral and/or injected TAT at birth are not usually vaccinated with tetanus toxoid until 4-6 months of age. However, recent evidence suggests that catabolic decay of antitoxin received by either route results in nonprotective titers in most foals by 2-3 months of age.[227] Also, up to 25% of foals receive suboptimal transfer of maternal antibodies so that even foals of recently vaccinated mares may have low levels of circulating TAT.[228]

These data suggest the following regimen for protection of foals against tetanus:

1. All foals of mares unvaccinated in the last 30 days of gestation or foals that have not acquired sufficient passive antibodies from colostrum should receive 1500 IU TAT at birth.

2. Tetanus toxoid should be administered at 2, 3 and 6 months of age, and then annually.

Tremor Syndromes

Ryegrass Staggers

Ryegrass staggers is a nervous syndrome characterized by tremors and ataxia that occurs in livestock of all ages.[171,229] It occurs most commonly in New Zealand but has also been reported in the US, England and Australia.[171,230] The disease generally affects horses grazing perennial ryegrass (Lolium perenne) pastures in mid-summer or fall. A wide range of pasture conditions has been associated with the staggers syndrome, including short-grazed dry pasture with scant green leaf, stubble shortly after removal of a hay crop, fresh regrowth pasture, or predominantly stemmy pasture.[171]

The clinical signs are those of a vestibulocerebellar disorder. Initially there are intermittent mild muscle tremors that progress to varying degrees of ataxia with a head nod, swaying, incoordinated gait and wide-based rocking stance.[171,229] Severely affected animals may stumble and fall, causing severe tetanic muscle spasms. If left undisturbed, recumbent horses usually recover and regain their feet within a short time. Excitement or blindfolding markedly exacerbates all signs. The condition is not usually fatal except where accidents

result in injury or drowning. Definitive neuropathologic changes are not seen at necropsy.[171]

The offending neurotoxin has not yet been identified but is thought to be a tremorgenic mycotoxin.[231] Earlier efforts to incriminate the ryegrass alkaloids perloline and halostachine were inconclusive.[171]

Careful removal of affected horses from pasture usually results in the resolution of signs in one week to several months. The use of a laxative-purgative at the time of removal may be appropriate. These animals should be placed in a flat area free of obstacles and handled as little as possible until they recover.

Paspalum Staggers (Dallis Grass Poisoning)

Paspalum staggers is clinically identical to ryegrass staggers and occurs in New Zealand, Australia, the US and Europe.[171] The signs are caused by toxin contained in the sclerotia (ergots) of Claviceps paspali that parasitize Dallis grass (Paspalum dilitatum).

Sympathetic Disorders

Horner's Syndrome

Damage to the sympathetic supply of the ocular structures results in Horner's syndrome.[232] This is evident as slight drooping of the upper eyelid (ptosis), constriction of the pupil (miosis), slight protrusion of the nictitating membrane, and enophthalmos due to sinking of the globe, all of which are ipsilateral. Vision, pupillary light, palpebral and corneal reflexes, and menace responses are unaffected. Depending upon the actual site of nerve damage, other ipsilateral signs may be seen including dilation of facial blood vessels, hyperemia of the nasal and conjunctival mucosae, and increased facial temperature and sweating.[232] These additional head signs are due to interruption of the sympathetic supply to other smooth muscles and glands of the head. Sweating, which may be only intermittent and temporary, is most obvious at the base of the ear, extending down the neck to about the level of the axis.

Subtle signs of Horner's syndrome are best detected by careful comparison of both sides of the face for any asymmetry. Anisocoria (unequal pupillary diameter) is most easily appreciated when the eyes are examined in a darkened area, and slight differences in facial temperature may be most obvious after the examiner's hands have been cooled by rinsing with alcohol.

Other signs associated with Horner's syndrome depend upon the location and size of the causative lesion(s). Sympathetic control of the head includes both central and peripheral components.[223,234] Upper motor neurons of the sympathetic nervous system descend from the brainstem in the cervical spinal cord (lateral tectotegmentospinal tracts) to synapse on preganglionic sympathetic cell bodies in the first 3 thoracic segments (T_1-T_3). Preganglionic fibers exit the spinal cord and pass back up the neck in the vagosympathetic trunk to synapse on postganglionic sympathetic neurons in the cranial cervical ganglion. Postganglionic fibers leave the cranial cervical ganglion, closely related to the caudodorsal aspect of the guttural pouch, to supply sympathetic innervation to the eyes and head.

Horner's syndrome has been associated with a large unilateral protozoal lesion in the cervical spinal cord and may result from any lesion of the descending sympathetic tracts in the brainstem and cervical or cranial thoracic spinal cord.[235] In addition to the above signs, damage to central sympathetic pathways causes sweating and increased temperature on the ipsilateral side of the body because the ipsilateral spinal cord sympathetic outflow is deprived of upper motor neuron influence.

Peripheral damage to pre- or postganglionic sympathetic fibers to the head commonly causes Horner's syndrome. Space-occupying cranial thoracic lesions, cervical trauma, irritant perivascular injections (vagosympathetic trunk), guttural pouch infections (cranial cervical ganglion) and periorbital disease are causes.[168,182,232,236]

It is useful to remember that the sympathetic supply to the cervical blood vessels and sweat glands is distributed with the cervical spinal nerves and is not derived from the cervical sympathetic trunk.[182]

Horner's syndrome is not a specific disease, but its recognition is helpful in defining the site of a lesion. With the aid of other signs the site can be determined and the primary process treated. With the exception of facial sweating, signs of Horner's syndrome are usually permanent, although not obviously harmful to the affected animal.

Spinal Malformations

Occipitoatlantoaxial Malformation

Occipitoatlantoaxial malformation (OAAM) is the term used to describe a group of congen-

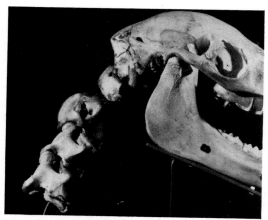

Fig 11. Right lateral view of the skull and first 4 cervical vertebrae from a newborn Arabian foal with OAAM. The hypoplastic atlas is fused to the occipital bones. The normally broad wings of the atlas are present as rudimentary peg-like processes. The atlantoaxial joint resembles a normal occipitoatlantal joint. Therefore, the assimilated atlas is occipitalized and the axis is atlantalized. The dens (not visible) is hypoplastic and the wings of the axis are broad.

ital disorders involving the occipital bones, atlas and axis. The basic malformations include fusion of the atlas to the occiput, hypoplasia of the atlas, hypoplasia of the dens, and modification of the atlantoaxial joint surfaces (Fig 11). There may be ventral luxation of the axis on the atlas, and some of the malformations include cervical scoliosis associated with an extra piece on the caudal axis.

At least 18 cases of OAAM have been reported in horses and are divided into 4 subtypes: familial OAAM in Arabians (11 cases), asymmetric OAAM (2 cases), OAAM with 2 atlases (1 case), and OAAM with asymmetric atlanto-occipital fusion (4 cases).[237-240]

Affected animals may manifest a wide variety of syndromes. Foals may be born dead because of severe compression of the medulla oblongata and cranial cervical spinal cord by the unstable craniovertebral bones during parturition. Foals may show tetraparesis or tetraplegia with milder compression of the CNS during parturition. Close inspection of the craniovertebral region often reveals a clicking noise when the head is moved. The clicking is presumably due to continual luxation—relocation of the axis and dens on the atlas, which is fused to the skull. Reduced atlanto-occipital movement can be detected in affected animals. The atlas is palpably abnormal and, in particular, the normally broad wings are reduced in size and can be palpated beneath the skin as

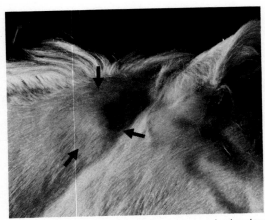

Fig 12. Close-up view of the right craniovertebral region of an Arabian yearling with OAAM and the wobbler syndrome. A bump is visible just caudal to the ear (arrows) and a bony, peg-like wing of the atlas was palpated at this site on each side. The animal had very restricted movement of the head on the neck.

small bony pegs (Fig 12). Some cases of OAAM are presented as wobblers, with progressive ataxia and tetraparesis in weanlings or yearlings. This is usually due to spinal cord compression caused by accumulation of fibrous tissue associated with the unstable atlantoaxial joint. Clicking sounds, and visible and palpable abnormalities may be found when the craniovertebral region is scrutinized. In addition, these young horses usually have an abnormal head and neck carriage, with the head held extended. One affected Arabian filly had abnormal head posture and a palpably abnormal atlas but no neurologic signs by 24 months of age; radiographs confirmed the presence of

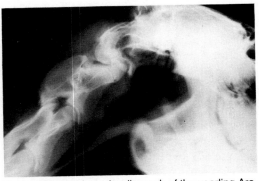

Fig 13. Plain left lateral radiograph of the yearling Arabian with OAAM shown in Figure 12, showing atlanto-occipital fusion, hypoplasia of the atlas and dens, and modification of the atlantoaxial joint. Ventral luxation of the axis on the atlas, with impaction of the dens on the body of the atlas, is also present.

OAAM. Horses with prominent asymmetry (subtypes 2 and 4) often have cervical scoliosis, which may be the only clinical sign.

Clinical diagnosis of an OAAM can be confirmed by radiography of the head and neck (Fig 13). It is extremely helpful to have radiographs of the same regions from normal horses of a similar age for comparison (Fig 14).

Surgical stabilization of the malformation may be considered in cases of OAAM to prevent further compression of the spinal cord. Fusion of the axis on the atlas, perhaps with a laminectomy of the atlas if the vertebral canal is severely compromised at that site, may be successful. Surgical interference is only palliative and results in further neck rigidity that may be unsightly and may promote malarticulations in the second through the seventh cervical vertebrae.

Careful dissection of the craniovertebral region at necropsy is required to accurately define the exact morphology of an OAAM (Fig 11). The entire vertebral column should be studied and, as with any congenital anomaly, all other organs should be scrutinized for coexisting malformation.

It is almost certain that OAAM is hereditary in Arabians and may have a simple autosomal recessive mode of inheritance.[237] Consequently, breeding affected animals and rebreeding their parents should be discouraged. The other subtypes of OAAM may be random malformations, although a genetic basis may exist.

Wobbler Syndrome

The wobbler syndrome, known in North America since at least 1938, is probably the most frequently seen neurologic syndrome in horses.[241] It occurs in many breeds of equidae, particularly light breeds and especially Thoroughbreds. Affected horses may be any age but are usually 6-24 months old and are most often rapidly growing males that are healthy in other respects. Neurologic signs consist of various combinations of ataxia, weakness and spasticity in the pelvic and sometimes the thoracic limbs. These signs may abate, remain static, fluctuate, or progress so much that the affected horse must be euthanized. These signs, which are essentially symmetric and reflect a spinal cord (or brainstem) disease, are collectively described as "wobbling."

Many wobblers have malformations of the cervical vertebrae associated with compression of the spinal cord, called cervical vertebral malformation. When the vertebrae and CNS are clinically and pathologically scrutinized in some wobblers, other causes are found for spinal cord (or brainstem) disease. Therefore, diseases such as vertebral trauma, degenerative myeloencephalopathy, protozoal myeloencephalitis, equine herpesvirus-1 myeloencephalitis, vertebral osteomyelitis and others have caused the wobbler syndrome. Unfortunately, the mechanism of damage to the spinal cord, let alone the exact cause of the lesion, frequently is not determined for many wobblers.

A wobbler is a (young) horse with signs of spinal cord disease that might be caused by a cervical vertebral malformation. Once a specific mechanism or etiology has been defined for a particular case, a more specific diagnosis can be made.

Reviews of the wobbler syndrome can be consulted for further information.[242,243]

Cervical Vertebral Malformation

Cervical vertebral malformation (CVM) is the term used to describe the bone and joint deformities and malarticulations in the cervical vertebrae of many wobblers. These bony lesions result in a focal compression-type myelopathy and signs of spinal cord disease.

Abnormalities in the cervical vertebrae have been known to occur in horses with the wobbler syndrome since at least 1939.[244] These malformations and malarticulations, particularly the intervertebral joint lesions, have been categorized and discussed in detail.[245-247] Similar joint lesions can exist in horses with no neurologic signs.[243,248,249] Closer attention was therefore given to the presence of a narrowed vertebral canal[250-252] Following further investigations, it was concluded that the most significant component of the malformation that resulted in compression of the spinal cord was stenosis of the cervical vertebral canal.[249,253] The fundamental importance of the sagittal diameter of the cervical vertebral canal in several cervical compressive myelopathies in humans, including spondylosis, is still widely accepted.[254-257]

Clinical Signs: Horses with ataxia due to CVM are usually of light breeds; Thoroughbreds are particularly affected. Both sexes are affected although there appears to be a higher frequency of affected males reported. Affected animals tend to be large for their age and breed. Young foals from a few months old to aged horses over 10 years old can be affected. The most frequent age at onset of neurologic signs is between 6 and 30 months. These young, rapidly growing horses tend to have

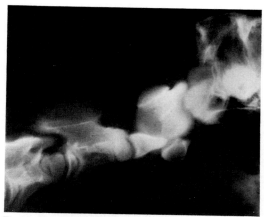

Fig 14. Plain left lateral radiograph of a normal neonatal foal for comparison with Figure 13.

vertebral canal stenosis, enlarged vertebral epiphyses and angular fixations between C_2 and C_5 as components of their malformation (Figs 15, 16).

A cluster of cases involved large horses that were worked hard, with ages ranging approximately from 5-10 years. The malformation in these adult horses may have some of the characteristics mentioned above. More often there are combinations of prominent vertebral canal stenosis and enlarged, arthrotic articular processes, most often involving C_5-T_1 (Fig 17).

Clinical evidence of ataxia, weakness and spasticity often begins acutely and is progres-

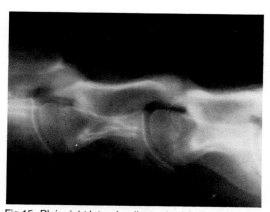

Fig 15. Plain right lateral radiograph of C_2-C_4 in a horse with cervical vertebral malformation. There is vertebral canal stenosis at the caudal end of C_3 and C_4 associated with enlargement of the caudal epiphyses (straight arrow). Notice also that the caudal limit of the roof of the vertebral canal within C_3 (curved arrow) extends well caudad. Any flexion of C_4 on C_3, with elevation of the cranial epiphysis of C_4, further compromises the space available for the spinal cord.

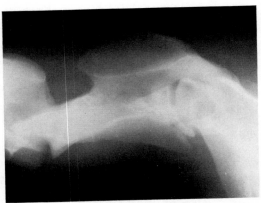

Fig 16. Plain right lateral radiograph of the flexed cervical vertebrae (C_1-C_3) in a yearling Quarter Horse colt with cervical vertebral malformation. This is a classic and profound form. There is angular fixation of C_3 and C_2, with limited movement at this joint, marked enlargement of the caudal epiphysis of C_2, and flattening of the cranial epiphysis of C_3. Of primary significance is the greatly reduced sagittal diameter of the vertebral canal measured at the caudal end of C_2, at the cranial end of C_3 and between C_2 and C_3 (Fig 11). The term flexion-fixation with luxation may be appropriate for this extreme type of malformation.

sive over a period of days to months. These signs frequently fluctuate, and the onset and fluctuation can be associated with injury such as a fall. In such cases it is difficult to determine if ataxia was present prior to the injury. Clinical signs may improve in some cases with residual ataxia remaining. It is possible that, with accommodation by the horse to a neurologic deficit, clinical signs could disappear if the spinal cord was not reinjured.

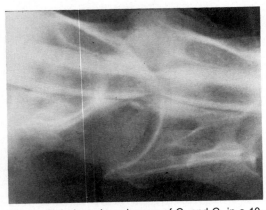

Fig 17. Right lateral myelogram of C_6 and C_7 in a 10-year-old Thoroughbred gelding with cervical vertebral malformation. There is stenosis of the cranial orifice of the vertebral canal within C_7 associated with very dense bone. Although there is some enlargement of the articular processes, this is not directly associated with the compressive myelopathy of this horse.

Physical examination usually reveals a well-grown horse, healthy in other respects. Affected young horses may have evidence of enlarged epiphyses of the long bones of the legs ("epiphysitis"). Signs of previous injury are occasionally seen. Some horses with prominent flexion—fixation at C_2-C_3 or C_3-C_4 have subtle but detectible cervical kyphosis and an abnormally rigid neck carriage.

Neurologic examination most often reveals various combinations of essentially symmetric ataxia, weakness and spasticity in the pelvic and usually the thoracic limbs (see Neurologic Examination section). These signs are related to pressure-induced damage to white matter tracts in the cervical spinal cord. Sometimes signs are asymmetric. In such cases, ataxia is often more prominent in the legs on one side and mild in the opposite legs. However, pelvic limb signs are almost always one grade worse then thoracic limb signs. This is consistent with most focal cervical lesions (see Neurologic Examination). As with most spinal cord diseases, signs can be exaggerated by walking the horse on a slope with the head elevated. This is particularly so for subtle spasticity in the thoracic limbs and for subtle ataxia in the pelvic limbs. Muscle atrophy, cervical pain and evidence of grey matter and spinal nerve root lesions, such as cutaneous hypalgesia and hyporeflexia of the neck, occur occasionally.

Therefore, wobblers with CVM can be clinically indistinguishable from so-called wobblers with other spinal cord diseases discussed below. The signalment, progression of signs, neurologic examination and particularly radiologic examination can be most helpful in the differential diagnosis of these diseases.

Diagnosis: Radiographic examination of the cervical vertebrae is the single most useful diagnostic aid in cases of CVM. It is also frequently misused and radiographs are often misread.[249,258]

Plain radiography is used in CVM cases to detect evidence of a narrowing (stenosis) of the vertebral canal. To improve objectivity, the minimum sagittal diameters and minimum flexed diameters of the cervical vertebral canal can be measured (Fig 18). Plain radiographs taken with the horse standing can be used to detect narrowing of the vertebral canal prior to obtaining radiographs in the recumbent, anesthetized horse when flexion and extension of the neck can aid in defining the maximal compromise to the vertebral canal. The values for the canal diameter for a particular wobbler can be compared with normal horses of similar size. If normal ranges are not available for the same radiographic technic used, the values in Table 3 or from other sources may be used. With experience, sites of canal stenosis can be detected readily on radiographs. However, by plotting individual horses' values on graphs drawn from the reference ranges, horses with stenosis can be identified more easily (Fig 19). Those horses with individual measurements that fall below the minimum range almost certainly have cervical vertebral stenosis. In addition, horses with values that form a curve that deviates downward within the smooth curve of reference ranges most probably have relative stenosis at that site. It must be remembered that extension of the caudal cervical vertebrae, and not flexion, may maximally compromise the canal at these sites. Also, if there is transverse compression of the spinal cord, as from a greatly enlarged articular process, the sagittal measurements may not be abnormal (although they more frequently are). Horses with unequivocal cervical vertebral stenosis should not be subjected to flexion and extension of the neck as these maneuvers will likely aggravate the spinal cord compression.

By consideration of the size of the horse, absolute sagittal diameters, shape of the measurement curves, and presence of enlarged articular processes, horses with CVM can be identified. These animals are then candidates for myelography, which is necessary to confirm compression of the spinal cord. If there has been considerable external injury, spinal cord compression can occur without definitive stenosis of the vertebral canal. Finally, the nature of a malformation and vertebral canal stenosis can change with time and growth of the horse. Therefore, the radiographic evaluation, including sagittal measurements, of a horse in which signs have been stable for months or years may be within normal limits. Examples of some of the plain radiographic characteristics of CVM are shown in Figures 15-17.

Positive-contrast myelography is the technic of choice to confirm the site and nature of spinal cord compression in cases of CVM.[259] Numerous agents have been used and currently the most acceptable are the nonionic, water-soluble agents, such as metrizamide (Amipaque: Winthrop). After the slow withdrawal of 20-40 ml CSF, 30-60 ml metrizamide are slowly instilled into the atlanto-occipital subarachnoid space. Metrizamide in water, with an iodine concentration of approximately

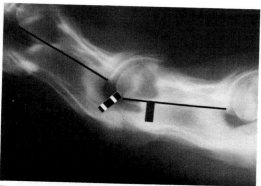

Fig 18. Plain right lateral radiograph of flexed cervical vertebrae in a normal horse. Horizontal black lines indicate the floor of the vertebral canal of C_3 and C_4. (The floor tends to be almost a straight line, with only minimal ventral concavity.) The heavy black vertical bar indicates the minimum sagittal diameter of the vertebral canal within C_4. The black and white bar indicates the minimum sagittal diameter of the vertebral canal between C_3 and C_4, also known as the minimum flexed diameter.

166 mg/ml, is isotonic with CSF and is well tolerated by horses.

Some muscle fasciculations and even seizure activity may be expected on recovery of horses from myelography.[260-261] These effects may be diminished by holding the horse's head and neck elevated while instilling the myelographic material over a 5-minute period. Continued elevation of the head for 5 minutes after

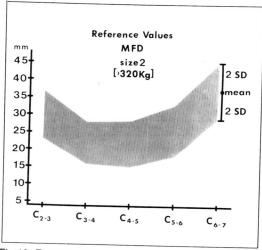

Fig 19. Example of the graphs that can be drawn from the reference values for the measurements of the minimum diameters of the vertebral canal. The shaded area in this graph indicates the 95.4% confidence limits for the minimum flexion diameter for horses weighing more than 320 kg. These graphs can reduce the subjectivity of radiographic diagnosis of cervical vertebral malformation with stenosis.

Table 3. Reference values of measurements from radiographs taken with the horse in lateral recumbency on the radiographic plate and with a 90-cm focal-film distance.[250] These ranges are for the minimum sagittal diameter and minimum flexed diameter (Fig 18) of the vertebral canal and for the minimum sagittal diameter of the myelographic dural space. These values are useful in identifying horses with CVM. Caution should be used when comparing values obtained with other radiographic technics.

| Radiographic Measurement | Body Size | Level in Cervical Vertebral Canal |||||||||||
		C_2	C_2-C_3	C_3	C_3-C_4	C_4	C_4-C_5	C_5	C_5-C_6	C_6	C_6-C_7	C_7
Minimum Sagittal Diameter	320 kg	20.8-26.8	—	18.1-21.5	—	16.7-20.7	—	17.3-22.1	—	18.3-23.9	—	19.8-26.1
	320 kg	22.1-31.3	—	18.5-25.9	—	17.7-24.9	—	18.7-26.1	—	19.0-29.1	—	22.2-32.6
Minimum Flexed Diameter	320 kg	—	19.3-29.7	—	13.4-22.0	—	13.2-22.5	—	16.1-25.7	—	21.6-36.7	—
	320 kg	—	22.8-36.5	—	15.6-27.8	—	14.8-28.2	—	17.9-32.9	—	28.5-45.6	—
Minimum Flexed Dural Space Diameter	320 kg	15.8-25.2	11.3-23.1	13.8-20.4	9.0-16.8	14.5-19.5	9.9-15.7	14.6-20.0	11.9-17.7	16.3-21.7	17.3-22.7	20.0-27.0
	320 kg	16.9-27.9	12.9-27.9	15.5-24.1	10.5-20.9	15.1-23.3	10.8-19.0	15.4-24.8	11.4-20.8	18.0-26.2	17.6-25.6	16.2-34.6

injection and leaving a patent spinal needle in the lumbosacral subarachnoid space also enhance caudal flow of the medium and probably improve the quality of the myelogram. Fever (104-107 F) is common within 6-24 hours following myelography. This is most likely associated with the aseptic leptomeningitis created, which can be detected by CSF analysis and histopathologic examination.[260]

Normal variations must be considered when interpreting equine myelograms.[250,259-261] Of most significance is the presence of indentations of the myelographic columns in normal horses. These subarachnoid encroachments are commonly demonstrated in the ventral myelographic column at the intervertebral spaces, especially at C_3-C_4, C_4-C_5 and C_5-C_6. During neck flexion these indentations become greater and can obliterate the ventral myelographic column. In addition, there is frequently a narrowing of the dorsal dye column at the cranial orifices of C_3-T_1. This is most prominent at C_6-T_1 and can be greatly exaggerated at these sites, particularly at C_7 and T_1, by full extension of the neck.

Classic CVM with stenosis can be demonstrated easily by myelography (Fig 17). Again, to decrease the subjectivity of interpretation, reference values for the sagittal diameter of the myelographic column (dural space) may be used for comparison (Table 3). As suggested above, horses with unequivocal spinal cord compression shown by myelography should not have their necks manipulated excessively. This is particularly so for neck flexion of horses with stenosis at C_2-C_5, and for neck extension of horses with stenosis at C_6-T_1.

Spinal cord compression due to CVM is occasionally not detected clearly on lateral myelograms. In such cases a ventrodorsal view is required (Fig 20). However, in most horses with transverse compression of the spinal cord associated with osteochondrosis or chronic degenerative joint disease of the articular processes, there is demonstrable sagittal stenosis of the vertebral canal (Figs 20, 21). Ventrodorsal views may help define other soft tissue compressions of the spinal cord, such as epidural cysts.

Analysis of CSF is not of great assistance in defining CVM. The changes seen are a reflection of compression of the spinal cord with small amounts of hemorrhage, and include slight xanthochromia and mild elevation of protein content (100-150 mg/dl). Infrequently there is a subtle mononuclear pleocytosis (8-20 cells/μl), and rarely erythrophagocytosis.

Needle electromyography performed under general anesthesia can indicate denervation (lower motor neuron disease) in animals with

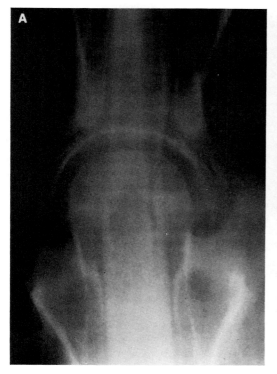

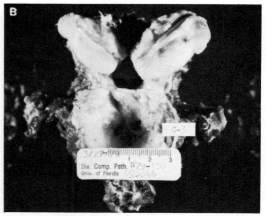

Fig 20. Ventrodorsal myelogram of C_3 and C_4 in a yearling Thoroughbred colt with the wobbler syndrome. The plain lateral radiographs taken in the neutral and flexed positions, and the minimum sagittal diameters of the vertebral canal were within normal limits. On the myelogram there is compression of the myelographic column from the right side at C_3-C_4. A caudal view of C_3 (B) reveals transverse stenosis of the vertebral canal associated with medial ingrowth of the articular processes, particularly on the right side. Extensive osteochondrotic lesions are present at the edges of the joint surfaces. The colt had acutely progressive, asymmetric, ataxic tetraparesis that was worse in the pelvic limbs than in the thoracic limbs and more evident on the left side. The compressive spinal cord lesion was more severe on the left side. This is an unusual example of cervical vertebral malformation in that compression of the spinal cord by only the medial ingrowth of articular processes without measurable dorsoventral stenosis of the vertebral canal occurs infrequently.

evidence of spinal cord grey matter and nerve root lesions.[250] This diagnostic aid can assist in defining the site(s) of spinal cord compression in horses with CVM in conjunction with myelography (see Chapter 19).

Necropsy Findings: Horses with CVM have one or more focal compression-type lesions in the cervical spinal cord. Such lesions may appear as flattening of the cord and histologically are characterized by swollen and disrupted axons, and phagocytosis of myelin in white matter. Mild hemorrhages are sometimes seen in the acute lesions. In the white matter of chronically affected animals there is continued degeneration of neuronal fibers, proliferation of capillaries with prominent fibrous coats and astrofibrosis. More severely affected horses also have neuronal necrosis, loss of cell bodies and sometimes astrofibrosis in the grey matter. Massive focal lesions also occur, with cavitating necrosis of white matter, particularly in lateral funiculi, and occasionally of grey matter. Markedly asymmetric lesions are found in those horses in which prominently asymmetric signs occur. Cranial to the focal lesion there is secondary degeneration of neuronal fibers (axons and myelin) in ascending tracts for variable distances, depending on the extent and age of the focal lesion. Caudal to the lesion there is secondary fiber degeneration in descending tracts. This fiber degeneration is the result of neuronal fibers being severed from their cell bodies by the focal lesion. It is most prominent in dorsolateral funiculi cranial to the lesion, and deep lateral and ventromedial funiculi caudal to the lesion (Fig 22).

The site of the focal lesion in CVM cases can be correlated with the gross findings from examination of the cervical vertebrae to define what caused the spinal cord compression. Dorsoventral stenosis of the vertebral canal is demonstrable in almost all cases (Figs 21, 23), although there are some exceptions (Fig 20). Vertebral canal stenosis may be evident at several sites but is most prominent at the site of spinal cord compression. In most cases of CVM there are other features associated with stenosis (Fig 23). Gross evidence of osteochondrosis and more chronic joint lesions, collectively described as degenerative joint disease, are

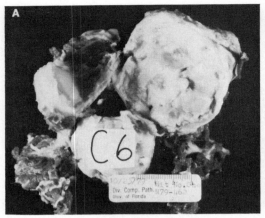
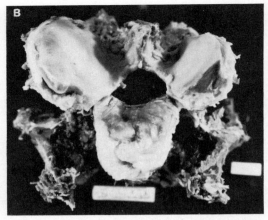

Fig 21. Cranial view of C₆ from 2 adult horses. The vertebra in (A), from a wobbler, has massive degenerative joint disease, particularly involving the left articular process.. Periarticular tissues encroach into an already stenotic vertebral canal, compressing the spinal cord at this site. This horse sustained an injury to its neck several months previously, which likely promoted the spinal cord compression. The horse from which the other vertebra (B) came did not have any neurologic signs or spinal cord lesions; yet there is moderate degenerative joint disease and asymmetry of the articular processes. Because there is ample space in the vertebral canal, medial protrusion of the articular surfaces did not compromise the spinal cord.

often striking in the vertebrae of horses with CVM (Figs 20, 21, 23).[246,250] This may be especially prominent at the site of spinal cord compression. However, these changes are also found, perhaps to a lesser extent, in horses that do not have compression of their spinal cords.[249,250,262] Enlarged epiphyses evident radiographically are demonstrated best on median sections of vertebrae (Figs 15, 23). Histologically there is evidence of osteochondrosis and sometimes osteopetrosis in the articular processes and physes of these vertebrae. Moreover,

Fig 22. Schematic diagram of the histopathologic lesions seen in cases of cervical vertebral malformation. A focal compression-type lesion in the cervical spinal cord, and secondary neuronal fiber degeneration in ascending tracts cranial to the lesion and in descending tracts caudal to the lesion occur. (Courtesy of the Cornel Veterinarian)

there are similar bone and cartilage lesions present in other sites in horses with CVM. Unaffected horses may also have similar but less pronounced bone lesions.[250]

Necropsy technic can be vital for confirmation of a diagnosis of CVM. Each cervical spinal cord segment must be clearly identified. The intact vertebral canal must be scrutinized. This necessitates a procedure such as disarticulation of the cervical vertebrae to harvest individual spinal cord segments. Absence of epidural fat is often noted at a site of vertebral canal stenosis. The presence of vertebral canal stenosis, enlarged articular processes and soft tissue masses that may compromise the vertebral canal can be confirmed. The postmortem identification of subtle degrees of vertebral subluxation or spondylolisthesis is difficult, if not impossible, to make. Definition of such a functional component of CVM, if it indeed occurs, is best made by quantitative dynamic radiography. This is unlike the profound flexion-fixation with luxation that can be demonstrated clearly by radiography and necropsy (Fig 16).

Pathogenesis: The pathogenesis of the focal spinal cord lesion in CVM is probably a combination of direct pressure-induced injury to neuronal fibers and their cell bodies, and ischemia resulting from alterations in spinal cord blood supply. Compression of the ventral vertebral venous plexus has been demonstrated radiographically in CVM[250] Some cases with greatly overgrown articular processes and cav-

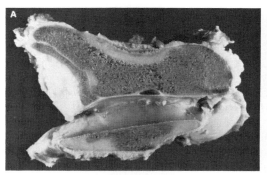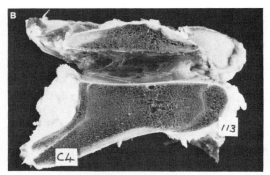

Fig 23. Median sections of C₄ from a horse with cervical vertebral malformation and spinal cord compression at C₄-C₅ (A), and from a control horse of similar age (B). Some characteristics of the malformation are evident when (A) is compared with (B). There is stenosis of the cranial orifice and particularly the caudal orifice of the vertebral canal. The latter is associated with enlargement of the caudal epiphysis, an irregular epiphyseal cartilagenous growth plate and even an area of petrotic bone in the metaphysis. In addition, the roof of the vertebral canal extends further caudad so that any flexion of the next caudal vertebra (C₅), with elevation of its cranial epiphysis, compresses the spinal cord further.

itating necrosis may have a component of compression of intervertebral vessels supplying the spinal cord.[263] However, compromise of the intervertebral vasculature by rootsleeve fibrosis and spasm, a purported mechanism of myelopathy in cervical spondylosis in humans, has not been reported in horses.[264-265]

The precise pathogenesis of the bone and joint lesions in CVM is not understood. It is becoming clearer, however, that this is a multifactorial disease with phenotypic expression depending on the interaction of many genetic and environmental factors. In fact, there are most likely multiple pathogenetic mechanisms that not only allow considerable variability in expression of the disease but may in the future be considered more precisely as several separate diseases. In light of the information available to date, it is convenient to consider the pathogenesis of CVM as follows. There probably is a genetic basis to CVM. Therefore, the genetically defined diameter of the cervical vertebral canal is of paramount importance. Additionally, as is the case in osteochondrosis, rapidly growing horses with relatively fine bones are affected.[266,267] Undoubtedly, selection pressures to attain a high-quality equine athlete have added to the genetic pool for predisposition to CVM. The proportion of the phenotypically expressed disease that is genetically determined is unknown.

To understand the weight of genetic input to the disease, CVM may be compared with enlarged epiphyses ("epiphysitis"), angular limb deformities and osteochondrosis. As is the case in these last conditions, there are associated nutritional and traumatic components.[267,268] High energy intake allows a rapid growth rate and a large size to be attained. In addition, excessive energy intake, and possibly imbalance of other nutrients, results in osteochondrosis of the articular surfaces and epiphyseal growth plates in the cervical vertebrae. These lesions develop at the time of maximum growth rate in the vertebral epiphyses that occurs just prior to closure of the epiphyseal growth plates.[269] Excessive weight-bearing on these articular processes and growth plates, and overt external trauma to the neck complicate the metabolic bone and cartilage disease present and promote development of degenerative joint disease in older horses. The role, if any, of degenerative intervertebral disc disease in the pathogenesis of CVM has yet to be determined.

With a multifactorial disease as proposed, it is very reasonable to have horses with some of the features of CVM but without phenotypic expression of the disease in the form of spinal cord compression. Only with these pathogenic mechanisms acting in concert may there be significant compromise of the vertebral canal and spinal cord compression.

Treatment and Prognosis: Horses with permanent signs of spinal cord disease do not make high-quality athletes, and wobblers are usually given a poor prognosis.[243] However, many ataxic mares have been used for breeding, and some horses with mild signs of the wobbler syndrome have returned to racing. In these cases, the type of spinal cord disease causing the signs is not usually documented.

The prognosis for wobblers with CVM depends on the severity of initial signs, chronicity of signs, the likelihood of recompression of the spinal cord, and the intended use of the horse. Many horses with moderate to marked neurologic signs associated with CVM are given conservative therapy. Frequently, this consists of paddock or stall rest and corticosteroid treatment for short periods. Most of these horses do not successfully return to work. In fact, the signs usually progress, especially if the horse is returned to training. Certainly this identifies these horses as unsuitable for use and they should not be passed in a purchase examination. The question of insurance liability has not been made clear. If there is an "unsuitable for intended use" clause in an insurance policy, there should be no problem. However, ambulatory horses with CVM are almost certainly not suffering sufficiently to necessitate humane destruction. If, on the other hand, the spinal cord compression is profound, and especially if the horse suffers falls from its incapacitation or if recumbency results, humane destruction is a viable alternative.

Of significance in determining prognosis is the recent interest in surgical intervention in cases of CVM.[270-272] In some cases surgery appears to halt further trauma to the spinal cord at the site of compression. However, at this time it is reasonable to state that in spite of these promising reports there is no proof that surgical therapy alone can result in a cure of the disease. Because of the likelihood that environmental factors, such as malnutrition and trauma, play a major role in the disease, any evaluation of surgical therapy should include comparison with control groups receiving conservative therapy aimed at controlling and correcting these environmental factors. In addition, any form of treatment of horses with confirmed CVM should only be undertaken after consideration of the probable genetic background of the disease.

Notwithstanding the above discussion, the types of surgery available and their potential indications in CVM warrant mention. Several surgical technics have been used to treat cervical spinal cord compression due to various causes in human and animals. These procedures consist of various combinations of decompression and immobilization-fixation. Despite early positive reports, the relative value of several of these technics for cases of CVM in dogs and for spondylosis and other compressive cervical myelopathies in humans is still somewhat controversial.[274-277] Broad conclusions on the applicability of surgical approaches to the treatment of CVM in horses, drawn mainly from these human and canine studies, include the following. Most surgical-steel stabilizing implants are not likely to withstand the tremendous forces acting in a horse's neck. Secondly, a ventral approach with intervertebral fusion using a cortical bone plug, as already used in horses with CVM, may primarily be indicated with compression of mainly the ventral myelographic column, and in horses in which the vertebral canal was maximally compressed upon flexion.[270-272] Such a technic may prevent further trauma to the spinal cord situated in a narrow vertebral canal and reportedly resulted in improvement and resolution of signs of wobbles in selected cases of CVM.[271] Dorsal decompressive laminectomy is a gargantuan undertaking in horses.[272,273] This last technic is primarily indicated with compression of mainly the dorsal myelographic column.

It must be restated that the effectiveness of these surgical procedures in treating horses with CVM, particularly in comparison with conservative measures to control environmental factors, is not known at this stage. Obviously, the ultimate goal must be to define the relative importance of each genetic and environmental factor discussed above, and to implement measures to prevent the phenotypic disease of CVM.

In summary, many wobblers have cervical vertebral malformation with compression of their cervical spinal cord. This results in ataxia, weakness and spasticity in the pelvic and usually the thoracic limbs. This developmental disease is characterized by static and dynamic stenosis of the vertebral canal. In association with this stenosis, there are various combinations of enlarged vertebral epiphyses, angular fixations, osteochondrosis and degenerative joint disease. Radiography, particularly myelography, can confirm the presence and site of spinal cord compression. Osteochondrosis, osteopetrosis and bone necrosis can be detected in the vertebrae, other bones and cartilage. A genetic component to the disease probably consists of a narrow vertebral canal and predisposition to the above bone and cartilage diseases. Signs are expressed when environmental factors, including excessive energy intake and excessive weight-bearing applied to the growing vertebrae, act in concert to further narrow and deviate the vertebral canal and compress the cervical spinal cord.

Equine Degenerative Myeloencephalopathy

Since at least 1974 it has been apparent that all equine wobblers did not have compression of their cervical spinal cord associated with CVM.[278] Instead some of these horses and zebras had, among other conditions, a diffuse spinal cord disease subsequently termed equine degenerative myeloencephalopathy (EDM).[279,280] The cause of EDM has not been elucidated.

Clinical Signs: The disease has been recognized in many northeastern states, and in Florida and California.[250] It affects young horses up to about 3 years of age. Both sexes and most light breeds (and zebras) have been affected. Single animals are usually affected, but at least 2 clusters of cases have been investigated. Although some of these cases have been related, no strong evidence for a hereditary basis of the disease has been forthcoming.

Physical examinations have been noncontributory and no head signs have been reported. Signs of symmetric ataxia, weakness and spasticity occur in all 4 legs, but no localizing findings are evident. These signs are usually insidious in onset with chronic progression, although some horses have an apparently acute onset of signs. Affected animals therefore show the wobbler syndrome. However, by a careful neurologic examination some horses with EDM may be differentiated from other wobblers with CVM (see Neurologic Examination section). After grading the total neurologic gait abnormality for horses with EDM, it is often apparent that the degree of abnormality is somewhat different than for most horses with CVM. Wobblers with CVM (or any focal cervical compressive lesion) most often have signs that are one grade more severe in the pelvic limbs than in the thoracic limbs. Horses with EDM frequently have equally severe signs in the thoracic and pelvic limbs. On occasion, the degree of gait abnormality in horses with EDM has been graded as profound in the pelvic limbs but very mild in the thoracic limbs. Also, of the basic components of a neurologic gait deficit (weakness, ataxia, spasticity and hypermetria), horses with EDM most often have marked weakness and ataxia.

Radiographic examination of the cervical vertebrae is helpful in ruling out stenosis of the vertebral canal and CVM. Some degree of articular process enlargement may be detected, just as it may in horses without spinal cord dis-

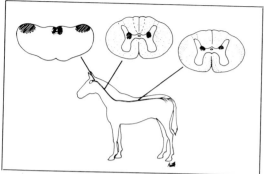

Fig 24. Schematic diagram of the histopathologic lesions in equine degenerative myeloencephalopathy.[259] Note the neuronal fiber degeneration (stippled areas) in most white matter funiculi, especially the dorsolateral and ventromedial tracts. There are also prominent lesions characterized by neuroaxonal dystrophy (black areas) in many sensory relay nuclear areas of the medulla oblongata and spinal cord. Compare with the lesions found in cervical vertebral malformation (Fig 23).

ease. Other diagnostic aids, including hematologic examination, serum chemistry determinations, CSF analysis and blood copper level determinations have contributed to the diagnosis of EDM by ruling out other possible causes. Therefore, the clinical diagnosis must be symmetric, ataxie tetraparesis in young light-breed horses. The definitive diagnosis can only be made by postmortem evaluation.

Since the cause of the disease is unknown and signs are generally progressive, horses with EDM are usually euthanized, although some affected horses have remained stable for a year.

Necropsy Findings: No significant gross findings are evident. Histologic lesions are apparently restricted to the CNS, although the peripheral nervous system has not been scrutinized.[250] Degenerative lesions occur throughout the spinal cord and caudal medullary white matter, and in many nuclei in the grey matter of the spinal cord and brainstem, thus the name of the condition (Fig 24).

Neuronal fiber degeneration is present in all funiculi of the spinal cord. This is most prominent in the dorsolateral (ascending spinocerebellar) tracts and the ventromedial (descending) tracts of the cranial cervical and midthoracic segments. An added component of demyelination can also be detected in these particular tracts. Neurochemical analyses have corroborated an added loss of spinal cord myelin lipids in EDM compared with spinal cord tissue from control horses and horses with other spinal cord diseases.

Grey matter lesions consist of prominent axonal swellings (spheroids), proliferation of glial cells, especially astrocytes, lipofuscin-like pigment accumulation and a loss of neuronal cell bodies. Spheroids are seen in various sizes and stages of disintegration, and have prominent vacuolation and fragmentation. Many brainstem and intermediate grey column spinal nuclei are affected. In particular, the lateral cuneate, cranial cervical intermediate column and thoracic nuclei have these lesions. The overall process occurring in the grey matter is regarded as a form of neuroaxonal dystrophy and probably represents the degeneration of terminal axons within affected nuclei, which are predominantly sensory relay proprioceptive nuclei.

Pathogenesis: Pathologically EDM is a degenerative disease characterized by neuroaxonal dystrophy and degenerative myelopathy. Possible etiologic mechanisms have been discussed, and these include toxic, nutritional, metabolic and hereditary processes.[250]

Induced vitamin E deficiency in rats shares many histologic features with EDM.[281] Several plant intoxications, including cycad palm (*Cycas* spp), locoweed (*Astragalus* spp and *Oxytropis* spp) and darling pea (*Swainsona* spp) toxicoses result in degenerative CNS lesions that include the formation of axonal spheroids.[282,283] It is interesting to note that the toxic effect of *Swainsona* spp is inhibition of a lysosomal enzyme, resulting in a lysosomal storage disease that mimics mannosidosis.[284] Many chemical poisonings result in degenerative lesions of the CNS somewhat similar to EDM.[285] These include organophosphate and carbamate compounds, which are related to many commonly used equine anthelmintics. Physiologic forms of neuroaxonal dystrophy have been related to malnutrition and aging without demonstrable neurologic signs.[286] In fact, mild neuroaxonal dystrophy and an associated accumulation of small amounts of lipofuscin-like pigment have been detected in normal horses, particularly within the lateral cuneate nucleus.[250,287] Also, several neoplastic-, chemotherapeutic- and metabolic-related forms of subclinical reactive neuroaxonal dystrophy are well recognized in humans.[288] Finally, hereditary neuroaxonal dystrophy is a well-recognized syndrome and morphologic disease in Suffolk sheep, cats and humans.[289-292]

Following consideration of the above comparisons, it is suggested that potential toxicoses, induced vitamin deficiencies and familial predisposition all be considered when cases of EDM are studied. In particular, a thorough epidemiologic investigation of all such factors may be the turning point in understanding the cause and, therefore, the possible treatment and prevention of EDM.

Miscellaneous Spinal Anomalies

In addition to cervical vertebral and occipitoatlantoaxial malformations, various other congenital and developmental anomalies of the vertebral column and spinal cord may result in signs of spinal cord disease. It must be emphasized that even though a vertebral malformation is detected, any signs of spinal cord disease can only be ascribed to that malformation if the whole neurologic evaluation is compatible. For example, a foal with lumbar spina bifida and stable paraparesis since it began walking is more likely to have an associated anomaly of the spinal cord (myelodysplasia), such as diplomyelia, meningomyelocele, meningocele or hydromyelia, rather than compression of the cord as a result of the bifida vertebral spine.[293] Animals with a neurologic deficit resulting from a vertebral column anomaly such as spina bifida or a butterfly-type vertebra would most likely have progressive signs of spinal cord disease once the animal is able to walk.[294]

Radiographic examination is necessary to confirm any of these malformations and myelography should confirm compression of the spinal cord.

Syringomyelia (central cavitation) at C_7-T_7 has been reported in a part-Thoroughbred filly.[295] A hopping gait, inability to turn easily and stiff rear limbs were noted at 6 weeks of age. Cervicothoracic scoliosis was also present.

Congenital deviations and contractures of the axial and appendicular skeleton occur in various combinations in foals. Affected foals are usually regarded as having the "contracted foal syndrome."[295-300] The malformations described are basically vertebral column contractures, limb contractures, hypoplastic vertebral articular processes, hypoplastic limb joint surfaces, asymmetry of the axial skeleton, asymmetry of the skull, and midline defects in the abdominal and thoracic cavities. Vertebral column defects include scoliosis, lordosis, kyphosis and torticollis. Affected foals may be ambulatory.[198,300] No ataxia, weakness or spasticity, as evidence of spinal cord disease, has been reported. One investigator believes the defects are based upon a primary hypoplasia of the joints although another has suggested that this hypoplasia may be secondary to the abnormal limb position.[295] The syndrome is probably analogous to arthrogryposis and talipes (clubfoot) in other species. In this regard the etiology is just as likely to be neuropathic or myopathic as it is to be primarily arthropathic.[301,302] Toxic, infectious, physical and possibly other processes that directly damage the ventral grey columns or the muscles of the foal *in utero* are thus potential causes of the syndrome.[303-305] Such mechanisms can result in contractures and fixations at birth. A newborn foal with flexion fixations (arthrogryposis) of the left pelvic limb has been studied.[306] Histologically this foal had a hypoplastic ventral grey column at L_4-S_2. The left side of the grey column contained about one-fourth the number of large motor neuronal cell bodies compared with the ventral grey column on the side of the unaffected limb. There was profound atrophy and fibrofatty atrophy of several muscle groups in the left rear limb.

Variations in the number of regional vertebrae and developmental vertebral ankyloses have been reported.[307-309] Morphologic variations, including cervical ribs and transposition of one or both ventral processes from the sixth to the seventh cervical vertebrae, have also been seen.[306] No neurologic signs have been ascribed to such malformations.

Acquired curvatures of the vertebral column have been associated with spinal cord compression. The etiology of these conditions of torticollis, scoliosis, lordosis and kyphosis is not always apparent. The causative mechanisms documented so far include trauma, muscle rupture with scarring, neurogenic muscle atrophy and nutritional myodegeneration.[310] To this list may be added severe thoracic disease, as evidenced by the development of profound lordosis of the thoracolumbar vertebral column in several young growing foals with severe pneumonia.[306] Whether this is an effect of positioning associated with pain, secondary alterations in collagen metabolism or some other mechanism is not known.

Infectious/Inflammatory Spinal Cord Diseases

Equine Protozoal Myeloencephalitis

Segmental myelitis was identified in Kentucky horses in 1964.[311] In 1970, a study of 52 cases of focal myelitis/encephalitis was reported.[312] Since that time, many horses with the same clinical and pathologic syndrome have been reported as affected by toxoplasmosis-like encephalomyelitis and protozoan encephalomyelitis.[313-317] Until the causative agent(s) is identified, it is accepted that all these disease entities are one, known as equine protozoal myeloencephalitis (EPM).[250,319-321]

Over 100 cases of EPM have been documented from northeastern, midwestern and southern states of the US. The disease is apparently confined to horses raised in continental America, that have spent some time east of the Rocky Mountains. It has not been reported elsewhere, although a similar syndrome, thought to be caused by *Toxoplasma gondii*, occurred in Brazil.[322] The prevalence of the disease is quite variable; however, where it occurs it is probably the third most frequent cause of spinal cord disease after spinal cord trauma and cervical vertebral malformation.

Many breeds of horses, particularly Standardbreds and Thoroughbreds, are affected by EPM. Animals are often affected at racetracks or on breeding establishments, and pleasure horses appear to be affected less frequently. Horses from 6 months to 16 years of age have been affected but are most often 1-6 years old at the onset of signs. More cases apparently occur in the spring and summer than at other times of the year. Although EPM must be regarded as an infectious disease, it is apparently not contagious from horse to horse. Because the disease occurs in clusters in certain areas and even on single farms over a period of several years, it is suggested that there is a common source of environmental or animal exposure. Two full sibling Quarter Horses have been affected within 1 month of each other.[321]

Cause: The putative agent of EPM is a sporozoon, with an apical complex, that almost certainly divides asexually by endopolyogeny, a characteristic of the Sarcosporidia group of coccidian parasites.[323]

Clinical Signs: The onset of signs is usually peracute or acute. Horses may stumble and fall during racing or training with no premonitory signs. Gait deficits that are usually interpreted as lameness are often seen early in the course of disease. Ataxia, weakness, recumbency, muscle atrophy and occasionally behavioral changes are other primary signs reported. The signs are progressive and almost all horses develop various degrees of ataxia, weakness and spasticity in one or more limbs, which reflects brainstem or spinal cord involvement. Signs can be symmetric in all limbs with no evidence of grey matter lesions; horses with such signs

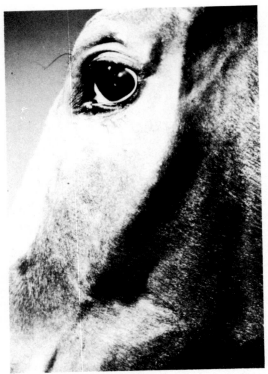

Fig 25. Left aspect of the head of a 5-year-old Thoroughbred gelding with masseter muscle atrophy. This horse also had atrophy of the temporalis and distal digastricus muscles on the left side. These lesions were the result of an equine protozoal myelitis (EPM) lesion in the motor nucleus of the trigeminal nerve in the brainstem. In addition, the horse had progressive ataxia, atrophy of the right half of the tongue, and atrophy of the right gluteal musculature. These additional signs were explained by other focal EPM lesions involving the hypoglossal nucleus, and the grey and white matter of the spinal cord at L_4-S_3.

matory CNS disease and evidence of lower motor neuron grey matter involvement, respectively. Samples of CSF collected from the lumbosacral site show some abnormality more frequently than samples collected from the atlanto-occipital site, probably because there are most often spinal cord lesions, especially involving caudal cervical, thoracic, lumbar and sacral segments. Also, samples from horses with large, active lesions that contain protozoal organisms are more likely to be abnormal than samples from horses with small, stable lesions that often may not contain visible protozoa. The CSF alterations found include a slight to moderate xanthochromia, a few hundred to a few thousand RBC and up to 100 WBC/μl CSF. Mononuclear cells predominate but neutrophils are also seen. The protein content is less frequently elevated and is usually not above 150 mg/dl.

Serum and CSF *Toxoplasma* indirect-hemagglutinating antibody (IHA) titers in horses with EPM have been consistently negative. One report indicated there may be higher IHA serum titers reactive against *Sarcocystis bovicanis* (*S cruzi*) in horses affected by EPM than in a control group.[250] More recently, an attempt to transmit *S bovicanis* to intact and corticosteroid-immunosuppressed horses was unsuccessful and there was no evidence of infection or seroconversion.[324]

Unfortunately, the only definitive means of diagnosing EPM at present is histologic observation of the putative agent within the CNS. Notwithstanding this, a diagnosis of EPM is entertained when typical lesions can be defined; such cases are designated EPM(−) in comparison to those in which the organisms are seen, which are designated EPM(+).[250]

Treatment and Prognosis: Several attempts have been made at treatment of horses with a clinical diagnosis of EPM.[250,325] Such treatment has been based upon the use of folic acid inhibitors that are used successfully for various protozoan infections, including toxoplasmosis, in humans and animals. A regimen used for 400- to 500-kg horses has included pyrimethamine tablets (Daraprim:Wellcome) at 100 mg daily, trimethoprim-sulfadiazine tablets (Tribrissen: Wellcome) at 2-3 mg/kg (trimethoprim) and 10-15 mg/kg (sulfadiazine), respectively, given BID (total daily dose of 24-36 mg/kg of the combination), and folic acid (Folvite:Lederle) at 75 mg given IM every 3 days. Use of this regimen has been continued for 1-2½ months and in

are being called wobblers. In many cases, however, especially as the disease progresses, markedly asymmetric signs with evidence of grey matter involvement and multifocal lesion sites become evident. Such signs include sensory deficits, focal sweating, monoplegia (single-limb paralysis), muscle atrophy, reflex loss and cranial nerve dysfunction. These signs are regarded as hallmarks of the disease, especially when evidence of multifocal lesions is present (Figs 25-27).

Diagnosis: There is no definitive antemortem diagnostic aid. Hematologic, serum chemistry, serologic and radiographic examinations are useful insofar as other diseases may be ruled out of the differential diagnosis. The use of CSF analysis and EMG studies can be helpful in confirming the presence of an inflam-

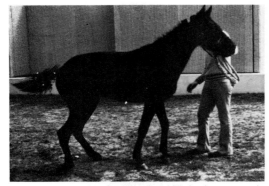

Fig 26. This yearling Standardbred filly had paraparesis worse in the right hindlimb than in the left. There was profound weakness in the right hindlimb, with constant knuckling of the fetlock and sinking of the pelvis as shown. A decreased panniculus response and depressed sensory perception were evident in the caudal lumbar region. When the animal was recumbent, the patellar reflex was poor in the left limb and almost absent in the right. These signs were caused by an equine protozoal myelitis lesion involving the grey and white matter from L_2-L_5; the lesion was more severe on the right side.

when a lesion is sectioned. Histologically, the inflammatory lesions consist of prominent lymphoid perivascular cuffing, and contain many macrophages, often eosinophils and occasionally multinucleate giant cells. Large necrotic areas with hemorrhage are present in acute and severe lesions, and astroglial scars occur with chronic lesions. Associated nonsuppurative meningitis is variably present. Consistent with the neurologic signs, lesions are often multifocal within the spinal cord, brainstem and sometimes the cerebrum and cerebellum. Asymmetry, and involvement of grey and white matter are also characteristic.

The organisms are seen singly and in groups, free in the tissue but most often within macrophages (Fig 28). Organisms have been seen in neurons, eosinophils and even within cell nuclei. Of potential significance in the etiopathogenesis of EPM is the fact that organisms have recently been detected within WBC contained in the lumen of intact capillaries within CNS lesions.[323] Parasitemia occurs in the life cycle of *Sarcocystis bovicanis* in calves, and hematologic multiplication and transmission of this disease by blood transfusion have been documented.[326]

several cases clinical signs have regressed so that horses have been used for breeding.

In addition to the caution expressed above concerning the lack of definitive clinical diagnosis in such cases, several other points concerning this type of therapy in horses must be mentioned. Neither pyrimethamine nor trimethoprim is licensed for use in horses in North America. Also, the dosages that have been used are at the low end of the ranges recommended for various severe infections in humans. Finally, it is absolutely arbitrary how long therapy should be continued without some diagnostic parameter, such as antibody titer, to monitor. Patients should be closely observed during therapy to detect severe leukopenia, anemia, thrombocytopenia or azotemia. In acutely progressive cases, drugs that tend to decrease edema formation in the CNS have been used with unknown effects. A test dose of mannitol at 0.25-0.5 g/kg may be given slowly IV and repeated if there is evidence of a clinical response. Some affected horses that have received corticosteroid therapy have had a rapid progression of signs. In several of these animals large numbers of protozoa were subsequently found in the CNS lesions. Consequently, it is advisable to not use corticosteroids to treat horses suspected of having EPM.

Necropsy Findings: Gross discoloration and softening are detected in fresh CNS tissue

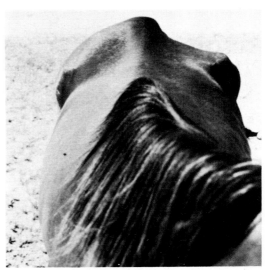

Fig 27. Cranial to caudal view of the back and rump of a 3-year-old Thoroughbred gelding with equine protozoal myelitis. Note the profound atrophy of the left gluteal and caudal longissimus lumborum musculature. Muscular atrophy was due to protozoal myelitis lesions in the grey matter at T_{18}-L_1 and at L_5-L_6 on the left side. The horse also had progressive tetraparesis and asymmetric ataxia. A separate lesion involving grey and white matter at C_1-C_6 accounted for the forelimb signs and probably the hyporeflexia and mild muscle atrophy of the caudal neck region on the right side.

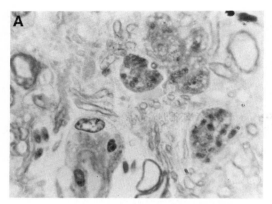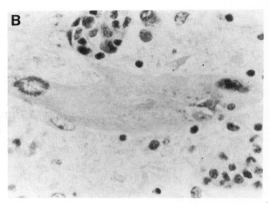

Fig 28. Photomicrographs (original magnification 1000X) of the putative sporozoan agent in equine protozoal myelitis. (A) The more typical groups of organisms can be seen in an area of degenerated myelin (right). At least 3 individual zoites are visible in the lower left corner. (B) An infected neuronal cell body is adjacent to a small vessel surrounded by lymphocytes and eosinophils (top center). Two different group forms and several individual zoites are evident in the right end of the neuron and a rosette form of the organism is present in the left end of the neuron.

In summary, EPM is a relatively frequent cause of progressive spinal cord and brainstem disease in light-breed horses in eastern North America. It can be diagnosed clinically with considerable certainty in many cases and is a potentially treatable disease. The causative agent is closely related to the known *Sarcocystis* spp, but definition of the life cycle and an accurate antemortem diagnostic test must be developed before therapeutic and preventive measures can be fully evaluated.

Spinal Infection and Inflammation

Equine Herpesvirus-1 Myeloencephalitis

Paresis following experimental equine herpesvirus-1 (EHV-1) infection was first reported in 1949.[327] Myeloencephalitis associated with EHV-1 infection has since been described in the US, Canada and Europe.[328-340]

Clinical Signs: There is no breed or sex predisposition to EHV-1 myeloencephalitis, although pregnant mares in early to mid-gestation may be more susceptible.[338,341] Foals may develop the disease, but cases have occurred more commonly in older horses. Although neurologic disease is a much less common sequela to EHV-1 infection than rhinopneumonitis, abortion or birth of weak foals, morbidity may be up to 100% among some groups of horses.[333,341]

Myeloencephalitis, like other diseases associated with EHV-1, occurs most commonly where there are aggregations of horses, as in racing, breeding or boarding establishments.

Signs of neurologic disease occur about 7 days after experimental EHV-1 infection by SC or nasal routes.[327,338,341] The onset of fever, with or without a cough and serous nasal discharge, often precede neurologic signs by several days. Respiratory disease may also be noted among horses in contact. Rarely, pregnant mares abort immediately before, during or some time after the development of neurologic signs, depending upon the stage of pregnancy. In many cases no antecedent disease is noticed.[340] Horses may be febrile (up to 106 F) at the onset of neurologic signs, and the fever may persist for several days.

There is a peracute onset of paresis and ataxia of the trunk and limbs. Gait abnormalities may be noticed initially in one or more limbs; typically the pelvic limbs are severely affected. Frequently signs are mildly asymmetric. Early involvement varies from subtle signs of clumsiness or stiffness during circling, to "dog-sitting" or recumbency. Characteristically, there is urinary incontinence and bladder distension at the onset, accompanied sometimes by vulval or penile flaccidity. Tail elevation, decreased tail tone, and perineal hypalgesia have been reported but are not consistent findings.[331]

In most horses with EHV-1 myeloencephalitis there is rapid stabilization of signs. Many horses begin to improve within hours, although the neurologic abnormalities in severely affected animals may continue to worsen for several days. If recumbency occurs it is usually within the first 24 hours, and paralysis may become so complete that the horse cannot lift its head from the ground. Even horses so affected are usually alert and have a good appetite. Clearcut clinical signs of brain disease are very rare, although a few cases of lingual, mandibular or pharyngeal paresis have been described.[322,340] Depression, when it occurs, is more likely to be due to complications of fever, secondary bronchopneumonia and recumbency than to primary brain disease.

Most horses with EHV-1 myeloencephalitis that remain standing recover completely. The time to recovery depends primarily upon the severity of the initial signs, and ranges from several days to more than 18 months. In those horses with protracted recovery, control of urination returns before gait abnormalities disappear.[333] Many horses that become tetraplegic with EHV-1 myeloencephalitis are euthanized, although there are reports of horses that stand again after being recumbent for several weeks. It is not clear whether spontaneous deaths that occur are directly due to EHV-1 infection, or to complications of paralysis and recumbency, such as dehydration, starvation, injury or secondary bacterial infection.

A particularly severe form of myeloencephalitis has occasionally occurred after use of a modified-live vaccine of monkey-cell origin. One report described tetraplegia in 3 horses 8-11 days after IM vaccination.[339] The vaccine has since been withdrawn from the market.

Diagnosis: Definitive diagnosis depends upon the demonstration of at least quadrupled serum-neutralizing (SN) or complement-fixing (CF) antibody titers between acute and convalescent sera. Horses in contact with affected animals, including those without clinical disease, may also have a significant rise in titer of antibodies to EHV-1.[341] There is apparently no correlation between the antibody titer and the severity of neurologic disease.[388]

Useful supporting evidence is xanthochromia and marked protein elevations (100-500 mg/dl) in samples of CSF. Cell numbers are usually normal.[338] Attempts to isolate the virus from CSF have been unsuccessful. The SN titers in CSF have not been consistently elevated in EHV-1 myeloencephalitis.[338]

The following procedures should be followed when EHV-1 myeloencephalitis is suspected. Serum from affected horses should be submitted to a diagnostic laboratory at the onset of disease (acute) and 10-14 days later (convalescent) for SN or CF titers. Paired sera from exposed horses should also be submitted for SN or CF titers. A CSF sample should be analyzed for color, protein and cell content. The CSF can be sent with serum for antibody titer determination and virus isolation. The brain of necropsied horses should be halved sagittally. Half

the brain and samples of spinal cord are fixed in formalin for histologic examination. The other half of the brain is refrigerated (not frozen) with samples of spinal cord, CSF and spleen, and submitted for virus isolation.[343] Nasopharyngeal swab samples and whole blood samples from affected and exposed horses may be submitted for virus isolation.[343]

Necropsy Findings: Grossly, a brownish patchy discoloration occurs in the spinal cord. Histologic lesions are usually scattered throughout the brain and particularly the spinal cord. Areas of ischemic and hemorrhagic infarction appear as edema and necrosis of parenchyma. These areas are often present in a radiating pattern around blood vessels. Such vessels, especially arterioles, often have swelling, necrosis and proliferation of the endothelium, swelling and hyaline necrosis of the intima, and a few mononuclear inflammatory cells. Perivascular cuffs of lymphocytes, plasma cells and macrophages occur in the meninges and parenchyma. Groups of such inflammatory cells associated with neuronal necrosis occur in the trigeminal ganglia. Lesions consistent with EHV-1 infection, and even intranuclear inclusions, may occur in other areas, such as the respiratory tract, thyroid gland and fetus.

In only a few instances has the virus been isolated from the brain or spinal cord of horses with the characteristic histologic findings of EHV-1 myeloencephalitis.[328,334,335] Isolation of virus from other tissues (except the fetus in pregnant mares) may also be difficult due to the high SN titer at the time of death.

Etiology and Pathogenesis: It has not yet been determined if EHV-1 myeloencephalitis is due to direct effect of the virus, to immune-mediated damage, or to some other cause. There is strong support for the theory of an immune-mediated disease but also evidence against that theory.[334,337,338] An alternative pathogenetic mechanism is direct spread of EHV-1 from infected WBC to endothelial cells in the CNS. There would be no extracellular phase, and endothelial cells could be infected in the presence of specific SN antibody.[338] The pathogenesis of EHV-1 myeloencephalitis may be clarified by studies using sensitive immunologic procedures, such as radioimmunoassay or immunofluorescence, to detect minute quantities of antibody or viral antigen.

There is no evidence for the existence of a separate neurotropic subtype of EHV-1 that might cause outbreaks of myeloencephalitis.

Treatment: Most horses with EHV-1 myeloencephalitis can recover if given adequate supportive treatment. The onset of recumbency is no reason for hasty euthanasia. Recumbent horses should be well bedded and encouraged to remain sternal if possible. Food and water may have to be fed by hand or nasogastric tube. Horses in lateral recumbency must be rolled to the opposite side regularly and often to help prevent development of decubiti. Administration of laxatives or enemas, or manual emptying of the rectum may be necessary. Secondary bacterial infections of the urinary or respiratory tract must be vigorously treated. Repeated urinary catheterization is unwise since it may introduce infection and urinary incontinence is seldom a limiting problem. However, recumbent horses with distended urinary bladders can develop cystitis that can rapidly become septic. Consequently, horses should be catheterized judiciously, given assistance to stand and posture for urination, and given appropriate antimicrobial therapy when necessary. In moderately affected horses, use of an abdominal sling may avoid the complications of prolonged recumbency.

The significance of spinal cord edema in the pathogenesis of EHV-1 myeloencephalitis is unknown but some veterinarians have reported a good response to early corticosteroid therapy.[341,342] Because of a profoundly depressant effect on lymphocytes, however, corticosteroids may be contraindicated in the presence of a cell-associated virus such as EHV-1.[341] Exogenous corticosteroids also may exacerbate secondary bronchopneumonia or cystitis.[340]

Levamisole has been used as an adjunct in the treatment of herpetic and some immune-complex mediated diseases in humans. This mode of therapy has not been evaluated in EHV-1 myeloencephalitis.[344]

Prophylaxis: Modified-live and inactivated, adjuvant-containing EHV-1 vaccines are commercially available. The efficacy of these vaccines in preventing EHV-1 myeloencephalitis has not been evaluated critically. In a small trial with a recently developed inactivated vaccine (Pneumabort-K:Fort Dodge), none of 11 vaccinated pregnant mares developed neurologic disease after EHV-1 infection, whereas 2 of 6 unvaccinated mares developed paresis.[345]

If the lesions of EHV-1 myeloencephalitis are immune-mediated, vaccination of infected horses may worsen the disease. Therefore, EHV-1 vaccines should not be used in horses with neurologic signs.

Vertebral Osteomyelitis and Epidural Empyema

Infection of the vertebrae and intervertebral discs, and purulent epidural infections may result in compression of the spinal cord, causing degrees of paraparesis or tetraparesis. These processes of vertebral osteomyelitis and epidural empyema most frequently occur as a result of septicemia. The frequency of septicemia and joint ill in horses is highest in the first month of life. The incidence of septicemia has been described as 10/1000 foals, with an associated mortality of 3.2/1000 foals.[346] It is now accepted that partial or complete failure of passive transfer of immunoglobulins via colostrum is the major reason for this.[346,347] This disease is quite rare because only a small proportion of foals with septicemia develop localized infections in the vertebral column and/or epidural space.

Cause: In a discussion on spinal abscesses and spinal cord compression in lambs, lesions were classifed according to the site of involvement;[348] the pathologic manifestations are likely the same in foals. The lesions described in lambs involved the costovertebral articulations, intervertebral articulations and vertebral canal floor. Such vertebral septic processes in food-producing animals are often associated with omphalophlebitis, traumatic reticuloperitonitis and tail-biting; specific arthritides due to *Brucella* and *Erysipelothrix* are also important in swine.[349,350]

Reports of vertebral osteomyelitis and epidural empyema in horses are not very frequent, although a similar, sometimes presumptive, association with septicemia is accepted.[346] The vertebral column and pachymeninges of horses are occasionally involved by direct spread from an inflammatory focus, such as a septic injection or an infected laceration, with resultant spinal cord compression.

Clinical Signs: Stiffness, reluctance to walk and reluctance to move the head, neck or back may occur prior to specific neurologic signs. A history or evidence of omphalitis, diarrhea, respiratory disease or swollen joints may signal possible sepsis. Ataxia, weakness and spasticity may appear in one or more limbs. These signs may have an acute onset or be steadily progressive. Asymmetry may be particularly prominent if there is nerve root or peripheral nerve involvement when lower motor neuron signs, such as profound weakness, areflexia and muscle atrophy, are present. Analgesia and localized sweating may help in localizing the site of the lesion. Palpation of the vertebral column may detect localized heat, pain and swelling. Systemic signs of sepsis, such as fever, polyarthritis, hypopyon, iritis, pulmonary abscesses and lymphadenopathy, should be searched for diligently. Hyperfibrinogenemia, hyperglobulinemia, monocytosis and leukocytosis are evidence of sepsis.

Diagnosis: Radiography of the appropriate vertebral segment is an aid to diagnosis.[250] If *Salmonella* is the cause of osteomyelitis, some of the characteristic radiographic features of this condition may be expected.[351] If an associated localized leptomeningitis is present, as occurred in less than half of the cases in one series of food-producing animals, pleocytosis and protein exudation may be expected on CSF analysis.[350] More often, results of CSF analysis are normal or consistent with spinal cord compression by revealing mild xanthochromia and mild elevation of protein content.[250]

Treatment: Successful management of discospondylitis in dogs and pyogenic vertebral osteomyelitis in humans involves concerted efforts to obtain cultures of the offending organisms and appropriate, long-term antimicrobial therapy.[352,353] This necessitates blood, urine, fecal, CSF, transtracheal aspirate and lesion biopsy cultures as indicated. A direct gram stain helps guide therapy. Samples should be submitted for aerobic and anaerobic culture.

Depending on results of sensitivity testing and the response of the patient, appropriate antimicrobial therapy may be required for 2-12 weeks. Because neonatal foals are most likely to have vertebral osteomyelitis caused by *Actinobacillus equuli*, *E coli* or beta-hemolytic *Streptococcus*, potassium penicillin G (25,000 IU/kg given IV QID) and kanamycin (5 mg/kg given IM TID) or sodium ampicillin (25 mg/kg given IV QID) may be appropriate initial therapy. Older foals may be infected by the same organisms, but *Salmonella* spp and *Corynebacterium equi* are also found.[354-356] Consequently, in these animals and in newborn foals in which *Klebsiella* infection is suspected, penicillin and gentamicin (2 mg/kg given IM QID) therapy may be more appropriate. Renal function should be monitored in foals receiving aminoglycosides. In older animals, almost any of these organisms may be present and coagulase-positive *Staphylococcus* spp, other *Corynebacterium* spp, *Actinobacillus lignieresi* and *Citrobacter* spp

have been encountered.[250,356,357] In such cases it is difficult to suggest a routine initial antimicrobial regimen without clues from the individual case history and physical examination; culture results are vitally important.

Vertebral osteomyelitis in adult horses may be caused by *Mycobacterium bovis* or *Brucella abortus*.[359,360] Multiple-site involvement, undulant fevers and weight loss may be associated with these syndromes. Treatment of tuberculosis patients is probably unwise and treatment of horses infected with *Brucella* with strain 19 vaccine must be tempered with consideration of the public health risks involved.

Another aspect of therapy of vertebral osteomyelitis and epidural empyema in horses is surgical exploration and drainage. This was successfully performed in a ram with tetraplegia secondary to osteomyelitis of C_3 and C_4, using a ventral approach, curettage of the lesion, dependent drainage, and topical and systemic antimicrobial therapy.[361] If neurologic signs have been rapidly progressive or if there is profound cord compression, indicated by recumbency, poor voluntary effort and hypalgesia caudal to the lesion, surgical relief of pressure on the spinal cord is probably required. Surgical drainage is also appropriate if large volumes of purulent material are present in association with damage to the spinal cord. Finally, surgical exploration, biopsy, culture and drainage are extremely helpful if antimicrobial therapy has been unsuccessful, particularly if no positive cultures have been obtained.

Prognosis: The prognosis for pyogenic vertebral osteomyelitis and epidural empyema is guarded, as in other forms of disseminated sepsis in horses. However, if patients can be treated before neurologic signs are marked, and if appropriate, long-term antimicrobial therapy is maintained, the outlook for improvement or resolution of neurologic signs may be fair to good.

Verminous Myelitis

Penetration of the spinal cord by wandering parasites may cause neurologic signs ranging from chronic, mild gait impairment to peracute quadriplegia and death. The severity of signs depends upon the number, size and species of parasites involved, the location of the lesion(s), and the extent of migration. *Strongylus vulgaris*, *Setaria* spp, *Hypoderma* spp and *Micronema deletrix* have been found in association with spinal cord damage. These parasites and their role in brain disease are also discussed under Verminous Encephalitis.

Clinical Signs: Strongylus vulgaris fourth-stage larvae occasionally enter the spinal cord, perhaps via nutrient arteries that arise segmentally from the aorta and via vertebral arteries.[362-364] The resulting neurologic disturbance is usually acute, often asymmetric, and referable to a single spinal cord lesion. The wandering larvae may die or migrate out of the spinal cord before causing extensive damage. Horses so affected may have residual, nonprogressive gait deficits. In other cases there is massive spinal cord destruction. In one instance an *S vulgaris* larva tunnelled the entire length of the spinal cord, causing progressive severe limb paralysis and death.[362]

Diagnosis: Spinal cord disease due to aberrant *S vulgaris* larval migration is difficult to distinguish clinically from other causes of acute ataxia and limb paresis such as protozoal myeloencephalitis, cervical vertebral malformation, trauma, EHV-1 myeloencephalitis and rabies. The results of CSF analysis are typical of CNS trauma, with xanthochromia, increased numbers of RBC, and mononuclear inflammatory cells. Although not always found, eosinophils in CSF samples are strong supporting evidence for a diagnosis of verminous myelitis. CSF should be collected from the atlanto-occipital and/or lumbosacral site, whichever is closer to the lesion.

Treatment: If verminous myelitis due to *S vulgaris* is suspected, high doses of anthelmintics with larvicidal properties may be used in an attempt to kill the parasite and halt progression of signs. Such anthelmintics include thiabendazole, at 440 mg/kg body weight daily for 2 days, and fenbendazole, at 60 mg/kg body weight daily for 2 days. Use of moderate doses of corticosteroids, such as dexamethasone at 0.25 mg/kg BID for several days, may be considered. The clinician must realize, however, that protozoal myeloencephalitis may mimic the syndrome of *S vulgaris* myelitis and such therapy may exacerbate the former.

The bovine filarioid nematode parasite, *Setaria digitata,* is reported to cause outbreaks of paralytic disease in horses, sheep and goats in Ceylon, Japan, Korea and India.[365] Infective larvae migrate to the spinal cord or brain after being deposited by vector mosquitos. Prophylaxis and early treatment with diethylcarbamazine citrate (40-100 mg/kg) produced promising results.[366]

A *Setaria* sp larva was recently identified in the cervical spinal cord of a horse from Indiana that had been euthanized because of progressive tetraparesis leading to recumbency.[367] There is one report of a *Hypoderma* spp larva penetrating the thoracic spinal cord of a horse.[368] Because of its large size, this parasite causes devastating damage as it migrates through the CNS. Therefore, in any case of suspected verminous myelitis, an organophosphate may be used (*eg*, trichlorfon at 40 mg/kg PO) in addition to the previously mentioned anthelmintics. Large numbers of *Micronema deletrix* organisms may invade the cervical spinal cord and meninges; however, signs of spinal cord disease are overshadowed by the fulminant encephalitis accompanying invasion of the brain. A single adult *Draschi megastoma* was found in the brainstem of a horse.[369] Such a parasite may migrate through the spinal cord.

Neuritis of the Cauda Equina

A distinct pathologic syndrome characterized by chronic inflammation of the extradural roots of the cauda equina is seen in horses and ponies of both sexes. Affected animals are usually mature or aged. The disease has not been reported to occur in foals or yearlings. Cases of neuritis of the cauda equina have followed outbreaks of respiratory disease.[370-373]

Clinical Signs: Because of the frequent multifocal or diffuse character of the disease, the name polyneuritis equi has been proposed. The presenting signs are quite variable, although usually referable to sacrococcygeal nerve root involvement. There is usually an insidious onset and progression over several weeks, although the signs may be noticed acutely by the owner. Often there is a recent history of rubbing and abrasion of the tail head and perineum, colic (due to obstipation), or hypersensitivity to pressure over the gluteal area. By the time veterinary attention is sought there is usually a well-demarcated area of cutaneous analgesia and areflexia involving the tail, perineum, gluteal area and penis (but not the prepuce). The tail hangs limply without tone and the anal sphincter, rectum, bladder urethral sphincter, and vulva or penis are paralyzed. This leads to fecal retention; feces may appear at the orifice of the flaccid, dilated anus. After 1-2 weeks there is marked atrophy of coccygeal muscles, urinary incontinence with bladder distension, and continual dribbling of urine from a gaping vulva or prolapsed penis, resulting in urine scalding of the perineum and legs. Appetite and vital signs are usually normal at this stage unless there is severe secondary cystitis.

Pelvic limb weakness may occur, especially as the disease progresses, due to inflammation of the sacral and even lumbar nerve roots and extension of the perineuritis to the lumbosacral plexus supplying the gluteal, sciatic and, rarely, the femoral nerves. Gait abnormalities are often subtle and asymmetric (at least initially), with slight swaying of the hips, stumbling and toe-dragging in the rear limbs. Depending on nerves affected, there may be atrophy of the gluteal, biceps femoris, or other muscles on one or both sides. Examination of CSF collected by lumbosacral puncture usually reveals moderate elevations in protein level and WBC numbers (mostly lymphocytes).[370]

Although signs of sacrococcygeal nerve root disease are most obvious, involvement of other nerve roots and peripheral nerves is not uncommon. Many affected horses also have cranial nerve deficits, including masseter atrophy and weakness (motor V), facial paralysis (VII), head tilt, nystagmus and staggering gait (VIII), tongue weakness (XII), difficult swallowing (IX, X), absent pupillary light reflex (III), and blindness (II).[370,372,374] Cranial nerves V, VII and VIII are most commonly affected, usually asymmetrically. There are rare reports of thoracic limb weakness and ataxia due to involvement of the nerve roots and nerves supplying the forelimbs.[370]

Treatment: Despite clinical fluctuations during the course of the disease, neuritis of the cauda equina is invariably progressive and fatal. However, regular manual evacuation of the rectum, catheterization of the bladder, and treatment of any urinary tract infection may prolong the life of the horse for many months. Treatment with various antibiotics, and systemic, epidural and subarachnoid administration of corticosteroids have been ineffective.

Necropsy Findings: Grossly, the epidural nerve roots of the cauda equina are discolored and coated in a thick, fibrous material. This perineural material extends intradurally and through intervertebral foramina, then along the lumbar, sacral and coccygeal nerves. Histologically there is a predominantly extradural inflammation, with hemorrhage and collagen deposition in the epineurium.

The lesions strongly suggest an infectious or immune-mediated mechanism, although all attempts at isolation of an etiologic agent or

determination of transmission of the disease have been unrewarding.[370,374]

Spinal Trauma

Equine practitioners probably see more cases of suspected spinal cord and brain trauma than any other neurologic disorder. At least 90 cases of vertebral trauma, with or without associated neurologic signs, are described in the literature.[374-385] In a 3-year study of fatal fractures in 125 horses at racing events in Britain, 23% of these fractures involved the vertebral column.[384] Approximately half involved the cervical vertebrae and the remainder the thoracolumbar vertebrae.

The incidence of injuries to the vertebrae is not known. However, in an evaluation of 2170 radiographic and necropsy referral cases, 16 fractures involved cervical vertebrae, 22 involved thoracolumbar vertebrae, and 4 involved sacral and coccygeal vertebrae.[378] Of the 42 fractures involving vertebrae, 21 horses had neurologic signs. All 21 horses sustained fractures of the vertebral body, arch and/or articular processes, whereas none of the 7 horses with fractured thoracic dorsal spinous processes had neurologic signs. From the cases described in the literature and general descriptions of vertebral fractures, as well as from the authors' personal experience, cervical vertebrae are more prone to fractures than the rest of the vertebral column.[381-389] The occipitoatlantoaxial region is most often involved with cervical trauma and the atlas may be the most frequently affected vertebral body.[374-377,379,382-384] Excluding fractures of the dorsal spinous processes that involve T_1-T_{12}, there are apparently several predisposed sites for thoracolumbar vertebral fractures.[377,378,380,381,384] These sites are the cranial thoracic (T_1-T_3), the mid-thoracic (T_9-T_{16}), and the lumbar vertebrae (T_{18}-L_6). These sites probably correspond to the anchor points of the spine, the site of most dorsoventral vertebral movement (T_{12}), and the site that bears the most weight.

Cervical vertebral fractures are probably more common in foals, whereas fractures in the thoracolumbar region are more prevalent in adults.[378,379,389] Horses in jumping events apparently sustain neck and back injuries quite frequently. The possibly increased susceptibility for back injury in heavily lactating brood mares could be related to vertebral osteoporosis.[378,384] Foals that pull back against a halter during handling and those that fall over back-

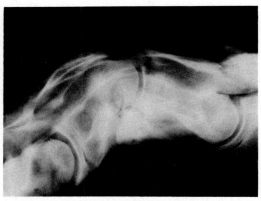

Fig 29. Radiograph of the cervical vertebrae of a mature Thoroughbred stallion that suffered a severe hyperflexion injury of the neck. Acute tetraplegia quickly resolved and, at the time the radiograph was taken, the stallion had a normal gait despite a slight cervical kyphosis. Multiple vertebral fractures have healed by apparent fusion of the fifth and sixth cervical vertebrae.

ward are more likely to injure the occipitoatlantoaxial region.[376,379,383] Any horse that rears up and falls may sustain head trauma. This is likely the mechanism for sacrococcygeal fractures, with damage to the cauda equina, all of which may occur simultaneously.[385] Younger horses, easily frightened by such things as thunderstorms, run into all sorts of objects and fall over while running, injuring their vertebrae and spinal cord. Cervical hyperflexion and hyperextension injuries result from such falls, and cranial thoracic and mid-back fractures result from striking solid objects (Figs 29, 30).[378]

Clinical Signs: An extremely important aspect of all cases of trauma to the vertebral col-

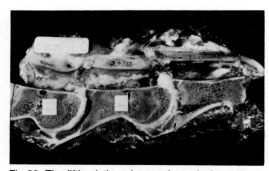

Fig 30. The fifth, sixth and seventh cervical vertebrae, shown here in median section, from a yearling Thoroughbred colt that sustained a hyperextension injury to the neck. There is dorsal luxation of C_5 on C_6, with a slightly displaced fragment off the ventral aspect of C_5. The spinal cord was moderately contused at the C_5-C_6 region, with resulting tetraplegia.

umn is whether or not neurologic signs are present. Surprisingly, not all horses with a fractured vertebral body, arch or articular process have signs of spinal cord disease. The syndromes that result are quite variable. Fractures of C_1-T_2 may result in degrees of tetraplegia or tetraparesis, with ataxia. Those of T_3-L_6 may cause paraplegia or paraparesis and ataxia. Fractures of the sacrum may produce urinary and fecal incontinence, and sometimes muscle atrophy and a gait abnormality in the pelvic limbs. Finally, fractures of the sacrum and coccygeal vertebrae may produce degrees of hypalgesia, hypotonia and hyporeflexia of the perineum, tail and anus.

Classically, neurologic signs appear suddenly at the time of injury. There also may be other signs due to the injury, such as lacerations or hemorrhage into and from body cavities, and particularly signs of pain and distress, including tachypnea, tachycardia, profuse sweating, mydriasis, and splinting or rigid posturing to protect body parts. Trauma patients may become frantic as a result of pain or the inability to stand. Such struggling can exacerbate trauma to the spinal cord. Sometimes there is a brief period of recumbency, followed by staggering for some time and then recovery from neurologic signs in hours to days. This can even occur with profound vertebral trauma. Such patients may still require treatment and/or rest. Neurologic signs may be delayed for hours or even days to months after an episode of trauma to the vertebral column.[378,379] Such cases usually involve various combinations of vertebral instability, progressive hemorrhage, callus formation and secondary degenerative joint disease involving damaged articular processes. All of these factors can produce delayed spinal cord trauma. The last 2 have resulted in the wobbler syndrome, with progressive signs of tetraparesis and ataxia in young horses.[379,390]

Diagnosis: It may be necessary to sedate a frantic horse with suspected spinal cord trauma to complete a physical examination. Diazepam at 0.1 mg/kg or xylazine at 1 mg/kg may be useful because of ease of administration, but chloral hydrate or pentobarbital may be more useful as longer-acting hypnotics. Evidence of respiratory difficulty, blood loss and gross instability of the limbs or neck must be attended to immediately. Signs of head trauma, longbone fracture and bleeding from body orifices should be searched for. A rectal examination should be performed whenever possible to assess retention of urine and feces and to palpate the pelvis, sacrum and caudal vertebral column (Figs 31, 32). Efforts should be made to reduce movement in all horses suspected of suffering spinal cord trauma.

A thorough neurologic examination should allow localization of the lesion(s) within the spinal cord. Horses with spinal cord trauma from C_1-T_2 usually have tetraparesis and ataxia or tetraplegia. A recumbent horse with a lesion at C_1-C_3 has difficulty raising its head off the ground in comparison with a horse recumbent as a result of trauma at C_4-T_2, in which the head and cranial neck may be lifted off the ground (Figs 33, 34). A paraplegic horse that "dog-sits" usually has a lesion caudal to T_2. Some degree of asymmetry may be present with spinal cord trauma but signs are almost always bilateral.

Localizing signs, such as hyporeflexia, hypotonia, sensory deficits and sweating, are extremely helpful findings (Figs 31, 33).[380] The level of hypalgesia on the neck or back indicates the cranial limit of a lesion. Partial depression of the local cervical responses may occur with mid-cervical and caudal cervical lesions. A depressed panniculus response over the trunk occurs frequently with caudal cervical-cranial thoracic spinal cord damage. A line of hyporeflexia may be evident along the trunk, approximating the cranial extent of a lesion. Particularly in the early post-trauma phase, a region of hyperesthesia may be detected just cranial to the lesion. Strip patches of sweating may occur when thoracolumbar spinal nerve roots are damaged. Excessive whole-body sweating, seen frequently in horses with a broken neck or back, may be due to pain and sympathetic discharge. Also, excessive sweating caudal to a profound spinal cord lesion may be expected from damage to the descending sympathetic spinal cord pathways. This may include sweating on the neck and Horner's syndrome if the lesion is cranial to the cranial thoracic segments.

If spinal shock, with suppression of all reflexes caudal to a massive spinal cord lesion, occurs in horses, it probably only lasts for minutes or hours. The Schiff-Sherrington phenomenon, with extensor hypertonia of the thoracic limbs, may occur after severe thoracic spinal cord damage. The important factor differentiating this from a severe cervical lesion is that in the former, voluntary effort and pain perception are good in the thoracic limbs, whereas in the latter, voluntary effort and pain perception are depressed (or absent) in all 4 limbs.

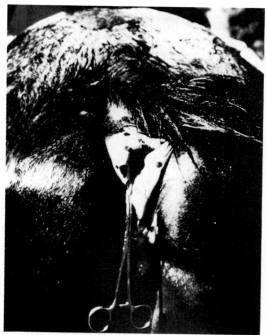

Fig 31. View of the tail, anus and perineum of a filly that suffered a fracture of the second sacral vertebra. Analgesia, areflexia and hypotonia were present in the tail, anus and perineal area, and there was fecal and urinary incontinence. These signs mimic those of neuritis of the cauda equina. An abnormal bulge, palpable on the ventral aspect of the sacrum, probably corresponded to the luxation at the fracture site.

At this stage of evaluation, an initial prognosis must be given; the outlook is guarded for all recumbent horses. However, much may be gained and little lost if final judgement is withheld for one to several hours, providing the horse is not suffering.[378,387] Considering the acute phase of experimental spinal cord trauma, the functional loss is far more profound

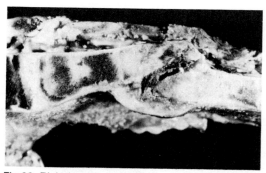

Fig 32. Right lateral view of the median section of the sacrum of the horse in Figure 31. (Courtesy of Dr G.P. Carlson)

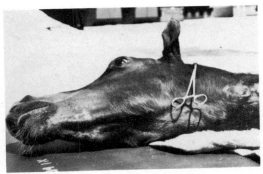

Fig 33. Ventral view of the head and neck of a tetraplegic 3-month-old Quarter Horse filly that sustained a neck injury while exercising on a mechanical walker. Signs of ataxia progressed to tetraplegia over 24 hours. The filly was unable to raise its head or neck up off the ground. There was a strip of analgesia on the neck caudal to the ears, as shown, with absence of the local cervical responses in this region, and hypalgesia of the whole body caudal to this site.

than that expected from the morphologic changes.[391-393] Consequently, if further damage is prevented, return of functional integrity can be remarkable, even in control animals receiving no therapy and in clinical equine patients (Fig 29).[378,382,394-396]

The most helpful aid in confirming a diagnosis of vertebral trauma is plain radiography.[375,376,378-380,382,383] However, this procedure does not directly evaluate the presence and extent of spinal cord trauma. Vertebral components may be in very different positions as compared with displacements that may have occurred at the time of injury. Although vertebral canal diameter is the most important component to evaluate, even this can give a false impression of the degree of spinal cord compromise (Fig 29).

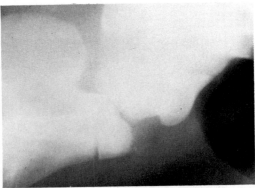

Fig 34. A fractured dens with atlantoaxial luxation was diagnosed radiographically. Lack of response to therapy and a bad prognosis necessitated euthanasia. Severe spinal cord contusion was confirmed at necropsy.

The possible combinations of epiphyseal separations, fractured vertebral bodies, luxations, separated articular pedicles and nondisplaced fractures are endless. However, the neurologic examination is usually of greater significance in determining prognosis and response to therapy, and radiographs are of more significance in deciding if surgery is indicated.

If there is a suggestion of increased intracranial pressure in a horse that may have sustained an injury, it is unwise to collect a large volume of CSF from the atlanto-occipital site because of the risk of caudal herniation of the occipital lobes of the cerebrum and the cerebellum. However, collection of CSF from horses with spinal cord trauma and no head signs is quite safe, particularly from the lumbosacral site. A CSF analysis is sometimes of great assistance in ruling out other causes of peracute spinal cord disease, such as EHV-1 myeloencephalitis, larval migration and protozoal myeloencephalitis. Firm evidence of subarachnoid hemorrhage, however, may not always be found on analysis of CSF from horses with spinal cord trauma; in fact, results of CSF analysis in such animals are often normal.

Electromyography can be valuable in helping localize the site of spinal cord trauma and can direct radiographic attention. Evidence of denervation of muscles only appears 5 or more days after the damage to the ventral grey matter. Prominent multifocal or diffuse denervation potentials found by electromyelography on a horse with spinal cord disease would be strong evidence for some (multifocal) mechanism other than injury.

Hematologic, chemical, serologic and other tests are more for differential diagnosis of spinal cord trauma cases, although a hematologic stress pattern, unconjugated hyperbilirubinemia, uremia, and chemical and enzymatic evidence of soft tissue and possibly bone damage may be expected in recumbent animals.

Treatment: The logical medical management of spinal cord trauma, based upon recent research into the pathophysiologic mechanisms involved, continues to be debated.[391,393,397-400] The initial events in spinal cord trauma are almost certainly mechanical.[392,394] The explanation of a profound functional loss from minimal anatomic derangement is possibly related to primary extrusion of K ions from cells, with an extensive local depolarization (block) of neurons.[391] An immediate systemic arterial pressor response is probably mediated by vascular and adrenergic receptors.[391] Suppression of this pressor response may markedly decrease the number of resulting spinal cord hemorrhages.[391,401,402] A dramatic change in spinal cord blood flow apparently occurs within 1-2 hours.[403] The rate at which spinal cord compression occurs is probably important; slow compression is associated with less permanent deficits than rapid compression to the same degree.[394] This leads to the suggestion that changes in blood flow are less important than primary mechanical factors, although time is probably important.[394]

It was reported that local catecholamine levels rose sharply in contused spinal cord and that anticatecholamine (alphamethyltyrosine, reserpine, levodopa, phenoxybenzamine) therapy drastically reduced the consequences of spinal cord trauma.[399] Other authors were not able to reproduce these results, although the role of vasoactive substances in spinal cord trauma has not been dismissed.[391,392,395,401,404,405]

One interesting hypothesis stated that platelet activation and resulting thrombi and emboli were a vital component of the cascade resulting in hemorrhage, edema and necrosis.[393] Suppression of platelet aggregation and block of vasospasm were thus logical treatment suggestions. Manipulation of vasoconstriction and clotting mechanisms with dimethyl sulfoxide and epsilon aminocaproic acid were purportedly very beneficial in spinal cord trauma.[397,398,405] However, in at least one controlled experiment, neither DMSO nor epsilon aminocaproic acid significantly improved the functional recovery of contused canine spinal cords.[400] Inasmuch as the clinical modulation of platelet function in spinal cord trauma patients is in its infancy, exciting results may be forthcoming. Also, recent interest has been revived in the use of compounds that decrease metabolic requirements, such as gamma hydroxybutyrate and barbiturates, and in loop diuretics, such as furosemide, in treatment of nervous system trauma.[404,407] The role of such therapy for spinal cord disease remains questionable.

A discussion of medical management of spinal cord trauma would be incomplete without reference to the use of hyperosmolar diuretics, such as mannitol, and glucocorticoids. A large proportion of spinal cord trauma patients of all species probably receive these compounds. Frequently used regimens vary from 20% mannitol given IV at 0.25-2 g/kg and dexamethasone given IV at 0.1-2.2 mg/kg, both repeated up to 4 times daily. There is little proof demonstrating the effectiveness of these compounds. Some reports suggest that, in experimental spinal cord trauma in dogs, these compounds were not very effective in protecting long-term spinal cord function.[396,397,406] It is possible, however, that glucocorticoids help reduce the severity of the damage in experimental spinal cord edema.[391]

There is not full agreement on the medical management of spinal cord trauma. The following remarks are based on the literature cited, on the experience of others and on personal experience with horses suffering from spinal cord trauma.[408,409] In the peracute stages, dexamethasone at 0.1-0.2 mg/kg may be given IV and repeated up to 4 times daily for 2-4 days. After the first 24-48 hours, the benefit of corticosteroids is probably reduced, and problems with decubital infections, cystitis, laminitis, delayed bone healing and occasional systemic infection can be so marked that their use is best avoided. If continued bleeding is suspected or if systemic blood pressure is likely to be elevated in the peracute phase following injury, 1-2 standard doses of furosemide are useful. The horse must be kept calm or sedated with chlorpromazine, acetylpromazine, chloral hydrate, pentobarbital or other agents. The use of 20% mannitol at 0.25-1 g/kg given IV and glycerol in water, given orally at 1 g/kg, has not been very successful in the authors' hands. Severe prerenal azotemia results from over use of furosemide and mannitol in recumbent patients. The effectiveness of DMSO in equine spinal cord trauma has been difficult to establish, although in acute cases the authors sometimes use 40% DMSO in 5% dextrose and water, given slowly IV at 1 g/kg at 12-hour intervals for up to 4 doses. Antibiotics are probably not required for vertebral fractures or spinal cord trauma but may be necessary to treat concurrent skin lesions, cystitis and pneumonitis, especially in recumbent patients. In the final analysis, if a dramatic improvement occurs in the specific neurologic deficits of a horse with spinal cord trauma after a particular treatment, consideration should be given to repeating that treatment.

External manipulation, external and internal fixation, and surgical decompression and fusion are types of therapy that have not been employed very extensively in horses suffering from vertebral damage. Manipulation of cervical vertebral luxations and torticollis, preferably under general anesthesia, with use of external support in the form of a cradle or neck cast, is a reasonable suggestion.[375,387,388] Great care must be taken when manipulating damaged vertebrae under anesthesia to prevent further spinal cord trauma. Excellent results were obtained with surgical immobilization of a fractured dens, with luxation of the axis, in a 3-week-old Appaloosa colt.[382] Complete remission of signs was obtained by surgical correction of a complete ventral luxation of the axis on the atlas in an 11-day-old Arabian colt.[410] The Appaloosa received oxytetracycline but no other drugs postoperatively and the Arabian colt received no drugs postoperatively.

Selection of candidates for surgery is vital. Surgery is probably indicated if a horse's neurologic condition deteriorates after appropriate medical therapy for spinal cord trauma, and decompression of the spinal cord and stabilization of luxations of fractures is feasible. The technics of cervical dorsal decompressive laminectomy described for horses may be modified for decompression of a spinal cord that is compromised by hematoma, displaced soft tissues or bone.[272,411] Surgical hardware often is not strong enough to withstand the forces within the middle of the equine cervical vertebral column. Therefore, intervertebral fusion may be a promising technic to stabilize fractures of the arch and articular processes of cervical vertebrae in horses, as it is in humans.[272,412,413] Other technics of vertebral plating, screwing, or wiring must be modified from standard small animal or human methods.

Prognosis: The prognosis for horses with spinal cord trauma associated with luxations or fractures of the vertebral body, arch or articular processes must remain guarded to poor for return to use.[378,379,387] Healing of such fractures frequently results in some degree of vertebral malalignment, sometimes with lordosis, kyphosis, scoliosis or torticollis (Fig 29).[379,388] Even after apparent healing and resolution of neurologic signs, delayed callus formation and degenerative changes in adjacent articulations can result in delayed permanent spinal cord compression.[379]

No simple rules can be given for the management of horses suffering from spinal cord trauma. In the authors' experience, 2 points are worthy of emphasis. First, thorough and repeated neurologic examinations are most helpful in arriving at a prognosis and evaluating progress of the case. Second, no individual medical or surgical therapeutic regimen is more singularly beneficial in healing spinal cord injuries than the passage of time.

Toxicity

Haloxon Toxicity

The occurrence of laryngeal paresis after use of the organophosphate anthelmintic haloxon has been reported in Australia and South Africa.[414,415] In the Australian incident, 11 foals given a haloxon paste preparation all developed some degree of acute laryngeal dysfunction, ranging from transient left-sided paresis to permanent bilateral paralysis.

In South Africa, the administration of a combination of haloxon and carbon disulfide has been linked to the occurrence of CNS lesions, especially in the brainstem and sacral spinal cord. These pathologic changes were associated with laryngeal paresis and, in severe cases, with paralysis of the esophagus, anus and bladder, and ataxia and weakness of the pelvic limbs. No lesions were produced when the drugs were used separately.

Vascular Spinal Cord Disease

Ischemic Myelopathy

Focal spinal cord infarction due to multiple fibrocartilaginous emboli has been reported in an 8-year-old Quarter Horse.[416] The fibrocartilaginous material was thought to originate from a degenerated intervertebral disc. The ischemic lesion involved both grey and white matter in the caudal cervical spinal cord and resulted in peracute quadriplegia.

Peripheral Neuropathies

Suprascapular Paralysis

Total paralysis of the suprascapular nerve causes atrophy of the supraspinatus and infraspinatus muscles within 1-2 weeks, resulting in prominence of the spine of the scapula ("sweeney").

Cause: Trauma is by far the most common cause of suprascapular paralysis. There is often a history of the horse striking an object or another horse with its shoulder. Other mechanisms, such as peripheral nerve neoplasms or abscesses that involve the C_6 nerve root or suprascapular nerve, could result in suprascapular paralysis. Lesions of the ventral grey matter at the C_6 spinal cord segment, such as equine protozoal myelitis, can produce this syndrome, although additional signs, such as pelvic limb ataxia, are usually present.

Clinical Signs: Frequently there is an initial decrease in the distance the affected leg is advanced and a slight dragging of the toe. The horse may stumble on the affected limb, particularly while trotting. Some abduction of the shoulder joint occurs during weight-bearing.[3,246,251] After several weeks there is marked atrophy of the suprascapular muscles, but there may be very little or no gait abnormality.[417] Some horses with prominent abduction or "popping-out" of the shoulder joint ("shoulder slip") circumduct the affected leg on protraction to avoid dragging the toe.[251] This degree of lateral luxation of the shoulder joint is variable and is probably due to the loss of lateral joint support afforded by the suprascapular muscles and tendons.[418] In traumatic neuropathy, the laxity may in part be due to damage to joint surfaces, joint capsule and other supporting tissues in the area.[251]

Severe trauma to or laceration of the cranial shoulder region may cause additional signs from damage to other nerves and muscles. With pectoral nerve involvement, the elbow is abducted, in addition to the shoulder, when the horse bears weight on the limb. Partial avulsion of other nerve bundles of the brachial plexus has occurred in a horse that suffered severe blunt trauma to the upper arm and shoulder. In addition to sweeney, there was abduction of the elbow (pectoral paralysis), a dropped shoulder (subscapular paralysis), inability to flex the elbow (musculocutaneous paralysis), and partial, proximal radial paralysis.

Treatment: Treatment of uncomplicated suprascapular nerve paralysis due to trauma is unnecessary if the horse is not used for performance. However, for cosmetic purposes and for horses expected to exercise satisfactorily, therapy should be considered at the time of injury and again in 2-12 weeks. Ideally the severed stumps of the nerve should be anastomosed if the suprascapular nerve is severed at the time of injury.[419,420] If this is not feasible because of related soft tissue trauma, the stumps of the nerve may be freed from adjacent tissues and identified using stainless steel sutures to allow exploration and anastomosis when other soft tissue healing is complete. It is reasonable to assume that at least the fibrous nerve sheath is still intact in cases of closed trauma resulting in suprascapular nerve paralysis. Under these circumstances, systemic administration of corticosteroids for a short time (*eg*, dexamethasone at 0.05 mg/kg given IM BID for 3 days) may be useful to suppress local swelling and inflammation that may further damage nerve fibers. Immediate application of ice packs to the area also should be considered.

Function returns in a period of days to weeks in cases of neurapraxia (concussion to the nerve). If there has been severance of axons (axonotmesis) or whole fibers (neurotmesis), with relative preservation of the endoneurium, perineurium and epineurium, the nerve fibers distal to the injury site undergo Wallerian degeneration and regeneration, and regrow down the distal fibrous framework at about 1 inch/month to reinnervate the atrophied muscles. Consequently, enough time should be allowed for this process to occur. However, allowance of too much time to elapse can result in permanent fibrosis and contracture of atrophied muscles. Therefore, if treatment of a horse with chronic, traumatically induced suprascapular paralysis is necessary, surgical exploration, with freeing of adhesions, removal of neuromata and possible reanastomosis, probably should be performed 8-12 weeks after injury.[421] Such delayed repair of compressed suprascapular nerves has resulted in full return of limb function and shoulder muscle mass. A technic for removing a section of scapula underlying the nerve, to aid in decompression, has been mentioned.[421] Technics for peripheral nerve surgery that should be applicable to horses are well described for dogs.[420]

Attempts at camouflaging signs of sweeney, such as injecting air under the skin of the shoulder or creating a foreign body reaction over the shoulder by implanting a coin, have been employed.[421] Results of such "treatments" are less than satisfactory.

Radial Paralysis

Failure to bear weight on a thoracic limb because of total radial paralysis reflects inability to extend the leg and flex the shoulder joint.[246,417,421] Affected horses have great difficulty getting up and down, and stand with the shoulder extended. The elbow, knee, fetlock and interphalangeal joints are flexed, and the dorsum of the toe rests on the ground.[418] The elbow is maintained in the "dropped" position during locomotion and the limb is advanced only half a stride, usually with the toe dragging; the horse collapses on the leg when forced to bear weight on it. With partial paralysis, the horse may be able to advance the leg by jerking the shoulder and arm craniad to support some weight, and may back up reasonably well.[246,418] This may reflect some function in the extensor carpi radialis and common digital extensor muscles.[418] Interestingly, horses with partial radial paralysis often can bear weight on the limb and paw the ground, especially if supported in a sling. This probably is due to function of the flexor muscles of the elbow (and musculocutaneous nerve), allowing elevation of the arm, passive striking of the ground, then flexion of the carpus and digits via ulnar and median innervation. Areas of analgesia of the skin of the leg have been defined in radial paralysis cases.[246] However, these are not easily defined in clinical cases and, if present, are likely to be extremely variable and subtle. Radial paralysis of more than 2 weeks' duration results in degrees of atrophy of the triceps, extensor carpi radialis, ulnaris lateralis and digital extensor muscles.

The radial nerve is well protected by surrounding muscle but can be damaged by direct trauma and prolonged lateral recumbency, particularly with malpositioning of the limb. The radial-type paralysis seen frequently in the dependent and occasionally the upper forelimb after anesthesia in lateral recumbency was thought to be the result of pressure on and stretching of the radial nerve.[422] This form of postanesthetic lameness is most probably the result of ischemic myopathy, with a component of ischemic neurapraxia (see Chapter 19).[423,424] Severe trauma to the cranial shoulder region may result in signs of radial paralysis as a component of presumed partial avulsion of the nerves of the brachial plexus, as described under suprascapular paralysis.[421] Fractures of the first rib can result in paralysis of the radial nerve and other nerves of the brachial plexus.

Radial paralysis may accompany humeral fractures. Function of this nerve should be evaluated prior to fracture repair because of the poorer prognosis that accompanies radial nerve damage.[421] If traumatic radial paralysis has occurred more than 5 days prior to evaluation, needle electromyography may be helpful in defining the extent of muscular denervation. The radial nerve should be examined at the time of any humeral fracture fixation, and appropriate debridement and reanastomosis performed as described under suprascapular paralysis. The forelimb should be placed in a light plaster cast to avoid trauma to the limb and flexion contracture.[421] Because the rate of regrowth of severed axons is about 1 inch/month, regrowth of more than about 12 inches cannot be expected since irreversible fibrotic contracture will likely intervene.

Tumors and abscesses in the cranial thorax and tumors of the brachial plexus and radial nerve may rarely result in radial paralysis. Spinal cord lesions, such as protozoal myelitis involving the caudal cervical and cranial thoracic ventral grey matter, can produce the syndrome, although additional signs of myelopathy are usually seen. Horner's syndrome may be expected with cranial thoracic grey matter or nerve root involvement.

Therapy is as described for suprascapular paralysis and described for other species.[420]

Musculocutaneous, Median and Ulnar Paralysis

Paralysis of any of these nerves rarely occurs as a singular event and the resulting syndromes are not well documented. However, brachial plexus injuries and spinal cord lesions involving grey matter of the brachial intumescence may cause signs related to involvement of some or all of these nerves. The nerves are well protected under the shoulder girdle and not often involved in long-bone fractures, although elbow fractures may affect the ulnar and median nerves.

The remarkable subtlety of alteration in gait with paralysis of the individual nerves after a period of adaptation (3 months) may in part be explained by crossing of fibers from one nerve to the other. Decussation occurs at least between musculocutaneous and median nerves.[417]

Section of the proximal musculocutaneous nerve results in a marked gait alteration that may disappear within 3 months.[417] Dragging of the toe is associated with decreased elbow flexion. Needle electromyography can disclose denervation potentials in the biceps and brachialis muscles. Partial sensory loss is expected in the skin of the cranial aspect of the knee and foreleg, probably down to the coronet.[417,425]

Median neurectomy results in a stiff gait in the limb, with dragging of the toe due to decreased flexion of carpus and fetlock, and hypalgesia of the medial aspect of the distal leg. Within 2 months there is little or no gait abnormality.[417]

Ulnar neurectomy results in a similar, though more pronounced, change in gait as in median neurectomy. There is decreased flexion of the carpus and fetlock, and the foot may be protected in a jerky fashion. There is said to be marked hypalgesia of the lateral aspect of the metacarpus and foot, and probably of the caudal aspect of the proximal leg.[417] The residual abnormalities in gait include stumbling on the limb and decreased flexion of the fetlock. Obvious atrophy of the digital flexors should be apparent. All these findings may be variable.[417]

Combined ulnar and median neurectomy apparently results in signs very similar to those of ulnar neurectomy alone.[417]

Therapy for paralyses of these nerves is the same as described for suprascapular paralysis, although aggressive therapy may be unnecessary because of the remarkable improvement of any gait alteration with the passage of time.

Femoral Paralysis

The femoral nerve innervates the major extensor muscles of the stifle and paralysis of this nerve results in inability to extend the stifle. Because of reciprocal flexion of the tarsus and digits when the stifle flexes, femoral nerve damage results in extensor paralysis, with the affected limb held in an overflexed position and the ipsilateral hip lower than the other. Essentially no weight is supported on the affected limb during locomotion.[3,246,418] If the horse is recumbent, the patellar reflex is depressed or absent, although there is a normal flexor reflex if the sciatic nerve is intact. There may be hypalgesia of the medial thigh if the lesion involves the saphenous nerve or the femoral nerve proximal to where this sensory branch divides off.[246,418] Ultimately there is atrophy of the quadriceps muscles.[421] The horse's gait abnormality may eventually improve, presumably by the action of the proximal abductor and adductor muscles fixing the stifle joint, allowing weight-bearing on the leg.[418]

The femoral nerve is well protected from external injury during its course but may be damaged by penetrating wounds in the caudal flank. Femoral paralysis has occurred with abscesses, tumors and aneurysms in the region of the external iliac arteries.[418] Fractures of the pelvis and femur may be associated with damage to the femoral nerve; integrity of the nerve should be determined before fracture repair is attempted in such cases.

Exertional rhabdomyolysis and postanesthetic myopathy syndromes may cause unilateral or bilateral extensor weakness in the pelvic limbs because of involvement of the quadriceps musculature (see Chapter 19). Overextension of the limb while the horse is recumbent may result in femoral paralysis.[421]

Spinal cord lesions of the ventral grey matter or nerve roots at L_4 and L_5 can result in femoral paralysis. Equine protozoal myeloencephalitis has caused this, although lesions and trauma also could do the same.

In spite of hope for improvement, the prognosis must be guarded unless the nerve can be repaired.[418] A light horse with unilateral femoral paralysis may get around satisfactorily without breaking down in the contralateral limb. Medical and surgical therapy are as defined under suprascapular paralysis.

Peroneal Paralysis

This branch of the sciatic nerve supplies the flexor muscles of the tarsus and extensor muscles of the digits. Paralysis thus results in extension of the tarsus and flexion of the fetlock and interphalangeal joints. At rest an affected horse holds the leg somewhat extended caudad, with the dorsum of the hoof resting on the ground. During locomotion the foot is dragged along the ground, then jerked caudad when an attempt is made to bear weight on the leg, after which the leg is pulled partly craniad again. This caudal jerking of the leg and sliding of the hoof on the ground may be repeated several times. If the leg is manually advanced and the toe extended, the horse can bear weight on the leg.[418] Hypalgesia reportedly occurs on the craniolateral aspect of the gaskin, hock and metatarsal regions.[246,418] Atrophy of the craniolateral aspect of the gaskin may be expected.

The peroneal nerve is most vulnerable to external injury where it crosses the lateral condyle of the femur. Injury from kicks by other horses and from lateral recumbency usually does not sever the nerve and many such cases eventually improve.

The limb should be supported and protected. Other aspects of therapy are as described for suprascapular nerve injury.

Tibial Paralysis

The tibial branch of the sciatic nerve innervates the gastrocnemius and digital flexor muscles. Paralysis causes the limb to be held with the tarsus flexed and the fetlock resting in a flexed or partly knuckled position. Consequently, the hip is held lower on the affected side. Flexion of the hock and extension of the digits is unopposed; therefore, the horse overflexes the limb when walking and the foot is raised higher than normal. In addition, controlled extension of the hock cannot occur at completion of the advancing phase of the stride and the foot is dropped straight to the ground. The overall stride is strikingly similar to that seen with stringhalt.[418] Atrophy of the gastrocnemius muscle and anesthesia of the caudal metatarsal region also occur.[246]

Tibial paralysis is very uncommon, partly because the nerve is well protected by the muscles and bones of the limb.

Sciatic Paralysis

The sciatic nerve supplies the main extensor muscles of the hip and flexor muscles of the stifle, and divides into the peroneal and tibial branches. Total sciatic paralysis results in a profound abnormality in gait and posture, mainly from flexor weakness. At rest the limb hangs behind the horse, with the stifle and hock extended and the fetlock and interphalangeal joints partly flexed and the dorsum of the hoof lying on the ground. During locomotion the foot is dragged or the lower limb is jerked dorsad and somewhat craniad by the flexor muscles of the hip and extensor muscles of the stifle (femoral nerve innervation). If the foot is manually advanced and placed on the ground ventral to the pelvis, the horse can support weight with some flexion of the hock and take a stride.[246,418] Atrophy of the caudal thigh and all of the limb distal to the stifle occurs.[246] Degrees of hypalgesia over most of the limb except for the medial thigh have been reported.[418]

The proximal sciatic nerve is well protected although, because of its close relationship with the pelvis, it may be damaged by fractures of the pelvis, especially of the ischium. In young foals, deep injection reactions caudal to the proximal femur and *Salmonella* osteomyelitis of the sacrum and pelvis have resulted in sciatic paralysis. Treatment of such primary problems may result in resolution of sciatic paralysis but the prognosis is bad, even with surgical anastomosis if the nerve is severed. This is because of the great distance over which nerve fiber regeneration must proceed. Support and protection should be given to the distal limb. Other aspects of therapy of peripheral neuropathies are covered above.

Syndromes of sciatic palsy and flexor weakness can occur with spinal cord lesions, such as equine protozoal myeloencephalitis affecting the L_5-S_3 ventral grey matter or nerve roots. Other signs, such as bladder paralysis, gluteal atrophy and degrees of extensor weakness, may also be present.

Other Pelvic Limb Peripheral Nerve Syndromes

The cranial gluteal nerve innervates the middle and deep gluteal muscles, making up the bulk of the rump of the horse, and the tensor fascia lata muscle. Gluteal atrophy, with a dramatic loss of bulk to the rump, occurs with cranial gluteal paralysis, along with a slight hollowing of the caudal flank region from atrophy of the tensor fascia lata muscle. Such a syndrome may occur with pelvic fractures but has been seen more commonly with equine protozoal myeloencephalitis lesions of the ventral grey horn L_6. A subtle to severe abnormality in the gait in the ipsilateral limb occurs, depending on the extent of the lesion.

Obturator nerve paralysis, with loss of adductor function in the pelvic limbs, is rare in horses.[246]

Coccygeal and Anal Paralysis

Variations of the syndrome of paralysis of the tail, anus, perineum, bladder and rectum occur with lesions of the sacrocaudal ventral grey column and nerve roots, cauda equina, and sacral and coccygeal nerves. Common causes include neuritis of the cauda equina, trauma to the sacral and caudal vertebrae, and cystitis and ataxia associated with ingestion of *Sorghum* grasses. These diseases have been discussed above under inflammatory, traumatic and toxic conditions of the spinal cord.

Peripheral Nerve-Muscle Disorders

Botulism

The signs of botulism are due to the actions of the extremely potent exotoxins elaborated by vegetative *Clostridium botulinum* organisms. These toxins interfere with the release of acetylcholine at nerve endings, causing widespread neuromuscular blockade and weakness.[426]

Clostridium botulinum is a gram-positive bacillus that requires anaerobic conditions for multiplication. Seven toxigenic serotypes are recognized, designated A to G, each producing toxins of slightly different composition and potency.[426] Types B, C and D have been incriminated in naturally occurring cases of equine botulism. *Clostridium botulinum* occurs commonly in soil and the intestinal contents of normal birds and mammals[426] The prevalence of each serotype in soil and intestinal contents varies greatly with geographic location.

The most common cause of botulism is the ingestion of preformed toxin in contaminated or spoiled feedstuffs.[426] Toxin can also be elaborated by *Cl botulinum* organisms in necrotic tissue (wound botulism, toxicoinfectious botulism), and there is some evidence that toxin can be produced by organisms in the GI tract of human infants.[427-430] Wound contamination (toxicoinfectious botulism) and ingestion of preformed toxin have caused botulism in horses.

Ingestion of Toxin: The type of toxin contaminating a feedstuff in a particular area often reflects the variety of *Cl botulinum* most commonly found in the local soil. Type-B toxin was identified in samples of potatoes and oats that caused outbreaks of botulism in horses in Israel and Canada, respectively.[431,432] In many countries of Europe, where the disease has been enzootic among horses, botulism due to type-C toxin is apparently most important (especially in France, Yugoslavia, Scandinavia and Spain), with type D occurring less frequently.[433] Many significant outbreaks in Europe have been traced to feed contaminated by the putrefied carcasses of cats, rodents or birds.[433-437] In Spain, 34 mules on 24 farms died with signs of botulism over 8 months. The source of toxin in these cases was a macerated cat skull found in a village granary. In a similar outbreak in Yugoslavia, 46 to 115 horses on one property showed signs of botulism after eating silage contaminated by a decomposed cat carcass; 29 of these horses died.[437] As little as 50-100 g of hay around such a carcass could be lethal if ingested by a horse.[434] One author found high levels of type-C toxin in feces of normal cats, and considered contamination of horse feed by cat feces a possible hazard.[436]

Regardless of the route of administration and the type of toxin, the clinical picture is rather consistent, varying only in severity. The mortality rate in naturally occurring cases has been estimated at from 69% to greater than 90%.[434,436,437] Death may occur within several hours of the appearance of clinical signs, or may take up to a week. One experimental horse showed typical signs of paralysis for 16 days before dying. Recovery may take weeks or even months but is complete if it occurs.

Locomotor abnormalities are usually noticed first. A slight drop in temperature may precede other signs. Affected horses move with a shuffling, stilted gait, drag their toes along the ground, and may stand with head and neck hanging below the horizontal position. Complete absence of facial expression creates a dull, sleepy appearance. Saliva frequently drools from the corners of the mouth (Fig 35). Although the appetite is unaffected, mastication and lingual movements may be so feeble that partly chewed food drops from the mouth. Difficulty in swallowing often causes water and

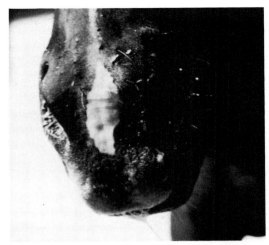

Fig 35. Adult horse with a botulism-like syndrome, showing the expressionless, flaccid muzzle and lips. Saliva drooling from the lips and food material in the nares are evidence of dysphagia. The nostrils fail to flare with inspiration.

feed material to exit the nostrils (Fig 35). There may be noticeable muffling of vocalization (dysphonia) and respiratory stridor, caused by dorsal displacement of the soft palate. Mydriasis and sluggish pupillary reflexes usually appear early in the course of the disease, as does flaccid paresis of the tongue.

Some affected horses turn to look at their flanks, suggesting the presence of abdominal pain. Often there is complete cessation of intestinal sounds and rectal examination may reveal dry, mucus-covered feces. Decreased tail tone may be noticed during rectal examination. The urinary bladder is often distended and there may be frequent passage of small amounts of urine, accompanied by penile protrusion and paralysis in males. Cattle with botulism have a high incidence of indicanuria, albuminuria and glycosuria.[438] Such changes would have diagnostic significance but have not been investigated in horses.

As weakness becomes more profound, there is muscular trembling and generalized sweating. Breathing becomes labored, with a prominent abdominal effort. Once adult horses with botulism become recumbent, they seldom rise again. Such horses soon become too weak to maintain a sternal position. Respiratory arrest and death occur after a variable period of lateral recumbency, during which there are weak paddling movements and increasing dyspnea. Skin sensation is normal throughout the disease, although spinal and cranial nerve reflexes are generally depressed. There are no abnormalities of sensorium, although weakness and lack of facial expression convey an impression of stupor. The clinical course in less severely affected animals may be complicated by the development of inhalation pneumonia or necrotic cystitis.

Botulinum toxin is very rarely detected in the serum of horses with naturally occurring botulism. However, toxin has been detected in the serum of several experimentally poisoned horses for several hours after the onset of clinical signs.[438]

Necropsy findings are generally unremarkable in cases of botulism. Toxin is occasionally demonstrated in liver or GI contents. It is important to remember that *Cl botulinum* organisms normally present in the intestine may elaborate toxin postmortem if sufficient putrefaction occurs. Only fresh or frozen samples should be submitted for toxin detection.

Toxicoinfectious Botulism: Toxicoinfectious botulism has recently been established as the probable cause of both the "shaker foal syndrome" and sporadic deaths in older horses.[429] The shaker foal syndrome has been enzootic in central Kentucky for more than 40 years. The disease most often affects fast-growing foals 2-4 weeks of age. Clinical signs are typical of botulism, as described in the previous section. There is initially a stilted gait, muscle tremor and inability to stand for more than a few minutes. There is palsy dysphagia, nasal reflux of milk, constipation, mydriasis, frequent urination and dyspnea. The mortality rate approaches 100%, with death usually occurring 1-3 days after the onset of signs.

In a series of 8 shaker foals, *Cl botulinum* type-B was isolated from foci of tissue necrosis in a variety of sites, including gastric ulcers, foci of hepatic necrosis, abscesses in the navel or lungs, and wounds in skin and muscle. Proliferation of *Cl botulinum* type-B organisms in these sites probably resulted in toxicoinfectious botulism. The shaker foal syndrome has since been reproduced by inoculation of *Cl botulinum* type-B spores into experimentally created areas of muscle necrosis.[439]

There may be a higher incidence of shaker foal syndrome in foals of mares fed an excessively nutritious diet and exposed to stress. High levels of glucocorticoids in the milk of such mares may facilitate dissemination of *Cl botulinum* organisms in the foal from the gut to areas of tissue necrosis.[429] Extremely small amounts of type-B toxin can be lethal in this situation, and attempts at detection of toxin in the sera of affected foals are unlikely to be successful. A 2-month-old foal had type-C toxicoinfectious botulism. In that case, the site of *Cl botulinum* infection was thought to be the colon, which was irritated by sand.[440]

Diagnosis: A definitive diagnosis of botulism, either ingested or toxicoinfectious, is seldom made ante mortem, but clinical signs are highly suggestive. Nevertheless, serum from horses with the first signs of disease should be frozen and submitted to a diagnostic laboratory for toxin detection. At necropsy, stomach and intestinal contents, feces, liver, suspect feed or carrion, and areas of tissue necrosis should be submitted for anaerobic culture and biologic assay for botulinum toxin. The results of such tests must be interpreted in light of the foregoing discussion.

Treatment: Death from botulism is usually due to respiratory failure. Unfortunately, prolonged artificial respiration of horses is not practical in most situations. It is conceivable, however, that respiratory support for an extremely valuable shaker foal could be provided in a sophisticated veterinary hospital. Less severely affected horses may need intensive support for several weeks during recovery. Placement of an indwelling nasoesophageal tube ensures adequate hydration and nutrition, and reduces the likelihood of aspiration pneumonia. Recumbent horses should be encouraged to remain sternal and, if possible, assisted to stand for short periods and posture for urination. Recumbent horses may require careful catheterization to prevent serious bladder distension and necrosis. Bacterial urinary and respiratory tract infections must be treated vigorously with appropriate antimicrobials. Aminoglycoside antibiotics, such as streptomycin and kanamycin, must not be used since they may potentiate muscle weakness.

Administration of a laxative, such as $MgSO_4$, is indicated to eliminate any toxin remaining in the intestine.

If toxicoinfectious botulism is suspected, as in a shaker foal, high levels of K penicillin (100,000-400,000 IU/kg body weight divided into 4 daily doses) may be given IV to destroy vegetative *Cl botulinum* organisms proliferating in necrotic tissue. However, use of antibiotics in humans with wound botulism is of questionable value. Wounds should be meticulously debrided and irrigated. Likewise, any abscess should be cultured and drained.

Specific serotherapy has been used for many years in Europe with moderate success.[433] One investigator reported a reduction in mortality rates from 90% to 25% due to use of specific antitoxin in field outbreaks of botulism.[436] Experimentally, survival rates have only been improved if massive IV doses (1000-2000 IU antitoxin/kg body weight) of specific antitoxin are used during the first few hours after the onset of clinical signs.[436] A bivalent homologous antitoxin against *Cl botulinum* types A and B is available in the US.[441] This product may be useful if used very early in the course of the shaker foal syndrome.

Use of drugs that may potentiate neuromuscular blockade, such as aminoglycoside antibiotics, tetracyclines and procaine penicillin, must be avoided. Edrophonium and other acetylcholine-potentiating drugs are used to help reverse the neuromuscular blockade of botulism in other species; the safety of their use in horses is yet to be determined. Neostigmine has often been used in horses with botulism-like syndromes. Doses vary from 2 mg IM to 20 mg in 500 ml 5% dextrose in water, given IV over 30 minutes. Parasympathomimetic effects are often seen but the value of such therapy in equine botulism is not certain.[442] However, such agents are probably worth trying to determine if the particular myasthenic syndrome is neostigmine-responsive.

Prevention: Very few challenge studies have been performed in horses vaccinated with botulinum toxoids.[443] Limited field use and results in other species indicate that effective protection can be achieved by yearly vaccination with adjuvanted botulinum toxoids.[436] Type-C toxoid is commercially available in the US.[441]

Postanesthesic Myasthenia

At least 3 horses have been encountered with a botulism-like syndrome immediately following general anesthesia. Difficult recovery from anesthesia, lack of facial expression, flaccid tongue, dysphagia, mydriasis and inability to elevate the head were the characteristic signs. Other signs of botulism, such as flaccid tail, reduced patellar reflexes, megaesophagus and even periods of several days of recumbency, were variably present. Whether this syndrome is a form of botulism or myasthenia resulting from neuromuscular blockade due to certain drug anesthetic agent combinations has not been determined. Each of the 3 affected horses totally recovered from the myasthenia within a month with supportive care.

Aortic Thrombosis

Thrombosis of the terminal aorta and iliac arteries may be associated with a variety of clinical signs, ranging from poor racing performance to peracute onset paraplegia, shock and death.[444-447] The severity of signs depends upon the degree of arterial occlusion and the rapidity of thrombus development. Intermittent claudication (lameness due to vascular compromise seen only during exercise) is the most common manifestation of partial aorta-iliac thrombosis.[445] This syndrome is discussed in more detail in Chapter 14.

The cause of this condition has not been determined in all cases, although migration by *Strongylus vulgaris* larvae is thought to be involved. Most cases of complete obstruction of the bifurcation of the aorta in humans, cats and dogs are secondary to embolization of large mural or valvular cardiac thrombi.[448,449] There is no evidence of an association between aortic obstruction and cardiac disease in horses. Several other predisposing causes suggested include previous strangles or influenza infections and nutritional and mechanical factors.

Profound neurologic deficits may accompany the other signs of aortic thrombosis in horses in which there is rapid occlusion of the terminal aorta and/or its branches without development of adequate collateral circulation. These horses usually become recumbent after a brief period of apparent distress marked by tachypnea, generalized sweating, and treading or kicking with the pelvic limbs.[446] There is complete paralysis of the pelvic limbs due to interference with muscular circulation. Hip flexion may be preserved in some horses. The hindquarters become cold and affected muscles may be firm palpation. Digital pulses are absent. Rectal examination may reveal an absent or decreased pulse in the terminal aorta and iliac arteries. Cutaneous analgesia may extend over the rump, pelvic limbs and tail. This is evidence of ischemic nerve damage.[3,446] Signs of shock develop quickly. One affected horse had multiple electrolyte derangements, renal failure due to myoglobinuria, and a clotting defect as terminal complications.[3] The prognosis is hopeless in such cases and euthanasia is indicated once the diagnosis is established.

Miscellaneous Neurologic Disorders

Granulomatous Ependymitis and Equine Infectious Anemia

Neuropathologic changes may occur during the course of equine infectious anemia (EIA) infection. These lesions include granular ependymitis, choroiditis and meningitis, with polymorphous lymphoreticular proliferations in the subependymal area of the ventricles and around vessels in the brain and spinal cord.[450,451] Neurologic signs are sometimes associated with such lesions.[451,452] One mare with EIA had behavioral changes, circling and gait alterations.[451] At necropsy, hydrocephalus was found in addition to the above changes. The CSF analysis showed elevations in protein content and lymphocytic pleocytosis.

Listeriosis

Encephalitis due to *Listeria monocytogenes* infection rarely has been documentated in horses.[453,454] *Listeria monocytogenes* was isolated from the brainstem of a 16-year-old Welsh pony gelding with signs of ataxia, weakness and deficits of cranial nerves V, VII, VIII and XII.[455] No immunologic deficiency was detected and there was no history of contact with ruminants or access to silage. A recent report described fatal listeria septicemia in an Arabian foal with combined immunodeficiency.[456] Presumably the infection in this foal was disseminated hematogenously to the CNS, where it affected meningeal and ependymal membranes, and associated brain and spinal cord parenchyma. Other forms of immunologic incompetence, such as steroid-induced immunosuppression, may enhance susceptibility of horses to listerial infections.

Epidural Extrasynovial Cysts

Epidural cysts may form adjacent to abnormal joints, especially between C_6-C_7 and C_5-C_6.[457,458] Redundant articular cartilage extends across the cranial dorsal arch, where it is infringed upon by an exuberant portion of the medial aspect of the caudal articular process of the next cranial vertebra. The associated cysts project into the vertebral canal from dorsal or lateral aspect and may compress the spinal cord. Significant (clinical) compression is most likely to occur if there already is relative narrowing of the vertebral canal at that site, as in cervical vertebral malformation.

Epidural cysts may be overlooked at necropsy if cervical vertebrae are disarticulated during removal of the spinal cord. Sagittal sectioning of the cervical vertebral column is more apt to preserve such structures, particularly if the section is made on the side opposite the cyst, as defined by myelography.

Acute Hematomyelia

Severe hemorrhage into the spinal cord and meninges occurred in 2 horses after anesthesia and surgery of 1-2 hours' duration in dorsal recumbency.[459] The hemorrhages were associated with massive venous distension throughout the grey matter and dorsal columns of the white matter. Early neuronal degeneration was present in these areas. Only the caudal thoracic and lumbosacral portions of the spinal cord were affected, resulting in total rear-limb paralysis anesthesia. The authors speculated that increased venous pressure within the spinal cord, as a result of dorsal recumbency, and decreased arterial pressure, due to halothane anesthesia, caused venous congestion, hypoperfusion, hypoxia and hemorrhage. The large size of the affected horses was thought to be a contributing factor.

References

1. Cook, WR and Jeffcott, LB, Newmarket, England: Personal communication, 1979.
2. Mayhew, IG. Cornell Vet **65** (1975) 500.
3. de Lahunta, A: Veterinary Neuroanatomy and Clinical Neurology. WB Saunders, Philadelphia, 1977.
4. Mayhew, IG *et al.* Cornell Vet **68** (Suppl 6) (1978) 44.
5. Nyland, TG *et al.* Am J Vet Res **41** (1980) 204.
6. Beech, J. J Am Vet Rad Soc **20** (1979) 22.
7. Klemm, WR: Applied Electronics for Veterinary Medicine and Animal Physiology. Charles C Thomas, Springfield, IL, 1976.
8. Redding, in Hoerlein: Canine Neurology. 3rd ed. WB Saunders, Philadelphia, 1978.
9. Grabow, JD *et al.* Am J Vet Res **30** (1969) 1239.
10. Parker, AJ *et al.* Am J Vet Res **35** (1974) 673.
11. Holliday, TA *et al.* Am J Vet Res **40** (1979) 326.
12. Henry, RW *et al.* Am J Vet Res **40** (1979) 1406.
13. Adams, RD: Diseases of Muscle: a Study of Pathology. 3rd ed. Harper & Row, Hagerstown, MD, 1975.
15. Harrison, in Hoerlein: Canine Neurology. 3rd ed. WB Saunders, Philadelphia, 1978.
16. de Lahunta, A: Veterinary Neuroanotomy and Clinical Neurology. 1st ed. WB Saunders, Philadelphia, 1977.
17. Bruner, DW and Gillespie, JH: Hagan's Infectious Diseases of Domestic Animals. 6th ed. Cornell Univ Press, 1977.
18. Byrne, RJ. Proc 3rd Int Conf Eq Inf Dis, 1972. p 115.
19. Hanson, RP. Proc 3rd Int Conf Eq Inf Dis, 1972. p 100.
20. Robin, Y *et al.* Ann Microbiol (Inst Pasteur) **125A** (1974) 235.
21. Nakamura, H. Eq Vet J **4** (1972) 155.
22. Goto, H. Eq Vet J **8** (1976) 126.
23. Timoney, PJ *et al.* Eq Vet J **8** (1976) 113.
24. Spertzel, RO. Proc 3rd Int Conf Eq Inf Dis, 1972. p 146.
25. Johnson, KM and Martin, DH. Adv Virus Res **19** (1974) 76.
26. Haring, M *et al.* Cir 322, Berkeley Agric Ex Sta, 1931.
27. Wong, FC and Drysdale, RA. Can J Pub Health **67** (Suppl 1) (1976) 21.

28. Kissling, RE and Chamberlain, RW. Adv Vet Sci **11** (1967) 65.

29. Sudia, WD and Newhouse, VF. Am J Epidem **101** (1975) 1.

30. Gibbs, EPJ. Eq Vet J **8** (1976) 66.

31. Galindo, P: Venezuelan Equine Encephalitis. Publ No 243, Pan Am Health Org, Washington, DC. p 249.

32. Rossdale, PD. Eq Vet J **4** (1972) i.

33. Taylor, WM and Bluff, E. JAVMA **161** (1972) 159.

34. Vanderwagen, LC et al. Am J Vet Res **36** (1975) 1567.

35. Ferguson, JA et al. Am J Vet Res **38** (1977) 425.

36. Rossdale, PD and Leadon, D. J Repro Fert (Suppl 23) (1975) 685.

37. Platt, H. Eq Vet J **5** (1973) 116.

38. Knight, HD. J Eq Med Surg **3** (1979) 175.

39. Stuart, BP et al. JAVMA **162** (1973) 211.

40. Jungerman, PR and Schwartzman, RM: Veterinary Medical Mycology. 1st ed. Lea & Febiger, Philadelphia, 1972.

41. Barron, CN. JAVMA **124** (1955) 125.

42. Dickson, J and Meyer, EP. Aust Vet J **46** (1970) 558.

43. McGrath, T. Am J Path **30** (1954) 651.

44. Irwin, CFP. Aust Vet J **33** (1957) 97.

45. Barclay, WP and de Lahunta, A. JAVMA **174** (1979) 1236.

46. Utz, JP et al. J Inf Dis **132** (1975) 368.

47. Jones, TC and Maurer, FD. Am J Vet Res **5** (1943) 15.

48. Rumbaugh, GE. JAVMA **171** (1977) 452.

49. Little, PB. JAVMA **160** (1972) 1407.

50. Little, PB et al. Am J Vet Res **35** (1974) 1501.

51. Fraser, H. Vet Rec **78** (1966) 608.

52. Orlander, HJ. Path Vet **4** (1967) 477.

53. Hadlow, WJ et al. Cornell Vet **67** (1977) 272.

54. Scharff, DK. VM/SAC **68** (1973) 791.

55. Stone, WM et al. J Parasit **56** (1970) 986.

56. Alstad, AD and Berg, EI. JAVMA **174** (1979) 264.

57. Ferris, DH et al. Am J Vet Res **33** (1972) 33.

58. Rubin, HL and Woodard, JC. JAVMA **165** (1974) 256.

59. Innes, JRM and Pillai, CP. Br Vet J **3** (1955) 223.

60. Fravenfelder, HC et al. JAVMA. In press, 1981.

61. Murphy, in Baer: The Natural History of Rabies. Academic Press, New York, 1975.

62. Crick, J and Brown, F. Vet Rec **99** (1976) 162.

63. Taylor, D. Vet Rec **99** (1976) 157.

64. US Dept Health, Education and Welfare: Rabies surveillance report. Ann summary, 1977-1978.

65. Parker, in Baer: The Natural History of Rabies. Academic Press, New York, 1975.

66. Baer, in Baer: The Natural History of Rabies. Academic Press, New York, 1975.

67. Ornelas, OV and Aranalde, GA. Southwest Vet **1** (1964) 13.

68. Baer, in Baer: The Natural History of Rabies. Academic Press, New York, 1975.

69. Marler, RJ et al. JAVMA **175** (1979) 293.

70. Bedford, PGC. Vet Rec **99** (1976) 160.

71. Glaess, AM. Southwest Vet **27** (1974) 283.

72. Owen, R. Vet Rec **102** (1978) 69.

73. Ferris, DH et al. Cornell Vet **58** (1968) 270.

74. Schroeder, WG. JAVMA **155** (1969) 1842.

75. Smith, LL and Clare, DA. Can Vet J **13** (1972) 193.

76. Carlson, GP, Davis, CA: Unpublished data, 1979.

77. Kissling, in Baer: The Natural History of Rabies. Academic Press, New York, 1975.

78. Schneider, LG. Zent Vet **16** (1969) 24.

79. Atanasiu, in Baer: The Natural History of Rabies. Academic Press, New York, 1975.

80. Austin, RJ. Can Vet J **17** (1976) 81.

81. Wilson, BJ et al. JAVMA **163** (1975) 1293.

82. Graham, R. Vet Med **31** (1936) 46.

83. Schwarter, LH et al. JAVMA **90** (1937) 76.

84. Biester, HE et al. Vet Med **35** (1940) 636.

85. Wilson, BJ and Maronpot, RR. Vet Rec **88** (1971) 484.

86. Badiali, L et al. Am J Vet Res **29** (1958) 2029.

87. MacCallum, WG and Buckley, SS. J Exp Med **6** (1901) 65.

88. James, LF et al. JAVMA **155** (1969) 525.

89. Harries, WN et al. Can Vet J **13** (1972) 141.

90. Staley, EE. VM/SAC **73** (1978) 1205.

91. James, LF and van Kampen, KR. JAVMA **158** (1971) 614.

92. Hartley, in Keeler et al: Effects of Poisonous Plants on Livestock. Academic Press, New York 1978.

93. Dorling, PR et al. Neuropath Neurobiol **4** (1978) 285.

94. O'Sullivan, BM and Goodwin, JA. Aust. Vet J **53** (1977) 446.

95. von Seiferle, E. Schweiz Archiv Tierheil **90** (1948) 615.

96. Gabel, AA and Koestner, A. JAVMA **142** (1963) 1397.

97. Gabel, AA et al. J Eq Med Surg **1** (1977) 221.

98. Cotchin, E and Baker-Smith, J. Vet Rec **97** (1975) 399.

99. Frankhauser, R et al. Bull Wld Hlth Org **50** (1974) 53.

100. Stater, EJ. Tierärztl Rdsch **45** (1939) 854.

101. Luginbuhl, H et al. Progr Neurol Surg **2** (1968) 85.

102. Henschen, in Henke-Lubarsch: Handbuch der speziellen pathologischen Anatomie und Histologie, Vol 13. Springer-Verlag, Berlin, 1955.

103. Grunberger, K. Dtsch Tierärztl Wschr **80** (1973) 49.

104. Steiner, K. Inaugural dissertation, Hannover, 1941.

105. Christensen, NE. Medlenbl Dansk Dyrloegef **29** (1946) 128.

106. Willis, LA: Pathology of Tumors. 3rd ed. Butterworth, London, 1960.

107. Eagle, RC et al. Vet Path **15** (1978) 488.

108. Gelatt, KN et al. Can Vet J **12** (1971) 53.

109. Folger, AF: To tilfaelde af retinaglion hos hesten. Aarskr Kongelig Vet. Landbohojskole, Copenhagen, 1919.

110. Finn, JP and Tennant, BC. Vet Path **8** (1971) 458.

111. Gmelin, W. Arch Prakt Tierheilk **51** (1924) 24.

112. Potel, K. Berl Munch Tierärztl Wschr **72** (1959a) 166.

113. Cotchin, E and Baker-Smith, J. Vet Rec **97** (1975) 399.

114. Courreges, P et al. Rev Cs Vet Armee **8** (1953) 156.

115. Louf, R. Rev Cs Vet Armee **9** (1954) 138.

116. Feldman, WH: Neoplasms of Domestic Animals. WB Saunders, Philadelphia, 1932.

117. Innes, JRM and Saunders, LZ: Comparative Neuropathology. Academic Press, New York, 1962.

118. Schellner, L. Tierärztl Umsch **39** (1933) 505.

119. Potel, K. Mh Vet Med **14** (1959A) 43.

120. Bertrand, I et al. Rev Neurol **67** (1937) 417.

121. Palmer, AC and Hickman, J. Vet Rec **72** (1960) 611.

122. Frauchiger, E and Fankhauser, R: Vergleichende Neuropathologie der Menschen und der Tiere. Springer Verlag, Berlin, 1957.

123. Laszlo, F. Dsch Tierärztl Wschr **47** (1940) 402.

124. Nobel, TA. Cornell Vet **45** (1955) 570.

125. Fankhauser, R et al. Dtsch Tierärztl Wschr **84** (1977) 81.

126. Squire, RA. Cornell Vet **54** (1964) 97.

127. Hobmaier, M. Mh Prakt Tierheilk **24** (1913) 456.

128. Runnells, RA and Benbrook, EA. JAVMA **104** (1944) 148.

129. Pick, M and Pueschner, H. Berl Munch Tierärztl Wschr **83** (1970) 249.

130. Traver, DS et al. JAVMA **170** (1977) 1400.

131. McGrath, JT. Proc 8th Ann Conv Am Assoc Eq Pract, 1962. p 157.

132. Peters, A. Vet J **65** (1909) 453.

133. Goldbert, W. Arch Prakt Tierheilk **51** (1924) 24.

134. Bisbocci, G. Nuova Ercolani **38** (1933) 381.

135. Waugh, SL et al. J Eq Med Surg **1** (1977) 311.

136. Reynolds, BL et al. JAVMA **174** (1979) 734.

137. Magnusson, H. Z Infekt-Kr Haustiere **17** (1916) 329,355.

138. Menzani, C. Clin Vet **54** (1931) 661.

140. Drew, RA and Greatorex, JC. Eq Vet J **6** (1974) 131.

141. Kelly, DF and Watson, WJB. Eq Vet J **81** (1976) 110.

142. Critchley, M and Ferguson, FR. Brain **51** (1978) 334.

143. Holz, K. Berl Munch Tierärztl Wschr **49** (1936) 114.

144. Uberreiter, O. Schweiz Arch Tierhilk **99** (1957) 51.

145. Tsiroyiannis, E et al. Ann Med Vet **102** (1958) 121.

146. Jubb, KVF and Kennedy, PC: Pathology of Domestic Animals. Academic Press, New York, 1970.

147. Moulton, JE: Tumors in Domestic Animals. Univ California Press, Berkeley, 1961.

148. Critchley, M and Ferguson, FR. Brain **51** (1978) 334.

149. Carlson, GP, Univ Calif: Personal communication, 1978.

150. Kelly, DF and Watson, WJB. Eq Vet J **8** (1976) 110.

151. Gilmour, JS and Fraser, JA. Eq Vet J **9** (1977) 40.

152. Baird, JD. Aust Vet J **49** (1973) 530.

153. Rossdale, PD and Leadon, D. J Repro Fert, Suppl 23 (1975) 685.

154. Palmer, AC and Rossdale, PD. J Repro Fert, Suppl 23 (1975) 691.

155. Palmer, AC and Rossdale, PD. Res Vet Sci **20** (1976) 267.

156. Rumbaugh, GE and Cundy, DR. J Eq Med Surg **1** (1977) 344.

157. May, CJ and Greenwood, RES. Vet Rec **101** (1977) 76.

158. Rossdale, PD et al. Vet Rec **99** (1976) 111.

159. Mahaffey, LW and Rossdale, PD. Lancet **1** (1959) 1223.

160. Rossdale, PD. Vet Clin No Am **1** (1979) 205.

161. Mayhew, IG and Ingram, JT. Proc 24th Ann Mtg Am Assoc Eq Pract, 1978, p 525.

162. de Lahunta, A: Veterinary Neuroanatomy and Clinical Neurology. 1st ed. WB Saunders, Philadelphia, 1977.

163. Hoerlein, BF: Canine Neurology. 3rd ed. WB Saunders, Philadelphia, 1978.

164. Einhorn, A and Mizrahi, EM. Am J Dis Child **132** (1978) 1121.

165. McGrath, JT. Proc 8th Ann Mtg Am Assoc Eq Pract, 1962. p 157.

166. Sheathers, AL. J Comp Path Ther **37** (1924) 106.

167. Getty, R. Sisson and Grossman's Anatomy of the Domestic Animals. 5th ed. WB Saunders, Philadelphia, 1975.

168. Firth, EC. Aust Vet J **53** (1977) 560.

169. Joyce, JR and Bratton, GR. VM/SAC **68** (1973) 619.

170. Williams, R et al. Proc Am Coll Vet Ophth **8** (1977) 101.

171. Mortimer, in Keeler et al: Effects of Poisonous Plants on Livestock. Academic Press, New York, 1978.

172. Cummings, JF et al. Acta Neuropath **46** (1979) 17.

173. Dorland: Illustrated Medical Dictionary. 25th ed. WB Saunders, Philadelphia, 1974.

174. Knight, AP. JAVMA **170** (1977) 735.

175. van Hertsch, V. Dtsch Tier Wschr **82** (1975) 473.

176. de Lahunta, A: Veterinary Neuroanatomy and Clinical Neurology. 1st ed. WB Saunders, Philadelphia, 1977.

177. Cook, WR et al. Vet Rec **83** (1968) 422.

178. Cook, WR. Vet Rec **78** (1966) 396.

179. Björklund, NE and Palsson, G. Nord Vet Med **22** (1970) 65.

180. Boucher, WB et al. JAVMA **145** (1964) 1004.

181. Cook, WR. Vet Rec **83** (1968) 336.

182. Owen, R. Eq Vet J **6** (1974) 143.

183. Hatziolos, BC et al. JAVMA **167** (1975) 51.

184. Wagner, PC et al. J Eq Med Surg **2** (1978) 355.

185. Cordy, DR. J Neuropath Exp Neur **13** (1954) 330.

186. Cordy, in Keeler et al: Effects of Poisonous Plants on Livestock. Academic Press, New York, 1978.

187. Gard, GP and de Sarem, WG. Aust Vet J **49** (1973) 107.

188. Young, S et al. JAVMA **157** (1970) 1602.

189. de Lahunta, A. Veterinary Neuroanatomy and Clinical Neurology. 1st ed. WB Saunders, Philadelphia, 1977.

190. Aronson, AL. Am J Vet Res **33** (1972) 627.

191. Holm, LW et al. JAVMA **123** (1953) 383.

192. Egan, DA and O'Cuill, T. Vet Rec **86** (1970) 736.

193. Knight, HD and Burau, RG. JAVMA **162** (1973) 781.

194. Willoughby, RA et al. Can J Comp Med **36** (1972) 348.

195. Goyer, RA and Rhyne, BC. Int Rev Exp Path **12** (1973) 1.

196. Willoughby, RA et al. Am J Vet Res **33** (1972) 1165.

197. Willoughby, RA and Brown, G. Can Vet J **12** (1971) 165.

198. de Lahunta, A. Proc Ann Mtg Am Coll Vet Int Med, 1979. p 10.

199. Sponsellar, ML. Proc 13th Ann Mtg Am Assoc Eq Pract, 1967. p 123.

200. Beech, J. Proc 22nd Ann Mtg Am Assoc Eq Pract, 1976. p 77.

201. Baird, JD and MacKenzie, CD. Aust Vet J **50** (1974) 25.

202. Dungworth, DL and Fowler, ME. Cornell Vet **56** (1966) 17.

203. Palmer, AC et al. Vet Rec **93** (1973) 62.

204. Bjorck, G et al. Zbl Vet Med A **20** (1973) 341.

205. Oliver, RE. N Zeal Vet J **23** (1975) 15.

206. Koch, P and Fischer, H. Tierärztle Umschau **7** (1952) 244.

207. Blood, DC et al: Veterinary Medicine. 5th ed. Lea & Febiger, Philadelphia, 1979.

208. Tillman, DB. Western J Med **129** (1978) 107.

209. Booth, NH and Pierson, RE. JAVMA **128** (1956) 257.

210. Gibbons, WJ. Cornell Vet **30** (1940) 533.

211. Donaldson, RS. Vet Rec (1977) 353.

212. Furste, W. J Trauma **16** (1976) 755.

213. Christensen, NA. Proc 2nd Int Conf Tetanus, 1966. p 455.

214. Mellanby, J and van Heyningen, WE. Proc 2nd Int Conf Tetanus, 1966. p 178.

215. Kryzhanovsky, GN. Proc 3rd Int Conf Tetanus, 1970. p 72.

216. Rie, MA and Wilson, RS. Ann Int Med **88** (1978) 653.

217. Owen, LN et al. Vet Rec **71** (1959) 61.

218. Sedaghatian, MR. Arch Dis Child **54** (1979) 623.

219. Sanders, RKM et al. Lancet (1977) 974.

220. Muylle, E et al. JAVMA **167** (1975) 47.

221. Lundavall, RL. JAVMA **132** (1958) 254.

222. Smithcors, JF. JAVMA **132** (1958) 303.

223. Heath, RB and Gabel, AA. JAVMA **157** (1970) 1486.

224. Odusote, KA et al. Trop Gorgr Med **28** (1976) 194.

225. Wintzer, HJ et al. Berl Munch Tier Wschr **88** (1975) 181.

226. Tennant, B. Proc 24th Ann Mtg Am Assoc Eq Pract, 1978. p 465.

227. Liu, IK. Vet Clin No Am. In press, 1981.

228. McGuire, TC et al. JAVMA **170** (1977) 1302.

229. Cunningham, IJ and Hartley, WJ. N Zeal Vet J **7** (1959) 1.

230. Shaw, JN and Muth, OH. JAVMA **114** (1949) 315.

231. Shreeve, BJ et al. Vet Rec **103** (1978) 209.

232. Smith, JS and Mayhew, IG. Cornell Vet **67** (1977) 529.

233. de Lahunta, A: Veterinary Neuroanatomy and Clinical Neurology. 1st ed. WB Saunders, Philadelphia, 1977.

234. Getty, R: Sisson and Grossman's The Anatomy of the Domestic Animals. 5th ed. WB Saunders, Philadelphia, 1975.

235. Mayhew, IG and de Lahunta, A, Cornell Univ: Unpublished data, 1977.

236. Firth, EC. Eq Vet J **10** (1978) 9.

237. Mayhew, IG et al. Eq Vet J **10** (1978) 103.

238. Watson, AG et al. Abst Anat Hist Embry **7** (1978) 354.

239. Whitwell, KE. Eq Vet J **10** (1978) 125.

240. Edland, H. Skandinavish Vet **36** (1946) 439.

241. Errington, BJ. Vet Bull **32** (1938) 152.

242. Beech, J. Proc 22nd Ann Mtg Am Assoc Eq Pract, 1976. p 79.

243. Binkhorst, GJ. Inaugural dissertation, Utrecht, 1976.

244. Dimock, WW and Errington, BJ. JAVMA **95** (1939) 261.

245. Rooney, JR. Cornell Vet **53** (1963) 411.

246. Rooney, JR: Clinical Neurology of the Horse. KNA Press, Kennett Square, PA, 1971.

247. Schebitz, H and Dahme, E. Proc 13th Ann Mtg Am Assoc Eq Pract, 1967. p 133.

248. Mechlenburg, G. Doctoral dissertation, Hannover, 1967.

249. Mayhew, IG et al. Cornell Vet **68**, Suppl 6 (1978) 1.

250. Wright, F et al. Vet Rec **92** (1973) 1.

251. Palmer, AC: Introduction to Animal Neurology. 2nd ed. Blackwell Scientific Publ, Oxford, 1976.

252. Dahme, E and Schebitz, H. Zbl Vet Med **17** (1970) 120.

253. Hebeler, W. Inaugural dissertation, München, 1977.

254. Jeffreys, RV. Acta Neurochirurg **47** (1979) 293.

255. Nurick, S. Br J Hosp Med (1975) 668.

256. Epstein, JA et al. J Neurosurg **51** (1979) 362.

257. Epstein, BS et al. Clin Neurosurg **25** (1978) 148.

258. Rendano, VT and Quick, CB. Mod Vet Pract **59** (1978) 921.

259. Rantanen, NW et al. Comp Cont Ed **3** (1981) S161.

260. Nyland, TG et al. Am J Vet Res **41** (1980) 204.

261. Beech, J. J Am Vet Rad Soc **20** (1979) 22.

262. Schulz, C et al. Dtsch Tier Wsch **72** (1965) 502.

263. Rovira, M et al. Neurorad **9** (1975) 209.

264. Gooding, MR. Lancet (1974) 1180.

265. Ashby, JG and Ayre, WB. Lancet (1975) 980.

266. Olsson, SE and Reiland, S. Acta Rad Scand, Suppl (1978) 299.

267. Stromberg, B. Eq Vet J **11** (1979) 211.

268. Lewis, LD. Proc 25th Ann Mtg Am Assoc Eq Pract, 1979. p 267.

269. Hertsch, B and Ragab, S. Berl Münch Tier Wsch **90** (1977) 172.

270. Wagner, PC et al. Vet Surg **8** (1979) 7.

271. Wagner, PC et al. Vet Surg **8** (1979) 84.

272. Wagner, PC et al. Comp Cont Ed **3** (1981) S192.

273. Stashak, TS. Paper presented at 116th Ann Mtg AVMA, Seattle, 1979.

274. Trotter, EJ et al. JAVMA **168** (1976) 917.

275. Hurov, LI. JAVMA **175** (1979) 278.

276. Mason, TA. Aust Vet J **53** (1977) 440.

277. Denny, HR et al. J Sm Anim Pract **18** (1977) 117.

278. Montali, RJ *et al*. Vet Path **11** (1974) 68.

279. Mayhew, IG *et al*. Proc 22nd Ann Mtg Am Assoc Eq Pract, 1976. p 103.

280. Mayhew, IG *et al*. JAVMA **170** (1977) 195.

281. Pentschew, A and Schwarz, K. Acta Neuropath **1** (1962) 313.

282. Hooper, in Keeler *et al*: Effects of Poisonous Plants on Livestock. Academic Press, New York, 1978.

283. Hartley, in Keeler: Effects of Poisonous Plants on Livestock. Academic Press, New York, 1978.

284. Dorling, PR *et al*. Neuropath Appl Neurobiol **4** (1978) 385.

285. Cavanaugh, JB. Br Med Bull **25** (1969) 208.

286. Seitelberger, F. Acta Neuropath **5** (1971) 17.

287. Puschner, H. Zbl Vet Med **18** (1971) 365.

288. Liu, HM. Acta Neuropath **42** (1978) 237.

289. Cordy, DR *et al*. Acta Neuropath **8** (1967) 133.

290. Woodward, JC *et al*. Am J Path **74** (1974) 551.

291. Martin, JJ *et al*. Acta Neuropath **45** (1979) 267.

292. Dorfman, LJ *et al*. Ann Neur **3** (1978) 419.

293. Leathers, CW *et al*. J Vet Orthoped **1** (1979) 55.

294. Mayhew, IG *et al*. Eq Vet J **10** (1978) 103.

295. Cho, Dy and Leipold, HW. Eq Vet J **9** (1977) 195.

296. Boyd, JS. Eq Vet J **8** (1976) 161.

297. Finnochio, EJ. VM/SAC **68** (1973) 125.

298. Rooney, JR. Cornell Vet **56** (1966) 172.

299. Rooney, JR. Clin Orthoped **62**(1969) 25.

300. Lerner, DJ and Riley, F. JAVMA **172** (1978) 274.

301. Leipold, HW *et al*. VM/SAC **68** (1973) 1140.

302. Drachman, DB *et al*. Arch Neur **33** (1976) 362.

303. Crowe, in Keeler *et al*. Effects of Poisonous Plants on Livestock. Academic Press, New York, 1978.

304. Hartley, WJ *et al*. Aust Vet J **53** (1977) 319.

305. Edwards, MJ. Adv Vet Sci **22** (1978) 29.

306. Mayhew, IG, Univ Florida: Unpublished data, 1980.

307. Stecher, RM and Goss, LJ. JAVMA **138** (1961) 248.

308. Stecher, RM. Am J Vet Res **23** (1962) 939.

309. Stecher, RM. J Mamm **43** (1962) 205.

310. McKelvey, WAC and Owen, R. JAVMA **175** (1979) 295.

311. Prickett, ME. Proc 14th Ann Mtg Am Assoc Eq Pract, 1968. p 147.

312. Rooney, JR *et al*. Cornell Vet **60** (1970) 496.

313. Cusick, PK *et al*. JAVMA **164** (1974) 77.

314. Eugster, AK and Joyce, JR. VM/SAC **71** (1976) 1469.

315. MacDonald DR and Cleary, DJ. Southwest Vet **23** (1970) 213.

316. Beech, J and Dodd, DC. Vet Path **11** (1974) 87.

317. Dubey, JP *et al*. JAVMA **165** (1974) 249.

318. Beech, J. VM/SAC **69** (1974) 1562.

319. Mayhew, IG *et al*. Proc 22nd Ann Mtg Am Assoc Eq Pract, 1976. p 107.

320. Traver, DS *et al*. JAVMA **170** (1977) 1400.

321. Traver, DS *et al*. J Eq Med Surg **2** (1978) 425.

322. Macruz, R *et al*. Rev Fac Med Vet Zootec Univ S Paolo **12** (1975) 277.

323. Simpson, CF and Mayhew, IG. J Protozool **27** (1980) 288.

324. Mayhew, IG and Fayer, R, Univ Florida: Unpublished data, 1979.

325. Mayhew, IG and de Lahunta, A, Univ Florida and Cornell Univ: Unpublished data, 1979.

326. Fayer, R. and Leek, RG. J Parasit **65** (1981) 890.

327. Manninger, R. Acta Vet Acad Sci Hun **1** (1949) 62.

328. Saxegaard, F. Nord Vet Med **18** (1966) 504.

329. Fankhauser, R. Schweiz Arch Tierheilk **110** (1968) 171.

330. Jackson, T and Kendrick, JW. JAVMA **158** (1971) 1351.

331. Bitsch, V and Dam, A. Acta Vet Scand **12** (1971) 134.

332. Moyer, WM and Rooney, JR. Proc 18th Ann Mtg Am Assoc Eq Pract, 1972. p 307.

333. Sprinkle, E. Norden News **50** (1975) 15.

334. Thorsen, J and Little PB. Can J Comp Med **29** (1975) 358.

335. Little, PB and Thorsen, J. Vet Path **13** (1976) 161.

336. Charlton, KM *et al*. Vet Path **13** (1976) 59.

337. Dinter, Z and Klineborn, B. Vet Rec **99** (1976) 10.

338. Jackson, TA *et al*. Am J Vet Res **28** (1977) 709.

339. Liu, IKM and Castleman W. J Eq Med Surg **12** (1977) 397.

340. Pursell, AT *et al*. JAVMA **175** (1979) 473.

341. Greenwood, RES and Simson, ARB. Eq Vet J **12** (1980) 113.

342. Platt, H *et al*. Eq Vet J **12** (1980) 118.

343. Crawford, TB. Proc 24th Ann Mtg Am Assoc Eq Pract, 1978. p 49.

344. Symoeus, J and Rosenthal, M. J Reticuloend Soc **21** (1977) 175.

345. Moore, RD and Koonse, HJ. Proc 24th Ann Mtg Am Assoc Eq Pract, 1978. p 75.

346. Platt, H. Eq Vet J **9** (1977) 141.

347. McGuire, TC *et al*. JAVMA **170** (1977) 1302.

348. Dodd, DC and Cordes, DO. N Zeal Vet J **12** (1964) 1.

349. Doige, CE. Can J Comp Med **44** (1980) 121.

350. Finley, GG. Can Vet J **16** (1975) 114.

351. Morgan, JP *et al*. J Am Vet Rad Soc **15** (1975) 66.

352. Kornegay, JN and Barber, DO. JAVMA **177** (1980) 337.

353. Frederickson, B *et al*. Clin Orthoped Rel Res **131** (1978) 160.

354. Platt, H. Br Vet J **129** (1973) 221.

355. Rossdale, PD and Leadon, D. J Repro Fert, Suppl 23 (1975) 685.

356. Rooney, JR. Mod Vet Pract **47** (1966) 43.

357. Chladek, DW and Ruth, GR. JAVMA **168** (1976) 64.

358. Evans, LH *et al*. JAVMA **153** (1968) 1085.

359. Kelley, WR *et al*. J Am Vet Rad Soc **13** (1972) 59.

360. Denny, HR. Eq Vet J **5** (1973) 121.

361. Palmer, AC and Hickman, J. Vet Rec **75** (1963) 213.

362. Little, PB. JAVMA **160** (1972) 1407.

363. Swanstrom, OG *et al*. JAVMA **155** (1969) 748.

364. von Pohlenz, J *et al*. Dtsch Tier Wochen **72** (1965) 510.

365. Innes, JRM and Pillai, CP. Br Vet J 3 (1955) 223.

366. Shoho, C. Vet Med 49 (1954) 459.

367. Frauenfelder, HC et al. JAVMA 177 (1980) 359.

368. Olander, HJ. Path Vet 4 (1967) 477.

369. Mayhew, IG et al. JAVMA. In press, 1981.

370. Cummings, JF et al. Acta Neuropath 46 (1979) 17.

371. Greenwood, AG et al. Eq Vet J 5 (1973) 111.

372. Bilinski, J et al. VM/SAC 72 (1977) 597.

373. Manning, JP and Gosser, HS. VM/SAC 68 (1973) 1162.

374. Baker, GJ. Eq Vet J 2 (1970) 37.

375. Funk, KA and Erickson ED. Can Vet J 9 (1968) 120.

376. Guffy, MM et al. JAVMA 155 (1969) 754.

377. Von Henkels P and Hug, HO. Berl Münch Tier Wschr 74 (1961) 141.

378. Jeffcott, LB and Whitwell, KE. Proc 22nd Mtg Am Assoc Eq Pract, 1976. p 91.

379. Lundvall, RL. Norden News (Summer, 1969) 6.

380. Mason, BJE. Eq Vet J 3 (1971) 155.

381. Moyer, WA and Rooney, JR. JAVMA 159 (1971) 1022.

382. Owen, R and Smith-Maxie, LL. JAVMA 173 (1978) 854.

383. Stone, DE et al. JAVAM 174 (1979) 1234.

384. Vaughan, JT and Mason, BJE: A Clinico-Pathological Study of Racing Accidents in Horses. Royal Veterinary College, Hatfield, Herts, England, 1976.

385. Wagner PC et al. Eg Vet J 1 (1977) 282.

386. Fessler, JF and Amstutz, HE. Textbook of Large Animal Surgery. Williams & Wilkins, Baltimore, 1974.

387. Hickman, J. Veterinary Orthopaedics. Oliver and Boyd, Edinburgh, 1964.

388. Lundvall, in Catcott: Equine Medicine and Surgery. 2nd ed. American Veterinary Publications, Santa Barbara, 1972.

389. Morgan, JP: Radiology in Veterinary Orthopedics. Lea & Febiger, Philadelphia, 1972.

390. Mayhew, IG et al. Cornell Vet 68 Suppl 6 (1978) 106.

391. Eidelberg, C. Rad Clin No Am 15 (1977) 211.

392. Griffiths, IR et al. Acta Neuropath 41 (1978) 33.

393. Nelson, E et al. Arch Neur 34 (1977) 332.

394. Kobrine, AI et al. J Neurosurg 51 (1979) 841.

395. Parker, AJ and Smith, CW. Res Vet Sci 16 (1974) 276.

396. Parker, AJ and Smith, CW. Res Vet Sci 21 (1976) 246.

397. Kajihara, K et al. Surg Neur 1 (1973) 16.

398. Mendenhall, HV et al. JAVMA 168 (1976) 1026.

399. Osterholm, JL. J Neurosurg 40 (1974) 5.

400. Parker, AJ and Smith, CW. Res Vet Sci 27 (1979) 253.

401. Rawe, SE et al. J Neurosurg 46 (1977) 350.

402. Rawe, SE et al. J Neurosurg 48 (1978) 1002.

403. Rivlin, AS and Tator, CH. J Neurosurg 49 (1978) 844.

404. Senter, HJ et al. J Neurosurg 50 (1979) 207.

405. St Němeček, P et al. Acta Neurochirurg 39 (1977) 53.

406. de la Torre, JC et al. Neur 25 (1975) 508.

407. Miller, SM et al. Bull NY Acad Med 56 (1980) 305.

408. de Lahunta, A: Veterinary Neuroanatomy and Clincial Neurology. WB Saunders, Philadelphia, 1977.

409. Holliday, in Catcott: Equine Medicine and Surgery. 2nd ed. American Veterinary Publications, Santa Barbara, 1972.

410. Holliday, TA, Univ Calif: Unpublished data, 1793.

411. Stashak, TS. Paper presented at 116th Ann Mtg AVMA, 1979.

412. Tunturi, T et al. Arch Orthoped Trauma Surg 94 (1979) 1.

413. Wagner, PC et al. Vet Surg 8 (1979) 7, 84.

414. Rose, RJ. Aust Vet J 54 (1978) 154.

415. Pienaar, JG. J So Afr Vet Assoc 48 (1977) 13.

416. Taylor, HW et al. Vet Path 14 (1977) 479.

417. Henry, RW. Master's thesis, Ohio State Univ, 1976.

418. Hickman, J. Veterinary Orthopaedics. Oliver and Boyd, Edinburgh, 1964.

419. Swaim, SF. JAVMA 161 (1972) 905.

420. Swaim, in Hoerlein: Canine Neurology. 3rd ed. WB Saunders, Philadelphia, 1978.

421. Adams, RD: Lameness In Horses. 3rd ed. Lea & Febiger, Philadelphia, 1974.

422. Rooney, JR. Cornell Vet 53 (1963) 328.

423. Trim, CM and Mason, J. Eq Vet J 5 (1973) 71.

424. White, in Robinson: Current Veterinary Therapy—Equine. WB Saunders, Philadelphia, 1982.

425. Blythe, LL and Kitchell, RL. Abstr Am Assoc Vet Anat 18 (1978) 10.

426. Smith, LD: Botulism. Charles C Thomas, Springfield, 1977.

427. Merson, MH et al. J Am Med Assoc 229 (1974) 1305.

428. Arnon, SS et al. J Am Med Assoc 237 (1977) 1946.

429. Swerczek, TW. JAVMA 176 (1980) 217.

430. Merson, MH and Dowell, VR. N Engl J Med 289 (1975) 1005.

431. Mitchell, CA et al. Can J Comp Med 3 (1931) 245.

432. Tamarin, R and Neeman, L. Refuah Vet 19 (1962) 48.

433. Jacquet, J. Bull Off Int Epiz 42 (1954) 473.

434. Muller, J. Bull Off Int Epiz 59 (1963) 1379.

435. Legroux, R et al. Ann Instit Pasteur 72 (1946) 545.

436. Botija, CS. Bull Off Int Epiz 42 (1954) 759.

437. Lapcevic, E. Bull Off Int Epiz 42 (1954) 507.

438. Egyed, MN. VM/SAC 68 (1973) 854.

439. Swerczek, TW. Am J Vet Res 41 (1980) 348.

440. MacKay, RJ and Berkhoff, GA. JAVMA. In press, 1981.

441. Jasmin, AM. VM/SAC 70 (1975) 797.

442. Steyn, DG. J So Afr Vet Assoc 21 (1950) 81.

443. White, PG and Appleton, GS. JAVMA 137 (1960) 652.

444. Tillotson, PJ and Kopper, PH. JAVMA 149 (1966) 766.

445. Azzie, MAJ. Eq Vet J 1 (1969) 113.

446. Mayhew, IG and Kryger, MD. VM/SAC **70** (1975) 1281.

447. Physic-Sheard, PW. Proc 24th Ann Mtg Am Assoc Eq Pract, 1978. p 127.

448. Ettinger, SJ: Veterinary Internal Medicine. WB Saunders, Philadelphia, 1975.

449. Beeson, PB and McDermott, W: Textbook of Medicine. 14th ed. WB Saunders, Philadelphia, 1975.

450. Luginbuhl, MW *et al.* Prog Neur Surg **2** (1968) 85.

451. McIlwraith, CW and Kitchen, DN. Cornell Vet **68** (1978) 238.

452. Tajima, M and Yamgina, S. J Jap Vet Sci **15** (1953) 37.

453. Belin, M. Bull Acad Fr **19** (1946) 176.

454. Grini, O. Norsk Vet Tidsskr **55** (1943) 97.

455. Robbins, J, Univ Florida: Unpublished data, 1981.

456. Clark, EG *et al.* JAVMA **172** (1978) 363.

457. Whitwell, KE. In Practice **2** (4) (1980) 17.

458. Gerber, H *et al.* Schweiz Arch Tierheilk **122** (1980) 95.

459. Schatzmann, U *et al.* Schweiz Arch Tier **121** (1979) 149.

22

The Eye

by K.N. Gelatt

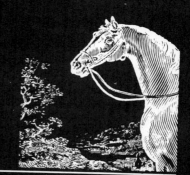

Significant advances in equine ophthalmology during the last decade have markedly improved diagnosis and treatment of ophthalmic conditions. However, certain ophthalmic diseases of the horse, such as equine recurrent uveitis, remain an enigma and will require considerable research efforts heavily concentrated in immunology. The successful treatment of ophthalmic disorders in horses requires a working knowledge of equine anatomy, physiology and ocular disease.

Equine eyes also have certain idiosyncrasies, in contrast to those of other species, and knowledge of these characteristics may be critical for resolution of certain equine ocular disorders. Most diagnostic procedures used in human and small animal ophthalmology are readily adapted for the horse. Future investigations must depend heavily on further refinement, as well as new diagnostic procedures, to investigate and document equine ophthalmic conditions.[1-20]

This chapter summarizes diseases of the equine eye and adnexa. Common diseases of the eye and periocular structures are presented with emphasis on clinical signs, specific treatments and prognosis.

OPHTHALMIC EXAMINATION

An adequate medical and visual history should be obtained from the owner or person responsible for the horse. Questions should be initially general and, as the problem becomes identified, should concentrate on areas pertinent to the visual system. Certain key questions are especially useful when obtaining a history during equine ophthalmic examination. The horse's performance and behavior as related to day and night vision should be ascertained. For instance, in the last several years,

a specific night blindness has been documented in the Appaloosa. Shying may indicate a significant visual problem of one or both eyes. The presence of blepharospasm, photophobia and ocular discharges should be evaluated.

Previous treatments administered for ophthalmic conditions and the response to therapy should be ascertained. Certain ophthalmic preparations, such as mydriatics, corticosteroids and decongestants, may mask significant ocular problems. For instance, intermittent conjunctivitis that reponds only transiently to topical antibiotic-corticosteroid preparations suggests nasolacrimal obstruction. Repeated attacks of blepharospasm, corneal edema, miosis and photophobia suggest recurrent uveitis.

An adequately sized room with reduced illumination is an important environment for examination of the horse. The animal is handled firmly but gently to facilitate examination. Animal and human traffic in the area should be restricted during ophthalmic examination to permit optimal observation of the patient. Most horses can be adequately examined without tranquilization, sedation or use of a twitch. I prefer to examine the horse as it stands in stocks, thereby permitting confinement of the animal, freedom of movement about the animal's forequarters and safety for the examiner. Tranquilization and/or sedation is used as a last resort when examining an aggressive and highly excited animal. However, the use of drugs may negate or impair certain diagnostic procedures in the evaluation of the patient's eye. For instance, administration of sedatives and tranquilizers reduces intraocular pressure 20-30% in the horse. Examination of the eye in bright sunlight is not recommended because the intense illumination may mask small opacities of the cornea and/or lens, and create interfering corneal reflections that impede thorough examination of deeper ocular structures.

Eyelid Akinesia

The orbicularis oculi muscle of the horse is a very powerful sphincter muscle that can close the palpebral fissure despite the examiner's attempts to retract the eyelids. Therefore, akinesia and in some circumstances local anesthesia of the eyelids are desirable to adequately examine the equine eye and occasionally facilitate certain types of therapy. Two basic groups of nerve blocks can be used in horses to facilitate ophthalmic examination. The auriculopalpebral nerve is blocked by infiltration of local anesthetic in the caudal aspects of the zygomatic arch. Frontal, lacrimal, zygomatic and infratrochlear nerve blocks provide adequate immobilization of the eyelid muscles and anesthesia of the eyelids.

Akinesia of the eyelids is satisfactorily produced by infiltration with local anesthetics of the auriculopalpebral nerve in the caudal aspects of the zygomatic arch.[21] Local anesthetic infiltrated in this area blocks most or all palpebral nerve fibers before they branch about the eye. The horse's head is held firmly and occasionally the upper or lower lip twitched. The skin dorsal to the caudal zygomatic arch is scrubbed and rinsed with alcohol. The bony groove in the ventral aspect of the temporal portion of the zygomatic arch can be usually palpated. A 20- to 22-ga hypodermic needle is inserted and directed dorsad. Before injection of 5-8 ml local anesthetic SC and subfascially, the needle position is checked by aspiration to prevent injection in the rostral auricular vein and artery. Successful nerve block is demonstrated by ptosis and slight eversion of the lower eyelid. Eyelid and ocular sensitivity are not affected (Fig 1).

Auriculopalpebral nerve block may occasionally result in local anesthetic gravitating ventrad to produce a temporary complete or nearly complete facial nerve block. Occasionally only partial akinesia of the upper eyelid results after a seemingly well-placed auriculopalpebral nerve block. Under these circumstances, the block is repeated more dorsal and rostral on the zygomatic arch.

The frontal, lacrimal, zygomatic and infratrochlear nerves may be blocked to provide akinesia and local anesthesia of the eyelids.[22] The frontal nerve and medial portion of the palpebral branch of the auriculopalpebral nerve are blocked by local infiltration of anesthetic in the supraorbital foramen and subcutaneous tissues immediately above this area. A 1-inch, 22-ga hypodermic needle is inserted directly into the foramen to a depth of 1-1.5 cm. Lidocaine HCl (5 ml) is injected partially into the foramen and the needle is withdrawn into the subcutaneous tissues, where additional anesthetic is injected.

To anesthetize the zygomatic nerve, the index finger is positioned on the ventral rim of the orbit against the supraorbital portion of the zygomatic arch. The hypodermic needle is placed medial to the finger and directed along the rim of the orbit, and 2 ml local anesthetic are injected.

The infratrochlear nerve is blocked by directing the hypodermic needle along the dorsal rim of the orbit just medial to the lateral canthus. Local anesthetic (2-3 ml) is injected just ventral to the rim of the orbit. The infratrochlear nerve is blocked by inserting the needle in a notch or irregularity of the dorsal rim of the orbit near the medial canthus. Local anesthetic (2-4 ml) is deposited in this area by deep injection slightly dorsal to the notch.

Of the above specific nerve blocks, the supraorbital and zygomatic types are recommended for ophthalmic examination and medication, and minor surgery of the eyelids. These nerve blocks have the disadvantage of necessitating manipulations near the eye. With the auriculopalpebral nerve block, the anesthetic is injected some distance from the eye.

Ophthalmic Examination

Ophthalmic examination in the horse involves evaluation of light-pupillary reflexes, the periocular and anterior segment of the eye, and the deep vitreous and ocular fundus. Light-pupillary responses are elicited in a semidarkened room with pupils in physiologic mydriasis. The light stimulus should have reasonable intensity and should be focusable. The light stimulus is directed into the temporal (lateral) and nasal (medial) retinal fields. Because the nasal retinal fibers decussate at the optic chiasma and the temporal fibers do not, additional information on the retina, optic nerves, optic chiasma, optic tracts and midbrain may be obtained. Light-pupillary reflexes are a rather crude test and do not imply the absence or presence of vision. Light-pupillary reflexes are subcortical and depend on the partial to complete integrity of the retina, optic nerve, optic chiasm, optic tract, pretectal and Edinger-Westphal nuclei, oculomotor and parasympathetic nerves, and the iridal sphincter musculature. Any disturbance in these respective afferent-efferent structures interferes with direct and consensual pupillary reflexes.

At this time, the examiner must decide which diagnostic procedures and drugs are required for the ophthalmic examination. These decisions may be critical since they involve irreversible steps. For instance, if the measurement of intraocular pressure is important, the use of tranquilizers and/or sedatives should be avoided because subsequent reduction in blood pressure may also reduce intraocular pressure 20-30%. Instillation of mydriatics may negate pupillary responses for several hours to even a few days. Instillation of a topical anesthetic may facilitate corneoconjunctival cytologic examination but precludes bacterial culture. Therefore, once the feasibility of these tests has been ascertained, the remainder of the ophthalmic examination is performed.

After evaluation of light-pupillary reflexes, 1% tropicamide (Mydriacyl:Alcon Laboratories) is instilled in both eyes for mydriasis and examination of deeper ocular structures. The mydriasis produced by tropicamide occurs in normal horses within 15-20 minutes and lasts approximately 8-12 hours. The use of atropine is not recommended because of its longer onset of action and prolonged duration of mydriasis, which may be 3-5 days in normal horses. Drug-induced mydriasis is essential to adequately evaluate the lens, vitreous and ocular fundus. Many focal paraxial cataracts may be easily missed if mydriasis is not routinely used.

The ophthalmic examination begins with the superficial structures and progresses to the ocular fundus. The orbit and adnexa are evaluated for deformities, size of the palpebral fissure, and relationship of the eyelids to the globe. The position of the nictitating membrane and presence or absence of ocular discharges are noted. Breed differences in frontal placement of the eye must also be considered, as in the Arabian breed. Focal enlargements of the orbit may result from trauma, systemic disease and neoplasia. The size and shape of the globes must be evaluated and compared. The average size of the adult equine globe is 43.7 mm craniocaudad, 47.6 mm at the vertical equator and 48.5 mm at the transverse equator. If discrepancies between the sizes of the globes occur, the dimensions of the globes may

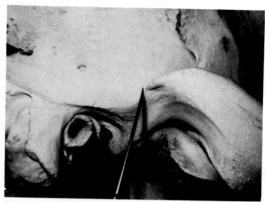

Fig 1. Auriculopalpebral nerve block. The local anesthetic is injected at the most dorsal or caudal groove of the temporal portion of the zygomatic arch.

be determined *in situ* by ultrasonography. The sensitivity of this system is ± 0.01 mm. Alternatively, the vertical and horizontal measurements of the corneas by calipers may provide useful information relative to the size of the globe with micro- and macrocornea. The position of the globe should be ascertained. Enophthalmia may indicate previous ocular inflammation, reduction of globe size and loss of orbital tissues. Exophthalmia may indicate a relative increase in size of the globe or retrobulbar tissues.

Eyelids are examined for abnormalities, such as ectropion, entropion, blepharitis, blepharospasm, congenital or acquired malformations and eyelid neoplasms. Illumination and some magnification are useful. Diffuse illumination with a penlight or otoscope with the speculum removed usually suffices. The cilia or eyelashes of horses are present only on the upper eyelids in a number of irregular rows. The upper eyelid has considerable motility but the lower lid is important in the retention and drainage of tears. The ability of the orbicularis oculi muscle to close the palpebral fissure is ascertained by lightly tapping the medial or lateral canthal areas. The eyelids should touch the globe, thereby preventing accumulation of tears and debris, and facilitating movement of tears to the nasolacrimal apparatus. The eyelid contours curve gently around the surface of the cornea; the orifices of the ducts of the tarsal or Meibomian glands are partially visible in the eyelid margin. A notch in the upper eyelids may indicate ocular hypotony, loss of retrobulbar contents or reduction in globe size.

The palpebral, fornix and bulbar conjunctivae are next examined. Topical anesthesia is occasionally used to examine the deeper aspects of the palpebral and fornix conjunctivae. While the ventral conjunctival fornix can be examined adequately by eversion of the lower lid, inspection of the upper conjunctival fornix, because of its greater depth, is partially achieved by direct observation and the remainder by digital probing of the area. If bacterial cultures are important, use of topical anesthetics before collection of specimens should be avoided because topical anesthetics and/or their preservatives reduce the recovery of organisms. Pigmentation, types of conjunctival exudates, hyperemia and other conjunctival abnormalities are evaluated. The ventral conjunctiva of horses is usually more hyperemic than the dorsal area and normally contains lymphoid follicles. Pigmentation is occasionally present on the lateral bulbar conjunctiva.

The palpebral (outer) and bulbar (inner) aspects of the nictitating membrane are inspected. The palpebral surface is examined by distorting the horse's eyelids vertically, causing the horse to retract the globe and protrude the nictitating membrane. The anterior mucous membrane of the nictitans is smooth and its leading margin is usually pigmented. At the base of the nictitans in the medial canthus is the caruncle, which has variable pigmentation, contains fine hairs and is occasionally the site for granulomas and neoplasms. The bulbar surface of the nictitating membrane normally contains limited numbers of lymphoid follicles and is examined under topical anesthesia with small thumb forceps grasping the leading margin and everting the structure. Nictitating membrane abnormalities include cartilage defects, protrusion, inflammation, hypertrophy, foreign bodies and neoplasia.

The nasolacrimal apparatus is evaluated by the presence of epiphora, staining of hair at the medial canthus, passage of fluorescein from the eye to the nose, nasolacrimal flush and dacryocystorhinography. The upper and lower lacrimal puncta are located about 8 mm from the medial canthus and are about 2 mm in diameter. The nasolacrimal duct opens at the mucocutaneous junction on the floor of the nostril. The most convenient clinical test for nasolacrimal patency is the fluorescein test, in which the dye is applied on the dorsolateral conjunctiva. Several minutes are permitted for the fluorescein to traverse the palpebral fissure, enter the nasolacrimal apparatus and emerge from the nasolacrimal duct. The test should be performed on both sides simultaneously and the times for fluorescein passage compared.

Intraocular pressure (IOP) is measured digitally through the upper eyelid or directly on the anesthetized cornea. More recent refinements for estimation of IOP in the horse have been achieved by the use of applanation tonometers. The Schiotz tonometer cannot be used in horses because the curvature of the equine cornea does not approximate that of the human cornea; the instrument must be positioned vertically on the center of the cornea to be accurate. The MacKay-Marg tonometer (Biotronics, Redding, CA) is reliable for estimating IOP in horses.[23,24] The instrument is not significantly adversely affected by corneal scarring or edema, deviations of the corneal curvature, and changes in ocular rigidity. In addition, the MacKay-Marg tonometer can be used horizontally in a horse, thereby permitting measurement of IOP in a standing unanesthetized horse. The mean IOP in horses, with only topical corneal anesthesia, is 28 mm Hg (SD ± 4 mm Hg). If sedation or tranquilization is used, IOP is reduced 15-20%.[24] While marked elevations in IOP are rare in horses, reduction in IOP (hypotony) is common with anterior segment inflammations.

The equine cornea is examined with diffuse and focal illumination, and with 2-20X magnification. The average adult equine cornea measures 33-34 mm horizontally and 26-27 mm vertically. The oval cornea is examined from both the direct and lateral positions. By inspection from at least 2 different angles, accurate localization of lesions within the corneal layers is facilitated. The otoscope with speculum removed or a focusable penlight combined with a binocular loupe is absolutely essential for adequately examining the cornea (Fig 2). The portable slit-lamp biomicroscope is unexcelled to accurately examine the cornea and remaining anterior segment of horses.

The cornea is covered with a thin preocular film that occasionally appears oil-like and normally very slightly retains fluorescein. Irregular white to grey lines may occur in the lateral and medial cornea adjacent to the limbus. These may represent abnormal insertions of the pectinate ligaments or peripheral anterior synechiae. The presence or absence of deep and superficial vascularization, pigmentation, foreign bodies, neoplasms, dermoids, scars and other lesions is noted. Large branching blood vessels in the anterior corneal stroma suggest superficial disease. Fine corneal blood vessels represent extensions of the vasculature of the deeper cornea and suggest involvement of the anterior uvea.

Evaluation of the cornea and its epithelial surface necessitates application of topical fluorescein, especially if ulceration is suspected. Fluorescein strips are recommended because fluorescein solutions are easily contaminated. The fluorescein strip is moistened with a drop of saline or artificial tear preparation placed directly on its tip and applied directly to the dorsolateral conjunctiva; the animal is permitted to distribute the fluorescein across the cornea. Direct contact of the fluorescein strip with the cornea should be avoided because it results in an unusually heavy deposit of the dye and may be falsely interpreted as an ulcer.

The anterior chamber is inspected for depth in the 4 quadrants, and for abnormal contents (blood, flare, cysts, parasites, and inflammatory and neoplastic cells). The anterior chamber is examined from the frontal and lateral aspects using magnification, and direct and oblique illumination. The aqueous humor normally contains protein at a level of 20-40 mg/dl; the increased protein content associated with inflammation creates a flare or cloudiness (aqueous flare) in the aqueous humor. The depth of the anterior chamber may be ascertained optically using slit-lamp biomicroscopy and in fractions of millimeters by ultrasonography. Anterior chamber paracentesis (keratocentesis) and subsequent examination for cells, proteins, bacteria and antibody titers may be indicated.

The iris, corpora nigrum and pupil are closely inspected since these structures are common sites for disease. The pupil is a uniform oval shape in adult animals; in newborn and young foals the pupil is round. Irregularities in the pupillary margin of the iris usually indicate posterior synechiae. Posterior synechiae may become obvious with drug-induced mydriasis, which further distorts pupillary shape. The normal iris has a dark-brown, rather smooth surface that curves gently anteriorly, with its central portion resting on the anterior lens surface. The corpora nigrum of horses is a mass on the upper pupillary margin and to a lesser extent on the lower margin. The irregular, nodular brown-black mass facilitates the light-regulating mechanism of the horizontally oriented oval pupil. Excessive size of the dorsal corpora nigrum may produce shying in horses and its atrophy is associated with iridocyclitis and recurrent uveitis.

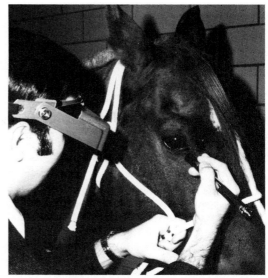

Fig 2. Examination of the external eye and adnexa with a penlight and head loupe.

Heterochromia iridis is a normal variation of iridal color that occurs in the palomino, light chestnut, grey and Appaloosa, and other spotted horses. The iris may be partially brown and blue, blue-white, or white with brown-black corpora nigrum.

The iris is examined with broad and focal beams of light and some magnification. An otoscope with speculum removed, focusable penlight and head loupe, or slit-lamp biomicroscope is used to examine the structure. The basal aspects of the iris and the iridocorneal angle are examined by gonioscopy.

The lens is divided clinically into anterior and posterior capsule, anterior and posterior cortex, and nucleus, and should be examined after drug-induced mydriasis. The lens axial region, through which most vision occurs, and the lens equator, in which most lens growth occurs, must also be evaluated. In daylight or in well-illuminated examination areas, the constricted pupil prevents examination of most of the lens except its axial region. When the horse is placed in a dark room, more of the lens can be evaluated; however, the amount of illumination must be increased with the use of magnification, which results in variable miosis. Therefore, drug-induced mydriasis is required to adequately examine the entire lens and its equator. The lens is examined by direct and oblique illumination and magnification, and portable slit-lamp biomicroscopy. The normal adult equine lens volume is about 3 ml, the di-

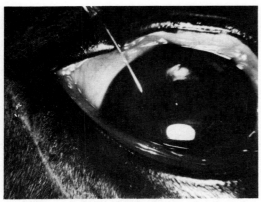

Fig 3. Anterior chamber paracentesis (keratocentesis) through the dorsolateral limbus.

ameter of its curvature is about 22 mm, and the axial length is 12 mm.[9]

Nuclear sclerosis of the lens becomes prominent as a horse ages. Refractive changes are usually noted at the junction of the lens nucleus and cortex when a horse reaches 5 years of age. Nuclear sclerosis in aged horses imparts a bluish color to the lens center that may be improperly termed cataract. In the evaluation of cataracts in the horse, every attempt should be made to localize the opacities. Determination of the anatomic position of the cataract facilitates prognostication as to the progression, regression or static nature of the cataract, and provides clues as to the cause.

The normal vitreous is a clear gel with optical properties that permit unaltered transmission of light from the lens to the ocular fundus. The anterior part of the vitreous is examined by direct and oblique illumination, magnification or slit-lamp biomicroscopy. The posterior aspects of the vitreous require direct and indirect ophthalmoscopy, or slit-lamp biomicroscopy using a Hruby lens. In foals and young horses, the normal vitreous is nearly totally gelatinous; as horses age, the vitreous deteriorates and some areas liquefy.

Vitreous abnormalities include persistent hyaloid vasculature, hemorrhage, infiltration with inflammatory cells, syneresis (liquefaction) and irregular degenerative strands. Consistency of the vitreous is ascertained by visualization of intravitreal abnormalities. If the vitreous has a gel consistency, the lesions oscillate slightly when ocular movement ceases but remain suspended within the structure. If the vitreous is liquefied (syneresis), the opacities move about during ocular movements and

gravitate ventrad when the eye is static. The presence of small strands within the vitreous in aged horses is probably a normal aging phenomenon. However, the presence of inflammatory or other cells within the vitreous is usually associated with intraocular inflammation.

Evaluation of the ocular fundus in horses is performed by direct and indirect ophthalmoscopy, slit-lamp biomicroscopy, ultrasonography, fluorescein angiography and electroretinography. The ocular fundus is divided arbitrarily into the tapetal fundus (tapetum lucidum), nontapetal fundus (tapetum nigrum), optic papilla, disc or nerve head, and retinal blood vessels. The variations in the normal ocular fundus among horses are discussed in the section on the ocular fundus.

Diagnostic Procedures

The increased availability and expansion of instrumentation for ophthalmic diagnostic procedures have improved diagnosis documentation and prognostication of diseases of the eye and periocular structures. In this section, many ophthalmic diagnostic procedures used in horses are described.

Anterior Chamber Paracentesis

Anterior chamber paracentesis (keratocentesis) is useful in selected patients for the treatment of hyphema and chronic iridocyclitis, and for diagnosis of certain anterior segment diseases. The use of keratocentesis to rapidly reduce intraocular pressure, treat hypopyon, and increase the secondary or plasmoid aqueous humor volume in horses is rarely indicated and not recommended.

Short-acting IV barbiturate anesthesia is necessary for keratocentesis. The anterior chamber is entered at the lateral or dorsolateral limbus with a 22-ga hypodermic needle and up to 1 ml aqueous humor is aspirated (Fig 3). An equal amount of sterile 0.9% saline or balanced salt solution (BSS: Alcon Laboratories) is injected to replace the aqueous humor and restore intraocular pressure to preparacentesis levels. The secondary aqueous humor that forms in horses after paracentesis is very high in protein content and contains fibrin that clots. Undesirable sequelae associated with keratocentesis include hyphema from touching the iris, introduction of foreign material, and trauma to the iris, cornea or lens.

Analysis of aqueous humor samples is indicated for the diagnosis and investigation of certain anterior segment diseases. In horses with

Leptospira titers and acute recurrent uveitis, antibody titers of the aqueous humor and serum may differ, depending on the stage of ocular disease. In acute attacks, serum and aqueous humor titers are about equal. In periods of relative quiescence or chronic inflammation in horses with leptospirosis-related recurrent uveitis, titers of antibodies to various *Leptospira* organisms are much higher in the aqueous humor than in serum.

Corneoconjunctival Cultures and Cytologic Examination

Corneoconjunctival cytologic examination and cultures are indicated in chronic, unusually severe and unresponsive external ocular infections. Topical anesthesia is used prior to collection of cytologic material but must be avoided prior to bacterial culture. The normal bacterial flora in horse eyes have not been ascertained but include predominantly *Staphylococcus, Streptococcus* and even *Pseudomonas*.

Dacryocystorhinography

The entire nasolacrimal apparatus can be outlined with radiopaque contrast material. Dacryocystorhinography is indicated when fluorescein passage, and nasolacrimal flushes and probing have failed. This method aids diagnosis and localization of congenital and acquired nasolacrimal obstructions. About 3-5 ml 40% iodized poppyseed oil (Lipiodol: Fougera) are injected in the upper or lower punctum until the radiopaque material emerges through the distal orifice of the nasolacrimal duct. Contrast dye may also be injected from both ends in cases of obstruction. Lateral and oblique lateral radiographs are most useful.

Direct and Indirect Ophthalmoscopy

Direct and indirect ophthalmoscopy are used to evaluate the ocular fundus. The advantages of direct ophthalmoscopy are use through miotic pupils, low cost, greater magnification for study of detail, and the ease with which this method is mastered. The ocular fundus image is real, upright and enlarged about 14-15 times (Fig 4).

Indirect ophthalmoscopy is neither superior nor inferior to direct ophthalmoscopy; the methods complement each other when properly used. The advantages of indirect ophthalmoscopy are ease of penetration of cloudy media, large field of view, ease of compensation for refractive errors, stereopsis with binocular models, and greater working distance between patient and examiner. Both methods supple-

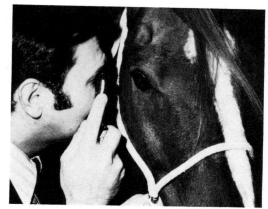

Fig 4. Direct ophthalmoscopic examination.

ment examination of the anterior segment of the eye (Fig 5).

A previous limitation of direct ophthalmoscopy was limited illumination; however, recent introduction of direct ophthalmoscopes with halogen illuminating systems has eliminated this problem. The more intensive illumination facilitates use of the instruments for examination of the anterior segment (with +4 to +6 lens) as well as the posterior segment. The halogen direct ophthalmoscopes may also be combined with a 10- to 20-diopter planoconvex lens positioned between the ophthalmoscope and the patient's eye to permit monocular indirect ophthalmoscopy, thereby expanding the use of the direct ophthalmoscope. I prefer direct ophthalmoscopy in horses because they are usually not alarmed by the instrument and the examiner is close enough to the horse to anticipate sudden movements before they occur.

Fluorescein Ophthalmic Stain

Fluorescein is used topically and parenterally as a diagnostic stain for ophthalmic problems. The compound is used topically in

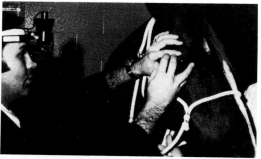

Fig 5. Indirect ophthalmoscopic examination.

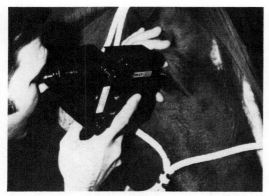

Fig 6. Fundus photography with the Kowa RC-2 camera.

determination of corneal epithelial integrity and patency of the nasolacrimal drainage apparatus. The water-soluble fluorescein does not penetrate the normal, lipid-selective corneal epithelium; however, in the presence of corneal ulceration and loss of this epithelial layer, fluorescein readily diffuses into the water-selective stroma and even into the anterior chamber in extensive ulcerations. Fluorescein passage is a fairly reliable test of nasolacrimal patency in horses. The use of ultraviolet or cobalt blue light to intensify the fluorescence facilitates detection of fluorescein passage.

Several years ago sodium fluorescein solution (10%, 10 ml) was used IV to ascertain integrity of the blood-aqueous barrier of the anterior segment. Inflammation of the anterior uvea results in a breakdown of the blood-aqueous barrier and permits rapid passage of

fluorescein into the aqueous humor. An intense, diffuse fluorescence of the aqueous humor or a fluorescent halo about the pupillary margin of the iris results. Experience has shown the IV fluorescein test for anterior segment inflammation is helpful but unreliable because false negatives occur. Other diagnostic procedures, such as slit-lamp biomicroscopy, are more reliable and informative.

External and Fundus Photography

External and fundus photography of normal and abnormal ocular conditions is used to record lesions and for teaching purposes. Several types of inexpensive close-up cameras with flash attachments are available for external photography. Alternatively, single-lens-reflex 35-mm cameras with a hand-held strobe or strobe mounted to the front of the lens can be used. The 50- to 120-mm medical macrolenses for 35-mm cameras are the most useful and versatile. For ocular fundus photography, the Kowa RC-2 and RC-3 medical cameras provide excellent photographs of equine intraocular structures (Fig 6). [25,26]

Only firm restraint is needed to photograph the eye and periocular structures of most horses. Flashes from strobe lights do not usually produce excessive struggling or excitement; however, the horse should be placed in stocks for convenience. Mydriasis is essential for lens and ocular fundus photography. If blepharospasm becomes inhibiting, auriculopalpebral or other eyelid nerve blocks can be employed. Tranquilization and/or sedation is necessary for intractable horses; use of xylazine at 0.5 mg/lb IV or 1 mg/lb IM is recommended in such cases for sedation for ophthalmic photography and examination.

Localization of Intraocular Opacities

Opacities in the anterior chamber, iris, lens and vitreous may be localized by parallax, the shadow test, determining the optical center of the eye, and slit-lamp biomicroscopy. The last 2 methods are preferred. In contrast to the eyes of small animals, in which the optical center of the eye is located in the caudal aspect of the lens nucleus, the center of the equine eye is at the posterior pole of the lens (Fig 7). Opacities anterior to the optical center of the eye move in the same direction as ocular movement. For instance, an anterior polar cataract moves to the right when the eye turns to the right. Opacities caudal to the optical center of the eye move opposite to the direction of ocular movement. For instance, a focal hemorrhage within the vitre-

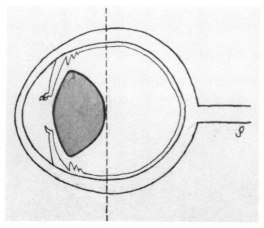

Fig 7. Localization of intraocular opacities based on the posterior pole of the lens as the center of rotation for the globe.

ous moves to the left when ocular movement is to the right. Small opacities in the posterior lens, *ie,* the posterior polar capsule and/or posterior polar subcapsular region, are frequently difficult to distinguish from changes in the anterior vitreous. Then, slit-lamp biomicroscopy provides a very reasonable, valid method to differentiate these 2 abnormalities.

Movement of ocular opacities may also provide clues about their position within the eye. Lesions within the lens, provided they are within the patellar fossa, remain stationary and stop after ocular movement. Vitreous opacities tend to oscillate and, if the vitreous is liquefied, settle or gravitate to the most ventral quadrant after ocular movement stops.

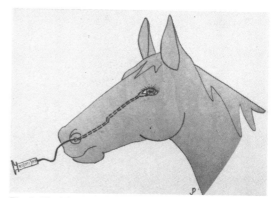

Fig 8. Flushing the nasolacrimal system after cannulating the distal orifice.

Nasolacrimal Flush

The nasolacrimal flush is used to determine patency of the nasolacrimal drainage apparatus. Most nasolacrimal obstructions involve the nasolacrimal duct and this technic re-establishes patency of the system. The orifice of the nasolacrimal duct is located on the floor of the nostril at the mucocutaneous junction. It can be cannulated with an 18-ga hypodermic needle, small male canine urinary catheter, small-diameter polyethylene tubing and various mastitis medication dispensers. Topical anesthetic ointment is rubbed 3 cm around the opening of the nasolacrimal orifice. The horse is twitched on the lower lip and the orifice is cannulated for approximately 1 cm. Sterile water or saline (5-10 ml) is injected retrograde with moderate pressure (Fig 8).

In the event nasolacrimal flushes cannot reestablish patency of the system, probing the upper lacrimal punctum with stiff polyethylene tubing during flushing may be necessary. Nasolacrimal flushing has also been recommended to medicate the eye and may be considered an alternative to the subpalpebral medication schemes discussed later.

Slit-Lamp Biomicroscopy

Slit-lamp biomicroscopy has been used in Europe for the study and diagnosis of ophthalmic conditions in horses since 1954.[27] Use of slit-lamp biomicroscopy in horses in the US is now becoming routine with the recent introduction of portable slit-lamp biomicroscopes. The Kowa SXL-1, SXL-2 and SXL-5 portable slit-lamp biomicroscopes provide for convenient examination of the anterior segment and lens. The horse is usually positioned within stocks to avoid unnecessary movement. The biomicroscope is reasonably light and can be manipu-

lated conveniently about the horse's eye. Biomicroscopy can detect minute evidence of disease of the cornea, anterior chamber, iris, lens and anterior vitreous, and can very accurately localize and determine the depth of ocular opacities. Photography with the slit-lamp biomicroscope in horses requires the use of larger table-mounted units, necessitating more restraint and sedation of the horse (Fig 9).

Tonometry

Tonometry is the estimation of intraocular pressure (IOP) and usually is performed digitally in the horse. The IOP is estimated by palpation of the globe with the first 2 fingers through the eyelid or directly on the anesthetized cornea. The digital method of estimation of IOP is crude, subjective and highly unreliable. With the recent introduction of applanation tonometers that can be used in a horizontal

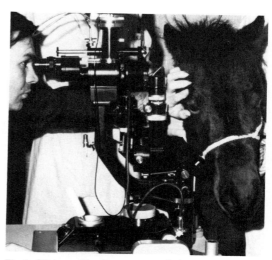

Fig 9. Slit-lamp biomicroscopy and photography.

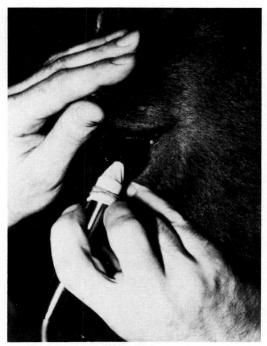

Fig 10. Applanation (MacKay-Marg) tonometry to estimate intraocular pressure.[24]

position, the estimation of IOP in horses has become accurate and reliable (Fig 10). The mean IOP of 6 horses was 25 mm Hg, using the electronic tonometer, topical anesthetic and tranquilizers.[24] In another study of 45 untranquilized horses, the mean IOP in the topically anesthetized eye was 28 mm Hg (SD ± 4 mm Hg).[24] Restraint agents, such as acepromazine and xylazine, produce ocular hypotony (reduced IOP). The reduction in IOP after xylazine administration is 30% and generally more uniform than that observed after acepromazine administration, which is 20%.[24]

Hypotony is commonly observed in horses with recurrent uveitis and other types of iridocyclitis. Glaucoma is rare in horses but its detection is aided by instrument tonometry.

Vision Testing

Ocular diseases in horses may slightly affect vision or cause total blindness. Because vision testing in horses is mostly subjective, assessment of vision may be inaccurate. Refractive errors can affect a horse's behavior and performance, and are measured by retinoscopy or estimated in diopters by direct ophthalmoscopy. Most horses are emmetropic (56%), but many are myopic (37%) and some are hyperopic (2%).[28] It has been suggested that wild horses

are hyperopic, and domestication and inbreeding have increased the frequency of myopia.

Like most other animals, horses have limited accommodation because of their large lens and poorly developed ciliary muscles. Accommodation may involve dynamic (changes in the lens because of ciliary body muscle activity) and static (relative irregularities or changes of ocular morphology) mechanisms. Because of their "ramp" retina, horses change focus predominantly by eye and head movement, which alters the axial length of images between the retina and cornea. The head is usually elevated for distant objects and lowered for near objects. The eye is rotated medial for near objects and lateral for distant objects. The field of vision for a horse with its head lowered is about 215°.

Two recent studies evaluated the "ramp" retina phenomenon in the equine eye.[29,30] The horse lacks the "area centralis." One study indicated refractive state shifts in the direction of hyperopia above and below the visual axis, with the shift greater below the axis than above it. Changes in lens-retina distance were greater below the axis than above it. Some dynamic but limited accommodative ability was evident in the living eye. Results of another study suggest horses have excellent vision for distant objects and, although they have relatively narrow binocular field of vision, pupil size facilitates lateral ocular observations. Altering head position produces emmetropic vision simultaneously; areas of blurriness and blindness occur at different focal areas in the same field of vision.

Vision testing is performed by moving the horse with considerable length of shank (to prevent direct following the owner or client) through an unfamiliar environment with obstacles of various sizes, shapes and contrast. We permit the animal to traverse the obstacles once, then cover each eye separately with a hood, blinder or bandage and repeat the experiment for each eye. The ocular movement, movement of the ears and head, and general behavior of the horse should be evaluated during the obstacle course. Blind horses are unusually alert, move their ears constantly, prance to compensate for irregularities in the ground, and stumble and/or collide with the obstacles. The results of vision testing in the obstacle course are correlated with the findings of ophthalmic examination.

Electroretinography is a method to electrophysiologically evaluate vision in horses and involves analysis of the outer retinal layers.

This test cannot determine the presence of vision but is an excellent method of evaluating generalized disorders of the outer retina. Night blindness in Appaloosas has been evaluated by electroretinography.

The visual evoked potential is an electrophysiologic test for vision that will have clinical application in future years. This method involves exposing the eye to various types of light stimuli and recording potentials at the level of the scalp over the occipital cortex. The method necessitates use of signal averagers and/or computers, which in recent years have become reasonably priced.

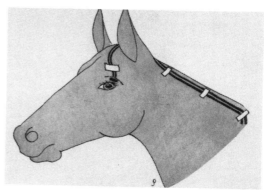

Fig 11. Subpalpebral medication. Tubing is implanted in the dorsal conjunctival fornix and extended to the withers.

Medication Technics

The horse, because of its size, powerful orbicularis oculi muscle and variable disposition, cannot be medicated as frequently as desired with ophthalmic solutions or ointments. In medicating the equine eye, it is often imperative that a certain dose of an ophthalmic preparation is applied periodically for transcorneal penetration. To achieve this, several schemes for continuous or intermittent medication of the equine eye were developed to deliver liquid preparations into the dorsal or dorsolateral conjunctival fornix.[31-33]

Subpalpebral Instillation

Intensive topical therapy is frequently desirable in severe ocular disease and postoperatively, and may be critical in influencing the eventual outcome. However, the instillation of medication may be very difficult in intractable horses or postoperatively. Subpalpebral instillation involves placement of various types of tubing into the dorsolateral conjunctival fornix to permit medication easily, reliably and at any frequency (Fig 11).

The advantages of subpalpebral instillation include: convenient administration of ophthalmic solutions; delivery of accurate drug dosage; relative safety for veterinarian, client and horse; feasibility of medication in case of complete temporary tarsorrhaphy or with the palpebral fissure open; reduced likelihood of the horse becoming shy about treatment and examination of the eye; and possibly reduced incidence of undesirable sequelae associated with frequent topical medication of the eyes.

Attempted instillation of an ophthalmic preparation may result in severe blepharospasm, protrusion of the nictitating membrane, retraction of the globe and possible transient increase in IOP. In the event of severe corneal weakening or intraocular surgery, this sequence may adversely affect the concurrent ocular condition.

Subpalpebral medication systems have few limitations. Those constructed from polyethylene or Silastic tubing are inexpensive. If focal eyelid swelling occurs around the subpalpebral tubing, the system should be checked carefully for leakage of ophthalmic preparations. In those subpalpebral systems with a footplate within the conjunctival fornix, the position of the footplate should be observed daily or palpated through the upper eyelid. The subpalpebral tubing may gradually migrate ventrad in the conjunctival fornix. If the subpalpebral tubing touches the limbus or cornea, an ulcer and/or granulation tissue result. Therefore, these systems must be inspected daily. Subpalpebral systems have been left in place in horses for as long as 8 weeks without adverse effects. Intensive topical treatment of an animal for this length of time is generally impossible with conventional methods.

A subpalpebral system may be constructed from medium-sized polyethylene or Silastic tubing, and is also available commercially (Becton-Dickinson, Rutherford, NJ). With polyethylene tubing, a small footplate is constructed by exposing the end of the tubing to heat. The polyethylene flares when warmed and contact of the flared area with a smooth flat surface, such as a stainless-steel table, results in immediate hardening and formation of a footplate 7-12 mm in diameter. With Silastic tubing, a thin Silastic sheet and Silastic glue are necessary to construct the tubing and footplate. The Silastic system is more resistant to damage and stretching without developing small leaks. Polyethylene tubing, if exces-

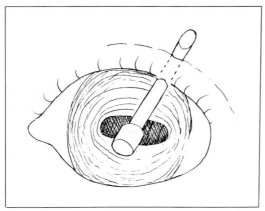

Fig 12a. Insertion of a large hub-less hypodermic needle into the dorsal conjunctival fornix and through the eyelid for placement of the subpalpebral system. A test-tube rubber stopper is used on the end of the needle to facilitate penetration of the eyelid.

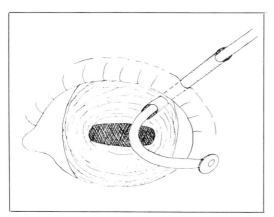

Fig 12b. Threading the subpalpebral tubing into the hypodermic needle.

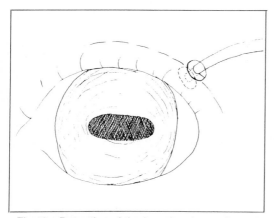

Fig 12c. Retraction of the hypodermic needle and final positioning of the subpalpebral tubing. A Silastic "washer" external to the eyelid skin secures the system.[33]

sively bent, may develop imperfections and even break.

Three continuous to intermittent medication systems have been reported for use in horses. In one system, polyethylene or Silastic tubing with a footplate is implanted in the dorsolateral conjunctival fornix. Another system uses a single piece of polyethylene tubing passing through the eyelid into the conjunctival fornix and through another perforation of the eyelids. Several holes are produced in the tubing within the conjunctival fornix. This method does not have a footplate to help retain the tubing. A third method recently suggested consists of retrograde flushing of medication into the eye via the nasolacrimal system; the primary disadvantage is the volume and cost of solutions necessary using this route.

We prefer a subpalpebral system constructed with Silastic tubing and a footplate, positioned in the dorsolateral conjunctival fornix. A 14-ga, hub-less hypodermic needle is inserted in the dorsal to dorsolateral conjunctival fornix to the outer surface of the eyelid (Fig 12a). Placement through the lid is facilitated by covering the blunt end of the needle with a rubber test-tube stopper. Sterile Silastic tubing is threaded into the needle lumen, and the needle and tubing are pulled through the lid. A single suture, Silastic washer, or ether-soaked adhesive tape is placed over or around the tubing as it exits the skin of the eyelid to maintain the corneal footplate in position and prevent movement within the conjunctival fornix (Fig 12c). The tubing can be extended to the forehead and side of the face or to the withers for administration. When continuous medication of the eye is essential, the system may be coupled to a small pump delivering 1-3 drops of ophthalmic medication to the eye hourly.

Ophthalmic Unsoundness

The basic criteria for ophthalmic unsoundness in horses have not been defined.[34,35] Certainly the visual demands of individual horses are paramount in determining ophthalmic soundness. The absolute need for optimal vision occurs in hunters and jumpers. Draft horses may have minor visual imperfections and still perform satisfactorily. Although Thoroughbreds and Standardbreds are raced with monocular vision, that practice is unsatisfactory and unsafe for the horse and rider/driver. The fundamentals for ophthalmic unsoundness in horses are defined below.

Blindness of one or both eyes constitutes unsoundness regardless of a horse's function. Horses have very limited binocular vision and an extensive monocular field. Loss of one eye (or both) is a severe visual handicap and such animals must be considered unsound. The globe may be reduced in size congenitally (microphthalmia) or may atrophy from disease, such as phthisis bulbi secondary to trauma, inflammation or surgery.

Strabismus constitutes an unsoundness in horses. In my experience, 2 kinds of strabismus occur in horses: esotropia and, more commonly, hypertropia. In both conditions, visual impairment is evidenced by stumbling, shyness, occasional falling and excitability. In hypertropia, the visual field of the horse is limited ventrad; this area is essential for satisfactory vision.

Corneal opacities may represent minor blemishes rather than unsoundness in the horse.[35] The significance of a corneal opacity is determined by the horse's function, and the extent and position of the opacity within the cornea. Dense central corneal opacities profoundly impair vision, especially during daylight, and constitute an unsoundness in horses. Opacities of the ventral cornea that are paracentral or within the visual field also constitute an unsoundness. Opacities of the dorsal, lateral and medial aspects of the cornea that are beyond the pupillary and visual axis are considered blemishes as long as the visual axis of the cornea is normal.

Heterochromia iridis is a condition in which the iris is a color other than brown. These colors commonly include blue and/or white, and are considered normal variants of iridal coloration. They do not represent an ophthalmic unsoundness or blemish. Albino horses, in which the irides are white and somewhat hypoplastic, may be photophobic in bright sunlight; such lesions must be considered a blemish.

Horses with evidence of past or present recurrent uveitis related to leptospirosis or onchocerciasis are unsound regardless of the animal's function. Horses with recurrent uveitis, regardless of etiology, suffer attacks intermittently. The intervals between attacks and their severity are not predictable. Recurrent uveitis can produce corneal opacities, cataracts, lens luxations, vitreous alterations, retinal detachment and chorioretinoneuropathies. Any of these lesions can seriously impair vision and produce blindness.

Cataracts of any type have been established legally as an unsoundness.[34] Those lens opaci-

ties within the polar areas of visual axis of the lens profoundly affect vision, especially in daylight when the pupil is constricted. Cataracts in the equator do not produce visual impairment but are considered an unsoundness because of their progressive nature. Although cataracts of the anterior capsule and cortex are not necessarily rapidly progressive, they also constitute an unsoundness because they frequently involve the visual axis. Cataracts of the posterior pole and the equatorial cortex are frequently associated with recurrent uveitis and are considered an unsoundness. Horses are the least able of species to compensate for lens opacities and have relatively impaired vision by early cataract formation. Therefore, cataracts of all types are an unsoundness.

Refractive errors are not commonly measured in horses; however, the animal's performance may be adversely affected by a marked difference in refractive errors between the eyes of an individual horse. A refractive error greater than 5 diopters between the eyes of a jumper/hunter is considered an unsoundness. This abnormality may result in the horse misjudging jumps, usually leaving early and landing early. The refractive error in the horse, as indicated in a previous section, may be roughly estimated by use of the direct ophthalmoscope to determine the optimum fundus focus of both eyes or more reliably by retinoscopy.

Vitreous floaters may adversely affect vision, depending on their size, shape and position in the vitreous cavity. These opacities, if extensive and within the visual axis, constitute an unsoundness in hunters and jumpers, and those horses in which vision is deemed critical. These opacities seem to relate directly to shyness and visual impairment. Vitreous opacities that remain suspended, are small and in the ventral vitreous are considered blemishes.

Certain ocular fundus abnormalities also constitute unsoundness. Optic nerve atrophy and exudative optic neuritis are unsoundnesses because they markedly impair vision and result in blindness. Peripapillary chorioretinopathy or chorioretinoneuropathy requires critical scrutiny in the determination of ocular soundness. When the abnormality appears to affect predominantly the choroid and retina but not the optic nerve, it may be considered a serious blemish. However, peripapillary chorioretinoneuropathy should be considered an unsoundness, regardless of the horse's function. Both conditions are frequently associated with the anterior segment lesions of recurrent

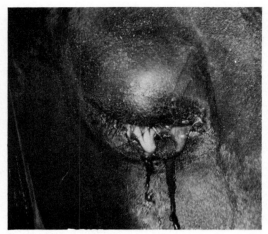

Fig 13. Orbital cellulitis.

uveitis and, as such, are certainly considered as unsoundness. Chorioretinopathies should be considered blemishes in most horses in the absence of visual impairment; however, involvement of the optic nerve (chorioretinoneuropathy) frequently impairs vision. Such animals should be considered unsound.

DISEASES OF THE ORBIT

Diseases of the orbit are infrequent in horses but necessitate thorough examination, diagnosis and treatment. Traditionally conditions of the orbit are divided into those that produce exophthalmos and those that produce enophthalmos. The orbital contents are increased in size in exophthalmia. The eye may be enlarged from glaucoma or the orbit may be infiltrated by a tumor. The eye is recessed or less apparent within the orbit in enophthalmia. The globe may be smaller or there may be partial loss of orbital tissues. Any associated damage to the globe requires additional consideration.

Orbital Trauma

Trauma to the orbit results from trailer accidents, fights, blows inflicted by the handler and contact with foreign objects. Trauma may occur more frequently in stallions and when many horses are maintained together. Simple to compound fractures of the orbit may involve the supraorbital process of the frontal bone and the zygomatic arch. These 2 bones are most susceptible to injury since they comprise the lateral orbital rim and wall. Damage to the globe is variable and influenced by the extent of trauma and displacement of fractures. Small fractures of these bones with minimal displace-

ment do not usually require surgery and heal without sequelae. Compound fractures with numerous fragments and extensive displacement necessitate thorough cleaning of the wound, removal of small bony fragments and fixation of large fragments with wires, screws or plates. Large doses of systemic antibiotics and topical treatment of the wound are indicated. The globe, extraocular muscles and retrobulbar fat also may be traumatized and require specific treatment.

The prognosis in simple fractures is usually good; however, compound fractures with considerable trauma to the orbit usually warrant a guarded prognosis because of possible damage to the globe and optic nerve, and infection of the bony and orbital tissues.

Orbital Cellulitis

Orbital cellulitis is an infection associated with injuries and infections of the sinus, teeth and other organs that extend into the orbit. Clinical signs usually develop in 24-48 hours and include severe swelling of the dorsolateral orbit and eyelids, filling and swelling of the orbital fossa, and evidence of pain and heat of the eyelids and orbital structures. The palpebral and bulbar conjunctivae are markedly hyperemic and chemotic, and mucopurulent exudates frequently discharge from the narrowed palpebral fissure. Exophthalmos and protrusion of the nictitating membrane are apparent. If ophthalmic examination is possible, hyperemia of the optic nerve head and papilledema may be present. Anorexia and low-grade fever are usually present. If diffuse within the orbit, the condition is classified as cellulitis. In time the inflammation may coalesce to form focal abscesses in the supraorbital fossa and the lateral to ventrolateral aspects of the orbit (Fig 13).

The prognosis in orbital cellulitis depends on the rapidity of diagnosis and the response to vigorous treatment with large doses of systemic antibiotics. Prolonged septic infection of the orbit may damage the extraocular muscles and orbital fat, and produce optic neuritis with subsequent atrophy. Fibrosis associated with resolution of the condition may interfere with extraocular muscle function and limit motility of the globe. Orbital fat may be destroyed in the inflammation and resorbed during healing; loss of this important space-occupying tissue results in variable enophthalmia. Systemic antibiotics, such as penicillin or tetracyclines, are useful against most organisms associated with orbital cellulitis when administered at maximum levels. Culture of orbital exudates and bacterial sensitivity tests aid selection of appropriate antibiotics. In the event of abscess formation, the pyogenic material is aspirated through a large-bore hypodermic needle or by lancing the most ventral area of the orbit.

In contrast to orbital cellulitis in cats and dogs, surgical drainage of orbital cellulitis in horses is not usually necessary. In the event the cellulitis fails to respond to high levels of systemic antiobiotics, drainage through the orbital floor should be attempted. The superior maxillary sinus is trephined in the standard manner and an opening is made through the sinus into the anterior floor of the orbit with a bone chisel. The pyogenic material is drained and the area lavaged locally with a combination of saline and antibiotics. In general, the more rapidly the orbital cellulitis responds to treatment, the better the prognosis for maintenance of vision. In the presence of extensive orbital swelling, diuretics are added to the parenteral antibiotics to reduce orbital edema and pressure on the globe. Topical antibiotics and, if necessary, mydriatics are indicated for the secondary iridocyclitis.

Exophthalmos may be associated with orbital neoplasms, which usually arise from adjacent periocular structures and the nasal and sinus cavities. Reported orbital neoplasms in the horse include lipoma, fibroma, squamous-cell carcinoma, fibrosarcoma, malignant melanoma, osteogenic sarcoma and malignant lymphoma. Although orbital neoplasms are rare in horses, orbital invasion by squamous-cell carcinoma from the nictitating membrane is the most frequent type. The clinical signs of orbital neoplasia are exophthalmos, strabismus, impaired globe motility and physical changes in the globe (Fig 14). Because of direct pressure on the globe, indentations of the ocular fundus and papilledema may be detectible by ophthalmoscopy. Tumors in the medial aspect of the orbit usually produce exotropia.

Enophthalmia

Enophthalmia results from reduction in orbital contents, including smaller than normal globes. Phthisis bulbi is common and is seen in 20-30% of horses presented for slaughter. Phthisis bulbi may result from trauma and prolonged or recurrent intraocular inflammation, with subsequent destruction of the ciliary body and ocular hypotony. Phthisis bulbi is evidenced by a small globe, protrusion of the nictitating membrane and a normal palpebral

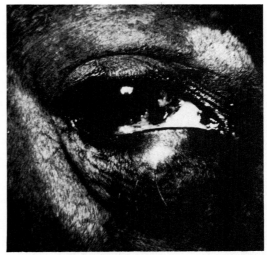
Fig 14. Involvement of the ventromedial orbit with malignant lymphoma.

fissure (Fig 15). Chronic mucopurulent or even follicular conjunctivitis may develop because of accumulation of material in the enlarged lacrimal lake between the eyelids and recessed globe. The cornea is usually vascularized, edematous and/or scarred and is translucent to completely opaque. The pupil is usually small and fixed, and cataracts may be present. There is no treatment for this condition.

Abnormally small globes occur in foals infrequently. The condition may be unilateral or bi-

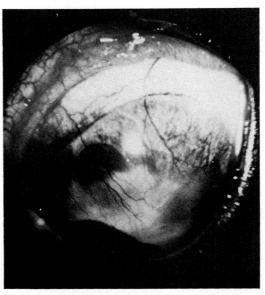
Fig 15. Phthisis bulbi (atrophy of the globe) secondary to corneal perforation.

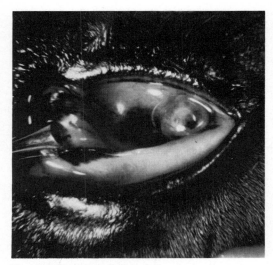

Fig 16. Microphthalmia in a foal.

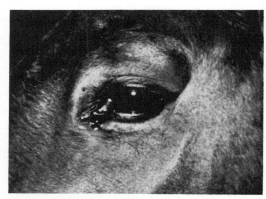

Fig 17. Horner's syndrome.

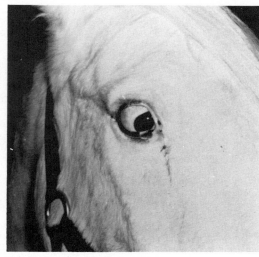

Fig 18. Convergent strabismus.

lateral and may vary from slightly smaller than normal globes to near anophthalmia.[36] Microphthalmia and congenital cataracts are the most frequent congenital anomalies in horses.[37] The condition is usually recognized in newborn foals, in which the palpebral fissure is usually smaller than normal and the nictitating membrane protrudes (Fig 16). Microphthalmia affects all breeds and has not been demonstrated as heritable in horses.

Horner's Syndrome

Another cause of enophthalmia is Horner's syndrome (see Chapter 21). Clinical signs of this sympathetic denervation of the eye and orbital tissues include ptosis, miosis, enophthalmia, hemilateral sweating (usually about the orbit and ear), and increased skin temperature of the affected facial, aural and cranial cervical region (Fig 17). It is important to recognize the subtle signs of Horner's syndrome. If accompanied by nasal exudates and especially hemorrhage, it may warrant examination of the guttural pouch.

Strabismus

Strabismus is rare in horses. In a survey of 5654 horses and mules, strabismus was detected only in mules at a frequency of 0.5% or 1 in 200.[4,5] Nearly all affected mules exhibited convergent strabismus (esotropia); the condition was not symmetric. Congenital strabismus also occurs in horses and is predominantly of the convergent type (Fig 18). Congenital strabismus was recently reported in Appaloosas, in which the condition is apparently congenital and exhibited by hypertropia (elevation of the globes dorsad).[41] Affected horses deviate the head as if to compensate for the abnormal visual axis, stumble and have a nervous temperament. In hypertropic Appaloosas, the condition is treated by surgical recession of the dorsal rectus muscle insertion or a combination of recession of the dorsal rectus muscle insertion and resection of the ventral rectus muscle insertion. Surgery results in rotation of the ocular axis to a more normal plane, and improves vision and behavior.

ORBITAL SURGERY

Surgical procedures of the orbit include orbitotomy, enucleation, exenteration and evisceration. Orbitotomy is surgical exploration of the retrobulbar space. Enucleation is excision of the globe from Tenon's capsule and is the most common orbital surgery performed in

horses. Exenteration is removal of the globe
and all orbital contents, and is reserved for extensive orbital neoplasia. Evisceration is removal of the lens, uveal tract, vitreous, retina
and occasionally the cornea, and insertion of a
prosthesis.

Enucleation

Enucleation is indicated in cases of phthisis
bulbi, with persistent conjunctivitis and pain,
absolute glaucoma, septic panophthalmitis,
extensive orbital and ocular trauma, with loss
of the globe's contents, and intraocular neoplasms. Enucleation is usually an elective procedure indicated when there is no possibility of
preserving the globe. The procedures for enucleation in horses are the subconjunctival and
the transpalpebral. In the subconjunctival
method, the globe is removed from Tenon's capsule through a limbal incision (Fig 19). In the
transpalpebral method, the bulbar, fornix and
palpebral conjunctivae, nictitating membrane
and globe are removed. The transpalpebral
procedure is especially useful for extensive
neoplasms of the cornea, conjunctiva and nictitating membrane.

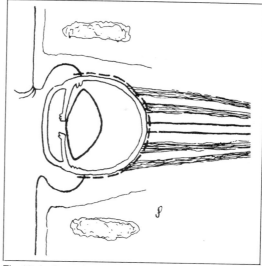

Fig 19. In the subconjunctival method of enucleation,
the incision is made between the sclera and bulbar
fascia (Tenon's capsule).

Enucleation is usually performed under halothane general anesthesia or after a combination of retrobulbar and palpebral nerve blocks
and the administration of IV chloral hydrate.
The latter method is not recommended because
of the advantages of recent refinements in inhalation anesthesia.

The eyelid hair is removed and the area is
scrubbed with surgical soap and water, and
rinsed with 0.9% sterile saline solution. After
the drapes are positioned, an eyelid speculum
retracts the eyelids and exposes the globe. The
nictitating membrane is grasped with serrated
thumb forceps and is protracted to expose its
base. Two heavy, curved hemostats, with their
tips slightly overlapping, are applied to the
membrane's base. Heavy, serrated scissors are
used to excise the nictitating membrane distal
to the hemostats, which are removed a few
minutes after resection. Hemorrhage from the
incision site is usually negligible.

The bulbar conjunctiva is incised with small
ophthalmic scissors near the limbus, usually
starting in the most exposed area and continuing for 360°. The globe is manipulated with
thumb forceps or a suture placed at the dorsolateral limbus. Dissection around the globe
separates Tenon's capsule from the sclera and
severs the extraocular muscle insertions. Hemostasis is controlled by carefully placed liga-

tures and electrocautery. The optic nerve and
surrounding posterior ciliary vasculature are
transected with heavy curved or enucleation
scissors for removal of the globe.

The edges of the bulbar conjunctiva are apposed with simple-interrupted or continuous 2-
0 chromic gut sutures. A penicillin solution is
injected through the bulbar conjunctiva into
the orbital space if infection was present or if
the area was contaminated during surgery.
The eyelid margins (the area where the hair
stops and the pigment begins) are incised for
360°, with special attention given to excision of
the proper amount at the medial canthus. The
eyelids are apposed with medium nonabsorbable synthetic sutures in a simple-interrupted
pattern.

In the transpalpebral method, the eyelids
are sutured shut or apposed with towel forceps.
The eyelids are incised at the junction of the
pigmentation and the beginning of the hair on
the eyelids. Dissection is continued 360° through
the lid substance to the palpebral conjunctival
submucosa and over the conjunctival fornices
(including the nictitating membrane) onto the
globe. The procedure continues in a similar
manner as described for the subconjunctival
method. Closure involves only the eyelids because the conjunctivae are excised.

Postoperative care after enucleation is usually minimal. Packing the orbit with sterile
surgical gauze or other material is not recommended. If infection occurs, the use of systemic

antibiotics is indicated for 5-7 days. Some hemorrhage may occur within the orbit from unligated blood vessels or following recovery from general anesthesia. If necessary, the orbit may be packed with ice to impede hemorrhage and swelling. Several months after enucleation, variable contraction of the orbital tissues results in a moderate, but not cosmetically unacceptable, concave appearance to the orbital rim and surface.

Use of orbital prostheses in horses has been investigated and may be indicated when cosmetic appearance is critical. Prostheses that replace the cornea and all ocular structures except the sclera have received only limited evaluation. The main adverse sequela is the development of infection between the prosthesis and the sclera, eventually resulting in extrusion of the implant. More recent ocular prostheses have been used in horses with moderate success and consist of a shell that is custom fitted over the existing phthisical and microphthalmic globes. The prosthesis is cosmetically acceptable, has a satisfactory retention rate, and seldom needs cleaning. The cooperation of an ophthalmic firm is necessary to acquire the proper size.

DISEASES OF THE EYELIDS

Congenital, traumatic and neoplastic lesions of the eyelids are common in horses. Reduction of the palpebral fissure size occurs infrequently, usually in conjunction with microphthalmia. Entropion, ectropion and dermoids occur occasionally in foals. When the conditions result in corneal and/or conjunctival damage, the eyelid anomaly should be corrected surgically.

Dermoids

Dermoids affect the eyelid margins, palpebral and bulbar conjunctivae, nictitating membrane and cornea. These congenital malformations are frequently pigmented and distinguished by large, coarse hairs on their surface. Dermoids should be excised and the resultant surgical defect repaired.

Entropion

Entropion in some foals may be managed medically for a few weeks with topical antibiotic ointments. In the process of rapid growth during the first few months of life, the eyelid defect gradually corrects itself. However, if irritation persists and the cornea is damaged, the entropion should be surgically corrected.

Surgical correction for entropion depends on the position and extent of the inversion, and if there is concurrent trauma and fibrosis.[42] Surgery is limited to the affected portion of the eyelid; the incision should be reasonably close to the eyelid margin to produce a normal contour and eliminate irritation. Entropion should not be overcorrected. The effects of postoperative scarring must be taken into consideration during surgery.

Entropion surgery is usually performed under inhalation anesthesia. The eyelid hair is removed and the surgical area is scrubbed with soap and water. Although many methods are available for the correction of entropion, the Holtz and Celsus procedures can be performed rapidly and provide satisfactory results. A section of skin and orbicularis oculi of the eyelids is excised, with the shape and extent of the excised section dependent on the position and severity of the entropion. Thumb forceps are positioned in the lateral canthus to elongate, straighten and provide tension on the eyelid for surgery. A Bard-Parker #15 scalpel blade is used to incise the eyelid skin and part of the thickness of the orbicularis oculi muscle. The eyelid skin and orbicularis oculi sections are separated and excised from the underlying poorly developed tarsus with a scalpel or ophthalmic scissors. Hemorrhage is controlled by hemostats or electrocautery; ligation of blood vessels is not recommended because ligatures may stimulate focal fibrosis. The skin and muscle are closed with simple-interrupted, medium nonabsorbable synthetic sutures.

Treatment after correction of entropion consists of ophthalmic antibiotic ointment applied 3-4 times daily for 7-10 days, after which time the sutures are removed. Success of the surgery can be evaluated in 4-6 weeks after healing is complete.

Eyelid Trauma

The eyelids of horses may be injured by foreign bodies, barbed wire, nails and other objects. Eyelid lacerations may be partial or complete, and vertical or horizontal to the eyelid margins. Lacerations of the eyelid margins are most important because they predominantly affect the cosmetic appearance and functional aspects of the eyelids. Although the eyelids are frequently lacerated, complete removal of eyelids is uncommon. Under most circumstances, correction of all eyelid lacerations is encouraged. Eyelid excision and excessive debridement of eyelid lacerations are not recommended because the eyelids are highly vascular and healing occurs even under the most difficult circumstances. Lacerations of the upper and lower eyelids usually involve the lateral half. Secondary blepharospasm may be so severe that an auriculopalpebral or other nerve block is necessary to examine the lacerated area and globe (Fig 20).

After administering a local anesthetic and tranquilizer, or a general anesthetic, the affected area is thoroughly cleaned with surgical soap and water, and liberally flushed with 0.9% sterile saline. The eyelid hair is removed by clippers or scissors and the area scrubbed again with surgical soap and water, and rinsed with 0.9% sterile saline. Because of the swelling of the lacerated area, 2 layers of sutures may be desirable for adequate apposition. The tarsoconjunctiva is apposed with simple-interrupted 2-0 chromic gut sutures that do not penetrate the palpebral conjunctiva. The outer muscle and eyelid skin layers are apposed with simple-interrupted, medium, nonabsorbable synthetic sutures. The eyelid margin should be slightly overcorrected or raised in the area of the laceration. After healing, this area usually becomes even with the remaining eyelid margin rather than notched. If the affected eyelid is retracted considerably, tarsorrhaphy is recommended to exert pressure from the opposite eyelid on the lacerated area.

Eyelid lacerations of several days' duration may be apposed in the same method described for acute lacerations. The edges of the wound are debrided minimally before apposition and closed in 2 layers. Incomplete or incorrect closure of eyelid lacerations may result in ectropion, entropion, exposure keratitis and cicatrix formation. Local malformations or defects may be corrected with blepharoplastic procedures described later in this section.

Systemic antibiotics are administered for several days after correction of eyelid lacerations. Topical antibiotics and, with excessive swelling, corticosteroids are also used. Corticosteroids do not appear to delay healing of the eyelids, perhaps because of vascularity of these structures. Topical and/or systemic corticosteroids may reduce eyelid swelling and pruritus. The horse may be cross-tied or have a neck cradle applied to prevent rubbing of the area.

Blepharospasm

Spastic contractions of the orbicularis oculi muscle are usually secondary to eyelid, conjunctival, corneal and intraocular irritation.

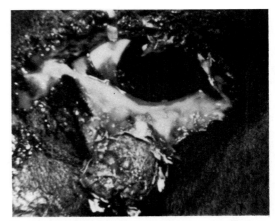

Fig 20. Lower eyelid laceration of 3 days' duration.

Blepharospasm associated with superficial ocular disease may be reduced for diagnostic reasons by instillation of topical anesthetics. However, prolonged use of topical anesthetics is not recommended because they reduce tear production, produce toxic changes in the corneal epithelium, and increase susceptibility of the cornea to self-inflicted trauma.

Blepharospasm associated with intraocular disease may be reduced diagnostically by the auriculopalpebral or other nerve blocks. The administration of mydriatics, such as atropine, produces iridocycloplegia. Spasms of the iridal sphincter and ciliary body musculature in intraocular inflammation appear to cause sufficient ocular pain to induce blepharospasm. Administration of atropine and other mydriatics markedly reduces pain and blepharospasm.

Blepharodermatitis

Eyelid inflammation is occasionally observed in horses with ringworm, eczema, mange or streptothricosis. Young horses are predominantly affected and the condition is treated in conjunction with the generalized skin disease.

Neoplasms

Eyelid neoplasms are common in horses and include predominantly squamous-cell carcinomas and sarcoids (fibrosarcoma and neurofibrosarcoma). Less frequently reported are fibroma, schwannoma, melanoma, mastocytoma, basal-cell carcinoma, adenoma, hemangiosarcoma and lymphosarcoma.[43-47]

Squamous-cell carcinoma is the most frequent ocular and periocular neoplasm in horses.[47-50] In a recent survey, 30% of all squamous-cell carcinomas affected the eye and its adnexa.[51] Squamous-cell carcinoma predomi-

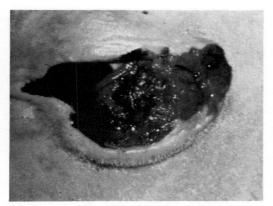

Fig 21. Squamous cell carcinoma of the lower eyelid and lateral canthus.

nantly affects older animals; average ages of affected horses are 8, 9.4 and 9.8 years. Squamous-cell carcinomas may occur more commonly in older white and palomino horses, however; additional studies are necessary for substantiation. Ocular squamous-cell carcinomas may affect the eyelids (20-30%), nictitating membrane (50-60%), and limbal area (20-30%).[47-50] Multiple lesions may occur within a single eye and associated adnexa, and 10-15% of affected horses have bilateral involvement. Squamous-cell carcinomas are locally invasive and have variable growth rates. They usually metastasize late in the disease; the metastatic rate ranges from 10-15%. Metastases in one study of affected horses involved the regional lymph nodes, salivary glands and thorax. Squamous-cell carcinomas of the nictitating membrane readily invade the orbit (Fig 21).

Squamous-cell carcinomas may be treated by surgical excision, radiation therapy or a combination of both. When radiation is the initial treatment, the mass should first be biopsied and examined microscopically to confirm the clinical diagnosis. Most squamous-cell carcinomas are reasonably sensitive to the various modes of radiation therapy and the predominant limiting factor to treatment is economics.[52-54] Surgical excision of squamous-cell carcinomas is commonly performed. When the nictitating membrane is involved, the structure is usually totally excised. With limbal squamous-cell carcinomas, the area is removed by superficial keratosclerectomy. The bulbar conjunctiva is reapposed to the limbus after tumor excision. Squamous-cell carcinomas infrequently invade intraocular tissues, necessitating enucleation. Excision of eyelid squamous-cell carcinomas requires repair of the surgical defect with blepharoplasty.

Equine sarcoids are locally aggressive subcutaneous tumors that may affect the eyelids.[55] They predominantly occur in younger horses (average age 4-5 years) and may involve multiple sites. Equine sarcoids recur one-third to one-half of the time following surgical excision, usually within 6 months of surgery. About one-third of all affected horses have multiple sarcoids. This apparently virus-induced tumor may depend on a delicate host-tumor relationship (Fig 22). The equine sarcoid is a subcutaneous tumor that affects predominantly the eyelids, rather than the conjunctiva and nictitating membrane. The tumor may proliferate through the skin as well as extend subcutaneously. The fascial layer of the eyelids connecting the tarsus to the orbital rim, ie, septum orbitale, is a reasonable tissue barrier to the extension of sarcoids into the orbit.

Treatment for equine sarcoid is by surgical excision, immunotherapy and cryotherapy. Equine sarcoids are not predictably sensitive to radiation therapy and that type of treatment is used infrequently. Surgical excision of equine sarcoids must involve a reasonably radical excision of the tumor and surrounding normal eyelid structures; the blepharoplastic procedures to reconstruct surgical defects are covered in the next section.

The variable surgical results and higher postoperative recurrence rate of equine sarcoids necessitate inclusion of other forms of therapy. Cryotherapy has been successfully employed in the treatment of this tumor.[57,58] Theoretically, ultracold therapy not only destroys neoplastic cells but also enhances host rejection of the tumor. Prior to cryotherapy, the affected area is prepared as for conventional surgery. At least 2 microthermocouple needles are positioned, one within the center of the tumor and one in the normal tissue lateral to the tumor margin or at its base. The normal surrounding tissues are covered with polystyrene plastic or Vaseline-impregnated gauze to minimize contact with the cryogen.

Cryotherapy involves liquid nitrogen sprayed onto or liquid nitrogen-cooled probes inserted directly into the mass. Recommended treatment includes 2 freezes in which the center of the tumor is lowered to -25 C (-13 F), with an interval between freezes to allow the tumor to attain pretreatment temperature. Two separate freezes are recommended to maximize tumor necrosis. The duration for freezing and thawing is directly influenced by the size and location of the mass. Tumor necrosis becomes apparent several days after cryotherapy. The mass becomes hyperemic and friable, exudates form on its surface, and it eventually sloughs. The healed surgical area is characterized by white hair and loss of pigment.

Immunotherapy has also been used to stimulate patient response to tumor-cell membrane antigens, causing rejection of the tumor. Use of autogenous and heterogenous vaccines for the treatment of equine squamous-cell carcinomas and sarcoids has yielded variable results. Of these 2 tumors, equine ocular sarcoid is particularly difficult to manage because of its usually low sensitivity to radiation and high recurrence rate (33-50%) within 3 years of excision. More recently, use of BCG vaccine (bacillus Calmette-Guérin), a potentiator of the cellular immune system, resulted in promising results for immunotherapy of equine ocular sarcoids.[56,59] Repeated intralesional injections (up to 4 times) of the vaccine produce remission of the tumor.

Sarcoids must be treated by radical excision and, if necessary, surgery and immunotherapy can be combined.

Blepharoplasty

Blepharoplastic procedures are used to reconstruct the eyelids following excision of neoplasms and cicatricial tissue to reasonably restore function and cosmetic appearance. These technics are used after removal of most extensive eyelid neoplasms without resorting to enucleation or exenteration. Squamous-cell carcinomas of the eyelids and palpebral conjunctiva are usually treated satisfactorily with blepharoplastic procedures. Surgery is occasionally combined with radiation therapy.

Blepharoplastic procedures include the sliding skin graft, tarsoconjunctival graft, whole-lid graft, pedicle skin graft, buccal graft for conjunctival defects, and combinations of these.[61] A sliding skin graft alone or combined with the tarsoconjunctival graft is used to repair most defects of the upper and lower eyelids and, with some modification, the lateral canthus. Repair of the medial canthal area requires pedicle skin grafts, tension-relieving incisions of the forehead skin, and sometimes autogenous skin grafts.

Blepharoplastic procedures usually provide optimal results for the lower eyelids because of the good resultant appearance and limited motility of those structures. The lower eyelids are

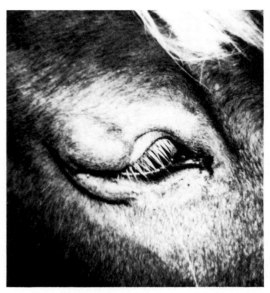

Fig 22. Sarcoid of the upper eyelid and lateral canthus.

a limited donor source for the upper eyelids; they do not have cilia. Whole eyelid grafts are used to restore lower lid defects by transplanting part of the upper lid.

The upper eyelid is the more mobile of the eyelids and has the greater effect on appearance. Function of the upper eyelids is absolutely essential for protection of the cornea and distribution of tears. The levator palpebrae superioris muscle is important in elevating the upper eyelids; severe damage produces ptosis.

The sliding skin graft is the basic blepharoplastic procedure.[60,61] The flap of skin is constructed slightly larger than the eyelid defect to compensate for cicatrization. Traction on the skin flap is minimized by adequate separation of the graft from the underlying subcutaneous tissue and, if necessary, countertraction with a temporary complete tarsorrhaphy.

Blepharoplastic procedures are usually performed under inhalation anesthesia. After clipping the eyelid hair, the area is washed with water and surgical soap. After draping, the neoplasm and 3-5 mm of adjacent normal eyelid are excised; hemorrhage is controlled by direct pressure and ligation (Fig 23a). The skin graft is then created by 2 slightly angled incisions twice the height of the defect. Angled incisions provide a graft slightly wider than the surgical defect (Fig 23b). Triangles of skin are excised at the base of the graft to prevent irregularities when the graft is moved into the defect. The skin graft is separated by blunt

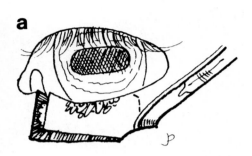

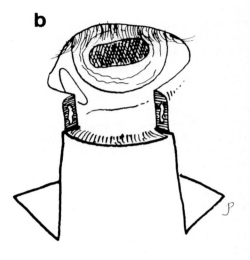

Fig 23a. Sliding skin graft. A full-thickness excision is made of the neoplasm in the lower eyelid.

Fig 23b. The length of the sliding skin graft is twice the height and slightly wider than the surgically created defect. Triangles of skin are excised to prevent irregularities in the skin when the graft is moved into the defect.

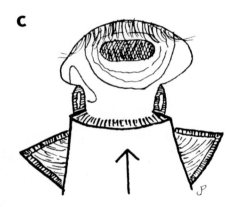

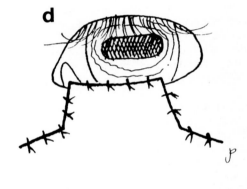

Fig 23c. The sliding skin graft is moved into the defect with minimal traction.

Fig 23d. The postoperative appearance of the sliding skin graft. The dorsal aspect of the skin graft is 2-3 mm above the adjacent eyelid margins.

dissection from the subcutaneous tissues to permit movement into the defect with minimal traction (Fig 23c). The graft is then shifted into the surgical defect until 2-3 mm of its free edge are above the adjacent eyelid margin. The graft and skin edges are apposed with simple-interrupted, medium, nonabsorbable synthetic sutures. The conjunctiva from the lower palpebral area and fornix is used to cover the bulbar (deep) portion of the skin graft; the conjunctiva is apposed with through-and-through sutures of 2-0 gut (Fig 23d).

Systemic and topical antibiotics are administered postoperatively for 7-10 days and a stockinette is applied to protect the eye between treatments. Both entropion and ectro-

pion occasionally occur after sliding skin grafts and usually result from inadequate separation of the graft from subcutaneous tissues.

Sliding skin grafts may be combined with tarsoconjunctival grafts following removal of extensive eyelid and conjunctival neoplasms. The sliding skin graft, as previously described, is constructed after the deeper tarsoconjunctival graft is completed and involves division of the opposite donor lid into tarsoconjunctiva and muscle-skin portions with an incision about 4 mm from the eyelid margin. The tarsoconjunctival graft is made similar to the skin graft but involves deeper tissues. It is slightly larger than the surgically created defect and is apposed with simple-interrupted absorbable sutures with the knots buried. The sliding skin graft is moved over the tarsoconjunctival graft and may involve the same lid or opposite lid, thereby providing opposing forces to minimize traction on the wound. Postoperative care after sliding skin and tarsoconjunctival grafts includes administration of systemic and topical antibiotics for 7-10 days; topical antibiotics are administered by the subpalpebral method. After 3 weeks the sutures are removed and the base of the tarsoconjunctival graft is excised. The defect in the donor eyelid is allowed to heal by secondary intention and the area is treated for an additional 2-3 weeks with a topical antibiotic-corticosteroid preparation.

Whole-eyelid grafts are used for treatment of broad but shallow defects of the lower eyelid. A portion of the upper eyelid can be rapidly transplanted to the lower lid to restore lower eyelid defects without adversely affecting the upper lid. A 10- to 15-mm strip of the upper eyelid margin containing the cilia is avoided to prevent adverse cosmetic results.

DISEASES OF THE NASOLACRIMAL AND TEAR SYSTEM

The nasolacrimal apparatus drains tears from the eye to the nose. The upper and lower lacrimal puncta are approximately 2 mm in diameter and about 8 mm from the medial canthus in the upper and lower eyelids. The respective canaliculi extend from each punctum and consolidate to form a poorly developed nasolacrimal sac. The nasolacrimal duct extends from the base of the sac and is reduced in diameter in its passage within the maxillary bone. It emerges in the turbinates with a prominent dilation at the level of the first premolar tooth and empties at the mucocutaneous junction of the nostril.

Diseases of the nasolacrimal apparatus usually result from obstructions at the base of the nasolacrimal sac and within the nasolacrimal duct. Congenital obstructions of the nasolacrimal duct in foals are usually associated with agenesis of the rostral portion a few centimeters caudal to its normal orifice at the mucocutaneous junction.[62,63] Affected foals have persistent epiphora that may not be detected until several months of age. Examination of the floor of the nostril reveals no nasolacrimal orifice (Fig 24). Passage of stiff nylon suture material from the upper punctum may help de-

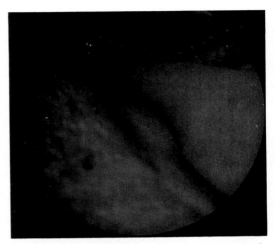

Fig 24. Congenital obstruction of the distal nasolacrimal duct in a foal associated with agenesis.

tect the most rostral extension of the nasolacrimal duct. A nasolacrimal flush through the upper punctum reveals the obstruction and may permit detection of fluid in its most rostral portion, which is frequently dilated.

Dacryocystorhinography can also be performed easily in foals under short-acting IV barbiturate anesthesia. Approximately 4-6 ml 40% iodinized poppyseed oil is injected through the upper lacrimal punctum, and lateral and oblique lateral radiographs of the skull are obtained. This procedure outlines the entire nasolacrimal apparatus and reveals any obstruction of the nasolacrimal duct. In most instances, the obstruction involves agenesis of the distal nasolacrimal duct and surgery can be performed through the nostril. With a small polyethylene tubing originating at the upper punctum in place, an incision is made directly over the anticipated distal opening of the nasolacrimal duct. If possible, the mucosa of the nasolacrimal duct is apposed to the nasal mucosa by simple-interrupted 4-0 chromic gut sutures. If the mucous membranes cannot be apposed, which is often the case, an indwelling catheter is positioned in the nasolacrimal apparatus for 3-6 weeks. Polyethylene tubing may be used for this purpose and footplates are constructed by heating both ends to retain the catheter with little chance of dislodgement. Topical antibiotic-corticosteroid preparations instilled in the eye egress down the nasolacrimal duct and do not significantly impair healing. If the agenesis is within the nasal cavity, construction of alternate drainage pathways might be considered into the maxillary sinus.

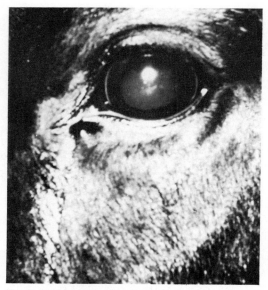

Fig 25. Epiphora due to nasolacrimal obstruction.

Nasolacrimal duct obstructions in adult horses are usually associated with conjunctivitis. Common clinical signs include persistent or intermittent epiphora and recurrent conjunctivitis (Fig 25). It is usually impossible to determine if the nasolacrimal obstruction was primary or secondary to the conjunctivitis. Once nasolacrimal obstruction develops, medical treatment of the conjunctivitis is unsuccessful until patency of the nasolacrimal apparatus is re-established. Obstruction of the nasolacrimal apparatus is usually at the base of the nasolacrimal sac or within the nasolacrimal duct by inflammatory cells, foreign material and inflammation of the duct. Fluorescein instilled in each eye simultaneously reveals the obstruction.

Once obstruction has been determined by lack of fluorescein passage, a retrograde nasolacrimal flush is performed from the nostril or alternatively through the upper punctum. The obstruction can be removed by forceful flushing with sterile 0.9% saline. If the system cannot be flushed by either route, the contents of the apparatus should be analyzed for crystals. Dacryoliths have been encountered in horses and require the use of various solutions, such as 0.5-1% edetate disodium (EDTA), to dissolve the crystals. After re-establishment of patency, the eye is treated topically for several days with antibiotic-corticosteroid solutions. Use of ophthalmic ointments after nasolacrimal flushing is not recommended because the base may reobstruct the nasolacrimal system.

Sinus and nasal neoplasms occur infrequently in horses. However, they may directly or indirectly affect the nasolacrimal apparatus and produce epiphora. Dacryocystorhinography may be used to determine the site of obstruction and facilitate determination of the presence and size of the neoplasm.

Tears are secreted by the lacrimal gland, gland of the nictitating membrane, Meibomian glands and the conjunctival goblet cells. The rate of aqueous tear production has been measured using the standard Schirmer tear test for humans, as well as a special modified test with #41 Whatman filter paper.[64,65] Deficiencies in tear production result in keratoconjunctivitis sicca. This condition is rare in horses and occurs predominantly after trauma.[66] The effects of reduced tear production are usually temporary. Damage to the cornea and conjunctiva can be minimized by frequent instillations of collyria, or artificial tear preparations and topical antibiotics.

DISEASES OF THE NICTITATING MEMBRANE

The nictitating membrane is a large appendix of the conjunctiva, an important protector of the eye and source of tears. The leading margin of the nictitating membrane is usually pigmented and lies immediately above the distal extension of the nictitating membrane cartilage. The caruncle is located at the base of the nictitating membrane at the junction of the upper and lower eyelids at the medial canthus. The caruncle has no useful function and is a raised 4- to 8-mm mass. It may be pigmented or nonpigmented and small, short hairs frequently arise from its surface.

Habronemiasis

Squamous-cell carcinomas and granulomas associated with *Habronema* spp may affect the caruncle. Horses in parts of the southern US are affected more frequently with the granulomas than with the tumors.[67] However, distinction between these 2 lesions may be difficult clinically and may require microscopic examination. *Habronema* granulomas on microscopic analysis may not include parts of the parasite; the predominating inflammatory cell is the eosinophil.

Habronema granulomas are treated topically with antibiotic-corticosteroid preparations and 0.025% isoflurophate ointment (Floropryl: Merck). The latter contains an organophosphate that kills the parasite. Large lesions can be reduced in size by cryotherapy, followed by topical treatment with the drugs mentioned above. Large lesions have also been treated experimentally by intralesional injection of 2-3 ml fenthion (Talodex: Diamond).

Congenital Anomalies

Congenital abnormalities of the nictitating membrane are rare in horses. The nictitating membrane may be hypoplastic, usually associated with microphthalmia. The nictitating membrane may also have adhesions to the bulbar conjunctiva, thereby limiting its movement. The adhesions appear to form prenatally and may represent failure of separation between the bulbar conjunctiva and the nictitating membrane or prenatal inflammation of these structures.

Protrusion

The nictitating membrane is concurrently affected in most conjunctival inflammations. Protrusion occurs commonly with tetanus and is associated with contraction of the retractor oculi muscles. Protrusion of the nictitating membrane is also common with severe ocular pain associated with corneal and intraocular diseases. The nictitating membrane often protrudes in phthisis bulbi or atrophy of the globe after extensive trauma and/or inflammation.

Trauma

The nictitating membrane is frequently affected by trauma. Minor injuries usually require only topical antibiotics to prevent secondary infection. Defects in the leading margin of the nictitating membrane do not usually necessitate surgical intervention unless the exposed cartilage contacts the cornea.

Neoplasia

Neoplasms of the nictitating membrane include adenoma, adenocarcinoma, malignant melanoma, chondroma and, most frequently, squamous-cell carcinoma. In several reports, the ratio of squamous-cell carcinoma incidence to that of all other lesions of the nictitating membrane is about 9:1 (Fig 26). Malignant tumors must be distinguished from hyperplasia and hypertrophy of the nictitating membrane and parasitic granulomas. Malignant neoplasms of the nictitating membrane are treated by local excision. Total excision of the structure is recommended with extensive involvement of both anterior and posterior aspects of the nictitating membrane by malignant neoplasms.

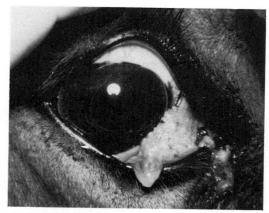

Fig 26. Squamous cell carcinoma of the nictitating membrane.

Total excision is preferred if the cartilage of the nictitans is involved and eroded by neoplasia. Local excision, with preservation of the nictitating membrane, is possible when the neoplasm extends from only the anterior surface of the nictitating membrane and can be easily elevated from the submucosa of this structure. Invasion of the orbit by squamous-cell carcinoma of the nictitating membrane occurs more readily than when this neoplasm originates from other conjunctival sites. Malignant tumors may be treated by surgery or radiation therapy. Radon implants are quite effectively used to treat squamous-cell carcinoma of the nictitating membrane.

Surgery of the Nictitating Membrane

Surgical procedures of the nictitating membrane include partial or complete excision because of neoplastic involvement, and use of the membrane as a patch for the treatment of corneal diseases. Surgery of the nictitating membrane may be performed after administration of a sedative and infiltration of local anesthetic at the base of the structure. Alternatively, surgery may be performed under short-acting IV barbiturate or inhalation anesthesia.

Tumors limited to the anterior surface of the membrane can often be excised without removal of the entire nictitans. The tumor margins must be accurately defined and the mass gently elevated from the submucosa of the nictitating membrane by infiltration of saline or local anesthetic beneath the mass. Small neoplasms can be removed with thumb forceps and curved scissors. The wound is allowed to heal by secondary intention. Development of excessive granulation is infrequent. Postoperative care consists of topical antibiotic-corticosteroid

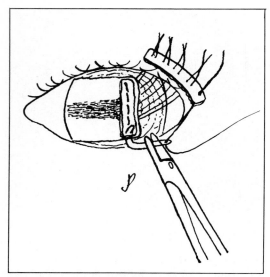

Fig 27. The nictitating membrane may be used to cover the weakened cornea. It is sutured to the dorsolateral eyelid with interrupted mattress sutures over rubber band stents.

preparations applied 2-4 times daily. Total excision of the nictitating membrane is accomplished by protraction of the structure as far as possible and excision at its base with heavy, serrated scissors. Hemostasis is achieved by electrocautery and/or direct pressure.

A nictitating membrane flap provides support to a cornea weakened by ulceration and partial thickness corneal lacerations, and after corneal surgery. The membrane may be sutured to either the dorsolateral conjunctival cul-de-sac and eyelid, or to the dorsolateral bulbar conjunctiva and episclera. The procedure is usually performed with short-acting IV barbiturate or inhalation anesthesia. Succinylcholine should not be used for restraint in horses with weakened corneas because it produces rapid, marked increase in intraocular pressure and it is not a general anesthetic. If deep corneal ulceration is present, perforation may occur if intraocular pressure is rapidly elevated by marked contraction of the extraocular muscles.

The nictitating membrane is attached to the upper eyelid and conjunctival cul-de-sac with 4-5 interrupted mattress sutures of medium nonabsorbable synthetic material. Intravenous drip tubing or a wide, flat rubber-band stent is used to distribute suture tension on both the nictitating membrane and eyelids (Fig 27). The flap is usually left in place 7-10 days, which is usually sufficient time for heal-

ing of corneal wounds. The nictitating membrane flap in horses is not as useful as in small animals because the larger structure in horses cannot be adequately maintained for more than 7-10 days. Tearing of sutures and/or the leading margin of the nictitating membrane may occur when this flap is used.

DISEASES OF THE CONJUNCTIVA

The conjunctiva is divided clinically into palpebral, fornix and bulbar parts. The palpebral conjunctiva forms the deep aspects of the eyelids and adheres rather tightly to the structures. The bulbar conjunctiva covers the distance between the fornix and the limbus, and is reasonably thin and moveable over the adjacent episclera. The ventral conjunctiva tends to be more hyperemic and contains more lymphoid follicles than its dorsal counterpart.

Congenital Lesions

Congenital abnormalities of the conjunctiva occur infrequently in horses and are usually exhibited as dermoids. The dermoids may span the conjunctiva, eyelid margin, nictitating membrane and cornea, and are treated by excision. The conjunctival wound is usually apposed to prevent formation of excessive granulation tissue, and the adherence and even migration of bulbar conjunctiva onto the corneal wound.

Conjunctivitis

Conjunctivitis is one of the more common ocular conditions seen in horses. The conjunctivitides are classified as acute, subacute and chronic, primary and secondary, and by the type of conjunctival exudate, ie, serous, mucous and purulent.

Primary conjunctivitis has been associated with *Moraxella* spp and the parasite *Thelazia californiensis*. The nonhemolytic diplobacillus *Moraxella* is similar but not identical to *M bovis*.[68] Swelling of the eyelids, hyperemia and inflammation of the conjunctiva, mucopurulent conjunctival exudates, and erosion of the eyelid margins characterize *Moraxella* conjunctivitis. Topical antibiotics effectively control the condition.

Conjunctivitis associated with *Thelazia californiensis* is characterized by chronicity, numerous lymphoid follicles, and seromucoid conjunctival exudates.[69] Under topical anesthesia, the white nematode (0.25 × 20 mm) may be located and removed by forceps. The

ventral bulbar conjunctival fornix and deep
fornix of the nictitating membrane should be
closely inspected to ensure total removal of the
parasites. Topical instillation of an anticholin-
esterase miotic, such as 0.25% demecarium
bromide (Humorsol: Merck), facilitates identification of the nematodes by inducing their
rapid movement and kills the parasites. *Thelazia californiensis* is distributed across the US
and is not limited to western states.

Secondary conjunctivitides are associated
with other ocular and systemic diseases.
Embedded foreign bodies result in mucopurulent conjunctivitis, blepharospasm and moderate pain. Treatment of the conjunctivitis is
successful only after identification and removal of the foreign body. Dust, dirt, microphthalmia, phthisis bulbi and nasolacrimal
obstructions result in secondary conjunctivitis.
Because of bacterial involvement, conjunctival
exudates are usually mucopurulent. Successful treatment of secondary conjunctivitides depends on removal of the primary cause.

Secondary conjunctivitides occur frequently
with systemic bacterial and viral conditions.
Equine influenza and rhinopneumonitis may
cause serous conjunctivitis that can become
mucopurulent with secondary bacterial infection. Equine viral arteritis is characterized by
palpebral edema, mucopurulent conjunctivitis,
photophobia, epiphora, keratitis and iridocyclitis. Strangles may cause mucopurulent conjunctivitis, hypopyon and iridocyclitis. Conjunctival abnormalities may also occur in various hemorrhagic conditions, such as anemia
and enterotoxemia.

Treatment of acute primary conjunctivitides
is usually by instillation of antibiotics and corticosteroids 4-6 times daily for 7-10 days; the
response is usually good. Chronic conjunctivitides respond more slowly to medication and
may require treatment for 4-6 weeks. Bacterial
culture and sensitivity tests are indicated to
facilitate proper choice of antibiotics for treatment of severe, chronic conjunctivitides.

Trauma

Trauma to the palpebral and bulbar conjunctiva is not uncommon and may be associated
with similar damage to the eyelids and globe.
Small conjunctival injuries are usually medicated with only topical antibiotics and heal by
secondary intention. Large conjunctival lacerations are usually repaired in association with
treatment of eyelid and globe injuries.

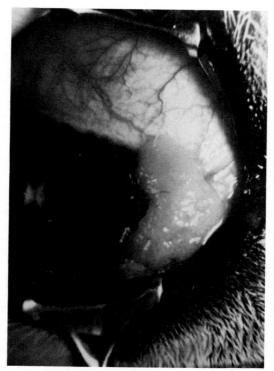

Fig 28. Squamous cell carcinoma of the dorsolateral
bulbar conjunctiva.

Neoplasia

Conjunctival neoplasms in horses include
squamous-cell carcinoma, sarcoid (fibrosarcoma and neurofibrosarcoma), adenocarcinoma, papilloma, lipoma, malignant melanoma
and others. The most common conjunctival
neoplasm is squamous-cell carcinoma, which
predominantly affects older horses. The most
common site of involvement is the dorsolateral
bulbar conjunctiva (Fig 28). Small conjunctival
tumors are usually satisfactorily treated by local excision. Excision involves the episclera
and/or cornea if necessary. Large conjunctival
defects resulting from excision of these tumors
are corrected with buccal mucous membrane
autografts. Squamous-cell carcinoma of the
conjunctiva may also be treated by radiation
therapy and cryotherapy.

Conjunctival flaps have been used infrequently in horses and may be adapted from
types used in small animals. The equine bulbar
conjunctiva is thin and quite friable, and usually tears under tension. Two useful types of
conjunctival flaps include the half-hood bulbar
conjunctival flap and the bridge conjunctival
flap. In both methods the bulbar conjunctiva is

sutured directly to the cornea to adequately position the flap over the weakened cornea. The bulbar conjunctiva adheres to the corneal defect over which it is sutured. The support offered by these conjunctival grafts is reasonable. Corneoscleral transposition is an alternative method in which adjacent cornea is moved into the weakened corneal ulcer site; this method is described in detail in the corneal ulcer section.

Conjunctival flaps are performed under short-acting IV barbiturate or inhalation anesthesia. The eyelids and cornea are prepared for aseptic surgery. For the half-hood bulbar conjunctival flap, the conjunctiva is incised 180° at the limbus in the region closest to the ulcer. The conjunctiva is separated from the deeper episclera by sharp-blunt scissor dissection. The bulbar conjunctiva is moved to the ulcerated area and secured by several 4-0 chromic collagen or other absorbable sutures apposing the leading margin to the cornea.

The bridge bulbar conjunctival flap is useful for treatment of ulcers of the central cornea. The bridge conjunctival flap is prepared using a strip of bulbar conjunctiva from the dorsolateral area, with both ends attached to the medial and lateral conjunctiva. This strip of bulbar conjunctiva should be at least 1½-2 cm wide to ensure vitality. The conjunctiva is moved into position and sutured to the cornea on its dorsal and ventral aspects; sutures are removed in 14-21 days. If the bridge bulbar conjunctival flap is too thin, the central area becomes necrotic from inadequate perfusion.

With both types of conjunctival flap, the conjunctiva is trimmed from the ulcer site 2-3 weeks after placement. The bulbar conjunctiva adheres to the ulcer site, thereby filling weakened corneal facets. The resultant leukoma is not unusually dense and is preferable to a perforated ulcer and anterior synechia. Topical antibiotics and corticosteroids are administered for 4-6 weeks to minimize corneal scarring after the flap is trimmed from the cornea.

DISEASES OF THE CORNEA

The cornea in normal adult horses measures 26-28 mm vertically and 32-38 mm horizontally.[9] The radius of curvature of the normal adult equine cornea is approximately 17 mm. Corneal thickness is quite variable but relatively thin for the globe size; its center is thinnest and may be as little as 0.56 mm thick. The equine cornea is affected by several specific diseases and by those of the external and periocu-

lar tissues, iris and ciliary body. Diseases of the cornea may be congenital, traumatic, inflammatory, degenerative or neoplastic.

Congenital Anomalies

Congenital abnormalities of the cornea include microcornea, melanosis, dermoids and iridocorneal angle anomalies. Microcornea usually occurs in conjunction with microphthalmia. However, reasonably normal-sized globes with corneas measuring less than 10 mm in diameter have been observed in a few foals and weanlings with visual impairment.

Congenital melanosis rarely affects the equine cornea. Pigmentation is usually central and involves the corneal epithelium and superficial anterior stroma. Neovascularization of the cornea is usually present, although the vessels may appear as ghost vessels by biomicroscopy. The pigmented area is usually present at birth or shortly thereafter and does not usually progress. Because foals are born with their eyelids open, corneal melanosis may result from intrauterine influences. The condition is treated successfully by superficial keratectomy.

Thin linear and band opacities occasionally occur in foals. These corneal lesions are apparently due to a thin, dense membrane; inflammatory sequelae are not usually evident. The anomaly is not progressive and the opacities are apparently due to edema immediately anterior to the defective Descemet's membrane.

Congenital iridocorneal angle anomalies occasionally affect the lateral and medial aspects of the limbal cornea. Slight opacities in this area are due to the more central attachments of pectinate ligaments from the base of the iris to Descemet's membrane. Congenital peripheral corneal opacities must be distinguished from those associated with peripheral anterior synechiae secondary to anterior segment inflammations. Congenital corneal opacities and angle anomalies do not progress and apparently do not predispose the horse to glaucoma.

Congenital dermoids sometimes affect foals and may be unilateral or bilateral. The ventral and lateral aspects of the cornea are most frequently affected. The dermoid may extend onto the adjacent bulbar conjunctiva, and infrequently to the nictitating membrane and palpebral conjunctiva. Dermoids are usually pigmented and must be distinguished from malignant melanomas. The surface of a dermoid is usually smooth and covered with long, irritating hairs. Although dermoids may be removed in foals by superficial keratectomy, some corneal scarring may persist. Because of

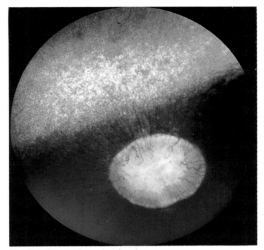

Fig C1. Normal ocular fundus.

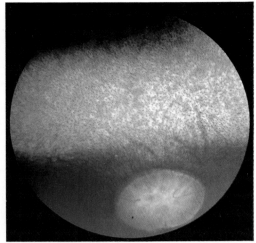

Fig C2. Normal ocular fundus of an aged horse.

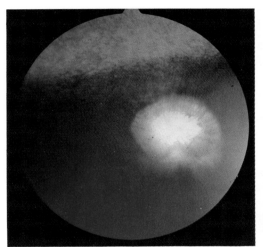

Fig C3. Normal ocular fundus with myelinization of the ventral optic nerve head.

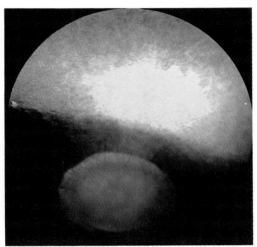

Fig C4. Normal ocular fundus with partial albinism of the tapetal and nontapetal fundi.

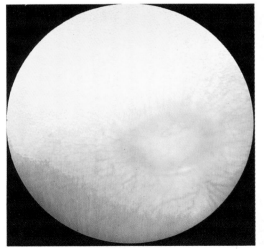

Fig C5. Normal albino ocular fundus.

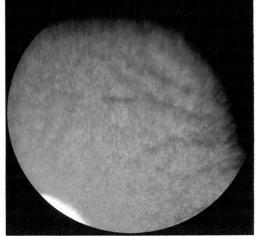

Fig C6. Converging pigment zones in the tapetal fundus indicating the exit of a vortex vein.

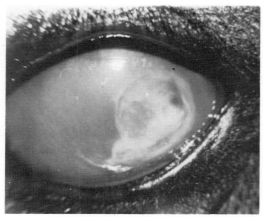

Fig 29. Corneal ulcer associated with *Pseudomonas aeruginosa* infection.

the tendency of the equine cornea to scar after superficial keratectomy, use of postoperative topical and, if necessary, subconjunctival corticosteroids is indicated once the surgical wound has epithelialized. Epithelialization of the corneal wound is ascertained by lack of fluorescein retention. If the dermoid extends from the cornea to the conjunctiva, the adjacent bulbar conjunctiva should be sutured to the limbus following excision to prevent sliding or migration onto the cornea and subsequent symblepharon formation. Histologically, dermoids have the same structures as normal eyelids.

Trauma and Ulceration

The horse, because of its nature and relatively susceptible and exposed eye, is predisposed to trauma to the cornea. Damage may be caused by blunt trauma, secondary corneal ulceration, foreign bodies and incomplete to complete corneal lacerations. Blunt corneal trauma may cause focal areas of corneal edema, and irregular and usually temporary breaks in Descemet's membrane associated with corneal indentation. Hyphema and secondary iridocyclitis may also occur concurrently. Management of this process is covered in the section on alterations of the aqueous humor.

Most corneal ulcers appear secondary to trauma, with subsequent bacterial and/or fungal involvement (Fig 29). Clinical signs of corneal ulceration include blepharospasm, epiphora, lacrimation, hyperemia and chemosis of the conjunctiva, conjunctivitis and secondary iridocyclitis. Corneal ulceration is determined by retention of topically applied fluorescein. The cornea does not normally re-

tain fluorescein because of its lipid-selective corneal epithelial barrier. If corneal epithelium is removed traumatically, fluorescein retention is detected by the use of cobalt blue or ultraviolet light. The central cornea is most frequently traumatized. Secondary bacterial and infrequently fungal infection may occur if the corneal lesion is not treated, if specific antibiotics are not administered or if the insult is treated with corticosteroids. Small traumatic lesions usually involve only the loss of corneal epithelium. These defects heal in 24-72 hours by local mitosis and migration of adjacent corneal epithelium.

Deeper traumatic corneal ulcers involving loss of epithelium and anterior stroma usually stimulate corneal neovascularization, which is exhibited by ingrowth of superficial branching vessels originating from the limbus. These blood vessels grow at the rate of 1-3 mm daily. Inflammatory cell and infrequently pigment cell infiltration may accompany neovascularization. Migration and mitosis of corneal epithelium seal the corneal barrier, and local fibroblastic activity within the stroma fills the defect. Stromal regeneration to fill the corneal facet and eventually restore the area to the normal curvature may require several weeks with deep corneal ulceration. The corneal epithelium is thicker than normal in these areas. Once the corneal ulcer has healed and the stroma is remodeled, neovascularization gradually recedes. However, these blood vessels can usually be detected by biomicroscopy as ghost vessels for months to years thereafter. In the event of additional trauma or ulceration to the cornea, the ghost vessels become rapidly patent and complete vascularization of the cornea occurs within a few days. Progression of corneal ulcers to Descemet's membrane is indicated as a clear area at the base of the ulcer that does not retain fluorescein (Fig 30). These ulcers frequently leak aqueous humor, which is indicated by the ventral flow of fluorescein from the corneal ulcer. Full-thickness corneal ulcerations cause rapid anterior movement of the iris and loss of aqueous humor through the ulcer. The incarcerated iris prolapse usually rapidly seals the corneal ulcer; intraocular pressure is restored but is subnormal. The amount of iris prolapsed depends on the size of the corneal defect. Panophthalmitis occurs only infrequently after corneal ulcer perforation, perhaps because of the continual outward seepage of aqueous humor through the early perforation and infiltration of the anterior segment of the eye with large numbers of inflammatory cells.

Clinical management of corneal ulceration is influenced by size, position, depth and duration of the ulcer, economics, temperament of the horse and the occasional necessity for surgical reinforcement of the weakened cornea by nictitating membrane and conjunctival flaps, tarsorrhaphy and corneoscleral transposition. Because of the ocular pain and irritation associated with these ulcers, the use of subpalpebral medication systems is often imperative. Unusually intense and chronic corneal ulcerations should be analyzed clinically by culture of the corneal defect before and after instillation of topical anesthetic and scraping the ulcer margins to detect possible bacterial and/or fungal involvement. Superficial corneal ulcers are usually treated by instillation of topical antibiotics and mydriatics 4-8 times daily. Antibiotics particularly effective in horses include neomycin-polymyxin B-bacitracin, chloramphenicol-polymyxin B, and gentamicin. These antibiotics possess broad antibacterial properties, including activity against *Pseudomonas* spp.[70] Mydriatics, such as 1-3% atropine, minimize pain associated with secondary iridocyclitis and dilate the pupil to minimize the possibility of posterior synechiae.

Deep corneal ulcerations require vigorous therapy and daily, if not more frequent, observation to determine ulcer progression or regression. In addition to antibiotics and mydriatics, use of 5% acetylcysteine (Mucomyst: Mead Johnson) should be considered to minimize damage from collagenase and/or other proteinases liberated by degenerating corneal tissues and certain bacteria, *eg, Pseudomonas* spp. Theoretically the excessive amount of collagenases in the corneal ulcer could cause progression of the ulcer in the absence of sepsis. Acetylcysteine must be prepared immediately before use and can only be refrigerated 1-2 weeks before it deteriorates, as evidenced by liberation of hydrogen sulfide.

Fulgal ulcers are rare in horses and usually associated with previous antibiotic-corticosteroid therapy.[71] Several fungal agents may be recovered from infected ulcers. Therapy of fungal ulcerations is difficult and requires specific antifungal drugs in addition to antibiotics to combat concurrent bacterial infections. Topical amphotericin B (1 mg/ml in distilled water) or 0.5% pimaricin (Natamycin:Alcon Laborato-

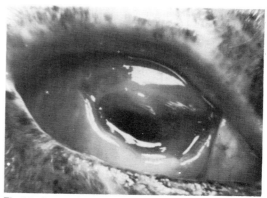

Fig 30. Central descemetocele.

ries) is effective in most fungal infections. Both drugs are relatively insoluble and have limited ability to penetrate the cornea.

Surgical intervention is essential if the corneal ulcer progresses or perforates. Deep corneal ulcers may be treated with bulbar conjunctival and nictitating membrane flaps, tarsorrhaphy and corneoscleral transposition. Surgical intervention should be initiated before perforation and iris prolapse occur, and requires IV barbiturate and/or inhalation anesthesia. The eyelids and external eye are prepared for surgery and the cornea is carefully cleaned with sterile dacron swabs or surgical cellulose sponges. At this time, bacterial and fungal culture of the ulceration should be performed (or repeated) to determine the reason for failure of medical therapy.

Tarsorrhaphy, and nictitating membrane and bulbar conjunctival flaps have been described in the previous section under conjunctiva and nictitating membrane. Corneoscleral transposition is a recently developed method for the treatment of corneal ulceration and involves sliding the superficial layers of adjacent cornea and sclera into the ulcerated area. The corneoscleral strip is sutured directly to the margins of the ulceration as well as the linear defect created in the adjacent conjunctiva. Use of simple-interrupted, two-thirds thickness sutures of 4-0 to 6-0 chromic collagen or other absorbable synthetic material is recommended. Movement of the sclera into the cornea results in gradual remodeling and minimal scar formation. Medical treatment after corneoscleral transposition is the same as for corneal ulceration. Suture removal is unnecessary because absorbable sutures are used.

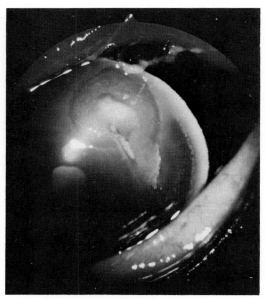

Fig 31. Partial-thickness corneal laceration following incomplete penetration by a foreign body.

Corneal ulcer therapy is continued until corneal epithelialization occurs, which is determined clinically by lack of fluorescein retention in the ulcer. Because corneal stroma regeneration is slow, initiation of topical, subconjunctival and systemic corticosteroid therapy should be delayed for several days to a few weeks. Once healing has occurred, as evidenced by regression of corneal neovascularization, corticosteroid therapy may commence to minimize corneal scarring. Affected eyes should be evaluated daily or every other day to detect any adverse effects or reulceration.

Chronic corneal ulceration occurs infrequently in horses and predominantly affects older animals. Chronic corneal ulceration in horses is fortunately superficial and perforation is unlikely as long as there is no secondary bacterial involvement. Cauterization of chronic corneal ulceration should be limited to topical application of a 3-5% aqueous iodine solution (USP) carefully manipulated on the corneal ulcer by sterile cotton or dacron swabs. Topical anesthesia and sedation may be necessary for chemical cauterization of chronic ulcers. The effect on the cornea is essentially that of "firing" and stimulates acute inflammation that eventually results in epithelialization of the ulcer. The use of broad-spectrum antibiotics and, if necessary, mydriatics is indicated following cauterization to ensure healing and prevent secondary infection.

Foreign Bodies

Foreign bodies infrequently injure and/or perforate the cornea. Thorns and splinters may partially or totally penetrate the cornea. Foreign bodies that completely penetrate the cornea may be removed by sedating the horse, applying local anesthesia or an auriculopalpebral nerve block, and using topical anesthesia on the cornea and conjunctiva. The foreign body is removed with thumb forceps or by vigorous flushing with collyria. The area should be gently scraped to remove all foreign material after removal of the main portion and treated with topical antibiotics 4-6 times daily. Mydriatics, such as 1-3% atropine combined if necessary with 10% phenylephrine, should also be used to combat secondary iridocyclitis.

If the foreign body has penetrated the cornea into the anterior chamber, it may be removed retrograde from its corneal site or through an adjacent limbal incision into the anterior chamber. The puncture site is closed with 4-0 to 6-0 chromic collagen or other synthetic absorbable suture placed through one-half to two-thirds the thickness of the cornea. The anterior chamber should be irrigated gently with a saline-potassium penicillin solution (1000-2000 IU/ml saline) to reduce the possibility of intraocular sepsis. Lavage of the cornea and anterior chamber with this mixture should be performed for 5-10 minutes and antibiotics should be administered systemically. If sepsis does not occur, the prognosis is usually good. The position and size of the resultant corneal scar also affect prognosis with regard to vision. Peripheral corneal trauma has less effect on vision than does central corneal trauma. The effects of secondary iridocyclitis and, occasionally, lens changes should also be considered.

Lacerations

Corneal lacerations occur most frequently in stallions and in ponies associated with children. Lacerations are usually classified as partial or full thickness (complete), puncture or linear, and peripheral or central.[72-74] Partial-thickness corneal lacerations are treated as contaminated corneal ulcers (Fig 31). If the corneal stroma is severely weakened, general anesthesia is used and the ulcer margins are apposed with 4-0 to 6-0 chromic collagen or other synthetic absorbable sutures placed through one-half to two-thirds the corneal thickness. Topical and systemic antibiotics, and mydriatics are administered 4-8 times daily for 1-2 weeks.

Puncture wounds of the cornea are treated similarly to corneal foreign bodies. The anterior chamber may be contaminated if the puncture is full thickness. Oval to round punctures may be sutured by alternating simple and horizontal mattress interrupted sutures. Although the postoperative cornea is markedly irregular, the globe may be saved. Small, paracentral puncture wounds may be corrected so that only a small corneal scar results and vision is preserved.

Corneal lacerations are usually full thickness and accompanied by iris prolapse. Extensive full-thickness lacerations may cause prolapse of the iris, ciliary body, lens and vitreous. Corneal laceration repair should be attempted since enucleation can be performed later if necessary. Most owners prefer the appearance of a shrunken globe to an absent one (Fig 32).

Signs of full-thickness corneal laceration include severe blepharospasm, lacrimation, epiphora, corneal edema, intraocular hemorrhage, collapsed anterior chamber and an obvious grey-yellow mass (prolapsed iris) protruding through the cornea. The prognosis depends on the temperament of the horse, duration, extent and site of the laceration, ease of surgical correction, involvement and possible loss of other intraocular structures, and postoperative complications. Corneal lacerations with associated iris prolapse of 1-12 hours' duration should be corrected by surgical intervention. Corneal lacerations with associated iris prolapse of several days' duration may be treated conservatively with a nictitating membrane flap or tarsorrhaphy. The result in cases of the latter type is a large adherent leukoma and not infrequently phthisis bulbi. A recently prolapsed iris can be safely replaced in the eye or excised with sharp iris scissors or electrocautery. The edges of corneal defect are apposed by simple-and/or horizontal-interrupted 4-0 to 6-0 chromic collagen or other synthetic absorbable sutures placed through one-half to two-thirds the corneal thickness. Integrity of the closure is tested by injection of saline and air into the anterior chamber through the wound or at the limbus with a cyclodialysis needle. The air bubble in the anterior chamber reduces the possibility of postoperative iridocorneal adhesions.

Postoperative treatment consists of mydriatics, systemic corticosteroids and large doses of topical and systemic antibiotics. Systemic corticosteroids should be administered because intraocular inflammation is usually severe. The

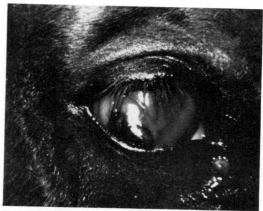

Fig 32. Full-thickness corneal laceration with iris prolapse.

need for vigorous topical medication requires the use of subpalpebral systems. The palpebral fissure is usually left open to permit daily inspection and, if necessary, changes in therapy.

Scars

Corneal scars are common in horses, especially following ulceration and trauma.[75] Prognosis is influenced by the size, position and depth of the corneal opacity, involvement of other tissues (most commonly adherence of iris), and contributing factors, such as ocular hypotony. If the corneal scar is large, central and reasonably dense, vision may be markedly impaired or absent. Many superficial corneal scars from trauma or healed ulcers gradually regress over several months. This process may be enhanced by the intermittent instillation of corticosteroids. After about a year, many corneal scars are detectible only by very close scrutiny of the cornea with light and some degree of magnification. Superficial central corneal scars that persist longer than 6 months may be removed by superficial keratectomy. However, the scar should be vigorously treated for 4-6 weeks with topical antibiotics and corticosteroids prior to excision. Neovascularization within the corneal scar indicates continued remodeling of the area. Surgical excision of the scar tissue should be delayed until such vessels regress.

Superficial keratectomy is indicated for the removal of superficial corneal scars, corneal and limbal neoplasms, dermoids, pigmentation and superficial dystrophy, and involves the removal of the corneal epithelium and anterior stroma in the affected area. General anesthesia is usually indicated.

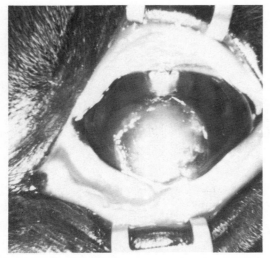

Fig 33. The postoperative appearance of the cornea after superficial keratectomy to remove a superficial central leukoma.

The eyelids and external eye are prepared for aseptic surgery. The lids are retracted by speculum or sutures and the globe stabilized by forceps or sutures. The periphery of the corneal lesion is incised with a #15 Bard-Parker or #64 Beaver scalpel blade held perpendicular to the cornea. A fine gritty texture is evident as the stromal tissue is incised. The edge of the corneal lesion is elevated with mouse-tooth forceps and the superficial stroma is excised with the scalpel held tangential to the cornea. Dissection within the corneal lamellae is continued to excise the lesion. The sterile corneal wound is treated as an ulcer with topical antibiotics and, if necessary, mydriatics. Once the

defect has epithelialized (fluorescein is no longer retained), an antibiotic-corticosteroid preparation is instilled for 2-4 weeks to minimize corneal scarring (Fig 33).

Corneal opacities associated with adherent leukomas (previous corneal perforations with iris prolapse) result in dense bluish-white scars not amenable to superficial keratectomy. If cosmetic improvement of a dense corneal leukoma and associated iris incarceration is necessary, the resultant corneal opacity may be tattooed black with a combination of platinum chloride and hydrazine after the outer layers of the cornea are removed by superficial keratectomy. Following corneal tattooing, the area is treated for several days as one would a corneal ulcer.

Corneal opacification may also be associated with glaucoma and the ocular hypotony associated with phthisis bulbi. A hypotonic cornea is characterized by neovascularization and linear irregularities representing folds in Descemet's membrane; there is no treatment. The corneal opacification associated with glaucoma is diffuse edema that dissipates once intraocular pressure returns to normal.

Degeneration

Corneal degeneration occurs rarely in horses; 2 distinct types have been noted. Peripheral, dense white corneal deposits occur infrequently and are usually accompanied by superficial corneal neovascularization. The abnormality may occur in diseased or apparently normal eyes. The chemical nature of the white deposits has not been determined but they may be a lipid (Fig 34).

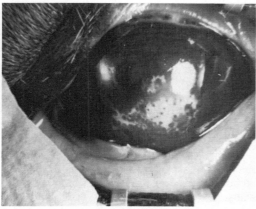

Fig 34. Superficial corneal degeneration. Note the white deposits of possible lipid material in the corneal stroma.

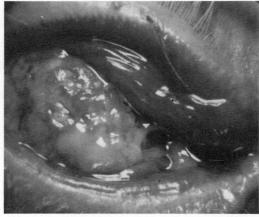

Fig 35. Squamous cell carcinoma of the cornea of an aged mare.

Punctate keratopathy occurs occasionally and is characterized by small, distinct, irregular lesions distributed throughout the anterior corneal stroma. These lesions may represent focal degeneration of the stroma, local cellular infiltration and the presence of *Onchocerca* larvae. Microscopic examination of corneas with punctate keratopathy has not been possible. Affected corneas do not retain fluorescein but may retain rose bengal stain.

Horizontal corneal irregularities, especially those of the ventral half, may occasionally be detected in horses during ophthalmoscopy and slit-lamp biomicroscopy. These corneal irregularities are apparently due to the uneven thickness of the corneal stroma and may be bilateral. These irregularities may cause astigmatism. Their cause is unknown.

Neoplasia

Corneal neoplasms are rare in horses.[76] Most arise at the limbus or from the adjacent bulbar conjunctiva. Papillomas and limbal squamous-cell carcinomas occur in horses. Local excision by keratosclerectomy is possible with limited corneal neoplasms. Enucleation should be considered if the eye cannot be adequately examined or intraocular infiltration by the neoplasm is apparent. Focal limbal squamous-cell carcinomas may also respond to treatment with radon implants. Preservation of the globe and, occasionally, maintenance of vision are possible if the lesion is excised (Fig 35).

ALTERATIONS IN THE AQUEOUS HUMOR

Changes in the aqueous humor result from trauma, inflammation, parasites and neoplasms. Although studies of the components of the equine aqueous humor have not been reported, the normal protein level is 15-30 mg/dl. Normal aqueous humor is optically clear. Increases in protein content and/or inflammatory cell numbers reduce that clarity and produce the Tyndall phenomenon. This phenomenon may be observed when a focused beam of light is directed from the lateral aspect of the eye and viewed frontally as it crosses the cloudy aqueous humor within the anterior chamber. Most changes in aqueous humor result from diseases of the anterior segment.

The earliest change in aqueous humor associated with anterior segment inflammation consists of elevated protein levels and inflammatory cell numbers. This phenomenon is referred to as aqueous flare and clinically is graded from +1 to +4 in severity. As the aqueous flare becomes more intense, it may result in hypopyon or the accumulation of purulent material in the ventral aspects of the anterior chamber. Hypopyon usually results from massive exudation of inflammatory cells from the iris and ciliary body into the aqueous humor. It appears as a light-yellow, irregular mass in the ventral anterior chamber and usually adheres to the ventral cornea and/or anterior iris. Other signs of iridocyclitis are also present. Hypopyon is usually aseptic and culture of the aqueous humor does not yield bacteria unless the cornea has been perforated or it is a young horse with terminal bacteremia. Culture of equine aqueous humor for viruses has not been reported.

Treatment of hypopyon is directed toward correction of the underlying iridocyclitis. Topical mydriatics, antibiotics and corticosteroids are administered to reduce anterior segment inflammation and associated exudation of proteins and inflammatory cells into the aqueous humor. Corticosteroids may also be administered subconjunctivally and systemically. Systemic antibiotics are also indicated in the presence of fever and/or leukocytosis. Removal of hypopyon by aspiration or irrigation of the anterior chamber is not advised unless intraocular pressure is increased by the condition. The secondary or plasmoid aqueous humor produced after anterior chamber paracentesis contains extremely high levels of proteins and fibrin. The resultant clot after anterior chamber paracentesis may be more extensive than before the procedure.

Parasites that may be found within the anterior chamber include immature stages of *Setaria digitata* and *Dirofilaria immitis*. The natural host for *S digitata* may be cattle and, in unnatural hosts such as the horse, immature parasites occasionally migrate to the anterior chamber. Treatment for *S digitata* infection of the anterior chamber can be medical (diethylcarbamazine) and/or surgical removal of the parasite.[77,78]

Traumatic hyphema occasionally occurs in horses, usually from blows to the head and eye.[79] The prognosis in traumatic hyphema in horses is guarded, which is in contrast to other species. Signs of iridocyclitis may be concurrent and include corneal edema, miosis, hypotony, blepharospasm, lacrimation, epiphora and photophobia. Traumatic hyphema is characterized by excessive amounts of fibrin, from iridocyclitis, that rapidly clots and gravitates

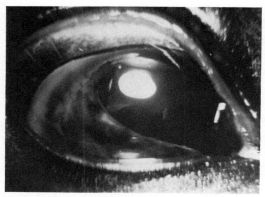

Fig 36. Fibrous membrane adhering to the iris and lateral peripheral cornea associated with previous hyphema and iridocyclitis.

ventrad. Other lesions of the iris, lens, vitreous and ocular fundus may also occur but usually cannot be detected until most of the hyphema has disappeared. In contrast to other species, horses may require 4-6 weeks for resorption of hyphema. Treatment is continued until intraocular inflammation and hyphema disappear.

Treatment for traumatic hyphema is directed at the underlying iridocyclitis. Hemorrhage within the anterior chamber seems to persist longer in horses than in other species. This may be related to the entrapment of RBC by fibrin in the aqueous humor. Persistence of fibrin may be related to its continued production by the inflamed anterior uvea and delayed breakdown related to possible changes in fibrinolysin. Reduction in aqueous fibrin facilitates the egress of RBC predominantly through the iridocorneal angle and reduces the tendency for fibropupillary membrane formation. Topical administration of mydriatics is indicated for the iridocyclitis. Mydriasis in horses with hyphema does not usually produce increased intraocular pressure. For the first 2 days, 10% phenylephrine is instilled at least 6 times daily. This sympathomimetic mydriatic produces mild mydriasis and vasoconstriction, which help stop intraocular hemorrhage. Once the hyphema has clotted, an additional parasympatholytic mydriatic, such as atropine, homatropine or cyclopentolate, should be instilled. The frequency of treatment is gradually reduced as the inflammation subsides. Corticosteroids are administered topically, subconjunctivally and parenterally to temper the iridocyclitis and reduce fibrin formation within the aqueous humor.

Several sequelae may follow traumatic hyphema and iridocyclitis. Fibrin in the aqueous humor may gradually remodel to become persistent fibropupillary membranes, resulting in cataracts and corneal leukomas. These bands usually attach the anterior surface of the iris to the caudal aspects of the cornea or the anterior lens capsule, and may cross the pupil to obstruct vision (Fig 36). Surgical removal of these bands may be necessary if vision is lost; however, the membranes are extremely strong and there are frequently concurrent corneal and/or lenticular pathologic changes. Corneal edema may result from direct trauma to the cornea, attachment of the fibropupillary membranes and formation of peripheral anterior synechiae. Phthisis bulbi may occur with destruction of the ciliary body.

Glaucoma

Glaucoma is rare in horses and usually associated with iridocorneal congenital anomalies, trauma or anterior uveal inflammation.[80,81] Lens luxation may occur in young animals subsequent to trauma or as a sequela to uveal inflammation, and may aggravate glaucoma. Rupture of the anterior hyaloid membrane associated with lens luxation and herniation of vitreous in the pupil may result in acute pupillary-block glaucoma.

Hydrophthalmos or buphthalmos is not as extensive in adult horses as other species. Enlargement of the globe is common in foals. Subluxation and anterior or posterior lens luxation also occur in horses. Most forms of glaucoma result from iridocorneal angle pathologic changes and lens luxations are probably secondary to the glaucomatous process.

Signs of glaucoma must be distinguished from iridocyclitis. Mydriasis, corneal edema, episcleral congestion, mild blepharospasm and a pale, slightly cupped optic nerve head characterize glaucoma. Intraocular pressure may be transiently elevated in early uveal inflammation; however, hypotony occurs as the disease progresses. Glaucoma secondary to uveal inflammation occurs infrequently and is probably related to extensive destruction of outflow pathways.

Treatment of glaucoma involves use of long-acting miotics to improve aqueous humor outflow through normal channels. Removal of displaced lenses may facilitate control of intraocular pressure by medical therapy and perhaps improve vision.

DISEASES OF THE IRIS AND CILIARY BODY

The irides of most adult horses are dark brown. The pupil is nearly circular in foals and during the first few weeks of life becomes oval and its long axis horizontal.[82] Light-induced pupillary reflexes are incomplete and sluggish in the first few weeks of life. The iris sphincter and dilator muscles are arranged differently in horses than in other species; the pupil constricts predominantly in the vertical axis rather than equally in all directions. Iridal dilator muscles are poorly developed in the lateral and medial aspects. In the dorsal and, to a lesser extent, ventral pupillary margins are dark-brown, irregular nodular structures called corpora nigra (granula iridis). The corpora nigra apparently facilitate pupillary function and increase effectiveness of the oval pupil by restricting passage of light. Although the ciliary body is not detectible clinically, its peripheral rostral aspects can be examined by gonioscopy. The iridal vasculature is composed of 3 arcades in the peripheral, central and pupillary margin areas. Incision and excision of the normal iris can be achieved with negligible hemorrhage; however, an inflamed iris may hemorrhage profusely after surgery.

Congenital Anomalies

Iridal congenital anomalies include pigmentation, hyperplasia of the corpora nigra, aniridia and persistent pupillary membranes. Heterochromia irides occurs infrequently in horses. Colors of the iris in heterochromia are usually combinations of brown, white and blue. Heterochromia may exist in one or both eyes and part or all of the iris ("walleye" or albinismus partialis). When the iris is nearly white with only pigmentation of the corpora nigra, the heterochromia is referred to as "glass eye" (albinismus totalis). Heterochromia is most frequently observed in white, spotted, palomino, Appaloosa and chestnut horses. Ocular conditions associated with heterochromia irides in horses have not been reported; in fact, the presence of heterochromia in horses is associated with a reduced frequency of recurrent uveal inflammation (Fig 37).

Heterochromia irides may also be inherited in white horses as the autosomal gene W that is lethal in homozygotes. Heterozygotes have pink skin and white coats, manes, tails and hooves, with occasional small spots of black in

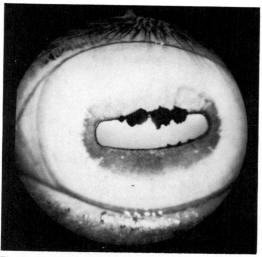

Fig 37. Heterochromia iridis (albinismus totalis).

the skin and hooves. Irides of these white horses may be pale blue, dark blue, brown or hazel. The fundic reflection may be red, associated with reduced pigmentation of the non-tapetal fundus.[83]

Hyperplasia of the corpora nigrum occurs infrequently. The structure may become exceedingly large and interfere with vision during bright sunlight. Affected horses may exhibit visual impairment and shyness. The condition is treated by careful excision of the corpora nigrum by aspiration or forceps.

Aniridia with associated cataracts is inherited as an autosomal dominant trait in Belgian horses. Clinical signs include a nearly absent iris and cataracts of varying types, positions and maturity. Vision in affected horses is usually poor or absent.[84]

Inflammation

Inflammation of the iris, ciliary body and choroid may be secondary to trauma, associated with systemic viral and bacterial diseases, or associated with anterior segment conditions, such as those of the cornea, lens-induced uveitis, and recurrent uveitis.[85,86] The first 3 types have been discussed in earlier sections. Lens-induced uveitis follows trauma and leakage of lens material, and extracapsular cataract surgery. Reaction of the equine eye to normal lens material is mild but more intense to cataractous lens material, especially from those that progress to hypermaturity. Surgery for cataracts in these cases requires vigorous medication to control the severe iridocyclitis.

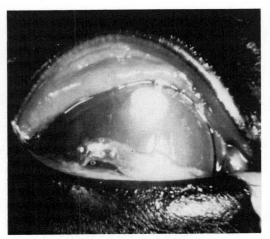

Fig 38. *Leptospira*-related recurrent uveitis.

Recurrent Uveitis

Equine recurrent uveitis is the most common intraocular disease complex of horses. The disease may occur in as much as 10% of the horse population. Recurrent uveitis has also been called recurrent iridocyclitis, moonblindness, periodic ophthalmia and recurrent iridocyclochoroiditis. The disease predominantly affects horses over 4 years of age and always affects both eyes of horses with brown irides. The severity of and time interval between attacks are quite variable. Stallions, geldings and mares are equally affected. This disease is not understood despite a reasonable amount of investigation. Results of recent investigations have divided recurrent uveal inflammations into at least 2 types with specific causes: recurrent uveal inflammation related to *Leptospira* and recurrent keratouveal inflammation related to *Onchocerca cervicalis*. However, there are undoubtedly other causes of recurrent uveal inflammation. Streptococcal infections warrant serious study. Recent advances in microbiology, ophthalmic pathology and immunology have made the feasibility of a comprehensive study of this disease complex more likely.

In 1947 a large number of horses with recurrent uveal inflammation exhibited high titers to *Leptospira*.[87] *Leptospira* titers in aqueous humor may be low in the initial few days of an attack and rise later. Aqueous humor titers to *Leptospira* in horses with relapses or chronic inflammations may be higher than those in the serum. Serum *Leptospira* agglutination titers of recently affected horses may be higher than those of the aqueous humor. Positive serologic reactions to the different *Leptospira* spp occur

in the serum of 70-95% of horses with recurrent uveitis and in 10-15% of apparently normal horses; however, detailed ophthalmic examinations in surveys of apparently normal horses were not reported.

The exact role of *Leptospira* in the pathogenesis of recurrent uveitis is not totally understood.[87-100] Horses with leptospirosis may have bilateral panuveitis and the virulent organism may be obtained from the aqueous humor. The early clinical signs may be missed in some horses initially exposed to *Leptospira*. Chronic and recurrent uveitis resulted after experimental ponies and horses were injected with *Leptospira*. Uveal inflammation was apparent 12-24 months after the acute illness.

Leptospira may also persist for a short period within the eye, presumably intracellularly. Perhaps an immune-mediated chronic inflammation is initiated after the initial exposure of the uveal tissues to *Leptospira*. Persistence of the organism within the uveal tract alters the response of ocular tissues to foreign antigens and results in persistent inflammation. Although clinically apparent attacks occur at irregular intervals, from a microscopic standpoint *Leptospira*-related uveitis is chronic and progressive. The confirmed presence of immunoglobulins within the iris and ciliary body of *Leptospira*-related recurrent uveitis patients supports the theory that this disease is, in part, an immune-mediated process.

Clinical signs of *Leptospira*-related recurrent uveitis are predominantly those of anterior segment inflammation. The entire uveal tract, including the choroid, is involved; however, the anterior segment inflammation may mask posterior segment changes. Clinical signs include lacrimation, blepharospasm, palpebral and bulbar conjunctival hyperemia (ciliary flush), miosis, ocular hypotony and photophobia. Corneal edema may occur within the first 2-3 days. An initial aqueous flare may progress to frank hypopyon; inflammatory cells and exudates may accumulate within the pupil and on the anterior lens capsule. The periphery of the cornea is invaded by deep and superficial corneal vessels. Posterior synechiae may develop within the first week (Fig 38).

Cataract formation involving the anterior and posterior cortices may develop. Cataracts associated with posterior synechiae affect the anterior lens capsule and underlying anterior cortex. Those of the caudal cortex are usually within the visual axis. Progression of these cataracts is influenced by the severity, length and number of recurrent attacks. The vitreous humor may become infiltrated with inflammatory cells and cyclitic membranes develop. Inflammatory cells within the vitreous may be evident in several days to a few weeks but require several months to exit. Vitreous syneresis (liquefaction) and formation of distinct strands may also occur (Fig 39).

Circumpapillary chorioditis, chorioretinitis and chorioretinoneuritis may occur. The initial lesion is inflammation and translucency of the retina adjacent to the optic nerve head. When these lesions become chronic, there is reduced pigmentation and pigment proliferation in the choroid and retina about the optic nerve head. The optic disc may also undergo segmental or complete atrophy in the inflamed area.

Retinal detachments may be associated with vitreous degeneration and lack of support by the formed vitreous, as well as subretinal exudates. Phthisis bulbi may eventually occur due to destruction of the ciliary body, resulting in ocular hypotony. Reduced eye size results in enophthalmia. The upper eyelids may develop an obvious notch associated with reduced globe size and orbital contents.

Leptospira-related recurrent uveitis may appear quiescent between clinical attacks; however, microscopic examination invariably reveals foci of inflammation in the uveal tract. Occasionally the veterinarian is asked to examine for soundness horses with *Leptospira*-related recurrent uveitis in periods of quiescence. Sequelae of uveitis are usually detectible. The iris may be less than a rich brown and slightly pigmented to grey. The corpora nigra are usually atrophied and occasionally absent. Small, brown deposits of iridal tissue, representing old posterior synechiae, may be present on the anterior lens capsule. Posterior synechiae, and anterior and posterior cataract formation may be evident. Fundic lesions of circumpapillary chorioretinopathy or chorioretinoneuropathy may be present. Vision may be adversely affected, depending on involvement of ocular tissues and the optic nerve (Fig 40).

The prognosis for *Leptospira*-related recurrent uveitis is poor but perhaps is not as unfavorable as previously reported. Prognosis is determined by severity of the inflammation, presence of ocular damage from previous attacks, and intraocular pressure. Ocular hypotony occurs with active recurrent uveitis; however, intraocular pressure should be reasonably normal between attacks provided the ciliary body has not been severely damaged. If

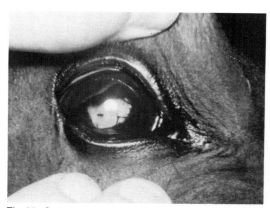

Fig 39. Complete mature cataract with posterior synechiae secondary to recurrent uveitis.

ocular hypotony is present but the presence of overt ocular inflammation cannot be ascertained, severe ciliary body damage has occurred. *Leptospira* titers should be monitored between attacks. Relapses occur at intervals as short as a few weeks to as long as several months to years later. Although variable, subsequent attacks are usually less severe.

Treatment for *Leptospira*-related recurrent uveitis consists of application of mydriatics to prevent synechia formation and suppression of uveal inflammation. Mydriatics, such as 1-3% atropine and 10% phenylephrine, are instilled hourly or 2-6 times daily until mydriasis results and 2-3 times daily thereafter. Fresh posterior synechiae frequently may be broken by

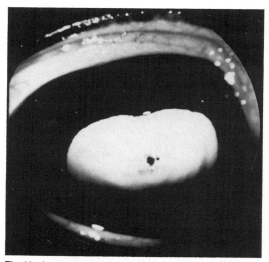

Fig 40. Appearance of the eye between recurrent uveitis attacks. Note the complete loss of the corpora nigrum and deposits of iridal tissues on the anterior lens capsule.

intensive mydriatic therapy; however, some iridal tissue may remain on the anterior lens capsule. Affected horses should be stabled in a darkened area to facilitate treatment and production of physiologic mydriasis. Placement of an affected animal in a bright environment usually results in severe blepharospasm and photophobia, and the animal usually instinctively seeks shade.

Topical, subconjunctival and systemic corticosteroids are administered to reduce uveal inflammation. A topical neomycin, polymyxin B and 0.1% dexamethasone preparation (Maxitrol: Alcon Laboratories) is administered 4-6 times daily. The subconjunctival corticosteroid of choice is methylprednisolone (Depo-Medrol: Upjohn); from 10-20 mg per site are injected into the dorsolateral bulbar subconjunctiva. This preparation provides anti-inflammatory activity for 7-10 days. Dexamethasone (5-20 mg) may also be mixed with the feed.

Systemic antibiotics are not usually administered unless leukocytosis or fever is present. Penicillin-dihydrostreptomycin administered in standard doses may be effective in horses with systemic signs of leptospirosis. Treatment by injection of foreign protein has been reported for this condition but is not recommended because large doses of exogenous corticosteroids provide more rapid anti-inflammatory activity when treatment must be vigorous. Also, the adverse reactions associated with foreign protein injections are avoided. The use of riboflavin and antihistamines is ineffective for this disease.

Prognosis in *Leptospira*-related recurrent uveitis is also influenced by the rapidity of the response to medical therapy and the prevention of undesirable sequelae, such as synechiae and cataract formation. The long-term use of systemic corticosteroids has been evaluated on a limited scale in horses with *Leptospira*-related recurrent uveitis. Because past studies indicated active uveal inflammation microscopically despite clinical quiescence, systemic corticosteroids may be used twice weekly to minimize and possibly prevent future clinical attacks. The doses of systemic corticosteroids required to effectively reduce microscopic ocular inflammation and minimize adverse effects of these drugs have not been ascertained.

Onchocerciasis

Ocular onchocerciasis was first reported in horses in 1939 when microfilariae of *Onchocerca cervicalis* were recovered from the eye of a horse with uveitis.[101] Subsequently several investigators observed the microfilariae of *O cervicalis* in eyes with recurrent uveitis.[102-107] Other investigators noted *O cervicalis* microfilariae occasionally may be observed in microscopically normal eyes and their relationship to the recurrent inflammation is incidental. However, the consensus of investigators dealing with this disease is that equine ocular onchocerciasis is a distinct type of recurrent uveitis incited by dying microfilariae within ocular tissues.

Onchocerca cervicalis is a white, thread-like worm living within the fibers of the ligamentum nuchae. The female is 30 cm by 400μ and the male 7 cm by 100μ. Microfilariae from the female migrate to the subcutis, where they are ingested by a midge, *Culicoides nubeculosus*, in which they develop to the infective stage in about 25 days. Infective microfilariae infect the horse subsequent to the bite of the midge. Ocular involvement with these migrating microfilariae appears to be coincidental. Microfilariae may enter the skin of the eyelids enroute to subcutaneous areas, predominantly in the ventral body. They may migrate into the palpebral conjunctiva and eventually to the limbus to enter the cornea and intraocular tissues. Migration of the microfilariae within the posterior and even anterior uvea may also be associated with hematogenous migration of the parasites. Clinical signs of equine ocular onchocerciasis vary from acute to chronic panuveitis, which may appear predominantly as recurrent anterior uveitis. The disease may also cause distinct limbal nodules, peripapillary patches of choroidal sclerosis, chorioretinopathy, chorioretinoneuropathy and skin lesions.

Horses with ocular onchocerciasis may have concurrent *Leptospira* titers in the serum and aqueous humor. Most affected horses are *Leptospira* negative. The microfilariae may be detected clinically by biopsy of the ventral to lateral bulbar conjunctiva, eyelid skin and skin of the ventral sternal area. Active microfilariae may be harvested by placing biopsy specimens in saline solution for 10-30 minutes. The supernatant of this preparation is filtered through a 5-μ millipore filter and stained with buffered Wright's stain. Conjunctival, corneal, eyelid and skin biopsies may also be fixed in 10% buffered formalin and examined by routine microscopy. The *O cervicalis* microfilariae are 60-70μ long, with a round head and pointed tail. With Wright's stain they have black dots over their entire body. Examination of micro-

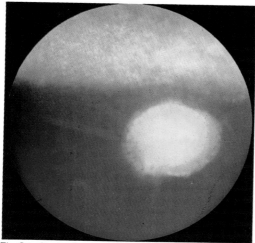

Fig C7. Ocular fundus with acute recurrent uveitis.

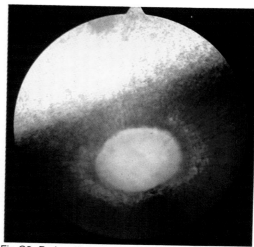

Fig C8. Peripupillary chorioretinopathy associated with recurrent uveitis.

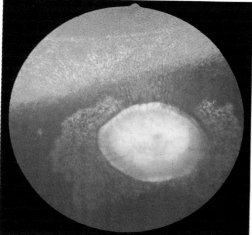

Fig C9. Extensive chorioretinopathy associated with recurrent uveitis.

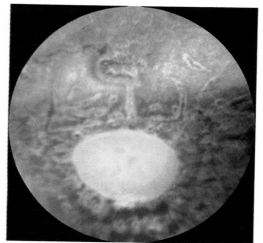

Fig C10. Chorioretinoneuropathy associated with extensive hemorrhage and trauma.

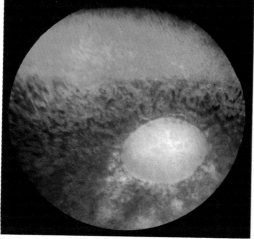

Fig C11. Retinal degeneration and optic nerve atrophy.

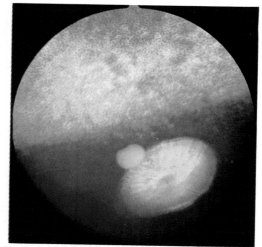

Fig C12. Astrocytoma of the peripheral optic nerve head.

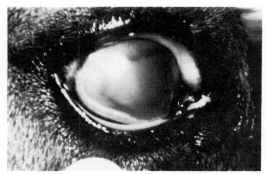

Fig 41. Recurrent keratouveitis associated with *On-chocerca cervicalis* microfilariae.

scopically positive biopsy specimens reveals mild to marked perivascular mononuclear inflammatory cell infiltration, with scattered eosinophils. The *O cervicalis* microfilariae may be observed in crossed, oblique and transverse sections.

Ocular onchocerciasis may appear clinically as acute and chronic inflammation, often coexistent within the same eye. The most distinguishing sign of *O cervicalis*-related uveitis is keratouveitis (Fig 41). Common signs of uveitis include epiphora, photophobia, blepharospasm, ocular hypotony and conjunctivitis. Small superficial, subepithelial white opacities 0.5-1 mm in diameter may occur within the cornea, usually near the lateral limbus. The adjacent bulbar conjunctiva may be hyperemic and chemotic. The iris may be inflamed and hypopyon may involve part of the anterior chamber. Pupillary and cyclitic membranes, posterior synechiae and cataracts may form. Active choroiditis or chorioretinitis may occur about the

optic nerve head, exhibited as multiple irregular, white foci.

Chronic ocular onchocerciasis also frequently has distinguishing clinical signs. Follicular conjunctivitis is frequently present as a characteristic change in the lateral bulbar region. Multiple small (0.5- to 1-mm), white nodules may appear on the surface of the lateral bulbar conjunctiva in contrast to the surrounding pigmentation. There may also be variably sized areas of focal vitiligo in the bulbar conjunctiva near the lateral limbus. The cornea may exhibit interstitial keratitis, with edema, deep neovascularization, pigmentation and disciform to linear opacities. A wedge-shaped area of sclerosing keratitis at the lateral limbus is especially noteworthy. The anterior chamber in the chronic inflammation may contain fibrin, inflammatory cells and infrequently microfilariae. Chronic iridal changes include focal areas of atrophy, increased pigmentation and posterior synechiae. Pupillary and cyclitic membranes are common. The lens is cataractous and frequently displaced from its patellar fossa. Circumpapillary lesions of the choroid, retina and optic nerve head also frequently occur. Alterations in the optic nerve vessels may occur.

Treatment of ocular onchocerciasis consists of administration of the microfilaricide diethylcarbamazine (Cypip: American Cyanamid), corticosteroids and mydriatics. Administration of diethylcarbamazine (2 mg/lb SID for 21 days) is avoided until the active uveitis is adequately controlled. Mydriatics, such as 1-3% atropine and 10% phenylephrine, induce pupillary dilation and minimize formation of posterior synechiae. These drugs are instilled as frequently as necessary to induce and maintain a widely dilated pupil. The use of topical, subconjunctival and systemic corticosteroids reduces the uveal response to the dying microfilariae. Once the active ocular inflammation is suppressed and clinical signs cease, diethylcarbamazine may be administered to kill the microfilariae. Diethylcarbamazine does not kill adult *Onchocerca* within the ligamentum nuchae; therefore, its effects are temporary. The administration of diethylcarbamazine throughout the summer months or quarterly to suppress microfilarial populations should be considered for affected horses.

Cysts

Iridal cysts may occur within the body of the equine iris and in the corpora nigra. Cysts of

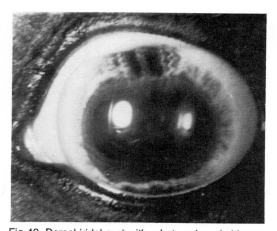

Fig 42. Dorsal iridal cyst with a heterochromic iris.

the iridal pigmented epithelium have been observed most frequently in ponies with heterochromia irides but also in ponies with brown irides.[108] The cysts may be bilateral or unilateral. Because the cysts are usually hollow, transillumination of the structures is usually possible. The cysts are evidenced clinically as focal enlargement of the iris which, after mydriasis, may markedly distort the pupillary aperture (Fig 42). The cysts may rupture spontaneously with intensive mydriatic therapy. The cause of iridal cysts in horses is unknown but may be congenital or associated with iridal atrophy. Treatment consists of removal of a small portion of the anterior wall. Spontaneous rupture of the cyst facilitates normal pupillary activity.

Neoplasia

Neoplasms of the iris and ciliary body are rare in horses.[109] Sarcoma, malignant melanoma and adenocarcinoma of the equine iris have been reported. Several cases of ciliary-body medulloepithelioma have been reported.[44,110] Malignant melanoma and sarcoid may also affect the choroid. Although uveal neoplasms are rare in horses, one should be highly suspicious of neoplasia in eyes with ocular inflammations that do not respond to intensive therapy, in glaucomatous eyes, and in eyes with overt pigmented or nonpigmented masses.

DISEASES OF THE LENS

The biconvex crystalline lens occupies the patellar fossa bounded anteriorly by the pupil, iris and posterior chamber, and posteriorly by the vitreous. The diameter of the normal adult equine lens is about 22 mm and the anteroposterior thickness is 11-12 mm. The volume of the normal adult lens is slightly more than 3 ml.[9] The anterior lens capsule is 60-90μ thick and the posterior capsule is 10-16μ thick. Nuclear sclerosis gradually occurs with aging and is evidenced as prominent refractive differences between the nucleus and cortex. As the horse becomes quite old, the lens becomes bluish; this should not be confused with cataract formation. The lens reacts to insult by death of cells and lens fibers, formation of opacities and occasional proliferation of the anterior lens epithelium.

Cataracts

Cataracts may be classified according to anatomic position within the lens (anterior capsule, anterior cortex, nucleus, posterior cortex, posterior capsule; axial and equatorial), by ma-

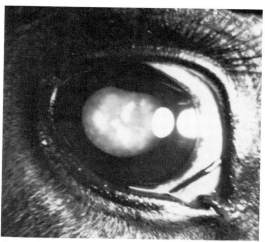

Fig 43. Complete, mature congenital cataract with microphthalmia.

turity (incipient, immature, mature and hypermature), by age (congenital, adult and senile) and by possible cause (congenital and/or inherited, associated with inflammation, trauma or other ocular anomalies, and as primary entities).

Examination of the equine lens must be performed with the pupil widely dilated. Small focal cataracts in the lens periphery cannot be visualized unless mydriasis is maximal. Diagnostic procedures used to determine the extent and position of the cataractous process within the lens include direct ophthalmoscopy, use of the posterior polar lens capsule as the ocular center of rotation, examination using focal, diffuse and oblique illumination, and slit-lamp biomicroscopy. Precise localization of opacities within the lens may assist in determining the possible cause and the prognosis.

Congenital cataracts may be divided into mature complete cortical, nuclear, "Y" and those associated with persistent hyaloid vasculature. Mature complete cortical congenital cataracts in foals usually produce blindness. However, because the foal closely follows its mother, visual impairment is frequently not detected until weaning. These cataracts are frequently bilateral and microphthalmia is present in about 50% of affected animals (Fig 43). The dense white cataract fills the entire pupil, even in mydriasis, and prevents visualization of the ocular fundus.

Nuclear congenital cataracts only involve the central part of the lens and appear as a focal opacity or concentric, irregular rings. There is usually sharp demarcation between the ca-

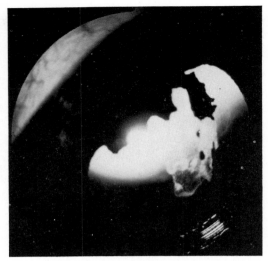

Fig 44. Anterior capsular and cortical cataract associated with posterior synechia involving the corpora nigrum.

taractous nucleus and the normal cortex. Progression of nuclear cataracts is unlikely; some may regress with age. Vision may be impaired, particularly during daytime, but drug-induced mydriasis usually facilitates vision.

The congenital "Y" cataract was first described in detail in 1959.[8] Cortical lens opacities appear as Y-shaped opacities in the anterior and posterior lens sutures. The cataract may result from increased lens ground substance or reduced lens fiber length and appear as vacuoles under magnification. The cataract usually does not progress.

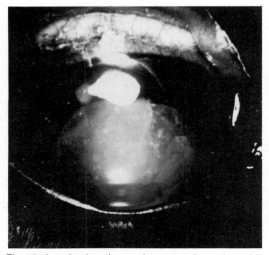

Fig 45. Anterior luxation and cataract formation with glaucoma in an aged Quarter Horse.

Posterior capsular and cortical cataracts occur with persistent hyaloid vasculature (tunica vasculosa lentis) and appear as irregular, concave opacities containing blood vessels. These cataracts are not usually progressive.

Congenital cataracts, sufficient to cause blindness in foals, may be removed by discission and aspiration, and by phacofragmentation. These surgical procedures are presented in the surgery portion of this section.

Cataracts may be associated with iridocyclitis, trauma, systemic diseases and recurrent anterior segment inflammation. Cataract formation is first evidenced by small vacuoles within the lens equator, and eventually involve the posterior and anterior lens cortices. Involvement of the lens is usually limited, and progression depends on the intensity and recurrence of anterior segment inflammation.

Pyramid-shaped cataracts may form directly beneath posterior synechiae (Fig 44). If the posterior synechiae are torn by intensive mydriatic therapy, progression of the cataract may be greatly slowed; however, small deposits of iridal tissue may remain on the anterior lens capsule. Complete mature cataracts associated with iridocyclitis may have a yellow color associated with deposits of cholesterol and/or Ca, as well as small amounts of iridal tissue on the anterior lens capsule.

Displacement

Lens luxation infrequently occurs in horses and is associated with glaucoma, aging, trauma, recurrent anterior segment inflammation and congenital anomalies. The displacement may be anterior (within the anterior chamber), posterior (displaced into the vitreous cavity) or a subluxation (within the patellar fossa, lacking part of its zonular attachments). Glaucoma development in eyes with displaced lens is dependent on the presence of other ocular disease and the effects of the lens and vitreous. Displacement of the vitreous anteriorly by the lens may result in pupillary block by the vitreous and subsequent rapid increase in intraocular pressure. Removal of the luxated lens by intracapsular methods may, in early cases, maintain vision and sometimes resolves the glaucoma. Horses with luxated lenses are frequently presented for an overt cataract without detection of the displacement. A luxated lens in horses appears to become more rapidly cataractous than in other species (Fig 45).

Cataract Surgery

Cataract surgery in foals has become commonplace during the last decade, but lensectomy is still not commonly performed in adults.[17,111-113] The operative procedure, preoperative and postoperative treatment, and success rate for cataract surgery have been detailed for foals and preliminary information has been reported for adult horses. Congenital, traumatic and primary cataracts can be successfully removed in horses. Removal of cataractous lenses from horses with recurrent anterior uveal inflammation can restore vision temporarily but does not prevent progression of the underlying uveal disease.

Four different surgical procedures have been used to remove cataractous lenses in the horse: discission and aspiration, phacofragmentation, extracapsular extraction and intracapsular extraction. Discission-aspiration and phacofragmentation are especially suited for soft cataracts in horses less than 3 years of age.[111,112] Extracapsular extraction involves removal of the anterior lens capsule and the lens substance, leaving the posterior lens capsule intact. The extracapsular technic is indicated for horses 3-6 years of age. Intracapsular extraction is recommended for horses more than 6 years of age, in which the lens is displaced, and involves removing the entire lens and capsules.

Careful selection of candidates for cataract surgery optimizes success rates. The patient should be physically able to withstand the rigors of general anesthesia and tolerant of handling several times daily. Intractable or vicious horses are rejected for cataract surgery until temperament problems are remedied. Topical antibiotics, corticosteroids and mydriatics are administered 2 days before surgery. Parenteral corticosteroids are administered the day prior to surgery. Approximately 1 hour before surgery, glycerol (1 ml/kg PO) is administered to reduce intraocular pressure and vitreous volume by lowering plasma osmolality. Use of carbonic anhydrase inhibitors, such as acetazolamide, has been recommended to reduce intraocular pressure in horses; however, use of osmotic agents is preferred because of their dual activity. General anesthesia with halothane is absolutely necessary for optimal results for cataract surgery. Use of retrobulbar nerve blocks or injections of saline to produce exophthalmos is not recommended because the equine sclera lacks rigidity and these methods may cause prolapse of vitreous through the pupil during surgery.

Preparation for surgery involves clipping the eyelid hair and scrubbing the periorbital skin with surgical soap and water before draping. The corneal and conjunctival surfaces are flushed with 0.9% sterile saline solution and any debris removed by sterile dacron swabs.

Soft cataracts in animals less than 3 years of age should be removed by discission-aspiration and phacofragmentation. With both methods, a 5-mm limbal-based conjunctival flap is prepared dorsad, often just ventral to the dorsal aspects of the leading margin of the nictitating membrane. A 3- to 7-mm limbal incision is made into the anterior chamber with a #11 Bard-Parker scalpel blade and the dorsal corpora nigra are removed by aspiration, phacofragmentation or serrated iris forceps. The main iridal substance is avoided during removal of this structure. A discission knife (Zeigler) is used to incise the anterior lens capsule in an X or Y shape and break the lens cortex and nucleus into large fragments while avoiding penetration of the posterior lens capsule. The anterior capsule and lens material are carefully removed by aspiration with a blunt 18- to 19-ga hypodermic needle and intermittent irrigation with 0.9% sterile saline solution. Intraocular pressure is maintained during the fragmentation and aspiration of the lens material with the phacofragmentation method. Intraocular pressure may be maintained at 10-15 mm Hg to prevent collapse of the anterior chamber and anterior displacement of the lens and vitreous.

The edges of the limbal incision are apposed with 1 or 2 interrupted modified McLean sutures of 4-0 chromic collagen or other synthetic absorbable material. The conjunctival flap is closed with continuous 4-0 chromic collagen or other synthetic absorbable sutures. The volume of the anterior chamber and preoperative intraocular pressure are restored by injection of 4-8 ml balanced salt solution.

Extracapsular and intracapsular cataract extractions differ only slightly from the preceding types. Because the methods are very similar, they are presented together. A 160-180°, 5-mm limbal-based conjunctival flap is made in the lateral quadrants by blunt-sharp dissection with ophthalmic scissors. The anterior chamber is entered with a #11 Bard-Parker scalpel blade and the limbal incision enlarged to approximately 160° with corneoscleral scissors. The dorsal corpora nigra are excised with iris scissors or serrated iris forceps. In extracapsular extraction, the anterior lens capsule is grasped with forceps or cryoprobe and as much as possible is removed. The remaining lens substance is removed by applying pressure at the external limbus with a muscle hook and sliding the lens material out

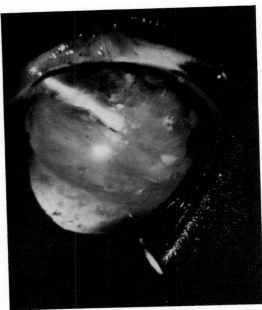

Fig 46. Aspiration of a congenital cataract in a foal.

the wound. Any remaining lens fragments may be flushed from the anterior chamber by gentle irrigation with balanced salt solution (Fig 46).

Intracapsular extraction may be accomplished with intracapsular forceps, erysiphake and cryoprobes. Alpha-chymotrypsin apparently does not produce zonulolysis in horses. After a 160-180° limbal incision, a single suture is placed across the center of the limbal incision to facilitate closure should complications, such as vitreous prolapse, occur during lens extraction. I prefer cryoextraction for the intracapsular method of removing most cataractous and luxated lenses from older horses (Fig 47). The cryoprobe is applied to the dorsal aspect of the anterior lens capsule, and the lens is gently pulled rostrad and tilted laterad and mediad to break the zonules. A muscle hook, applied at the external ventral limbus, is used to push the lens dorsad as traction is exerted with the cryoprobe to slide the lens from the eye. The preplaced suture is then tied to close the limbal incision.

Limbal incisions in both the intra- and extracapsular methods are closed with 8-12 modified McLean sutures of 4-0 to 6-0 chromic collagen or other absorbable synthetic material. Balanced salt solution is used to restore the anterior chamber volume and intraocular pressure to preoperative values. The conjunctival flap is apposed with continuous 4-0 chromic collagen or other synthetic absorbable sutures.

Because of the frequency of medication required, a subpalpebral system is used routinely in all patients subjected to cataract surgery. Postoperative treatment is directed predominantly at controlling iridocyclitis and minimizing sequelae. Topical antibiotics, corticosteroids and mydriatics are administered from 4-8 times daily, and parenteral antibiotics and corticosteroids are also administered the first few days to control the iridocyclitis. Topical treatment must often be continued 2-4 weeks.

Success of restoring vision is 70-85% in young horses with congenital cataracts, using the discission-aspiration and phacofragmentation methods. I prefer to operate on foals with congenital cataracts as early as possible to minimize the possibility of sensitization of the eye to the lens material. Young foals are also amenable to frequent handling with minimum harm to the animal and nursing personnel. The success rate with the extracapsular and intracapsular methods in adult horses is approximately the same as for young foals; however, the number of animals amenable to this type of surgery is limited. Animals with primary cataracts or cataracts secondary to trauma are the best candidates for cataract surgery and have vision restored rapidly after surgery. Vision is evident in young foals immediately after surgery and appears the same as in normal horses in later life. These animals may be maintained with other animals and have not demonstrated any visual deficits when compared to performing horses. Postoperative funduscopic examination frequently requires some dioptric focus by the direct ophthalmoscope (+3 to +6 diopters). Evaluation of foals in obstacle courses and pastures suggests satisfactory vision. Older horses seem to adapt more slowly after cataract surgery and perhaps not as well as foals. This phenomenon in adult animals requires additional study.

DISEASES OF THE VITREOUS BODY

The equine vitreous is normally a clear gel occupying the space bounded rostrad by the lens and posterior chamber, and in the remaining directions by the retina and pars plana portion of the ciliary body. Slit-lamp biomicroscopy is the best clinical method for detailed studies of the vitreous.

The vitreous body is examined clinically by slit-lamp biomicroscopy, and direct and indirect ophthalmoscopy. Because the vitreous is normally a clear gel, opacities are considered abnormal. Opacities suspended within the vitreous move opposite to the direction of movement of the anterior segment and oscillate slightly when ocular movement ceases. In the event the vitreous becomes liquefied (syneresis), opacities move opposite to the direction of movement of the anterior segment and gravitate ventrad when ocular movement ceases.

Persistence of the hyaloid vasculature (tunica vasculosa lentis) is rare in foals (Fig 48). The vasculature is commonly present at birth but usually regresses in the first 2 weeks of life. It appears as faint branches just caudal to the posterior lens capsule, tending to coalesce near the pole of the lens. However, remnants of the hyaloid vasculature in yearlings and older horses may appear as irregular, branching fine strands immediately caudal to the posterior lens capsule or as irregular and often incomplete filaments in the vitreous between the lens and optic nerve head. Distinction between posterior capsular cataracts and remnants of the hyaloid system may be quite difficult clinically and is critical in soundness examinations. This distinction is best achieved by slit-lamp biomicroscopy.

Because the vitreous permits unaltered transmission of light to the ocular fundus, opacities, such as blood, inflammatory cells, strands and neoplastic cells, interfere with light transmission and may be detected during ophthalmoscopy and biomicroscopy. Regression requires 2-6 months once inflammatory cells and blood infiltrate the vitreous. Some liquefaction of vitreous usually results as a sequela of previous inflammation and/or trauma.

Inflammatory cells suspended within the vitreous appear as tiny particles that reflect direct light or as dark structures with retroillumination. Inflammatory cells in the vitreous are a common sequela of recurrent uveal inflammation and usually enter the vitreous after severe attacks to remain for several months. Filamentous networks may also be present in the vitreous.

Vitreous opacities may also be associated with aging and ocular inflammation. These opacities may appear in the vitreous as specks, threads or filaments, and occur in 15% of weanlings, 26% of yearlings and as many as 90% of horses over 10 years of age.[4] Differentiation of vitreous opacities resulting from ocular inflammation and those from age is often difficult. Vitreous opacities associated with recurrent inflammation are cellular and usually

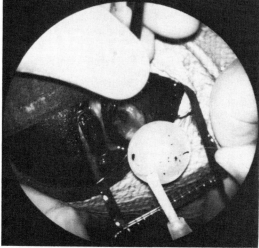

Fig 47. Cryoextraction of a cataract in an aged horse (intra-capsular method).

extensive. However, one should not totally rely on vitreous opacities but should also observe for other sequelae, such as cataracts and iridal changes.

Synchysis scintillans has been observed in horses, especially in aged animals. The vitreous becomes liquefied and contains refractile bodies that may be cholesterol. These crystals appear as minute yellow bodies that move freely in the vitreous with movements of the head and eye. When ocular movements cease, the crystals settle gradually to the most ven-

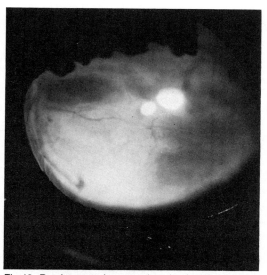

Fig 48. Persistent tunica vasculosa lentis with posterior cortical cataract formation in a weanling.

tral aspects of the vitreous chamber. Affected horses usually have no visual impairment but may exhibit excessive head movement.

DISEASES OF THE FUNDUS

The ocular fundus is ophthalmoscopically divided into retinal blood vessels, optic nerve head (disc or papilla), tapetal fundus and nontapetal fundus.[115-117] Interpretation of ocular fundus findings depends on knowledge of the variations of the ocular fundus in normal and disease states. Mydriasis produced by instillation of 1% tropicamide ensures adequate visualization of the entire ocular fundus. The horse should be examined in a dark stall under drug-induced mydriasis for optimal results.

A normal neurosensory retina is transparent. Different colors of the ocular fundus are derived from the retinal pigmented epithelium, tapetum fibrosum and pigment within the remaining choroidal layers. Because of limited retinal vasculature, most of the equine retina depends on metabolites diffusing from the choroid.

Forty to 60 retinal blood vessels emerge from the optic nerve head and extend into the retina for only 1-2 disc diameters. Because of their small size and color similarity, arterioles and venules usually cannot be differentiated. Vessels usually traverse the retina in nearly straight lines but may be quite tortuous on the surface of the optic nerve head. The optic nerve head is situated in the nontapetal fundus, although the tapetal fundus may occasionally touch the dorsal aspects of the optic nerve head. The surface of the optic nerve head is slightly irregular and its margins may be 1 diopter above the surrounding ocular fundus. The optic nerve head is round to oval and light to dark orange. In older horses an irregular light-yellow to white fibrous framework is usually apparent on the surface of the optic nerve head.

The roughly triangular tapetal fundus varies from light yellow to blue-green but is usually yellow-green. White and light-colored horses usually have a light-yellow tapetal fundus. The blue-green tapetal fundus occurs most frequently in black or grey horses. Fine black dots ("stars of Winslow") are distributed throughout the tapetal fundus in a uniform manner and represent penetration of the tapetum fibrosum by small choroidal vessels. Spots or elongated strips of pigmentation may appear in the normal tapetal fundus. Converg-

ing lines of pigmentation in the dorsomedial and dorsolateral fundus represent sites where vortex veins exit the globe.

Irregular thinning, white scleral crescents, reduced pigmentation and prominent choroidal vessels may be present in the tapetal and nontapetal fundus immediately dorsal to the optic nerve head. Partial to total albinism may be present in the tapetal and nontapetal fundus. Albinoid areas of the tapetal fundus are light yellow, with red stars of Winslow. Demarcation between the albinotic fundus and the usually yellow-green tapetal zone is distinct. Albinism may also involve the nontapetal fundus to result in a diffuse brown-red appearance. There is no detectible pigment within the nontapetal fundus and underlying choroidal vessels can be visualized. In light chestnut, palomino, grey and Appaloosa horses, the large choroidal blood vessels may be visualized as lines throughout the nontapetal fundus, which is referred to as a tigroid nontapetal fundus.

Pigmentary Disturbances

Pigmentary disturbances are frequent in the nontapetal fundus. Focal areas of reduced pigmentation are common around the posterior pole dorsal to the optic nerve head. Small islands of tapetal zones may be present as a result of reduced pigmentation, especially in the peripapillary region between the tapetal and nontapetal fundus. Foci of reduced pigmentation may be detected in horses of any age. These zones may be small or large and usually have a cobblestone appearance. There is no pigment proliferation in these areas, which distinguishes the areas of inflammatory origin that exhibit both areas of reduced pigment and hyperpigmentation. Irregular, radiating translucent zones are occasionally present on one or both sides of the optic nerve head. These light-grey zones may represent small amounts of myelin or increased retinal thickness adjacent to the optic nerve head.

Chorioretinitis

Peripapillary or circumpapillary chorioretinitis and chorioretinoneuritis are part of the ocular fundus abnormalities in recurrent uveal inflammation. These diseases may resolve but leave areas of focal degeneration. In active peripapillary chorioretinitis, the retina appears slightly raised and edematous, and exudates on the margins of the optic disc may protrude into the vitreous. This abnormality in ophthalmoscopically inactive peripapillary chorioretinopathy is characterized as a butterfly-like zone of reduced pigmentation and pigment proliferation. The optic nerve may be involved. When affected, the margin of the optic nerve head may have a dense peripapillary area of pigment; affected areas of the optic nerve head may also be pale to white. The retinal blood vessels in the area may be normal, greatly reduced in number or absent.

A specific chorioretinoneuropathy associated with severe acute blood loss and trauma has been reported.[118] The affected horses were blind, and had bilateral and nearly identical ocular fundic abnormalities. The horses were presented 1-6 months after the onset of blindness, which was directly related to bilateral optic nerve atrophy. The optic nerve heads were small, white and devoid of blood vessels. Focal areas of reduced pigmentation and pigment proliferation were scattered throughout the nontapetal fundus. Lesions in the tapetal fundus were focal, elongated strips of hyperreflectivity and pigment proliferation. Microscopic examination of affected globes failed to reveal extensive numbers of inflammatory cells. Affected retinas had focal degeneration with migration and hypertrophy of the retinal pigmented epithelium and extensive optic nerve atrophy. The condition may result from temporary ischemia associated with severe blood loss. Because retinal and optic nerve tissues are predominantly neural, cell death occurs rapidly and in a more or less irregular fashion, probably due to the distribution of choroidal blood vessels. The condition did not respond to large doses of systemic corticosteroids.

Retinal Detachment

Retinal detachment is usually associated with recurrent uveal inflammation and trauma. Because the retina lacks blood vessels, except around the optic nerve head, a detachment must be closely examined at its attachment at the optic nerve head and at its peripheral region near the ora serrata. Unilateral retinal detachments produce blindness in the affected eye and may not be obvious unless the horse's good eye is covered during visual testing. There have been no reports of successful treatment in horses.

Night Blindness

Night blindness has been observed predominantly in the Appaloosa. The ocular fundi of night-blind horses are normal. Visual testing under reduced illumination and by electroretinography indicates extensive loss of scotopic (rod) vision. Impaired day vision also occurred in some horses. Night blindness in Appaloosas may be an inherited condition.[119,120]

Optic Nerve Hypoplasia

Optic nerve hypoplasia has occurred in foals.[121,122] Because foals are usually with the mare for the first several months of life, congenital blindness may not be apparent until weaning. Optic nerve hypoplasia has occurred in foals with other ocular anomalies, including microphthalmia, cataracts and retinal detachment. The optic nerve heads in affected individuals are slightly smaller than normal, white and devoid of most to all retinal blood vessels. Pupillary reflexes to light are greatly diminished or absent. Testing of affected animals in an obstacle course usually results in collision with most objects. The animal may be easily excited, tends to prance and constantly moves its ears. There is no treatment.

Papilledema

Papilledema may be associated with retrobulbar inflammation, orbital neoplasms, retrobulbar hemorrhage, meningitis, internal hydrocephalus and increased intracranial pressure. The optic nerve surface is raised above the ocular fundus 3-10 diopters and the retinal blood vessels are congested. Edema and congested small vessels occur on the optic nerve head and peripapillary ocular fundus. This condition must be distinguished from optic neuritis.

Exudative Optic Neuritis

Exudative optic neuritis has been observed in horses for nearly a century.[123-125] Affected horses become acutely blind, and ophthalmoscopically have multiple wavy, mobile excrescences and hemorrhages on the optic nerve head. The condition is frequently bilateral. Response to systemic corticosteroid administration is variable. Optic nerve atrophy may eventually result.

Optic Nerve Atrophy

Atrophy of the optic nerve head and nerve occurs most frequently as a sequela to recurrent uveal inflammation. The pupil is usually unresponsive to light stimulation and vision is markedly impaired or lost in affected eyes. The optic nerve head is small and white, and retinal blood vessels usually disappear.

Neoplasia

Optic nerve neoplasms occur rarely in horses, but medulloepithelioma and neurofibroma have been reported.[126-128] Masses on the optic nerve head have also occurred in aged horses without signs of visual impairment. Ophthalmoscopically they may involve the surface and margins of the optic nerve head. The masses are single, usually unilateral, light yellow to orange, smooth and raised 2-4 diopters above the ocular fundus surface. Microscopic studies in one horse revealed an astrocytoma.[129] The mass, limited to the edge of the optic nerve head and protruding into the vitreous, was predominantly astrocytic glial cells, with a few microcytes. Another report of 2 horses with unilateral ocular nerve masses indicated the presence of proliferative neuropathy.[130] Ophthalmoscopically the masses were similar to those in the horse of the first report but had blood vessels on their surface. Histologically the lesions consisted of fat-like cells and tortuous blood vessels with heavy deposits of collagen in their walls. The masses involved the optic nerve head surface and extended into the optic nerve substance.

References

1. Nicolas, E: Veterinary and Comparative Ophthalmology. H and W Brown, London, 1914.

2. Jakob, H: Tierärztliche Augenheilkunde. Schoetz, Berlin, 1920.

3. Errington, BJ and Shipley, WD. Vet Bull 35 (1941) 96.

4. Errington, BJ. JAVMA 108 (1941) 115.

5. Errington, BJ. Vet Med 37 (1942) 16.

6. Formston, C. Vet Rec 68 (1956) 984.

7. Smythe, RH: Veterinary Ophthalmology. 2nd ed. Ballière, Tindall and Cox, London, 1958.

8. Überreiter, O. Adv Vet Sci 5, Academic Press, New York, 1959.

9. Prince, JH et al: Anatomy and Histology of the Eye and Orbit in Domestic Animals. Charles C Thomas, Springfield, 1960.

10. Smythe and Lundvall, in Catcott: Equine Medicine and Surgery. American Veterinary Publications, Santa Barbara, 1963.

11. Roberts, EJ. Vet Rec 76 (1964) 137.

12. Ammann, K: Eye diseases in the horse. In Veterinary Encyclopedia, Vol II. Medical Book Co, Copenhagen, 1968.

13. Komar, G and Szutter, L: Tierärztliche Augenheilkunde. Paul Parey, Berlin, 1968.

14. Cox, JE. Vet Rec 84 (1969) 526.

15. Gelatt, KN. Okla Vet Med Assoc J 21 (1969) 6.

16. McDonald, DR. Southwest Vet 23 (1970) 15.

17. Gelatt, KN. Proc 17th Ann Mtg Am Assoc Eq Pract, 1971. p 323.

18. Gelatt, KN: Diagnostic Procedures of Comparative Ophthalmology. 2nd ed (special supplement). AAHA, South Bend, 1974.

19. Gelatt, KN: Veterinary Ophthalmic Pharmacology and Therapeutics. 2nd ed. VM Publishing, Bonner Springs, Kansas, 1978.

20. Gelatt, KN et al. J Eq Med Surg 1 (1977) 13.

21. Rubin, LF. JAVMA 144 (1964) 1387.

22. Manning, JP and St. Clair, LE. VM/SAC 71 (1976) 187.

23. Cohen, CM and Reinke, DA. JAVMA 156 (1970) 1884.

24. McClure, JR et al. VM/SAC 71 (1976) 1727.

25. Barnett, KC and Keeler, CR. Vet Rec 80 (1967) 624.

26. Gelatt, KN and Henry, JD. Mod Vet Pract 50 (1969) 40.

27. Überreiter, O. Wien Tierärztl Monatsschr 43 (1956) 1.

28. Cottier, R. Arch Wiss Prakt Tierheilk 78 (1943) 395.

29. Sivak, JG and Allen, DB. Vision Res 15 (1975) 1353.

30. Knill, LM et al. Am J Vet Res 38 (1977) 735.

31. Gelatt, KN. Vet Med 62 (1967) 1165.

32. Martin, B and Severin, G. Proc 14th Ann Mtg Am Assoc Eq Pract, 1968. p 324.

33. Gelatt, KN. J Eq Med Surg 3 (1979) 141.

34. Rubin, LF. Proc 9th Ann Mtg Am Assoc Eq Pract, 1963. p 121.

35. Craven, JR. Eq Vet J 3 (1971) 141.

36. Gadd, JD and Hoover, R. Proc 8th Ann Mtg Am Assoc Eq Pract, 1962. p 275.

37. Priester, WA. JAVMA 160 (1972) 1504.

38. Hatziolos, BC et al. JAVMA 167 (1975) 51.

39. Smith, JS and Mayhew, IG. Cornell Vet 67 (1977) 529.

40. Firth, EC. Eq Vet J 10 (1978) 9.

41. Gelatt, KN and McClure, JR, Jr. J Eq Med Surg 3 (1979) 240.

42. Peiffer, RL, Jr et al. VM/SAC 72 (1977) 1219.

43. McFadyean J. J Comp Path Therap 66 (1933) 186.

44. Blodi, FC and Ramsey, FK. Am J Ophth 64 (1967) 627.

45. Priester, WA and Mantel, N. J Nat Cancer Inst 47 (1971) 1333.

46. Cotchin, E. Eq Vet J 9 (1977) 16.

47. Lavach, JD and Severin, GA. JAVMA 170 (1977) 202.

48. Runnells, RA and Benbrook, EA. Am J Vet Res 3 (1942) 176.

49. Koch, SA and Cowles, RR. VM/SAC 66 (1971) 327.

50. Gelatt, KN et al. JAVMA 165 (1974) 617.

51. Strafuss, AC. JAVMA 168 (1976) 61.

52. Burger, CH. No Am Vet 36 (1955) 371.

53. Silver, IA and Cater, DB. Acta Radiol 2 (1964) 226.

54. Lewis, RE. Proc 10th Ann Mtg Am Assoc Eq Pract, 1964. p 217.

55. Strafuss, AC et al. VM/SAC 68 (1973) 1246.

56. Wyman, M et al. JAVMA 171 (1977) 449.

57. Farris, HE et al. VM/SAC 71 (1976) 325.

58. Lane, JG. Eq Vet J 9 (1977) 127.

59. Murphy, JM et al. JAVMA 174 (1979) 269.

60. Gelatt, KN. JAVMA 151 (1967) 27.

61. Milne, FJ. Proc 10th Ann Mtg Am Assoc Eq Pract, 1964. p 326.

62. Lundvall, RL and Carter, JD. JAVMA 159 (1971) 289.

63. Hjorth, P. Nord Vet Med 23 (1971) 260.

64. Williams, R et al. Proc Ann Mtg Am Coll Vet Ophth, 1977. p 101.

65. Marts, BS *et al.* J Eq Med Surg **1** (1977) 427.
66. Joyce, JR and Bratton, GR. VM/SAC **68** (1973) 619.
67. Joyce, JR *et al.* VM/SAC **67** (1972) 1008.
68. Hughes, DE and Pugh, GW. Am J Vet Res **31** (1970) 457.
69. Grant, B *et al.* VM/SAC **68** (1973) 62.
70. Gelatt, KN. VM/SAC **69** (1974) 1309.
71. Mitchell, JS and Attleberger, MN. VM/SAC **68** (1973) 1257.
72. Severin, GA. Proc 12th Ann Mtg Am Assoc Eq Pract, 1966. p 45.
73. Wyman, M. JAVMA **153** (1968) 1703.
74. Gwin, RM *et al.* J Eq Med Surg **1** (1977) 413.
75. Keller, WF *et al.* JAAHA **9** (1973) 252.
76. Überreiter, O and Köhler, H. Tierärztl Monatsschr **50** (1963) 70.
77. Ahmed, SA and Gupta, BN. Indian Vet J **42** (1965) 140.
78. Jemelka, ED. VM/SAC **71** (1976) 673.
79. Gelatt, KN. VM/SAC **70** (1975) 475.
80. Brannen, HS. Southwest Vet **19** (1966) 237.
81. Gelatt, KN. VM/SAC **68** (1973) 261.
82. Barnett, KC. J Repro Fert Suppl **23** (1975) 701.
83. Pulos, WL and Hutt, FB. J Hered **60** (1969) 59.
84. Eriksson, K. Nord Vet Med **7** (1955) 773.
85. Jones, TC. JAVMA **155** (1969) 315.
86. Searl, RC. Vet Med **63** (1967) 426.
87. Heusser, H *et al.* Schweiz Med Wschr **78** (1948) 756.
88. Yager, RH *et al.* JAVMA **117** (1950) 207.
89. Wood, RM and Davis, GR. Am J Ophth **33** (1950) 961.
90. Heusser, H. Schweiz Arch Tierheilk **94** (1952) 296.
91. Witmer, R *et al.* Schweiz Arch Tierheilk **95** (1953) 419.
92. Schebitz, H. Berl Münch Tierärztl Wschr **67** (1954) 29.
93. Bryans, JT. Cornell Vet **55** (1955) 16.
94. Robert, SJ. JAVMA **133** (1958) 189.
95. Roberts, SR. JAVMA **141** (1962) 229.
96. Roberts, SR. Am J Ophth **55** (1963) 1049.
97. Morter, RL *et al.* Proc 68th Ann Mtg US Livestock Sanitary Assoc, 1964. p 147.
98. Cross, RSN. Vet Res **78** (1966) 8.
99. Morter, RL *et al.* JAVMA **155** (1969) 436.
100. Williams, RD *et al.* Invest Ophth **10** (1971) 948.
101. Iyer, PRK. Indian J Vet Sci Anim Husb **8** (1938) 3.
102. Böhm, LK and Supperer, R. SF Ost Akad Wiss **161** (1952) 9.
103. Böhm, LK and Supperer, R. Wien Tierärztl Monatsschr **41** (1954) 129.
104. Dimic, J *et al.* Wien Tierärztl Monatsschr **46** (1959) 374.
105. Cello, RM. Proc 8th Ann Mtg Am Assoc Eq Pract, 1962. p 123.
106. Cello, RM. Eq Vet J **3** (1970) 1.
107. Fischer, CA. Proc Ann Mtg Am Coll Vet Ophth, 1976. p 105.
108. Rubin, LF. JAVMA **149** (1966) 151.
109. Saunders, LZ and Barron, CN. Cancer Res **18** (1958) 234.
110. Bistner, SI. Cornell Vet **64** (1974) 588.
111. Gelatt, KN *et al.* JAVMA **165** (1974) 611.
112. Gelatt, KN and Kraft, WE. Vet Med **64** (1969) 415.
113. Van Kruningen, HJ. JAVMA **145** (1964) 773.
114. Andrasic, N *et al.* Zbl Vet Med **10A** (1963) 566.
115. Gelatt, KN and Finocchio, EJ. Vet Med **65** (1970) 569.
116. Barnett, KC. Eq Vet J **4** (1971) 1.
117. Gelatt, KN. JAAHA **7** (1971) 158.
118. Gelatt, KN. J Eq Med Surg **3** (1979) 91.
119. Witzel, DA *et al.* J Eq Med Surg **1** (1977) 226.
120. Witzel, DA *et al.* J Eq Med Surg **1** (1977) 383.
121. Strunjak, Z. Vet Arch **11** (1941) 236.
122. Gelatt, KN *et al.* JAVMA **155** (1969) 627.
123. Bayer, J. Bildliche Darstellung des Gesunden und Kranken Auges Unserer Haustiere. Braumuller, Wien (1890) plate IX.
124. Roesti, W. Arch Tierheilk **77** (1941) 81.
125. Kovacs, AB. Magyar Allat Lap **26** (1971) 65.
126. Hieronymi, E. Monatssch für Prakt Tierheilk **25** (1914) 54.
127. Hamm, K. Wien Tierärztl Monatsschr **46** (1959) 117.
128. Eagle, RC *et al.* Vet Path **15** (1978) 488.
129. Gelatt, KN *et al.* Can Vet J **12** (1971) 53.
130. Saunders, LZ *et al.* Vet Path **9** (1972) 368.

23

The Reproductive System

by A.C. Asbury

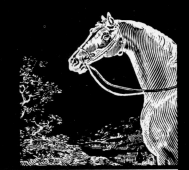

Equine reproductive problems represent challenges, satisfactions and frustrations to the veterinarian. Perhaps no other domestic species is as subject to the whim of humans and the vagaries of management as the horse. An arbitrary breeding season that suits the calendar rather than the reproductive cycle is a prime example. Obstacles such as long estrus periods with unpredictable ovulation time, failure to cull animals past their reproductive prime, and lack of selection for breeding efficiency all add to the challenge.

The practitioner who can use knowledge of equine reproductive physiology, develop clinical proficiency and realistically assess management problems can expect a truly rewarding experience with reproductive work. In the face of snowballing scientific knowledge, the art and skill of practice remain an integral part of this aspect of veterinary medicine.

REPRODUCTIVE SYSTEM EXAMINATION: THE MARE

History

Obtaining a valid breeding history of an individual mare can be the most rewarding aspect of the entire evaluation procedure; yet history-taking is often slighted because of the difficulties involved. Owners or their representatives often lack the specific information required to define the history properly. Records, when available, may be sketchy. Since improper management is often the principal cause of infertility, an in-depth history is essential. When physical causes of the problem fail to materialize later in the examination, finding a clue in the history may save much time and effort in effecting a solution.

The ideal breeding history consists of a sequential, year-by-year account of the mare's entire breeding career. It should include the background of the mare in the years before the animal was bred, ie, the number of years in race or show training. Starting the history with the date of the first foal may be misleading for the occasional mare that was bred several seasons before conceiving and delivering a live foal.

Known abortions, possible early embryonic deaths, twinning and neonatal deaths should be documented. A total list of live foals, their sires and foaling dates is imperative. Particular note should be taken of the most recent seasons foals were produced regularly. Detailed records for these years, including teasing and breeding data, are invaluable since they may reveal cyclic patterns. Short cycles, suggesting uterine infection, and prolonged diestral patterns, suggesting endocrine dysfunction, should be noted.

Veterinary treatment history, including culture data, treatment schedules and routine prophylactic measures, should be evaluated. First-hand communication with practitioners and management personnel who have previously attended the mare often yields useful information. As examples, the ease with which estrus was detectible, restraint necessary to produce signs of estrus, and other "personality" traits may save further trial and error efforts.

Knowledge of the stallions to which the mare was bred for all seasons is helpful, including any years the mare went barren. When stallions of known marginal fertility are involved, this information is valuable. Information pertaining to stallion fertility is often closely guarded; however, serious students of various breeds may examine published records of numbers of foals produced per crop and, balancing this with stallion popularity, can make some objective deductions about fertility.

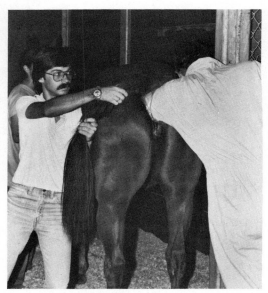

Fig 1. The stall doorframe protects the examiner during genital examination.

Possibly the one aspect of a breeding history that is most helpful in evaluating a mare's record is the level of management to which the animal has been subjected in the past. Such information is often difficult to sort out since the disgruntled owner of a barren mare tends to place all the blame on prior management. Careful questioning often points to deficiencies severe enough to solve the whole problem. Sometimes moving a mare to an establishment with a reputation for careful teasing, close supervision and good breeding technic is all that is required.

General Physical Appraisal

A brief physical assessment of each mare should be a routine part of the reproductive examination. The objectives of this procedure are to detect problems that could interfere with fertility and to take appropriate steps.

Extremes in body condition, from debilitation to obesity, may affect fertility. Feeding or management changes, dental treatment or parasite control may be indicated. Organic disease as a cause of poor condition must be considered and treated.

Early in the breeding season, barren or maiden mares may be encountered with a long winter haircoat and lack of "bloom." These signs correlate well with anestrus that persists into spring. Regardless of corrective measures

undertaken, informing the owner that a delay in cycling should be expected pays dividends in client relations.

Mares with acute or chronic injuries from racing or showing occasionally experience depressed fertility. Long-term, unrelenting pain can adversely influence appetite, condition and attitude. Special handling of these cases should be recommended early.

Experienced practitioners can detect subtle abnormalities in a mare during examination. Behavioral quirks and disposition may warrant special handling or teasing technics. Awareness of the condition of the animal as a whole is as important in reproductive management as detection of specific genital problems.

Examination of the Reproductive Tract

Four procedures should be included in a complete examination of the mare's reproductive tract: examination of the external genitalia and related areas; rectal palpation of the internal genitalia; visual examination of the cervix and vagina; and direct palpation of the cervix, vagina and occasionally the endometrium. Additional aids that may be employed are uterine culture, endometrial biopsy and visual inspection of the endometrium. All or parts of this examination may be indicated in the evaluation of the case or in subsequent examinations to determine the optimum time for breeding.

Inspection of the external genitalia should include the entire perineal area as well as the tail and buttocks, where signs of vaginal discharge may be noted. The vulva is best evaluated during estrus, when relaxation and elongation are greatest. The examination is directed toward loss of integrity of the vulva, which allows aspiration of air and fecal matter into the vagina. Conformation defects and loss of labial tone are the chief causes.[1]

The dorsal commissure of the vulva should be no more than 4 cm dorsal to the pelvic floor.[2] Greater distances predispose to cranial horizontal tipping. The relationship of vulvar length to the angle of declination is important regarding pneumovagina and contamination.[3] Positive identification of mares that aspirate air can be accomplished by uniform lateral pressure with the hands on each side of the labia and listening for the characteristic "windsucking" that follows.[2]

By parting the labia, the color and moisture of the vaginal vestibule can be assessed. True

estrus produces a glistening pink to red mu-
cusa. Anestrus generally is reflected by a pale,
dry mucosa; dark-red or muddy colors suggest
inflammation.[2] When the labia are spread
enough to allow air into the vestibule, an intact
vulvovaginal sphincter should be observed in
the normal mare. This functional closure prevents contamination of the cranial vagina and
is notably absent in the chronic windsucker.

Rectal palpation of the internal genitalia,
while the most difficult part of the examination, is often the most rewarding. The technic
requires considerable experience to master, yet
is essential to the management of reproductive
problems in mares. It can be accomplished successfully in a variety of settings, with simple
or elaborate facilities and with a wide range of
restraint technics. In selecting an approach,
the key objective is safety of the mare, examiner and handlers.

Many mares are examined in box stalls (Fig
1). The preferred technic is to restrain the mare
with a twitch or lip chain and place the hindquarters in the corner where the stall door
opens. The operator can then stand enough to
one side to gain protection from the door frame.

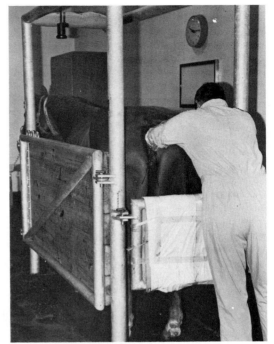

Fig 2. Use of stocks during genital examination.

Examination stocks offer the advantage that
less restraint is generally needed so that mares
are more relaxed for the procedure (Fig 2).
Stocks should be viewed critically for design
that predisposes to injury. Overhead braces are
dangerous for animals that rear. Sides could
cause injury if a leg is thrown over or if the
mare attempts to jump out. A rear door protects the operator but is hazardous if the mare
squats suddenly during examination. The front
of the chute should be open, allowing a quick
exit forward in case of trouble.

Mares can be accustomed to examination in
the open. In this case the handler and examiner work from the same side. The right-handed
palpator stands at the mare's left hip initially,
grasps the base of the tail with the left hand,
and proceeds slowly and deliberately to introduce the palpation hand into the rectum (Fig
3). Once the examination is underway, the operator can move safely to a point close behind
the left hindquarter. Muscular movements
preparatory to kicking can be anticipated when
close contact with the mare is maintained. Restraint in the form of a twitch or lip chain can
be supplemented by a front leg strap. Hobbles
and sidelines offer the potential for entanglement and overexcitement.

Chemical restraint in the form of tranquilizers or sedatives for reproductive examinations is generally too unpredictable to be
reliable. Xylazine, in fact, may cause a greater
tendency to kick when the rear of the mare is
examined. In horses that absolutely require

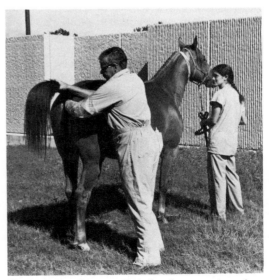

Fig 3. Appropriate position for the operator when
beginning a rectal examination in the open.

some sedation, a moderate dose of chloral hydrate is the preference of the author.

The actual technics of rectal palpation have been well described.[4-6] Mares require a gentle approach. Guarding against trauma to the rectal mucosa must always be kept in mind. Tenesmus or peristaltic contractions should never be overcome by counterpressure.

Probably the biggest hurdle the beginning palpator must overcome is gaining sufficient relaxation of the rectum to allow complete examination of the ovaries, uterus and cervix. One hint helpful to most beginners is to extend the arm further into the rectum than necessary and then pull back the rectal wall, which tends to go slack. Ample lubrication and sleeves free from irritating seams are essential.

The genitalia should be examined systematically, using the same routine for each examination. Both ovaries, the entire uterus and the cervix can be palpated readily. A suggested routine is to first locate the ovary opposite to the hand of palpation. Completely evaluate that ovary and next proceed to the tip of the uterine horn on that side. Follow the uterus across its length with the fingers bent over the cranial margin so the ventral aspect can be assessed, and finish at the second ovary. After completely examining that ovary, move the hand back to the midline and palpate the cervix by compressing it ventrad against the pelvic floor.

Ovarian Palpation

The entire surface of the ovary must be palpated to identify landmarks and important structures. This is done by holding the ovary against the palm by pressure from the middle and ring fingers on the opposite side. The thumb, index finger and middle finger may then explore the pole of the ovary lying in the hand. Still in the same position, the greater curvature or center of the ovary is palpated with the thumb and apposing fingers. The opposite pole is best evaluated by turning the entire ovary 180° on its mesovarial attachment and repeating the process above.

Identification of the cranial and caudal aspects of the ovary is aided by locating the free edge of the mesovarium, which attaches to the ovary on its cranial half. The ovulation fossa, a sharp indentation in the ovarian stroma, should be medial and slightly ventral when the ovary is in cranial-caudal alignment. It is important to note the exact position of structures to aid evaluation of subsequent changes.

Two functional structures of the ovary can be identified by rectal palpation: the follicle and the corpus hemorrhagicum (CH). Follicles are fluid-filled, symmetric structures that, as they mature, tend to project above the ovarian surface. A shoulder tends to form around the base of the follicle as it grows, increasing in its angle as ovulation approaches.[2] The turgidity of the follicle generally changes with maturity, progressing from firm and thick-walled to very fluctuant and thin-walled.

The important changes to consider in predicting time of ovulation are size, projection from the surface and turgidity. None of these parameters is absolute. Small ovaries, as found in young mares, are prone to ovulate smaller follicles than large ovaries of multiparous mares. Occasionally a follicle that is still firm and tense ovulates with no prior change in turgidity. All the criteria for maturity must be correlated, and changes noted during sequential examinations are most helpful. One author modestly stated, "With experience one is able, on one examination, to be right in more than 50% of the cases in deciding whether ovulation will occur within 3 days."[7]

To be of greatest value, sequential examinations must be accompanied by recording size and turgidity data in some numeric fashion. Follicle size can be estimated in fingerwidths, millimeters or inches. Prior knowledge of the width of finger tips or the distance from finger tips to the various phalangeal joints is necessary before assigning numbers to structures. Some subjective method of assigning values for turgidity is also helpful. All data must be recorded for later comparison.

An example of data recorded by the author's method of evaluation follows:

5/14/80 RO 80 x 50 x 50 mm   FR, AP, 40, #3
         LO, 50 x 40 x 40 mm   NSS

Explanation:
On May 14 the mare had a right ovarian size of 80 mm (length), 50 mm (height) and 50 mm (width). There is a 40-mm (diameter) follicle on the cranial pole, which is softening somewhat (#1 = firm, #4 = very fluctuant). The left ovarian size is also given. NSS = no significant structures.

By setting up one's own parameters of evaluation and devising a simple scheme for abbreviation, a great deal of data can be recorded in a line or 2. Another useful scheme of follicle description has been presented.[2]

Determination of the time of ovulation is an extremely important aspect of the reproductive examination. Since the ovum is viable only for a few hours (probably 8) after ovulation, many unnecessary breedings can be eliminated with this information. Collapse of the follicle is generally assumed to be the time of ovulation. Typically this collapse is felt as a crater or pit at the location of the follicle. When palpating this crater, the mare responds to the local pain involved by tensing the flank muscles on that side or raising the leg somewhat.

The borders of the crater are sharp and the cavity feels empty for about 8 hours. As the hemorrhage organizes into a clot to form the CH, the mushy consistency of the cavity becomes progressively firmer by 24 hours. After 24 hours the crater may redistend with clot and serum to suggest the presence of another follicle. The consistency of the CH in this stage has been likened to that of a ripe plum and the size is almost invariably smaller than the original follicle. These changes are best evaluated by repeated examination. When initially presented with a mare that has ovulated 24-48 hours previously, some confusion between follicle and CH may occur. Consideration of other estral signs is helpful in these cases.

The mature (5 days postovulation) corpus luteum (CL) is seldom detectable by rectal palpation. Retraction deep into the ovarian stroma occurs rather quickly. The equine practitioner must rely on the signs associated with elevated blood progesterone levels to suggest the presence of a functional CL. These signs are discussed later in the chapter.

Uterine Palpation

Pregnancy examination by rectal palpation is considered in a separate section. In palpation of the nonpregnant uterus, the examiner should attempt to define the size, tone, consistency and general conformation of the organ, and follow this assessment with a detailed examination for abnormalities. The initial impression is best gained by cupping the fingers over the cranial brim of the uterus, with the palm on the dorsal aspect, and by sliding the hand from the tip of one uterine horn to the other.

Uterine size is estimated by circling the organ with the index finger and thumb, and calculating the diameter of each horn and the body. Previous calibration of the diameter of the circle by the finger to various points on the thumb is helpful in making these measure-

ments.[2] The postpartum uterus normally has a disparity of size between the previously gravid horn and its counterpart for up to 30 days.

Evaluation of uterine tone is helpful in determining the stage of the estrous cycle. The effect of progesterone on the uterus is to increase tissue density, causing a tubular, compact feeling when palpated. In some areas this effect suggests induration or rigidity.

The tubularity of diestrus progresses to relaxation in proestrus and estrus. Circulating estrogens produce uterine edema, spreading the tissues of the endometrium and myometrium. The palpator detects this edema as a soft thickening of the uterus. There is also the impression that the thickened wall could be compressed easily between the fingers. Those practitioners with experience in palpating the bovine uterus must condition themselves to the differences between estral tone in the 2 species.

In anestrus the uterus becomes flaccid, thin-walled and often quite indistinct. Endometrial atrophy is the prominent anatomic feature of this stage. Beginning palpators may experience difficulty in tracing the entire uterus in anestrus due to thinning of the wall.

During the general evaluation of the uterus, specific changes in conformation and consistency should be noted. Particular attention should be given to enlargements of the ventral aspect of the uterus in the area of the junction of the horn and body. These sacculations may indicate myometrial and endometrial atrophy, or diffuse lymphatic stasis or lacunae.[2] Abnormal fluid accumulations in the uterine lumen are best detected in this manner. Areas with notable differences in consistency, either firmer or softer than the uterus as a whole, are critical to subsequent diagnostic procedures, particularly endometrial biopsy.

Deep palpation of the uterus often reveals subtle lesions that may be missed on the general examination. Deep digital pressure is exerted between the thumb and forefingers while the entire uterus is explored in a systematic manner. Endometrial folds normally feel like small ridges as they slip through the fingers. These are prominent during estrus and less distinct in anestrus. Areas devoid of endometrial folds suggest fibrotic lesions or denuding of that area of endometrium. Endometrial cysts as small as 2-3 mm often can be detected. The procedure should never be attempted if there is any possibility of pregnancy.

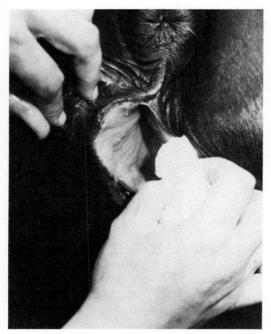

Fig 4. Cleaning the labia prior to vaginal procedures.

Cervical Palpation

By compressing the cervix against the pelvic floor, its size and consistency can be evaluated. The effects of estrogens and progesterone on the cervix are similar to those on the uterus. Estrogens produce cervical softening, shortening and edema. The maximal effect during estrus produces a cervix so soft it flattens readily with pressure. The diestral cervix is long, tubular and readily palpated. Early pregnancy produces diestral changes discussed under pregnancy examination.

In anestrus the cervix becomes soft and indistinct. Other clues, such as ovarian inactivity and changes in the speculum examination, are often necessary to confirm anestrus.

Vaginoscopic Examination

The entire vagina and external cervical os can be inspected visually through a vaginal speculum, allowing dilation of the vagina with air, and viewing with a bright light source. The degree of cervical relaxation and the character of uterine, cervical and vaginal secretions can be evaluated. Anatomic and traumatic abnormalities of the area are also easily detected.

Preparation of the mare for vaginal examination requires restraint in a suitable location, preferably out of direct sunlight. The tail should be wrapped and the perineal area carefully washed with a nonirritating soap. After ample rinsing, the labia should be blotted dry and clean moist cotton used to wipe the inner edges of the labia (Fig 4). In many examination procedures the speculum examination is followed by a uterine culture and/or biopsy. Aseptic preparation of the vulva takes on greater significance in these cases to prevent uterine contamination.

The metal trivalve (Caslick's) speculum or one of the tubular types is satisfactory for vaginal examinations. Standards of practice today require a separate sterile instrument for each examination, which makes the disposable plastic or cardboard tube or a glass tubular speculum more practical. The latter are readily made from heat-resistant glass tubing cut to 35- to 38-cm (14- to 15-inch) lengths and firepolished. These specula are easily cleaned, individually autoclaved, pass easily into the cranial vagina and permit maximum visualization (Fig 5).

Vaginoscopic examinations help determine the stage of the estrous cycle if used in conjunction with teasing and rectal palpation. In estrus, the cervix progressively softens and drops toward the floor of the distended vagina. At the time of maximal relaxation, the cervix appears completely flattened on the vaginal floor, especially in multiparous mares. Maiden and younger mares usually have a lesser degree of softening.

Estrogen secretion by the developing follicle also produces edema, mucus secretion and hyperemia of both the cervical and vaginal mucosa. Early in estrus it is common for the external cervical os to have edematous folds of mucosa, which resolve as ovulation approaches. The degree of mucus secretion correlates well with follicular development and appears as an increasing shine of the cervical and vaginal mucosal surfaces. Estrogens also enhance the blood supply to the reproductive tract to cause hyperemia, which is manifested as a pink color of all visible surfaces. Judging the degree of hyperemia is important in evaluating the cervix and vagina for inflammatory and physiologic changes. Artifactual reddening can be produced quickly by air in contact with the tissues, so evaluation must be made shortly after dilation of the vagina.

In diestrus or under the influence of progesterone, characteristic vaginoscopic changes are also evident. The cervical and vaginal surfaces become pale and dry, and often a heavy, sticky mucus is present. The color of the membranes is typically grey, with a yellowish cast.

The external cervical os projects into the cranial vagina from high on the wall and is tightly contracted. The appearance of the cervix correlates well with its elongated shape and firm consistency on rectal examination.

The gonadal steroids, estrogen and progesterone, produce specific visual clues in the speculum examination. Total lack of steroid production likewise results in a typical picture. Inactive ovaries are commonly found in winter anestrus and in conditions of gonadal dysgenesis. Cervical and vaginal color in anestrus is blanched, almost white. The cervix becomes atonic and flaccid, and often gapes open to reveal the uterine lumen. Blood vessels are scarce on the vaginal wall and little hyperemia occurs after exposure to air.

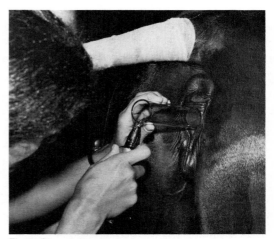

Fig 5. Glass tube used as a vaginal speculum.

Vaginoscopic examination is an essential procedure for detecting pathologic or anatomic variations. Inflammatory changes, such as mucosal hyperemia and suppurative exudates, often can be discovered visually. Additionally, persistent hymen, urine pooling, rectovaginal defects and other conditions affecting fertility may be discovered or confirmed with a speculum. These disorders are considered in detail in subsequent sections.

Once the health of the genital tract has been established, routine vaginoscopic examinations may be deleterious in a breeding program. Repeated exposure of the vagina, cervix and uterus to air, with its accompanying contaminants, may produce unnecessary irritation and inflammation. This is a major consideration in older mares with lowered resistance to contamination. It is a good practice after every vaginal dilation to express vaginal air by rectal compression of the distended genital tract. Strict adherence to this program reveals the fact that many mares with a relaxed cervix experience uterine distension with air after speculum examination.

Manual Examination of the Vagina, Cervix and Uterus

Evaluation of the mare's genital tract is incomplete without manually exploring the vaginal and cervical lumen. In selected cases, intraluminal palpation of the uterus is also indicated. Aseptic technic is essential in these procedures, both in preparation of the mare and in hand and arm protection. A sterile, shoulder-length glove is ideal, but a practical alternative is a clean plastic sleeve with a sterile surgeon's glove applied over it. Lubrication should be with a sterile, water-soluble product.

When the gloved hand is introduced into the vagina, the labia should be parted to reduce contamination.

Vaginal lesions overlooked in the speculum examination are rarely detected by palpation, although minute rectovaginal defects may be felt more easily than seen. The key organ in direct palpation is the cervix. By carefully dilating the external os and then palpating the entire cervical canal, it is possible to locate lacerations and adhesions not evident on vaginoscopy. The same technic is employed in passing instruments or catheters into the uterus.

When prior rectal examination suggests gross lesions in the uterine lumen, direct palpation of the endometrium may be helpful. The cervix must be carefully dilated to admit the gloved hand, a procedure that is possible during estrus in many mares. Occasionally the administration of estrogens, such as estradiol cypionate (ECP:Upjohn), 12-24 hours prior to examination is necessary to gain full cervical relaxation. By progressively introducing more fingers into the cervix and with steady pressure, the uterine lumen is entered.

With the hand in the uterus, such lesions as intraluminal adhesions, endometrial cysts, neoplasms or other palpable changes may be detected. Abnormalities of the uterine wall may be found by palpating the uterus with one hand in the lumen and other in the rectum. Epidural anesthesia may be helpful in this procedure.

It is fortunate that the disorders in question here are more common in older, multiparous mares. Intraluminal palpation may not be feasible in maiden or primiparous animals. Since

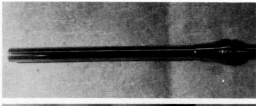
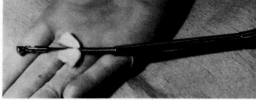

Fig 6. Knudsen sampler in retracted position (upper) and with swab exposed (lower). The entire instrument is 75 cm long.

some endometrial irritation is inevitable, intraluminal palpation should probably be reserved for those mares with reproductive problems.

Diagnostic Aids

A variety of diagnostic procedures is available to support physical findings in the reproductive examination of mares. In addition, some can provide prognostic information about the fertility potential of the individual. The most useful aids are culture, endometrial biopsy, endometrial cytologic examination and fiberoptic examination of the uterus.

Culture of the Reproductive Tract: Probably no procedure in reproductive practice stirs such a divergence of opinion and is accomplished under such a broad spectrum of technics as culture of the mare's genital tract. At issue is the significance of cervical vs uterine cultures and at what stage of the cycle is culturing most valuable. Instrumentation varies from the traditional wire loop to sophisticated instruments with guarded swabs. Cultures are either made through a speculum or by manual insertion to the desired location.

If the objective of the culture is to evaluate the status of the uterus and confirm a diagnosis of endometritis, a true uterine culture should be attempted. It should be taken only from the uterus without any of the number of potential sources of extraneous bacteria. Environmental contamination and contaminants from the vulva or vagina are all potential sources of bacteria that can muddle the interpretation of results.[2] To eliminate these sources we must select a good site for examining the mare, prepare the

animal for aseptic examination and use an instrument that samples only the uterus.

Several commercial culture instruments provide varying degrees of protection of the swab as it passes into the uterine lumen. The author's choice of culture instruments, which stands out from all commercial and homemade contrivances, is the Knudsen endometrial sampler (Jacoby, Stockholm) (Fig 6). This device is initially expensive and somewhat of a chore to prepare but yields the most reliable information of all instruments tried. A fairly large cotton swab can be used to assure absorption of a significant amount of uterine fluid. The swab is absolutely guarded as it passes into the uterine lumen and as it emerges back through the cervix. The instrument can be passed through a glass speculum during estrus or inserted with a gloved hand.

The ideal time in the estrous cycle to obtain a uterine culture is the subject of much debate.[8] In my opinion, the best time to recover uterine organisms is the first day of standing estrus, even if the cervix is not fully relaxed. At this time glandular secretions from the endometrium are increasing, making a moist swab easier to obtain, and the full flushing action of estrus has not yet taken place. During diestrus the endometrium is often dry, making bacterial recovery more difficult. The technic of culturing in the winter, during anestrus and prior to the breeding season, must be questioned since the chances for missing bacteria associated with chronic endometritis are greatest at this time.

Special circumstances indicate sampling parts of the reproductive tract other than the uterus. Experience with the organism producing contagious equine metritis and in some cases *Klebsiella* has shown that these bacteria may concentrate in the caudal vagina, urethral opening, clitoral fossa and clitoral sinuses.[9,10] Sampling these portions of the tract is indicated when infections of those areas is suspected. Otherwise a true uterine culture is the most reliable diagnostic procedure when endometritis is a consideration. Cervical and uterine cultures correlate well when significant exudate exits the cervix from the infected uterus, but in these cases it is just as easy to obtain a uterine swab as a cervical one.

The laboratory technic for obtaining meaningful uterine cultures is critical. The clinician must know which bacteria are present and in what quantity to interpret the culture. Any steps, therefore, that reduce the chances of isolating an organism or change the numbers recovered are pitfalls leading to judgement errors.

Uterine swabs ideally are plated directly on the final medium for culture. This method gives positive correlation between numbers of organisms on the swab and numbers of colonies on the plate. The time allowable between taking the sample and plating it depends upon the moisture of the swab. Bacteria are lost as the swab dries and any method that delays drying, such as refrigeration or adding sterile saline to the swab, helps extend bacterial viability. When many mares are examined at one farm over a prolonged period, it is advantageous to streak culture plates on location.

Transporting or storing swabs in nutrient broth increases the chances of proliferation of a few contaminating bacteria, which makes quantitation impossible. Stabbing swabs into semisolid holding medium may reduce the numbers of organisms on the swab and necessitates plating the entire holding medium, which is inaccurate and inconvenient.

Growing and identifying the organisms that cause endometritis are fairly simple. Advanced microbiologic technics are not required except in special situations, such as in cases of contagious equine metritis. The practitioner should be able to make therapeutic decisions in most cases by grossly inspecting colonies and making gram stains. Plating on blood agar and one selective gram-negative medium is adequate, although more sophisticated multiple diagnostic plates are available commercially. Plates are incubated at 37 C (98.6 F), preferably in a candle jar to provide microaerophilic conditions, and inspected daily. An indication of the number of colonies must be included in the laboratory report. Pure cultures are more significant than mixed ones.

The following organisms, in significant numbers and in fairly pure cultures, must be considered pathogenic: beta-hemolytic streptococci, hemolytic E coli, Pseudomonas spp, Klebsiella spp, and Monilia (Candida) spp. The degree of inflammation detected upon physical examination and by other diagnostic aids heavily influences the opinion as to the origin of disease. Other organisms, when isolated repeatedly, are occasionally suspect in the presence of inflammation. However, alpha-hemolytic streptococci, staphylococci and various enteric organisms other than those listed generally should be viewed as contaminants.

It is strongly recommended that the clinician either perform or closely supervise microbio-

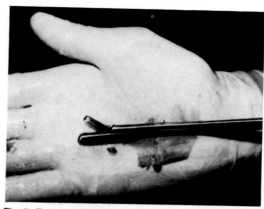

Fig 7. Endometrial biopsy instrument, with the jaws open.

logic examinations in a reproductive practice. No laboratory report can convey the same information that an experienced practitioner can obtain by examining cultures. A commercial laboratory can be used to identify organisms when necessary since identification is essential to proper interpretation.

Endometrial biopsy: Attempts to correlate endometrial histologic findings with infertility and fertility potential have been made over the last 25 years.[11-15] Standards of biopsy specimen procurement, processing and interpretation have been established to make this procedure an integral part of reproductive examination.[16,17]

Uterine biopsy must be considered only as an adjunct to the entire examination procedure and should never be undertaken without first completing a physical examination of the tract as described. Absolute assurance that the mare is not pregnant is obviously essential since the biopsy procedure invariably produces abortion.

Deep palpation of the uterus to detect physical abnormality enhances the value of endometrial biopsy. In the absence of clinically detectible pathologic changes, a single endometrial sample is representative of the entire endometrium.[18]

Logical candidates for endometrial biopsy are barren mares with any clinically evident abnormality of the reproductive tract, failure to conceive after repeated beddings to a stallion of known fertility, history of early embryonic death, and history of cyclic failure during the breeding season. Those mares presented for fertility evaluation as a part of a prepurchase examination should also have a uterine biopsy.

The technic for obtaining and processing biopsy specimens has been described elsewhere.[17]

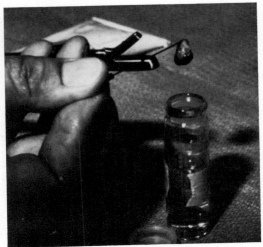

Fig 8. Lifting tissue specimen from the basket of the biopsy instrument with a small-gauge needle.

The instrument of choice is a 70-cm alligator punch with a basket 20 x 4 x 3 mm made expressly for the purpose (Pilling, Fort Washington, PA) (Fig 7). After proper preparation of the mare, as described earlier under vaginoscopic examination, the instrument is introduced into the uterine lumen with a gloved hand. The tip is guarded carefully as it passes through the cervix to protect against cervical trauma.

When the basket of the instrument is located well inside the uterine lumen, the hand is withdrawn from the vagina and inserted in the rectum. The instrument is then directed to the uterine area chosen for the biopsy. In the presence of previously detected focal lesions, multiple biopsies are indicated, including the area

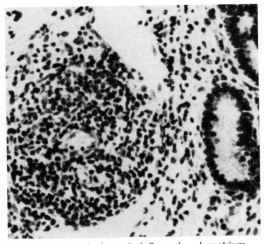

Fig 9. Lymphocytic focus in inflamed endometrium.

in question as well as a portion of endometrium that feels normal. In the absence of palpable focal lesions, the base of either horn should be sampled.

The safest approach to obtaining the biopsy is to turn the instrument on its side and press a portion of endometrium between the side walls of the punch with the index finger. If the uterus is pushed into the front of the 20-mm basket, there is a chance of cutting through the entire uterus and possibly the rectal wall.

Removal of the specimen from the basket is best done with a small-gauge hypodermic needle as gently as possible (Fig 8). Rough handling usually disrupts the luminal epithelium. The tissue should be placed immediately in fixative. Cellular detail and tissue integrity are best preserved with Bouin's fixative for 12-24 hours, with replacement of the Bouin's solution by 80% ethanol or 10% formalin after that time. The fixed tissue should then be trimmed for embedding so that sections are cut perpendicular to the endometrium. Paraffin-embedded sections are best stained with hematoxylin and eosin for routine examination.

It is advantageous for the clinician to interpret endometrial biopsies. Total familiarity with the clinical picture helps correlate biopsy findings with the rest of the data. With minimum study, most practitioners can learn to identify basic physiologic changes associated with cyclic phenomena and the significant pathologic changes related to infertility and early embryonic death. A summary of these changes is presented below. The reader is referred to other sources for more detail.[11,15-19]

The characteristic histologic changes evident in endometrial biopsy in relationship to stages of the estrous cycle are presented in Table 1 and Figures 11-13. Significant pathologic changes in endometrial biopsies are inflammation, fibrosis and lymphatic stasis. To be of diagnostic and prognostic value, these changes must be characterized and quantitated.

Endometrial inflammation is evidenced by increased numbers of inflammatory cells in foci or diffused in various areas of the lamina propria. The cellular infiltrate is classified as to the predominant cell type. Acute inflammations contain mostly polymorphonuclear neutrophils (PMN) and interpretation must take into account the physiologic appearance of PMN during the estrogenic phase of the cycle. Most commonly seen in chronic endometritis is infiltration of lymphocytes, accompanied by

Table 1. Histologic Findings Related to Stage of Estrous Cycle

Stage of Cycle	Luminal Epithelium	Glandular Density and Patterns	Other
Proestrus	low columnar	increasing edema may push glands into clumps	
Estrus	tall columnar (Fig 11)	decreased density due to edema	margination of neutrophils in smaller veins and capillaries
Diestrus	variable; generally low, cuboidal early and increasing in height as estrus approaches	density increased due to reduction of edema and glandular proliferation (Fig 12)	
Anestrus	cuboidal, atrophic	glandular atrophy, reduced density, glandular ducts arranged in straight lines (Fig 13)	glandular epithelium low and cuboidal; glandular lumens may contain trapped secretions

varying degrees of plasma cell and macrophage infiltration (Fig 9).

Endometrial fibrosis most commonly occurs around the glands and appears in response to inflammation, glandular damage or to other undefined causes (Fig 10). Periglandular fibrosis may interfere with gland function to the extent that glandular support of the early conceptus is altered, resulting in early embryonic death.[17] Excellent correlation exists between mares with severe periglandular fibrosis and those that conceive but fail to sustain pregnancy beyond 70-80 days.[17,20]

Lymphatic stasis appears on biopsy as large, fluid-filled spaces lined with endothelial cells. When widespread and accompanied by a palpable jelly-like consistency of the uterus, this lesion is correlated with reduced fertility. Since large areas of edema may be artificially produced during biopsy, care must be taken in identifying these as lymphatics.

When these basic pathologic changes are observed, they should be evaluated for severity and distribution.[17] This allows mares to be categorized into 3 diagnostic and prognostic groups, which are the key to sensible use of the information:[17,19]

Category I includes mares with an endometrium compatible with conception and capable of supporting a foal to term. Pathologic changes, if present, are slight and widely scattered. No endometrial atrophy or hypoplasia is present during the physiologic breeding season.

Category II includes mares with an endometrium that reduces the chance for conception and pregnancy maintenance, but with

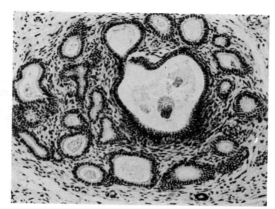

Fig 10. Nest of glands due to periglandular fibrosis. Note dilation of the glands.

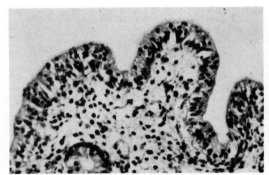

Fig 11. Tall columnar epithelium as seen during estrus. A diffuse lymphocytic infiltrate is also present.

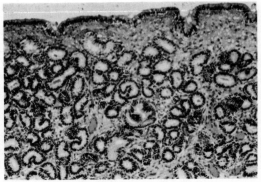

Fig 12. Gland density associated with diestrus.

reversible or only moderate pathologic changes. Endometrial changes may include combinations of any of the following: slight to moderate, diffuse cellular infiltrations of superficial layers; scattered, frequent inflammatory or fibrotic foci throughout the entire lamina propria; scattered, frequent periglandular fibrosis of individual gland branches of any degree of severity; 3 or fewer nests of gland branches per low-powered field in 5 fields (fields 5 mm in diameter); and widespread lymphatic stasis without palpable changes in the uterus.

Category III includes mares with an endometrium that reduces the chances for conception and pregnancy maintenance, with essentially irreversible lesions. The endometrium may contain any of the following changes: widespread periglandular fibrosis of any degree of severity, with 5 or more nests in an average low-power field; widespread, diffuse, severe cellular infiltration of superficial layers; lymphatic stasis accompanied by palpable changes in the uterus; endometrial atrophy or hypoplasia with gonadal dysgenesis; and pyometra accompanied by endometrial atrophy or widespread, diffuse, severe infiltration.

Mares in category I have a 70% or better chance for producing a live foal. Mares in category II have a 50-70% chance for production, dependent on other management considerations. Mares in category III have less than a 10% chance for continued production. Care should be taken in pronouncing a mare sterile on the basis of single or multiple biopsies. The occasional exception can be embarrassing.

In addition to prognostic value, biopsies can aid assessing the presence or absence of endometritis when clinical and cultural findings are inconclusive.

Endometrial or Cervical Cytologic Examination: The equine uterus responds to irritants, such as bacterial pathogens, by mobilizing neutrophils, which migrate through the endometrium and enter the uterine lumen.[17] A high correlation between PMN numbers recovered by uterine or cervical swabs and cases of endometritis has been reported.[13,21] This cellular response can be detected by smearing uterine swabs or cervical mucus onto a slide, staining the smears and examining for the presence of PMN. Using the same swab used to sample the uterus, smear it after inoculation of the medium to provide quick verification of the presence of inflammation.

Examination of smears of mucus or exudate collected on the speculum after routine vaginoscopy is an excellent screening technic.[21] Air-dried smears can be stained with a rapid cytologic stain (Diff-Quik:Harleco).

Significant numbers of PMN suggest that endometritis exists. More than one PMN per 5 240X fields has been suggested as the dividing line between physiologic and pathologic numbers of cells.[13] In fact, PMN are numerous in most cases of endometritis (Fig 14).

In the author's experience, nearly half of the mares examined by biopsy and culture show histologic evidence of endometritis without bacteriologic recovery of a pathogen. Examination for PMN provides a quick and inexpensive way to identify these mares early. The technic may also be helpful when a slow-growing, fastidious agent, such as the contagious equine metritis organism, is involved.[22]

Fiberoptic Examination of the Uterus: A potential diagnostic aid in detection of uterine abnormalities is visual inspection of the lumen through a flexible fiberoptic instrument. The technic has not gained widespread acceptance

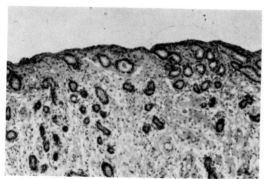

Fig 13. Gland density associated with anestrus. Note the linear arrangement of the gland ducts.

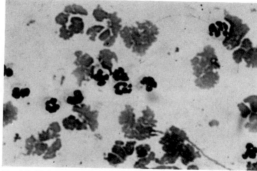

Fig 14. Polymorphonuclear leukocytes on slide streaked with culture swab.

but should be considered when palpable changes in the uterus need further identification or when other diagnostic procedures fail to indicate a cause of infertility.[11]

Any flexible instrument suited for examination of the equine upper respiratory tract is adequate for uterine examination. There must be a capability for inflation of the uterus. Unfortunately, the biopsy instruments in these endoscopes do not provide an endometrial sample large enough for meaningful evaluation.

Ideally the fiberoptic instrument should be sterilized with ethylene oxide prior to uterine use. A practical alternative is to thoroughly clean the working end of the instrument with povidone iodine solution (Povidol:National) by repeated washings. Prolonged immersion may damage instruments with failing seals.

The endoscope is passed through the cervix with the gloved hand as described previously. The hand remains in the vagina to extend or retract the instrument and one or more fingers remain in the cervical canal to seal it for inflation purposes. There is some advantage in selecting mares in diestrus for this, since inflation is more easily maintained with a tight cervix.

When the tip of the endoscope is in the uterine lumen, inflation allows examination of the body of the uterus and identification of the bifurcation. The latter appears as a vertical pillar especially evident as inflation of the horns commences and should not be confused with an intraluminal adhesion. The endoscope is then advanced down each uterine horn to systematically observe all of the endometrium.

Typical lesions found with endoscopy are cystic structures, adhesions and textural and color changes of the endometrium. In a recent study, 40 mares with a history of infertility were palpated rectally, examined endoscopi-

cally and had uterine biopsies taken.[23] Endoscopy revealed lymphatic cysts, polyps and other nodules in 14 mares, intraluminal adhesions in 8, and areas of color change in 6. Endometrial biopsy was more efficient than endoscopy alone in detecting pathologic uterine changes; however, endoscopy was a useful diagnostic aid.

Pregnancy Diagnosis

The ability to diagnose pregnancy early and accurately is fundamental to any successful equine reproductive program. Among compelling economic and physiologic needs to detect pregnancy before 40-50 days are: the very short physiologic breeding season artificially imposed by the calendar; the myriad reasons that mares fail to show estrus following service; long gestation, which allows little time to breed the mare back and to keep the animal in annual production; and the costs of owning horses, with the obvious penalties imposed by lowered reproductive efficiency. This list barely scratches the surface of reasons why the practitioner must be able to answer the question: Is the mare pregnant?

Manual examination of the reproductive tract per rectum is the accepted method of pregnancy diagnosis. In all but a few selected circumstances this is the most accurate, rapid and economic method of determining normal, abnormal or multiple pregnancy. When the mare is confirmed nonpregnant, rectal examination may suggest the reasons for failure and indicate required corrective steps.

The reader is referred to an especially helpful description of manual examination for pregnancy.[4] The technic, facilities and restraint for rectal examination have been described earlier in this chapter.

Uterine Changes in Pregnancy

As early as 17 or 18 days postovulation, certain changes in uterine tone and consistency suggest pregnancy.[24] Increases in thickness and tone of the uterine wall at this time are produced by progesterone secreted by the CL. Tone and thickness are greater than that produced by progesterone in mid-diestrus, probably because the progesterone effect is cumulative. However, pregnancy cannot be diagnosed on the basis of uterine tone and thickness. Mares are notorious for persistence of the CL spontaneously without conception or even breeding.[25]

To confirm pregnancy, the actual conceptus in its chorionic vesicle must be identified with certainty. At this very early stage of pregnancy (17-18 days), the vesicle may be apparent to the examiner as a distinct, fluid-filled, spherical structure on the ventral aspect of the uterus, usually at the base of either horn. Since the vesicle is only about 2.5 cm in diameter at this stage, considerable proficiency is required to define it.[24] Some normal "curling" of the base of the uterine horn occurs during prolonged progesterone influence. A common error in early pregnancy examination is to mistake this curled horn for the chorionic vesicle.

The conceptus grows slowly, with the vesicle reaching 3 cm in diameter at 25 days and 4-4.5 cm at 30 days. Recognition of the vesicle requires the same approach until 50 days or later. Palpation of the ventral aspect of the uterus is required, with the fingers bent over the cranial margin to reach well under the uterine body and horns. Little dorsal distension occurs during this period. The approximnate sizes of the chorionic vesicle through 90 days are presented in Table 2.

In the early development of skills in rectal examination for pregnancy, it is reasonable for the beginner to concentrate on the 35-45 day examination. At this time the chorionic vesicle is large enough to be readily recognized as the fingers slide along the underside of the uterus. Both margins of the vesicle should be quite distinct, making an abrupt junction with the non-gravid portion of the uterus. The sensation of fluid under slight tension is important and is interpreted as a "live" feeling.

A common error at this stage is not extending the fingers back far enough under the edge of the uterus, thus missing the vesicle. Another possibility for confusion is to mistake the bladder for a chorionic vesicle. If care is taken to explore the total tract continuously from one ovary to the other, the entire uterus can be pal-

Table 2. Size and Shape of the Chorionic Vesicle in Early Pregnancy.[5]

Days of Gestation	Vesicular Size and Shape		
16	1.8-2.2 cm	(¾-⅘")	pigeon egg (round)
20	2.6-3.2 cm	(1-1¼")	bantam egg (slightly oval)
25	3.0-3.8 cm	(1¼-1½")	pullet egg (slightly oval)
30	4.2-4.5 cm	(1½-1¾")	small hen egg (oval)
35	4.4-5.9 cm	(1¾-2¼")	large hen egg (oval)
40	5.7-6.9 cm	(2¼-2¾")	turkey egg (oval)
45	7.6-5.0 cm	(3 x 2")	goose egg
50	8.9-6.3 cm	(3½ x 2½")	orange (oval)
60	13.3 x 8.9 cm	(5¼ x 3½")	small melon (oval)
90	23 x 14 cm	(9 x 5½")	small football (oval)

pated and this error avoided. Examination of mares bred back at foal heat can be confusing when the formerly pregnant horn has not yet completely involuted.

Cooperation from the mare, in terms of rectal relaxation, is a factor in the ease with which the diagnosis is made. It is infinitely better to admit some doubt about the mare's status and re-examine the animal at a later date than to guess in the fact of an incomplete examination.

All serious equine practitioners should strive to gain experience in pregnancy diagnosis at 35-38 days or less. This time coincides with the onset of pregnant mare's serum gonadotrophin (PMSG) secretion by the endometrial cups. Should some pregnancy abnormality, such as twins, be diagnosed, it is helpful to make decisions about therapeutic abortion before PMSG levels are significant (see discussion on therapeutic abortion).

From 50-90 days of gestation, the chorionic vesicle enlarges rapidly and assumes an oval shape as it spreads through the uterine lumen. During this period, depending on the age and past foaling history of the mare, the uterus extends over the pelvic brim and becomes too large and heavy to retract and delineate completely. From the time the uterus attains this position until the fetus can consistently be palpated (120-150 days), positive pregnancy diagnosis becomes somewhat more difficult.

The first step in examining such mares is to grasp one ovary and the broad ligament and, with traction, attempt to elevate the uterus into the pelvic cavity. A nonpregnant uterus can be elevated enough to allow palpation of its entirety. A pregnant uterus fails to respond to the pressure, but the attachment of the ligament to the tip of the uterine horn can be felt.

The hand is then placed flat on the dorsal surface of the uterus and its fluid content confirmed by ballottement. If the uterine wall feels thin and viable, and if the fluid is watery, a positive diagnosis of pregnancy can be made. A condition that might be confused with pregnancy at this stage is pyometra, which is associated with a thick, doughy uterine wall and much less resiliency of the fluid contents.

Due to the relatively large volume of fluid in relation to fetal size, positive identification of the fetus is inconsistent before 120 days. After that time, ballottement as described above results in the fetus floating up in the fluid and contacting the hand. Positive identification of the fetus confirms the diagnosis.

From about 150 days until birth the fetus can be readily located by rectal examination.

Cervical Changes Detected by Rectal Examination

Supportive evidence of early (17-20 days) pregnancy in mares is obtained by carefully palpating the cervix, in conjunction with uterine palpation.[26] The cervix responds to progesterone in essentially the same manner as the uterine wall, and often more dramatically. A typical cervix in early pregnancy is elongated, tubular and very firm. When palpated through the rectum it often seems to extend into the uterine lumen and into the cranial vagina. Cervical tone and consistency seem to be more exaggerated than during diestrus. This exaggeration is felt by some practitioners to be a more consistent and significant finding than uterine tone and consistency.

The same precautions should be observed when correlating cervical changes with pregnancy as mentioned for uterine changes. Spontaneous persistence of the CL without pregnancy produces similar findings. Pregnancy must be confirmed by identifying the chorionic vesicle.

In mares that fail to return to estrus at the appropriate interval after breeding, the presence of an estrogen-dominated cervix may be a helpful negative finding. If softening and relaxation of the cervix are detected rectally, efforts to detect estrus should be intensified.

Ovarian Changes in Pregnancy

Ovarian activity is of no help in pregnancy diagnosis. Since the CL of the mare is enveloped in ovarian stroma within a short time after ovulation, it cannot be palpated as supportive evidence of pregnancy. Follicular activity during early pregnancy must be understood to avoid confusion. The mare typically develops large follicles that ovulate during the first few months of gestation. No negative evidence of pregnancy should be interpreted when large preovulatory follicles are palpated. The role of secondary follicles and CL formation are discussed under the physiology of gestation.

Twin Pregnancy

Twinning is highly undesirable in mares and is considered by some to be the largest cause of abortion.[27] When abortion does not occur it is extremely rare for either surviving foal to be large and strong enough to have commercial value. Lack of uterine capacity to support 2 fetuses is the apparent cause of the problem.

The diagnosis of twin pregnancy is a crucial one since most owners elect to terminate the pregnancy. If the mare is to be rebred in the same season after termination of the pregnancy, it is essential to make that decision before serum PMSG levels are elevated (38 days) or the mare will not recycle before 120 days from the original conceptions.[28] This puts added pressure on the practitioner to make an accurate early assessment.

Twins can usually be detected by identifying 2 distinct chorionic vesicles during rectal examination. There are enough exceptions to this statement, however, to make a negative statement hazardous. Few veterinarians certify mares to be carrying single foals on the basis of rectal palpation. The disparity is due to the location of the twin fetuses in the uterus. When the chorionic vesicles develop well apart, eg, in opposite horns, there is a palpable separation between them until about 50 days; sequential examinations reveal development of both. Some mares carry twins that cannot be palpated as such. In these cases it is likely that both vesicles developed closely side by side.

There is a temptation, when 2 vesicles of disproportionate size are found, to convince oneself that the smaller embryo will not survive and that the mare will carry and give birth to only one foal. It is the author's experience that in every case where twin vesicles were identified, a problem with twinning was a reality.

Once past the 50 or 60 day point, rectal examination is useless to confirm twin pregnancy. Since many mares are sold while pregnant, both buyer and seller would benefit from definitive certification of a single-foal pregnancy. Fetal electrocardiography has been suggested as a diagnostic aid that could indicate single or double heartbeats.[29] A study on the limitations of fetal electrocardiography raises doubts as to the reliability of this technic.[30]

Vaginal Examination in Pregnancy

Changes evident by vaginoscopy may support the diagnosis of pregnancy but should never be substituted for positive criteria. In early pregnancy, much as in diestrus, the cervix is very tight and protrudes into the vaginal vault high on the wall. The cervix and vagina are typically pale and sometimes yellowish. A heavy, viscous mucus is evident on the external cervical os, vaginal walls or both. Any of these changes are compatible with diestrus, particularly if persistent.

Vaginal examination may help when uterine tone and consistency are difficult to assess and when large follicles are palpated on the ovaries. Failure to find the vaginal and cervical changes of estrus can help eliminate the possibility that the mare is in heat.

A valid use of the vaginoscope in pregnancy examination exists when the chorionic vesicle is difficult to define by rectal palpation. By dilating the vagina with air through a speculum, the uterus may be pushed into a position more favorable for rectal exploration.

Laboratory Tests for Pregnancy

When vicious or intractable mares are presented for pregnancy examination or when the size of the animal precludes safe rectal palpation, laboratory tests for pregnancy can be helpful. The current popularity of miniature breeds of horses underscores the need for accurate laboratory tests. Practitioners with limited experience in physically examining the reproductive tract may find laboratory tests valuable as a supplement to rectal palpation.

The presence of a circulating PMSG in mares between 40 and 140 days of gestation is the basis for the procedures with the greatest clinical use. Two characteristics of PMSG secretion must be understood to use the tests for gonadotrophins: the time limits of measurable levels of PMSG in serum and the continuation of secretion by the endometrial cups following early fetal death.[28]

Although some mares may produce PMSG in detectable levels from as early as 40 to as late as 150 days of gestation, variations in time and test sensitivity suggest that the presence of PMSG should be considered significant from 45 to 110 days.[31,32] Peak serum levels of PMSG occur between 50 and 70 days.[32] If tests at either

end of the range are negative, the possibility of undetectable levels should be considered.

The most serious reservation in using the presence of PMSG as a determination of pregnancy is the fact that PMSG persists after fetal loss. Once formed, the endometrial cups secrete PMSG through their normal life span. Should embryonic death occur after 40 days, positive PMSG levels indicate pregnancy where no viable fetus exists.[28]

Immunologic Test for PMSG: The hemagglutination inhibition (HI) test is the quickest, most practical method of PMSG detection. The presence of gonadotrophin in the serum inhibits the agglutination of RBC coated with gonadotrophin in the presence of PMSG antibody. This test is available in kit form (MIP Test: Diamond) and results are read in 2 hours.

Biologic Tests for PMSG: The effect of PMSG on the reproductive tract of various laboratory animals is the basis for a number of valid assays for the gonadotrophin.[34] The most practical and inexpensive bioassay involves injecting 0.5-1.0 ml test serum SC into 21-day-old female mice. Saline-injected mice serve as controls. Levels of PMSG of 1 unit/ml test serum cause enlargement and congestion of the mouse uterus at 72 hours in comparison with controls.

A comparison of the HI, mouse inoculation and gel diffusion tests showed excellent accuracy with the first 2 tests.[33] The sensitivity of mouse inoculation is not enough of an advantage to overcome the practicality of the HI test. If the limitations of PMSG testing in general are observed, the commercial HI test is a highly satisfactory laboratory test for pregnancy in the mare.

Urinary Estrogens: From about 150 days of gestation to near term, the fetus and placenta of the pregnant mare produce estrogens in large quantities, which are excreted in the urine. Simple laboratory tests for these estrogens, such as the Cuboni test, or modifications of it are reliable indicators of pregnancy. These procedures are little used since rectal palpation from 150 days on is simple and fetal parts are readily palpable during this period. For the remote circumstance when rectal examination is impossible and a definitive pregnancy diagnosis is required, the procedure for the Lunaas modification of the Cuboni test is presented.[35] One ml of the urine to be tested is diluted with 10 ml distilled water in a 100-ml flask. After 15 ml concentrated sulfuric acid are added, the mixture is allowed to stand 3-5 minutes and is cooled. A strong, narrow-beamed light is shined through the mixture in a darkened room. Light-green fluorescence is evident in a positive sample. It is helpful to compare a known negative urine as a control when interpretation of fluorescence is questionable.

THE ESTROUS CYCLE

To manage normal mares for maximum fertility and to implement corrective measures in abnormal mares, it is essential to understand the basic elements of equine reproductive physiology. The estrous cycle is an interplay of anatomic, endocrine and behavioral events that must be synchronized for ovulation to occur. There are normally wide variations in events within the cycle, particularly related to season, and aspects of reproductive function not seen in other domestic species. These characteristics must be put in proper perspective and, where possible, used to best advantage.

After years of limited activity, equine reproductive research is currently attracting funding and competent investigators, with the result that new basic and applied information is increasing the pool of knowledge in this area. The advent of the International Symposia in Equine Reproduction has brought much of the current information together.[36,37] A recent text on equine reproductive physiology is highly recommended.[38]

Seasonal Aspects of the Estrous Cycle

Most mares are seasonally polyestrous and experience peak reproductive efficiency in late spring, summer and early autumn. To synchronize birth with favorable climatic and nutritional conditions, animals with a near-year gestation must breed during those periods.

The most important factor controlling seasonality is photoperiod or daylight length. Increasing photoperiod initiates the complex endocrine interactions leading to ovulation. Decreasing photoperiod dampens the system and eventually stops ovulation in most mares. The moderation of winter climate and natural production of more high-quality feed are also undoubtedly involved in improving reproductive function as daylight lengthens.[39]

The estrous cycle can be divided into 3 phases: the ovulatory phase, or the time from the first ovulation of spring until the latest one in autumn; the anovulatory phase, or period of complete inactivity (winter anestrus); and the transitional phase, or intermediate stage between anovulatory and ovulatory phases. This occurs both in spring and in autumn as the endocrine function of the mare rises and falls and is characterized by increasing or decreasing ovarian activity, erratic behavior and the absence of ovulation.

A study involving large numbers of mares showed that nearly all of them ovulated immediately after the summer solstice.[40] The ovulatory rate dropped to below 20% in winter. Peak reproductive efficiency, therefore, was attained at a time when the artificially designated breeding season was ending. In those breeds that use a January 1 birthdate for all animals and discriminate against foals born during the summer, most of the breeding season occurs before most mares are in the ovulatory phase of the cycle.

The anatomic, endocrine and behavioral nature of each phase of the cycle is distinctly different. The practitioner must be able to categorize and manage each mare with respect to the degree of reproductive efficiency exhibited. For example, many unproductive breedings can be avoided during the early spring by recognizing a mare as in the transitional phase. Full sexual receptivity may be evident in the mare's reactions to the stallion, yet ovarian activity is not developed to the point where ovulation is possible.

The clinically significant physical changes, hormone interactions and behavioral responses of the estrous cycle are illustrated by a "typical" mare progressing from winter anestrus, through the transition and into the ovulatory period:

Anovulatory Phase

In response to the diminished photoperiod of winter and other related factors governing seasonality, the anovulatory mare is best described as sexually dormant. The ovaries and tubular tract are atrophied. The ovaries are small, smooth and firm, and there is no detectible follicular activity and no functional tissue from previous CL.

Lacking the stimulus of gonadal estrogens and progesterone, the uterus becomes atonic and thin-walled. Lack of uterine definition may make palpation per rectum difficult. Uterine changes include glandular atrophy and compaction of the stroma due to the absence of edema. The cervix is similarly flaccid and difficult to palpate. Inspection of the cervix through a speculum reveals a pale, dry organ that is often relaxed, sometimes to the point of gaping open. The vaginal tract is also quite pale and without evident secretions. Distension with air produces little hyperemia or engorgement of superficial blood vessels.

The endocrine functions that govern cyclicity are essentially shut down during the anovulatory phase. Shortened photoperiod, acting through the pineal mechanism, may interrupt release of gonadotrophin-releasing hormone (GnRH) by the hypothalamus.[41] Seasonal differences in GnRH levels in various portions of the hypothalamus have been described.[42] Lacking hypothalamic stimulation, the anterior pituitary gland fails to produce significant amounts of either follicle-stimulating hormone (FSH) or leuteinizing hormone (LH). Reduced levels of gonadotrophins are responsible for ovarian inactivity, with resulting lack of estrogen and progesterone secretion by the gonads.

The behavioral patterns of seasonal anestrus are less specific and less predictable than endocrine function. Most mares are passive to mildly resistant in the presence of a stallion. It is not unusual, however, for a mare in deep anestrus to be sexually receptive to the point where the animal will accept the stallion at any time. In the absence of follicular development, this behavior seems paradoxical. It is possible that minute amounts of steroid hormones produced by the adrenal glands could be responsible.

Endocrinologically, anestral mares are quite similar to ovariectomized mares. Very small doses of exogenous estrogens cause sexual receptivity in both. For this reason, spayed mares make excellent teasers for semen collection because they can be predictably induced into the behavioral estrus with small doses of estrogenic hormones. In addition, good cervical relaxation can be achieved in anestral mares if necessary.

Since deep winter anestrus may persist into the artificially defined breeding season, great benefit would result from the initiation of cyclicity at an earlier time. To date, the only successful method to accelerate the process is the use of artificial lighting to lengthen the photoperiod. This program must be started about 2 months before results can be expected. The clinician faced with a mare still in deep anestrus in February, March or April can do little other than wait for the seasonal changes to exert their effects. Economic pressures may force practitioners to attempt therapeutic measures, such as hormone treatment. As long as the mare is dormant, these efforts will fail. Trials

with GnRH and progesterone, while encouraging in mares in shallow anestrus and transition, have not benefited mares in deep anestrus.[43,44] The use of FSH and/or LH in any form is similarly unrewarding.

Transitional Phase

The changeover to a fully functional ovulatory phase is gradual in most mares that have undergone a winter anovulatory phase. This transition is characterized by re-establishment of endocrine function, erratic sexual behavior and follicle development without ovulation. Therefore, the transition is a continuation of the period of infertility, which often coincides with the time when it would be extremely beneficial to breed mares for early foals. Managing transitional mares becomes a major concern for practitioners during spring months.

The physical changes evident in the reproductive tract during the transitional phase of the estrous cycle are primarily ovarian. Follicles develop, often in multiples, to a size and consistency well short of a preovulatory condition, and then regress. Little pattern is noted in this development and if examinations are performed sporadically, the impression is of static ovaries.

Increasing follicular activity causes the ovaries to enlarge considerably from their size during anestrus. There is a noticeable change in consistency as multiple small follicles begin to grow. A springy resilience is evident on deep palpation, in contrast to the dense, firm consistency noted during the anovulatory phase. A great variability is noted in transitional mares in the number and types of follicles palpated. Commonly many small (10- to 15-mm) follicles are clustered on the ovarian surface, suggesting bunches of grapes. These small structures stay firm and are barely distinguishable in consistency from the ovarian stroma. As the season progresses, most mares develop 1-2 larger follicles that slowly progress to 20-25 mm, stay quite firm and then slowly regress. In the period immediately preceding the first ovulation, one follicle typically develops to 35-40 mm, then slowly matures, gradually enlarges and softens until it ovulates. This process may take several weeks.

During the period ovarian activity is increasing, little physical change can be detected in the tubular reproductive tract. The uterus tends to stay thin-walled and flaccid during the transition due to relatively low levels of ovarian hormones produced. As follicular activity increases, some changes are noted on palpation, probably due to estrogen-induced edema. These changes are minimal and not helpful in predicting when true cyclicity will start.

Endocrine patterns of transition are related to increasing release of FSH from the anterior pituitary, without significant amounts of LH production. Luteinizing hormone tends to remain at the same low basal levels that exist during the anovulatory phase until the ovulatory phase commences.[45]

The reasons for FSH release from the pituitary without a similar LH pattern are not clear. Perhaps differences in release patterns or quantity of GnRH may be responsible. Estrogens interacting with GnRH also play a part in the initial LH surge.[46]

With recurrent stimulation from FSH but in the absence of LH, gonadal steroid production is limited to the estrogens. Until the first ovulation, with ensuing CL formation, there is no significant progesterone production. It is interesting that the endometrial glands do not proliferate or begin active secretion until they are exposed to progesterone. Since conception is common at the first ovulation, the glands obviously commence their function very shortly after their first exposure to progesterone.

Behavioral patterns during transition are erratic. Prolonged periods of full sexual receptivity are usual as follicular development progresses. Examination of these transitional mares that show strong estral signs without imminent ovulation is particularly helpful to the breeder. Many unnecessary breedings during the early season can be avoided by careful ovarian palpation. The benefits of conserving the stallion and avoidance of excessive contamination of mares during this unproductive stage of the cycle are obvious.

Some transitional mares are behaviorally anestral during the period of follicular development. Others respond to the teaser with no correlation to ovarian status, showing receptivity and resistance in no definable pattern.

The management of mares that have not started ovulating when the breeding season is well under way is particularly frustrating. Owners paying board bills tend to lose their objectivity when several months elapse and their mares are not yet bred. Patient explanations of the nature of seasonality seem to lose their effect as April progresses. Artificial lighting is the best solution, but must be instituted at least 60 days before results are seen.

Some benefit in hastening the onset of the ovulatory phase of the cycle has been shown experimentally by the use of GnRH injections in conjunction with progesterone therapy.[43] The technic is not well adapted to a practical situation but further trials may produce workable programs for use of these compounds.

An empirical scheme, using only progesterone on mares that remain transitional late in the spring, has been employed by the author. A dose of 150 mg progesterone in oil is administered IM daily for a week. In those mares exhibiting persistent estral signs, there is generally a change to rejection of the teaser by the third or fourth day of treatment. Following termination of progesterone treatment, a significant number of mares return to estral behavior, develop a normal follicle and ovulate. It is difficult to estimate the true effect of this program, since at this time of the season mares are due to start ovulating regardless of treatment. Nevertheless, the numbers of mares ovulating shortly after this treatment appear more than coincidental.

Attempts at using prostaglandins on mares in the transitional period invariably fail due to the absence of a functional CL. Prostaglandin therapy is described elsewhere in the text.

The transitional period after the ovulatory phase of the cycle receives little attention from owners or clinicians, as the breeding season does not correspond with this period of waning reproductive function. Decreasing photoperiod in the autumn has a similar effect on the mare as the increasing photoperiod in spring. Behavior and ovulation become more erratic as the ovulatory season nears its end.

After the last ovulation, it is not uncommon for a follicle to develop to a large size and then fail to ovulate or regress. These so-called "autumn" follicles have been mistakenly referred to as "cystic follicles." They are not pathologic and disappear spontaneously, often weeks or months later.

Ovulatory Phase

In most mares in temperate zones, seasonal influences produce a definable period of fertility. By using ovulation as the event necessary for fertility, a physiologic breeding season can be precisely defined between the first and last ovulations. During this ovulatory phase the mare establishes a cycle that, in comparison with that of other domestic species, is a model of inconsistency. Acceptance of these inconsistencies as variations within normal limits is

Table 3. Mean Length of Components of the Estrous Cycle[38]

	No. of References	Composite Mean (days)	Range of Means (days)
estrus	26	6.5	4.5- 8.9
diestrus	10	14.9	12.1-16.3
estrous cycle	18	21.7	19.1-23.7

the only way to approach broodmare management and maintain sanity. Mares "normally" ovulate without showing estral behavior, show estral signs without ovulating, undergo prolongation of CL life span for a couple of months, or split heats with an 8- to 10-day interovulatory interval, just to suggest a few possibilities.

The following definitions apply to this discussion: The *estrous cycle* is the period from one ovulation to the next, when signs of estrous behavior accompany ovulation. *Estrus* is a period of sexual receptivity. *Diestrus* is the period from the end of one estrus to the beginning of the next estrus, characterized by formation of a functional CL.

The length of the individual components and the total estrous cycle vary greatly (Table 3).[38] Variation is well correlated with season, with most variability at the onset and the end of the ovulatory phase. Therefore, the length of estrus is shortest during the peak of the ovulatory season and corresponds with the peak of fertility. The effects of season on estrous cycle length and on estrus in 11 mares is detailed in Table 4.[47]

From these data it should be apparent that much closer management is required to breed mares at the optimal time early in the season than at its peak. In the following example, assume that sperm viability is 48 hours in the mare and that ovulation occurs 24 hours before the end of estrus. Without palpation for follicle development, if breeding commences on the second day of estrus, 3 breedings are necessary to adequately expose mares with an 8- to 9-day estrus. Mares with a 4-day estrus must only be bred once.

The basic endocrine, physical and behavioral elements of the estrous cycle are presented in simplified form in Table 5. Some areas from the table are discussed below.

Early Estrus: In response to GnRH release from the hypothalamus, the anterior pituitary releases FSH, which in turn stimulates follicle development. The resulting estrogen production from these growing follicles initiates the physical and behavioral changes of early estrus.

Late Estrus: As follicle maturation approaches, a large preovulatory surge of estrogens produces a positive feedback on the pituitary, precipitating a rise in LH levels. In contrast to females of other species, mares have a prolonged surge in LH levels that often lasts for 7-8 days and usually peaks after ovulation (Fig 15). Since it is common for multiple follicles to develop during estrus, this long exposure to LH may account for the large number of multiple ovulations that occur.

Ovulation: In its embryologic development, the cortex of the equine ovary folds at its hilus and becomes surrounded by medullary tissue.

Table 4. Seasonal Effect on Estrous Cycle Length and Duration of Estrus[47]

	Avg. Cycle Length (days)	No. of Cycles	Avg. Duration of Estrus (days)	No. of Estrus Periods
January	32.3	22	5.06	18
February	34.4	20	6.69	13
March	26.1	25	8.38	26
April	21.9	28	7.26	29
May	19.5	39	5.72	28
June	21.1	31	4.47	28
July	24.6	28	4.70	20
August	20.4	27	4.75	24
September	20.6	32	4.44	27
October	20.5	35	4.53	31
November	24.8	25	5.70	27
December	30.4	21	7.23	22

**Table 5. Basic Endocrine, Physical and Behavioral Changes
During the Estrous Cycle**

Stage of Cycle	Endocrine Changes		Physical Changes		Behavioral Changes
	Pituitary	Gonadal	Ovary	Tubular Tract	
early estrus	FSH rise	estrogen rise	follicle develops	uterine edema, cervical relaxation	beginning receptivity
late estrus	LH surge	estrogen peak	follicle matures	maximum uterine edema and cervical relaxation	strong receptivity
ovulation	LH near peak	estrogen fall begins, progesterone rise begins	follicle collapses, fresh "crater" palpable	uterine compaction, cervix still relaxed	variable, usually still receptive
early diestrus	LH fading	progesterone climbing	CH palpable	firm uterine tone	rejects stallion
mid-cycle	FSH rise	progesterone peaks	may detect follicular activity, CL may be palpable	maximum uterine tone, cervix firm, tubular	rejects stallion
late diestrus		luteolysis: rapid demise of CL causes progesterone fall	no palpable changes	early softening of uterus	rejects stallion

Mechanically this arrangement only allows ovulation through the hilar area or ovulation fossa. Follicles are palpated on the general ovarian surface, but the follicle collapses at ovulation and forces the ovum through its tract to the ovulation fossa.[48]

The time of ovulation in relationship to estrus varies. It is virtually impossible to predict ovulation time only from the duration of estrus. One report indicated that only 46% of the mares studied ovulated on the day prior to the end of estrus, and nearly 12% ovulated 3 days before the end of heat.[47] Very few mares (1.4%) ovulated after sexual receptivity had ceased.

Ovulation usually occurs during evening or night hours, with approximately 75% of mares ovulating between 4 PM and 8 AM.[49] The incidence of multiple ovulations reportedly varies from 14.5% to 42.8%.[40,50] The incidence was 25.5% in one study, but 1 of 11 mares had a 73.5% incidence and may have distorted the incidence figure. Elimination of this mare drops the incidence to 20%.

Endocrine changes following ovulation are quite rapid in most mares, and physical and behavioral changes follow very shortly. Some luteinization probably occurs prior to ovula-

tion; however, estrogen levels drop drastically when the follicle collapses and the CL develops quickly. The resulting changeover in estrogen:progesterone ratio causes rapid cessation of estral behavior. At this point, progesterone rather than estrogen has the dominant effect on behavior and the physical character of the tubular genitalia.

Early Diestrus: Development of the CL to the point of maximum progesterone production takes a number of days. The most important period of CL maturation is that time when the CL is responsive to prostaglandins, either endogenous or exogenous. The CL is refractory to luteolysis by prostaglandins for 5 days after the end of estrus.[51] In most mares this can be interpreted as 4 days after ovulation. This information weighs heavily on clinical judgement regarding the use of prostaglandins to manipulate the cycle.

Mid-Cycle: In mid-diestrus there is a normal surge in FSH release from the pituitary that causes some follicle development. These follicles may be detected when the ovaries are palpated at this stage of the cycle. Seldom are follicles of preovulatory size noted at this time, and other clinical signs of diestrus, ie, good

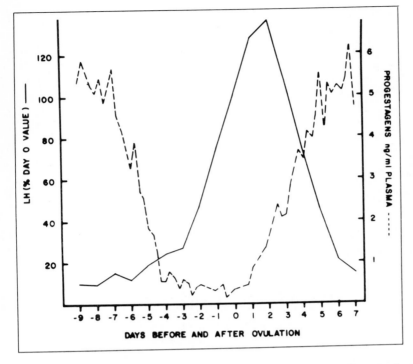

Fig 15. Levels of LH in plasma, demonstrating the prolonged LH surge in mares. [From J Repro Fert Suppl 23 (1975) 155]

uterine tone and firm cervix, indicate clearly these follicles are not associated with a return to estrus.

It is entirely possible, however, that regression of the CL can occur prematurely and mid-cycle follicles can develop in association with declining progesterone and increasing sexual receptivity. Fertile ovulations can occur during these so-called "split heats." The necessity for teasing mares continuously between heat periods is therefore obvious. Split heats were noticed in 5% of the estrous cycles observed in one study.[47]

Late Diestrus: The physiology of late diestrus, resulting in demise of the CL and return to estrus, is closely associated with the uterus. The mare's uterus, as in other species, is involved in maintaining the CL.[52] A luteolytic factor, now known to be prostaglandin F_2 alpha, is produced by the endometrium and travels via the systemic circulaton to the ovary, where it abruptly terminates the CL. Many other workers have shown that prostaglandin F_2 alpha or its analogs similarly lyses the CL when administered by injection.[51,53]

The uterus must first recognize a signal indicating "not pregnant," which undoubtedly involves complex biochemical interchanges between the conceptus and the maternal reproductive tract. Lack of that information results in prostaglandin release within the last day or 2 of diestrus. The resulting CL lysis is rapid; progesterone levels decline sharply (Fig 16). Removal of the physiologic brake of progesterone dominance allows the cycle to repeat.

The Use of Artificial Light

Manipulation of the seasonality of the mare was first suggested in 1947 and practical applications of a gradually increasing photoperiod were reported in 1968.[55] Mares were confined at night and subjected to extended periods of light from artificial sources. The length of lighting was increased over several months so that total daily light exposure reached 17-19 hours by early May. The chief advantage of this program was to significantly advance the onset of the ovulatory season to better coincide with the man-made breeding calendar. Since that time many trials with artificial lighting have proven its advantages. In one study, exposure of mares to 16 continuous hours of light caused ovulation 85 days earlier than in unlighted control mares.[56]

Artificial lighting is a highly useful management tool and is undoubtedly the most effective way to align the physiologic breeding season with the calendar. A 200-watt incandescent bulb is adequate to light a stall. Lighting should be started at least 2 months before the

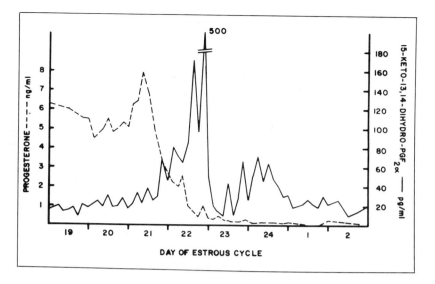

Fig 16. Decline in levels of circulating progesterone in response to prostaglandin release.[68]

first ovulations are expected. No disadvantages are seen in using 16 hours of light daily as compared with gradually increasing periods of light.

The cost of keeping barren mares in stalls for several months may be too expensive for use in all operations. However, lighting programs have been successfully used in paddock situations and appear to be equally effective with confinement programs.

Mares should be kept on the artificial light program until they are obviously pregnant or until natural daylight length approximates the artificial scheme. Groups of mares in lighted paddocks are best kept in the same groups to avoid disturbances in "pecking order."

Artificially decreasing daylight length has the same effect as natural shortening of photoperiod. Autumn transition and anestrus can be induced in about 2 months of decreasing daylight length. The only application of such programs is for investigative use.

THE NONPREGNANT MARE

Estrous Cycle Irregularities

The following cyclic abnormalities pose a clinical challenge to the practitioner. Some of the problems must be approached with management changes, eg, improved teasing procedures. Others may be handled medically and a final group, eg, diestral ovulation, need merely be understood to effect proper solutions.

Behavioral Anestrus During the Breeding Season

The mare that cycles and ovulates but fails to show detectible signs of heat is classified as behaviorally anestral. The principal factors responsible for virtually all of these cases are inadequate estrus detection and psychic factors that prevent display of sexual receptivity.

The primary objective in these mares is to demonstrate that they are cycling and ovulating. Periodic rectal and vaginal examinations at no more than 5-day intervals are the best approach. it may be helpful to monitor circulating progesterone levels where practical.

Once cyclicity is established, the mare should be followed closely until signs of full estrus appear. At this point, variations of the teasing procedure may be tried and defects in the teasing program can be pinpointed.

If there is convincing evidence that all possible teasing methods fail to produce the desired response and that other mares on the premises are being teased properly, a presumptive diagnosis of psychic anestrus can be made. Psychic factors usually involve very nervous maiden mares and foaling mares that are overly protective of their foals. Most of these mares can be bred naturally using various forms of restraint or by varying the location of the attempted breeding. Foals should be in close proximity to the mare or entirely separated. Tranquilization may be helpful. Allowing the teaser to actually mount the mare once or twice can be especially useful. An occasional mare is too dangerous to breed without risking injury to the stallion, mare or handler and

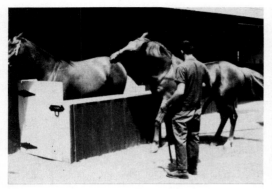

Fig 17. Teasing individual mares in a chute.

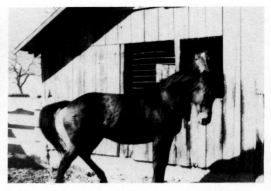

Fig 18. In this method of group teasing, mares in a pasture have access to the stallion in the shed.

must be passed. Artificial insemination, where allowed, is an obvious solution in these cases.

Once bred, the mare must be followed closely to detect either return to estrus or pregnancy. It is common, however, for these mares to show estral behavior freely in subsequent cycles.

Veterinarians can provide a valuable service to their clients by evaluating the teasing program. There are as many ways to tease mares as there are breeding establishments. Selecting the proper approach or combination of methods that suits the farm layout and personnel is a challenge. Observation and recording data are 2 essentials of a successful teasing program. The more familiar the personnel become with the idiosyncrasies of individual mares, the more effective job they can do. It is an advantage, therefore, to have the same people tease mares when possible.

It is usually most productive to handle each mare individually, teasing them in stalls, over a teasing board or loose (Fig 17). Variations in restraint and approach should be continuously tried. Supplemental procedures, such as group teasing, can be helpful. A stallion can be penned where mares are free to approach on their own (Fig 18). With proper control, some stallions can be led into or near fields of mares. It must be remembered that some mares do not show estrus on their own initiative and these loose teasing methods must be considered adjuncts to a careful individual teasing program.

Some breeders have success with stallions running loose with mares. Either a pony stallion too small to breed mares or some mechanical alteration to prevent coitus is employed. A surgical technic to produce retroversion of the penis caudad has produced useful teaser stallions.[57] Vasectomized stallions are not accept-

able teasers to run with mares. Repeated intromission, even without fertile ejaculates, creates too much irritation and contamination in most mares.

Excellent discussions of teasing methods are recommended to the reader for more detail.[38,58]

Prolonged Diestrus

Mares may fail to return to estrus after a normal ovulatory cycle for a number of reasons. If the mare was bred, the logical cause could be normal pregnancy or conception, with early embryonic death. In unbred mares, abnormal uterine contents, as in pyometra or mucometra, might prevent the release of prostaglandins from the endometrium. Another possibility is that the mare actually recycled normally but estrous signs were not displayed or detected.

A number of well-documented cases of true spontaneous persistence of the CL have been reported in mares with normal uteri.[25] In 7 of 11 mares followed clinically and by daily plasma progestin determinations, 11 cases of prolonged diestrus due to CL persistence occurred in a 2-year period.[47] Duration of the prolonged luteal phase ranged from 35-95 days.

The causes of such prolonged luteal function must be related to inadequate luteolysis by prostaglandins and appears to be a failure of the uterus to produce this luteolytic substance. In the cases studied, CL function, as measured by progesterone production, was similar to that in hysterectomized mares.[25] After the initial peak plasma progestin levels, a gradual decline was noted over the entire extended luteal phase. A rapid drop in progestin levels to baseline levels was noted just prior to the onset of estrus (Fig 19).

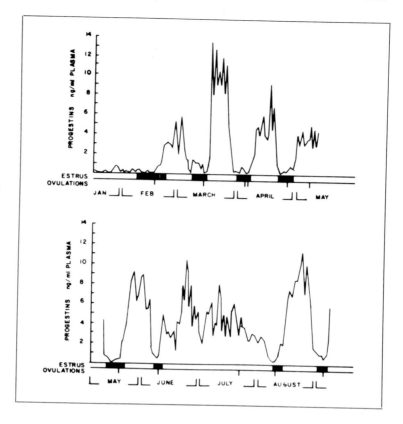

Fig 19. Normal estrous cycle profile, demonstrating spontaneous prolongation of diestrus from June into August.[25] Note the diestral ovulation.

Many cases of spontaneous persistent CL can be recognized by clinical examination. In mares with a reliable history of failure to return to estrus, signs of persistent progesterone effect on the uterus and cervix should be sought. Excellent uterine tone and a firm, elongated cervix can be detected in a high percentage of affected mares. The presence of well-developed follicles should not distract from the diagnosis.

Treatment of prolongation of the luteal phase of the cycle is directed at luteolysis. Administration of prostaglandin or one of its analogs, or indirect stimulation of natural luteolysis by uterine infusion is the logical choice. A detailed discussion appears below.

Diestral Ovulation

Ovulation in the presence of a functional CL, without signs of estrus, is relatively common in cycling mares. These ovulations are frequently detected if mares in diestrus are examined regularly. In one study, 64 examples of diestral ovulation were observed in 10 of 11 mares during a 2-year period.[47] Evidence of the normalcy of these ovulations is shown by a mare that conceived, carried and delivered a foal after artificial insemination in conjunction with diestral ovulation.[59]

Ovulation during diestrus can prolong diestrus. Complete luteolysis does not occur if normal prostaglandin release occurs when a new CL forms as a result of recent diestral ovulation. The immature CL (4 days from ovulation or less) is unaffected by prostaglandin and contributes more progesterone in the face of destruction of older CL. The same circumstances may be responsible for failure of exogenous prostaglandin therapy.

Pseudopregnancy

The term pseudopregnancy has been applied to most conditions resulting in prolonged diestrus in mares. The most common usage is for mares that are bred, fail to return to estrus and are subsequently found open. Pseudopregnancy and spontaneous CL persistence are used synonymously. Mares rarely remain behaviorally anestral for a period similar to gestation, show abdominal enlargement and lactate at the time of expected parturition. Two such cases have been observed by the author.

A true pseudopregnancy may not be a clinical entity in the mare and the term should be abandoned. Instead, a more specific diagnosis of one of the causes of prolonged diestrus should be made.

Prostaglandin-Induced Luteolysis

Prostaglandin F_2 and a variety of synthetic prostaglandin analogs have been shown as effective luteolytic agents in mares since the early 1970's.[51,53,60] In these and other studies, compounds administered directly into the uterus or by SC or IM injection resulted in rapid demise of the CL and subsequent return to estrus. Prostaglandins have since become valuable therapeutic tools for equine reproductive practice as luteolytic agents, both to terminate diestrus and to induce early abortion.[61] They are also useful in the induction of parturition.[52] Indications for the clinical use of prostaglandins include interrupting prolonged diestrus due to a spontaneous persistent CL, interrupting prolonged diestrus when diestral ovulation prevents normal return to estrus, changing the distribution of estrus in groups of mares booked to the same stallion to avoid overbreeding, shortening the interovulatory interval when breeding is passed or missed (as in twin ovulation, passed foal heat, etc), shortening the interovulatory interval when diagnostic or therapeutic procedures require cervical relaxation, synchronizing estrus in donor and recipient mares for embryo transfer, terminating pregnancy at up to 38 days of gestation, treatment of mismating, and treatment of those cases of pyometra that cause persistent CL. These indications all use the luteolytic action of prostaglandins. The use of prostaglandins in induction of labor is discussed separately.

Since the only effect of prostaglandins on the estrous cycle is to cause CL lysis, it may seem elementary to state that a mature (4 days or older) CL must be present before results are evident. Yet there are practitioners who, under pressure from owners, continue to use prostaglandins when there is no logic for their use. Transitional mares that have yet to ovulate by early spring obviously cannot benefit from prostaglandin therapy. We must educate breeders that these drugs do not "bring mares into heat" but only remove the progesterone brake from cycling mares.

In contrast to cows, which respond to prostaglandin-induced luteolysis with a fairly precise and predictable interval to ovulation, mares are notoriously variable in their response. The most important factor in this variability is the follicular status of the ovary at the time of administration of the drug.[63] Those mares with large follicles at the time of treatment had the greatest variability in response. When follicles 40 mm in diameter or larger were present, the follicle regressed about 33% of the time and a newly developed follicle was ovulated later. In the remaining mares, ovulation occurred in that large follicle to produce shorter than normal intervals from treatment to ovulation. In fact, some mares ovulated 24-72 hours after treatment, with only brief displays of estrus.[64] Less variation occurs in mares with smaller follicles on the day of treatment. The average time between treatment and ovulation in such mares is about 6 days.

This information stresses the importance of careful assessment of ovarian status when the decision is made to treat a mare with prostaglandin. If large follicles are present, careful teasing and palpation should follow daily to identify estrus and impending ovulation.

Variations in response to prostaglandin treatment also include partial and complete failure of luteolysis. In a study of 66 cycles during which a prostaglandin analog was administered in the presence of 6-day-old CL, only 65% of the mares responded with complete luteolysis. Incomplete luteolysis, with progesterone levels that failed to drop to levels that would allow estrus to occur, was apparent 26% of the time. Incomplete luteolysis and subsequent recovery of CL function occurred 6% of the time, and no luteolysis was apparent in 3%.[65] The doses in this study were those recommended by the drug manufacturer. Whether these figures are representative of large populations or not, it is obvious that practitioners must expect some treatments to fail to produce luteolysis, even when all the proper criteria for prostaglandin use are observed.

Prostaglandins available for clinical use are the natural compound and a number of synthetic analogs. Natural prostaglandin F_2Alpha (Prostin F_2Alpha:Upjohn) and the analog prostalene (Synchrocept:Diamond) are currently the only such drugs marketed in the US. Fluprostenal (Equimate:ICI) is marketed in many other countries and is expected to be available in the US in the near future.

The usual luteolytic doses for these compounds in light breeds of horses (400-500 kg) are: prostaglandin F_2Alpha 5-10 mg IM; prostalene, 2 mg SC; and fluprostenol, 250 μg IM. The chief differences in these compounds are in the adverse effects produced, none of which are serious when the drugs are used at levels recommended for luteolysis. Sweating, increased GI motility and slight posterior ataxia are the main adverse effects noted. Adverse effects are more evident following use of the natural compound than when analogs are administered. Slight to profuse sweating is evident in most mares treated with natural prostaglandin and usually ends in 30-45 minutes. Experience with both the natural and synthetic products has led to the conclusion that the presence or absence of adverse effects is not a significant factor in drug selection.

For many years veterinarians have recognized that infusion of the uterus with fluids results in a return to estrus and ovulation in many mares. It is now recognized that this treatment causes natural prostaglandin release from the endometrium due to irritation from the infusion. Regression of the CL follows quickly, with the resulting progesterone drop and return to estrus.[66]

If the same criteria are observed as for exogenous prostaglandin therapy, uterine infusion will give the same results. Warm saline solution (250-500 ml) should be aseptically infused through the cervix either by gravity or with slight pressure. There is obviously some disadvantage to uterine infusion vs prostaglandin injection in terms of convenience and time, but there are occasional indications for its use.

The knowledge that uterine infusion or irritation terminates CL function has another significance. Once the CL is mature, administration of medications into or manipulation of the uterus should be avoided if CL maintenance is desired. Early pregnancy can be terminated easily with uterine infusion as early as 5-6 days postovulation. Diagnostic procedures that produce significant endometrial trauma, such as biopsy or uterine flushing, similarly shorten CL life span. The significance of irritation caused by endometritis in altering cycle length is discussed later.

Anestrus During the Ovulator Season

If anestrus is defined as a cessation of reproductive function, which includes lack of follicle development and ovulation, it is unlikely that this phenomenon would occur during the peak stimulation of long photoperiod. Prior to the advent of practical endocrine assays, it was difficult to understand a complete interruption of function during the physiologic breeding season. Occasional mares were encountered that underwent ovarian atrophy and loss of uterine tone similar to those seen in winter anestrus.

Recent studies in which endocrine function and clinical signs were monitored have shown that a period of true anestrus, with complete absence of luteal function, is not a rare occurrence during the ovulatory season.[47] When the situation occurs in one out of a group of normally cycling mares, it is difficult to establish a cause. Large numbers of mares suffering an interruption of cyclicity at the same time, however, may be affected by nutritional factors. One such instance was associated with a dry spell and failure of pasture grasses even though supplemental feeding was more than adequate.[67] Further investigation into factors affecting reproductive function is needed.

The diagnosis of true anestrus in spring and summer requires the physical findings described above plus periodic assays for circulating progesterone. Some circumstantial evidence may be gained from failure of mares to respond to prostaglandin therapy. There is no logical treatment for such mares other than waiting for cyclicity to return, whatever the etiology may be.

Lactational anestrus, as seen in other animals such as beef cows, apparently does not occur in mares. The great majority of foaling mares cycle quite efficiently during the period that corresponds with peak lactation. Individual cases of true anestrus in postpartum mares should not be attributed to lactation.

Shortened Interestrus Interval

The discussion of cyclic irregularities to this point has dealt with extended periods without estrus, whether undetected or organic. The opposite situation, when estrus occurs more frequently than normal, is a variation that deserves mention. Shortened interestrus intervals may be completely normal in some mares or may be associated with some uterine abnormality, specifically inflammatory disease.

In mares with normal uteri, a premature return to estrus is not unusual. As previously discussed, some mares experience CL failure in mid-diestrus, allowing a mid-cycle follicle to develop and ovulate. This split heat does not always occur midway between estrus periods. Some mares ovulate, promptly go out of heat and 2 or 3 days later show strong receptivity again, develop a follicle and ovulate.

When managing such mares for maximum fertility, it is safe to assume that conception has failed or that an embryo will not survive the endocrine environment associated with return to estrus. Mares should be rebred on the split heat. The best explanation for this pattern is that a CL has failed to become established from the first ovulation and the resulting progesterone drop allows another cycle to start. Breeding of these mares can be missed if teasing is not carried out systematically throughout the entire cycle.

A shortened interestrus interval may, however, signal a uterine problem. One of the best clues of endometritis is premature return to estrus. Documentation of prostaglandin release, resulting in shortened diestrus in mares with uterine infections, has been presented.[68] It is logical that if saline infusions cause enough irritation to trigger a shortened cycle, the inflammatory response to a bacterial infection should be more than adequate to provide the same stimulus.

Shortened intervals are much more likely to occur with acute infections than with chronic ones. Contagious equine metritis, for example, produces transient but acute inflammation, and shortened interestrus intervals occur in most cases.[69] Once a bacterial infection becomes chronic, the occurrence of shortened cycles diminishes markedly.

If degenerative endometritis exists, prostaglandin release may be interfered with, causing longer interestrus intervals.

Ovulatory Failure

Once the ovulatory phase of the estrous cycle is established, it is unusual for mares to show signs of estrus, develop follicles and then fail to ovulate.[47] Such failure is characteristic of transitional mares, both before and after the ovulatory season. It is common, however, for the first few ovulations of the season to occur at the end of very long estrus periods, with follicles persisting for many days before ovulation. In these cases it may become important to a breeding program to hasten the onset of ovulation with drugs that supplement natural production of LH.

Human chorionic gonadotrophin (HCG), an LH-rich product of the human placenta, is the most efficient agent for inducing ovulation in mares. Doses of 1500-2000 IU cause ovulation within 48 hours of injection, even when administered very early in estrus.[70] Therefore, HCG can be used to great advantage to correlate breeding with ovulation. A workable scheme is to give HCG by IV injection on the afternoon of the day prior to the scheduled breeding.

Because the large molecular size of the protein in HCG causes antibody production in recipient mares, anaphylactic reaction is a possibility when subsequent doses are given. However, the author has not observed such reactions. Concern that antibody might cause refractory response after repeated injections has been expressed.[71] A recent study showed, however, that although antibody could be demonstrated in some mares, there was no interference with ovulation when HCG was given at each estrus throughout the entire ovulatory season.[72]

Before use of HCG to induce ovulation, careful consideration must be given to the presence of multiple follicles, even seemingly insignificant ones. The additional LH stimulation provided by HCG may result in more multiple ovulations than usual and an increased chance of twinning.

Infectious Causes of Infertility

Endometritis

Primarily at the time of breeding and during parturition, the mare is subjected to gross bacterial contamination of the reproductive tract. Healthy mares respond to these insults with an efficient defense mechanism to allow subsequent normal pregnancy. When the competence of the system is compromised, the contaminating organisms may establish themselves to produce a protracted inflammatory process that can interfere with fertility. Bacterial endometritis is perhaps the most significant cause of reduced reproductive performance in mares.

An efficient protective system exists in the mare's uterus. Semen cultures from stallions indicate that large numbers of bacteria are present in semen, even when meticulous hygienic measures are employed to collect semen, without extraneous contamination. Many potentially pathogenic organisms can be recovered from the semen of stallions with normal fertility.[73] Semen is deposited directly into the uterus at coitus. The glans penis of the stallion acts like a plunger and, with the cervix of the mare greatly relaxed in estrus, the negative pressure in the uterus causes intrauterine deposition of the entire ejaculate.[74]

Bacteria and inflammatory by-products must be removed from the uterus if the embryo is to survive when it reaches the uterine lumen 4-5 days after fertilization. Higher conception rates in young, healthy mares are circumstantial evidence for the uterine defense mechanism. More convincing is conception at the first postpartum estrus or "foal heat," when semen deposition may follow postpartum inflammation by as little as 5-6 days.

Inoculation of large numbers of pathogenic bacteria into the uterus of young healthy mares results in a rapid inflammatory response, followed by a return to normal in a few days. The same inoculations into mares with a history of endometritis and infertility produces a less intense and more persistent inflammatory response. Clinical signs of inflammation and positive uterine cultures last for prolonged periods.[75,76]

The uterine response to bacterial contamination is probably cellular and noncellular. The cellular aspect is principally neutrophilic, with migration of neutrophils through the endometrium and into the uterine lumen, where phagocytosis and intracellular lysis of bacteria occur. In the studies referred to above, the cellular response in healthy mares was rapid and intense, with large numbers of neutrophils mobilized and then quickly reduced in number. In mares with impaired cellular reaction, neutrophils were fewer in number but persisted longer. This association with prolonged low-grade inflammation is the basis for using neutrophil numbers in the endometrial smear as a diagnostic aid in evaluating endometritis.

The noncellular aspects of uterine resistance are less clearly understood. Immunoglobulin secretion from the uterus may be a significant factor and the presence of these proteins in the endometrium and uterine lumen has been reported.[77] Other factors are being investigated, such as differences in chemotaxis between normal and abnormal mares, and direct inhibition of bacteria by noncellular uterine secretions.[78]

Unless trauma occurs, most mares apparently lose their ability to combat bacterial contamination gradually, so that fatigue of the immune system, rather than failure of the system, is responsible for most genital tract infections. The many factors involved can be grouped into 2 syndromes: prolonged and uninterrupted irritation of the genitalia, and intermittent, repeated irritation.

In the case of continuous irritation, there is anatomic failure of the normal barriers that prevent aspiration of air and contaminants into the reproductive tract. In healthy mares there are 3 major functional sphincters that maintain the integrity of the tract: the vulvar sphincter, comprised of the labia, constrictor muscles of the vulva and the perineal body; the vestibular sphincter, a natural closure at the vulvovestibular junction activated by the constrictor muscles of the vestibule; and the cervix which, even when completely relaxed, lies collapsed and acts as a valve to protect the uterus.

Loss of integrity of any of the 3 sphincters can lead to failure of the entire anatomic protective system. By far the most likely sequence, however, starts with failure of the vulvar sphincter. Contamination of the caudal vagina then causes the vestibular sphincter to fail and finally the cervix loses its ability to protect the uterine lumen.

The causes of failure of the anatomic protective system are multiple and interrelated. Aging, poor body condition and multiple parturitions are the principal underlying factors that result in stretching and disruption of sphincter muscles, loss of support for the entire reproductive tract, and sagging of the viscera. All of these changes may be involved in producing abnormal perineal angle, loss of labial and vulvar tone, and thinning of the perineal body. Pneumovagina results and can exist in varying degrees from caudal pneumovagina to pneumouterus. A concurrent source of continuous irritation may be cranial reflux of urine, with pooling in the fornix of the vagina and eventual bathing of the uterine lumen due to urine flow through the cervix. The continuous irritation of the tubular genitalia by air, fecal contaminants and sometimes urine may be a major source of fatigue of the normal uterine defense mechanism, leading to endometritis.

Another source of failure of uterine immunocompetence is repeated contamination of the tract in the absence of obvious anatomic change. Although aging is a likely contributory factor, the physical changes associated with aging may not be evident. Changes in the endometrium at the cellular level may be involved. In any event, some mares suffer fatigue of the uterine defense mechanism through repeated exposure to irritants and organisms. The source may be multiple breedings, normal or abnormal parturition, genital tract manipulation and examination with contaminated instruments, or the use of irritant drugs.

Natural service produces physical irritation of the tubular organs in addition to bacterial contamination. Vaginoscopic examination shortly after coitus reveals gross inflammatory changes that appear too quickly to be the result of bacterial multiplication. Every exposure of the uterus to irritants produces an inflammatory response. After a certain number of these responses, it is logical that the system loses some efficiency, either through fatigue or organic change. As mares approach the point where defense mechanisms become marginal, management programs, such as breeding with minimum contamination and irritation, may greatly extend their productive lives.

Parturition is another prime source of uterine irritation and contamination. During and after normal foaling, circumstances favor bacterial invasion of the vagina and uterus. The physical trauma of delivery adds another insult. Any abnormality of parturition, particularly involving manual intervention, compounds the problem. Proper foaling management can reduce the insult to the defense mechanism and is discussed in detail under parturition.

Endometritis in the mare is essentially a bacterial infection. The principal organisms involved are common opportunistic skin, soil and fecal organisms that become established in the uterus when natural defenses fail. Occasionally yeasts and less often fungi are incriminated in the disease process, and may appear after prolonged antibiotic therapy for bacterial endometritis. Other agents, such as viruses, mycoplasma and protozoa, have not been identified as causes of uterine infection in mares.

The criteria for establishing a causal relationship between a bacterial agent and endometritis should include repeatable uterine cultures of that organism in large numbers and in reasonably pure form, and some evidence of inflammation, either physical or by the diagnostic aids described earlier. Although 19 pathogenic bacteria have been isolated from mares with endometritis, almost 80% of the recoveries involved 4 organisms.[79] Most investigators agree that beta-hemolytic *Streptococcus E coli, Pseudomonas* spp and *Klebsiella* are the major pathogens involved.[5]

Streptococcus zooepidemicus is the beta-hemolytic streptococcus associated with the greatest number of uterine infections and caused more than 66% of the infections in mares in one study.[80] Approximately 25% of all barren mares are infected with streptococci.[5] The organism is a common skin saprophyte on the external genitalia of stallions and mares, and is introduced in pneumovagina, breeding, foaling and by human intervention. Streptococci can be recovered from the genitalia in virtually all mares after natural service or parturition, but its establishment as a pathogen depends on the efficacy of the mare's defense system in removing contaminants.

Escherichia coli is incriminated less frequently than streptococci and, according to some studies, is a rather minor factor in producing endometritis.[80] In the author's experience, *E coli* is the second most common pathogen and is almost always associated with the anatomic defects that predispose mares to pneumovagina and fecal contamination. At the time of parturition, ample opportunity exists for *E coli* contamination, since defecation usually accompanies the second stage of labor.

Pseudomonas aeruginosa infections of the endometrium are apparently increasing in frequency in recent years as compared with early reports.[79-81] The resistance of *Pseudomonas* to antibiotic therapy is significant. Once established, *Pseudomonas* endometritis is difficult to reverse. The bacteria are often present in large numbers in the ejaculates of stallions, many of which have normal fertility when bred to healthy mares.[73] Exposure of mares with marginal resistance to such contaminated semen may result in a high incidence of infection.

Klebsiella pneumoniae is another organism that may be transmitted by coitus. *Klebsiella* infection may be a true venereal disease, implying infection in the stallion rather than mere passive transfer of bacteria.[80] However, this hypothesis is the subject of some disagreement. Experimental infection of mares with *Klebsiella pneumoniae* capsule type 68 has shown that the organism persists in the caudal vagina and clitoral fossa, which could be a factor in contaminating the stallion during coitus.[10] Some farms have experienced a high incidence of *Klebsiella* endometritis in mares bred to stallions that shed the organism. *Klebsiella* also produces a stubborn inflammation in the uterus which, when well established, presents serious problems in treatment.

Miscellaneous bacteria are occasionally incriminated in uterine infections in mares, including *Staphylococcus* spp, *Corynebacterium* spp, *Enterobacter* spp, *Proteus* spp, *Pasteurella* spp and others. Some reports incriminate *Staphylococcus aureus* as a significant pathogen, while others relegate it to a minor position.[79,80] If clinical signs of infection accompany the recovery of these bacteria, they must be regarded as significant. However, such circumstances are quite rare.

Fungi and yeasts are potential pathogens in the etiology of endometritis. Occasional recoveries of these organisms from clinically normal

Table 6. Diagnostic Criteria for Endometritis

Physical Examination	Uterine Culture	Endometrial Biopsy	Endometrial Smear	Diagnosis and Comments
gross inflammation and/or discharge	pathogen isolated repeatedly	significant inflammation	many neutrophils	endometritis
inconclusive physical findings	pathogen isolated repeatedly	significant inflammation, probably chronic	many neutrophils	endometritis, probably chronic
	no growth	significant inflammation	many neutrophils	endometritis, failed to isolate causal organism; reculture
	pathogen or nonpathogen isolated repeatedly	insignificant or no inflammation	no or few neutrophils	normal endometrium, culture results from contamination
no signs of inflammation	no growth	no inflammation	no or few neutrophils	normal endometrium

mares can be disregarded. However, there are cases in which obvious signs of inflammation are evident and the yeast *Candida* spp, especially *Candida albicans*, is reportedly cultured. There is almost always a history of repeated antibiotic therapy for bacterial endometritis. Identification of the presence of yeasts and fungi is important because further antibiotic therapy enhances their growth. *Candida* grows readily on media used for routine microbiologic culture. Identification is aided by examining wet mounts or stained smears of the organism for the typical budding pattern of yeast.

Since the bacteria causing endometritis are essentially opportunistic contaminants, it is reasonable that mixed infections may occur. The diagnosis of such multiple pathogens by cultural methods may be difficult due to overgrowth of plates by one organism. If treatment is instituted to reduce the levels of one organism, others may proliferate if the antibiotic used has only a limited spectrum. The use of a selective medium to encourage the growth of gram-negative organisms and suppress gram-positive ones is sound laboratory practice. Mixed infections are detected more easily when these media (EMB or McConkey's agar) are used in conjunction with nonselective media.

The diagnosis of endometritis should be made after consideration of predisposing factors, the mare's general physical condition, examination of external and internal genitalia, and culture and diagnostic study results. By considering all these criteria, it is less likely that a maiden mare with normal conformation will be diagnosed as infected on the basis of a few streptococci on a culture plate. At the same time, an older barren mare will not be declared sound for breeding on the basis of a negative culture and no physical examination.

Since treatment for endometritis is time-consuming, expensive and entails some risk, it is important to be certain of the diagnosis before proceeding with therapy. A summary of the criteria for diagnosis is presented in Table 6. Refer to the initial part of this chapter for detail on culture, and endometrial biopsy and cytologic examination.

Management of endometritis in mares must be aimed at correction of contributing causes, such as anatomic defects, reversing the inflammatory process by elimination of causal organisms, and managing the mare to avoid recurrent infection. The anatomic aspects of treatment are covered in the section on surgical procedures for correction of pneumovagina.

Reversing the uterine inflammatory process may be as simple as correcting the anatomic defect. Infertility due to endometritis secondary to pneumovagina may be spontaneously resolved after a Caslick operation or vaginoplasty. The natural defense mechanisms in these mares are restored by elimination of the continued irritation from air and external con-

Table 7. Percentage of Sensitivity of 4 Common Endometrial Pathogens[79,82]

	Streptococcus zooepidemicus	E coli	Pseudomonas aeruginosa	Klebsiella pneumoniae
ampicillin	100[a]/100[b]	80/0	0/0	3/0
chloramphenicol	100/100	100/100	7/3	100/76
polymyxin B	3/NT[c]	99/100	100/100	100/100
erythromycin	99/100	1/NT	0/NT	0/NT
gentamicin	86/99	100/100	100/94	100/100
kanamycin	7/0.3	95/83	0/3	83/76
neomycin	3/0	82/59	0.4	69/51
nitrofurantoin	89/NT	89/NT	0/NT	54/NT
nitrofurazone	NT/100	NT/99	NT/2	NT/65
penicillin G	100/99	0/0	0/0	0/0
triple sulfa	10/0	51/74	0/37	29/78
streptomycin	3/0	31/8	0/0	19/8
tetracycline	75/18	75/27	0/0	65/27

a—reference 79
b—reference 82
c—not tested

taminants. The bacterial infection is eliminated by the mare without assistance.

The Caslick operation is the most important procedure in the treatment of pneumovagina and infertility due to infection of the genital tract in mares.[5] Once pneumovagina is corrected, the mare must be kept sutured for the rest of its productive life. Incision and reclosure for breeding and foaling are necessary, and a delay in resuturing of no more than a few days may be enough to allow reinfection.

In the interest of time and in the face of severe and protracted cases of endometritis, it is often necessary to remove the causal organisms and speed uterine recovery. Antibiotics provide the logical therapeutic approach to this objective. There are many unanswered questions about dosage, route of administration and frequency of treatment with antibiotics. Although there are complications resulting from antibiotic use, years of production have been added to the lives of many mares as a result of antibiotic therapy.

Most practitioners feel that local treatment or intrauterine infusion is preferred to systemic antibiotic therapy. Fifty percent of equine practitioners surveyed called systemic therapy useless and another 32% felt that antibiotic injections were only occasionally helpful in treating endometritis.[82] In fact, little definitive information is available to support or refute these impressions. Therapeutic tissue levels in the endometrium must be established and the systemic doses necessary to produce these levels calculated to properly address the problem.

The duration of effective levels of antibiotic in the uterus after intrauterine infusion has been studied in cows and mares.[83,84] Chloramphenicol instilled in normal mare uteri is quickly absorbed, attains peak serum levels in 45 minutes, and declines to nondetectible levels in 12 hours. It is common to administer intrauterine antibiotics at 24- to 48-hour intervals; however, there may be some advantage to increasing the frequency of these treatments.

Selecting the proper antibiotic for the specific organism involved in the uterine infection is generally based on antibiotic sensitivity testing. It is possible that in vitro and in vivo efficacy may not be the same. For example, most cultures of Pseudomonas show in vitro sensitivity to polymyxin B, yet few cases of Pseudomonas endometritis respond well to polymyxin B therapy. Nevertheless, the antibiotic sensitivity test is the only rational guide to antibiotic selection. Sensitivities of the 4 common pathogens to the most widely used antibiotics are presented in Table 7.[79,82]

If the intrauterine route is chosen, it is necessary to use drugs and vehicles that are noninjurious to the endometrium. The safest approach is to use water-soluble antibiotics administered in a suitable volume of sterile saline to assure distribution throughout the uterus. Most of a 250-ml infusion should stay in the uterine lumen. Some suggested doses of antibiotics for intrauterine administration are given in Table 8.[20,82]

Infusions should be administered with sterile equipment and proper aseptic preparation of the mare. Catheters can be passed through the cervix and into the uterine lumen with a speculum or manually. The use of self-retaining catheters to avoid repeated introduction of instruments into the uterus has not found much acceptance among equine practitioners.

Local antibiotic therapy for bacterial endometritis may result in some complications. The most perplexing problem occurs when treatment for one pathogen allows proliferation of another that is often more difficult to manage than the original. A common example of this is a streptococcal infection that, after treatment with the appropriate antibiotic, results in a *Pseudomonas* or a yeast infection. The possibility exists in these cases that a mixed infection existed initially and antibiotic use merely allowed development of the secondary infection. Penicillin is a prime offender in these cases. *Pseudomonas* is typically resistant to penicillin, and *Candida* and other yeasts actually proliferate in its presence.

Another explanation is that accidental introduction of the second organism occurred during the course of treatment for the primary infection. Whatever the etiology, these problems with antibiotic therapy are frustrating, time-consuming and expensive. An entire breeding season can pass while sequential pathogens are treated. These situations emphasize the necessity for an accurate diagnosis of endometritis and the use of antibiotics only in those cases requiring treatment.

Another troublesome problem associated with local antibiotic therapy is treatment failure. If bacterial numbers are not adequately reduced, resistant organisms may survive, requiring the use of different drugs. A sequence of treatments is likely to follow. Many of these mares end up with stubborn secondary (or tertiary, etc) infections.

Drug hypersensitivity is another possible complication of antibiotic use. Although these reactions are relatively rare in horses, serious allergic problems may follow intrauterine infusion, especially with penicillin and related compounds.

The use as a lavage of some nonantibiotic solutions in large volumes may be indicated when exudates accumulate in the uterus. Great care must be exercised in selecting antiseptics for uterine irrigation. Chlorhexidine solution (Nolvasan:Fort Dodge) is highly irritating to the mucosa of the entire reproductive tract. Even very dilute solutions may cause severe reactions and ensuing endometrial, cervical

Table 8. Suggested Single-Treatment Doses of Antibiotics for Intrauterine Therapy[20,82]

ampicillin[a]	3 g
chloramphenicol[b]	2-3 g
gentamicin[c]	1-2 g
kanamycin	1-2 g
neomycin	4 g
potassium penicillin	3-5 million IU

a—water-soluble preparation
b—oral solution
c—if small volume is used, add 1 ml 7½% NaHCO$_3$ solution per 50 mg gentamicin

and vaginal adhesions. Strong irritants, such as Lugol's solution, are contraindicated as uterine medication. Even the so-called "tamed" or povidone iodine preparations may irritate some uteri unless diluted to 1:10 or more.

Treatment of well-established yeast and fungal infections may be difficult. Antibiotics, of course, are not indicated. Of the antifungals, nystatin and amphotericin B suspensions have been used. The author has had some success with infusions of 50 mg amphotericin B (Fungizone:Squibb) in 200 ml water daily for 5 days. Yeast infections occasionally become completely refractory to any treatment and cause permanent endometrial damage that results in sterility.

Once active endometrial inflammation has been controlled by surgical or medical means, great care must be taken to prevent recurrence. Reduced genital tract contamination is the obvious key to managing mares with a history of endometritis. Some alternative to natural service usually is indicated because the massive uterine contamination associated with natural breeding will likely cause reinfection.

Artificial insemination, when permitted by the breed registry, is the first choice in managing the breeding of such mares. The use of semen extenders containing antibiotics effectively minimizes bacterial contamination. Even breeding with raw semen has an advantage over natural service in that the physical irritation of coitus is avoided and the volume of semen can be limited to the amount necessary for fertilization.

In breeds in which artificial insemination is not permitted, some reduction of bacterial contamination can be achieved by other means. Antibiotic treatment of the uterus before and after breeding may be helpful. In prebreeding treatments, care must be taken to avoid spermicidal levels of antibiotic in the uterus at the time of breeding. Intrauterine antibiotics infused postovulation are directed at returning the uterine environment to normal prior to the descent of the embryo at 4-5 days. Treatments on postovulation days 1 and 2 are indicated.

An alternative approach to managing natural service in mares with a tendency for reinfection is the "minimum contamination technic" for natural service.[85] Semen extenders with antibiotics are infused into the uterus prior to service in volumes large enough to coat the entire uterine lumen, cervical canal and vagina. The stallion then breeds the mare and the ejaculate is deposited directly in the extender.

Details of artificial insemination, semen extender and the minimum contamination technic are presented in the discussion of the stallion.

No matter what approach is selected to control bacterial contamination, limiting the number of breedings is essential to success with these problem mares. Careful management to determine the optimal breeding time is indicated. The use of HCG to shorten the interval to ovulation is especially useful.

Vaginitis and Cervicitis

Inflammation of the cervix and vagina of mares seldom occurs separate from endometritis. In the early stages of pneumovagina, it is possible to detect vaginal hyperemia and some degree of exudate without concurrent uterine inflammation. It is usually just a matter of time until endometritis follows as an extension of vaginal and cervical involvement. A grossly inflamed cervix without signs of significant vaginal irritation indicates the same degree of inflammation in the uterus.

When pneumovagina is responsible for only vaginitis and cervicitis, a rapid return to normal should follow correction of the anatomic defect. If there is no evidence of air aspiration, consideration should be given to the possibility that irritating substances or contaminated equipment have been introduced into the vaginal tract.

A serious sequel to severe cervical inflammation or trauma, such as that produced by dystocia or obstetric manipulation, is cervical fibrosis. The mare's cervix responds to such insults with the formation of adhesions that may either obliterate the cervical canal or interfere with its proper closure, depending on the degree and location of fibrosis. Vaginal adhesions are less common but may result from the same causes as cervical fibrosis.

Treatment of cervical adhesions is generally unrewarding. In early cases, frequent manipulation may break down scar tissue and application of bland topical preparations or antibiotic-corticosteroid ointments may retard reformation or adhesions. Some chronic cases have been corrected by using self-retaining devices in the cervical canal to prevent scar reformation. It is not unusual, however, in chronic cases to be unable to locate the former lumen of the cervical canal. These mares obviously have an extremely grave prognosis for future fertility.

Practitioners must be aware of the hazards of cervical trauma. Instruments should be well guarded by gloved fingers when introduced through the cervical canal and lubrication should always be employed when any vaginal or cervical manipulation is attempted.

Venereal Diseases

Contagious Equine Metritis: In 1977 a previously unrecognized, highly contagious venereal infection was described in Thoroughbreds in England.[86] The disease was characterized by a mucopurulent vulvar discharge and reduced fertility in mares, but no clinical signs in stallions. Initially no consistent organisms were identified in cultures of samples from infected mares, but an intensified effort led to isolation of the causal agent, a gram-negative coccobacillus not readily classified.[87] This organism was inoculated into test mares and produced the same clinical signs.

Contagious equine metritis (CEM) spread quickly among about 250 mares and 23 stallions on 29 premises before breeding was halted in Newmarket.[88] A short time later it was confirmed in Ireland where, retrospectively, it had occurred the previous season. In the fall of 1977 the disease was confirmed in Australia and in 1978 was diagnosed in the US and the European continent. The US outbreak was linked directly to 2 stallions imported from France in 1977.

The CEM organism, tentatively named *Hemophilus equigenitalis*, is a slow-growing fastidious bacterium. Microaerophilic conditions are necessary for its growth and special media are helpful. These characteristics account for the difficulty in isolating it from the first field cases. The organism can survive for long periods on the external genitalia of stallions and in the caudal vagina and clitoral area of mares. Venereal transmission is, therefore, especially efficient.

The clinical signs of CEM in the mare are those of acute endometritis in about 70% of exposed animals. Vulvar discharge may be evident 2-3 days postinsemination or may not be evident until a premature return to estrus occurs in 8-10 days. The exudate is typically mucoid, grey-white and profuse, although some variation has been noted. Clinical signs of inflammation are evident and the presence of neutrophils in uterine swab samples is especially helpful in screening mares.[22] The endometritis of CEM is of fairly short duration. However, after the acute signs resolve, the mare is left as an asymptomatic carrier of the organism for long periods. Experimental inoculation produced carrier mares from which the agent was intermittently recovered for many weeks.[89] In these cases, the clitoral sinuses and fossa were the best sources of the organism.[9]

Not all mares experience acute infection after exposure. Some are infected without any clinical signs and may conceive and foal with the bacteria present in the caudal vagina and clitoral area.

Clinical signs in stallions are absent and the male's role is that of an asymptomatic carrier. The organism resides on the penis, in the urethral diverticulum, and in and around the prepuce, where it can persist for many months.

The diagnosis of CEM is made by culture and identification of *H equigenitalis*. This presents problems due to the organism's fastidious nature and propensity to reside in areas where a multitude of contaminants complicate its isolation. Original culture technics incorporated streptomycin in the media to inhibit contaminants, but a streptomycin-sensitive strain of *H equigenitalis* has been recognized.[90] The organism grows best on Eugon's chocolate agar in 5% CO_2 and may take 5 days to grow on plates to the point of recognition.

A transient rise in humoral antibody levels has been noted in mares with CEM. From 7-8 to about 45 days postinfection these antibodies can be detected by agglutination and complement-fixation tests.[90-93] Serologic tests are helpful in screening mares exposed to suspect stallions.

The control of CEM has been directed at preventing spread of the disease. Quarantine measures and breeding restrictions have been successfully confined recent outbreaks. In the US the disease is reportable and appropriate governmental agencies should be notified of any suspicious situations (see Chapter 10).

Topical treatment of affected stallions has been quite successful. Thorough scrubbing of the entire penis and prepuce with chlorhexidine scrub, followed by a liberal coating of the entire area with nitrofurazone ointment, is recommended. This procedure is repeated daily for 5 days. Particular attention is paid to the urethral diverticulum. A high percentage of affected stallions treated in this manner have been cleared of the organism. Subsequent cultures are indicated to determine the result of the procedure.

Treatment of mares has not been as effective as that of stallions. The acute endometritis seems to resolve itself with or without antibiotic therapy. About 20% of infected mares remain asymptomatic carriers regardless of treatment.[94] Mares with continually positive cultures should not be considered for further breeding until cultures are negative. Some have remained positive for over a year. A recent suggestion that the clitoral sinuses of carrier mares be surgically excised to eliminate the site of persistence of the organism may have some merit.

A positive aspect of the appearance of CEM has been the increased awareness of the necessity for hygienic procedures in breeding horses. Overall improvement in management and observation could lead to improved fertility in all breeding operations.

Equine Coital Exanthema: Equine coital exanthema (ECE) is a disease of the external genitalia caused by a herpesvirus antigenically different from equine herpesvirus-1 (EHV-1) or rhinopneumonitis virus.[95-97] Although it is primarily regarded as a venereal disease, ECE may be transmitted by grooming, veterinary instruments and possibly insects.[98]

The lesions appear on the vulva of mares and on the penis and prepuce of stallions. Initial vesicles progress rapidly to pustules and then to shallow necrotic ulcers (Fig 20). Edema, tenderness and painful urination are exhibited by mares in the acute stages. Lesions may spread from the vulva to the surrounding perineal skin. Stallions in heavy service may be reluctant to breed, and lesions on the glans penis and urethral process may remain inflamed until breeding is interrupted. Intranuclear inclusion bodies can be demonstrated histologically in tissues obtained from lesions.

Healing occurs in 7-10 days in the absence of secondary bacterial infection. The effect on fertility is apparently negligible. In natural outbreaks the virus has not been associated with

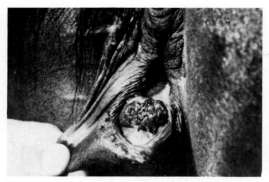

Fig 20. Perineal lesion caused by coital exanthema.

abortions. Respiratory disease as a part of the syndrome has been suggested after experimental inoculation of horses with the virus.[96]

Dourine: Dourine is a venereal trypanosomal disease caused by *Trypanosoma equiperdum.* Enzootic in some tropical countries, the disease was last observed in the US on the Papago Indian reservation in southern Arizona in the 1950's.

Dourine is a chronic systemic infection that begins with swelling of and discharge from the external genitalia, and progresses to emaciation, paralytic disorders and death in over 50% of cases.[5,99] During the course of the infection, typical raised "plaques" appear on the skin.

Infected animals are identified by the complement-fixation test, which has been the basis for eradication of the disease.

Pyometra

Pyometra, the accumulation of pus in the uterus, is an occasional sequel to endometritis and sometimes cervicitis. The exact mechanisms responsible for this problem are not clearly understood. If cervical obstruction due to fibrosis prevents expulsion of uterine contents, the cause seems logical. Often, however, no signs of cervical occlusion are evident.

Pyometra sometimes results in an altered estrous cycle due to prolonged luteal phase, as also seen in cows. Other mares may show estrus, often on a regular basis.[100] Neither pattern appears related to mechanical obstruction of drainage through the cervix.

Culture of the fluids in pyometra cases may yield any of the common bacterial or fungal agents responsible for endometritis. Occasionally the fluid is sterile. Systemic signs of disease are not evident. Occasional slight variations in the hemogram, such as mild neutropenia or anemia, have been reported.[100]

Once established, pyometra is a difficult problem to manage. Deep, chronic inflammatory changes in the endometrium are evident and endometrial atrophy is common when fluid accumulation persists for any significant time. Endometrial biopsy is clearly indicated as a prognostic step before attempting treatment.

Therapy for pyometra involves mechanical evacuation of the retained pus and use of appropriate intrauterine antibiotics. The exudates may be viscous enough to require repeated washing and drainage for their removal. However, fluid accumulation tends to recur and, even with diligent treatment, the prognosis for future fertility is poor.

Those mares that show estrus and expel some pus during that time have a somewhat better prognosis for a return to breeding. Endometrial atrophy seems less pronounced in these cases. If severe cervical adhesions occur in chronic cases of pyometra, the prognosis is essentially hopeless. Intraluminal uterine adhesions frequently develop as a complication to this type of pyometra.

Noninfectious Causes of Infertility

Early Embryonic Death

Early embryonic death is failure of the conceptus to reach the size and age that allows its detection by pregnancy examination. Those mares detected as pregnant but failing to foal are discussed in the section on abortion even though some such cases could be technically classified as embryonic loss.

When conception occurs and the embryo fails to establish itself to the point where it is clinically recognizable, it is usual to regard this situation as infertility. Prior to 18-25 days postovulation, there is no practical means of determining the presence of a viable embryo. Failure to return to estrus is not very good evidence in mares because of their predisposition to prolonged luteal activity without pregnancy.

As embryo transfer procedures in horses are developed, there may be more data on embryo survival. For now, practitioners must look upon the mare bred to a fertile stallion at the proper time but failing to become pregnant as a case of failure of fertilization or early embryonic death. In the absence of known abnormalities it seems logical that some of these fall into the latter category.

If fertilization occurs and the ovum or sperm is genetically abnormal, development may be interrupted very early. Cleavage of the blastocyst beyond the 2- to 4-cell stage is necessary for it to descend the oviduct to the uterus. Arrest of cleavage has been verified experimentally as a cause of failure of embryos to reach the uterine lumen.[101] Unfertilized ova do not descend to the uterus and are retained in the oviduct.[102] Genetic abnormalities must be a factor in embryonic death at later stages when the conceptus is in the uterine lumen, but little is known of the incidence of such failures.

A factor in embryo survival that can be modified to some degree on a practical basis is the uterine environment at the time of blastocyst descent. When endometritis is present to any degree, the possibility exists that bacteria, their by-products and by-products of inflammatory response may alter the biochemical environment of the uterus.

There is evidence, albeit based on uncontrolled observation, that the uterine environment can be modified by local therapy. Since at least 4 days are required for the passage of the fertilized ovum down the fallopian tube, medication can be safely infused into the uterus following ovulation during that time. Even in mares with no evidence of active endometritis but a history of chronic infection, there may be an advantage to such postbreeding treatment. The use of water-soluble antibiotics, specific where possible, is indicated in such cases.

Nutrition of the mare during early pregnancy may be a factor in early embryonic death. A high incidence of pregnancy failure at 25-31 days of gestation has been suggested due to lack of nutrients.[103] Conception and development to 25 days was not affected by malnutrition, nor was embryonic viability after 31 days. Other effects of nutrition on fertility are essentially those that alter the estrous cycle and have been discussed previously.

Developmental Anomalies

Gonadal Dysgenesis: Abnormal numbers of chromosomes in mares, resulting in infantile reproductive organs and infertility, have been reported.[104-106] Characteristic clinical findings include extremely small ovaries with no functional germinal tissue, an infantile uterus often consisting of no more than a thin band of tissue, a flaccid cervix, and essentially normal external genitalia. Most affected individuals are smaller than normal but otherwise phenotypically normal. Various breeds are represented in the 26 cases described.

The chromosomal variations in these cases, as determined by karyotype, are mostly those involving one missing X chromosome (63X). The probable origin of this defect is the genetic process of nondysfunction or error in chromosome division, which may occur during the meiotic division of either gamete or in mitosis after fertilization. Other karyotypes reported are 63X/64XX, 63X/64XY, 65XXX, 64XY and one case of autosomal deletion. Although the physical findings in these mares seems enough to dismiss their potential fertility, karyotyping is essential to confirm the diagnosis because not all mares with hypoplastic ovaries are chromosomally abnormal or infertile.

The similarity of the 63X mare to the 45X Turner syndrome in humans has led to the term for such mares as "Turner mares." In humans there are other physical changes not seen in mares, such as "webbing" of the neck and some cardiac defects. Endocrine profiles of affected mares reveal very low estrogen and progesterone levels, and in some cases higher than normal LH levels. Lack of estrogen feedback to the hypothalamus is suggested as a reason for elevated LH levels.

The behavior of most mares with gonadal dysgenesis is typical of those in winter anestrus or of ovariectomized mares. Passive behavior or some sexual receptivity is generally evident.

Practitioners should understand that gonadal dysgenesis may exist if an infantile genital tract is discovered. It is helpful to confirm or refute the diagnosis with chromosome determinations since mares with true dysgenesis are sterile. A shortage of laboratories capable of accurately performing equine karyotyping is a drawback. Many suspicious cases are not examined in the laboratory. More awareness of the condition may encourage development of more facilities to make this diagnosis.

Hermaphroditism: True hermaphroditism, characterized by gonads resembling those of both sexes, has not been observed in horses. Male pseudohermaphroditism is encountered occasionally. Such animals have internal testes, masculine behavior, and external genitalia suggestive of the female, but with a large protruding clitoris containing the urethra. Various chromosomal mosaic patterns have been associated with male pseudohermaphroditism.

Reproductive Tract Tumors

Ovarian Tumors: Granulosa-cell tumors are the most common ovarian neoplasm of the mare and are by far the most clinically significant. The production of steroid hormones by

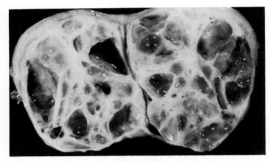

Fig 21. Sectioned granulosa-cell tumor, showing multicystic configuration.

these tumors results in changes in sexual behavior, suppression of contralateral ovarian function and infertility.

Behavioral changes are the most frequent suggestion that a granulosa-cell tumor exists. Three types of behavior are recognized in affected mares: aggressive masculine activity in the presence of other animals, continuous or irregular estral behavior, and anestral behavior. A recent study of mares with hormone-secreting tumors showed that behavioral patterns were best correlated with testosterone production by the affected ovary.[107] Plasma levels of testosterone above 100 pg/ml were noted in mares with stallion-like characteristics. Below that level, either estral or anestral behavior was seen. Extremes of masculinization with granulosa-cell tumor may result in teasing, mounting and copulatory movements, male vocalization, and the development of male secondary sex characteristics.

Ovarian tumors may be suspected after physical examination to determine the cause of infertility of anestrus. Rectal palpation reveals an enlarged and abnormally firm affected ovary. Even before the tumors reach a grossly abnormal size, a high index of suspicion exists when the ovulation fossa of that ovary is obliterated by early tumor growth. The character of the contralateral ovary is helpful in assessing the presence of a hormone-secreting tumor. Atrophy and complete inactivity of the opposite gonad, especially during the physiologic breeding season, is characteristic.

In early cases, sequential evaluations are helpful in detecting growth in the suspect ovary and monitoring inactivity in the unaffected ovary. Evidence that the contralteral ovary is producing follicles and ovulating is enough to rule out granulosa-cell tumor. Since other ovarian neoplasms are extremely rare,

the most likely differential diagnosis is ovarian hematoma.

An ovarian hematoma may result from continued hemorrhage into the follicular cavity following ovulation. These ovaries may grow to enormous size before regressing. The consistency of the hematoma is usually less dense than that of a granulosa-cell tumor and the ovulation fossa is usually still palpable in most cases. The most significant aid in separating tumor from hematoma is the opposite ovary, with normal function continuing in the case of ovarian hematoma. A 35-cm hematoma was discovered in a heavily pregnant mare during a routine examination by the author.

Treatment of mares with secreting ovarian tumors must be surgical removal if future fertility is the objective. When surgery is not elected, the owner should be informed of potential future problems with ovarian size, discomfort and even hemorrhage due to ruptured ovarian ligaments. Metastasis is extremely rare, with one case out of 78 reported in one study.[108] Surgical considerations and technic are considered separately.

The gross appearance of granulosa-cell tumors is reasonably consistent. The diameter may vary from 6-40 cm but most are 10-20 cm wide.[107-108] On section, multiple cystic structures and a yellowish stroma between cysts are evident (Fig 21). Cysts may contain blood, blood-tinged fluid, or most often straw-colored, serum-like fluid.[107]

Some histologic variations may be noted among tumors and within the same tumor. In addition to granulosa cells, parts of some neoplasms consist of theca cells. It has been suggested that these secreting tumors be referred to as granulosa-theca-cell tumors.[107]

The prognosis for fertility following successful removal of a granulosa-cell tumor is favorable. In 42 of 57 mares followed after surgery, cycles were re-established in 2-16 months, with a mean of 8.5 months. In the same study, 30 of 39 mares produced live foals.[108] If ovariectomy is performed during the winter, the interval to subsequent cycles is usually delayed by the natural seasonality of the mare. Several mares in the author's experience have had fertile cycles within a month of surgery performed during the physiologic breeding season.

A variety of nonsecreting ovarian tumors in mares has been reported, but all are extremely rare. Teratoma, cystadenoma, cystadenocarcinoma and melanoma are among such nonsecreting neoplams. Individual assessment of size and potential threat to the mare must be made in these cases.

Tubular Tract and External Genitalia Tumors: Neoplasia of the mare's tubular reproductive tract is an insignificant cause of infertility. Lesions are rarely discovered in the uterine wall, cervix and vaginal wall. Of these, the leiomyoma is most frequently mentioned. These tumors cause infertility only when large enough to mechanically interfere with conception and pregnancy. Some atrophy of the endometrium overlying uterine wall leiomyomas has been reported.[17]

Squamous-cell carcinoma occasionally develops in the perineal region, particularly at the mucocutaneous junction on the labia. Irritation, secondary infection and mechanical interference with breeding are possible ways these lesions could contribute to infertility. Melanomas in the perineal region of grey mares may also develop to the point of mechanical interference.

Miscellaneous Causes of Infertility

Cystic Disorders of the Uterus

In some older multiparous mares, the accumulation of fluid in the lymphatics of the endometrium and myometrium produces palpable changes in the uterus. These lymphatic lacunae are evident in endometrial biopsies of affected mares and may cause infertility.[109] The uterus in these cases feels heavy and "doughy," with most of the enlargement noted ventrad at the junction of the horns and body.

Extreme cases of lymphatic stasis may cause nonglandular, lymph-filled endometrial cysts. These cysts are usually palpable as distinct vesicles in the uterine wall and may reach several centimeters in size.

It is difficult to determine the effect of lymphatic stasis and cysts on fertility. Since this syndrome usually occurs in older mares with other problems, it may be impossible to evaluate. Very few of these mares conceive and maintain pregnancy.[17] Some improvement can be noted on palpation when these mares are treated repeatedly with hot (50 C) saline infusions of 500-1000 ml. Larger cysts may be perforated and drained in an effort to increase the functional area of the endometrium.

Cystic distension of the endometrial glands has been described.[109] These lesions are essentially microscopic and recognizable only by biopsy. Many of these cysts are apparently the result of periglandular fibrosis interfering with endometrial gland secretion. When significant areas of endometrium are involved, the prognosis for maintaining pregnancy is poor. Such mares should be evaluated in the same manner as for periglandular fibrosis.

Infertility from Trauma

Most accidents resulting in disruption of the reproductive tract of mares are associated with parturition and are discussed in a later section.

Vaginal rupture breeding is occasionally encountered, particularly when small maiden mares are bred to large stallions. Perforation occurs in the vaginal fornix adjacent to the cervix. If the stallion ejaculates during this situation, semen is deposited intraperitoneally and causes severe irritation and pain.

If copious hemorrhage is noted when the stallion dismounts, a ruptured vagina should be suspected. Vaginoscopic examination confirms the damage. Treatment is directed at controlling the subsequent acute colic pain; systemic antibiotics are indicated to prevent peritonitis. Affected mares should be kept standing for 48 hours to prevent prolapse of viscera through the perforation. Vaginal tears heal rapidly and most affected mares can be rebred at the subsequent estrus.

The use of a breeding roll between the stallion and mare restricts the depth of penile intromission and prevents vaginal rupture.

THE PREGNANT MARE

The Physiology of Pregnancy

Fertilization

In the optimum situation, fully capacitated, viable spermatozoa are present in the oviduct at the time of ovulation, and fertilization occurs promptly. Breeding mares after ovulation is detected becomes decreasingly productive in a matter of hours. Whether this is a function of spermatozoal capacitation time, ovum viability or both is not known. The net result is that by about 8 hours postovulation, breeding does not result in pregnancy.

Spermatozoal viability in the mare's reproductive tract is surprisingly long. Variations occur with individual stallions, but a 5-day interval from breeding to ovulation and conception is not unusual. The survival time for spermatozoa in the mare is thought to be 48 hours. Most successful breeding programs are based on alternate-day breeding.

Oviductal Transit

The fertilized ovum takes approximately 5 days to traverse the oviduct and enter the uterine lumen. Cleavage of the zygote to a specific stage is necessary for its final delivery into the uterus.[101] Infertile ova from previous ovulations, as well as fertilized eggs in which cleavage has been arrested, are retained in the oviduct.[102]

Transit time from ovulation to migration of the embryo into the uterus coincides with the time required for maturation of the corpus luteum. Progesterone levels are peaking and the endometrial glands are actively secreting nutrients for the embryo in time for its arrival.

Preimplantation

The embryo remains essentially unattached to the endometrium from the time of its descent into the uterus until about 40 days of age. During this time it is suspended or held by uterine tone and migrates to the site of future implantation, usually at the base of either uterine horn. Movement of the conceptus from one horn to another can occur in early pregnancy or even after 40 days in some cases.[110]

A gradual transition occurs from simple contact between the chorion and endometrium at about 40 days to final maturation of the placental structures (microcotyledons) at about 150 days.[111] Morphologic studies suggest that the microcotyledons are advanced enough by 100 days for some movement of substances across the placental junction.[112]

The period from descent of the embryo into the uterus until 100 days of gestation can be classified as a preimplantation period. Embryonic survival during this period depends on the yolk sac, which has essentially disappeared at 40 days, and on endometrial glandular secretions directly absorbed by the opposing chorionic surface. Abnormalities of a significant number of endometrial glands could interfere with this support system. There is a high correlation of glandular and periglandular lesions with embryonic death at 40-100 days.[17]

Endometrial Cups

Secretory structures, the endometrial cups, develop in the uterus as a result of interaction between fetal and maternal tissues. Pregnant mare serum gonadotrophin (PMSG), a glycoprotein with significant FSH activity and some LH activity, is produced by the endometrial cups. Although the exact role of PMSG in early pregnancy has not been determined, the presence of the compound has major clinical significance to the practitioner.

At 37 and 38 days of pregnancy, trophoblast cells from the chorionic girdle invade the endometrium and differentiate into mature secretory cup cells capable of PMSG production.[113,114] The endometrial tissues respond to the invasion by developing extensive vascular and connective tissue components adjacent to the cup cells and by an inflammatory response to the foreign cells. The result is about a dozen glandular structures arranged in a circular pattern in the base of the uterine horn. This corresponds to the site of origin of the umbilical cord as the fetus develops.

Large amounts of PMSG, secreted by the endometrial cups, are detectible in the serum as early as day 38, peak near day 60, and gradually disappear by days 120-140. The life span of the cups is determined by the response of the maternal tissue to the foreign fetal tissue. The inflammatory reaction results in eventual sloughing of the cups, which begins around day 70 and is complete when PMSG disappears from the blood.[115] The sloughed cup tissue is trapped by the overlying placental membrane, forming the allantochorionic pouches.[116] These structures may be completely resorbed by late pregnancy but can occasionally be found by close inspection of the placenta at parturition.

The classic concept of the role of PMSG in pregnancy evolved shortly after the discovery of the hormone. When it became evident that ovulation occurs during early pregnancy, a logical assumption followed that gonadotrophin was responsible for follicle development, ovulation and formation of secondary corpora lutea.[117] In light of evidence that the ovary is not necessary for the maintenance of pregnancy after days 50-70, the older concept is no longer completely acceptable.[118] The luteotrophic action of PMSG is apparently important.[119] Also, the autoimmunologic actions of PMSG may be more important than its gonadotrophic effects.[115]

The practitioner can take advantage of some of the clinical implications associated with the presence of PMSG in pregnant mares. As previously discussed under pregnancy examination, PMSG is a useful indicator of pregnancy. Once formed, the endometrial cups persist to their normal limit of hormone production whether pregnancy is maintained or not. False-positive PMSG tests for pregnancy are thus a possibility in mares that abort after 40 days.

The estrous cycle is blocked by PMSG for the duration of life of the endometrial cups. Once pregnant beyond 38-40 days, mares do not return to estrus until 110-130 days from the original ovulation date. Abortion, whether from natural causes or induced, does not alter this course. Neither luteolytic doses of prostaglandins nor saline infusions are beneficial in restoring the cycle in mares with functional cups. Therapeutic abortion cannot be induced with normal regimens of prostaglandin therapy between 40 and 120 days.

It becomes imperative, then, for the clinician to advise the client that once the endometrial cups are established, the mare will not resume cycling until the end of the natural course of PMSG secretion. If twins are detected past 38 days and therapeutic abortion is elected, little chance exists that the mare can be rebred in the same season. The early diagnosis of pregnancy by manual examination thus becomes more important.

On occasion it may be useful to employ one of the PMSG tests to determine cup function. In mares diagnosed as pregnant and subsequently found open, the prognostic value of knowledge of the establishment of endometrial cups should be evident.

Implantation and Placentation

The ultimate physical relationship between the chorion and the endometrium is developed from about 100-150 days of gestation. Formation of the functional placental exchange unit, the microcotyledon, marks the onset of complete fetal support by the uterus. The microcotyledons, about 1 mm in diameter, consist of multiple folds of chorionic epithelium (trophoblast) that interdigitate with corresponding endometrial crypts lined with endometrial epithelium.[120] Thousands of these microcotyledons make up the junction of the chorion and endometrium. They are barely visible as velvety projections from the surface of the chorionic side of the placenta at parturition. Between the microcotyledons a small space exists into which the endometrial glands continue to secrete. The equine placenta can be classified as epitheliochorial, diffuse and microcotyledonary. The epitheliochorial junction makes large-molecule transfer to the fetus impossible. The equine fetus, therefore, acquires no antibodies by placental transfer from the dam.

The relationship of the mature fetal membranes is illustrated in Figure 22. The chorioallantois attaches to the entire endometrial surface except for a small area adjacent to the cervix, which is devoid of microcotyledons

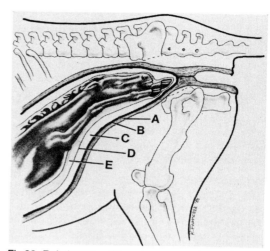

Fig 22. Relationship of the components of the placenta. A. Uterus. B. Chorioallantois. C. Allantoic space. D. Amnion. E. Amniotic space.

(cervical star). Immediately inside the allantoic side of this membrane is the allantoic space, which functions as a mechanical barrier and as a reservoir for urinary wastes that empty from the urachus. Allantoic fluid is transparent, watery and amber, and at term ranges from 8-18 L in volume.[5] Floating free in the allantoic space is the hippomane, an amorphous, rubbery structure best described as an allantoic calculus.

The amnion, or allantoamnion, is the membrane encasing the fetus. The amnionic membrane is whitish, translucent and thin. Blood vessels appear prominently between the allantoic and amniotic layers. There is no attachment of the amnionic membrane to the chorioallantoic membrane except at the base of the umbilical stalk. The equine fetus is thus very mobile in the uterus and delivery may occur without amniotic rupture. Amnionic fluid occupies the space between the allantoamnion and the fetus. Normally 3-7 L of clear, colorless and somewhat viscous fluid are present. Small white plaques may occur over parts or all of the amnionic membrane. There is no known significance to these plaques.

The umbilical cord is comprised of an allantoic portion and an amnionic portion. It contains the 2 umbilical arteries and one umbilical vein, the urachus, which opens into the allantoic space, and the tiny remnant of the yolk sac. The umbilical cord of horses is rather long, ranging from 50-100 cm, further contributing to mobility of the fetus.[5] Fetal movement during pregnancy results in some twisting of the cord. Careful evaluation should precede conclusions that an abnormally twisted umbilicus contributed to fetal death.

Hormonal Events in Pregnancy

Some of this material is based on evidence that is not entirely conclusive but represents current concepts still subject to further investigation. An excellent in-depth review of this subject has been published.[38]

Anterior Pituitary

At 10- to 11-day intervals during early pregnancy, FSH surges occur similar to those during the estrous cycle. These surges correspond to periods of follicular growth, particularly at or about days 24 and 38.[121,122] Rising LH levels in relationship to ovulation in pregnant mares are less impressive than those occurring during estrus.[121] Although some confusion results from LH assays attempted in the presence of PMSG, LH is more efficient than PMSG in binding to receptor sites on the equine ovary.[123]

Pituitary hormones are of little consequence during mid-pregnancy and late pregnancy. The ovaries become inactive and atrophied during those periods as other sources of steroid hormones come into play.

Posterior Pituitary

Oxytocin is discussed later in conjunction with its role in initiating parturition.

Ovary

As follicles develop during early pregnancy, they produce estrogens as do those of cycling mares. Progesterone levels tend to override the estrogenic effects on the reproductive tract and on behavior. It is not unusual, however, for pregnant mares to exhibit signs of estrus, although rarely to the point where mounting and breeding are possible. These mares almost always have large follicles in early pregnancy.

Progesterone, which is necessary for the maintenance of pregnancy, arises from the primary and secondary corpora lutea, and is critical until days 50-70, when pregnancy is no longer dependent on the corpus luteum.[124] Progesterone levels in the blood rise abruptly after the initial ovulation, fall somewhat by day 10 or 12, and then peak again as secondary corpora lutea are formed around day 38.

Early Embryo

Estrogens and androgens are produced by the conceptus as early as day 10.[125] These hormones probably play a role in the early mater-

nal recognition of pregnancy, as well as in the process of attachment and implantation.

Endometrial Cups

The role of these structures in production of PMSG has been discussed previously (see Physiology of Pregnancy).

Placenta and Fetus

The combination of fetus and placenta (fetoplacental unit) makes significant contributions to the endocrine patterns of pregnant mares. Of particular concern is the production of progesterone and other progestins by the fetoplacental unit in time to supplement the fading source of progesterone by the ovaries. For a short time prior to day 60, a small amount of circulating progesterone is produced by the fetoplacental unit. At about the same time, other progestins, notably 5-alpha pregnane, can be detected in the blood and subsequently increase to a level higher than that of progesterone throughout pregnancy.[126] Since the equine placenta can metabolize various progesterone precursors, circulating levels of progesterone may not reflect values in the fetoplacental unit. During the last month of gestation, progesterone and progestin levels rise dramatically and remain elevated until after parturition.

Fetal Gonads

During the second half of gestation, the fetal gonads increase greatly in size, primarily due to proliferation of the interstitial cells. The maximum size is attained at 180-200 days of pregnancy, at which point the fetal gonads are larger than the dam's ovaries. The gonads gradually reduce in size from this point until parturition. The growth and reduction of these fetal organs correspond closely to the levels of estrogens present in the mare's urine. The fetal gonads are the principal source of conjugated and unconjugated estrogens produced in heavily pregnant mares. Fetal gonadectomy, with subsequent maintenance of pregnancy to term, results in a dramatic decrease in estrogen levels in the dam.[127] Progesterone levels are unaffected. The role of estrogens in late pregnancy may relate to late fetal development and to the sequence of events that trigger parturition.

Urinary estrogens from pregnant mares have been the basis of estrogen production by the pharmaceutical industry for years. They provide the practitioner with another chemical test for pregnancy in mid- to late gestation.

Abnormalities of Gestation

Abortion

Embryonic death, prior to the time when pregnancy can be determined, has been discussed previously in the section on infertility. Abortion, as considered here, is any embryonic or fetal loss from the point of recognizable pregnancy to parturition. Horses apparently suffer a higher incidence of fetal loss than other domestic species, with a range of 5-15%.[5] Some aspects of equine reproductive anatomy and physiology that may contribute to the problem are late implantation, diffuse placentation and a simple cervix. Many potentially pathogenic organisms contaminate the uterus during breeding and foaling. If remnants of these populations remain after conception, the organisms may proliferate and cause endometritis, placentitis and subsequent abortion. Abortion rates are higher in older mares, a fact that correlates with lowered uterine resistance, higher incidence of periglandular fibrosis, and a variety of other factors.[128]

Many equine abortions, especially those in early gestation, are only detected when apparently pregnant mares show signs of estrus or are routinely re-examined for pregnancy. Recovery of pathogens from the uterus of these mares is seldom possible and endometrial biopsy may not be contributory.

Diagnostic reliability in determining the cause of abortion is highest when fresh, late-term fetuses and placentae are examined by qualified pathologists in well-equipped laboratories. Even under these conditions, it is optimistic to expect a specific answer in more than half of the cases presented.

Viral Causes: Equine herpesvirus-1 (EHV-1) and equine viral arteritis virus (EVA) are important causes of abortions. The more widespread and significant of these is EHV-1. It produces respiratory infections, neurologic disorders and late-term abortions in mares. Abortion storms in the densely populated horse country of central Kentucky resulted in the characterization of a specific disease as the cause in 1936.[129,130] During the ensuing 40 years, EHV-1 remains the most significant infectious cause of equine abortions.

The mobility and concentrations of horses today and the characteristics of the EHV-1 virus keep exposure to the agent at a consistently high level. Virtually all sucklings, weanlings and yearlings raised in groups contract the respiratory disease. Since immunity is short-lived, repeated infections keep the virus constantly available to animals of breeding age, which may not have clinical signs of the respiratory component of the infection.

The possibility that EHV-1 infection is perpetuated by carriers or a natural reservoir has been suggested.[131] Another characteristic of herpesviruses in other species is their tendency to latency and subsequent recrudescence.[132] This has not been conclusively demonstrated in horses but may help explain the long intervals between respiratory infections and abortion. Abortions following shipping or other stress tend to support the concept of latency.

Abortion occurs when EHV-1 invades the fetus, causing respiratory tract infection, fetal viremia, and focal liver necrosis. The period of highest susceptibility is the second half of gestation, with 90% of abortions induced by EHV-1 occurring between 8 months and term.[5] Fetal death usually precedes abortion by a very short time; fetuses infected late in gestation may be born alive and survive for 1-2 days.

The diagnosis of EHV-1 abortion is based on gross and microscopic changes in the aborted fetus and by virus isolation. Aborted fetuses are fresh and free from postmortem autolysis at delivery. Gross necropsy findings vary and include pleural and peritoneal effusion, petechial hemorrhages throughout the upper and lower respiratory tract, pulmonary edema, and focal hepatic necrosis. Significant gross changes are not observed in the placenta. Microscopic lesions include focal hepatic necrosis, inflammatory changes in the respiratory tract, and intranuclear inclusion bodies in the liver, bronchial epithelium, thymus and occasionally the lymph nodes. The identification of intranuclear inclusion bodies is the basis for most diagnoses of EHV-1 abortion. However, failure to identify these structures does not rule out the virus as a cause of abortion. Demonstration of inclusion bodies becomes more difficult as fetuses and foals survive the infection for longer periods of time before death. Intranuclear inclusion bodies are seldom found in affected late-term foals or those born alive.

Definitive diagnosis of EHV-1 abortion is by virus isolation, which is best achieved in tissue culture. The technics are time-consuming, expensive and not always reliable, but may be essential to instigation of appropriate control measures. Most laboratories prefer an intact fresh fetus for virus isolation, with liver and thymus tissue the preferred organs for the source of EHV-1.[133] Serologic changes are not helpful in diagnosing EHV-1 abortion because rising titers in mares occur too long before abortion to be of value.

Development of a satisfactory control program for the prevention of abortion due to EHV-1, suitable for each farm, should be the equine practitioner's objective. A variety of vaccination regimens are available and the decision of which, if any, to use depends on the exposure potential, general management of young animals and breeding stock, and ability of the management to carry out recommendations precisely. Regardless of the vaccination program used, pregnant mares should not be stressed or allowed prolonged contact with younger horses, and additions of new animals to the herd should be minimized.

Emphasis on the management aspects of controlling EHV-1 abortion should never be relaxed, regardless of the vaccines used. The transient nature of immunity, conferred by vaccination or natural exposure, must always be considered. Long-distance shipment of heavily pregnant mares is a particularly common source of stress. The stress of transportation, coupled with adaptation to a new environment, is enough to overcome the benefits of any control program. Chapter 2 contains a discussion of vaccination against EHV-1.

Equine viral arteritis is a severe systemic and respiratory infection of low incidence. The EVA virus is in the same family as those that produce the viral encephalitides of horses. Affected animals may experience fevers to 41.1 C (106 F), depression, respiratory distress, ocular signs and dependent edema. During the acute stages of the disease, the virus may invade the fetus of mares in the second half of gestation; fetal death and abortion follow in a few days.

Abortion may occur in as many as half of affected mares.[5] Since fetal death precedes expulsion by a few days, autolysis of the fetus is a common finding. Gross lesions in the fetus may be confused with those found in EHV-1 infection; petechial hemorrhage may be the predominant finding. No inclusion bodies are found histologically, but necrotic lesions in small arteries may suggest EVA. Although the diagnosis can be confirmed by isolating the virus from aborted fetuses, serologic changes may be a more practical diagnostic aid. Since abortion follows the acute infection in the mare, a rapid antibody response should be evident in acute and convalescent sera. The pathology laboratory at the University of Kentucky in Lexington is equipped to measure EVA antibody.

Equine viral arteritis is controlled by isolation of affected horses. The disease is spread by droplet inhalation and requires direct contact. No commercial vaccines are available, although a modified-live virus vaccine has been developed.[134] Immunity following natural infection is prolonged.

Bacterial Causes: Mares may abort as a result of bacterial infection of the endometrium, placenta or fetus. *Streptococcus zooepidemicus* is most often associated with bacterial endometritis. Other potential pathogens include *E coli, Pseudomonas* and *Klebsiella*. The mechanism of abortion due to these bacteria appears to be survival of a small population of pathogens that entered the uterus at breeding. During the course of gestation, more often early than late, the bacteria multiply and cause inflammatory changes in the endometrium and placenta. Fetal death and abortion occur when enough placental area is involved to compromise fetal support. An alternative mechanism is bacterial invasion of the uterus via the cervix during pregnancy. Although the equine cervix is a relatively simple tubular structure, it is effectively sealed by heavy, viscous mucus.

The evidence supporting the first mechanism is circumstantial. Many mares that suffer abortions due to bacterial causes have a history of endometritis caused by the same organism. Abortions of this type are more often diagnosed in older mares with spotty production records and declining uterine immunocompetence.

When freshly recovered fetuses and placentae are examined, the most striking gross findings are inflammation and necrosis of the placenta. Edema of the fetal membranes is common, and suppurative exudates may still cling to the chorionic surface of the chorioallantois. Fetal lesions are usually masked by autolytic changes. Recovery of the pathogenic bacteria in relatively pure culture and in large numbers from the fetus and placenta is the basis for the diagnosis. Bacteria can usually be recovered from the stomach contents, heart blood, spleen, liver or thymus. Cultures obtained from the mare's uterus during the first few days after abortion may also be helpful.

Bacterial abortion is essentially controlled by preventing endometritis in barren mares. Attention must be given to the anatomic changes of the external genitalia that predispose to loss of integrity, contamination and persistent endometritis. The short breeding season often necessitates breeding mares that have not completely recovered from bacterial infections. These mares represent the group at highest risk for subsequent bacterial abortion.

Abortions have been associated with rising titers to *Leptospira pomona* and fever but with no confirming recovery or identification of the organism in aborted fetuses.[135] The clinical significance of leptospirosis as an abortigenic disease in mares is questionable.[136]

Other organisms incriminated as a cause of bacterial abortion include mycoplasmas and *Brucella abortus*. Mycoplasma has been isolated from aborted equine fetuses but its role in producing abortion is still unclear.[137,138] *Brucella abortus* has also been isolated from aborted fetuses.

Mycotic Causes: Abortions associated with placental lesions caused by fungi occur in significant numbers in various horse-breeding areas. Fungi proliferate at the junction of chorion and endometrium to produce placentitis. Disruption of the chorionic attachment results in fetal death and abortion. The principal agents involved in mycotic abortion are *Aspergillus* and *Mucor*.[139]

Typical gross findings in aborted fetuses and placentae include greatly thickened, irregular areas on the chorion, occasional lesions on the amnion, and rarely plaques on the fetus itself. Fungi can be readily demonstrated by direct smear from the chorionic lesion. Fungal cultures further help identify the causal agent.

The route of infection in mycotic placentitis and abortion has not been established. Secondary infections by yeasts and fungi are common in mares with a history of endometritis treated vigorously with antibiotics. It is conceivable that remnants of these endometrial fungal infections could persist during pregnancy to eventually produce placentitis. Intranasal and hematogenous routes of infection by fungi have not been demonstrated in horses. Some practitioners note that the incidence of mycotic abortion is higher in mares stabled in dusty quarters. Horses in some subtropical climates seem to have more mycotic abortions than those in drier parts of the country.

Abortion due to placental lesions, such as those produced by fungal agents, may be preceded by premature lactation. Chorionic separation undoubtedly plays a role in this phenomenon.

Prevention of mycotic abortion probably lies in determining those mares at risk prior to breeding and, if necessary, treating the uterus to remove any mycotic organisms present.

Noninfectious Causes: Twinning is the most significant noninfectious cause of abortion. In areas where abortion induced by EHV-1 infection is controlled effectively, twinning may be the most important cause of all equine abortions.[128] The incidence of twinning is reported as 1-2%. This figure is undoubtedly low due to the fact that many twin abortions are not recognized as such and are not reported. On one farm, 20 sets of twins were aborted from 199 mares in one season. The true incidence probably lies between these 2 extremes.

There is undoubtedly a large discrepancy between the number of mares experiencing multiple ovulations and those conceiving twins and carrying them to the point where they may be recognized. Early embryonic loss of one conceptus would be the most logical explanation for this difference. Careful examination of the placenta from apparent singleton foals may reveal fetal remnants or structures confirming the fact that twin conceptions did occur. The so-called "amorphous globosus" is a ball of bony tissue connected to the placenta by an umbilical stalk.

Twin foals are seldom carried to term because of the limitation of uterine size. Live twin foals delivered at term are invariably smaller than normal. Inadequate endometrial space for chorionic attachment is the cause of retarded growth in these cases and more commonly the cause of premature death of one twin, which then leads to abortion of the pair. Careful observation of mares during mid- and late pregnancy may reveal premature lactation for only a few days. This sign suggests that twin fetuses are being carried and that one fetus has died. In most cases, abortion of both fetuses follows within a few weeks.

Some twin conceptions can be confirmed prior to day 60 by rectal palpation. After both uterine horns become distended from 60 days to term, it is virtually impossible to diagnose twins by physical means. A reliable practical method of diagnosing twin pregnancy in midgestation would be extremely beneficial to the equine industry. Many broodmares change hands through auction sales in the fall of the year and many unsuspecting buyers take home mares that subsequently abort twins. Little recourse is available to these buyers and in many cases the sellers are obviously unaware of the situation.

The equine practitioner is constantly frustrated by attempts to control twinning in mares. Probably the largest single factor favoring twin conceptions is that spermatozoa survive in the reproductive tract of the mare for many days following breeding or insemination. Twinning is a greater threat in mares bred by stallions with great spermatozoal longevity.

One means of reducing the incidence of twinning is by not breeding mares with multiple preovulatory follicles. However, since the number of mares that ovulate more than one follicle is significantly higher than the number of twins conceived, a good argument against this technic can be made. The alternative to passing an estrus in which 2 ovulations seem imminent is to follow the mare closely and hope that one follicle will ovulate at least 12 hours prior to the second. Since ovum longevity rarely exceeds 8 hours postovulation, it is possible to breed the mare on the second follicle when such an interval exists between ovulations. It is advisable, however, to ensure ovulation of the second follicle by an injection of HCG in these cases.

Management of twin pregnancies by terminating the life of one embryo is a subject of considerable controversy. Various reports suggest that one embryonic vesicle may be either crushed or destroyed by aspiration. Some practitioners are convinced this is a reliable technic. In the author's experience, such methods have been consistently unsuccessful, resulting either in death of both embryos or survival of both. One recent study suggested the possible alternative of premedicating the mare with antiprostaglandin drugs prior to aspiration of one vesicle.[140] Meclofenamic acid was used in 1-g doses for 3 days prior to treatment. A 16-ga needle was then inserted into the vesicle per vaginum and the fetal fluid aspirated. In all cases, collapse of the fetal sac could be detected by rectal palpation. None of the mares so treated continued to term with a singleton pregnancy, but survival of one fetus for a significant number of days after treatment indicates that this technic deserves further investigation.

Endocrine Causes: Any disruption of the finely tuned interaction of endocrine events in early pregnancy could conceivably lead to embryonic loss. Failure of the corpus luteum to become established or failure of the uterus to recognize pregnancy and maintain luteal function are examples of such abnormalities. Once pregnancy is established to the point where it can be diagnosed, however, there are no documented hormonal causes for abortion in mares. Considerable controversy still exists regarding the role of adequate levels of progesterone produced by the corpus luteum, secondary corpora lutea or the fetoplacental unit in maintaining pregnancy in some individuals. Circumstantial evidence based on supplementation of progesterone to mares with known histories of early abortion, resulting in maintenance of pregnancy, have perpetuated the confusion.

Traditional schemes for administering exogenous progesterone have used doses of 250-500 mg repositol progesterone at intervals of 10-30 days. Research into the catabolism of repositol progesterone in ovariectomized mares indicates that doses of this magnitude are rapidly eliminated from the circulation and could not be responsible for continued physiologic levels of progesterone.[141] To maintain circulating progesterone levels above 1 ng/ml plasma, progesterone in oil must be injected daily in doses of 100-200 mg. To maintain these same blood levels, weekly doses of 2 g repositol progesterone were necesary.[142] These trials were conducted on ovariectomized mares from which no progesterone contribution was available from the ovaries or a pregnant uterus. While it is impossible to rule out the traditional progesterone support scheme as effective in mares whose natural progesterone production is marginal, it appears highly unlikely that an occasional small dose of progesterone is a valid means of preventing early abortion in mares.

Physical Causes: The most significant physical causes of pregnancy failure in mares are endometrial changes that alter uterine ability to support the embryo to the time of placentation. Glandular secretions are extremely important in the nourishment of the equine conceptus because placental development is slow. Until 100-150 days, when sufficient interchange occurs between endometrium and chorion, glandular secretion of proteins appears to be critical. Certain alterations in the physical character of the endometrium correlate very highly with embryonic death during the period of glandular support.[17]

Fibrotic changes around the glands themselves most severely restrict glandular function. Periglandular fibrosis is the prime offender in interference with gland function. Other lesions, such as severe, deep inflammatory changes and lymphatic stasis, accompanied by palpable uterine changes, seem to be involved in the same process. The reader is referred to the section on Examination for details on obtaining and interpreting an endometrial biopsy, which is a reliable prognostic tool.

Probably the most widely used excuse for undiagnosed equine abortion is alleged trauma to the mare while pastured with other animals. Virtually every owner can recall a time a few days previously when mares were kicking at each other, running excessively or otherwise inflicting physical damage upon themselves. Although severe injury, such as slipping and falling, or severe compression of the abdomen late in pregnancy can cause expulsion of the fetus through the easily dilated cervix, most other alleged traumatic events are probably not the cause of abortion. The protective mechanisms involved in the developing fetus are sufficient to ensure that minor traumatic encounters do not disrupt pregnancy.

Torsion of the umbilicus may cause fetal death. Careful examination of the entire placenta in all cases of abortion reveals a small percentage of cases in which the umbilical cord has been twisted to the point of causing severe edema and occlusion of blood vessels. The long umbilical stalk of the fetus and the free-floating character of equine pregnancy lend themselves to this condition.

Induction of Abortion

On occasion the practitioner is called upon to therapeutically abort mares that have conceived twins, have become pregnant from inadvertent breedings, or have recently been purchased as athletes but are pregnant. Pregnancy may be terminated from shortly after breeding up until approximately 4 months of gestation without danger to the dam.

Mismating occurs occasionally when teaser animals gain access to paddocks of mares or when mares are inadvertently bred to the wrong stallion. The ideal procedure in such cases is to examine the mismated mare immediately and repeat examination until the time of ovulation can be determined. Injection of prostaglandin 5-6 days after ovulation causes regression of the corpus luteum and a return to estrus.

Prostaglandins may be used to abort mares successfully up until the time of the formation of the endometrial cups, ie, at 36 days or less. Once pregnancy has proceeded to the point where PMSG levels are rising, the method of choice for therapeutic abortion is manual dilation of the cervix and irrigation of the uterus with large volumes of sterile saline. Strict asepsis is required to minimize uterine contamination.

At 4-5 months of gestation and beyond, the risks of uterine damage, dystocia, retained placenta and other complications increase. Although abortion may be induced in mid-term by cervical dilation or later in gestation by oxytocin injection, conservative veterinarians discourage this practice. In terms of future production of the mare, it is often wise to allow the mare to foal naturally rather than interfere.

Torsion of the Uterus

The suspension of the equine uterus from the broad ligaments attached to the dorsolateral body wall makes torsion of the gravid uterus unlikely. The cause of uterine torsion in mares is not known, although severe trauma and violent rolling may play a role. Signs of abdominal discomfort in mares late in pregnancy suggest uterine torsion as a consideration in the differential diagnosis. Colic signs may be mild to severe and related to tension on the broad ligaments or pressure on the uterine wall. Secondary GI disturbances may result from the altered position of the displaced uterus. Necrosis of the uterus, with subsequent rupture, may occasionally result in extrauterine pregnancy.

Rectal examination can help detect uterine torsion. The most diagnostic findings are those related to tension and position of the broad ligaments. In the typical clockwise torsion of the uterus, the left broad ligament is stretched across the dorsal aspect of the uterus from left to right and the right broad ligament disappears ventrad down the right body wall toward the right ovary. The fetus is usually displaced craniad by torsion in the uterine body; occasionally this twisting can be palpated just cranial to the cervix. Vaginal signs of uterine torsion are inconclusive. In cases of torsion of 180° or more, the cranial vagina may have signs of twisting to the point where the cervix cannot be palpated readily nor observed through a speculum.

Although uterine torsion in mares can be corrected by rolling in a manner similar to that used for cows, the basic approach to correction is surgical.[143,144] In simple uterine torsions without complications of tissue necrosis, the objective is to return the uterus to normal position and allow pregnancy to continue to term. Many cases managed in this manner result in eventual normal delivery. Correction of uterine torsion in mares at term often results in immediate delivery of a normal foal. When possible, a standing flank laparotomy is the most logical approach. Simple 180° torsions can often be corrected through this approach simply by rolling the twisted uterus back into normal position. More complex cases, particularly those with secondary bowel involvement, may require paramedian or midline approaches.

When uterine torsion has resulted in uterine rupture and escape of the fetus into the peritoneal cavity, the prognosis is obviously grave. Occasionally these cases are managed successfully by removing the fetus and closing the defect in the uterus. However, the formation of adhesions or other damage to the abdominal viscera typically results in loss of the mare.

Rupture of the Prepubic Tendon

Very rarely in light breeds of horses, the additional burden of a heavy, pregnant uterus causes separation of the ventral abdominal musculature from its attachment to the pelvis by the prepubic tendon.[5] The sudden appearance of a ventral displacement of the caudal abdomen with accompanying edema suggests prepubic tendon rupture. This may be confused with physiologic edema that precedes parturition. Some mares develop massive areas of edema from the udder craniad, occasionally involving both rear legs as well. Careful physical examination can distinguish physiologic edema from prepubic tendon rupture.

Management of mares with a ruptured prepubic tendon consists of mechanical support of the abdomen, when possible, until parturition. Restriction of exercise and diet are also of value in reducing abdominal mass. The objective in prepubic tendon rupture is to maintain the mare until a live foal can be delivered. This may be a valid indication for induction of parturition at the appropriate time.

Hydroallantois

Hydroallantois is rare in mares. A rapid, abnormal enlargement of the abdomen during late pregnancy was associated with abnormalities of the chorioallantoic membrane in a series of mares.[145] Spontaneous abortion occurred in 4 of 8 cases and therapeutic abortion was indicated in the other 4. A total of 120-220 L allantoic fluid was expelled upon rupture of the chorioallantoic membrane. Examination of the allantoic side of the membrane revealed edema and cystic changes.

Hydrops Amnion

Hydrops amnion, associated with fetal abnormality, is not recognized in mares.

Parturition

Normal Parturition

The mare normally delivers the foal rapidly, efficiently and usually at night. Survival of horses in the wild is partially dependent upon a quick delivery and early mobility of the foal. For these reasons, parturient mares, left to their own devices, seek a secluded and suitable site for delivery and encourage their offspring to stand, nurse and travel with minimal delay. Management of domesticated horses should allow this normal sequence of events to occur as undisturbed as possible.

The length of gestation in horses is extremely variable. The generally accepted average gestation length for light breeds is 335-342 days, with a range of 305-365 days.[146] Donkeys, and mares carrying mule foals have slightly longer gestation periods than do mares.[5] Mares bred late in the spring tend to have shorter gestation periods than those bred in February or March. The age of the mare apparently has no effect on gestation length. Male foals are carried a significantly longer period than female foals.

The clinical significance of the great variability in gestational length in horses relates to the final maturation processes in the fetus prior to delivery. When induction of labor or cesarean section is elected, much of the success of the procedure lies with the assurance that the fetus is sufficiently mature to survive. The indications of impending parturition are just as variable as gestation length. While some mares typically show mammary development, production of colostrum and relaxation of ligaments just prior to delivery, others leak milk for several days before parturition, and still others, notably maiden mares, foal with no outward signs of impending parturition.

The biologic events in the initiation of parturition are complex, interrelated and not completely understood. Mares deliver foals in the face of high circulating levels of progesterone and estrogen. The levels of these hormones fall drastically in the hours just preceding parturition. Circumstantial evidence suggests that the fetal adrenal gland is a key organ in the initiation of parturition. The adrenal glands of fetuses enlarge dramatically immediately preceding parturition, and circulating levels of corticosteroids are progressively higher in fetuses as delivery is approached. Corticosteroids apparently do not cross the placental barrier in either direction, which is supported by the fact that normal exogenous doses of corticosteroids do not induce parturition in mares.[147,148] Regardless of the endocrine events, prostaglandin F$_2$alpha is a key initiator of contractions of uterine musculature. Oxytocin also plays an active role in the control of contractions involved in delivery of the foal.

Outward signs in the mare during the days and weeks preceding parturition are somewhat variable. Most mares reduce their physical activity in the last weeks prior to parturition, often separating themselves from the group and apparently seeking isolation. Many reduce their feed intake, particularly of roughage. Signs of impending parturition include relaxation of the sacrosciatic ligaments, elongation of the vulva, and mammary changes. Probably the most reliable sign is udder development and the appearance of colostrum, which often manifests itself as beads of wax-like material at the teat orifices ("waxing up"). Because these signs are subject to extreme variability, many a night can be spent observing a mare with wax on its teats, milk in its udder, and relaxed ligaments.

The actual delivery process has arbitrarily been classified into 3 stages of labor. The first stage is the initial uterine contraction, which lasts until the chorioallantoic membrane ruptures ("breaking water"). The second stage is active expulsion of the fetus, and the third stage is expulsion of the fetal membranes. During the first stage of labor, uterine contractions are evidenced by restlessness, walking, frequent urination, slight to moderate sweating and an anxious attitude. At this point mares still maintain some control over the birth process. Distractions or untoward external influences cause mares in the first stage of labor to postpone parturition for some time, even days.

The fetus plays an active role in positioning itself for delivery. Movements by the fetus probably occur during stage 1 or the phase of initial uterine contractions. The fetal position prior to delivery is dorsopubic rather than dorsosacral. The foal lies in the uterus on its back, with the forelegs folded over the chest and the head in a variety of positions. During the first stage of labor, the fetus extends the forelegs and head, and appears to be reaching for the birth canal. Further uterine contractions cause rotation of the forelimbs and head into the dor-

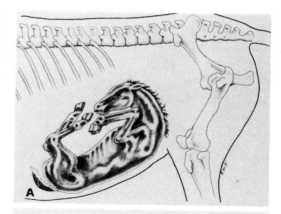

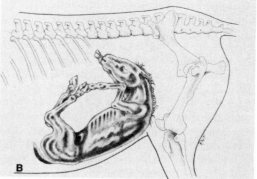

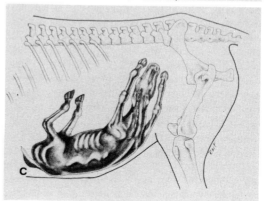

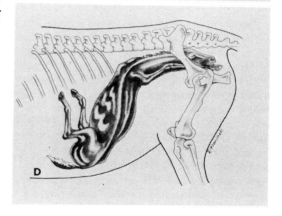

Fig. 23. Fetal rotation during early labor. The fetus changes from a dorsopubic to a dorsosacral position, and actively places its forelegs and head in the normal posture.[153]

sosacral presentation, while the rear portions of the foal remain dorsopubic. A gradual rotation occurs as contractions progress and the forelimbs and head enter the birth canal (Fig 23).[149] In the terminal phases of stage 1, uterine contractions are sufficient to force the fetus, membranes and fluid against the allantochorionic membrane in the area of nonattachment adjacent to the cervix. The membrane ruptures at this point, allowing the escape of the allantoic fluid to the outside.

Stage 2 of labor is rapid, averaging 12-15 minutes, and commences with the release of allantoic fluid. Most mares become laterally recumbent for stage 2 and abdominal contractions begin. The fetal forelimbs, still encased in the amnionic membrane, appear at the vulva first. With each abdominal contraction, the foal progesses a bit further caudad, with the tip of the muzzle evident when the forelegs have cleared the vulva by 10-15 cm. At this point the shoulders of the foal have entered the birth canal and particularly violent contractions move the shoulders through the maternal pelvis. Another concerted effort is made as the hips enter the birth canal. Delivery is accomplished very quickly once the hips clear the maternal pelvis. It is typical for the entire foal to be delivered before the amnionic membrane ruptures. Movement of the forefeet and head of the foal tears the amnion. The umbilical cord remains attached even after the entire foal has cleared the vulva. Significant amounts of blood are transferred from the placenta to the foal at this time following delivery. The umbilical cord ruptures spontaneously, due either to movement of the foal or the mare. The point of rupture is a spot about 50 mm from the foal's body. Depending on the exertion necessary for delivery of the foal, the mare tends to lie in lateral recumbency for a few minutes after delivery unless disturbed.

The third stage of labor or the expulsion of the fetal membranes may take place while the mare is still in lateral recumbency. It is not unusual for the entire placenta to be passed within 10 minutes of delivery. Retention of the membranes for up to an hour or more after delivery is normal. Continued uterine contractions are manifested as abdominal discomfort during the third stage of labor. Some mares lie back down, roll with some degree of violence, and otherwise exhibit signs of abdominal pain. Experience dictates when this postpartum pain reaches abnormal proportions and some complication of parturition has occurred.

Management of Foaling

The economics of the horse-breeding business dictate that mares be observed during the foaling process to detect any abnormalities. The most natural and probably most successful foaling management scheme would be to turn mares out in large clean pastures and allow the process to proceed without human intervention. Since limitations of space, adverse weather conditions and general concern for the welfare of the mare and foal seldom allow for such natural management, observation of mares is the norm. To observe mares in the days prior to foaling and during the foaling process, they must be maintained in a central facility for optimal use of stable personnel. On most farms pregnant mares are grouped by expected foaling date in smaller paddocks adjacent to foaling quarters. As mares deliver their foals, they are removed from the nursery and the next candidates replace them. Unfortunately, this scheme guarantees concentration of parasites, bacteria and other contaminants that add to the risks against raising healthy foals.

Where climatic situations allow, mares can foal outdoors and still be supervised. Portable paddocks can be used and moved regularly to clean areas of pasture. Large, outdoor foaling pens can be meticulously cleaned and rebedded between foalings. Most managers house mares inside barns where climate can be controlled and observation is easiest. Foaling stalls should be roomy, well ventilated, easily cleaned, and reserved only for foaling rather than for holding mares awaiting parturition.

Outside interference from visitors and interested spectators should be discouraged and only personnel dealing directly with the foaling should be in the foaling barn. Some large commercial operations have experimented with artificial flooring in the foaling stall, such as rubber mats or synthetic material, to reduce bacterial contamination of the mare in the immediate postpartum period. Unfortunately, many mares are reluctant to lie down in an unbedded stall and the advantages of cleanliness are often overcome by the disadvantages of prolonged labor.

Feeding mares near parturition should take into account the natural withdrawal of most mares from high roughage intake. Occasional mares continue to consume hay to capacity up until the time of foaling. Large amounts of roughage in the large bowel of mares is apparently related to higher incidents of colonic and cecal damage during foaling.

The preparation of the mare prior to foaling is a subject of some debate. Wrapping the tail and washing the perineal area are necessary in some foaling schemes. Leaving the mare totally undisturbed has the advantage that less disturbance ensures a more natural delivery. A compromise is to clip the long tail hairs of heavily pregnant mares distad to a level ventral to the ventral commissure of the vulva to reduce postpartum contamination of the birth canal.

In caring for the mare in the immediate postpartum period, great caution should be exercised that the mare is not disturbed or disrupted in the natural birth process. When foaling is apparently proceeding without complication, the dam and foal should be left alone as much as possible. Rushing into the stall, as soon as the foal is born, to wash the mare's udder, disinfect the foal's navel and administer prophylactic medication disturbs the dam and offspring.

The most serious questions arise as to when human intervention is necessary in the foaling process. Minimal intervention and disturbance are indicated during stage 1 since mares may arrest the foaling process if seriously disturbed. Until stage 1 is completed and the chorioallantoic membrane is ruptured, there is no logical reason for intervention. Up until this point, the fetus is becoming positioned for expulsion and the cervix has not been fully dilated. During the entire course of stage-1 labor, the mare should be quietly observed, with a minimum amount of light in the stall to make the observations.

A new attitude should prevail when stage 2 commences and the foal is being expelled. If 10 minutes of strenuous labor, with vigorous abdominal contractions, produce no signs of the forelimbs, rear limbs or head at the vulva, problems may rightfully be expected. At this point, using the maximum aseptic technic permitted by the situation, manual exploration of the birth canal should be undertaken. If both forefeet can be detected in the birth canal, followed by the tip of the muzzle, the mare should be allowed to continue attempts to deliver the foal. If strenuous abdominal contractions fail to produce evidence of impending delivery within the next 10 minutes, assistance in delivery is probably indicated (see Dystocia).

Induction of Parturition

Medical, surgical and management situations arise that make elective induction of parturition in mares advantageous. Medical induction of labor and delivery has been extensively practiced since the 1970s. Regimens using oxytocin injection, oxytocin in combination with estrogens, and prostaglandin analogs have been used with success.[150-152] An excellent review of various methods for inducing parturition has been published.[153]

Indications

The indication for inducing parturition at term is essentially any situation in which the health of the mare or foal is threatened and in which prompt delivery improves the prognosis for the dam and/or the foal. This can be broadened to include those situations in which management is inadequate to supervise normal delivery and the presence of a veterinarian at the time of delivery would be an asset. Induction of labor might be advantageous in cases of intractable colic in a mare due to foal, prepubic tendon rupture, extensive loss of colostrum prior to delivery, premature separation of the chorioallantoic membrane, and failure of a mare to proceed with normal labor after the initial stages have begun. Inducing labor as a pure convenience for the management is somewhat questionable, since this involves risks that may not be present under normal circumstances.

Selection of Candidates

The selection of mares for induction of parturition involves some critical criteria. By far the most important of these is the presence of milk or colostrum in the udder. Colostrum or milk is not present in the udder unless the foal has attained sufficient maturity to ensure its survival. Induction based purely on the stage of gestation, without consideration of mammary development, may result in dysmature foals with a survival rate lower than expected, and the possibility the dam may not have sufficient milk. A second criterion, somewhat less critical than mammary development, is gestational age. Although the length of gestation is extremely variable in horses, a safe rule to apply to induction candidates is a minimum of 320 days of gestation. Less important criteria include relaxation of the sacrosciatic ligaments and relaxation of the cervix. The last 2 can be overlooked if the length of gestation is adequate and there is milk in the udder.

Technic

Although fluprostenol, a prostaglandin analog, is an efficient drug for the induction of labor, only oxytocin will be considered here.[156]

Oxytocin has been used in a single large IM dose (100-120 IU), multiple smaller IM or IV doses, or by drip infusion in a dilute saline solution. The author's choice is the last method and experience has suggested that slow IV drip of oxytocin more closely duplicates oxytocin levels in the physiologic process of labor and delivery.

An oxytocin solution is made by adding 100-120 IU oxytocin to 1 L normal saline. Ideally, an indwelling catheter is placed in the jugular vein to minimize the chance of extravasation during the procedure. The solution is administered at a rate approximating 1 L/hour. Signs of the first stages of labor, such as sweating, abdominal discomfort and nervousness, occur within 10-15 minutes of administration. Most mares rupture the chorioallantois within 20-30 minutes from the onset and proceed promptly with second-stage labor. It is unusual for normal mares not to produce a foal within 45-50 minutes of initiation of treatment.

Once labor has proceeded to the point at which delivery is assured, administration of oxytocin can be stopped. Should the mare initiate second-stage labor without presenting the forefeet and head into the birth canal, prompt examination to ascertain the position of the fetus is in order. The fetus, which before the initiation of treatment has been in a dorsopubic position, is usually in the normal position as described under normal parturition. It is relatively simple, however, to correct minor abnormalities of posture in the early stages of induction, before the mare begins vigorous abdominal contractions.

Complications with induction of labor by oxytocin administration have been no greater than those experienced with normal delivery. The incidence of retained placenta associated with induction of parturition appears to be no higher than in normal parturition.

It should be re-emphasized that induction of parturition cannot be successfully accomplished in mares by administration of normal doses of glucocorticoids.[148] Although massive doses of dexamethasone given for several consecutive days induce parturition, complications, such as dysmaturity, retained placenta and dystocia, are significant using this technic.[153]

Dystocia

Although the incidence of difficult birth is low in mares as compared with other species, problems associated with dystocia, when it does occur, are generally severe. All of the participants in this situation are generally anxious and the pressure upon the equine practitioner to solve the problem quickly can be immense.

Various characteristics of equine parturition affect the management of dystocia cases. One of the most influential aspects is the prime factor. Knowledge that in normal situations the total process of parturition can be completed within 30 minutes adds to the pressure of handling abnormal cases. Placental separation occurs in a relatively short time once labor commences and fetal hypoxia and death are common in prolonged, difficult parturition.

The expulsive efforts made by mares during second-stage labor makes management of dystocia particularly difficult for the operator. It is virtually impossible to maintain the arm in the birth canal with the fetus when a mare applies full pressure by abdominal press. Also, the stimulation of examination and attempted corrective procedure seems to increase the mare's efforts. Repulsion and mutation of malpositioned fetuses can become impossible when mares attempt to expel the arm of the operator and uterine contents at the same time.

An additional factor in the management of equine dystocia is the response of the reproductive tract to trauma. The uterus, cervix and vaginal mucosa of the mare are especially vulnerable to trauma involved in obstetric procedures. Application of instruments should be made with great discretion and every effort made to minimize physical damage to the reproductive tract. The uterus, vagina and especially the cervix respond with dramatic fibrosis to any handling other than the most gentle.

The temperament of mares, particularly those during parturition, makes their management more of a problem than in females of other species. Primiparous mares are especially unpredictable, being at once in pain, frightened and unfamiliar with the procedures taking place.

The causes of dystocia can be classified as either fetal or maternal. The overwhelming majority of cases relate to fetal causes.

Fetal Causes: The most common cause of equine dystocia is abnormal presentation, position or posture of the fetus. As mentioned earlier, the live fetus plays an active role in positioning itself for delivery. Failure of the

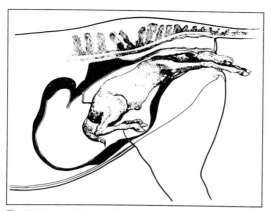

Fig 24. Lateral view of a fetus in the normal anterior dorsosacral position, with the forelimbs and neck fully extended.

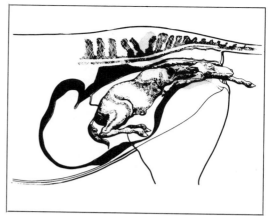

Fig 25. Lateral view of a fetus in an anterior dorsosacral position, with the right carpus flexed.

foal to be presented normally immediately suggests some abnormality or death of the fetus.

Compounding the problem of postural and position abnormalities is the length of limbs of equine fetuses. A minor abnormality, such as a foreleg retained at the carpus, becomes a major obstacle when the length from the carpus to the foot is considered.

Most fetuses are in anterior presentation during labor (Fig 24). The most common postural abnormalities are retention of one or both forelimbs or deviation of the head (Figs 25, 26). The long neck of the foal may seriously impede correction of a retained head. Posterior presentations are relatively uncommon. When they do occur, one rear limb may be retained or, in the case of a true breech presentation, both rear limbs are retained at the hip (Fig 27).

Transverse presentations fortunately are extremely rare and have been related to bicornual development of the fetus during gestation.[154] Transverse presentation is an indication for cesarean section.

Another fetal cause of dystocia is twin fetuses. Often the delivery of twins, particularly with one or both dead, results in a tangle of limbs and heads to the extent that delivery of either fetus is impossible without assistance. In all cases of dystocia, the operator should consider the possibility that more than one fetus is present.

Disparity of fetal size and maternal pelvic diameter can cause dystocia. Dystocia due solely to fetal size is unusual if the maternal pelvis is of normal dimensions. The size of the dam's uterus exerts a great influence on the size of the fetus.[155] The size of the sire of the

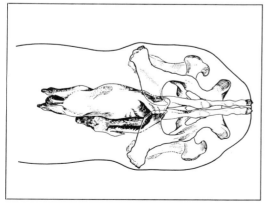

Fig 26. Dorsal view of a fetus in an anterior dorsosacral position, with the head deviated to the right.

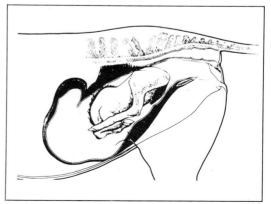

Fig 27. Lateral view of a fetus in the posterior dorsosacral breech position.

fetus is a very minor part of the determination of foal size.

Miscellaneous fetal causes of dystocia include fetal monsters, with hydrocephalus the most common abnormality observed, and premature delivery of the chorioallantoic membrane. In the latter case, the presence of chorioallantoic membrane in the birth canal impedes passage of the fetus.

Maternal Causes: The maternal causes of dystocia in mares are essentially those of inadequate pelvic size or pelvic abnormality. The primary factors that influence pelvic size are age, nutrition and general development of the mare. The practice of breeding 2-year-olds that are not adequately developed at the time of breeding is a leading cause of maternal dystocia due to inadequate pelvic size.

Pelvic abnormality is probably more significant as a maternal cause of dystocia. Old injuries, such as ilial or acetabular fractures and other compressing injuries to the pelvic girdle may result in limitation in the size of the birth canal. Examination prior to the time of breeding should identify those animals that could present delivery problems. If the pelvic abnormality is sufficient to cause suspicion of pending dystocia, preparations should be made for elective cesarean section.

Another maternal cause of dystocia is uterine inertia. Affected mares begin to labor but are unable to deliver the foal due to failure of the uterus to sustain contraction or due to failure of the mare to make the necessary expulsive efforts. Prime causes of uterine inertia are weakness and debilitation, and metabolic or systemic disease.

Torsion of the uterus has been previously discussed.

Treatment

The satisfactory management of equine dystocia requires restraint to provide safety to the personnel and animals involved and prompt correction of the problem if a live foal is to be delivered. Asepsis and adequate lubrication are prerequisites. Minimal mechanical interference is a rule and proper postpartum care is essential.

Upon arriving at the scene, the practitioner must rapidly assess the situation, decide the safest approach to examination and correction of the problem, and make best use of the personnel available to assist him or her. Examination of mares in stocks and chutes should be avoided whenever possible since manipulation during the examination and corrective proce-

dures usually causes mares to lie down. Such movement can result in injury to the fetus. In such cases the procedure must be interrupted until the mare is stimulated to stand again or is extracted from the stock. Probably the safest overall location for obstetric procedures is in the stall. Exceptionally difficult mares can be backed to the stall door and the operator can proceed with some degree of safety by standing behind the door frame.

Use of physical restraint is advisable. Application of a twitch, war bridle or other device by knowledgeable personnel can be invaluable. Too many practitioners overlook the advantage of taking a moment to place a sideline on a fractious mare. Properly applied, the sideline restricts the mare's ability to kick, yet provides stability during the procedure.

The tendency to use chemical restraint must be tempered by consideration for viability of the fetus. Tranquilizers may adversely affect the foal's survival in prolonged procedures. The use of narcotics and barbiturates may be hazardous to survival of the foal. Use of xylazine alone is of questionable value in obstetric procedures because some animals may become sensitive to manipulation of the rear quarters while appearing to be well sedated by the drug.

Epidural anesthesia is an asset in many cases. The difficulties of administering epidural anesthesia quickly and effectively to the mare must be considered in the decision to use this type of restraint. Often the time involved in achieving good epidural anesthesia could be better used in other methods of management of the problem.

Short-term general anesthesia may be indicated when minor postural abnormalities are discovered and expulsive efforts make correction of these abnormalities impossible. The use of a xylazine-ketamine combination provides 10-15 minutes of good relaxation, with some degree of anesthesia. This procedure has proved helpful when only simple corrective measures are necessary to alleviate the dystocia. Xylazine is administered IV at 1 mg/kg. After the xylazine takes effect, ketamine is given IV at 2 mg/kg. Most mares lie down smoothly with little apprehension and provide the operator with the required time to make the minor corrective manipulation.

Longer-term general anesthesia has become an asset to management of serious dystocia in mares. General anesthesia with halothane provides profound muscular relaxation of skeletal muscles and the myometrium. A rather low level of halothane anesthesia is often sufficient to to allow repulsion and correction of the dystocia.

During induction of halothane anesthesia, particular attention should be paid to the status of the foal. If the foal is still alive, anesthesia may be induced with only IV glyceryl guaiacolate. Most light-breed mares can be intubated after IV administration of 1-2 L 5% glyceryl guaiacolate. If the foal is already dead, the addition of a barbiturate to the glyceryl guaiacolate solution may be of benefit.

The greatest advantage of halothane anesthesia in managing serious dystocias is the time saved should conventional procedures fail to produce the foal. The mare is already anesthetized for the eventuality of cesarean section. In fact, if adequate help is available during the obstetric procedure, preparations can begin for a cesarean section should the obstetrician fail to deliver the foal.

Obstetric procedures useful in managing dystocia are mutation, forced extraction, fetotomy and cesarean section. During any of these procedures the emphasis of the operator should be placed on asepsis, adequate lubrication, rapid assessment of the problem, and minimal use of traumatic instruments.

Mutation: Mutation is the correction of abnormal presentation, position and posture of the fetus. Probably the most important aspect of this procedure is repulsion. To correct even the most simple postural abnormality, the fetus must be repelled craniad to a point allowing correction of abnormal placement of a limb or the head. Great care should be taken, when returning a retained limb to its normal posture, to guard the uterine wall and cervix against trauma. Even though the fetal foot is coated with a soft gelatinous material, the abrupt return of a forelimb to its normal position can lacerate the uterus, cervix or vagina.

Forced Extraction: Once mutation is complete, forced extraction may be necessary, depending on the status of the mare and size of the foal. Obstetric chains may be placed on the forelimbs of the fetus by slipping a loop of the chain over the foot, with the loop in the dorsal position. In cases of retention of the head, an obstetric chain may be passed behind the poll and through the mouth to direct movement of the head during the extraction process. Obstetric snares may be of value but emphasis should be placed on protecting the mare's reproductive tract. Blunt eye hooks may be of value to maintain corrective posture of the head.

The amount of traction required to deliver the equine fetus with maximum safety to both dam and foal is that which can be applied by no more than 2 people pulling on obstetric chains or ropes. Traction should be applied in conjunction with the maternal expulsive effort. The fetal extractor should not be used in managing obstetric problems in mares. It is relatively easy with the fetal extractor to exert sufficient pressure to damage the fetus or maternal pelvis, with subsequent nerve paralysis.

Forced extraction occasionally results in delivery of the cranial portions of the foal but subsequent hip lock. Rotation of the equine fetus during delivery does not preclude the occurrence of hip lock as in bovine dystocia cases. A helpful hint in managing hip lock is to place a rope halter on the foal's head and apply traction to the head, with the subsequent traction transmitted down the vertebral column rather than along the skin as when traction is placed on the forelimbs.

Fetotomy: Dismemberment of a dead fetus to allow delivery is generally discouraged in equine dystocias because of the trauma resulting from use of fetotomy instruments. In general, if delivery can be accomplished by means of a single fetotomy incision, the procedure is valid. Total fetotomy is contraindicated in mares. The prognosis for fertility of mares in which extensive fetotomy procedures have been performed is guarded to poor due to the inevitable lacerations and scarring of the reproductive tract.

Cesarean Section: Cesarean section has become a valid obstetric procedure in the management of difficult dystocias in recent years. Improvement in aseptic surgical technic and general anesthetic methods have made cesarean section a routine surgical procedure.

If the need for cesarean section is evident prior to the end of gestation, timing of the operation is critical. The same criteria used for induction of parturition should be applied to mares selected for elective cesarean section. Maturity of the foal is a prime consideration. Signs of milk in the udder, adequate stage of gestation, and ligament relaxation are all indications of fetal maturity. Probably the safest approach to deciding when to perform an elective cesarean section is to wait for the mare to actually begin labor. This procedure, of course, requires constant supervision of the mare during the last weeks of gestation.

In nonelective or emergency cesarean section, the decision to perform surgery should be made as soon as possible. The longer the mare is in labor and the longer the foal is dead, the less chance the mare has for recovery. An early decision to perform surgery is critical if a serious dystocia is encountered that cannot be rapidly resolved by ordinary obstetric procedures.

The postsurgical formation of adhesions between the uterus and adjacent abdominal structures should be considered. Palpation of the uterus per rectum should commence by the second or third postsurgical day to evaluate uterine involution and to determine and reduce the formation of intra-abdominal adhesions. Details on the surgical procedure are included in a separate section.

Postpartum Complications

Retained Placenta

Expulsion of the fetal membrane is normally accomplished within 1½ hours of delivery of the foal.[5] Failure to completely expel the placenta by 3 hours may be considered abnormal.[156] By 8 hours postpartum, bacteria in the uterus are replicating in a log phase and proliferation of potentially toxic organisms reaches significant levels shortly thereafter. The bacteria, by-products of tissue breakdown and debris, create the potential for several serious sequelae to retained placenta. It is critical, therefore, to manage mares with a retained placenta as emergencies. Treatment should be instituted prior to 8 hours postpartum and continued until danger of bacterial metritis and septicemia has passed and the membrane has been completely delivered.

The principles of proper treatment for retained placenta are to promote intact expulsion of all membranes and control bacterial growth in the uterus. The use of oxytocin to enhance uterine contraction, with subsequent expulsion of the placenta, is successful in many cases. If oxytocin is administered early and successfully causes passage of the membranes, it may not be necessary to manually medicate the uterus. For this reason, it is highly desirable to attempt oxytocin therapy early after retained placenta has been defined.

The methods of administration of oxytocin vary and the choices are similar to those described for induction of labor. Single large doses may be given IM, smaller multiple doses administered at intervals, or a single large dose in saline administered via IV drip. Uterine contractions are evident within minutes of administration and are manifested as abdominal discomfort, sweating and mild colic in some cases. The placenta may be delivered within 15-20 minutes of administration.

Careful aseptic exploration of the uterine lumen should be undertaken in mares that fail to deliver the placenta promptly after several attempts with oxytocin or in cases in which the placenta has not been passed within 8 hours. This examination should be made with a sterile rectal sleeve, covered by a sterile glove and lubricated with a sterile lubricant. The degree of adherence of the chorion to the endometrium should be assessed at this time. Membranes lying free in the uterine lumen should be brought to the outside to add to the traction on the retained portions of the placenta. At the time of examination, antibiotics should be distributed through the uterine lumen.

Manual stripping of the chorion from the endometrium is hazardous. Rough handling of the retained placenta and vigorous manual removal may result in significant scarring of the endometrium and prevent future pregnancy. Hemorrhage at the time of manual removal is an additional complication.

Refractory cases of retained placenta must be managed by local administration of antibiotics at least twice daily and by systemic antibiotic therapy. When the uterus is medicated, the remaining attachment should be re-evaluated and any free membrane brought to the outside.

Explanation to the owner for this conservative therapy is important. Cases of retained placenta have been managed in this manner for up to 6 days with no apparent ill effects.

An alternative treatment regimen involves redistension of the intact allantoic space with 10-12 L warm, mild antiseptic solution.[157] The intact chorioallantoic membrane is identified at the vulva, a stomach tube introduced within its margin and the solution pumped gently into the space. The opening of the membrane is then ligated and the intact membrane repelled into the pelvic cavity. The apparent effect of this treatment is to reinitiate spontaneous uterine contraction, resulting in delivery of the entire retained membrane. This treatment is likely to be successful because the pressure created in the vagina and pelvic cavity initiates release of oxytocin.

All membranes should be carefully examined after expulsion in cases of retained placenta or after normal parturition. Spreading the chorioallantoic portion on the ground allows the clinician to discover if the placenta has been passed intact. Large defects in the membrane indicate that portions are still retained, and treatment should be continued to manage bacterial growth.

Metritis-Laminitis-Septicemia Complex

A serious sequela to retained placenta or any gross contamination of the uterus during foaling is acute metritis, with concurrent laminitis and/or septicemia. This syndrome is potentially lethal and should be managed vigorously. The signs of acute metritis may commence as early as 10-12 hours postpartum. Fever and elevated pulse and respiratory rates are noted, and the animal quickly becomes severely depressed. The mucous membranes appear muddy to purple, and any vaginal discharge is reddish-brown and foul smelling. Rapidly progressive laminitis may be evident early in the course of the disease and can become severe enough to cause sloughing of the hooves.

Management of this postpartum infection is aimed at reducing bacterial growth, removal of the fluid accumulated in the uterus, and general support of the systemic problems. Some success may be obtained by siphoning the fluids from the uterine lumen by introducing a large-bore stomach tube, keeping the uterine wall away from the tube's orifice, and allowing the fluids to run by gravity to the outside.

In acute metritis, the uterus is especially prone to sequestering fluid and exudate, and the removal of fluid should be repeated as often as necessary. Antibiotics should be instilled in the uterus and systemic antibiotic therapy instituted. Supportive fluid therapy is indicated in severe cases. Attempts to prevent laminitis should be instituted early, including use of phenylbutazone and forced exercise. Some practitioners are convinced that antihistamines are beneficial in these cases.

Despite vigorous attempts to treat acute metritis and its associated complications, many affected mares die.

Postpartum Colic

Abdominal pain following delivery of a foal is normal in most mares. Uterine contractions that persist after foaling and expulsion of the membranes is evidenced by some degree of discomfort, occasional rolling, and mild signs of distress. Judgment of the severity of this postpartum pain is involved in the consideration of other more serious causes of colic.

Causes of severe postpartum colic include inversion of the tip of one uterine horn, hemorrhage from a ruptured vessel in the broad ligament, and trauma to portions of the large colon.

In the normal involution process, the tip of one uterine horn can invaginate upon itself due to the slack in the broad ligament, trapping the uterine wall or the uterine wall and ovary. Spasms of the myometrium around the inversion cause severe, unrelenting pain. Because this pain cannot be controlled with medication, analgesic therapy is a practical means of differentiating uterine horn inversion from normal postpartum pain.

Inversion of the tip of the uterine horn may be corrected manually by way of the uterine lumen. Occasionally it may be necessary to distend the uterus with fluid to correct the inversion. In extreme cases, general anesthesia, with its associated relaxation of the myometrium, may be necessary to correct this disorder.

Uterine Prolapse

Prolapse of the uterus may follow dystocia, retained placenta or normal delivery, particularly in multiparous mares. Uterine prolapse should be treated as an emergency situation because mares are particularly predisposed to shock and hemorrhage under such circumstances. Treatment of shock is as essential as replacing the prolapse.

Cleansing and replacement of the prolapsed uterus should be attempted as soon as possible, with particular attention to minimizing trauma to the exposed endometrium. Epidural anesthesia greatly facilitates replacement by reducing straining. Administration of oxytocin after replacement of the prolapsed organ speeds involution.

Hemorrhage may occur as a result of stretching of the broad ligaments following uterine prolapse. The combination of shock, hemorrhage, and contamination and/or trauma to the uterus results in failure of treatment in a significant number of cases.

Uterine Rupture

Rupture of the uterus may occur in serious dystocia or may go unrecognized when it occurs early in second-stage labor. In the latter case, suggestion of uterine rupture may not be evident until the mare has developed significant peritonitis some hours after foaling. The uterine wall should be explored manually following successful management of serious dystocia or in mares that have undergone prolonged and difficult labor.

The uterus usually ruptures on the dorsal aspect of the body of the organ and is probably associated with penetration by the feet of the foal. The uterus may rupture spontaneously, considering the violence with which some mares fall to the ground during the early portions of second-stage labor.

Attempts should be made to repair the wound as soon as possible after recognition of the rupture. Rough apposition of the margins of the wound may be accomplished by blind suturing through the birth canal, although this approach is extremely difficult. Laparotomy, preferably through a flank incision is the next logical step.

Whether uterine rupture is recognized and repaired immediately or is not diagnosed until peritonitis develops, peritoneal lavage should be performed as a supportive measure. Infusion of the peritoneal cavity with large volumes of warm, sterile fluid containing antibiotics should be followed by ventral drainage of this fluid. This method of treatment of peritonitis is preferred over conventional systemic antibiotic therapy.

Postpartum Hemorrhage

Blood vessels in the broad ligaments may rupture following parturition, particularly in older mares. The resulting hemorrhage slowly dissects into the broad ligament. As hemorrhage progresses, it extends beneath the uterine serosa and may proceed uninterrupted until the mare dies from blood loss.

The clinical signs of postpartum hemorrhage into the broad ligaments are those of colic, as tension increases on the broad ligament and the uterine serosa stretches. These colic signs often go unobserved because normal parturition has preceded the event and mares are assumed to be in satisfactory condition. The mare is usually discovered to be weak, extremely anemic or dead.

Hemorrhage into the broad ligament can be diagnosed by rectal palpation of the uterus and ipsilateral broad ligament and ovary. Palpation causes extreme discomfort and enlargement of the uterus suggests the extent of hemorrhage.

Conservative treatment appears to be as successful as heroic attempts. Confinement of the mare to a dark, quiet stall and minimizing any disturbances are probably as successful as other methods of management. Little success is achieved with blood transfusions, fluid therapy or plasma replacement.

Another type of postpartum hemorrhage is rupture of large, intra-abdominal blood vessels

during parturition. These mares die quickly and the diagnosis is confirmed at necropsy.

Perineal and Rectovaginal Injuries

Primiparous mares are particularly susceptible to injury to the reproductive tract and associated structures during parturition. The prominence of the vaginovestibular sphincter and remnants of the hymen in mares foaling for the first time is responsible for most of these injuries. The feet of the foal may encounter this tissue barrier and not proceed through the birth canal. Abdominal expulsive efforts at this point cause laceration of the dorsal vagina and other tissue. Various rectovaginal and perineal injuries are discussed in the surgical section.

Alert observation by attendants at foaling may prevent serious vaginal and perineal injuries. If entrapment of the forefeet of the foal is suspected, immediate examination and correction of the problem may result in normal delivery. One or both of the forefeet and/or the head may be presented through the anus when rectovaginal perforation has occurred. Prompt repulsion of the foal craniad into the uterus and redirection of the limbs may result in normal delivery and prevent third-degree laceration.

The temptation to repair perineal and rectovaginal lacerations immediately after they occur should be resisted. Universal failure of surgical apposition of these tissues in the fresh state is due to the ensuing edema and inflammation. A 3- to 6-week interval should pass before repair is attempted. The prognosis for future fertility in mares that have been treated successfully is good. Most mares rid themselves of the fecal contamination of the uterus spontaneously after the defect is repaired.

Large-Bowel Trauma

The large bowel may be traumatized if parturition occurs when the large bowel is full of ingesta or distended with gas. Expulsive efforts are severe enough to rupture portions of the large bowel that become entrapped in the birth canal. The cecum is the most likely organ to be ruptured, apparently due to intra-abdominal pressure. The large colon and possibly even the rectum may be damaged in a variety of degrees during the foaling process.

Rupture of the cecum or large colon results in signs of severe peritonitis rather quickly. Abdominocentesis is an important diagnostic tool in such cases; the mare should be destroyed if feces is discovered in the peritoneal cavity. Less dramatic are those cases in which the large bowel is damaged but not ruptured. The ensuing necrosis may result in slowly developing peritonitis due to diffusion of organisms through the damaged gut wall.

Although treatment of rupture or severe trauma to the large bowel is virtually impossible, some preventive measures prior to foaling are logical. Although most mares voluntarily restrict their roughage intake within a few days of parturition, some do not. This is particularly true when mares are managed in groups that compete for feed. It is a good management practice to reduce the quantity of hay fed to all mares in the last days prior to parturition.

Cervical Laceration

The cervix may be lacerated during normal parturition or subsequent to dystocia. Evaluation of these lacerations is difficult in the widely dilated cervix even though cervical damage may be suspected during assistance in delivery. All mares suspected of sustaining cervical lacerations should be examined at a suitable interval postpartum.

Severe lacerations of the cervix are difficult to repair. Descriptions of surgical procedures on the cervix should be consulted but a generally unfavorable prognosis for future fertility should be rendered for all mares sustaining major cervical damage.

Miscellaneous Postpartum Complications

Eversion or prolapse of the urinary bladder is an occasional sequela to parturition.[158] The extreme relaxation of tissues in the pelvic area predisposes the mare to eversion of the bladder during or immediately after parturition. If diagnosed early, urinary bladder eversion can be managed effectively by cleansing and replacing the organ following epidural anesthesia. Prolonged exposure of the prolapsed bladder may result in irreversible damage.

A rare postpartum metabolic disorder may be recognized in mares on a marginal plane of nutrition. Low dietary intake of Ca, as may be present under range conditions, may predispose mares to hypocalcemia and result in eclampsia syndrome several weeks postpartum. Eclampsia may be confused with tetanus due to the spastic muscular contractions and trembling involved. The most significant distinguishing feature is the lack of prolapse of the nictitating membrane in eclampsia. Response to IV Ca therapy is satisfactory and correction of dietary deficiencies is indicated.

Reproductive Management of Mares

The prime objective in managing an equine breeding program is delivery of adequate numbers of viable spermatozoa into the genital tracts of healthy mares at an appropriate time to ensure the maximum opportunity for fertilization. The major obstacles to attaining this objective are: failure to properly coordinate the physiologic breeding season of horses with the breeding calendar imposed by various breed registries; failure to properly detect estrus and determine the optimum time for breeding; failure to identify and correct reproductive abnormalities of mares; and failure to deliver viable semen.

These obstacles must be properly addressed to achieve a program yielding maximum fertility. Further management is then required to maximize the foaling rate and minimize neonatal loss. The following section summarizes problems encountered in reproductive management of mares.

Management of Foaling Mares

Following the prolonged suppression of pituitary and ovarian function imposed by gestation, the mare responds with a dramatic fertile cyclic state after foaling. The first postpartum estrus ("foal heat") occurs very quickly and, coupled with rapid uterine involution, the mare is able to conceive within a very few days after parturition. Following foal heat, most mares continue to cycle at a normal interval. The first few postpartum cycles are among the most predictable events in the mare's reproductive life.

Although foal heat is an entirely physiologic event, much controversy exists over the value of breeding mares at this time. There is concern over higher incidences of embryonic death and abortion following conception at this first estrus. Additional belief that breeding mares during foal heat may influence subsequent cycles adds to the confusion. A comprehensive study involving a large number of foaling mares over a 3-year period has been published.[159] The following data are from this study. In 470 foaling mares, 97% had ovulated by 20 days postpartum and 43% had ovulated by day 9. The mean interval from foaling to first ovulation was 10.2 days, with a standard deviation of ± 2.4 days. The effect of season on foaling mares was evident in the interval to the first ovulation. Mares foaling in January and February showed a 33% incidence of ovulation by day 10; 55% of mares foaling in March had ovulated by then, and mares foaling in April and May had 65% and 83% ovulation rates, respectively, by the tenth day. The seasonal effect on foaling mares has been largely overlooked. Use of artificial lighting for pregnant mares during the winter may be worth considering.

The same study indicated that conception rate, foaling rate and pregnancy loss were not significantly different among mares bred at the first estrus and those bred at subsequent heats. There were variations among years and among farms, but the cumulative totals were remarkably similar.

A significant advantage was shown in the interval from foaling to conception in mares bred during foal heat over those not bred until subsequent cycles. A difference of 18 days was realized by the former group. The information from this study indicates an advantage to breeding during foal heat, particularly in mares that foal late.

Estrus detection in mares suckling foals presents potential problems. The protective nature of some mares may be such that they may not exhibit estral behavior when approached by a teaser stallion. This is a problem in mares with their first foal at foot. All the resources of the teasing personnel are needed to note behavioral changes in such mares. Restraint in various forms may be of value. The presence or absence of the foal and its location during teasing are variables to consider.

Failure to detect estrus by the expected time is an indication for routine examinations of the reproductive tract to monitor changes. Mares reluctant to exhibit estrus are a problem in detection of a return to estrus after breeding. Knowledge of the time of ovulation is helpful in predicting the time for return to estrus.

A complete genital examination is indicated for all foaling mares prior to the first postpartum breeding. The most appropriate time for such an examination is during the first day on which signs of estrus are strong. Assessment of uterine involution by size is probably the least critical portion of the examination. Cervical or vaginal damage sustained during delivery is best detected by vaginoscopy and manual palpation of the vaginal area. Suspicious exudates of uterine origin may be noted at this time.

Any dystocia, retained placenta, persistent purulent exudate, or physical damage to the reproductive tract is a valid reason for not breeding during foal heat. Therapeutic or corrective measures should be initiated as soon as possible to improve the chances of conception on the next heat.

Uterine or vaginal discharges must be carefully evaluated during the early postpartum period. Blood may be retained in the uterus until the first estrus and is seen as a mucoid, chocolate-brown discharge. Uterine treatment is seldom indicated by the presence of this material. Uterine cultures may be used to confirm the presence of pathogens when purulent exudate is noted in the presence of inflammation. However, cultures taken during foal heat should be viewed with discretion since some normal residue of organisms is invariably evident.

Breeding procedures for foaling mares should be aimed at minimal trauma and contamination, particularly during foal heat. The uterus is particularly sensitive to undue stress at that time. Every effort should be made to minimize the number of natural services. Artificial insemination, when permitted, is a definite aid to increasing conception rates in these mares.

Management of Maiden Mares

As a group, maiden mares should have the highest degree of potential fertility. Assuming normal reproductive development, they have the best resistance to bacterial contamination and tolerate marginal breaches of management better than barren mares. Problems with maidens relate to estrus detection, breeding and adjustment to life as a broodmare.

Often young mares are nervous and unfamiliar with breeding routines, especially teasing and natural service. Psychic factors may prevent normally cycling maidens from exhibiting estrus, and great patience is required to determine the proper time for breeding. Forcibly restraining mares for teasing and breeding may establish habits that adversely influence their entire reproductive life. A determined, firm but low-key approach to handling such mares is the method of choice. Tranquilization is sometimes indicated to adapt maidens to a routine, particularly for a first natural service. However, use of tranquilizers should not be a substitute for schooling.

Fillies with extensive athletic careers or show-circuit backgrounds may be difficult to convert to broodmares. Medication administered during athletic training has been said to be a deterrent to future fertility. While there is no doubt that prolonged use of glucocorticoids, anabolic steroids or similar compounds may delay the onset of fertile cycles, there is a tendency for farm personnel to use prior medication as an excuse for reproductive failure of any kind.

After long periods of confinement, rigidly scheduled training or other established routines, many maiden mares deteriorate in condition upon retirement to the breeding farm. Special handling, feeding and close observation alleviate this problem somewhat. Turning a nervous filly out into a large pasture with mature barren mares almost guarantees the filly will receive physical punishment, psychic abuse and inadequate nourishment.

A complete reproductive examination on all maiden mares prior to breeding is advisable. Attention should be directed to the size and normalcy of the ovaries and uterus during rectal palpation. The pelvic canal should be explored for size and any impingement by old traumatic episodes. The vaginal examination should, in addition to routine inspection, be used to evaluate remnants of the hymen that might cause problems in breeding. Most persistent hymens are simply treated by stretching or incision. Totally imperforate hymens are rare. Such hymens can trap mucus and uterine secretions in the cranial vagina.

Uterine cultures of maiden mares may be required before breeding on some farms. The chance of endometritis occurring in a maiden mare is remote. In the absence of clinical signs of inflammation, a positive culture should be viewed skeptically.

Occasionally young mares have pneumovagina and concurrent vaginitis, cervicitis and even a vulvar discharge. Such cases respond quickly to a Caslick's operation.

Breeding maiden mares by natural service presents a challenge even to experienced horsemen. The unpredictability of the mare poses a potential for injury to the stallion, mare and attendants. After suitable restraint is applied, it is wise to allow a teaser stallion to mount the mare a few times prior to breeding the mare with the proper stallion. A breeding roll, which limits intromission, is advisable when breeding small mares to large stallions.

Management of Barren Mares

The causes of infertility and their correction have been previously discussed. Reproductive management of barren mares represents the major challenge to the equine practitioner engaged in breeding work. Emphasis should be on careful assessment and reassessment of the mare to define the problem.

Management of mares with a history of endometritis should stress the need for as few breedings as possible. Artificial insemination or technics associated with minimal contamination should be used when possible.

Artificial lighting is an especially useful aid in managing barren mares. The more ovulatory cycles available during the breeding season, the greater the chance of returning the mare to production.

References

1. Caslick, EA. Cornell Vet 27 (1937) 178.
2. Greenhoff, GR and Kenney, RM. JAVMA 167 (1975) 449.
3. Pascoe, RR. J Repro Fert Suppl 27 (1979) 299.
4. Dimock, WW. Ky Agr Expt Sta Circular #61, December, 1947.
5. Roberts, SJ. Veterinary Obstetrics and Genital Diseases. 2nd ed. Author, Ithaca, NY, 1971.
6. Witherspoon, DM. Proc 23rd Ann Mtg Am Assoc Eq Pract, 1977. p 15.
7. Day, FT. Vet Rec 83 (1957) 1258.
8. Panel Discussion. Proc 24th Ann Mtg Am Assoc Eq Pract, 1978. p 190.
9. Simpson, DJS and Eaton-Evans, WE. Vet Rec 102 (1978) 19.
10. Stratton, LG et al. J Repro Fert Suppl 27 1979) 317.
11. Brandt, GW and Manning, JP. VM/SAC 66 (1969) 977.
12. Knudsen, O and Sollen, P. Nord Vet Med 13 (1961) 449.
13. Knudsen, O. Cornell Vet 54 (1964) 415.
14. Ressang, A. Proefschrift, Utrecht, Breukelen, 1954.
15. Tobler, EE. VM/SAC 61 (1966) 779.
16. Kenney, RM. Proc 23rd Ann Mtg Am Assoc Eq Pract, 1977. p 105.
17. Kenney, RM. JAVMA 172 (1978) 241.
18. Bergman, RV and Kenney, RM. Proc 21st Ann Mtg Am Assoc Eq Pract, 1975. p 355.
19. Kenney, RM. Proc Ann Mtg Soc Therio, 1978. p 14.
20. Asbury, AC, Gainesville, FL: Unpublished data, 1979.
21. Gadd, JD. Proc 21st Ann Mtg Am Assoc Eq Pract, 1975. p 362.
22. Wingfield-Digby, NJ. Eq Vet J 10 (1978) 167.
23. Mather, EC et al. J. Repro Fert Suppl 27 (1979) 293.
24. Van Niekerk, CH. J So Afr Vet Assoc 36 (1965) 53.
25. Stabenfeldt, GH et al. Eq Vet J 6 (1974) 158.
26. Solomon, WJ. Proc 17th Ann Mtg Am Assoc Eq Pract, 1971. p 73.
27. Jeffcott, LB and Whitwell, KE. J Comp Path 83 (1973) 91.
28. Allen, WR. Eq Vet J 2 (1970) 64.
29. Colles, CM et al. Eq Vet J 10 (1978) 32.
30. Buss, DD and Asbury, AC, Gainesville, FL: Unpublished data, 1979.
31. Cole, HH and Hart, GH. Am J Physiol 93 (1930) 57.
32. Day, FT and Rowlands, IW. J Endocrin 2 (1940) 255.
33. McCaughey, WJ et al. Eq Vet J 5 (1973) 94.
34. Cowie, AT. Joint Publication No. 13, Commonwealth Agr Bur, Weybridge, England, 1948.
35. Lyngset, O. Vet Rec 77 (1965) 218.
36. Anon. Proc 1st Int Symp Eq Repro, 1974. p 1.

37. Anon. Proc 2nd Int Symp Eq Repro, 1978. p 1.

38. Ginther, OJ: Reproductive Biology of the Mare. McNaughton & Gunn, Ann Arbor, 1979.

39. Belonje, PC and Van Niekerk, CH. J Repro Fert Suppl **23** (1975) 167.

40. Osborne, VE. Aust Vet J **42** (1966) 149.

41. Sharp, DC et al. J Repro Fert Suppl **27** (1979) 87.

42. Strauss, SS et al. J Repro Fert Suppl **27** (1979) 123.

43. Evans, MJ and Irvine, CHG. Biol Repro **15** (1976) 477.

44. Evans, MJ and Irvine, CHG. J Repro Fert Suppl **27** (1979) 113.

45. Garcia, MC and Ginther, OJ. Endocrin **98** (1976) 958.

46. Garcia, MC and Ginther, OJ. Am J Vet Res **36** (1975) 1581.

47. Hughes, JP et al. Proc 18th Ann Mtg Am Assoc Eq Pract, 1972. p 119.

48. Witherspoon, DM and Talbot, RB. JAVMA **159** (1970) 1452.

49. Hughes, JP et al. JAVMA **161** (1972) 1367.

50. Warszawsky, LF et al. Am J Vet Res **33** (1972) 19.

51. Allen, WR and Rowson, LEA. J Repro Fert **33** (1973) 529.

52. Ginther, OJ and First, NL. Am J Vet Res **32** (1971) 1687.

53. Douglas, RH and Ginther, OJ. Res Prostaglandins **2** (1972) 265.

54. Burkhardt, J. J Agric Sci **37** (1947) 64.

55. Loy, RG. Proc 14th Ann Mtg Am Assoc Eq Pract, 1968. p 159.

56. Kooistra, LH and Ginther, OJ. Am J Vet Res **35** (1975) 1413.

57. Belonje, CWA. J So Afr Vet Assoc **27** (1956) 53.

58. Rossdale, PD and Ricketts, SW: The Practice of Equine Stud Medicine. Baillere Tindall, London, 1974.

59. Hughes, JP and Stabenfeldt, GH. JAVMA **170** (1977) 733.

60. Noden, PA et al. Fed Proc Am Soc Exp Biol **32** (1973) 229.

61. Kooistra, LH and Ginther, OJ. Am J Vet Res **37** (1976) 35.

62. Jeffcott, LB and Rossdale, PD. Eq Vet J **9** (1977) 208.

63. Loy, RG et al. J Repro Fert Suppl **27** (1979) 299.

64. Hughes, JP and Loy, RG. Proc 24th Ann Mtg Am Assoc Eq Pract, 1978. p 173.

65. Kiefer, BL et al. J Reprod Fert Suppl **27** (1979) 237.

66. Neely, DP et al. Am J Vet Res **40** (1979) 665.

67. Pashen, RL and Allen, WR. Vet Rec **99** (1976) 362.

68. Neely, DP et al. J Repro Fert Suppl **27** (1979) 181.

69. David, JSE et al. Vet Rec **101** (1977) 189.

70. Loy, RG and Hughes, JP. Cornell Vet **56** (1966) 44.

71. Sullivan, JJ et al. JAVMA **162** (1973) 895.

72. Roser, JF et al. J Repro Fert Suppl **27** (1979) 173.

73. Hughes, JP et al. Cornell Vet **57** (1967) 53.

74. Millar, R. Aust Vet J **28** (1952) 127.

75. Peterson, FB et al. Proc 15th Ann Mtg Am Assoc Eq Pract, 1969. p 279.

76. Hughes, JP and Loy, RG. Proc 15th Ann Mtg Am Assoc Eq Pract, 1969. p 289.

77. Kenney, RM and Khaleel, SA. J Repro Fert Suppl **23** (1975) 357.

78. Asbury, AC and Halliwell, REW, Gainesville, FL: Unpublished data, 1980.

79. Shin, SJ et al. J Repro Fert Suppl **27** (1979) 307.

80. Dimock, WW and Edwards, PR. Bull 286, Ky Agr Exp Sta, 1928.

81. Hughes, JP et al. Cornell Vet **56** (1966) 53.

82. Conboy, HS. Proc 24th Ann Mtg Am Assoc Eq Pract, 1978. p 165.

83. Kendrick, JW. Report to Calif Milk Adv Bd, Davis, CA, 1978.

84. Threlfall, WR. Proc Ann Mtg Soc Therio, 1979. p 45.

85. Kenney, RM et al. Proc 21st Ann Mtg Am Assoc Eq Pract, 1975. p 327.

86. Crowhurst, RC. Vet Rec **100** (1977) 476.

87. Platt, H et al. Vet Rec **101** (1977) 20.

88. Powell, DG. Eq Vet J **10** (1978) 153.

89. Timoney, PJ et al. Eq Vet J **10** (1978) 148.

90. Swerczek, TW. J Repro Fert Suppl **27** (1979) 361.

91. Benson, JA et al. Vet Rec **102** (1978) 277.

92. Croxton-Smith, P et al. Vet Rec **103** (1978) 275.

93. Bryans, JT and Hendricks, JB. J Repro Fert Suppl **27** (1979) 343.

94. Knowles, RC et al. Mod Vet Pract **59** (1978) 819.

95. Pascoe, RR et al. Aust Vet J **44** (1968) 485.

96. Bryans, JT. Proc 14th Ann Mtg Am Assoc Eq Pract, 1968. p 119.

97. Girard, A et al. Can J Comp Med **32** (1968) 603.

98. Gibbs, EPJ and Morris, JM. Eq Vet J **4** (1972) 74.

99. Udall, DH: The Practice of Veterinary Medicine. 6th ed. Author, Ithaca, NY, 1954.

100. Hughes, JP et al. J Repro Fert Suppl **27** (1979) 321.

101. Betteridge, KJ et al. J Repro Fert Suppl **27** (1979) 387.

102. Van Niekirk, CH and Gerneke, WH. Onderstepoort J Vet Res **33** (1966) 195.

103. Van Niekirk, CH. J So Afr Vet Assoc **36** (1964) 61.

104. Hughes, JP et al. J Repro Fert Suppl **23** (1975) 385.

105. Chandley, AC et al. J Repro Fert Suppl **23** (1975) 377.

106. Trommershausen-Smith, A et al. J Repro Fert Suppl **27** (1979) 271.

107. Stabenfeldt, GH et al. J Repro Fert Suppl **27** (1979) 277.

108. Meagher, DM et al. Proc 23rd Ann Mtg Am Assoc Eq Pract, 1977. p 133.

109. Kenney, RM and Ganjam, VK. J Repro Fert Suppl **23** (1975) 335.

110. Bain, AM and Howey, WP. J Repro Fert Suppl **23** (1975) 541.

111. Samuels, CA et al. J Repro Fert Suppl **23** (1975) 575.

112. Ginther, OJ: Reproductive Biology of the Mare. McNaughton & Gunn, Ann Arbor, 1979.

113. Allen, WR et al. Anat Rec **177** (1973) 485.

114. Allen, WR and Moor, RM. J Repro Fert Suppl **20** (1972) 313.

115. Allen, WR. J Repro Fert Suppl **23** (1975) 405.

116. Clegg, MR *et al*. Endocrin **54** (1954) 448.

117. Cole, HH *et al*. Anat Rec **49** (1931) 199.

118. Holtan, DW *et al*. J Repro Fert Suppl **27** (1979) 457.

119. Squires, EL *et al*. Proc Am Soc Anim Sci, 1978.

120. Steven, DH and Samuel, CA. J Repro Fert Suppl **23** (1975) 579.

121. Evans, MJ and Irvine, CHG. J Repro Fert Suppl **23** (1975) 193.

122. Irvine, CHG and Evans, MJ. Proc Int Cong Anim Repro Art Insem, 1976. p 372.

123. Stewart, F and Allen, WR. J Repro Fert Suppl **27** (1979) 431.

124. Squires, EL and Ginther, OJ. J Anim Sci **40** (1975) 275.

125. Flood, PF *et al*. J Repro Fert Suppl **27** (1979) 413.

126. Holtan, DW *et al*. J Anim Sci **37** (1973) 315.

127. Pashen, RL and Allen, WR. J Repro Fert Suppl **27** (1979) 499.

128. Platt, H. J Comp Path **83** (1973) 199.

129. Dimock, WW and Edwards, PR. Cornell Vet **26** (1936) 231.

130. Dimock, WW. JAVMA **96** (1940) 665.

131. Doll, ER and Bryans, JT. JAVMA **142** (1963) 31.

132. Burrows, R and Goodridge, D. Proc 24th Ann Mtg Am Assoc Eq Pract, 1978. p 17.

133. Crawford, TB. Proc 24th Ann Mtg Am Assoc Eq Pract, 1978. p 49.

134. McCollum, DH. JAVMA **155** (1969) 318.

135. Little, RB *et al*. Vet Med **45** (1950) 104.

136. White, FH, Univ Florida: Personal communication, 1980.

137. Langford, EV. Vet Rec **94** (1974) 528.

138. Moorthy, ARS *et al*. Aust Vet J **52** (1976) 385.

139. Mahaffey, LW and Adam, NM. JAVMA **144** (1964) 24.

140. Pascoe, RR. Eq Vet J **11** (1979) 64.

141. Ganjam, VK *et al*. J Repro Fert Suppl **23** (1975) 177.

142. Hawkins, DL *et al*. J Repro Fert Suppl **27** (1979) 211.

143. Bowen, JM *et al*. Vet Rec **99** (1976) 495.

144. Wheat, JD and Meagher, DM. JAVMA **160** (1972) 881.

145. Vandeplassche, M *et al*. Vet Rec **99** (1976) 67.

146. Hintz, HF *et al*. J Eq Med Surg **3** (1979) 289.

147. Nathanielsz, PW *et al*. J Repro Fert Suppl **23** (1975) 625.

148. Drost, M. JAVMA **160** (1972) 321.

149. Jeffcott, LB and Rossdale, PD. J Repro Fert Suppl **27** (1979) 563.

150. Purvis, AD. Proc 18th Ann Mtg Am Assoc Eq Pract, 1972. p 113.

151. Hillman, RB. J Repro Fert Suppl **23** (1975) 641.

152. Rossdale, PD *et al*. Vet Rec **99** (1976) 26.

153. Jeffcott, LB and Rossdale, PD. Eq Vet J **9** (1977) 208.

154. Vandeplassche, M. Eq Vet J **12** (1980) 45.

155. Walton, A and Hammond, J. Proc Royal Soc **125** (1938) 311.

156. Sager, FC. JAVMA **115** (1949) 450.

157. Burns, SJ *et al*. Proc 23rd Ann Mtg Am Assoc Eq Pract, 1977. p 381.

158. Walker, DF and Vaughan, JT. Bovine and Equine Urogenital Surgery. Lea & Febiger, Philadelphia, 1980.

159. Loy, RG. Vet Clin No Am (Lg Anim) **2** (1980) 345.

FEMALE UROGENITAL SURGERY
by P.T. Colahan

Caslick's Procedure

The Caslick's operation prevents aspiration of irritants, air and fecal material into the genital tract by reducing the vulvar cleft.[1-5]

Technic: The procedure is performed by restraining and tranquilizing the mare in stocks or a doorway. The tail is wrapped and the rectum manually emptied to reduce defecation during the procedure. The vulva and perineum should be thoroughly scrubbed, but use of irritating antiseptics should be avoided on these delicate tissues. The labial margins are then infiltrated with local anesthetic (lidocaine or mepivacaine) using a 22-ga or smaller needle. The tissues should be distended sufficiently to stretch the skin along the labial margins. An 8-mm strip of mucosa and skin is then removed along the mucocutaneous junction with sharp scissors. Care should be taken to ensure that an uninterrupted raw surface is obtained from 1 cm ventral to the pelvic floor to and including the dorsal commissure. The raw edges of the right and left labia are then sutured together. Various suture patterns, including simple-continuous, interrupted and vertical mattress, have been used successfully.[2,4,5] All are effective if carefully placed no more than 8 mm apart. Size 2-0 nonabsorbable monofilament (nylon or polypropylene) is the preferred suture material.[2,4,5]

At the time of foaling and possibly at the time of breeding, the vulvar cleft must be reopened and resutured to prevent laceration of the vulva.[4-6] It is important, therefore, that no more than an 8- to 10-mm strip of mucosa and skin be removed from the stretched labial margin during the initial procedure so that, with repetition of the procedure, excessive scarring and loss of plasticity of the tissues do not occur.[2,4] Removal of a strip narrower than 8 mm may lead to gaps between the healed labia, especially at the dorsal commissure.[2]

An alternative to complete surgical opening of the vulvar cleft for breeding has been used.

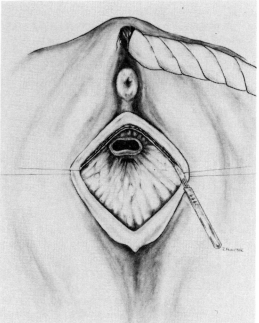

Fig 28. Incision along the mucocutaneous junction at the dorsal commissure.

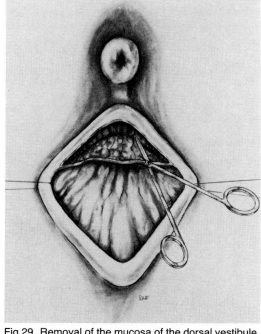

Fig 29. Removal of the mucosa of the dorsal vestibule.

The ventral aspects of the adhered labia can be protected by a single suture of umbilical tape placed high enough to allow intromission. This is commonly called a "breeding stitch."[4-6] In general it is not possible to adequately protect the vulva in this manner and still allow intromission by the stallion. The suture also poses some danger of trauma to the stallion's penis. The usefulness of the breeding stitch is therefore limited.

Perineal Reconstruction

Perineal body reconstruction restores the integrity of the vestibular sphincter.[5,7] The diameter of the vestibule is surgically reduced and the perineal body enlarged dorsoventrad and craniocaudad. The vulvar and vestibular sphincters can become incompetent due to repeated stretching during foalings or second-degree lacerations.[3,5,7] If sphincter function cannot be restored by the Caslick's procedure, surgical reconstruction of the perineal body is indicated.

Technic: As for any of the standing perineal surgical procedures, preparation of the mare for surgery must include restraint in stocks with an adequate rear gate or kickboard. Some degree of tranquilization is usually necessary.

Epidural anesthesia is preferred but local infiltration can also be used. The tail is wrapped so that all hair is covered and tied out of the way. The rectum is thoroughly evacuated manually and a tampon of rolled cotton or gauze sponges placed in the rectum to prevent expulsion of feces into the surgical field during the procedure. The perineum and vulva are thoroughly scrubbed. The tail, buttocks and stocks are then draped out of the surgical field.

Retraction is obtained with 2 stay sutures of umbilical tape in the vulva or with long-jaw Balfour retractors. An incision is made along the mucocutaneous junction of the labia and the dorsal commissure (Fig 28). A triangular section of mucosa is then dissected submucosally from the dorsum and dorsolateral aspects of the vestibule. The apex of the mucosal triangle is located at or near the vestibulovaginal junction and the base at the mucocutaneous junction of the labia. This triangular section is then removed (Figs 29, 30). Care must be used in the submucosal dissection not to enter the rectum. If the rectum is entered, the defect should be closed with sutures that invert the rectal mucosa into the rectum and the dissection continued. The incised edge of the mucosa of the right side of the vestibule is then sutured

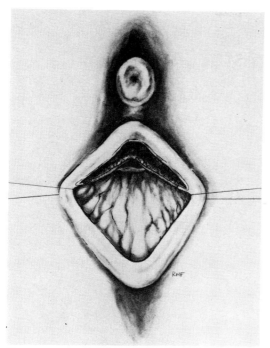

Fig 30. Surgical site after completed dissection.

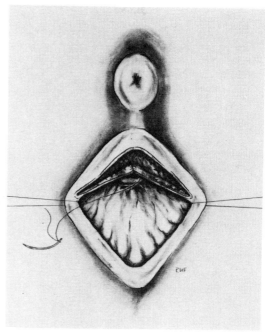

Fig 31. Apposing the mucosal edges with simple-continuous sutures.

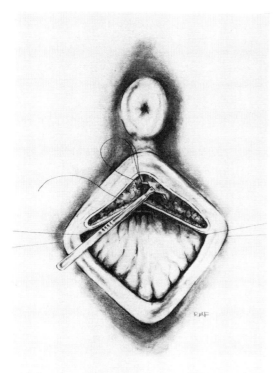

Fig 32. Closing the deep layers of the perineal body.

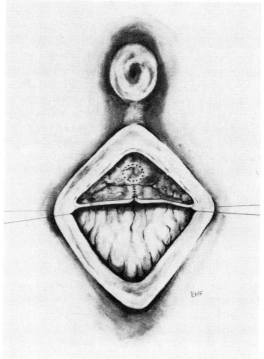

Fig 33. Alternative closure of the mucosal and deep layers.

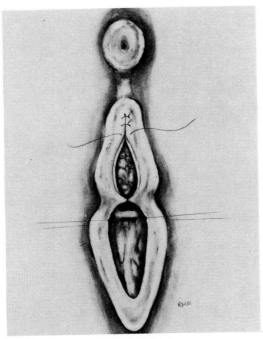

Fig 34. Closure of the perineal skin.

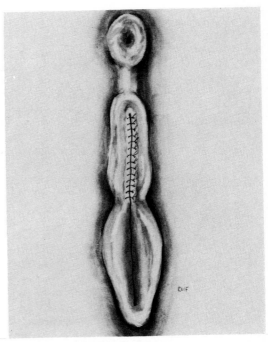

Fig 35. Completed reconstruction.

to the incised edge of the left side of the vestibular mucosa with a simple-continuous pattern of 0 polypropylene (Fig 31). The raw surfaces dorsal to this suture line are apposed with simple-interrupted "quilting" sutures of gut or polypropylene (Fig 32). Suturing must precede from deep layers to superficial layers, alternating first the continuous line in the mucosa, then the "quilting" sutures above (Fig 33). The skin of the perineum and vulva are closed as for Caslick's procedure (Figs 34, 35). Complete healing of the deep tissues takes 4-8 weeks and complete sexual rest is mandatory during that time.[5,7]

Urethral Extension

Urethral extension was developed to reduce irritation to the genital tract due to pooling of urine in the cranial vagina.[8] The procedure is designed to surgically create a mucosal tube from the urethra to the mucocutaneous junction so that urine is voided to the exterior rather than into the vestibule.

Technic: Following restraint and preparation as described for perineal body reconstruction, the bladder is catheterized with a 30-Fr Foley catheter to prevent urine flow during the procedure. Retraction is provided by Balfour retractors or umbilical tape stay sutures in the

vulva. The membranous transverse fold over the urethra is grasped with forceps and split into dorsal and ventral layers with a scalpel. This incision is then continued caudad along the ventrolateral aspect of the vestibule (Fig 36). The incision is stopped about 1 cm from the mucocutaneous junction of the labia, and the mucosa is undermined dorsad and ventrad to create 2 mucosal layers (Fig 37). Sufficient dissection is necessary to allow the edges of these layers to be readily pulled to the midline. The mucosal layers are then apposed right side to left side with 3 separate suture lines to create a mucosal tube that lengthens the urethra.

The ventral mucosal layers are apposed using a continuous horizontal or vertical mattress pattern of 2-0 polypropylene (Fig 38). The dorsal raw surfaces are apposed and the cut edge everted ventrad. This suture line must be carefully placed so that a complete seal is obtained. Urine leaking through this layer dissects between and through the dorsal layers and leads to fistula formation.

The ventral suture line is oversewn with a simple-continuous pattern of 2-0 polypropylene placed in the submucosal tissue between the dorsal and ventral layers (Fig 39). The dorsal shelves are then apposed using a continuous vertical or horizontal mattress pattern of

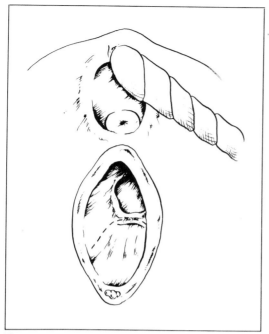

Fig 36. Site of excision.

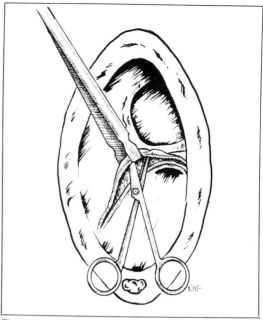

Fig 37. Creation of 2 mucosal flaps after the initial incision.

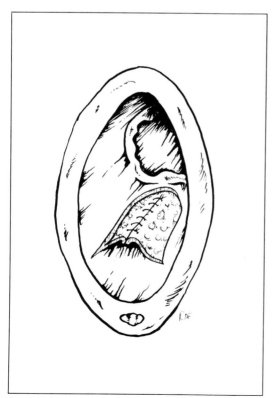

Fig 38. Ventral mucosal flaps apposed with inverting continuous vertical mattress sutures.

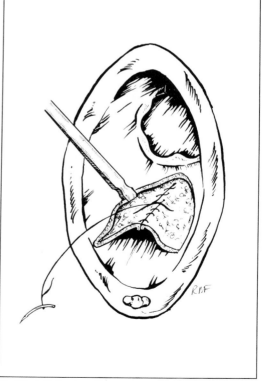

Fig 39. Initial suture line oversewn with simple-continuous sutures.

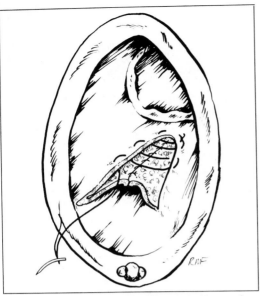

Fig 40. Dorsal mucosal flap apposed with everting continuous horizontal mattress sutures.

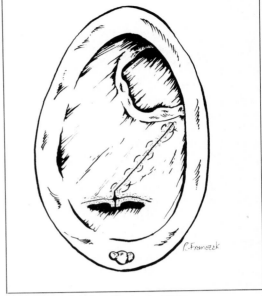

Fig 41. Completed urethral extension.

2-0 polypropylene (Fig 40). The mucosa of this layer is everted dorsad (Fig 41). The Foley catheter is removed after completion of surgery, and tetanus prophylaxis, antibiotic and anti-inflammatory therapy are administered.

Continued urine pooling due to fistula formation has been a complication and the success in repairing these fistulae has been variable. Mares with scarring of the vestibular walls or atrophic, thin, inelastic vestibular mucosa are unrewarding candidates for this procedure.

Another surgical procedure, urethroplasty, has been described to treat vesicovaginal reflux.[9] In this technic, the transverse membranous fold over the urethra is moved caudad 4-5 cm, in effect moving the urethra caudad. Success with this procedure has been variable.

Ovariectomy

The most common indication for ovariectomy in mares is removal of an ovarian tumor.[4,5,10-13] Bilateral ovariectomy is performed occasionally for elimination of estrus in mares not valued for breeding or to modify aggressive or nymphomaniac behavior.[5,12,14] Removal of both ovaries from normal mares has been performed via colpotomy in the standing mare under tranquilization and epidural anesthesia, using a chain ecraseur.[4,5,14] Alternatively, a flank approach in the standing position involves use of an ecraseur or emasculator.[4,5,11]

Unilateral ovariectomy for removal of tumors can also be performed under local anesthesia via either approach. However, the increased vascularity of the tumescent ovaries dictates thorough ligation of engorged vessels in the ovarian stump, which can be extremely difficult or impossible in the standing animal. Excessive traction on the ovary to obtain exposure of the ovarian vessels causes intense pain and may cause the mare to rear or fall.

General anesthesia facilitates delivery of the tumor from the abdomen and exposure of the vascular stump. The approach under anesthesia is dictated by the size of the tumor and the width of the paralumbar fossa.[4,5,11] Large tumors are more readily removed in dorsal recumbency via a ventral midline or paramedian approach caudal to the umbilicus.[4,5,11-13]

Vaginal Approach: A prerequisite for vaginal ovariectomy is a noninfected reproductive tract. Presurgical preparation should include fasting for 24 hours, tranquilization, epidural anesthesia, manual emptying of the rectum, preparation of the tail and perineum, and restraint in stocks. The vagina should be lavaged with a warm, mild antiseptic to stimulate aspiration of air into the vagina. The solution is evacuated after the vagina balloons.

Using aseptic technic, a 3-cm incision is made in the vaginal mucosa on the dorsolateral aspect (2 o'clock) of the vaginal fornix with a scalpel or hard-back knife. The vaginal wall is then penetrated with straight Mayo or other blunt scissors. This must be done quickly and forcibly so the peritoneum is penetrated and does not separate from the vaginal wall. Incision at this location avoids the rectum and median fold of the fornix dorsad, the urogenital artery at the 3 o'clock position, the urethra and bladder ventrad, and the pelvic flexure on the left lateral aspect. Penetrating any of these structures would cause serious, if not fatal, consequences. This incision is then bluntly enlarged with the fingers sufficiently to allow partial introduction of the cupped hand. Manual enlargement allows entry of the hand into the peritoneal cavity.

Local anesthesia of the ovarian pedicle helps prevent kicking or falling during ecrasement. This is accomplished by soaking a gauze sponge, to which a yard of umbilical tape is attached, in lidocaine or mepivacaine and holding the sponge on the pedicle for a minute. Following anesthesia of the pedicle, the chain ecraseur is introduced into the abdomen and the loop placed carefully around the overian pedicle. Extreme care must be taken not to include any segments of small intestine, mesentery or small colon within the loop. The loop is then tightened, checked for inclusion of bowel or mesentery, and the pedicle swiftly crushed and the ovary removed. The procedure is then repeated on the contralateral ovary. Finally, the vagina is manually cleaned of blood.

The mare is given antibiotics before, during and after surgery. Tetanus prophylaxis is also given. Close observation for 8-12 hours is essential to detect colic or signs of intra-abdominal hemorrhage, such as pulse elevation or weakness. The mare should be cross-tied for 48 hours to prevent recumbency and eventration through the vaginal incision. Exercise should be limited to hand-walking. After 10-14 days, a vaginal examination should be performed to inspect the vaginal incision.

Ventral or Standing Flank Approaches: The standing flank ovariectomy is performed through a grid incision in the paralumbar fossa. Local anesthesia of the pedicle and use of a chain ecraseur are the safest methods. Emasculators have been used, but the risk of damaging bowel or mesentery is greater than with the ecraseur due to the open jaws of the emasculator.

Because of the greatly increased blood supply and large size of ovarian tumors, removal is usually performed under general anesthesia via a flank or ventral approach.[4,5,11-13] The choice depends on the size of the ovary, age and physical condition of the mare, space available in the flank, and the surgeon's preference of positioning. A high incidence of postanesthetic complications, including paralysis, myositis and wound dehiscence, has been attributed to a decrease in arterial pressure when tension is placed on the ovarian pedicle, but this has not been proven[11,12] In general, careful consideration should be given to removal of a tumor 10-12 cm in diameter or larger through a flank incision.

The flank, ventral paramedian or midline incision is made routinely. Once the abdomen is opened, delivery of a large tumor can be facilitated by large stay sutures placed in the tumor or by needle aspiration of cystic tumors. The vessels of the pedicle must be carefully ligated after delivery of the tumor. Because the vasculature is enlarged in tumescent ovaries, difficulty is frequently encountered in dissecting the vessels, particularly the large veins from the surrounding tissue of the pedicle. The vessel walls tear easily, resulting in considerable hemorrhage. Double transfixation ligation of segments of the pedicle with #2 gut provides the best hemostasis. These sutures should be overlapped so that no vessels escape ligation. As portions of the pedicle are ligated, clamps can be placed on the ovarian side of the pedicle and the pedicle severed. This provides added exposure to the pedicle. After the ovary is removed, the stump is carefully evaluated for hemorrhage and the cut edges oversewn to prevent formation of adhesions. When hemostasis is absolute, the abdomen is closed routinely.

Cesarean Section

The general indications for cesarean section include relief of dystocia and delivery of a live foal, relief of dystocia when the risks of fetotomy are greater than surgery, and facilitation of correction of an immutable uterine torsion. These conditions arise when a live foal cannot, with assistance, be rapidly and atraumatically delivered. In the case of a dead foal, cesarean section is indicated when delivery requires more than 2 fetotomy incisions.[5,15,16]

The most common types of dystocia that necessitate cesarean section are transverse presentation due most commonly to bicornual gestation, oversized fetus, fetal malposition with accompanying uterine injury, fetal malposition with uterine involution or fetal emphysema, deformed or narrow pelvis in dam, and severe illness of the mare at term.[5,15,16]

When these or other indications for cesarean section are present, rapid initiation of surgery is essential. Delay prior to cesarean delivery endangers the life of the foal.[16] Also, prolonged or traumatic attempts to reposition the foal risk damage to the genital tract and endanger the life and fertility of the mare, as well as the life of the foal.[15] When the foal is dead, removal by fetotomy should be limited to 2 or less incisions.[15] A fetotomy requiring multiple incisions, even by a practiced individual, results in extensive damage to the genital tract and, in particular, the cervix.[15] Fertility is greatly reduced post-fetotomy due to cervical adhesions or cervical patency.[15]

The development of inhalation anesthesia and postoperative supportive therapy has greatly increased the survival rates of mares subjected to cesarean section.[5] This has made surgical intervention in equine dystocia appropriate in many cases in which fetotomy had formerly been the only treatment available. Selection of an anesthetic regimen depends on the status of the foal. If the foal is dead or its survival is not a consideration, the selection should be based solely on the condition of the mare, availability of agents, and preference of the anesthetist.[5,15-17] Depression of the foal's cardiovascular, nervous and, most importantly, respiratory function by tranquilizers or large doses of anesthetics should be avoided. A protocol using guaiafenesin induction, endotracheal intubation and maintenance on low levels of halothane is effective and reasonably safe.[5,15,16] Infiltration of local anesthetic at the surgical site helps control pain so that halothane levels can be reduced. Positive-pressure ventilation is invaluable in maintaining blood O_2 levels and preventing an increase in blood CO_2 levels.

The length of the period between induction and delivery of the foal is critical. Although they do so at various rates, all anesthetics commonly used in horses cross the placental barrier. Reducing the exposure time of the foal reduces their effect on the foal. Also, anesthesia, particularly anesthesia in dorsal recumbency, depresses the cardiovascular system of the mare. This reduces the blood supply to the uterus and foal, producing hypoxemia and acidosis. Shortening the time prior to delivery also reduces these effects.

Technic: The surgical approaches for cesarean section are the low flank (Marcenac), paracostal and ventral midline (see Laparotomy in Chapter 13).[5,16] The low flank approach offers the best exposure to the uterus and is done in lateral recumbency. The mare is placed in right lateral recumbency, with the rear limbs slightly extended caudad. The skin is incised starting at the mid-costal arch and extending caudoventrad to the medial aspect of the fold of the flank. The deep abdominal fascia lies superficially to the external abdominal oblique muscle and the fibers lie perpendicularly to the incision. The external abdominal oblique muscle and aponeuroses, which parallel the skin incision, are incised. The internal oblique aponeurosis runs perpendicularly to the incision and is separated bluntly in the direction of its fibers. The fibers of the transverse abdominal muscle run obliquely to the incision and also must be separated. The peritoneum is then located through retroperitoneal fat and incised to open the abdominal cavity.[5,16]

The paracostal incision parallels the costal arch 10 cm caudad. It does not provide as extensive exposure of the caudal abdomen as the Marcenac technic.[5]

The most popular approach for cesarean section in North America is the ventral midline, with the mare in dorsal recumbency.[5] The incision is begun just cranial to the mammary gland and extended craniad as far as necessary. The incision is carried through, in succession, the skin, superficial abdominal fascia, deep abdominal fascia, united tendons of the external and internal abdominal oblique aponeurosis, fascia transversalis and peritoneum. This approach offers excellent exposure, with minimal hemorrhage.

Regardless of the approach used, after the abdomen is opened the horn of the uterus containing the limbs is delivered through the incision. The uterus is incised over the greater curvature, avoiding the major vessels of the uterus. This incision should be large to avoid tearing the uterus when the foal is delivered. The fetus is grasped by the limbs and delivered. Care must be taken to avoid spillage of uterine contents into the abdomen. If the foal is alive, a pause of several minutes allows for return of blood from the placenta to the foal. The umbilical cord can then be ligated and cut. The placenta is delivered if it readily separates from the uterus. Otherwise it is freed from the incision site and the edges of the uterine incision sutured with gut in a continuous interlocking pattern. This suture line compresses the vessels in the uterine wall and prevents hemorrhage.[5,15,16] The uterus is then closed with 2 layers of gut in a continuous inverting suture line. Care should be taken not to include the undelivered placenta in any suture line. The uterus and abdomen are then cleaned of blood, lavaged and replaced in the abdomen. The abdomen is then closed routinely.

Systemic antibiotics should be given before, during and after surgery. Tetanus prophylaxis should also be given. Fluids or plasma should be administered as needed. Administration of 50 IU oxytocin in 1 L sterile saline via IV drip over 1 hour to treat a retained placenta is advisable.[5,16] Light daily exercise and systemic treatment for laminitis should also be undertaken.[5] Rectal palpation of the uterus at 3 and 5 days helps prevent formation of adhesions.[15]

The results of cesarean sections indicate an overall survival rate of 81% for the mare and 30% for the foal.[15,16] For the mare this varies from 61-100%, depending on the cause of the dystocia. Survival rates for the foal greatly increase with early initiation of surgery and appropriate anesthesia.[15,16]

The predominant cause of death of mares subjected to cesarean section is uterine hemorrhage, which underscores the importance of the coaptive suture in the incised uterine margins. Other fatal complications include incisional herniation, peritonitis, laminitis, shock and fractures incurred during recovery.[16] The incidence of retained placenta is 80%.[16] Vigorous attempts at removal of the placenta intraoperatively can result in extensive uterine damage. It is vital that the placenta not be included in any of the uterine suture lines so that when separation occurs it can be expelled.

The conception rate for mares subjected to cesarean section is only about 50%. Of those that conceive, about 25% abort.[16] These decreases in conception and foaling rates have been ascribed to uterine adhesions, scarring in the uterine wall, and endometrial destruction.[16] Comparisons with fertility rates after fetotomy indicate lower fertility after fetotomy (38% overall) as well.[16] Although the survival and fertility rates are poor in cases of immutable dystocia considered for cesarean section, there is no viable alternative.

Uterine Torsion

Torsion of the uterus causes 5-10% of all serious dystocias in mares.[15] Reports vary concerning the prevalence of the direction of the rotation (clockwise vs counterclockwise) and the extent of the rotation (180-360° or more).[17,18] Most cases occur near the end of pregnancy (last month), but can occur anytime in the last 4 months of pregnancy.[17,18] Rectal examination

is usually diagnostic and reveals the broad ligaments pulled taut over and under the uterus, torsion of uterine body or vagina, or dorsopubic position of the fetus.[5] Surgical correction is indicated upon diagnosis. Attempts at correction by rolling have an increased risk of rupture of the uterus.[5,17]

Surgical correction is undertaken through a flank incision in the standing position. The selection of side depends upon direction of rotation. It is considered safer to reduce the torsion by elevation from beneath and repulsion of the fetus rather than by traction applied by grasping the fetus through the uterine wall. Pulling on the uterus and fetus incurs a greater risk of uterine rupture.[5]

The survival rates in a series of 42 cases of uterine torsion were 61% for mares and 31% for foals. Certainly the prognosis can be improved with early diagnosis and immediate surgical correction. Common causes of the mare's death are uterine rupture and vascular compromise of the uterus, including irreversible thrombosis, hematoma and severe venous congestion. Mares with rupture of the uterus and escape of the fetus into the peritoneal cavity have survived with proper surgical and supportive care.[18]

Rectovaginal Injuries

Laceration of the vagina usually occurs when the foal is delivered with a forelimb over its head or neck, causing trauma to the vestibule and/or perineum during delivery. Damage to the vestibule can also occur because of improper assistance at delivery or, rarely, due to delivery of an exceptionally large fetus. The injuries suffered are rectovestibular or perineal lacerations and rectovestibular fistulas.

If the foal's foot penetrates the dorsal vestibular wall and the ventral rectal wall but is replaced by an assistant or the foot naturally falls back into the vestibule during relaxation of the abdominal press, a rectovaginal or rectovestibular fistula results. A perineal laceration results if the foal's foot traumatizes the mucosa and the perineum during its passage.

Perineal Lacerations: Perineal lacerations are classified according to the severity of damage. First-degree lacerations involve only the mucosa and dermis of the dorsal commissure of the vulva.[4,5] These injuries are readily repaired by a simple Caslick's procedure.[5]

Second-degree lacerations involve the constrictor vulvae and other musculature of the perineal body.[19] Healing in most cases of second-degree laceration does not result in re-union of these muscles and effective return of the constrictor function of the vulva. Consequently, air and feces can be aspirated into the vulva and vagina, resulting in chronic irritation, inflammation and infertility. A Caslick's procedure to reduce the vulval orifice does not, in many cases, prevent the contamination completely since it does not rebuild the sunken perineum. Surgical reconstruction of the perineal body as previously described is necessary. It has been proposed that second-degree lacerations are of greater economic significance than third-degree lacerations because they insidiously reduce fertility.[5]

Third-degree perineal lacerations involve the wall of the rectum and vagina, musculature of the perineal body, perineal septum and anal sphincter.[19] Third-degree injuries are most common in primiparous mares. The foal's extended hoof catches on the low angular fold of the hymen at the vaginal vestibular junction. As the foal is delivered, the hoof penetrates deeper into the tissue of the dorsum of the vestibule and lacerates it. The prominence of the hymen in primiparous mares increases the chance of the hoof initially catching on it. [5]

Several methods for repair of third-degree lacerations have been published.[2-4,20-27] Any of these procedures can be used successfully to repair rectovaginal lacerations if a few basic principles are rigidly followed. Strong suture material, which maintains its strength for a minimum of 10-14 days in tissue, must be used. Tension on the suture line must be minimized by adequate dissection of the tissues to allow for apposition without tension. Maximum apposition of tissues involved allows for a thicker, stronger shelf between the rectum and vestibule after healing. It also ensures a seal between the rectum and vestibule to prevent fecal contamination and fistula formation. The stool must be reduced in volume and maintained in a soft consistency to facilitate passage by the surgical site. If this is not accomplished, postoperative pain leads to rectal impaction and dehiscence of the suture line. Methods to accomplish this include feeding lush green grass pasture, pelleted rations, danthron, laxatives, including mineral oil and magnesium sulfate in the feed or by stomach tube, and wet bran mashes.[2,5,20,21,23,25-28] Even prolonged fasting has been recommended to reduce passage of feces. Reservations have been expressed concerning the last method since prolonged fasts predispose animals to enteritis and diarrhea.[5] In general, a 24-hour fast reduces stool passage during the operative and immediate postoperative period. Surgery should not be attempted until the stool is of proper consistency.

The surgical procedure is most easily performed with the mare standing in stocks. It has been performed in dorsal recumbency under general anesthesia, but the abdominal viscera push caudad into the pelvic canal and make exposure difficult. Also, tilting the head ventrad to allow for surgical exposure places the weight of the viscera on the diaphragm and compromises ventilation. The procedure is easily performed in the standing position with tranquilization and epidural anesthesia; the complications of general anesthesia are of sufficient seriousness that it is indicated only in intractable mares. Tranquilization is necessary in most cases to relieve anxiety and decrease the mare's movement during surgery. Acepromazine is usually used and, if necessary, sedation with chloral hydrate or a chloral hydrate-magnesium sulfate combination also can be used.[5] Xylazine and morphine can be used in combination, but xylazine has a diuretic effect and can cause micturition during the procedure.[5,29]

The tail is wrapped after tranquilization and restraint of the animal in stocks. The epidural site is surgically prepared and epidural anesthesia administered. The tail is tied out of the way of the surgical field and the rectum is manually evacuated. The perineum is thoroughly scrubbed and the vestibule and rectum swabbed with a mild antiseptic solution. Any excessive fluid remaining in the rectum or vagina after this swabbing should be sponged out.

Balfour retractors with 3½- or 4½-inch jaws provide good retraction of both superficial labial and deeper vestibular and rectal tissues. However, they tend to slip out of position and must be held in place by sutures placed in the skin over the tuber ischii, or by an assistant. Alternatively, stay sutures of large-diameter, nonabsorbable material can be placed in the labial and perineal tissue. These sutures may be held by an assistant or anchored to the skin over the tuber ischii. Stay sutures do not slip but occasionally do not provide adequate retraction of deeper vestibular or rectal tissue. Manual retraction of these by an assistant may be required.

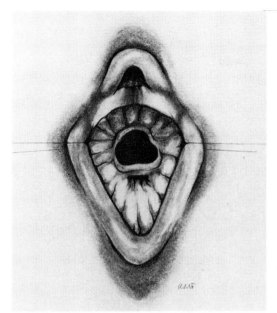

Fig 42. Third-degree perineal laceration.

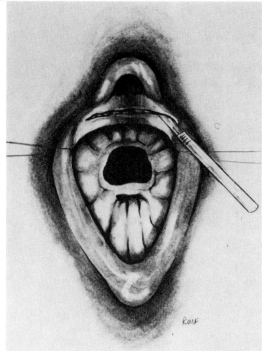

Fig 43. Splitting the septum between the vestibule and the rectum.

The first phase of repair of third-degree lacerations is reconstruction of the rectovestibular septum. The second stage is reconstruction of the perineal body and perineum. Although many methods of repair have been described, the variations generally involve timing of the phases of the surgery or the suture material or pattern used. The 6-bite pattern of large nonabsorbable sutures knotted in the vagina, the 4-bite pattern of large nonabsorbable sutures knotted in the rectum, and the multiple suture line patterns of absorbable or nonabsorbable material will be described here.[2,5,20,21,27]

In phase one, the shelf remaining craniad between the vestibule and rectum is split in a frontal plane (Figs 42, 43). Using sharp and blunt dissection, the shelf is separated craniad for 1-2 inches (Fig 44). This dissection is then carried caudad to the cutaneous perineum along the junction of the rectal and vaginal mucosa. This dissection of the lateral junctions between the remaining rectal and vaginal tissue must create 2 flaps of tissue that can be brought together and sutured without tension.

If the suture pattern to be used is a 6-bite pattern knotted on the vaginal side, dissection should create a thicker rectal flap than vaginal flap. If the suture pattern is to be a 4-bite suture pattern knotted on the rectal side, dissection should create a more substantial vaginal flap. If a multilayer suture pattern is to be

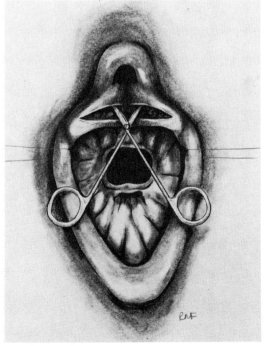

Fig 44. Dissecting to create flaps to reconstruct the septum between the vestibule and the rectum.

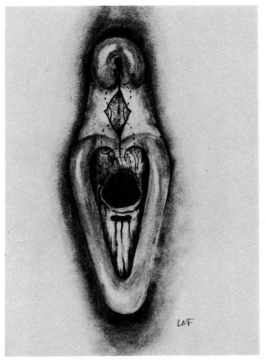

Fig 45. Placement of the 6-bite suture pattern knotted in the vestibule.

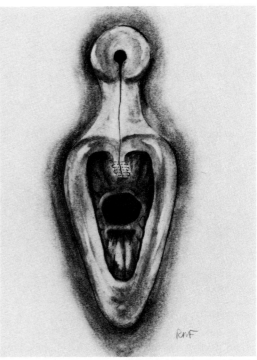

Fig 46. Placement of continuous horizontal mattress sutures in the vaginal mucosa prior to placement of the 4-bite suture.

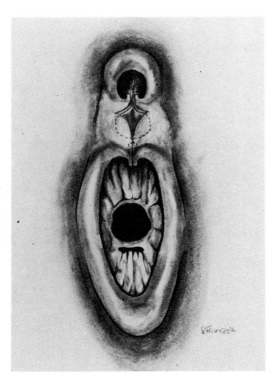

Fig 47. Placement of the 4-bite suture pattern knotted in the rectum.

used, dissection should create flaps of sufficient thickness on both the vaginal and rectal sides to allow for placement of deep bites in the 2 submucosal lines. In all patterns the submucosal and perivaginal tissues provide support.

Hemorrhage is usually not extensive, particularly if blunt dissection is used. However, persistent bleeders should be ligated. Continued bleeding postoperatively can lead to hematoma formation and failure of the reconstruction.

Heavy, noncapillary, nonabsorbable synthetic suture material and a heavy Martin's uterine half-circle cutting needle are used in the 6-bite vertical suture pattern for repair of phase one. The suture is passed through the left vaginal flap 3 cm from the edge, emerging in the dissected plane. A deep bite is taken in the left rectal flap starting 3 cm from the edge. The needle should not penetrate the rectal mucosa and should emerge from the submucosa at the edge of the flap. A deep bite is taken in the right rectal flap, entering at the edge and emerging from the submucosa 3 cm from the edge in the dissected plane. This again should not penetrate the rectal mucosa. The suture is passed through the right vaginal flap 3 cm

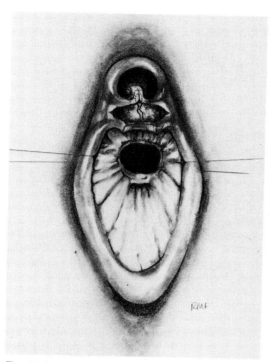

Fig 48. Placement of inverting suture in the rectal submucosa.

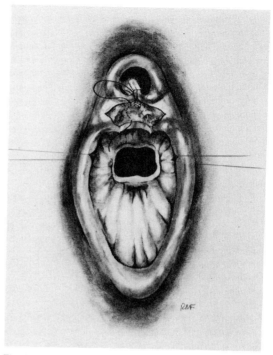

Fig 49. Placement of heavy reinforcing suture in the perivaginal-perirectal tissue.

from the edge. A shallow bite is taken 0.5 cm from the edge, passing the suture from the mucosal surface of the flap back to the bisected surface. The suture is passed through the left vaginal flap from the cut surface to the mucosal surface 0.5 cm from the cut edge, and is then pulled tight and knotted in the vagina so the rectal edges are everted. No suture should be palpable on the rectal surface. Sutures are placed in this manner 1.5 cm apart out to the musculature of the perineal body (Fig 45). The ends are left 10 cm long to facilitate removal.[5]

In the 4-bite knot-in-the-rectum method, suturing is begun with a continuous horizontal mattress pattern of #1 gut in the edge of the vaginal mucosa for 4-5 cm (Fig 46). A purse-string suture of #3 gut is placed in the space created by splitting the intact cranial shelf between the rectum and vagina. The flap is apposed and the pocket that tends to form at the beginning of the suture line is obliterated with 2-3 of these sutures placed 1-2 cm apart. If this pocket is not obliterated, feces accumulate at this point and can lead to fistula formation. When the caudal margin of the split, intact shelf is reached and apposition is begun, the 4-bite (modified Lembert) pattern is begun (Fig

47). A deep bite is placed in the perivaginal tissue of the thick vaginal flap on the right. A shallow bite is placed in the vaginal submucosa on the right and another shallow bite is placed in the vaginal submucosa on the left. A deep bite is placed in the heavy connective tissue of the right vaginal flap. Tightening this suture causes the vaginal tissues to invert and the rectal mucosa to come into closer apposition. When reconstruction reaches the end of the continuous horizontal pattern initially placed in the edge of the vaginal mucosa, the suture pattern is continued caudad another 5 cm. The main 4-bite suture pattern can then be continued caudad also. These 2 suture lines are continued alternately to the cutaneous perineum. In this method, no attempt is made to suture the rectal submucosa or mucosa. The apposition of a thick vaginal flap and the clot that forms on the rectal surface seals the suture line and prevents leakage. As the wound heals, granulation tissue replaces the clot and the rectal mucosa grows across the granulating bed to complete healing on the rectal surface.

Various repair technics involving a number of separate suture lines have been described.[2,27] They generally involve a continuous mattress

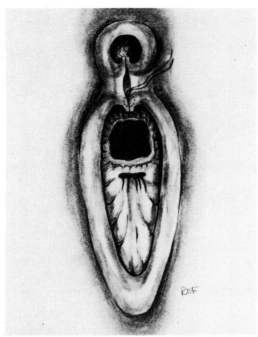

Fig 50. Placement of inverting suture in the vaginal submucosa.

pattern of absorbable or nonabsorbable sutures placed in the rectal and vaginal submucosae (Figs 48, 50). These initial suture lines are reinforced by one or more suture lines of heavier material placed with deep bites in the perirectal and perivaginal connective tissue (Fig 49). Absorbable and nonabsorbable sutures in interrupted and continuous patterns have been used for these reinforcing sutures. Due to the limited space available for suturing, it is essential to place the separate suture patterns simultaneously by alternating from one suture line to the next. If suturing is not done in an alternating manner, those suture lines completed first prevent access for placement of subsequent sutures.

The second phase of repair, reconstruction of the perineal body, follows reconstruction of the septum between the vestibule and the rectum. Some surgeons complete both phases at the same time, while others delay the second phase until the rectovestibular septum is healed.[2,4,5,20,21,25,27,28] The latter requires 2-3 weeks after completion of the first phase. Delaying the second phase allows feces to pass more readily since the anal sphincter is not intact. This helps prevent rectal impaction and dehiscence of the suture line.

Surgical repair of the perineal body and anal sphincter resembles reconstruction of the peri-

neal body after second-degree laceration. Two triangular areas of mucosa and skin overlying the muscle of the perineal body and anal sphincter are dissected from the level of the external anal sphincter ventrad to the level of the dorsal commissure. The rectal and vaginal mucosae are apposed at the margin with simple-interrupted sutures of 0 or 00 nylon or polypropylene. The freshened surfaces between the margins are apposed with simple-interrupted sutures of 0 or 00 gut, polyglycolic acid or polypropylene.

Rectovaginal Fistulas: Two methods have been described for repairing rectovaginal fistulas. One is to cut the anal sphincter and the perineal body, and repair the resulting third-degree laceration by one of the methods described.[25] Repair of a fistula by this method is not recommended. The only advantage obtained is to allow exposure for repair. A major disadvantage is the loss of support for the repaired tissue provided by the perineum and perineal body. The method that preserves the anal sphincter and perineal body obtains exposure by splitting the perineum in a transverse manner.[2,5,30]

Following the same preparation as for a third-degree laceration, the perineum is incised in the frontal plane (Fig 51). The perineal body is then bisected transversely so the anus and rectum are separated from the vulva and vestibule. This dissection is carried craniad to the fistula and 3-5 cm beyond. When the dissection is complete, 2 fistulas can be viewed in the dissected plane (Fig 52). One fistula on the dorsal aspect of the dissected plane communicates with the rectum, and the fistula on the ventral aspect of the dissected plane communicates with the vagina. These 2 fistulas are then closed using a modified-Lembert pattern of 0 or #1 chromic gut or polypropylene. The suture is passed into the rectal submucosa beginning 2 cm from the margin of the fistula, emerging near the fistula margin. The suture is passed into the right margin of the rectal fistula and emerges 2 cm from the margin (Fig 53). Tying this suture brings the submucosal tissues into apposition and everts the margin of the rectal fistula into the lumen of the rectum. This suture pattern is continued, placing the sutures 1-1.5 cm apart until the rectal fistula is closed (Fig 54).

The rectal repair can be closed in a transverse manner as well. Since the peristaltic stress on the rectum is at right angles to the long axis of the bowel, sutures placed parallel with the long axis, ie, suturing the fistula in a

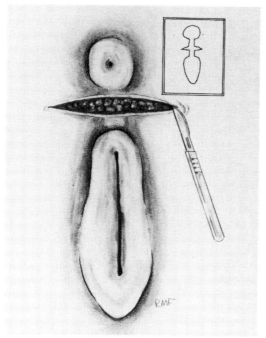

Fig 51. Incision of the perineal body in a frontal plane. Inset shows the relationship of the direction of the openings into the vagina and rectum.

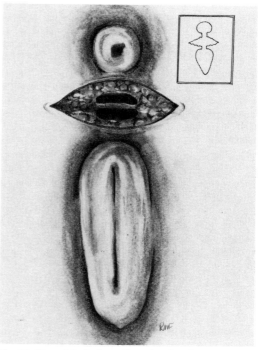

Fig 52. Completed dissection showing fistulas. Inset shows flaps created by dissection.

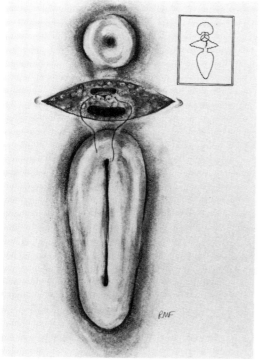

Fig 53. Placement of inverting suture in the rectal submucosa. Inset shows the effect of the suture.

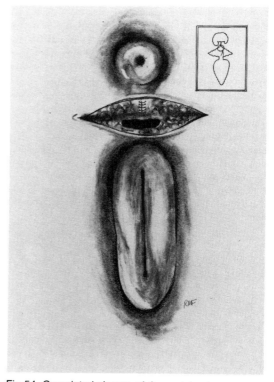

Fig 54. Completed closure of the rectal submucosa.

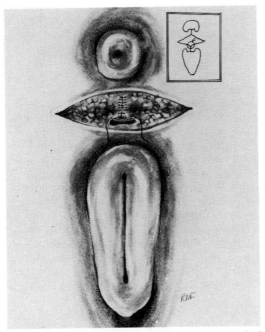

Fig 55. Placement of inverting sutures in the vaginal submucosa. Inset shows the effect of the sutures.

transverse rather than a craniocaudal direction, have less stress on them and less tendency to fail.[5,30] However, closing the rectal side of the fistula in a transverse manner using sutures oriented craniocaudad can be very difficult, given the exposure provided by the perineal dissection. Closing the rectal fistula with sutures oriented perpendicularly to the long axis of the bowel can be successful despite the stress placed on them by rectal peristalsis if the sutures are close together and adequate bites in the connective tissue of the submucosa are taken. Suturing in this manner is much easier.

In either method of suturing, these sutures should be placed approximately 1 cm apart. The vaginal fistula is sutured after the rectal fistula is closed. The suture is passed into the vaginal submucosa 2 cm from the margin of the fistula, emerging near the margin of the fistula on the left. The suture is placed from near the margin of the vaginal fistula on the right, emerging 2 cm from the fistula laterad (Fig 55). When the suture is tied, the vaginal submucosa is apposed and the fistula margin is inverted into the vagina (Fig 56). After both fistulae are closed, the space between the rectal tissue and vaginal tissue is closed with simple-interrupted sutures of 0 gut or polypropylene

to obliterate the deadspace of the dissection (Figs 57, 58). The skin of the perineum is then closed with nonabsorbable suture in a vertical mattress or simple-interrupted pattern (Fig 59).

Alternatively, if the rectovaginal septum is thin, the deadspace created by dissection can be packed with gauze.[30] In this case, the perineal skin is loosely sutured to hold the packing in place while the defect granulates. A thicker septum is obtained by healing the dissection in this manner. However, this is usually not necessary. This technic requires daily repacking and cleaning of the perineum until healing is complete.

Continuation of the laxative diet is essential for 14 days after repair of a rectovaginal laceration or fistula. Mineral oil or other effective laxatives should be given if constipation occurs. Gentle manual evacuation or gentle enemas may be given if the rectum becomes impacted but the success of the repair is greatly compromised if these efforts are vigorous or must be repeated.

Tetanus prophylaxis is mandatory and use of antibiotics has been advocated.[5] Considering the inevitable contamination in this region and the high incidence of anaerobic bacteria in the feces, use of penicillin is justified. However, a great advantage for using antibiotics has not been demonstrated. If antibiotics are used, administration should begin several hours prior to surgery so that effective blood levels are present at the time of surgery. Administration should be continued for at least 48 hours postoperatively.

Sutures should be removed in 14 days from repairs in which nonabsorbable sutures have been used and the suture ends have been left exposed. Natural breeding should be delayed for 3 months, but artificial insemination can be undertaken 6-8 weeks postoperatively.

References

1. Caslick, EA. Cornell Vet **27** (1937) 178.
2. Delahanty, DD. JAVMA **153** (1968) 1563.
3. Peck, GK. Vet Med **47** (1952) 359.
4. Vaughan, in Oehme and Prier: Textbook of Large Animal Surgery. Williams & Wilkins, Baltimore, 1974.
5. Vaughan, in Walker and Vaughan: Bovine and Equine Urogenital Surgery. Lea & Febiger, Philadelphia, 1980.
6. Crowhurst, RC and Caslick, W. No Am Vet **27** (1946) 761.
7. Gadd, JD. Proc 21st Ann Mtg Am Assoc Eq Pract, 1975. p 362.
8. Brown, MP *et al.* JAVMA **173** (1978) 1005.

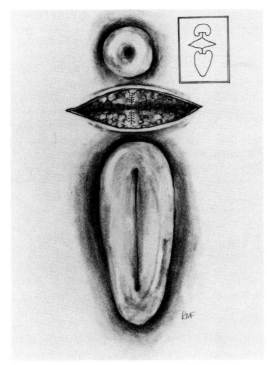

Fig 56. Completed closure of the vaginal submucosa.

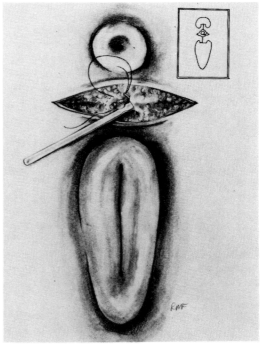

Fig 57. Closure of the space between the vagina and rectum. Inset shows the location of the suture.

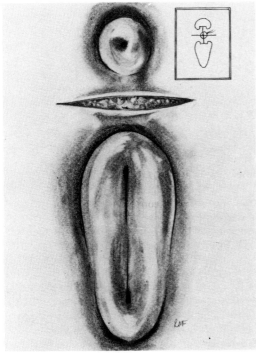

Fig 58. Closure completed to the subcutaneous level. Inset shows closure of the dissection.

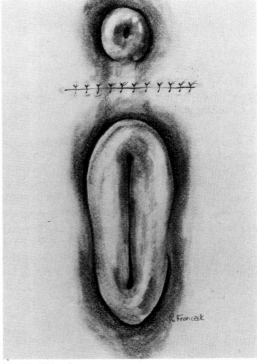

Fig 59. Skin closure.

9. Monin, T. Proc 19th Ann Mtg Am Assoc Eq Pract, 1973. p 99.

10. Clark, TL. J Repro Fert **23** (1975) 331.

11. Meagher, DM *et al*. Proc 23rd Ann Mtg Am Assoc Eq Pract, 1977. p 133.

12. Pearson, H *et al*. Eq Vet J **7** (1975) 131.

13. Stickle, RL *et al*. JAVMA **167** (1975) 148.

14. Williams, WL: Veterinary Obstetrics. Author, Ithaca, NY, 1909.

15. Vandeplassche, M. Eq Vet J **12** (1980) 45.

16. Vandeplassche, M *et al*. Proc 23rd Ann Mtg Am Assoc Eq Pract, 1977. p 75.

17. Vandeplassche, M *et al*. Eq Vet J **4** (1971) 105.

18. Wheat, JD and Meagher, DM. JAVMA **160** (1972) 881.

19. Habel, RE. Cornell Vet **43** (1953) 249.

20. Aanes, WA. JAVMA **144** (1964) 485.

21. Aanes, WA. Proc 19th Ann Mtg Am Assoc Eq Pract, 1973. p 225.

22. Arthur, GH: Veterinary Reproduction and Obstetrics. 4th ed. Williams & Wilkins, Baltimore, 1975.

23. Farquharson, J. No Am Vet **24** (1943) 220.

24. Fowler, ME. Proc 6th Ann Mtg Am Assoc Eq Pract, 1960. p 105.

25. Heinze, CD and Allen, AR. Vet Scope **11** (1) (1966) 12.

26. Straub, OC and Fowler, ME. JAVMA **138** (1961) 659.

27. Stickle, RL *et al*. Vet Surg **8** (1979) 25.

28. Wheat, JD, Univ Calif: Personal communication, 1977.

29. Klein, LV and Baitjer, C. Vet Anesth **1** (1974) 2.

30. Bemis, HE. No Am Vet **11** (1930) 37.

THE STALLION
by R.E. Larsen

Reproductive Anatomy

The scrotum of the stallion is thin-skinned, with the underlying tunica dartos closely adherent. The scrotum is not as pendulous as in ruminants and may not be immediately apparent on visual examination due to the ability of the horse to retract the testes against the inguinal region. The testes lie in the scrotum horizontally, with the long axis parallel to the vertebral column. The head of the epididymis is closely attached to the testis at the cranial pole. The body of the epididymis passes over the dorsal surface of the testis. The tail of the epididymis is loosely attached to the caudal pole of the testis. The ductus deferens lies along the dorsal surface of the testis, medial to the body of the epididymis, and joins the spermatic cord bundle as a separate structure covered by its own fold of visceral vaginal tunic.

The spermatic cord, comprised of the testicular artery, vein, lymphatics and nerves, and covered by the visceral layer of vaginal tunic,

enters the craniodorsal aspect of the testis. The 2 ductuli deferenti expand into a tubular ampullary gland region approximatly 10 cm cranial to their convergence in the pelvic urethra. In intact males, the ampullae may be 3-5 times the diameter of the ductuli deferenti or 1.5-2 cm wide.

The seminal vesicles are located at the most cranial, dorsolateral aspect of the pelvic urethra. They are responsible for the formation of gel, contribute protein to the seminal plasma, and are the major source of citrate. The glucose and sorbitol in the ejaculate presumably are produced mainly by the seminal vesicles. In contrast to many other species, horses produce almost no fructose in semen.[1]

The prostate is a paired organ just caudal to the seminal vesicles on the lateral aspects of the pelvic urethra. Prostatic fluid in the stallion is not well characterized but probably is the source of a mostly ionic solution containing various enzymes. The bulbourethral glands are the most caudal accessory gland, located just cranial to the point at which the urethra bends around the ischial arch. Their total contribution to the ejaculate is small compared with that of the prostate or seminal vesicle.

Breeding Soundness Examination

Breeding soundness examination is generally oriented toward making a prediction of a stallion's fertility. However, with the exception of identifying animals with such low sperm cell output that fertility is unlikely, quantitative prediction cannot be easily made. Breeding soundness involves more than adequate semen parameters. Ophthalmic, musculoskeletal and behavioral problems should also be considered.

Physical Examination of the Genitalia

Physical examination should include palpation of the scrotal contents, rectal examination of the male accessory gland structures, and observation of the penis and prepuce during erection and washing preparatory to semen collection. The testes of the stallion lie horizontally in the scrotum, with the tail of the epididymis on the most caudal aspect. This orientation predisposes the stallion to 180° torsion of the testis. The body of the epididymis, which is often not firmly attached to the testicular surface, may be palpated as a discrete structure that can be manipulated to the lateral surface of the testis. The tail of the epididymis can be easily distinguished from the head by its rubbery or fluid-filled tone and the marked degree of protrusion. The vascular bundle of the spermatic cord can be identified on the cranial dorsal aspect of the testis. The tail and body of the epididymis are often unattached to the testis itself and may be freely movable in the caudal aspect of the scrotum.

During examination for torsion of the testis, the orientation of the spermatic cord insertion on the dorsum of the testis and identification of the tail of the epididymis are assessed for definitive diagnosis. Each testis should be examined with 2 hands, one hand holding the testis while the other traces the epididymis. Each testis is then examined with one hand alone, grasping the spermatic cord and following it to the testicular surface to verify which pole of the testis is being entered by the spermatic cord bundle.

Phenothiazine tranquilizers are often used to relax the retractor muscles of the penis for effective flaccid protrusion of the penis during examination and therapy. A number of cases of paralysis of these muscles and inability to retract the penis have been reported in stallions and geldings following administration of tranquilizers.[2] These preparations should be used with an awareness of the potential risk which, while small, carries with it disastrous consequences. Amputation of the penis may be the only viable therapeutic solution.

Scrotal width, rather than scrotal circumference, is used as an indicator of normal testicular development and potential for spermatozoa production (Table 9). Scrotal width is more highly correlated with amount of testicular parenchyma and sperm production than with the sperm cell output, which is measured in the ejaculate.[3] This is due to variability in total cells appearing in successive ejaculates and to losses during collection.[4] Despite this variability, scrotal width can still be used as an indicator of sperm-producing capacity. If a stallion has a scrotal width less than 2 standard deviations from the mean for its age, below-average sperm cell output can be expected.

Rectal palpation of the pelvic urethra, prostate, bulbourethral glands, seminal vesicles and ampullae is performed, with greatest emphasis on the seminal vesicles. The prostate is not easily distinguishable on palpation from the surrounding tissue of the pelvic urethra. The bulbourethral glands are small and located well caudad and not closely attached to the pelvic urethra. The seminal vesicles are small paired structures projecting from the craniolateral surface of the pelvic urethra.

Table 9. Testicular Size in Stallions of Different Ages[3]

Age	Mean Scrotal Width + 2 SD
2-3 years	96 ± 15 mm
4-6 years	100 ± 15 mm
7 years	109 ± 15 mm

These normally small, collapsed bladder-like structures are difficult to palpate as discrete organs unless they contain fluid or are thickened due to inflammation. Because they accumulate fluid, the seminal vesicles may distend up to 7 cm long and 5 cm wide, particularly during sexual excitement. Massage during sexual excitement causes passage of the fluid into the urethra. In some cases it may drain from the penis as this is done. The ampullae and ductuli deferenti are readily identified on rectal palpation. Tracing the course of the ductus deferens may aid in locating testes retained in the inguinal region of the abdomen.

Extreme caution should be exercised in deep rectal palpation of the stallion. In general, stallions are rarely palpated and do not submit to the manipulative procedure to the same degree as do mares. The pelvic male accessory sex glands may be located with "wrist-deep" palpation. Examination of this area poses little risk when done with care.

Semen Examination

Timing of semen collections for evaluation following sexual rest or inactivity is an important consideration. Some investigators feel that examination of 10 ejaculates, over a period of weeks or months, is necessary for adequate evaluation to predict the level of fertility. The opportunity for this degree of thoroughness is seldom available; 2 collections at a 1-hour interval in one day is a more practical approach.[5,6] This allows a comparison of sperm cell numbers in the ejaculate between the 2 collections. If the second ejaculate contains approximately 50% of the number of cells present in the first ejaculate, the collections may be considered representative of typical ejaculates.[7] Ideally, daily collection for 7 days provides a good estimate of the sperm-output capacity for a stallion for that time of year. After 7 days of collection, sperm cell numbers in one ejaculate approach the daily output.[8]

Semen evaluation is best performed on an ejaculate collected with an artificial vagina (AV). Two hard-shell water-jacket models are available (Figs 60, 61). A more flexible rubber and leather model (NASCO, Fort Atkinson,

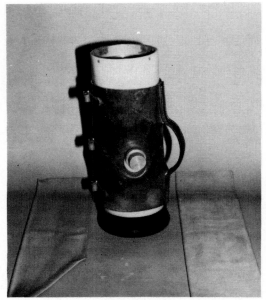

Fig 60. Plastic-shelled "Colorado model" artificial vagina with 2 rubber liners. One liner creates an inner water jacket and the other directs semen into the collection vessel.

WI) is also available. Each model has its own advantages, but in most stallions any can be used effectively. The inner temperature of the AV is regulated to approximately 44 C (111.2 F). Different stallions may prefer temperatures ranging from 40.5-47 C (104.9-116.8 F). The collection container may be a plastic bag or a plastic jar. Use of filters (Lane, Denver, CO) in the AV offers the advantage of gel re-

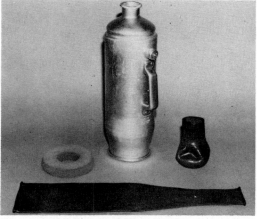

Fig 61. Aluminum "Japanese or Nishikawa model" artificial vagina with single liner and foam doughnut, which fits into the distal end of the water jacket.

moval during collection and more rapid evaluation of gel-free semen (Fig 62). The gel may alternatively be removed after collection by pouring the semen through gauze or milk-filter material or by aspiration from the surface of the semen sample with a syringe. An insulating cover should be used over the collection container attached to the AV to prevent chilling of the ejaculate and death of spermatozoa due to cold shock.

The stallion is teased and allowed to maintain an erection for examination and washing of the penis and prepuce. As the stallion mounts the mare, the penis is deflected to the side and the AV presented to the penis (Fig 63). The stallion should be allowed to accomplish part of the penetration of the AV with his own thrusting. Following the initial thrusts, the stallion stands fairly still for the ejaculatory contractions. The operator can evaluate the progress of the ejaculation by maintaining hand contact with the proximal portion of the penis and feeling the urethral contractions on the ventral surface of the penis. A normal ejaculation consists of at least 6-7 waves passing through the urethra.

Critical semen parameters for evaluation include sperm cell concentration, total number of sperm cells in the ejaculate, volume, motility and morphology.[9] Sperm cell stress tests have also been used and involve evaluation of motility after semen stands for varying periods under different conditions.

While minimal acceptable standards for total cells in the ejaculate are not universally defined, the following considerations have been used as guidelines. When semen is collected after one week of sexual rest, the stallion should have the potential to ejaculate 4×10^9 sperm in his first ejaculate between April and July.[10] Daily sperm output after 7 days of daily collection should be at least $1\text{-}3 \times 10^9$.[11,12] Sperm production depends to a certain extent on the season. Sperm output during the winter months is approximately one-half of that seen during the summer.[7,13] Use of a hemocytometer after semen dilution is a practical method of determining sperm cell concentration, from which total cells in the ejaculate may be calculated. Spectrophotometric methods and electronic cell counters work well but require a degree of standardization that may not be practical for many clinical practices doing limited numbers of breeding soundness examinations. Their usefulness (particularly the spectrophotometer) in active stud farm operations using artificial insemination is well recognized.

The volume of the ejaculate is generally not a critical factor in stallion fertility. Volume must be measured to calculate total sperm numbers but probably does not influence fertility independent of sperm numbers. Acceptable fertility has been achieved following artificial insemination with as little as 0.6 ml semen, providing sperm cell numbers are adequate.[14] In some semen evaluation systems that use 2 ejaculates taken an hour apart, one of the criteria for representativeness of the ejaculates is an approximately equal volume for each sample.[10] However, in one study the volume of the first ejaculate was considerably greater than the second during the months of May-July.[15] Volume may also be influenced by the stallion's response to AV temperature and pressure, and by his willingness to mount and breed the mare in the presence of the handlers and semen collection team.

In the same evaluation scheme using 2 ejaculates, a criterion for representativeness is motility of spermatozoa in the second ejaculate equal to or greater than that of the first.[10] Motility is considered normal when above 60% immediately after ejaculation and above 10% after the sample stands for 6 hours at 22 C (71.6 F). Other schemes for motility evaluation include extending semen 1:3 with 7% glucose and storing for 48 hours at 4 C (39.2 F).[16] Spermatozoa must maintain oscillatory movements for that period to be rated as "good" potential fertility. An alternative scheme involving measurement of initial motility in 0.430 osmolar egg yolk-glucose extender has been used in correlation of fertility and motility.[9]

Smears of semen for microscopic examination are prepared in the same manner as blood smears but must be made on a prewarmed slide. Smears are stained with Williams' or Giemsa stain. Samples too dense to evaluate individual cells should be diluted with warm normal saline. Negative staining with India ink or eosin-nigrosin "live-dead" stain, a more common approach to the morphologic evaluation of spermatozoa, should be performed on warm slides with gel-free semen. This procedure involves placing one drop of stain on a glass slide, mixing a minute amount of semen at the tip of a pipette or wooden applicator stick with the stain, and slowly spreading the drop in the manner of a blood smear. This provides a dark background against which spermatozoa may be viewed for morphologic assessment.

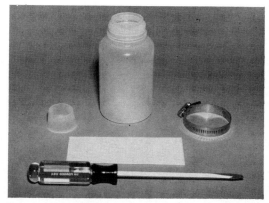

Fig 62. Plastic bottle with accessories for fitting milk-filter material to separate gel, and clamp for attaching bottle to rubber liner.

Since the live-dead staining qualities of eosin-nigrosin stain are inconsistent, this type of stain is best used only as a background against which cells are viewed. A raw semen smear should be stained with Geimsa, Wright's or other stain for observation of inflammatory and immature cells from the testis.

It is difficult to rank the importance of the different abnormalities seen in stallion sperm. The critical parameter in morphologic evaluation is probably percentage of normal cells. However, a simple assessment of percentage of normal sperm cells in the ejaculate and total normal cells is of more value than assessing the percentage of various anomalies. For reference and legal purposes, records should be kept on incidence of each type of abnormality observed in each semen evaluation.

Statistical methods of estimating minimal numbers of normal motile spermatozoa necessary for conception predict that as few as 10×10^6 cells could produce a pregnancy.[9] Artificial

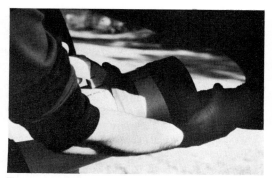

Fig 63. Intromission of penis into the artificial vagina during mount of the mare.

insemination studies have produced acceptable fertility with 100 x 10^6 normal motile cells from some stallions.[16] It is not likely that conception rates can be increased over that obtained with 500 x 10^6 cells by the insemination of even higher numbers of normal motile cells.[17] Unfortunately, when sperm concentration has been reduced to low numbers by depletion or low sperm production, other factors, such as questionable ejaculation or aberrant maturation, may further reduce potential fertility.

Reproductive Tract Disease

Bacterial Contamination of Semen

Stallion semen, even in clinically normal, fertile stallions, may be heavily contaminated with microorganisms. However, infection and inflammation are less common in the reproductive tract of stallions. The mean bacterial population in undiluted semen from normal stallions was 573,000/ml in one study.[18] Commonly detected aerobic organisms include *E coli, Klebsiella* sp, nonhemolytic and beta-hemolytic *Streptococcus, Pseudomonas aeruginosa, Staphylococcus* sp, *Corynebacterium* sp, *Proteus* sp and fungi.[19] Particular attention has been paid to those stallions shedding *Klebsiella* sp and *Pseudomonas* sp in semen. Because most of these stallions have normal fertility, the strain of the organism and the resistance to infection of the mare being bred are probably the important considerations in reproductive failure related to bacteria in semen.

Klebsiella can be recovered from the nostrils, prepuce, pre-ejaculatory secretions, body surface and feces of some stallions. In most cases, there is difference in conception rate between stallions shedding *Klebsiella* and the general population of stallions.[20] However, certain stallions carry strains of the organism, notably type 5 and type 68, that cause purulent vaginitis and endometritis in mares.[20-22] Few stallions chronically shedding *Klebsiella* have been assessed for the location of the bacteria, but colonization of the mucosal surfaces of the bladder and prostate without actual tissue invasion has been reported.[21]

The use of studs shedding *Klebsiella* involves antibiotic therapy, test matings, sanitary technics for artificial insemination, and natural mating after intrauterine infusion of the mare with semen extenders containing antibiotics. *Klebsiella* is difficult to eliminate from the semen with systemic antibiotic therapy of the stallion. Since the bacterium is apparently a surface contaminant in most cases rather than a tissue invader, all but the most aggressive therapeutic regimens are unlikely to completely eliminate the organism. Gentamicin at 4.4 mg/kg for 34 days has been used to eliminate *Klebsiella* from semen but care must be taken in evaluation of ejaculates during therapy.[23] Samples must be recultured after treatment to adequately evaluate therapeutic effects. The West German Thoroughbred breeding industry operates under the following regulations: (a) mares may only be served if free of *Klebsiella*; (b) on a test basis, clinically normal stallions shedding *Klebsiella* may serve healthy mares, which are then examined clinically and bacteriologically 10 days after mating. The stallion is considered free of pathogenic *Klebsiella* and may be used without restriction if at least 10 mares are serviced without infection; and (c) stallions with clinical signs of *Klebsiella* infection or causing infection in test mares are quarantined.[20]

Pseudomonas was isolated from the urethra or semen of 33.7% of stallions in one survey.[24] None of the stallions harboring *Pseudomonas* had gross pathologic changes in any part of the genital tract. There was no pus in the semen, although *Pseudomonas* is occasionally cultured from stallions shedding pus in the semen. Because certain stallions cause venereal infection of the uterus and infertility, it must be assumed that pathogenic strains of the organism in semen and reduced endometrial resistance in the mare contribute to reproductive failure. Most stallions with *Pseudomonas* in the reproductive tract have conception rates comparable to those not carrying the organism.[24,25] The organism has been eliminated from semen in some cases with gentamicin at 4.4 mg/kg for 10-20 days.[23] The control of uterine infection is probably best achieved through use of procedures for minimum contamination at breeding.

A technic causing minimum contamination during natural service consists of wrapping the mare's tail with gauze and pulling it to the side to keep hair from the vulvar region. The vulva is thoroughly scrubbed 3 times with povidone iodine, warm water and cotton, with a rinse after each scrub. The stallion is teased to full erection and the penis washed with warm soapy water, using absorbent cotton or paper towels. Multiple rinses remove the soap residue. Just before mounting is permitted, the uterus of the mare is filled to overflowing with a warm semen diluent containing antibiotics (see section on artificial insemination). Use of 100-300 ml diluent allows a portion to flow out of uterus to coat the cervix and vagina.[19] The stallion is then allowed to cover the mare and ejaculate into the extender containing antibiotics.

While mycoplasmas and yeasts have been isolated from semen, their role in pregnancy loss and infertility due to venereal transmission has not been well established.[26,27]

Equine Coital Exanthema

The etiologic agent of equine coital exanthema (ECE) is a herpesvirus distinct from equine herpesvirus-1 and cytomegalovirus.[28-30] This infectious venereal disease causes vesicles, pustules and ulcers on the external genitalia of infected mares and stallions. Spread of the disease is mainly by genital contact, although occasional animals develop lesions unexplained by mating or direct contact with affected animals.[30] Antibodies to ECE are detected mainly in horses used for breeding and rarely in horses under 2 years of age, which suggests that transmission by means other than genital contact is uncommon.

Lesions initially appear as weeping blisters on the glans penis and prepuce, and progress to circumscribed inflamed areas 0.5-1.5 cm in diameter. The penis and prepuce may be painful and edematous.

In one outbreak, susceptible mares bred to an infected stallion had reduced conception rates for that mating.[32] However, conception rates are apparently not reduced following recovery. Mares uninfected after breeding to an affected stallion had normal conception rates.[32]

Treatment is oriented toward cleansing the penis and prepuce, reducing inflammation, and prevention of secondary bacterial infections. Lesions typically heal 10-14 days after onset. Infected animals carry and excrete the herpesvirus after clinical recovery.

Seminal Vesiculitis

Seminal vesiculitis is the most commonly diagnosed abnormality of the accessory sex glands. At sexual rest, normal seminal vesicles are empty bladder-like organs that are difficult to palpate rectally. Enlarged seminal vesicles with a hardened, "meaty" texture indicate seminal vesicular disease. Diagnosis is by bacteriologic and cytologic examination of the ejaculate and by rectal palpation. In many cases, the inflammation resolves to the extent that, while enlarged and hardened glands may be present, no abnormality in the ejaculate can be identified. In most cases the animal continues to produce adequate seminal plasma volume.

Bacterial culture and cytologic evaluation may also be done on fluid collected after sexual excitation. Collection of seminal vesicular secretions for culture is accomplished by urethral catheterization. A 100-cm human decompression tube with an inflatable rubber cuff is passed up to the pelvic urethra for collection of specimens for bacteriologic examination. The seminal vesicles are then compressed per rectum and samples of both right and left vesicle collected separately for evaluation.[33]

Organisms associated with seminal vesiculitis in stallions are *Staphylococcus aureus*, *Pseudomonas aeruginosa*, and beta-hemolytic *Streptococcus*. Other organisms are involved but few studies have been done on horses with this condition. In bulls, abscesses and foci of infection in other areas of the body affect the seminal vesicles by hematogenous spread. Congenital anomalies in anatomic orientation between ampullae and seminal vesicles may predispose to infection.[34,35]

Treatment of seminal vesiculitis is with an antibiotic selected on the basis of sensitivity testing. Even then, organisms in the seminal vesicles are not easily reached by most agents. Difficulties related to permanently eliminating the bacteria have led to surgical removal of the affected gland.[36-38] Removal of one or both seminal vesicles reduces semen volume and citric acid content of the ejaculate but does not affect total sperm cell output and motility.[38]

Hemospermia

Hemospermia, blood in the ejaculate, is associated with reduced fertility in stallions. Reduced fertility is apparently related to the presence of RBC in semen rather than to serum constituents.[39] It is often seen in stallions booked to large numbers of mares. Bacterial urethritis is the most common cause but it may also be caused by urethral strictures, trauma to the glans penis, and seminal vesiculitis. Urethral scarification and strictures can result from the continued pressure of an improperly sized stallion ring. Affected stallions may exhibit pain on mounting and breeding, and require several mounts for a service. Diagnosis of hemospermia is best done with collection of semen by AV. It is difficult to determine if the mare or the stallion is the source of blood following natural service.

Further diagnostic tests should be considered to localize the lesion when RBC are observed grossly or microscopically. Collection of semen with an open-ended artificial vagina and fractionation of each jet of ejaculate can provide evidence for the source of blood. Blood clots incorporated into the gel suggest seminal vesiculitis. Frank drops of whole blood suggest physical trauma to the distal urethra or the penile surface. The erect penis should be examined for evidence of lesions from trauma. Fiberoptic endoscopic examination of the urethra may reveal ulceration, prolapsed vessels, inflammation, or strictures from scarification, neoplasia or granulation tissue. Subischial urethrotomy has been advocated for more complete endoscopic examination of the pelvic and subischial portions of the urethra. Radiographic examination by barium and air double-contrast technic can identify space-filling lesions and erosions. Culture and cytologic evaluation of urethral swabs or scrapings are also useful.

Treatment is directed at resolution of the lesion. Sexual rest is all that is required in some cases. Systemic and local antibiotic therapy following sensitivity testing is used to treat bacterial urethritis. When urethrotomies have been performed for diagnostic or therapeutic reasons, medicated urethral inserts may be placed in the urethra through the open incision. Surgical correction of strictures and prolapsed vessels has been accomplished by ventral midline exposure of the urethra. Suturing involves only the fascial planes, with both the urethral epithelium and skin apposed only by the underlying sutures.[40] Cauterization of the urethra with silver nitrate should be avoided since it may cause scar formation, strictures and granulation. Methenamine given PO and diluted formaldehyde given IV have been used to control chronic hemospermia in certain cases.[41]

Neoplasia

Penile Tumors: The most common neoplasm of the equine penis is squamous-cell carcinoma. Squamous-cell carcinoma occurs mainly in adult horses and has no breed predilection.[42] One survey revealed that 45% of all squamous-cell carcinomas occur on the penis or prepuce.[43] The tumor is slow to invade the penis and regional nodes, although penile invasion and metastasis to the superficial inguinal nodes ultimately occur.[42] Surgical excision has generally been the treatment of choice, often involving penile amputation and removal of lymph nodes.[44]

Granulomas caused by parasitic larval infestation of the spirurid stomach worm *Habro-*

nema are often seen during the summer and in warmer geographic areas, and must be distinguished from squamous-cell carcinoma. The urethral process, glans penis and preputial ring are the usual sites of deposition of larvae by flies acting as intermediate hosts.[45,46] The characteristic multiple caseous granules found throughout the granulomatous tissue represent masses of dead eosinophils. Diagnosis is made by demonstration of larvae on microscopic examination of tissues.[45]

Treatment of habronemiasis is directed toward inactivation of larvae with systemic and topical organophosphates. Trichlorfon or ronnel has been incorporated into topical dressings and also used systemically. Ronnel may be administered by mouth or stomach tube daily for 21 days at 10 mg/lb or at 45 mg/lb once every 2 weeks. Trichlorfon can be administered IV at 10 mg/lb after dilution in 2 L saline. This solution should be given slowly and antidotes, such as atropine and pralidoxime chloride, should be available in case of adverse reactions.[47]

Testicular Tumors: Interstitial-cell tumors occur in equine testes as firm, tan nodules. There may be some question as to whether lesions represent neoplasia or hyperplasia. Interstitial-cell tumors may be a source of excess or abnormal steroid production. Some horses with this type of tumor are vicious.[48] However, no connection has been made between abnormal behavior and presence of this type of neoplasia.

Sertoli-cell tumors are rarely seen in horses. This type of tumor tends to develop in retained rather than descended testes.

Seminomas are found in descended or retained testes and are the most commonly diagnosed testicular tumor of aged stallions.[48] These grey, lobulated tumors are soft and have a glistening cut surface.[48,49] Some seminomas exhibit malignant behavior.[50] Diagnosis is often made when the affected testis becomes larger than the other. The affected testis may shrink in response to the presence of the tumor until the mass of neoplastic tissue becomes larger than the previous testicular size. Unilateral castration is the treatment of choice in unilaterally affected stallions.

Teratomas are uncommon and usually occur in a retained testis. Teratomas are composed of tissue derived from embryonic endoderm, mesoderm and ectoderm. Bone or hair follicles and shafts within affected testes are common. Rather than cryptorchidism predisposing the animal to the development of teratomas, it is thought that teratoma development prevents testicular descent.[42] Subcapsular cysts are a common feature of teratomas. Cyst expansion may progress to the point that drainage is required to permit delivery of the cryptorchid testis by inguinal approach.[51] Size and shape of enlarged cystic testicular teratomas may create difficulty in recognizing the structure on rectal palpation. Diagnosis is made at cryptorchidectomy.

Genital Injuries

Penile injury most often occurs from kicks by the mare during breeding, movement of the mare after intromission, laceration by breeding stitches in the vulva of the mare, or contact with external objects by the erect penis during mounting of an unrestrained mare.[47,52] Hematoma or traumatic posthitis may result if the erect penis is kicked during the mount or dismount. The penis often is retracted into the swollen prepuce and the prepuce is prolapsed.[45] Replacement of tissues to their normal anatomic location facilitates venous and lymphatic drainage, and reduces edematous swelling. This may be possible with massage and bathing with a mild antiseptic solution. Alternative cold and warm water sprays may assist in reducing edema. Suspensory devices to support the weight of the edematous penis and prepuce are also helpful, particularly when exercise is used as an adjunct to therapy. When paraphimosis of both the penis and prepuce occur, use of a mesh "stallion supporter" is important as the initial step in edema control.[47]

Most hematomas and ruptures of penile erectile musculature are due to trauma to superficial vessels or to the corpus cavernosum penis. Rupture of the corpus spongiosum penis, with urethral obstruction, has been described.[53] Most bleeding lesions are due to cuts on the external surface of the penis, often caused by tail hairs of the mare. Traumatic rupture of the corpus cavernosum penis, with external hemorrhage, may occur after severe bruising.[54]

The etiology of orchitis and epididymitis is rarely determined except on necropsy or unless due to trauma. Penetrating wounds introduce infectious agents, which may cause swelling and abscesses. No specific agent causing orchitis or epididymitis has been described. Blunt trauma, such as from a kick, may result in hematocele formation. Sterile drainage and culture of fluid contents may provide a diagnosis. Treatment may require unilateral castration to restore normal spermatogenesis following

the irritation and local temperature rise caused by a lesion if only one testis is involved.[55]

Spermatogenesis and passage through the epididymis require approximately 60 days in stallions.[56,57] Evaluation of fertility should be performed after that period following cessation of treatment for any testicular lesion.

Migration of strongyle larvae occasionally causes adhesions between the tunics. These may be incidental findings on routine castrations.[47,48] The significance of aberrant parasitic migration in testicular or epididymal inflammation has not been established.

Vascular lesions in the spermatic cord may be due to varicocele formation or thrombosis. Equine infectious anemia (EIA) or equine arteritis viruses can cause lesions in testicular vessels. Focal areas of testicular infarction may be a sequela of EIA.[47]

Mating Behavior

Libido, as measured by reaction time during semen collection, changes with season.[7] The total period of visual contact with the mare until copulation is shortest from May to August and longest during winter. This is also true for the number of mounts required for service. Overall number of mounts per service is approximately 1.4.[58] Reaction time and mounts per service are reduced during a second mating or semen collection one hour after the first. The previous ejaculation evidently serves as a stimulus for a more rapid response on the second breeding attempt. This effect dissipates and is not seen if mating or collection is performed 24 hours later.[59]

After mounting and intromission, an average of 7 intravaginal thrusts are required to cause ejaculation.[58] Studies with open-ended artificial vaginas have demonstrated that pressure and friction on the shaft of the penis by the circular musculature of the vaginal vestibular wall and the vulva stimulate ejaculation rather than pressure on the glans penis. Emission of semen begins about 10 seconds after vaginal penetration and consists of an average number of 8 seminal jets during the next 8 seconds. Pelvic thrusting causes gradual enlargement of the glans penis until, just before emission of the first jet of semen, the mushroom-like engorgement or "belling" of the glans is maximal.

The first 3 jets of semen contain 80% of the spermatozoa ejaculated. Penile detumescence begins during the following urethral contractions. Semen at that time contains clearer, more mucinous accessory sex gland secretions. The first jet of semen is ejaculated at the highest pressure and subsequent jets are under lower pressure, with gradual decline of erection and partial withdrawal of the penis. It is likely that the high-pressure sperm-rich jets are ejaculated directly through the cervix since the penis is at maximum penetration at that time, with the enlarged glans penis pressed against the cranial vagina and cervix. The loss of erection during later stages of ejaculation may result in a portion of the ejaculate being deposited in the vagina.

During the ejaculatory phase of the mount, stallions typically cease thrusting and stand relatively quietly over the mare. The tail twitches during the emission of semen and is often used as an indication of successful ejaculation during natural breeding. However, this sign and urethral pulsation, which may be palpated in the proximal shaft of the penis, may occasionally occur without ejaculation. For this reason, many stud managers examine dismount samples for the presence of spermatozoa regardless of signs of ejaculation.

Ejaculatory disturbances and vices of stallions are encountered often enough to warrant special effort and forethought during training and routine use of stallions. Young stallions, in particular, may develop poor breeding habits. In studies done with stallions of all ages, there was a tendency in the nonbreeding season for longer reaction times, increased numbers of mounts for ejaculation, and a greater tendency for biting and striking the mare before and during the mount.[60] This behavior tended to persist in 2- and 3-year-old stallions even after sexual rest and a more normal breeding schedule; older stallions reverted back to their former acceptable mating behavior. Excessive use of young stallions should be avoided. A 2-year-old should not breed more than 5-10 mares during the first season. Rough handling, in isolation, forced breeding of certain mares, excessive collection for semen evaluation during the winter, and excessive use as a teaser may all lead to abnormal behavior.[15]

Stallions injured during copulation may become reluctant to breed or may develop abnormal ejaculatory responses. Genital or musculoskeletal pain causes abnormal response to breeding similar to those seen with purely psychological causes. Causes of breeding failure have been classified as failure to attain or maintain an erection because of inability

or poor libido; incomplete intromission and pelvic thrusting due to pain or poor libido; dismount at onset of ejaculation due to pain or psychologic association of ejaculation with previous injury; failure to ejaculate in spite of successful intromission and prolonged erection; and necessity for longer than normal sexual rest between ejaculates (stallion maintains good libido but cannot ejaculate unless rested for a few days). Stallions may fit into more than one category.

Therapy is directed toward observation of sexual responses while allowing the stallion to act independently. Semen is collected by AV when a given situation produces a favorable response.[60] Gentle retraining and correction are initiated after several collections under desirable conditions. Several days or weeks of observation may be necessary. Affected stallions should be allowed to observe other stallions during mating or semen collection. They may be used to tease mares in heat as long as an active interest is demonstrated. A particular mare arousing a stallion's interest can be placed in an adjacent paddock.

Drugs may be used when necessary to reduce inflammation and pain. Training to mount a dummy only slightly higher than the stallion's thorax was effective with one stallion.[61] This reduced pain and pressure on the stallion's hindlimbs during mounting and thrusting, and eliminated fear of injury.

Pilocarpine and ephedrine have been used with limited success in an attempt to restore smooth muscle and nerve response within the genitalia.[62] Results of amphetamine and atropine use are not encouraging.

Some stallions urinate during ejaculation, probably due to the stimulation of nerve fibers serving the tissues involved in ejaculation and urination. Reproductive performance in these stallions suffers when the ejaculate is contaminated with urine but is not affected when semen is ejaculated without urination. The simplest solution is to wait for urination and then immediately perform the mating or semen collection.[63] Collection of each seminal jet individually with an open-ended AV may also allow selection of uncontaminated fractions for insemination.

Testosterone is necessary for the development and maintenance of good breeding behavior.[11] Secretion of testosterone is influenced by photoperiod. Blood testosterone levels during the winter were elevated in stallions under extended artificial lighting periods as compared with those in control stallions under natural lighting.[59] However, although elevated blood testosterone levels were associated with reduced stimulation time (increased libido) in stallions under prolonged photoperiod, they did not necessarily produce increased spermatozoa output or seminal volume.[59] Under normal conditions, stallions in the northern hemisphere have lowest testosterone levels between October and January and the highest in May.[64] Volumes of first ejaculates during May, June and July are double those of the non-breeding season. Highest spermatozoa output is in July as expected due to the delay of 60 days for spermatogenesis and epididymal transit time following hormonal stimulus.[64]

While relatively low blood levels of endogenous testosterone can maintain normal sexual behavior and spermatogenesis, augmentation with injectable androgens is very unlikely to have a beneficial effect. Testosterone propionate administered to normal stallions at 200 mg/kg every 2 days reduced total numbers of spermatozoa ejaculated, sperm cell motility and scrotal width by 90 days of treatment.[65] Libido was not enhanced. This effect is related to inhibition of LH secretion. Exogenous androgens have a negative-feedback effect on the hypothalamus and pituitary, reducing LH production and secretion, and reducing testicular production of testosterone. Extremely high and potentially toxic doses of exogenous androgens would be necessary to overcome this effect.

Single blood testosterone determinations are not useful to predict fertility or mean blood testosterone levels. Blood testosterone levels fluctuate widely throughout the day and are subject to diurnal variation. Blood testosterone levels are highest at 8:00 AM and lowest at 8:00 PM.[66] The effect of this diurnal variation on behavior has not been determined. In any case, even the mean blood level of testosterone may not reflect the fertility of a stallion. Subfertile animals often have testosterone levels in the normal range (0.4 - 5.2 ng/ml for single samples, 1.68 - 2.92 ng/ml for the mean of multiple samples).[64,66,67]

Mating behavior is maintained even with very low levels of testosterone. Stallions may continue apparently normal breeding, with ejaculation of sperm-free semen, even after castration. The inclination and ability to mate may be lost the fall and winter following castration. There has been some concern about the fertility of matings after castration due to the fact that spermatozoa may be stored in the ductus def-

erens for considerable periods after castration and may appear in the ejaculate. Studies of ejaculates from geldings indicate that all sperm cells are nonmotile by 7-8 days postcastration and fertility after this period is highly unlikely.[68]

Masturbation in stallions is generally thought of as abnormal behavior and is treated by application of rings or ribbons to the penis, or by attaching an irritating surface, such as a brush, on the ventral body wall or cranial to the prepuce where the erect penis will contact it. The use of stallion rings may be related to occasional urethral lesions (see Hemospermia). Treatment with these technics may prevent masturbation but stallions well adjusted to normal mating seldom masturbate to the extent that libido is reduced. There is little evidence that sperm cell reserves are actually reduced by masturbation, but occasional reports suggest that some stallions may reduce sperm output for breeding if allowed to masturbate between breedings.

Artificial Insemination

The status of artificial insemination (AI) in horses has not progressed technically at the same rate seen in cattle because of reluctance to approve AI with fresh or frozen semen by certain breed registries (notably in Thoroughbreds), the need for multiple inseminations due to the character of the equine estrous cycle, and difficulties encountered in storing equine semen in the fresh or frozen state. However, AI is now commonly used with Quarter Horse and Standardbred mares, and conception rates obtained with raw or extended unfrozen semen are not inferior to those obtained naturally.

Semen for use with AI should be collected with an AV. The use of condoms negates certain advantages that AI provides under ideal conditions. Use of the AV permits collection with minimal bacterial contamination and allows filtration of the gel with minimal loss of sperm cells. The gel absorbs spermatozoa and filtration after mixing adds another step in semen handling during which sperm cells may be damaged or lost due to retention on additional filters and containers. Use of a specialized, shortened AV also permits collection of the ejaculate in fractions when extension or freezing technics call for collection of only sperm-rich semen.[58,63,69]

Raw semen should be used for AI as soon after collection as possible. Semen should be maintained at 30-35 C (86-95 F) until use and protected from rapid drops in temperature. Semen is placed in the uterus by passing a gloved hand, guarding the end of a plastic pipette, into the vagina and inserting the pipette through the cervix. Insemination volumes are 4-10 ml, although smaller volumes are not detrimental to fertility if adequate numbers of normal sperm cells are in that volume. In general, at least 100 million normal motile cells should be infused into the uterus. The more conservative approach is to use 500 million normal cells. Higher numbers of cells apparently do not enhance conception rates. Because of this and to reduce the number of seminal microflora introduced into the uterus, semen in excess of that required for delivery of 500 million cells is often discarded.

Reduction of microflora introduced into the uterus is an advantage of using semen extenders containing antibiotics. Another reason for use of semen extenders is that semen in the liquid state can be stored for longer than the few hours that raw semen permits. The extender, at semen temperature, is added to semen immediately after collection.[70,71] Ratios of extender to semen are usually between 1:1 and 4:1 or involve the addition of a set number of cells to a predetermined volume, *eg*, 500 million motile cells to 10 ml extender.[17] The basic protective component in most extenders is milk or egg yolk. Both have been successfully used for many years; however, milk-based extenders have been preferred for liquid storage. Yolk is detrimental to the maintenance of motility if semen is centrifuged for concentration of cells and removal of excess seminal plasma.[72] Table 10 details preparation of semen extenders.

After extension, semen is cooled to 5 C (41 F) over a 2-hour period. Although fertility may be retained for up to 3 days in diluents such as cream-gel extender, there is a significant reduction in fertility when semen is stored for 24 hours.[17,73] For this reason, many artificial insemination programs consist of collection, extension and insemination on an every-other-day basis. Semen is used on the day of collection rather than on the following day.

Addition of glycerol does not enhance the fertility of stored equine semen because of a toxic effect. Even when glycerol must be added for freezing equine semen, the addition is just before freezing to minimize the time of contact.[74]

Cream-gel extender has been used with such good results that there is some reluctance to switch to other formulations. However, once semen is mixed with this extender, it is very dif-

Table 10. Semen Extenders

Cream—Gelatin Extender: (100) ml)
1. Dissolve 1.3 g Knox gelatin in 10 ml distilled water. Sterilize.
2. Add half-and-half cream heated to 92 C for 10 minutes to make 100 ml. Do not boil or allow to exceed 95 C.
3. Add 20 mg gentamicin sulfate and 50 mg polymyxin B sulfate to give 200 µg/ml and 500 µg/ml, respectively.
4. Freeze in 10-ml to 50-ml quantities.

Skim-Milk Extender: (100 ml)
1. Heat skim milk to 92 C for 10 minutes. Do not boil or allow to exceed 95 C.
2. Follow steps 3 and 4 as in Cream-Gelatin Extender.

Minimum Contamination Technic Extender: (100 ml)
1. Add 2-4 g Sanalac powdered milk (Beatrice Foods) and 4.9 g glucose to 90 ml distilled sterile water.
2. Add 7.5 g NaHCO$_3$ to 100 ml distilled sterile water for a stock solution.
3. Add 2 ml of the 7.5% NaHCO$_3$ stock solution to the Sanalac-glucose solution.
4. Add 100 mg gentamicin sulfate to the Sanalac-glucose solution.
5. Add distilled sterile water up to 100 ml.

ficult to microscopically evaluate motility. Skim milk has been used with equal success in same-day insemination programs and has the advantages of allowing microscopic observation of cells and being simple to prepare.[75] In either case, a volume of raw semen containing 500 million sperm cells should be added to 10 ml of the extender. This comprises one insemination dose unless the number of mares requires further splitting. Under good conditions, total cell numbers may be reduced to 100 million. When semen must be stored for 24 hours prior to use, 100 million spermatozoa are not sufficient to maintain maximum reproductive efficiency and more sperm cells should be used.

Semen may be centrifuged to concentrate sperm, minimize dilution damage during extension, remove seminal plasma, remove some of the microflora in semen from stallions shedding large numbers of bacteria, and reduce insemination volume in stallions with dilute ejaculates. Fertility is not depressed by centrifugation at 310 G for 3-5 minutes.[72]

The minimum contamination technic for AI involves washing and centrifugation of semen from stallions shedding pathogens.[19] Collection is as sanitary as possible, allowing the pre-sperm fraction to be ejaculated, thus flushing the urethra before application of the AV. Semen is evaluated and immediately placed in an equal volume of antibiotic-containing extender. Centrifugation for 3 minutes produces a soft pellet. The supernatant is removed and the pellet resuspended in the appropriate amount of extender for the number of mares to be bred. The semen is then held for at least an hour before insemination to allow time for antibacterial action of the extender.

Antibiotics are generally added to semen extenders to prevent multiplication of bacteria during semen storage and to reduce the number of potentially pathogenic bacteria. The minimum contamination technic is oriented mainly to the handling of problem stallions and mares. Stallions may be chronic shedders of pathogenic strains of *Klebsiella, Pseudomonas* or other organisms causing endometritis, and certain mares cannot withstand the challenge of even the normally innocuous bacteria introduced during a natural service. Antibiotics with no effect on sperm motility when used at effective levels in extenders, include gentamicin sulfate, lincomycin, nalidixic acid, polymyxin B sulfate and sodium penicillin G. Antibiotics that reduce sperm motility include streptomycin sulfate, kanamycin and erythromycin.[76]

Equine semen has been successfully frozen by a variety of methods. However, no one method has proven completely satisfactory. One of the main problems has been the apparent loss of longevity of frozen-thawed semen in the uterus; good conception rates are obtained only when insemination is within 12 hours of ovulation.[77] The toxic effects of glycerol apparently contribute at least partially to the reduction in fertility seen with the use of frozen-thawed semen.

References

1. Mann, T. J Repro Fert Suppl 23 (1975) 47.
2. Whittle, BA and Crooks, JL. Vet Rec 101 (1977) 312.
3. Thompson, DL et al. J Repro Fert Suppl 27 (1979) 13.
4. Pickett, BW et al. JAVMA 165 (1974) 708.
5. Van Duijn, Jr, C and Hendriske, J. Report 897. Institut voor Veeteeltkundig Ondezoek Schoonoord, 1968.
6. Pickett, in Morrow: Current Therapy in Theriogenology. WB Saunders, Philadelphia, 1980.
7. Pickett, BW et al. J Anim Sci 43 (1976) 617.
8. Sullivan, JJ and Pickett, BW. J Repro Fert Suppl 23 (1975) 29.
9. Kenney, RM et al. Proc 17th Ann Mtg Am Assoc Eq Pract, 1971. p 53.
10. Kenney, RM. Proc 21st Ann Mtg Am Assoc Eq Pract, 1975. p 336.
11. Pickett, BW. Proc Ann Mtg Soc for Therio, 1978. p 32.
12. Amann, RP et al. J Repro Fert Suppl 27 (1979) 1.
13. Pickett, BW et al. J Repro Fert Suppl 23 (1975) 25.
14. Pickett, BW et al. Proc 5th Ann Mtg Nat Assoc Artific Breeders, 1974. p 47.
15. Pickett, BW and Voss, JL. Proc 18th Ann Mtg Am Assoc Eq Pract, 1972. p 501.
16. Bielanski, W. J Repro Fert Suppl 23 (1975) 19.
17. Demick, DS et al. J Anim Sci 43 (1976) 633.
18. Simpson, RB et al. Proc 21st Ann Mtg Am Assoc Eq Pract, 1975. p 225.
19. Kenney, RM et al. Proc 21st Ann Mtg Am Assoc Eq Pract, 1975. p 327.
20. Merkt, H et al. J Repro Fert Suppl 23 (1975) 143.
21. Crouch, JRF et al. Vet Rec 90 (1972) 21.
22. Stratton, LG et al. J Repro Fert Suppl 27 (1979) 317.
23. Hamm, DH. J Eq Med Surg 2 (1978) 243.
24. Hughes, JP et al. Cornell Vet 57 (1967) 53.
25. Hughes, JP and Loy, RG. Eq Vet J 7 (1975) 155.
26. Moorthy, ARS et al. Aust Vet J 53 (1977) 167.
27. Von Sonnenschein, B et al. Dtsch Tierärztl Wschr 85 (1978) 389.
28. Pascoe, RR et al. Aust Vet J 48 (1972) 99.
29. Pascoe, RR and Bagust, TJ. J Repro Fert Suppl 23 (1975) 147.
30. Gibbs, EPJ, and Roberts, MC. Eq Vet J 4 (1972) 74.
31. Bagust, TJ et al. Aust Vet J 48 (1972) 47.
32. Bitsch, V. Acta Vet Scand 13 (1972) 281.
33. Cooper, WL. Proc Ann Mtg Soc for Therio, 1979. p 1.
34. Blom, E. Nord Vet Med 31 (1979) 193.
35. Blom, E. Nord Vet Med 31 (1979) 241.
36. Klug, VE et al. Dtsch Tierarztl Wschr 86 (1979) 182.
37. Klug, E et al. J Repro Fert Suppl 27 (1979) 61.
38. Von Deegen, E et al. Dtsch Tierarztl Wschr 86 (1979) 140.
39. Voss, JL. Proc Ann Mtg Soc Therio, 1976. p 93.
40. Voss, JL and Pickett, BW. J Repro Fert Suppl 23 (1975) 151.
41. Voss, JL and Wotowey, JL. Proc 18th Ann Mtg Am Assoc Eq Pract, 1972. p 103.
42. Cotchin, E. Eq Vet J 9 (1977) 16.
43. Strafuss, AC. JAVMA 168 (1976) 61.
44. Scott, EA. JAVMA 168 (1976) 1047.
45. Vaughan, et al, in Oehme and Prier: Textbook of Large Animal Surgery. Williams & Wilkins, Baltimore, 1974.
46. Drudge, in Catcott: Equine Medicine and Surgery. 2nd ed. American Veterinary Publications, Santa Barbara, 1972.
47. Walker, DF and Vaughan, JT: Bovine and Equine Urogenital Surgery. Lea & Febiger, Philadelphia, 1980.
48. McEntee, K. Proc Ann Mtg Soc for Therio, 1979. p 80.
49. Knudsen, O and Schantz, B. Cornell Vet 13 (1963) 395.
50. Becht, JL et al. JAVMA 175 (1979) 292.
51. Stick, JA. JAVMA 176 (1980) 211.

52. Lieux, in Catcott: Equine Medicine and Surgery. 2nd ed. American Veterinary Publications, Santa Barbara, 1972.

53. Firth, EC. JAVMA **169** (1976) 800.

54. Pascoe, RR. Aust Vet J **47** (1971) 610.

55. Gygax, AP *et al.* Eq Vet J **5** (1973) 128.

56. Swierstra, EE *et al.* J Repro Fert Suppl **23** (1975) 53.

57. Swierstra, EE *et al.* J Repro Fert **40** (1974) 113.

58. Tischner, M *et al.* J Repro Fert **41** (1974) 329.

59. Thompson, DL *et al.* J Anim Sci **44** (1977) 656.

60. Pickett, BW and Voss, JL. J Repro Fert Suppl **23** (1975) 129.

61. Kenney, RM and Cooper, WL. JAVMA **165** (1974) 706-707.

62. Rasbech, NO. J Repro Fert Suppl **23** (1975) 123.

63. Nash JR, JG *et al.* JAVMA **176** (1980) 224.

64. Berndtson, WE *et al.* J Repro Fert **39** (1974) 115.

65. Berndtson, WE *et al.* J Repro Fert Suppl **27** (1979) 19.

66. Sharma, OP. Biol Repro **15** (1976) 158.

67. Cox, JE *et al.* Eq Vet J **5** (1973) 85.

68. Shideler, RK *et al.* J Repro Fert Suppl **27** (1979) 25.

69. McCarthy, PF *et al.* Proc Ann Mtg Soc for Therio, 1979. p 5.

70. Pickett, BW *et al.* Proc 20th Ann Mtg Am Assoc Eq Pract, 1974. p 155.

71. Pickett, BW and Voss, JL. J Repro Fert Suppl **23** (1975) 95.

72. Pickett, BW *et al.* Fert Ster **26** (1975) 167.

73. Allen, WR *et al.* Eq Vet J **8** (1976) 72.

74. Sullivan, JJ. Cryobiol **15** (1978) 355.

75. Pickett, in Morrow: Current Therapy in Theriogenology. WB Saunders, Philadelphia, 1980.

76. Back, DG *et al.* J Anim Sci **41** (1975) 137.

77. Pace, MM and Sullivan, JJ. J Repro Fert Suppl **23** (1975) 115.

SURGERY OF THE MALE GENITALIA
by C.D. Heinze

Castration[1]

Indications

Horses are castrated for various reasons. One is to increase the animal's tractability, particularly that of a vicious or "studdish" horse. A gelding performs much better than a stallion, whether used for racing or as a draft horse. This is especially true when the animal is used with or near mares. After castration, many dangerous stallions are handled much more easily. Preventing certain secondary sexual characteristics, such as an overdeveloped crest, may be desirable in many animals. Poorly bred or inferior animals should be castrated to avoid transmission of unwanted characteristics. Testicular disease, cryptorchidism and inguinal herniation are indications for castration.

General Considerations

Castration is one of the most common surgical procedures performed on horses. The surgery can be done with the horse standing, in lateral recumbency or in dorsal recumbency, with the legs flexed. Restraint procedures include use of local anesthetics, sedatives, tranquilizers, a combination of these, and general anesthetics. The surgical technics are classified as "open" or "closed," depending on whether the tunica vaginalis is incised. Although personal preference largely determines the technic used, the horse's age, breed, and disposition, the assistance available, and the owner's wishes are factors that influence the veterinarian's decision. No single technic is ideal for all situations. Most horses are castrated between 1 and 2 years of age.

A thorough physical examination should precede surgery. Infectious diseases, anemia and unthriftiness caused by parasitism or malnutrition are reasons for postponing surgery until they have been corrected. An inguinal hernia or cryptorchidism will delay or at least alter the surgical procedure.

Prior to surgery and any local injections, the scrotum and sheath should be thoroughly cleaned with surgical soap. If there is a ring on the penis, it should be removed. An antiseptic is applied liberally to the scrotal area to complete the preparation.

Restraint Methods

Although the fastest and simplest method of castration is with the horse standing, the surgeon runs the greatest risk of personal injury with this method. Shetland ponies, mature stallions used for breeding, and intractable horses should not be castrated while standing.

If analgesia of the surgical area is achieved, a twitch is all the physical restraint needed. If a local anesthetic is not given, a tail rope used as a sling, in addition to a twitch and a sedative, is required for most horses. The surgeon usually stands on the left side of the horse making body contact in the flank region.

Alternatively, the horse can be cast in lateral recumbency after administration of a muscle relaxant. A combination of xylazine and ketamine provides adequate analgesia and muscle relaxation for castration in lateral recumbency. Recovery is prompt and smooth. The upper rear limb is placed in a sideline and secured in flexion.

The surgery also can be performed easily and safely with the horse under general anesthesia and in lateral recumbency. The upper rear limb is secured in flexion with a sideline to assure the surgeon's safety in case anesthesia is light and to provide access to the surgical site. A minimum of assistance, usually only one person, is needed; the horse requires 20-40 minutes to recover from anesthesia.

Casting the horse on its back and tying both hindlegs in full flexion provides the greatest safety for the surgeon. This technic may require more assistants than the previously described methods. It also takes more time and subjects the horse to the greatest risk of injury. The stress of casting can be minimized, however, if adequate sedation or muscular relaxation is obtained prior to casting the horse and tying the limbs. The dorsal recumbent position facilitates handling of surgical complications should they develop.

Tranquilizers and Sedatives

Tranquilizers and sedatives administered IV are useful for standing castration on unruly horses, when animals are to be cast, and for all horses to be given a general anesthetic. Acepromazine maleate, at 3 mg/100 lb body weight, has proved satisfactory for tranquilization.

Chloral hydrate, alone or in combination with other drugs, is generally used to sedate a horse. For standing castration, a mixture of 30% chloral hydrate and 25% magnesium sulfate, injected IV at 5 ml/100 lb body weight, provides satisfactory sedation. For unruly horses and those to be castrated without inducing local analgesia, sedation is superior to tranquilization.

Short-Term General Anesthesia

Xylazine is administered IV at 1 mg/kg body weight and a suitable interval is allowed for the drug to take effect. Ketamine is then administered IV at 2 mg/kg. Horses typically lie down without undue struggling and can be maintained in recumbency for the 10-12 minutes required for the procedure.

Glyceryl guaiacolate, in combination with barbiturates, provides somewhat longer anesthesia when more complicated surgery is anticipated. Glyceryl guaiacolate is administered IV through a 10- or 12-ga needle at 5 g/100 lb body weight, not exceeding an initial dose of 60 g. The guaiacolate is added to a 5% solution of dextrose (usually 1 L solution). Many veterinarians prefer to add 1-2 g, depending on the size of the horse, of a thiobarbiturate to this mixture. Administering the solution from a special plastic container, on which digital pressure can be applied, speeds administration of this large volume of fluid. Most, if not all, of the calculated dose can be given before the animal is recumbent by using such a container. The injection site is clipped, scrubbed and infiltrated SC with 2-3 ml lidocaine to facilitate passage of the large needle.

Longer-Term General Anesthesia

Cryptorchid castration, inguinal herniorrhaphy or other complicated castrations may require general anesthesia for prolonged periods. These cases are best handled by induction, intubation and inhalation anesthesia.

Local Analgesia

Using a 22-ga needle and a local anesthetic in a 10-ml syringe, the scrotal skin is anesthetized with a series of linear injections ½ inch lateral to the median raphe. Injection of 8-10 ml on each side of the raphe anesthetizes an area large enough for 2 incisions.

The simplest method of anesthetizing the deeper structures is to infuse 10 ml local anesthetic directly into each testis, using the same syringe and a 2-inch, 18-ga needle. The deeper structures may also be anesthetized by injecting the anesthetic into the highest part of the inguinal area, where the spermatic cords can be palpated and immobilized between the thumb and forefinger. With the same syringe and needle, each cord is injected in a fanlike manner with 10 ml anesthetic.

Another method of anesthetizing the deep structures is to pass 5-inch, 18-ga needle through the testis and inject 3 ml anesthetic dorsal to it. The needle is then inserted to its full length into the caudal side of the spermatic cord and an additional 7 ml are injected. This is repeated on the opposite side. Reasonable care should be taken to ensure that the needle is not passed into the venous pampiniform plexus or spermatic artery on the cranial side of the cord because the ensuing hematoma would complicate the surgery.

Instruments

Because most veterinarians are right-handed, the following descriptions and illustrations are designed for a right-handed surgeon. The equipment needed includes an emasculator (I prefer a Reimer), a #4 Bard-Parker handle and #20 blade (recumbent position), a #3 Bard-Parker handle and #12 blade (standing position), scissors, several Ochsner forceps, and a pair of sterile gloves (Fig 64).

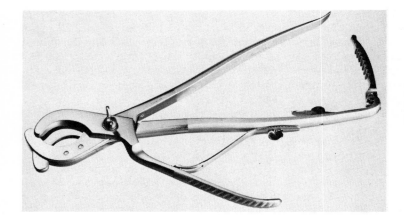

Fig 64. The Reimer emasculator.

Technic

Standing: After the scrotal area is repainted
with an antiseptic, the surgical site is checked
to determine that analgesia is complete and
the nose twitch is applied. The surgeon stands
on the left side of the horse, making body contact in the flank area and, with his left hand,
immobilizes the testes in the scrotum. With the
scalpel held in the right hand and the point of
the blade directed upward and backward, bilateral incisions are made through the skin,
dartos and scrotal fascia ½ inch lateral to the
medial raphe. Each incision is made boldly in
a craniocaudal direction and extended through
the tunics enclosing the testis.

A curved Ochsner forceps is applied to the
pampiniform plexus of each testis to control
hemorrhage. The tunica vaginalis of one testis
is grasped with another Ochsner forceps to assist in holding the serous sac when freeing it
from the scrotal tissue and inguinal canal area.
By blunt dissection, the parietal layer of the

tunica vaginalis is then freed from the surrounding tissue well into the inguinal canal.

While applying tension with the left hand to
the structures to be excised, the emasculator,
held in the right hand, is placed around the
tunic and cord above the forceps, partially
closed, guided into the inguinal canal, and
locked in position to crush the contained structures (Fig 65). The scrotal veins should not be
injured during this manipulation. The cutting
blade is then closed to complete the excision.
The emasculator is in place while the opposite
testis and adjacent structures are prepared for
excision. The second testis is then emascu-
lated. The emasculator should be left in place
in the closed position for a minimum of 60 seconds on each cord. All subcutaneous tissue that
tends to prolapse through the wound edges
should be removed with scissors.

The order in which the testes are prepared
and excised is a matter of personal preference,
but most surgeons prefer to remove the near

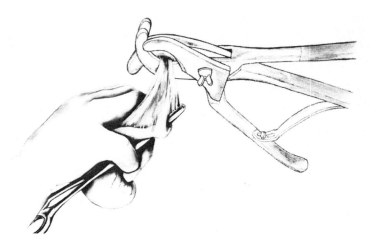

Fig 65. As tension is applied to
the structures in the left hand,
a Reimer emasculator is placed
around the tunics and cord
above the Ochsner forceps in
the inguinal canal and locked
in position.

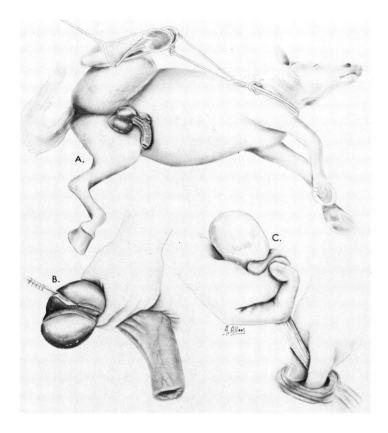

Fig 66. Closed technic for castration. With the horse positioned for surgery (A), 2 incisions are made bilateral to the median raphe of the scrotum (B). The testis is held with the right hand while the tunica vaginalis communis is freed with the left (C).

testis first. A modification of this technic involves making the near incision, completing the surgery on that side, and then repeating the procedure on the far side. Another method is to make only one incision in the median raphe and to remove both testes through it.

Some surgeons prefer not to use a tranquilizer because it relaxes the penis, thus causing interference at the surgical site. Many prefer to incise the scrotal ligament, a fold of the tunica vaginalis attached to the tail of the epididymis, to permit removal of a greater length of the spermatic cord.

Prior to removing the emasculator from each cord, a large Ochsner forceps may be applied to the pampiniform plexus and allowed to remain in place until the following day. This prevents much postoperative bleeding.

Recumbent: The horse is placed on its left side, with the upper leg secured in flexion (Fig 66). The scrotum and sheath are thoroughly cleaned with surgical soap and antiseptic is liberally applied to the scrotal area. The testes are immobilized in the scrotum with the left hand. The skin, dartos and scrotal fascia over

each testis are incised ½ inch lateral to the median raphe.

In the closed technic, the left testis and spermatic cord contained within the parietal layer of the tunica vaginalis are bluntly dissected from the surrounding tissues well into the inguinal canal. While applying tension with the left hand to the structures to be excised, the emasculator, held in the right hand, is placed around the tunica vaginalis and cord, and partially closed to crush the contained structures. The scrotal veins should not be injured while doing this. The cutting blade is closed to complete the excision. The emasculator is allowed to remain in place while the right testis and adjacent structures are prepared for excision. The emasculator should be left closed for a minimum of 60 seconds after each cord is severed. Each skin incision is then lengthened in a cranial direction until it is 4-6 inches long, depending on the size of the horse. All subcutaneous tissue that might prolapse through the wound edges is removed.

In the open technic, the tunica vaginalis is freed from surrounding tissues as in the closed method. The tunica vaginalis communis is

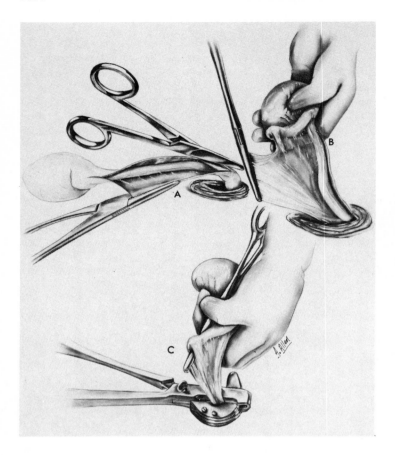

Fig 67. Open technic for castration. The tunica vaginalis communis is split (A). In a lateral view, the vas deferens passes from the tail of the epididymis in the fold on the medial surface of the mesorchium (B). The tissues are removed with a modified White emasculator (C).

then split with scissors, grasped with an Ochsner forceps, and divided as previously described (Fig 67).

Alternatively, the primary skin incision can be made deeply enough to cut through the tunica vaginalis communis into the testis. Ochsner forceps are placed on each tunic and the structures are freed and divided as previously described.

The advantage of the closed technic is that it greatly diminishes the possibility of septic material being introduced into the peritoneal cavity during surgery. Its main disadvantage is that contraction of the cremaster muscles, in a semiconscious animal, may complicate immobilization of the testis within the serous sac and subsequent dissection of the tunica vaginalis communis from the surrounding fascia.

Some veterinarians prefer the open technic because it permits positive identification of all structures to be excised and the tunic covering the ends of the incised cord. This theoretically diminishes the possibility of cord infection.

Ligation of the spermatic artery and vein should be considered for hemostasis in animals with enlarged vessels, such as aged stallions and those with testicular tumors. This is essential when an emasculator other than the Reimer type is used on these stallions. When the vessels are to be ligated, the open technic is used to exteriorize them. A ligature of #3 chromic catgut is transfixed high enough on the cord so it will not be disturbed during the emasculation.

Aftercare

Tetanus antitoxin is administered to all horses not previously immunized with toxoid. The horse is confined and observed for the first hour after surgery to minimize the chances of complications and to be sure that it recovers from anesthesia properly. Starting the next day, the horse is exercised twice daily, 20 minutes each time, for 2 weeks. Animals turned out on pasture should be checked daily to make sure they are exercising sufficiently to control postoperative swelling and edema.

Cryptorchidectomy

Indications

Cryptorchidism usually is unilateral, with more than 50% of the cases occurring on the left side. The undescended testis is removed because cryptorchids are undesirable as breeding animals and generally act more "studdish" than normal stallions.

When a testis is retained in the inguinal canal, it occasionally is difficult to palpate if it is high in the canal the and horse is standing. When the animal is recumbent and under general anesthesia, however, there is usually sufficient relaxation to enable palpation of the testis. If a definite diagnosis of cryptorchidism cannot be made before surgery, it is better to prepare for a cryptorchidectomy than for a standard castration.

Technic

After inducing general anesthesia, the horse is placed in lateral recumbency, with the affected side up. Anesthesia is then maintained with an inhalant anesthetic. When a surgical level of anesthesia has been established, the animal is rolled into dorsal recumbency at a 15° tilt, with the affected side up. The legs are flexed and supports are placed around the animal to maintain the position. Ropes are not used nor needed. The skin over the affected side, including the scrotal area, is prepared for surgery.

An incision of sufficient length to accommodate the surgeon's hand is made with a scalpel through the skin and fascia over the inguinal ring. By blunt dissection with the hands, the tissue is separated over the external inguinal ring. The large blood vessels encountered during this dissection should be handled carefully to avoid hemorrhage. A hand is passed through the external inguinal ring into the inguinal canal to carefully separate the tissues within the canal down to the internal ring.

The vaginal process, which lies over the internal ring, is penetrated with a finger to enter the peritoneal cavity. The processus vaginalis is a tough layer of peritoneum and is not easily penetrated. When doing this, care should be taken to preserve the conformation of the internal ring. After inserting the index finger into the peritoneal cavity, the testis or epididymis often can be palpated. It may be necessary to insert a second finger before either of these structures can be grasped and retracted into the canal. When neither the testis nor epididymis can be identified, the caudal edge of the vaginal ring is searched for the attachment of the gubernaculum testis. It is about 3/16 inch in diameter in many young stallions. When located, the gubernaculum is retracted through the vaginal ring into the inguinal canal; it is followed by the epididymis. Gentle traction on the epididymis draws the testis against the internal ring.

Small retained testes readily pass through the ring; larger ones must be manipulated carefully to stretch the internal inguinal ring before they pass. Abnormally large cystic or neoplastic testes require enlargement of the internal ring before they can be withdrawn.

If the gubernaculum testis is rudimentary or has shrunken to the point that it is unidentifiable, the entire hand must be inserted into the peritoneal cavity for a more complete search. The hand is fanned back and forth gently to move the intestines about and then is held still for a moment. When the hand is closed, the testis often is within the fingers. Because a piece of intestine containing a fecal ball may be grasped instead of the testis, it may be necessary to repeat this procedure several times before the testis is clearly identified.

When the testis and epididymis have been brought outside the abdominal wall, they are removed in the usual manner. If abdominal contents tend to protrude through the internal inguinal ring and into the inguinal canal, the internal ring should be closed with several simple-interrupted sutures of #1 chromic catgut. The external ring is closed in a similar manner and the edges of the skin incision are apposed with interrupted sutures of Vetafil. The skin sutures are left with 2-inch tails so they can be easily grasped when removed on the tenth postoperative day.

The remaining testis is removed as in the usual castration. Horses with 2 retained testes are rolled into a 15° tilt on the opposite side and the procedure is repeated.

Aftercare

After surgery, the horse is placed in a darkened, well-bedded stall or recovery room. Starting the following day, it is exercised twice daily for 20-30 minutes to control swelling at the surgical site.

Tetanus antitoxin is administered to all horses not previously immunized with toxoid. A therapeutic level of antibiotics is established and maintained during the first 3 postoperative days; it is continued for 2 additional days if there was a break in aseptic technic.

Comments

A modification of the above technic has been reported.[2] After the internal inguinal ring has been adequately exposed, a 10-inch curved sponge forceps is passed through the inguinal canal to grasp the processus vaginalis. This is accomplished by placing one hand in the canal, with the index finger against the vaginal process, and inserting the forceps with the other hand down to the area. The index finger is moved aside and the forceps is pushed through the internal ring, stretching the vaginal process inwardly. The handles of the forceps are opened slightly and then closed to grasp the membrane and withdraw it through the internal ring. By rolling the membrane, the small cordlike gubernaculum testis can be palpated through the vaginal process. When this has been done, the vaginal process is torn to grasp the gubernaculum. The procedure from this point is as previously described.

When the spermatic cord is too short to perform emasculation in the usual way, an ecraseur or long hemostat is used to clamp it prior to severing the cord with scissors.

When the testis is cystic, the fluid often can be removed through a needle attached to a rubber tube. This is difficult if the cystic portion is compartmentalized like a honeycomb.

Many veterinarians prefer to pack the inguinal canal instead of closing it with sutures because it is easier and faster. Care should be taken to avoid placing any part of the pack in the peritoneal cavity, however, because intestines may adhere to it. Several sutures through the skin keep the pack in place. After 24 hours, the skin sutures and pack are removed.

When an inhalation anesthetic is not used, a glyceryl guaiacolate-thiobarbiturate mixture can be given to induce general anesthesia. Use of this mixture is recommended because the initial injection produces anesthesia of sufficient duration to complete the operation, and recovery is reasonably prompt and without undue struggling. Deep narcosis, instead of surgical anesthesia, is maintained with IV anesthetics when additional time is needed to complete the operation. In this situation, the upper rear limb is placed in a sideline and secured in flexion. Double sidelines or casting equipment are needed when cryptorchidism is bilateral.

Retained testes occasionally cannot be successfully removed via the inguinal approach. Paramedian or flank laparotomy is indicated in such instances (see Chapter 13).

References

1. Heinze, CD. JAVMA **148** (1966) 428.
2. Adams, OR. Proc 11th Ann Mtg Am Assoc Eq Pract, 1965. p 295.

INDEX

INDEX

1404

O